Brief Contents

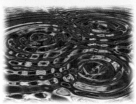

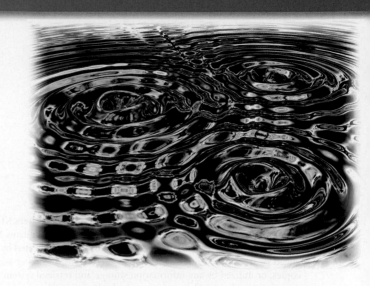

Psychiatric Nursing
CONTEMPORARY PRACTICE

Fifth Edition

ENHANCED UPDATE

Mary Ann Boyd, PhD, DNS, RN, PMHCNS-BC

Professor Emerita
Southern Illinois University Edwardsville
Edwardsville, Illinois

Clinical Faculty
St. Louis University
St. Louis, Missouri

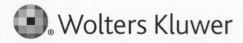

Philadelphia • Baltimore • New York • London
Buenos Aires • Hong Kong • Sydney • Tokyo

Publisher: Lisa McAllister
Acquisitions Editor: Patrick Barbera
Marketing Manager: Dean Karampelas
Product Development Editor: Helen Kogut
Editorial Assistant: Dan Reilly
Production Project Manager: Cynthia Rudy
Design Coordinator: Joan Wendt
Illustration Coordinator: Jennifer Clements
Manufacturing Coordinator: Karin Duffield
Prepress Vendor: Aptara, Inc.

5th edition, Enhanced Update

9 8 7 6 5 4 3 2 1

Printed in China.

ISBN 978-0-06-000037-0.

Cataloging-in-Publication Data available on request from the publisher.

LWW.com

To my husband James with love and sincere appreciation and gratitude.

Contributors

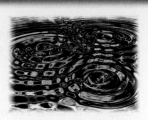

Beverly Baliko, PhD, RN
Associate Professor
College of Nursing
University of South Carolina
Columbia, South Carolina
Chapter 40: Caring for Survivors of Violence

Ann R. Bland, PhD, PMHCNS/NP-BC
Admissions Nurse
Holly Hill Hospital
Raleigh, North Carolina
Chapter 27: Borderline Personality Disorder

Andrea C. Bostrom, PhD, PMHCNS-BC
Professor
Kirkhof College of Nursing
Grand Valley State University
Grand Rapids, Michigan
Chapter 22: Schizophrenia

Mary R. Boyd, PhD, RN
Associate Professor
College of Nursing
University of South Carolina
Columbia, South Carolina
Chapter 40: Caring for Survivors of Violence

Stephanie Burgess, PhD, APRN, FNP-BC
Associate Dean for Nursing Practice & Clinical Professor
College of Nursing
University of South Carolina
Columbia, South Carolina
Chapter 40: Caring for Survivors of Violence

Jeanne A. Clement, EdD, PMHCNS-BC, FAAN
Associate Professor Emeritus
College of Nursing
The Ohio State University
Columbus, Ohio
Chapter 12: Cognitive Interventions in Psychiatric Nursing

Sheri Compton-McBride, MS, RN
Director of Clinical Acquisitions and Instructor
School of Nursing
Southern Illinois University Edwardsville
Edwardsville, Illinois
Chapter 32: Sleep–Wake Disorders

Catherine Gray Deering, PhD, APRN, BC
Professor
Clayton State University
Morrow, Georgia
*Chapter 15: Mental Health Promotion for Children
    and Adolescents*
*Chapter 34: Mental Health Assessment of Children
    and Adolescents*

Peggy El-Mallakh, PhD, RN
Assistant Professor
College of Nursing
University of Kentucky
Lexington, Kentucky
Chapter 5: Mental Health Care in the Community

Judith M. Erickson, PhD, PMHCNS-BC
Dean
Harriet Rothkopf Heilbrunn School of Nursing
Long Island University
Long Island, New York
*Chapter 26: Anxiety, Obsessive-Compulsive, Trauma, and
    Stressor-Related Disorders*

Cheryl Forchuk, RN, PhD
Associate Director of Nursing Research
University of Western Ontario
Lawson Health Research Institute
Arthur Labatt Family School of Nursing and Department
    of Psychiatry
London, Ontario
Chapter 9: Communication and the Therapeutic Relationship

Vanya Hamrin, RN, MSN, APRN, BC
Associate Professor
School of Nursing
Vanderbilt University
Nashville, Tennessee
*Chapter 34: Mental Health Assessment of Children and
    Adolescents*

Kimberlee Hansen, RN, MS, NP
Nurse Practitioner
Jefferson Barracks Division
VA St. Louis Health Care System
St. Louis, Missouri
*Chapter 28: Antisocial Personality and Other Personality and
    Impulse-Control Disorders*

Emily J. Hauenstein, PhD, LCP, MSN, RN
Professor and Associate Dean for Research
School of Nursing
University of Rochester
Rochester, New York
Chapter 21: Suicide Prevention

Peggy Healy, MSN, RN-BC, PMHN
Program Manager, Mental Health Clinic
VA St. Louis Health Care System
St. Louis, Missouri
Chapter 36: Mental Health Assessment of Older Adults

Gail L. Kongable, RN, MSN, FNP
Nurse Practitioner, Family Medicine of Albemarle
University of Virginia
Charlottesville, Virginia
Chapter 42: Caring for Medically Compromised Persons

Ruth Beckmann Murray, EdD, MSN, RN, N-NAP, FAAN
Professor Emerita
Doisy College of Health Sciences, School of Nursing
St. Louis University
St. Louis, Missouri
Chapter 38: Caring for Persons Who Are Homeless and Mentally Ill

Nan Roberts, MSN, PMHCNS-BC
Advanced Practice Nurse
St. Charles, Missouri
Chapter 23: Schizoaffective, Delusional, and Other Psychotic Disorders

Victoria Soltis-Jarrett, PhD, PMHCNS-BC, PMHNP-BC
Associate Clinical Professor and Coordinator of the PMHNP Program
University of North Carolina at Chapel Hill
Chapel Hill, North Carolina
Chapter 29: Somatic Symptom and Related Disorders

Georgia L. Stevens, PhD, APRN, PMHCNS-BC
Director
P.A.L. Associates
Partners in Aging and Long-Term Caregiving
Washington, D.C.
Chapter 17: Mental Health Promotion for Older Adults

Roberta Stock, MSN, PMHCNS-BC
Advanced Practice Nurse
Community Treatment, Inc.
Jefferson County Missouri Community Mental Health Centers
Crystal City, Missouri
Chapter 23: Schizoaffective, Delusional, and Other Psychotic Disorders

Sandra P. Thomas, PhD, RN, FAAN
Professor and Chair, PhD Program in Nursing
University of Tennessee
Knoxville, Tennessee
Chapter 19: Management of Anger, Aggression, and Violence

Barbara Jones Warren, PhD, RN, CNS-BC, PMH, FAAN
Professor, Clinical Nursing
Specialty Director, Psychiatric and Mental Health Nursing
National Institutes of Health/American Nurses Association Ethnic/Racial Minority Fellow
The Ohio State College of Nursing
Columbus, Ohio
Chapter 24: Depression

Jane H. White, PhD, PMH-CNS, BC
Vera E. Bender Professor of Nursing and Associate Dean for Research and Graduate Programs
School of Nursing
Adelphi University
Garden City, New York
Chapter 30: Eating Disorders

Deborah McNeil Whitehouse, DSN, APRN, BC
Dean
College of Health Sciences
Eastern Kentucky University
Richmond, Kentucky
Chapter 27: Borderline Personality Disorder

Rhonda K. Wilson, MS
Quality Manager
Chester Mental Health Center
Chester, Illinois
Chapter 41: Caring for Persons With Mental Illness and Criminal Behavior

Richard Yakimo, PhD, PMHCNS-BC, N-NAP
Assistant Professor
University of Missouri—St. Louis
College of Nursing
St. Louis, Missouri
Chapter 16: Mental Health Promotion for Young and Middle-Aged Adults
Chapter 38: Caring for Persons Who Are Homeless and Mentally Ill

Reviewers

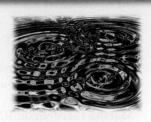

Pamela Adamshick, PhD, RN, PMHCNS-BC
Associate Professor of Nursing
St. Luke's School of Nursing
Moravian College
Bethlehem, Pennsylvania

Mary J. Baukus, MS, MA, RN
Master Faculty Specialist
Bronson School of Nursing
Western Michigan University
Kalamazoo, Michigan

Annette L. Becker, MS, RN
Assistant Professor
Utica College
Utica, New York

Marilynn Berg, MEd, BScN, RN
Faculty
Grant MacEwan University
Edmonton, Alberta, Canada

Cynthia Bostick, PhD, PMHCNS-BC
Lecturer
California State University
Carson, California

Linda G. Brown, PhD(c), MNS, RN-BC
Assistant Professor
Department of Undergraduate Nursing
School of Nursing
Hampton University, College of Virginia Beach
    Campus
Virginia Beach, Virginia

Catherine B. Burke, RN, MS
Retired Nursing Professor
Kankakee Community College
Kankakee, Illinois

Cindy Burkhardt, DNP, RN, PMHNP-BC
Assistant Professor
School of Nursing
The University of Texas at Houston
Houston, Texas

Barbara Champlin, PhD, RN
Associate Professor
St. Catherine University
St. Paul, Minnesota

Darlene M. Copley, RN, MS, APRN-BC
Associate Professor
Department of Nursing Science
St. Cloud State University
St. Cloud, Minnesota

Gail A. Cummings, MSN, PMH-APRN
Assistant Professor of Psychiatric Nursing
Lehigh Carbon Community College
Schnecksville, Pennsylvania

Janet Curley, RN, MA, MEd
Assistant Professor
Alfred State College
Alfred, New York

Jan Dalsheimer, MS, RN, CNE
Associate Clinical Professor
Texas Woman's University
Dallas, Texas

Julie Donalek, DNSC, CNS-BC
Assistant Professor
DePaul University
Chicago, Illinois

Diane C. Ebken, MS, RN, CNE
Instructor in Nursing, Senior Lecturer
School of Nursing
The Pennsylvania State University
University Park, Pennsylvania

Laurie Galatas, MN, RN
Associate Clinical Professor
College of Nursing
Texas Woman's University
Dallas, Texas

Nickole Marie George, PhD, MSN, BSN
Assistant Professor
The University of Pittsburgh-Johnstown
Johnstown, Pennsylvania

Marsha Gerdeman, RN, MS
Associate Professor
Rhodes State College
Lima, Ohio

Debra Gottel, MHS, BSN
Instructor
College of Nursing
University of South Florida
Tampa, Florida

Dianne Groll, RN, BA, BScH, MSc, PhD
Assistant Professor
Department of Psychiatry
Queen's University
Kingston, Ontario

Nancy Kostin, MSN, RN
Associate Professor of Nursing
Madonna University
Livonia, Michigan

Mary F. Leveillee, MS, RN
Director, Undergraduate Studies
College of Nursing
University of Rhode Island
Kingston, Rhode Island

Lou-Ann H. Martinez, RN, MS, APRN, BC
Professor of Nursing
Polk Community College
Winter Haven, Florida

Terran Mathers, RN, BA, DNS
Faculty, Associate Professor
Division of Nursing
Spring Hill College
Mobile, Alabama

Marie Messier, MSN, MEd, BSN, RN
Associate Professor of Nursing
Germanna Community College
Locust Grove, Virginia

Nancy Miller, MS, RN
Nursing Instructor
Minneapolis Community and Technical College
Minneapolis, Minnesota

Shirley Kelley Misselwitz, MSN, RN
Associate Professor of Nursing
West Liberty University
West Liberty, West Virginia

Marilyn Mouradjian, RN, MSN
Full-Time Adjunct Faculty
Psychiatric/Mental Health Nursing
Oakland University
Rochester, Michigan

Sue Myers, RPN, AdvPsychNurs, BSW, MV/TEd
Program Head, Psychiatric Nursing
Saskatchewan Institute of Applied Science and
   Technology
Regina, Saskatchewan

Susan A. Newfield, PhD, RN, PMHCNS-BC
Associate Professor
Health Sciences Center, School of Nursing
West Virginia University
Morgantown, West Virginia

Glenda Nickell, RN, MSN
Instructor of Clinical Nursing
University of Missouri
Sinclair School of Nursing
University of Missouri
Columbia, Missouri

Bonnie Noll-Nelson, DNP, RN
Professor of Nursing
Mount Aloysius College
Cresson, Pennsylvania

Sudha C. Patel, BSN, MN, MA, DNS RN
Assistant Professor
University of Louisiana at Lafayette
Lafayette, Louisiana

Olimpia Paun, PhD, PMHCNS-BC
Associate Professor
Rush University College of Nursing
Chicago, Illinois

Leandra M. Price, RN, BSN, MSN, CNS, DNP
Assistant Faculty
Eastern Kentucky University
Richmond, Kentucky

Miley O. Pulliam, RN, ADN, BSN, MSN
Associate Degree Nursing Instructor
McLennan Community College
Waco, Texas

Sandra D. Robinson, RN, BA, BSN, MS
Associate Professor
Antelope Valley College
Lancaster, California

Kathryn Schroeder-Bruce, MSN, PMHNP-BC
Associate Professor of Clinical Nursing
University of Rochester
Rochester, New York

Mary Shoemaker, RN
Instructor
Morehead State University
Morehead, Kentucky

Patti Skorupka, PhD, APRN, BC
Assistant Professor
School of Nursing
Duquesne University
Pittsburgh, Pennsylvania

Margaret M. Slusser, PhD, RN, PMHCNS-BC
Chairperson and Associate Professor
Department of Nursing and Health
Division of Science and Health Care
DeSales University
Center Valley, Pennsylvania

Ardith L. Sudduth, PhD, FNP-BC
Assistant Professor
University of Louisiana at Lafayette
Lafayette, Louisiana

Susan G. Szczesny, MS, RN, BC, NP
Instructor
College of Nursing
Wayne State University
Detroit, Michigan

Martha J. Thie, EdD, MSN, BSN
Associate Professor Emerita of Nursing
University of Indianapolis
Indianapolis, Indiana

Joyce Vogler, DrPH, MSN, APRN-BC
Associate Professor
School of Nursing and Dental Hygiene
University of Hawaii
Honolulu, Hawaii

Mary E. Weyer, EdD, APN, CNS
Professor
Elmhurst College
Elmhurst, Illinois

Jean Yockey, MSN, FNP-BC, CNE
Associate Professor
University of South Dakota
Vermillion, South Dakota

Kirstyn K. Zalice, MSN
Clinical Assistant Professor
School of Nursing and Allied Health
Robert Morris University
Moon Township, Pennsylvania

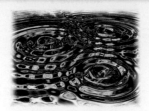

Preface

The role of psychiatric–mental health nursing continues to expand as the demand for qualified mental health professionals increases. At the same time, nurses in other health care areas and settings are increasingly being asked to care for persons with mental health problems and disorders. Nursing faculty are expected to prepare students to care for individuals with psychiatric problems in all health care settings.

In the fall of 2013, the American Psychiatric Association published its long awaited fifth revision of the mental disorders diagnostic taxonomy that changed the names of several mental disorders and assigned others to new categories. Then in June 2014, the new *Psychiatric-Mental Health Nursing Scope & Standards of Practice* was published. In order to equip nursing faculty and students with the latest scope and standards and mental disorders taxonomy, we made the decision to enhance the fifth edition of *Psychiatric Nursing: Contemporary Practice* using the new *Scope & Standards* and *DSM-5* taxonomy. In addition, this enhanced, updated edition includes up-to-date research findings within our changing social world, such as the increase in adolescent use of marijuana that coincided with its legalization in many states, as well as other evidence-based studies. Mental health promotion and prevention of mental disorders also continue to be emphasized.

The pedagogical features of previous editions, including NCLEX Notes, Nursing Care Plans, Critical Thinking Questions, Fame & Fortune highlights, and summaries of entertainment videos offer opportunities for students to challenge the stigma associated with mental disorders.

Our goal is to prepare nursing leaders who challenge the status quo, partner with their patients in the delivery of care, and use the latest evidence in their nursing practice.

TEXT ORGANIZATION

Early chapters of *Psychiatric Nursing: Contemporary Practice, Fifth Edition, Enhanced Update* introduce students to mental health care in contemporary society. Recovery and its 10 components are presented in Chapter 2 and set the stage for recovery-oriented nursing practice. As the building blocks for the future chapters, the first three units present the conceptual underpinnings and principles of psychiatric–mental health nursing. Units 4 and 5 present mental health promotion and prevention content, including very comprehensive chapters on stress

and mental health and suicide prevention. Unit 6 presents the care of persons with mental disorders, including an explanation of the impact of the *DSM-5*. The last three units focus on the care of children, older adults, and special populations including those who are homeless or medically compromised.

The text presents complex concepts in easy-to-understand language with multiple examples and explanations. Students find the text easy to comprehend, filled with meaningful information, and applicable to all areas of nursing practice.

PEDAGOGICAL FEATURES

The fifth edition of *Psychiatric Nursing: Contemporary Practice, Enhanced Update* incorporates a multitude of pedagogical features to focus and direct student learning:

- **Expanded Table of Contents** allows readers to find and refer to concepts from one location.
- **Learning Objectives, Key Terms,** and **Key Concepts** in the chapter openers cue readers on what will be encountered and what is important to understand in each chapter.
- **Summary of Key Points** lists at the end of each chapter provide quick access to important chapter content to facilitate study and review.
- **Critical Thinking Challenges** ask questions that require students to think critically about chapter content and apply psychiatric nursing concepts to nursing practice.
- **Movies** list current examples of movies that depict various mental health disorders and that are widely available on DVD for rent or purchase. Viewing points are provided to serve as a basis for discussion in class and among students.

SPECIAL FEATURES

- **NCLEX Notes** help students focus on important application areas to prepare for the NCLEX.
- **Emergency Care Alerts** highlight important situations in psychiatric nursing care that the nurse should recognize as emergencies.
- **Fame and Fortune** features highlight famous people who have made important contributions to society despite dealing with mental health problems. In many

instances, the public remained unaware of these disorders. The feature emphasizes that mental disorders can happen to anyone and that people with mental health problems can be productive members of society.

- **Diagrams, illustrations, and photos** colorfully illustrate the interrelationship of the biologic, psychological, and social domains of mental health and illness.
- **Nursing Management of Selected Disorders** sections provide an in-depth study of the more commonly occurring major psychiatric disorders.
- **Nursing Care Plans,** based on case scenarios, present clinical examples of patients with a particular diagnosis and demonstrate plans of care that follow patients through various diagnostic stages and care delivery settings.
- **Interdisciplinary Treatment and Recovery Plans (ITPs)** are linked with their respective nursing care plans in several chapters. ITPs are used extensively in practice.
- **Research for Best Practice** boxes highlight today's focus on evidence-based practice for *best practice,* presenting findings and implications of studies that are applicable to psychiatric nursing practice.
- **Therapeutic Dialogue** boxes compare and contrast therapeutic and nontherapeutic conversations to encourage students by example to develop effective communication skills.
- **Psychoeducation Checklists** identify content areas for patient and family education related to specific disorders and their treatment. These checklists support critical thinking by encouraging students to develop patient-specific teaching plans based on chapter content.
- **Clinical Vignette** boxes present reality-based clinical portraits of patients who exhibit the symptoms described in the text. Questions are posed to help students express their thoughts and identify solutions to issues presented in the vignettes.
- **Using Reflection** boxes provide examples of how the nurse uses reflection to interpret a clinical situation in the nurse–patient relationship.
- **Drug Profile** boxes present a thorough picture of commonly prescribed medications for patients with mental health problems. Examples include lorazepam (Ativan), an anxiolytic, and mirtazapine (Remeron), an antidepressant. The profiles complement the text discussions of biologic processes known to be associated with various mental health disorders.
- **Key Diagnostic Characteristics** summaries describe diagnostic criteria, target symptoms, and associated findings for select disorders, adapted from the *DSM-5* by the American Psychiatric Association.
- **Nursing Diagnosis Concept Maps** help students learn to organize complex patient data into a meaningful nursing diagnosis and visually link key concepts of a disorder to in-practice examples.

- **Patient education**, **family**, **and emergency icons** highlight content related to these topics to help link concepts to practice.

TEACHING/LEARNING PACKAGE

To facilitate mastery of this text's content, a comprehensive teaching and learning package has been developed to assist faculty and students.

- prepU : Adaptive Learning | Powered by prepU provides students with the practice they want and need—at their own pace and based on their level of understanding linked to the content of this text. ISBN: 978-1-4698-9049-4
- Lippincott CoursePoint **Lippincott CoursePoint is a fully adaptive and integrated digital course solution for nursing education.** CoursePoint synthesizes adaptive learning tools and content with an electronic version of the text and a wide array of integrated learning aids—all in one convenient location. ISBN: 978-1-4698-9476-8

Instructor Resources

Tools to assist you with teaching your course are available upon adoption of this text on thePoint at http://thepoint.lww.com/Boyd5eUpdate.

- The **Test Generator** lets you put together exclusive new tests from a bank containing hundreds of questions to help you in assessing your students' understanding of the material. Test questions link to chapter learning objectives. This test generator comes with a bank of more than 775 questions.
- An extensive collection of materials is provided for each book chapter:
  - **Pre-Lecture Quizzes** (and answers) are quick, knowledge-based assessments that allow you to check students' reading.
  - **PowerPoint Presentations** provide an easy way for you to integrate the textbook with your students' classroom experience, either via slide shows or handouts. Multiple-choice and true/false questions are integrated into the presentations to promote class participation and allow you to use i-clicker technology.
  - **Guided Lecture Notes** walk you through the chapters, objective by objective, and provide you with corresponding PowerPoint slide numbers.
  - **Discussion Topics** (and suggested answers) can be used as conversation starters or in online discussion boards.
  - **Assignments** (and suggested answers) include group, written, clinical, and Web assignments.
  - **Case Studies** with related questions (and suggested answers) give students an opportunity to apply their knowledge to a client case similar to one they might encounter in practice.

- An **Image Bank** lets you use the photographs and illustrations from this textbook in your PowerPoint slides or as you see fit in your course.
- A sample **Syllabus** provides guidance for structuring your course.
- **Access to All Student Resources** is also provided.

Student Resources

An exciting set of free resources is available to help students review and apply important concepts. Students can access these resources on thePoint. at http://thepoint. lww.com/Boyd5eUpdate using the codes printed in the front of their textbooks.

- **NCLEX-Style Review Questions** for each chapter help students review important concepts and practice for NCLEX.
- ⚙ **New online video series,** *Lippincott Theory to Practice Video Series: Psychiatric–Mental Health Nursing,* includes videos of true-to-life patients displaying mental health disorders, allowing students to gain experience and a deeper understanding of mental health patients. The video series allows viewing of complete patient interviews and also gives the opportunity to

view snippets of those interviews, for closer analysis or classroom discussion. Theory to Practice topics such as Depression, Eating Disorders, and Addiction make up some of the innovative videos to help students in their course and beyond.

- ⚙ **Watch & Learn Video Clip** on cognitive functions is included from *Lippincott Video Guide to Psychiatric–Mental Health Nursing Assessment.*
- ⚙ **Practice & Learn Activities** offer case studies related to therapeutic communication, antidepressants, and dementia from *Lippincott Interactive Case Studies in Psychiatric–Mental Health Nursing.*
- M⚙VIE viewing **GUIDES** highlight films depicting individuals with mental health disorders and provide students the opportunity to approach nursing care related to mental health and illness in a novel way.
- **Clinical Simulations** on schizophrenia, depression, and the acutely manic phase walk students through case studies and put them in real-life situations.
- **Journal Articles** provided for each chapter offer access to current research available in Wolters Kluwer journals.

Mary Ann Boyd, PhD, DNS, RN, PMHCNS-BC

Acknowledgments

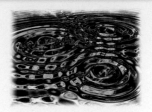

This text is a result of many long hours of diligent work by the contributors, editors, and assistants. Psychiatric nurses are constantly writing about and discussing new strategies for caring for persons with mental disorders. Consumers of mental health services provided directions for nursing care and validated the importance of nursing interventions. I wish to acknowledge and thank these individuals.

Betsy Gentzler of Wolters Kluwer was an extraordinary partner in this project during the development of the original revision. I want to especially acknowledge her attention to detail and her commitment to the completion of this edition. She provided direction, support, and valuable input throughout this project. Helen Kogut was also an extraordinary partner during revision of this update. Helen brought a broad knowledge base and extreme patience during the whole update process.

Contents

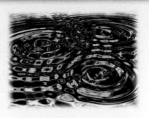

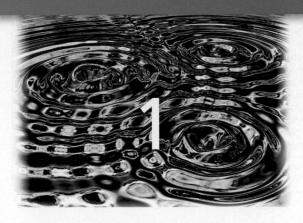

1

Psychiatric–Mental Health Nursing and Evidence-Based Practice

Mary Ann Boyd

KEY CONCEPTS

- psychiatric–mental health nursing
- evidence-based practice

LEARNING OBJECTIVES

After studying this chapter, you will be able to:

1. Identify the dynamic scope of psychiatric–mental health nursing practice.

2. Relate the history of psychiatric–mental health nursing to contemporary nursing practice.

3. Discuss the importance of evidence-based psychiatricmental health nursing practice in all health care settings.

4. Outline the evolution of recovery in mental health care.

5. Discuss the impact of recent legislative and policy changes in the delivery of mental health evidence.

KEY TERMS

- asylum • deinstitutionalization • institutionalization • moral treatment • neurosis • psychoanalysis
- psychosis

Everyone experiences emotional and mental health issues at some time in their lives. During periods of illness and stress, mental health issues often become overwhelming to individuals and their families. Every nurse has an opportunity to provide effective mental health interventions, no matter the practice site. Nurses in acute care settings are likely to care for persons in mental health crises because medical problems are treated before any mental health issues (e.g., physical injuries from a suicide attempt are treated before the underlying depression). Like anyone else, people with psychiatric disorders seek health care for their medical illnesses. The stress of the medical illness can also exacerbate psychiatric symptoms.

The practice of psychiatric–mental health nursing is dynamic, challenging, and rewarding.

> **KEYCONCEPT** Grounded in nursing theories, **psychiatric–mental health** nursing is defined as the "nursing practice specialty committed to promoting mental health through the assessment, diagnosis, and treatment of behavioral problems, mental disorders, and comorbid conditions across the lifespan. Psychiatric–mental health nursing intervention is an art and a science, employing purposeful use of self and a wide range of nursing, psychosocial, and neurobiological evidence to produce effective outcomes" (American Nurses Association, American Psychiatric Nurses Association, International Society of Psychiatric–Mental Health Nurses 2014, pg 1).

BOX 1.1

Psychiatric–Mental Health Nursing's Phenomena of Concern

Phenomena of concern for psychiatric-mental health nurses are dynamic, exist in all populations across the lifespan and include but are not limited to:
- Promotion of optimal mental and physical health and well-being
- Prevention of mental and behavioral distress and illness
- Promotion of social inclusion of mentally and behaviorally fragile individuals
- Co-occurring mental health and substance use disorders
- Co-occurring mental health and physical disorders
- Alterations in thinking, perceiving, communicating, and functioning related to psychological and physiological distress
- Psychological and physiological distress resulting from physical, interpersonal, and/or environmental trauma or neglect.

- Psychogenesis and individual vulnerability
- Complex clinical presentations confounded by poverty and poor, inconsistent, or toxic environmental factors
- Alterations in self-concept related to loss of physical organs and/or limbs, psychic trauma, developmental conflicts, or injury
- Individual, family, or group isolation and difficulty with interpersonal relations
- Self-harm and self-destructive behaviors including mutilation and suicide
- Violent behavior including physical abuse, sexual abuse, and bullying
- Low health literacy rates contributing to treatment non-adherence

---

Psychiatric nurses care for patients with a wide range of emotional problems and mental disorders (Box 1.1). These nurses, specializing in mental health nursing, are not only experts in caring for persons with a primary diagnosis of a mental disorder but also for those with self-concept and body image issues, developmental crises, co-occurring disorders, end-of-life changes, and emotional stress related to illness, disability, or loss. It is a psychiatric nurse who is called when violence, suicide, or a disaster erupts. In this text, the terms *psychiatric nursing* and *psychiatric–mental health nursing* are used interchangeably. The standards of practice are discussed in Chapter 6.

THE PAST AND PRESENT

Psychiatric nursing has a history that can be traced back to the early days of nursing practice. Today the specialty has developed into one of the core mental health professions with an emphasis on evidence-based practice.

Early Founders

The roots of contemporary psychiatric–mental health nursing can be traced to Florence Nightingale's holistic view of a patient who lives within a family and community. She was especially sensitive to human emotions and recommended interactions that today would be classified as therapeutic communication (see Chapter 9). For example, this early nursing leader's intervention for reducing anxiety about an illness was to encourage independence and self-care (Nightingale, 1859).

Linda Richards, the first trained nurse in the United States, opened the Boston City Hospital Training School for Nurses in 1882 at McLean Hospital, a mental health facility (Cowles, 1887) (Box 1.2). Employees of McLean

were recruited into the nursing program to learn to provide physical care for patients with mental disorders who developed medical illnesses. In 1913, Effie Taylor integrated psychiatric nursing content into the curriculum at Johns Hopkins' Phipps Clinic. Taylor, like Nightingale before her, encouraged nurses to avoid the dichotomy of mind and body (Church, 1987). The first psychiatric nursing textbook, *Nursing Mental Disease*, was written by Harriet Bailey in 1920. Gradually, nursing education programs in psychiatric hospitals were phased into mainstream nursing education programs (Peplau, 1989).

Emergence of Modern Nursing Perspectives

As psychiatric–mental health nursing developed as a profession in the 20th century, modern perspectives of mental illness emerged, and these new theories profoundly shaped mental health care (see Units ii and iii). In 1952, Hildegarde E. Peplau published the landmark work *Interpersonal Relations in Nursing* (1952). This publication introduced psychiatric–mental health nursing practice to the concepts of interpersonal relations and the therapeutic relationship. Peplau conceptualized nursing practice as independent of physicians. The use of self as a nursing tool was outside the dominance of both hospital administrators and physicians.

Peplau also contributed to educational programs for psychiatric nursing, developing a specialty training program in psychiatric nursing—the first graduate nursing program—in 1954 at Rutgers University. Subspecialties began to emerge, focusing on children, adolescents, and older adults.

In 1967, the Division of Psychiatric and Mental Health Nursing Practice of the American Nurses Association (ANA) published the first *Statement on Psychiatric Nursing Practice*. This publication was the first official sanction of

History of Psychiatric–Mental Health Nursing

1882 First training school for psychiatric nursing at McLean Asylum by E. Cowles; first nursing program to admit men

1913 First nurse-organized program of study for psychiatric training by Euphemia (Effie) Jane Taylor at Johns Hopkins Phipps Clinic

1914 Mary Adelaide Nutting emphasized nursing role development

1920 First psychiatric nursing text published, *Nursing Mental Disease* by Harriet Bailey

1950 Accredited schools required to offer a psychiatric nursing experience

1952 Publication of Hildegarde E. Peplau's *Interpersonal Relations in Nursing*

1954 First graduate program in psychiatric nursing established at Rutgers University by Hildegarde E. Peplau

1963 *Perspectives in Psychiatric Care* and *Journal of Psychiatric Nursing* published

1967 *Standards of Psychiatric–Mental Health Nursing Practice* published; American Nurses Association (ANA) initiated the certification of generalists in psychiatric–mental health nursing

1979 *Issues in Mental Health Nursing* published; ANA initiated the certification of specialists in psychiatric–mental health nursing

1980 *Nursing: A Social Policy Statement* published by the ANA

1982 *Revised Standards of Psychiatric and Mental Health Nursing Practice* issued by the ANA

1985 *Standards of Child and Adolescent Psychiatric and Mental Health Nursing Practice* published by the ANA

1987 *Archives of Psychiatric Nursing and Journal of Child and Adolescent Psychiatric and Mental Health Nursing* published

1994 *Statement on Psychiatric–Mental Health Clinical Nursing Practice and Standards of Psychiatric–Mental Health Clinical Nursing Practice* published

1996 Guidelines specifying course content and competencies published by the Society for Education and Research in Psychiatric–Mental Health Nursing

2000 *Scope and Standards of Psychiatric–Mental Health Nursing Practice* published

2003 A second advanced practice role, Psychiatric–Mental Health Nurse Practitioner, was delineated

2014 *Psychiatric–Mental Health Nursing: Scope and Standards of Practice* was revised to reflect the expanding role of psychiatric–mental health nurses practicing in a recovery-oriented environment.

a holistic approach of psychiatric–mental health nurses practicing in a variety of settings with a diverse clientele, emphasizing health promotion as well as health restoration. Since 1967, there have been several updates of the official practice statement that reflect the expansion of the role of psychiatric nurses with a delineation of functions.

Over the past century, psychiatric nursing practice expanded from the hospital to the community. Today in the United States, many nursing graduate degree programs offer specializations in psychiatric–mental. Psychiatric nurses sit on corporate boards; serve in the armed forces; lead major health care initiatives; teach in major universities, and care for young and old people, families, and disadvantaged and homeless individuals. Psychiatric nursing is truly a versatile and rewarding field of nursing practice (Fig. 1.1).

Evidence-Based Practice and Current Psychiatric Nursing

Evidence-based practice is the standard of care in psychiatric nursing and mental health care. Clinical decisions that lead to high-quality patient outcomes are based on research and evidence-based theories, clinical expertise, and patient preferences and values. By combining data from various sources such as expert opinion, patient data, and clinical experiences, the nurse is able to be objective yet open to new ideas. For example, using epidemiological data helps nurses identify high-risk groups for suicide; for example, white, divorced males over the age of 85, but evidence from clinical experiences also show that middle-aged adults with depression are also at risk for suicide.

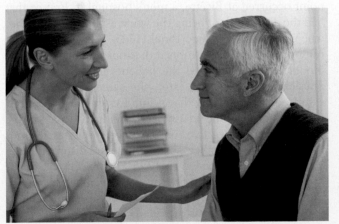 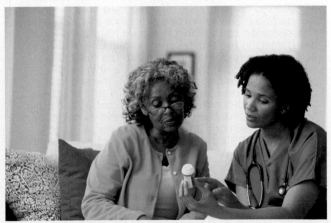

FIGURE 1.1 Contemporary psychiatric–mental health nursing is a versatile and rewarding field of practice.

> **KEYCONCEPT** **Evidence-based practice** is a problem-solving approach to the delivery of health care that integrates the best evidence from well-designed studies and patient care data, and combines with it with patient preferences and values and nurse expertise (Melnyk et al., 2009).

In an evidence-based approach, clinical questions are defined; evidence is discovered and analyzed; the research findings are applied in a practical manner and in collaboration with the patient; and outcomes are evaluated. One of the first steps is seeking out a mentor who can help through the evidence-based process because this approach requires using literature search skills, followed by careful reading and critiquing of the current studies and seeking the advice experts in the field. A nurse might start with a clinical question such as are group cognitive therapy nursing interventions effective in increasing the likelihood of continuing treatment following discharge from the hospital. The nurse and mentor will narrow the question and begin a critique of the literature. Even though the process results in directions for practice, the nurse will face many challenges. See Box 1.3.

BOX 1.3

Research Evidence for Best Practice: **Challenges of Conducting Evidence-Based Research**

Beebe, L., Adams, S., & El-Mallakh, P. (2011). Putting the "Evidence" in evidence-based practice: Meeting research challenges in community psychiatric settings. Issues in Mental Health Nursing, 32(8), 537–543.

THE QUESTION: How are the system-, clinician-, and client-related research barriers in community psychiatric settings overcome?

METHODS: Barriers in implementing nursing research were identified by three nurse researchers. They described how the strategies they used to overcome these barriers to continue with their research.

FINDINGS: In Dr. Beebe's study, the challenge was transportation to the study site. She reported how she identified participants who needed assistance and included transportation costs within her grant. Dr. Adams identified barriers in the timely communication with new residents who were being recruited into the study. She addressed this issue by building partnerships with agency staff members and supporting the two case managers in increasing their availability to the subjects. She also provided a small, financial incentive to the participants. Dr. El-Mallakh found barriers in clients' comprehension, memory, and decision-making skills. She also found low literacy and education in her population. She tailored her interaction with the participants to recognize these deficits.

IMPLICATIONS FOR NURSING: Barriers to conducting research that supports evidence-based practice will exist but can be overcome. Generating evidence is important in order to provide the best care to our patients.

EVOLUTION OF MENTAL HEALTH RECOVERY

Throughout history, popular beliefs of the time served as the basis for understanding and treating people with mental illnesses. Prehistoric healers practiced an ancient surgical technique of removing a disk of bone from the skull to let out the evil spirits. In the early Christian period (1–100 AD), when sin or demonic possession was thought to cause mental disorders, clergymen treated patients, often through prescribed exorcisms. If such measures did not succeed, patients were excluded from the community and sometimes even put to death. Later in the medieval era (1000–1300 AD), contaminated environments were believed to cause mental illness. Consequently, individuals were removed from their "sick" environments and placed in protected asylums. Table 1.1 provides a summary of historical events and correlating perspectives on mental health during the premoral treatment era (800 BC to the colonial period).

Moral Treatment and Asylums

As evidence mounted that insanity was an illness and recovery was a possibility, existing primitive physical treatments, such as venesections (bloodletting) and gyrations (strapping patients to a rotating board), began to be viewed as either painful or barbaric. With neurobiologic science not advanced enough to offer reasonable treatment approaches, a safe haven, or **asylum**, was considered the best option for treatment. In the moral treatment period (1790–1900), **moral treatment**, that is, the use of kindness, compassion, and a pleasant environment, was adopted. Individuals with mental disorders were routinely removed from their communities and placed in asylums, which was thought to be best for their safety and comfort.

Despite the good intentions that may have been at the root of the moral treatment movement, within the asylums, patients were often treated inhumanely. A turning point occurred at Bicêtre, a men's hospital in France that had the distinction of being the worst asylum in the world, when physician Philippe Pinel (1745–1826) ordered the removal of the chains, stopped the abuses of drugging and bloodletting, and placed the patients under the care of physicians. Three years later, the same standards were extended to Salpêtrière, the asylum for female patients. At about the same time in England, William Tuke (1732–1822), a member of the Society of Friends, raised funds for a retreat for members who had mental disorders. The York Retreat was opened in 1796; restraints were abandoned, and sympathetic care in quiet, pleasant surroundings with some form of industrial occupation, such as weaving or farming, was provided (Fig. 1.2).

(text continues on page 6)

Table 1.1	PREMORAL TREATMENT ERA	
Period	**Beliefs About Mental Illness**	**Mental Health Care**
Ancient Times to 800 BCE	Sickness was an indication of the displeasure of deities for sins. Viewed as supernatural.	Persons with psychiatric symptoms were driven from homes and ostracized by relatives. When behavioral manifestations were viewed as supernatural powers, the persons who exhibited them were revered.
Periods of Inquiry: 800 BCE to 1 CE	Egypt and Greek periods of inquiry. Physical and mental health viewed as interrelated. Hippocrates argued abnormal behaviors were due to brain disturbances. Aristotle related mental to physical disorders.	Counseling, work, music were provided in temples by priests to relieve the distress of those with mental disorders. Observation and documentation were a part of the care. The mental disorders were treated as diseases. The aim of treatment was to correct imbalances.
Early Christian and Early Medieval: 1–1000 CE	Power of Christian church grew. St. Augustine pronounced all diseases ascribed to demons.	Persons with psychiatric symptoms were incarcerated in dungeons, beaten, and starved.
Later Medieval: 1000–1300	In Western Europe, spirit of inquiry was dead. Healing was taken over by theologians and witchdoctors. Persons with psychiatric symptoms were incarcerated in dungeons, beaten, and starved. In the Middle East, Avicenna said mental disorders are illnesses.	First asylums built by Muslims. Persons with psychiatric symptoms were treated as being sick.
Renaissance: 1300–1600	In England, insane were differentiated from criminal. In colonies, mental illness were believed to be caused by demonic possession. Witch hunts were common.	Persons with psychiatric symptoms who presented a threat to society were apprehended and locked up. There were no public provisions for persons with mental disorders except jail. Private hospitalization for the wealthy who could pay. Bethlehem Asylum was used as a private institution.
Colonial: 1700–1790	1751: Benjamin Franklin established Pennsylvania Hospital (in Philadelphia)—the first institution in United States to receive those with mental disorders for treatment and cure.	The beginnings of mental diseases viewed as illness to be treated.

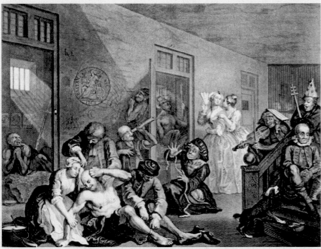

Interior of Bethlehem Asylum, London

(Continued)

Table 1.1	PREMORAL TREATMENT ERA (*Continued*)	
Period	Beliefs About Mental Illness	Mental Health Care
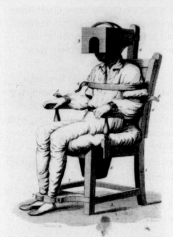 The Tranquilizer Chair of Benjamin Rush. A patient is sitting in a chair, his body immobilized, a bucket attached beneath the seat. From U.S. National Library of Medicine. *Images from the History of Medicine,* Washington, DC: National Institutes of Health, Department of Health and Human Services.	1773: First public, free-standing asylum at Williamsburg, Virginia. 1783: Benjamin Rush categorized mental illnesses and began to treat mental disorders with medical interventions, such as bloodletting, mechanical devices.	

In the United States, the Quakers were instrumental in stopping the practice of bloodletting; they also placed great emphasis on providing a proper religious atmosphere (Deutsch, 1949). The Quaker Friends Asylum was proposed in 1811 and opened 6 years later in Frankford, Pennsylvania (now Philadelphia), to become the second asylum in the United States. The humane and supportive

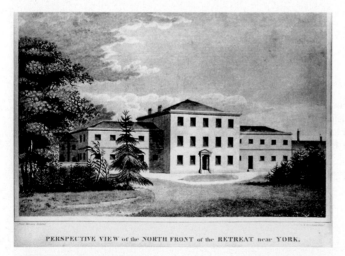

PERSPECTIVE VIEW of the NORTH FRONT of the RETREAT near YORK.

FIGURE 1.2 The perspective view of the north front of the retreat near York. (From U.S. National Library of Medicine. *Images from the history of medicine.* Washington, DC: National Institutes of Health, Department of Health and Human Services.)

rehabilitative attitude of the Quakers was seen as an extremely important influence in changing techniques of caring for those with mental disorders. As states were founded, new hospitals were opened that were dedicated to the care of patients with mental disorders.

Even with these hospitals, only a fraction of people with mental disorders received treatment. Those who were judged dangerous were hospitalized; those deemed harmless or mildly insane were treated the same as other indigents and given no public support. In farm communities, as was the custom during the first half of the 19th century, poor and indigent individuals were often auctioned and bought by landowners to provide cheap labor. Landowners eagerly sought them for their strong backs and weak minds. The arrangement had its own economic usefulness because it provided the community with a low-cost way to care for people with mental illness. Some states used almshouses (poorhouses) for housing mentally ill individuals.

Public Funding, Dorothea Dix, and State Hospitals

Hospitals for individuals with mental illness were few because of financing; there were no funding mechanisms to support these large institutions. The first step in resolving the funding problem was defining responsibility—that is, which agency would be responsible for paying for care. In 1828, Horace Mann, a representative in the Massachusetts state legislature, saw his plea that the "insane are wards of the state" become a reality. State governments were mandated to assume financial responsibility for the care of people with mental illnesses.

After states were designated as being financially responsible for the treatment of their residents with mental illnesses, the next step was ensuring that each state appropriated funds. Dorothea Lynde Dix (1802–1887), a vigorous crusader for the humane treatment of patients with mental illness, was responsible for much of the reform of the mental health care system in the 19th century. Her solution was state hospitals. She first influenced the Massachusetts legislature to expand the Massachusetts State Hospital. Then, through public awareness campaigns and lobbying efforts, she managed to convince state after state to build hospitals. At the end of Dix's long career, 20 states had responded directly to her appeals by establishing or enlarging state hospitals (Box 1.4).

Institutionalization and Its Outcomes

In state hospitals, **institutionalization**, the forced confinement of individuals for long periods of time in large facilities, became the primary treatment for more than 50 years (1900 to 1955). Institutions had little more to offer than food, clothing, pleasant surroundings, and perhaps some means of employment and exercise. Outcomes of institutionalization were consistently negative. Thousands of people were warehoused within the walls of institutions for months and years with little hope of reentering society. Patients were socially isolated from their families and normal community life. The medical superintendent's major concern was the day-to-day operation of the large, aging physical structures. Untrained attendants who had little understanding of mental illnesses were responsible for the care, which was often cruel and inhumane. There were few educated nurses. Patients suffered adverse physical and psychological effects. There were few trained mental health providers. Early institutions eventually evolved into self-contained communities that produced their own food and made their own clothing. Institutionalization was a dismal failure.

Women had a particularly difficult time and often were institutionalized at the convenience of their fathers or husbands. Because a woman's role in the late 1800s was to function as a domestic extension of her husband, any behaviors or beliefs that did not conform to male expectations could be used to justify the claim of insanity. Women were literally held prisoner for years. In the asylums, women were psychologically degraded, used as servants, and physically tortured by male physicians and female attendants (Bly, 1887).

The relatively primitive and often misguided biologic treatments were unsuccessful. For example, the use of

---

BOX 1.4

Dorothea Lynde Dix

At nearly 40 years of age, Dorothea Dix, a retired school teacher living in Massachusetts, was solicited by a young theology student to help in preparing a Sunday School class for women inmates at the East Cambridge jail. Dix led the class herself and was shocked by the filth and dirt in the jail. She was particularly struck by the treatment of inmates with mental disorders. It was the dead of winter, and no heat was provided. When she questioned the jailer about the lack of heat, his answer was that "the insane need no heat." The prevailing myth was that people with mental illnesses were insensible to extremes of temperature. Dix's outrage initiated a long struggle in the reform of care.

An early feminist, Dix disregarded the New England role of a Puritan woman and diligently investigated the conditions of jails and the plight of the mentally ill. During the Civil War, she was appointed to the post of Superintendent of Women Nurses, the highest position held by a woman during the war.

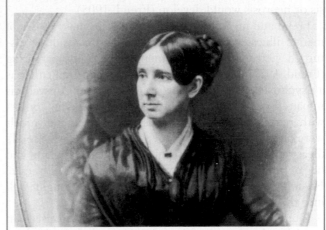

Dorothea Lynde Dix. (From U.S. National Library of Medicine. *Images from the history of medicine*. Washington, DC: National Institutes of Health, Department of Health and Human Services.)

---

hydrotherapy, or baths, was an established procedure in mental institutions. Warm baths and, in some instances, ice cold baths produced calming effects for patients with mental disorders. However, this treatment's success was attributed to the restraint of patients during the bath rather than the physiologic responses that hydrotherapy produced. Baths were then applied indiscriminately and used as a form of restraint rather than a therapeutic practice.

In 1908, Clifford Beers (1876–1943), who recovered from a mental disorder and became an advocate of humane treatment, published an autobiography, *A Mind That Found Itself*, depicting his 3-year hospitalization experience. He was beaten, choked, imprisoned for long periods in dark, dank, padded cells, and confined for many days in a straightjacket. By 1909, Beers formed a National Committee for Mental Hygiene. Through the committee's advocacy efforts, other mental health services were initiated, such as child guidance clinics, prison clinics, and industrial mental health care.

Freud's Contribution

At the same time that the institutionalization movement was gaining strength, Sigmund Freud (1856–1939) and the psychoanalytic movement of the early 1900s exerted influence on the mental health community. Freud, trained as a neuropathologist, developed a personality theory based on unconscious motivations for behavior, or drives. According to the Freudian model, normal development occurred in stages, with the first three—oral, anal, and genital—being the most important. Infants progressed through the oral stage, experiencing the world through symbolic oral ingestion; through the anal stage, in which toddlers develop a sense of autonomy through withholding; and on to the genital stage, in which a beginning sense of sexuality emerges within the framework of the oedipal relationship. If there was any interference in normal development, such as psychological trauma, psychosis or neurosis would develop (Freud, 1905).

Freud and his followers believed the primary causes of mental illnesses were psychological and a result of disturbed personality development and faulty parenting (Freud, 1927). Mental illnesses were categorized either as a **psychosis** (severe) or neurosis (less severe). A psychosis impaired daily functioning because of breaks in contact with reality. A neurosis was less severe, but individuals were often distressed about their problems. Soon, Freud's ideas represented the forefront of psychiatric thought and began to shape society's view of mental health care. Freudian ideology dominated psychiatric thought well into the 1970s.

Intensive **psychoanalysis**, therapy that focused on repairing the trauma of the original psychological injury, was the Freudian treatment of choice. However, psychoanalysis was costly and time consuming and required lengthy training. Few could perform it. Thousands of patients in state institutions with severe mental illnesses were essentially ignored.

Freud's view of mental illness as a psychological disorder gained credibility. He was a prolific writer who reported that his patients improved through psychoanalysis and interpretation of dreams (Freud, 1900). His outcomes were not judged by contemporary standards or subjected to meta-analysis processes. Today psychoanalysis remains as a treatment option for a select group of patients who have the cognitive abilities to discuss and understand complex psychological concepts.

National Action

During World War II (1939–1945), mental illness was beginning to be seen as a problem that could happen to anyone. Many "normal" people who volunteered for the armed services were disqualified on the grounds that they were psychologically unfit to serve. Others who had already served tours of duty developed psychiatric and emotional problems related to their wartime experiences. Today these problems are recognized as a distinct disorder: posttraumatic stress disorder (see Chapter 27).

In 1946, the National Mental Health Act created a six-member National Mental Health Advisory Council that established the National Institute of Mental Health (NIMH), which was responsible for overseeing and coordinating research and training. Under the Act's provisions, the federal government also provided grants to states to support existing outpatient facilities and programs to establish new ones. Before 1948, more than half of all states had no clinics; by 1949, all but five had one or more. Six years later, there were 1,234 outpatient clinics. During the same time period, the Hill–Burton Act provided substantial federal support for hospital construction, which expanded the number of psychiatric units in general hospitals.

Impact of Psychopharmacology

Psychopharmacology revolutionized the treatment of people with mental illness. Initially, barbiturates, particularly amobarbital sodium (Amytal sodium), were tried for treating mental diseases in the 1930s (Malamud, 1944). When chlorpromazine (Thorazine) was introduced in the 1950s, the mental health community was rather hopeful that a medication had been discovered to cure severe mental illness. In reality, the phenothiazines were the first of many antipsychotics to be developed (see Chapter 11). The medications calmed the patients and reduced some of the symptoms. With calmer patients and fewer symptoms, the negative effects of living in a restrictive and coercive institutional environment became evident.

A New National Objective: Community Treatment

In 1961, *Action for Mental Health*, a report of the Joint Commission on Mental Illness and Health Commission, called for larger investments in basic research; national personnel recruitment and training programs; one full-time clinic for every 50,000 individuals supplemented by general hospital units and state-run regional intensive psychiatric treatment centers; and access to emergency care and treatment in general, both in mental hospitals and community clinics. The funding for the construction and operation of the community mental health system would be shared by federal, state, and local governments. The ideas expressed in the report clearly shifted authority for mental health programming to the federal government and were the basis of the federal legislation, the *Mental Retardation Facilities and Community Mental Health Centers Construction Act*, signed into law by John F. Kennedy in 1963. Unfortunately, this act funded only some of the approaches proposed by the Commission and did not support the operation of state-run regional intensive psychiatric centers.

The supporters of this 1963 legislation believed the exact opposite of what Dorothea Dix believed during the previous century. That is, instead of viewing an institution as a peaceful asylum, institutionalization was viewed as contributing to the illness. If patients were moved into a "normal" community-living setting, it was believed that the symptoms of mental disorders could easily be treated and eventually would disappear. Thus, **deinstitutionalization**, the release of those confined to mental institutions for long periods of time into the community for treatment, support, and rehabilitation, became a national movement.

The inpatient state hospital population fell by about 15% between 1955 and 1965 and by about 59% during the succeeding decade. The 2,000 projected community mental health centers (CMHCs) that should have been in place by 1980 never materialized. By 1990, only about 1,300 programs provided various types of psychosocial rehabilitation services, such as vocational, educational, or social-recreational services (International Association of Psychosocial Rehabilitation, 1990).

Deinstitutionalization: A Failed Approach

There is no evidence that the majority of persons discharged from state hospitals benefited from CMHC services. The CMHCs, by and large, ignored the legions of people with serious mental illnesses and instead focused on the treatment of alcoholism and drug addiction. Individual psychotherapy, the primary treatment offered in most centers, was insufficient for those who needed other types of treatment, housing, and vocational opportunities. By the 1990s, deinstitutionalization was considered a failure.

CONTEMPORARY MENTAL HEALTH CARE

Millions of adults and children are disabled by mental illness every year. Compared with all other diseases, major depressive disorder, anxiety disorder, and drug use disorders rank in the top eight conditions responsible for chronic disability in the United States (U.S. Burden of Disease Collaborators, 2013). Government initiatives are attempting to increase the public's understanding of mental disorders and related issues.

In 1999, *Mental Health: A Report of the Surgeon General* summarized evidence for the treatment of mental illness. As the first report addressing mental health by the Office of the Surgeon General, two main findings were presented (U.S. Department of Health and Human Services [U.S. DHHS], 1999):

- The efficacy of mental health treatments is well documented.
- A range of treatments exists for most mental disorders.

The following year, another landmark report, *Report of the Surgeon General's Conference on Children's Mental Health: A National Action Agenda*, was published. This report highlights consensus recommendations for identifying, recognizing, and referring children to services; increasing access to services for families; and using evidence for evaluating treatment services, systems of care, and financing (U.S. Public Health Service, 2000).

In 2003, the *President's New Freedom Commission on Mental Health* recommended that the mental health system be transformed. The report identified six goals as the foundation for transforming mental health care in the United States into a consumer-centered, family-centered, and recovery-oriented system (Box 1.5) (New Freedom Commission on Mental Health, 2003).

In 2010, the *Patient Protection and Affordable Care Act* was passed that provided more people with access to affordable, effective treatments for their mental health needs. This law also prevents insurance companies from excluding people because of pre-existing conditions. The intent of this legislation is to put the consumers of mental health care back in charge of their care. No longer can mental health care be denied funding.

Recovery and the Consumer Movement

Recovery from mental illness is realistic and now a worldwide goal. Consumers are demanding that mental health services receive the same support and attention as other health services. The traditional medical model, which is viewed as autocratic and paternalistic, is being replaced by a collaborative model whereby mental health professionals work in partnership with consumers to help rebuild their lives. Consumer advocacy efforts have led to the implementation of recovery philosophy and practices

---

BOX 1.5

U.S. Goals in a Transformed Mental Health System

Goal 1 Americans understand that mental health is essential to overall health.
Goal 2 Mental health care is consumer and family driven.
Goal 3 Disparities in mental health services are eliminated.
Goal 4 Early mental health screening, assessment, and referral to services are common practice.
Goal 5 Excellent mental health care is delivered, and research is accelerated.
Goal 6 Technology is used to access mental health care and information.

Source: New Freedom Commission on Mental Health. (2003). *Achieving the promise: Transforming mental health care in America* (p. 8). DHHS Publication No. SMA-03-3831. Rockville, MD: U.S. Department of Health and Human Services.

(see Chapter 2). In this text, the terms *consumers* and *patients* are used interchangeably.

National Mental Health Objectives

The vision of *Healthy People 2020* is to have a society in which all people live long and happy lives. The overarching goals of *Healthy People 2020* are to

- Attain high-quality, longer lives free of preventable disease, disability, injury, and premature death.
- Achieve health equity, eliminate disparities, and improve the health of all groups.
- Create social and physical environments that promote good health for all.
- Promote healthy development and healthy behaviors across every stage of life (U.S. DHHS, 2010).

The mental health goal is to improve mental health through prevention and by ensuring access to appropriate, quality mental health services. Three new mental health issues have emerged in the past decade: physical and mental trauma experienced by military members and veterans, large-scale psychological trauma in communities caused by natural disasters, and the understanding and treatment of older adults with dementia and mood

disorders. Objectives focusing on mental health and mental disorders provide guidance for all health care professionals (Box 1.6).

The challenge for psychiatric nursing is to work toward these goals through direct practice, advocating for persons with emotional and mental disorders, and improving the social and physical environments of care.

BOX 1.6

Mental Health and Mental Disorders Objectives for the Year 2020

MENTAL HEALTH STATUS IMPROVEMENT
- Reduce the suicide rate.
- Reduce suicide attempts by adolescents.
- Reduce the proportion of adolescents who engage in disordered eating behaviors in an attempt to control their weight.
- Reduce the proportion of persons who experience major depressive episodes.

TREATMENT EXPANSION
- Increase the proportion of primary care facilities that provide mental health treatment onsite or by paid referral.
- Increase the proportion of children with mental health problems who receive treatment.
- Increase the proportion of juvenile residential facilities that screen admissions for mental health problems.
- Increase the proportion of persons with serious mental illness who are employed.
- Increase the proportion of adults with mental health disorders who receive treatment.
- Increase the proportion of persons with cooccurring substance abuse and mental disorders who receive treatment for both disorders.
- Increase depression screening by primary care providers.
- Increase the proportion of primary care physician office visits that screen youth ages 12 to 18 years for depression.
- Increase the proportion of homeless adults with mental health problems who receive mental health services.

Source: U.S. Department of Health and Human Services. (2010). *Healthy people 2020.* Retrieved July 7, 2014, from http://www.healthypeople.gov.

SUMMARY OF KEY POINTS

- Every practicing nurse cares for persons with an emotional or mental disorder. Every nurse needs basic psychiatric nursing knowledge and skills.

- Psychiatric–mental health nursing is a specialized area of nursing that promotes mental health through applying the nursing process. Psychiatric nurses care for people with a wide range of emotional problems and mental disorders.

- The need for psychiatric–mental health nursing was recognized near the end of the 19th century when Linda Richards opened the Boston City Hospital Training School for Nurses in 1882. Today psychiatric nursing is recognized as one of the core mental health professions.

- Evidence-based practice is the standard of care in psychiatric nursing and in the mental health field. Historically, popular beliefs about the source of mental illnesses and treatment served as evidence.

- Over time, most treatment approaches, including institutionalization and deinstitutionalization, did not result in positive outcomes.

- Freud contributed to the psychoanalytic understanding of personality development and showed the strength of psychoanalysis. However, the psychoanalytic model was not effective in the treatment of people with severe mental illnesses.

- The U.S. Surgeon General's reports, the President's New Freedom Commission on Mental Health, and the goals of *Healthy People 2020* continue to highlight the need for resources for the care of persons with mental illness.

- The Patient Protection and Affordable Care Act prevent third-party payers from excluding people from insurance coverage for pre-existing disorders.

- Today consumers of mental health services insist on building partnerships with providers in order to recover from mental illness. The traditional medical model is being replaced by a collaborative approach in which consumers and mental health care providers develop a partnership in recovery-oriented care.

CRITICAL THINKING CHALLENGES

1. Discuss whether the problems of these patients should be addressed by a psychiatric nurse:
   a. A 32-year-old recently divorced woman with obesity and diabetes, who recently lost her job and can no longer pay for her medications.
   b. A 25-year-old veteran whose war injuries have left him paralyzed from the waist down.
   c. An 86-year-old woman whose husband recently died and now must move to a nursing home.
2. Give three examples of changes in nursing practice based on new evidence.
3. Present an argument for the moral treatment of people with mental disorders.
4. Identify common themes in the 1999 *Mental Health: A Report of the Surgeon General*, the President's New Freedom Commission of Mental Health Report, and *Healthy People 2020: National Health Promotion and disease Prevention Objectives*.

MOVIES ***One Flew Over the Cuckoo's Nest:*** 1975. This classic film stars Jack Nicholson as Randle P. McMurphy, who takes on the state hospital establishment. This picture won all five of the top Academy Awards: Best Picture, Best Actor, Best Actress, Best Director, and Best Adapted Screenplay. The film depicts life in an inpatient psychiatric ward of the late 1960s and increased public awareness of the potential human rights violations inherent in a large, public mental system. However, the portrayal of electroconvulsive therapy is stereotyped and inaccurate, and the suicide of Billy appears to be simplistically linked to his domineering mother. This film depicts the loss of patients' rights and the use coercion and punishment in mental institutions before the deinstitutionalization movement.

VIEWING POINTS: This film should be viewed from several different perspectives: What is the basis of McMurphy's admission? How does Nurse Ratchet interact with the patients? How are patient rights violated?

I Never Promised You a Rose Garden: 1977. This movie, now available on DVD, stars Kathleen Quinlan as Deborah Blake, a 16-year-old young woman who is institutionalized for her mental illness. Her treatment in the institution was typical of the 1960s. In this film, the therapeutic relationship between Deborah and her physician was considered ideal.

VIEWING POINTS: How were patients, especially adolescent girls with emotional problems, treated in the 1960s? How would Deborah's treatment be judged today?

References

American Nurses Association, American Psychiatric Nurses Association, International Society of Psychiatric–Mental Health Nurses, and. (2014). *Psychiatric–mental health nursing: Scope and standards of practice. 2nd Edition.* Silver Spring, MD: Nursebooks.org.

Bailey, H. (1920). *Nursing mental diseases.* New York: Macmillan.

Beers, C. (1908). *A mind that found itself.* New York: Longmans, Green, & Co.

Bly, N. (1887). *Ten days in a mad-house.* New York: Ian L. Munro.

Church, O. (1987). From custody to community in psychiatric nursing. *Nursing Research, 36*(10), 48–55.

Cowles, E. (1887). Nursing reform for the insane. *American Journal of Insanity, 44*(176), 191.

Deutsch, S. (1949). *The mentally ill in America.* London: Oxford University Press.

Freud, S. (1900). Interpretation of dreams. In J. Strachey, A. Freud, A. Strachey, & A. Tyson (Eds.), (1953). *The standard edition of the complete psychological works of Sigmund Freud* (Vol. IV). London: Hogarth Press.

Freud, S. (1905). Three essays on the theory of sexuality. In J. Strachey, A. Freud, A., Strachey, & A. Tyson (Eds.), (1953). *The standard edition of the complete psychological works of Sigmund Freud* (pp. 135–248). London: Hogarth Press.

Freud, S. (1927). The ego and the id. In E. Jones (Ed.), (1957). *The international psycho-analytical library, N. 12.* London: Hogarth Press.

International Association of Psychosocial Rehabilitation Services. (1990). *A national directory: Organizations providing psychosocial rehabilitation and related community support services in the United States.* Boston, MA: Center for Psychiatric Rehabilitation, Boston University.

Malamud, W. (1944). The history of psychiatric therapies. In J. K. Hall, G. Zilboorg, & H. Bunker (Eds.), *One hundred years of American psychiatry* (pp. 273–323). New York: Columbia University Press.

Melnyk, B. M., Fineout-Overholt, E., Stillwell, S. B., & Williamson, K. M. (2009). Igniting a spirit of inquiry: An essential foundation for evidence-based practice. *American Journal of Nursing, 109*(11), 49–52.

New Freedom Commission on Mental Health. (2003). *Achieving the promise: Transforming mental health care in America (Publication No. SMA-03-3831).* Rockville, MD: Department of Health and Human Services.

Nightingale, F. (1859). *Notes on nursing: What it is and what it is not.* London: Harrison & Son.

Peplau, H. (1952). *Interpersonal relations in nursing.* New York: Putnam.

Peplau, H. (1989). Future directions in psychiatric nursing from the perspective of history. *Journal of Psychosocial Nursing and Mental Health Services, 27*(2), 18–21.

U.S. Burden of Disease Collaborators. (2013). The state of US health, 1990–2010: Burden of diseases, injuries, and risk factors. *The Journal of the American Medical Association.* doi:10.1001/jama.2013.13805

U.S. DHHS. (1999). *Mental health: A report of the surgeon general.* Washington, DC: U.S. Department of Health and Human Services, Substance Abuse and Mental Health Services Administration, Center for Mental Health Services, National Institutes of Health, National Institute of Mental Health.

U.S. DHHS. (2010). *Healthy people 2020.* Retrieved from http://www.healthypeople.gov.

U.S. Public Health Service. (2000). *Report of the Surgeon General's Conference on Children's Mental Health: A national action agenda.* Washington, DC: Department of Health and Human Services.

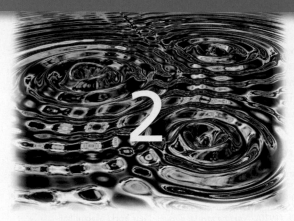

Mental Health and Mental Disorders
Fighting Stigma and Promoting Recovery

Mary Ann Boyd

KEY CONCEPTS

- mental health
- mental disorders
- stigma
- recovery
- wellness

LEARNING OBJECTIVES

After studying this chapter, you will be able to:

1. Relate the concept of mental health to wellness.

2. Identify the rationale for promoting wellness for people with mental health challenges.

3. Differentiate the concepts of mental health and mental illness.

4. Discuss the significance of epidemiological evidence in studying the occurrence of mental disorders.

5. Describe the consequences of the stigma of mental illness on individuals and families.

6. Identify recovery components and their role in the treatment of mental illness.

KEY TERMS

- cultural syndrome • DSM-5 • epidemiology • incidence • label avoidance • mental disorder • mental health
- point prevalence • prevalence • public stigma • rate • self-stigma • social change • syndrome

To understand health and illness in any practice area, nurses need a basic understanding of mental health and its relationship with wellness. This chapter discusses concepts of mental health and wellness, the diagnosis of mental disorders, how the stigma of mental illness can be a barrier to treatment, and the importance of focusing on recovery from mental illness.

MENTAL HEALTH AND WELLNESS

Mental health is conceptualized by the World Health Organization (WHO) as a state of well-being in which the individual realizes his or her own abilities, can cope with life's normal stresses, can work productively and fruitfully and can make a contribution to society. A person cannot be healthy without being "mentally" healthy, but it is possible to be mentally healthy and have a mental

or physical disorder (World Health Organization [WHO], 2013a). Mental health is essential to personal well-being, interpersonal relationships, and contributing to the community.

> **KEYCONCEPT** **Mental health** is the emotional and psychological well-being of an individual who has the capacity to interact with others, deal with ordinary stress, and perceive one's surroundings realistically (adapted from American Nurses Association, American Psychiatric Nurses Association, International Society of Psychiatric–Mental Health Nurses, 2014).

Related to the concept of mental health, wellness is defined as a "purposeful process of individual growth, integration of experience, and meaningful connection with others, reflecting personally valued goals and strengths and resulting in being well and living values"

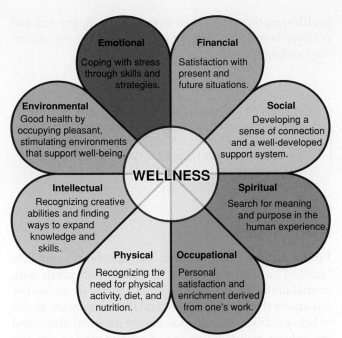

FIGURE 2.1 Eight dimensions of wellness. Adapted from Swarbrick, M. (2006). A wellness approach. *Psychiatric Rehabilitation Journal, 29*(4), 311–314. (U.S. DHHS, SAMHSA, 2010)

(McMahon & Fleury, 2012). Wellness involves having a purpose in life, being actively involved in satisfying work and play, having joyful relationships, having a healthy body and living environment, and being happy (U.S. Department of Health and Human Services, Substance Abuse & Mental Health Services Administration [U.S. DHHS, SAMHSA], 2010) (see Fig. 2.1). Mental health problems significantly impact the process of wellness: Many people with mental health problems die decades earlier than the general public from preventable diseases (Schuffman, Druss, & Parks, 2009; Whiteford et al., 2013). Poverty, unemployment, underemployment, trauma, and lack of education, common in people who have mental health issues, often prevent the achievement of wellness (U.S. DHHS, SAMHSA, 2010).

OVERVIEW OF MENTAL HEALTH DISORDERS

Mental disorders can disrupt mental health and result in one of the most common causes of disability. In this text, the terms "mental disorder" and "mental illness" will be used interchangeably.

> **KEYCONCEPT** **Mental disorders** are clinically significant disturbances in cognition, emotion regulation, or behavior that reflect a dysfunction in the psychological, biological, or developmental processes underlying mental dysfunction. They are usually associated with distress or impaired functioning (American Psychiatric Association [APA], 2013).

A mental illness or mental disorder is a **syndrome**, a set of symptoms that cluster together that may have multiple causes and may represent several different disease states that have not yet been defined. Unlike many medical diseases, mental disorders are defined by clusters of behaviors, thoughts, and feelings, not underlying biologic pathology. Laboratory tests are not generally used in diagnosing mental disorders.

The landmark study *Global Burden of Disease 2010* found an alarming impact of mental and behavioral disorders on health and productivity in the world. Depression is one of the leading disease burdens in middle- and high-income countries such as the United States. By 2030, depression is projected to be the leading burden worldwide (WHO, 2013b). In the United States, 1 in 4 adults, or 57.7 million people, has a diagnosable mental disorder in any given year (National Institute of Mental Health, 2013).

Evidence for this very high occurrence of mental disorders is established through epidemiological research. **Epidemiology**, the study of patterns of disease distribution and determinants of health within populations, contributes to the overall understanding of the mental health status of population groups, or aggregates, and associated factors. Epidemiological studies examine associations among possible factors related to an area of investigation, but they do not determine causes of illnesses. The Centers for Disease Control and Prevention (CDC) tracks and reports mental health epidemiological data. Throughout this book, epidemiological data are included in discussions of mental health problems and mental disorders. See Box 2.1 for an explanation of terms.

Diagnosis of Mental Health Conditions

Mental disorders are organized and diagnosed according to the criteria published in the *Diagnostic and Statistical Manual of Mental Disorders–5* (*DSM-5;* APA, 2013). The current *DSM-5* system contains subtypes and other specifiers that further classify disorders. Although the *DSM-5* specifies criteria for diagnosing mental disorders, there are no absolute boundaries separating one disorder from another, and disorders often have different manifestations at different points in time.

In a mental disorder, alterations in behaviors, thoughts, and feelings are unexpected and are outside normal, culturally defined limits. If a behavior is considered normal within a specific culture, it is not viewed as a psychiatric symptom. For example, members of some religious groups "speak in tongues." To an observer, it appears that the individuals are having hallucinations (see Chapter 22), but this behavior is normal for this group within a particular setting.

The amount of disability or impairment in functioning is an important consideration when assessing a person with a mental disorder. A person's ability to understand,

---

BOX 2.1

Epidemiologic Terms

In epidemiology, certain terms have specific meanings relative to what they measure. When expressing the number of cases of a disorder, population rates, rather than raw numbers, are used.

Rate is the proportion of the cases in the population when compared with the total population. It is expressed as a fraction, in which the numerator is the number of cases and the denominator is the total number in the population, including the cases and noncases. The term *average rate* is used for measures that involve rates over specified time periods:

$$Rate = \frac{Cases\ in\ population}{Total\ population\ (cases\ and\ noncases)}$$

Prevalence refers to the total number of people who have the disorder within a given population at a specified time regardless of how long ago the disorder started.

Point prevalence is the basic measure that refers to the proportion of individuals in the population who have the disorder at a specified point in time (*t*). This point can be a day on the calendar, such as April 1, 2012, or a point defined in relation to the study assessment, such as the day of the interview. This is also expressed as a fraction:

$$Point\ prevalence\ rate = \frac{Cases\ at\ t}{Population\ at\ t}$$

Incidence refers to a rate that includes only *new* cases that have occurred within a clearly defined time period. The most common time period evaluated is 1 year. The study of incidence cases is more difficult than a study of prevalent cases because a study of incidence cases requires at least two measurements to be taken: one at the start of the prescribed time period and another at the end of it.

---

communicate, and get along with others is important in the recovery process. If symptoms impair an individual's ability to independently perform self-care and daily activities, recovery will be more difficult. The WHO Disability Assessment Schedule 2.0 is an instrument that can be used for measuring the amount of impairment that the individual experiences.

Some disorders are influenced by cultural factors (see Chapter 3), and others are considered **cultural syndromes** that represent a specific pattern of symptoms that occur within a specific cultural group or community (APA, 2013). There is little research that reliably describes cultural syndromes, but there are two conditions, *ataque de nervios* and *susto*, that are frequently reported in small number of persons (Razzouk, Nogueira, & Mari Jde, 2011) (Box 2.2).

Stigma

Stigma, one of major treatment barriers facing individuals with mental health problems and their families, was highlighted in the President's New Freedom Commission on Mental Health *Report* in 2003. People with mental

health symptoms have been stoned to death, hanged, and publicly humiliated. Stigma leads to community misunderstanding, prejudice, and discrimination.

KEYCONCEPT **Stigma** can be defined as a mark of shame, disgrace, or disapproval that results in an individual being shunned or rejected by others. Public stigma, self-stigma, and label avoidance are three types of stigma people with mental illnesses experience.

Public Stigma

Public stigma occurs after individuals are publicly "marked" as being mentally ill. When individuals with mental illness act or say things that are odd or unusual or tell others that they have a mental illness, they are at risk of being publicly identified as having a mental illness and are subject to prejudice and discrimination. Common stereotypes include being dangerous, unpredictable, and incapable of functioning independently. People with mental illness are sometimes treated as if they are responsible for their disabilities and are inaccurately accused of being weak or immoral (Corrigan, Morris, Michaels, Rafacz, & Rüsch, 2012). Stigmatization robs individuals of work, independent living, and meaningful relationships (see Fame & Fortune, p. 16).

The media often perpetuates negative stereotypes of persons with mental health issues. Films are especially important in influencing the public perception of mental illness because the media tend to be especially effective in shaping opinion in situations in which strong opinions are not already held. Although some films present sympathetic portrayals of people with mental illness and professionals who work in the field of mental health (e.g., *Beautiful Mind, Benny and Joon, The Soloist*), many more

---

BOX 2.2

Cultural Syndromes: Frequently Reported Cultural Syndromes in Latin America and the Caribbean

Ataque de nervios: frequents episodes of loss of control, uncontrollable crying, tremors, and severe anxiety and sadness with somatization symptoms including muscle and headache, nausea, loss of appetite, insomnia, fatigue, and psychomotor agitation. Reported among women over 45 years old, with little education, and who have experienced a loss (such as a divorce) or acute distress.

Susto: fright characterized by symptoms of psychomotor agitation, anorexia, insomnia, fever, diarrhea, confusion, apathy, depression, and introversion following an emotional trauma or witnessing a traumatic experience.

(Razzouk et al., 2011.)

FAME & FORTUNE

Barret Robbins (1973–)

NFL Center

PUBLIC PERSONA

Barret Robbins was a shining football star when he played at Texas Christian University and was a member of the Phi Kappa Sigma fraternity. He was drafted by the Oakland Raiders in the second round of the 1995 draft. He became one of NFL's best centers and was elected to the Pro Bowl in 2002.

PERSONAL REALITIES

Barret Robbins was first diagnosed with bipolar disorder after his disappearance 2 days before Super Bowl XXXVII when he was hospitalized after a mania-driven drinking binge. He had been hospitalized for depression during college. Since the time he lost his career, he has been on a very rocky road to recovery. He has been arrested, shot, and separated from his family. He was recently released from a period of jail following an assault on a police detective release from a treatment facility ("Miami Beach Det. Reveals Details About Run-In With Ex-NFL Star," http://miami.cbslocal.com/2012/09/24/miami-beach-det-reveals-details-about-run-in-with-ex-nfl-star/). He is hopeful that he will be able to stay on his medication and away from substances to regain his life.

FAME & FORTUNE

Thomas Eagleton, LL.B (1929–2007)

U.S. Senator from Missouri (1968–1987)

PUBLIC PERSONA

Thomas Eagleton was born in St. Louis, Missouri. He graduated from Amherst College in 1950 and Harvard Law School in 1953. He was elected circuit attorney of St. Louis and Attorney General of Missouri in 1960. He was elected to the U.S. Senate in 1968 and served in the Senate for 19 years. He was instrumental in the Senate's passage of the Clean Air and Water Acts and sponsored the Eagleton Amendment, which halted the bombing in Cambodia and effectively ended American involvement in the Vietnam War. He was active in matters dealing with foreign relations, intelligence, defense, education, health care, and the environment. He served in public office for more than 30 years, wrote three books, and held the title of Professor of Public Affairs at Washington University in St. Louis. The U.S. Courthouse in downtown St. Louis was named for him.

PERSONAL REALITIES

Thomas Eagleton was nominated to run for vice president at the 1972 Democratic Party convention with George McGovern as the presidential candidate. After the convention, Mr. Eagleton's hospitalization and treatment for depression was revealed. He was replaced on the Democratic presidential ticket within a few weeks.

Source: *The Biographical directory of the United States Congress, 1774–present.* Retrieved March 8, 2007, from http://bioguide.congress.gov/scripts/biodisplay.pl?index = E000004.

do not. People with mental illness are portrayed most often as aggressive, dangerous, and unpredictable. Films such as *Friday the 13th* (1980) and *Nightmare on Elm Street* (1984) perpetuate the myth that all people who leave psychiatric hospitals are violent and dangerous. Movies such as *The Exorcist* (1973) suggest to the public that mental illness is the equivalent of possession by the devil. These films in part account for the continuing stigma of mental illness.

When people with mental illnesses or emotional problems are stigmatized by society, they are often ostracized by the society in which they live. The stigma associated with all forms of mental illness is strong but generally increases the more an individual's behavior differs from the cultural norm.

Mental health treatment and providers are also objects of stigma. In films, psychiatric hospitals are often portrayed as dangerous and unwelcoming places, such as in *The Snake Pit* (1948), *One Flew Over the Cuckoo's Nest* (1975), *Instinct* (1999), *Twelve Monkeys* (1995), *Sling Blade* (1996), *Girl, Interrupted* (1999), *Don Juan Demarco* (1994), *A Beautiful Mind* (2001), and *Analyze That* (2002). Nurses are dressed in white in contrast to the dark, gloomy surroundings, and patients have little to do other than to walk the halls of the institution, acting odd. Psychiatrists, psychologists, and other health professionals who work with people with mental illnesses are often portrayed as "arrogant and ineffectual," "cold-hearted and authoritarian," "passive and apathetic," or "shrewd and manipulative" (Wedding, Boyd, & Niemiec, 2009).

One of the best ways to counteract the negative effects of stigma is to have contact with the stigmatized group (Corrigan et al., 2012). Another way is to use nonstigmatizing language. Just as a person with diabetes mellitus should not be referred to as a "diabetic" but rather as a "person with diabetes," a person with a mental disorder should never be referred to as a "schizophrenic" or "bipolar" but rather as a "person with schizophrenia" or a "person with bipolar disorder." Using words such as "psycho," "nuts," "funny farm," and "maniac" reinforces negative images of mental illness. Jokes that depict people with mental illness as stupid, dangerous, or incompetent perpetuate negative myths.

Self-Stigma

Self-stigma occurs when negative stereotypes are internalized by people with mental illness. Patients are aware of the public's negative view of mental illness and agree with the public's perceptions. They begin to believe that they are unpredictable, cannot become productive members of society, or have caused their illness. As a result of the application of the negative stereotype to self, they have low self-esteem (Corrigan et al., 2012).

Label Avoidance

Label avoidance, avoiding treatment or care in order not to be labeled as being mentally ill, is another type of stigma, and one of the reasons, that so few people with mental health problems actually receive help (Ciftci, Jones, & Corrigan, 2013). By avoiding treatment, they avoid the stigma of mental illness. For example, negative views of mental illness by several of the Asian cultures influence the willingness of its members to seek treatment. They may ignore their symptoms or refuse to seek treatment because of the stigma associated with being mentally ill (Ciftci et al., 2013; Lee et al., 2009).

RECOVERY FROM MENTAL ILLNESS

Recovery is the single most important goal for individuals with mental disorders (U.S. DHHS, SAMHSA, 2009). The following definition of recovery was released following a lengthy consensus process that began in 2010 and involved government agency officials, experts, consumers, family members, advocates, researchers, managed care representatives, and others.

> **KEYCONCEPT** **Recovery** from mental disorders and/or substance use disorders is a process of change through which individuals improve their health and wellness, live a self-directed life, and strive to reach their full potential (U.S. DHHS, SAMHSA, 2012).

Recovery-oriented treatment is based on the belief that mental illnesses and emotional disturbances are treatable and that recovery is an expectation. There are four dimensions that support recovery, including *health* (managing disease and living in a physically and emotionally healthy way), *home* (a safe and stable place to live), *purpose* (meaningful daily activities and independence, resources, and income), and *community* (relationships and social networks). Consumers and families have real and meaningful choices about treatment options and providers. In recovery-oriented care, the

---

BOX 2.3

Research for Best Practice: **Nurse and Patient Recovery Skills**

Aston, V. & Coffey, M. (2011). Recovery: What mental health nurses and service users say about the concept of recovery. *Journal of Psychiatric and Mental Health Nursing, 19(3),* 257–263.

THE QUESTION: How do nurses and consumers view recovery-oriented care?

METHODS: Data were collected from a group of consumers and another group of nurses. Open-ended questions guided the discussions, which took place at a local drop-in center and day hospital. Data were recorded and underwent a rigorous process of analysis

FINDINGS: Four recovery-oriented practice themes emerged that impact both consumers and nurses. The first theme was the meaning of recovery. Both groups were uncertain of the in-depth meaning of recovery. The second theme was semantics, that is, the use of language to describe recovery and its process. Both groups found the word "recovery" difficult to associate with mental health but could not come up with a better term. The nurses were also unclear about their role within recovery. The third theme was therapeutics—specifically relationships between nurses and patients. Both the nurses and patients described difficulty in developing a collaborative relationship with each other because they were accustomed to the typical dependent nurse–patient relationship. The last theme related to the concept of a journey. Recovery is usually described as a journey, but not everyone will go through the journey. However, those who go through the journey describe it as a long and winding road.

IMPLICATIONS FOR NURSING: Traditional views are not easily changed. Being involved in decision making helps the patient transition from a dependent-driven relationship to a collaborative recovery-oriented one. Lack of information and training along with working in rigid task-oriented systems create frustration and lack of role clarity for both the nurse and the consumer.

---

person with a mental health problem develops a partnership with a clinician to manage the illness, strengthen coping abilities, and build resilience for life's challenges (Box 2.3).

Mental health recovery benefits not only the individual and family but also society by ultimately reducing the global burden of mental health problems. Recovery is guided by 10 fundamental principles; see Box 2.4.

Individuals with mental illnesses can regain mental health with the support of families, mental health providers, and society. The contributions of these individuals strengthen communities and support the overall health of a nation.

BOX 2.4

Guiding Principles of Recovery

Recovery emerges from hope: The belief that recovery is real provides the essential and motivating message of a better future—that people can and do overcome the internal and external challenges, barriers, and obstacles that confront them.

Recovery is person-driven: Self-determination and self-direction are the foundations for recovery, as individuals define their own life goals and design their unique path(s).

Recovery occurs via many pathways: Individuals are unique with distinct needs, strengths, preferences, goals, culture, and backgrounds including trauma experiences that affect and determine their pathway(s) to recovery. Abstinence is the safest approach for those with substance use disorders.

Recovery is holistic: Recovery encompasses an individual's whole life, including mind, body, spirit, and community. The array of services and supports available should be integrated and coordinated.

Recovery is supported by peers and allies: Mutual support and mutual aid groups, including the sharing of experiential knowledge and skills, as well as social learning, play an invaluable role in recovery.

Recovery is supported through relationship and social networks: An important factor in the recovery process is the presence and involvement of people who believe in the person's ability to recover; who offer hope, support, and encouragement; and who also suggest strategies and resources for change.

Recovery is culturally-based and influenced: Culture and cultural background in all of its diverse representations including values, traditions, and beliefs are key in determining a person's journey and unique pathway to recovery.

Recovery is supported by addressing trauma: Services and supports should be trauma-informed to foster safety (physical and emotional) and trust, as well as to promote choice, empowerment, and collaboration.

Recovery involves individual, family, and community strengths and responsibility: Individuals, families, and communities have strengths and resources that serve as a foundation for recovery.

Recovery is based on respect: Community, systems, and societal acceptance and appreciation for people affected by mental health and substance use problems—including protecting their rights and eliminating discrimination—are crucial in achieving recovery.

(U.S. DHHS, SAMHSA, 2012)

SUMMARY OF KEY POINTS

- Mental health is the emotional and psychological well-being of an individual. To be mentally healthy means that one can interact with others, deal with daily stress, and perceive the world realistically. Mental disorders are health conditions characterized by alterations in thinking, mood, or behavior and are associated with distress or impaired functioning.

- Epidemiology is important in understanding the distribution of mental illness and determinants of health within a given population. The rate of occurrence refers to the proportion of the population that has the disorder. Incidence is the rate of new cases within a specified time. Prevalence is the rate of occurrence of all cases at a particular point in time.

- Stigma toward mental illness can be viewed in three ways. Public stigma marks a person as having a mental illness. When a person with a mental illness shares the public's negative view of mental illness, self-stigma occurs. If a person with a mental illness does not seek treatment because of fear of being labeled "mentally ill," label avoidance occurs.

- The *DSM-5* organizes psychiatric diagnoses according to behaviors and symptom patterns.

- Cultural syndromes are specific disorders found within a particular locality or culture. There is little research on the syndromes, but *ataque de nervios* and *susto* are well documented.

- Mental health recovery is the single most important goal for the mental health delivery system. Recovery is viewed a process of changes through which individuals improve their health and wellness, live a self-directed life, and strive to reach their full potential.

CRITICAL THINKING CHALLENGES

1. A person who is seeking help for a mental disorder asks why the individual's physical health is important to the nurse.
2. Compare the meaning of the epidemiological terms *prevalence*, *incidence*, and *rate*. Access the CDC's website (www.cdc.gov), and identify major mental health problems in the United States.
3. Examine the description of people with mental illness in the media, including television programs, news, and newspapers. Are negative connotations evident?
4. Examine how family and friends describe people with mental illness. Do you think their description of mental illness is based on fact or myth? Explain.
5. Explain the three forms of stigma and give examples.
6. Discuss the negative impact of labeling someone with a psychiatric diagnosis.
7. Using the components of mental health recovery as a framework, compare the goals for a person with schizophrenia with those with a medical disease such as diabetes.

Beautiful Dreamers: 1992, Canada. This film is based on a true story about poet Walt Whitman's visit to an asylum in London, Ontario, Canada. Whitman, played by Rip Torn, is shocked by what he sees and persuades the hospital director to offer humane treatment. Eventually, the patients wind up playing the townspeople in a game of cricket.

VIEWING POINTS: Observe the stigma that is associated with having a mental illness.

References

American Psychiatric Association. (2013). *Diagnostic and statistical manual of mental disorders* (5th ed.). Arlington, VA: Author.

American Nurses Association, American Psychiatric Nurses Association, & International Society of Psychiatric–Mental Health Nurses. (2014). *Psychiatric–mental health nursing: Scope and standards of practice.* 2nd edition. Silver Spring, MD: American Nurses Association.

Ciftci, A., Jones, N., & Corrigan, P. W. (2013). Mental health stigma in the Muslim community. *Journal of Muslim Mental Health, 7*(1), 17–31.

Corrigan, P. W, Morris, S. B., Michaels, P. J., Rafacz, J. D., & Rüsch, N. (2012). Challenging the public stigma of mental illness: A meta-analysis of outcome studies, *Psychiatric Services, 63*(10), 963–973. doi:10.1176/appi.ps.005292011

Lee, S., Juon, H. S., Martinez, G., Hsu, C. E., Robinson, E. S., Bawa, J., et al. (2009). Model minority at risk: Expressed needs of mental health by Asian American young adults. *Journal of Community Health, 34*(2), 144–152.

McMahon, S., & Fleury, J. (2012). Wellness in older adults: A concept analysis. *Nursing Forum, 47*(1), 39–51.

National Institute of Mental Health. (2013). The numbers counts: Mental disorders in American. Retrieved June 18, 2014, from http://www.nimh. nih.gov/health/publications/the-numbers-count-mental-disorders-in-america/index.shtml

President's New Freedom Commission Mental Health. (2003). Achieving the promise: Transforming mental health care in America—Final report (DHHS Publication No. SMA-03–3832). Retrieved June 30, 2009, from http://www.mentalhealthcommission.gov/report/FinalReport/toc.html

Razzouk, D, Nogueira, B, & Mari Jde, J. (2011). The contribution of Latin American and Caribbean countries on culture bound syndromes studies for the ICD-10 revision: Key findings from a working in progress. *Revista Brasileira de Psiquiatria, 33*(suppl. 1), S5–20.

Schuffman, D., Druss, B. G., & Parks, J. J. (2009). State mental health policy: Mending Missouri's safety net—Transforming systems of care by integrating primary and behavioral health care. *Psychiatric Services, 60*(5), 585–588.

U.S. DHHS, SAMHSA. (2009). Transforming mental health care in America: Federal action agenda—First steps. Retrieved June 18, 2014, from http://www.samhsa.gov/federalactionagenda/NFC_FMHAA.aspx

U.S. DHHS, SAMHSA. (2010). The eight dimensions of wellness (Publication No. SMA12-4568). Retrieved from http://store.samhsa.gov/product/ SAMHSA-s-Wellness-Initiative-Eight-Dimensions-of-Wellness/SMA12-4568

U.S. DHHS, SAMHSA. (2012). SAMHSA's working definition of recovery updated. Retrieved June 18, 2014, from http://blog.samhsa.gov/2012/03/23/defintion-of-recovery-updated/#.U4MD_kAQOuY.

Wedding, D., Boyd, M. A., & Niemiec, R. (2009). *Movies and mental illness* (3rd ed). Göttingen, Germany: Hogrefe & Huber.

Whiteford, H. A. Degenhardt, L., Rehm, J., Baxter, A. J., Ferrari, A. J., Erskine, H. E., et al. (2013). Global burden of disease attributable to mental and substance use disorders: Findings from the Global burden of Disease Study 2010. *Lancet. 382*(9904), 1575–1586.

WHO. (2013a). *Comprehensive mental health action plan 2013–2020. Sixty-six World Health Assembly, Agenda Item 13.3.* Geneva, Switzerland: Author.

WHO. (2013b). *Depression. A hidden burden.* Geneva, Switzerland: Author. Retrieved June 18, 2014, from http://www.who.int/mental_health/management/depression/flyer_depression_2012.pdf?ua=1

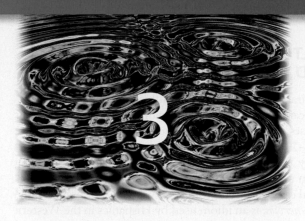

3

Cultural and Spiritual Issues Related to Mental Health Care

Mary Ann Boyd

KEY CONCEPTS

- culture
- cultural competence
- spirituality

LEARNING OBJECTIVES

After studying this chapter, you will be able to:

1. Discuss the ways that cultural competence is demonstrated in psychiatric nursing.

2. Describe the beliefs about mental health and illness in different cultural and social groups.

3. Differentiate concepts of religion and spirituality.

4. Discuss the role of spirituality and religiousness in persons with mental illness.

5. Discuss the beliefs of major religions and their role in shaping views on mental illnesses.

KEY TERMS

- acculturation • cultural explanations • cultural identity • cultural idiom of distress • linguistic competence
- religiousness

All cultural groups have sets of values, beliefs, and patterns of accepted behavior, and it is often difficult for those of one culture to understand those of another. This is especially true regarding mental illness—whereas some cultures view it as a condition for which the ill person must be punished and ostracized from society, other cultures are more tolerant and believe that family and community members are key to the care and treatment of mentally ill people. Nurses' and patients' religious backgrounds and cultural heritages may be different, so it is important for nurses to understand clearly the thinking and perspectives of other cultures and groups.

This chapter examines cultural and social mores of various cultural and religious groups. Understanding cultural and religious beliefs and the significance of spirituality is especially important when caring for people with mental health problems. These beliefs and practices can define and shape the experience of being mentally ill and

influence the willingness to seek care. Treating mental disorders is intertwined with people's attitudes about themselves, their beliefs, values, and ways.

> **KEYCONCEPT** **Culture** is not only a way of life for people who identify or associate with one another on the basis of some common purpose, need, or similarity of background but also the totality of learned, socially transmitted beliefs, values, and behaviors that emerge from its members' interpersonal transactions.

Cultures are dynamic and continually changing. When immigrants arrive in the United States with their own cultures, they begin to adapt to their new environment. **Acculturation** is the term used to describe the socialization process by which minority groups learn and adopt selective aspects of the dominant culture. Their culture changes as a result of the influences of the new environment. Eventually, a new minority culture evolves that is different than the native culture and also different from the dominante culure, which in turn is transformed by the new residents.

Everyone has a **cultural identity**, or set of cultural beliefs with which one looks for standards of behavior. Because culture is broadly defined, many people consider themselves to have multiple cultural identities. The dominant culture for much of the U.S. history, has been based on the beliefs, norms, and values of white Americans of Judeo-Christian origin. Even though the United States is rapidly changing, most health care professionals are primarily products of an education system of white American culture. All persons and organizations function within a culture.

CULTURAL AND LINGUISTIC COMPETENCE

Psychiatric–mental health nurses have an obligation to be culturally and linguistically competent to provide quality care. There are several definitions of cultural and linguistic competence, but there is a general consensus that cultural and linguistic competence involves an adjustment or recognition of one's own culture in order to understand the culture of another person. **Linguistic competence**, the capacity to communicate effectively and convey information that is easily understood by diverse audiences, is an important part of cultural competence (Goode & Jones, 2009). A nurse who is culturally competent understands and appreciates cultural differences in health care practices and similarities within, among, and between groups.

> **KEYCONCEPT** **Cultural competence** is a set of academic and interpersonal skills that are respectful of and responsive to the health beliefs, health care practices, and cultural and linguistic needs of diverse patients to bring about positive health care outcomes (U.S. Department of Health and Human Services [U.S. DHHS], 2013).

Cultural competence is demonstrated in several ways. Valuing patients' culture beliefs and recognizing the need to bridge language barriers are essential behaviors. There are linguistic variations within cultural groups as well as cultural variations within a language group. Speaking the same language does not guarantee shared meaning and understanding. Communication may be adversely affected when patients are unable to fully express themselves in English. Understanding the impact of literacy levels is integral to providing culturally competent care. Demonstrating an understanding that literacy levels contribute to the interpretation of personal, psychological experiences is critical (U.S. DHHS, 2013).

CULTURAL AND SOCIAL FACTORS AND BELIEFS ABOUT MENTAL ILLNESS

Cultural beliefs and practices influence how patients communicate and manifest their symptoms, cope with their illnesses, and receive family and community support. The *DMS-5* differentiates **cultural idiom of distress**, a commonly used term or phrase that describes the suffering within a cultural group from **cultural explanations**, perceived causes for symptoms (APA, 2013). For example, the term, *nervios*, is an idiom used by Hispanics in the Western Hemisphere that explains a wide range of somatic and emotional symptoms such as headache, irritability, nervousness, insomnia, and difficulty concentrating. The term *susto*, (extreme fright causing the soul to leave the body) is believed to be the cause of a group of varied symptoms including appetite disturbance, sleep problems, low self-worth among people in Central and South America.

Social factors also contribute to the development of mental disorders. Ethnic and racial minorities in the United States live in a social environment of inequality that increases their exposure to racism, discrimination, violence, and poverty, which contribute to the experience of their illnesses (U.S. DHHS, 2013). Racially and ethnically diverse groups are less likely to receive mental health services and more likely to receive poorer quality care. Poverty is found in all cultural groups and is present in other groups, such as older adults, people with physical disabilities, individuals with psychiatric impairments, and single-parent families. In the United States, one third of people living below the poverty line are single mothers and their children; 27.2% of African Americans live below the poverty level, as do 25.6% of Hispanic Americans and 9.7% of white Americans (DeNavas-Walt, Proctor, & Smith, 2013). Currently in the United States, the poverty guidelines for a family of four is a yearly income of $23,283 or less in the 48 mainland states; $29,440 or less in Alaska; and $27,090 or less in Hawaii (U.S. Census, 2013).

Families living in poverty are under tremendous financial and emotional stress, which may trigger or exacerbate mental problems. Along with the daily stressors of trying to provide food and shelter for themselves and their families, their lack of time, energy, and money prevents them from attending to their psychological needs. Often, these families become trapped in a downward economic spiral as tension and stress mount. The inability to gain employment and the lack of financial independence only add to the feelings of powerlessness and low self-esteem. Being self-supporting gives one a feeling of control over life and bolsters self-esteem. Dependence on others or the government causes frustration, anger, apathy, and feelings of depression and meaninglessness. Alcoholism, depression, and child and partner abuse may become a means of coping with such hopelessness and despair. The homeless population is the group most at risk for being unable to escape this spiral of poverty.

BOX 3.1

Cultural Competence and Mental Health

- Learn about the patient's country of origin before assessment.
- Conduct a thorough social and cultural assessment.
- Demonstrate genuine interest in and respect for the individual.
- Educate patients about mental health issues, including available treatments, benefits of obtaining services, and contributions and abilities of individuals with a mental illness.
- Do not assume that all individuals of a racial or ethnic group are the same.
- Being quiet and lack of eye contact may be culturally appropriate and may indicate shyness, not depression or another mental illness.
- Tailor interventions to the individual; one intervention does not work for everyone.

Adapted from Acosta, H. (2009). *Hispanic mental health: Do and don'ts when working with Hispanics in mental health.* Retrieved on July 16, 2009, from http://www.culturally competentmentalhealthnj.org.

Hispanic Americans

The number of Hispanic Americans living in the United States has been gradually increasing, and this group is now the largest minority in the United States. From 2000 to 2008, there was a 75% increase in population, from 35.3 to 53 million, representing 17% of the U.S. population. Countries of origin include Mexico (65%), Central and South American (16%), Puerto Rico (8%), and Cuba (4%). Hispanic populations are largest in urban areas, such as New York, Chicago, Los Angeles, San Francisco, and Miami–Fort Lauderdale (U.S. Census Bureau, 2013).

Studies indicate that Hispanic Americans tend to use all other resources before seeking help from mental health professionals. Reasons for this are unclear, but barriers for treatment include beliefs that mental health facilities do not accommodate their cultural needs (e.g., language, beliefs, values), cost of care, and concerns regarding immigration status (Lee, Laiewski, & Choi, 2014; Kalthman, de Mendoza, Gonzales, & Serrano, 2013) (Box 3.1).

African Americans

In 2012, the estimated population of African Americans was 44.5 million, or 12.8% of the United States population (U.S. Census Bureau, 2013). Although African Americans share many beliefs, attitudes, values, and behaviors, there are also many subcultural and individual differences based on social class, country of origin, occupation, religion, educational level, and geographic location. Many African Americans have extensive family networks in which members can be relied on for moral support, help with child rearing, provide financial aid, and help in crises. In many African American families, older members

are treated with great respect. But African Americans with mental illness suffer from the stresses of double stigma—not only from their own cultural group but also from longtime racial discrimination. To make matters worse, racial discrimination may come from within the health community itself (Box 3.2).

Several studies show that diagnoses and treatment for African Americans often are racially biased (Eack, Bahorik, Newhill, Neighbors, & Davis, 2012). African Americans are disproportionately diagnosed as having schizophrenia when compared to other groups. Evidence suggests that the overdiagnosis in research studies may be related to whether the interviewer perceived that the patient was honest in reporting symptoms. A trusting, open, and collaborative therapeutic relationship during the diagnostic process is essential in order to conduct a meaningful assessment (Eack et al., 2012).

Asian Americans, Polynesians, and Pacific Islanders

In 2012, more than 18.9 million (4.4% of the U.S. population) Asian Americans, Polynesians, and Pacific Islanders lived in the United States, and this group represents one of the fastest growing minority populations in the United States. This large multicultural group includes Chinese,

BOX 3.2

Research for Best Practice: **African American Men and Women's Attitudes, Stigma and Coping**

Ward, E. C., Wiltshire, J. C., Detry, M. A., & Brown, R. L. (2013). *African American men and women's attitude toward mental illness, perceptions of stigma, and preferred coping behaviors.* Nursing Research, 62(3), 185–194.

THE QUESTION: What are the attitudes toward mental illness, perceived stigma, and preferred coping behaviors related to seeking treatment of mental illness in African American women?

METHODS: An exploratory, cross-sectional survey design was used. Community-dwelling African Americans (n = 272) age 25 to 85 years rated their beliefs, coping preferences, and perceived stigma associated with seeking treatment for mental illness.

FINDINGS: The findings suggested that these participants understood some of the causes of mental illness, identified many of the symptoms of mental illness, and believed that treatment controlled the mental illness. Their attitudes suggested that they were not very open to acknowledging psychological problems and were concerned about the stigma associated with mental illnesses. While somewhat open to mental health services, they preferred religious coping, especially in the older and middle-aged participants.

IMPLICATIONS FOR NURSING: The nurse should consider the impact of stigma on the willingness to seek treatment for mental illness. There is a need for psychoeducation interventions designed to increase openness to psychological problems and reduce stigma.

Filipino, Japanese, Asian Indian, Korean, Vietnamese, Laotian, Cambodian, Hawaiian, Samoan, and Guamanian people. Most Chinese, Japanese, Korean, Asian Indian, and Filipino immigrants have migrated to urban areas; the Vietnamese have settled throughout the United States (U.S. Census Bureau, 2013).

Generally, Asian cultures have a tradition of denying or disguising the existence of mental illnesses. In many of these cultures, it is an embarrassment to have a family member treated for mental illness, which may explain the extremely low utilization of mental health services. Only 17% of those experiencing problems seek care (Lee et al., 2009).

Asian Americans may experience a culture-bound syndrome, such as neurasthenia, which is characterized by fatigue, weakness, poor concentration, memory loss, irritability, aches and pains, and sleep disturbances. Associated with the Korean culture, *hwa-byung*, "suppressed anger syndrome," is characterized by subjective and expressed anger, sensations of heat, and feelings of hate (Lee et al., 2012). Research regarding specific mental health problems in Asian cultures is sparse, but various data suggest that rates of suicide within Native Hawaiian adolescents are higher than those of other adolescents in the United States (Suicide Prevention Resource Center, 2013).

Native Americans

In 2012, the estimated population of Native Americans was more than 6.3 million people, over 1% of the U.S. population (U.S. Census Bureau, 2013). Native American cultures emphasize respect and reverence for the earth and nature, from which come survival and comprehension of life and one's relationships with a separate, higher spiritual being and with other human beings. Shamans, or medicine men, are central to most cultures. They are healers believed to possess psychic abilities. Healing treatments rely on herbal medicines and healing ceremonies and feasts. Self-understanding derives from observing nature; relationships with others emphasize interdependence and sharing.

Traditional views about mental illnesses vary among the tribes. In some, mental illness is viewed as a supernatural possession, as being out of balance with nature. In certain Native American groups, people with mental illnesses are stigmatized. However, the degree of stigmatization is not the same for all disorders. In tribal groups that make little distinction between physical and mental illnesses, there is little stigma. In other groups, a particular event, such as suicide, is stigmatized. Different illnesses may be encountered in different Native American cultures and gene pools.

Women of Minority Groups

Women within minority groups may experience more conflicting feelings and psychological stressors than do men in trying to adjust to both their defined role in the minority culture and a different role in the larger predominant society. Compared to men, more Asian American women suffer from depression, yet are less likely than white women to seek out mental health care (Appel, Huang, Ai, & Lin, 2011).

Rural Cultures

Most mental health services are located in urban areas because most people live near cities. Those living in rural areas have limited access to health care which leads to fewer people being diagnosed with a mental health problem. Even though rural residents are less likely than urban residents to have mental health diagnoses or receive mental health care, the suicide rate is higher in the rural areas with firearms most commonly used (Searles, Valley, Hedegaard, & Betz, 2013). Rural areas are also diverse in both geography and culture. For example, access to mental health for those in the deep South is different from access for those with the same problems in the Northwest. Treatment approaches may be accepted in one part of the country but not in another. Suicide rates are higher in rural areas when compared to urban areas.

SPIRITUALITY, RELIGION, AND MENTAL ILLNESS

Both spirituality and religion are factors that may influence beliefs about mental illness and impact treatment and recovery.

> **KEYCONCEPT** **Spirituality** develops over time and is a dynamic, conscious process characterized by two movements of transcendence (going beyond the limits of ordinary experiences): either deep within the self or beyond the self. Self-transcendence involves self-reflection and living according to one's values in establishing meaning to events and a purpose to life. Transcendence beyond self is characterized by a feeling of connection and mutuality to a higher power (Vachon, Fillon, & Achille, 2009).

Related but different than spirituality, **religiousness** is the participation in a community of people who gather around common ways of worshiping. Spirituality can be expressed through adhering to a particular religion. Religious beliefs often define an individual's relationship within a family and community. Many different religions are practiced throughout the world. Judeo-Christian thinking tends to dominate Western societies. Other religions, such as Islam, Hinduism, and Buddhism, dominate Eastern and Middle Eastern cultures (Table 3.1). Because

Table 3.1	MAJOR WORLD RELIGIONS AND BELIEF FORMS		
Source of Power or Force (Deity)	**Historical Sacred Texts or Beliefs**	**Key Beliefs or Ethical Life Philosophy**

Buddhism

Buddha Individual responsibility and logical or intuitive thinking Buddhist subjects include: • *Lamaism* (Tibet), in which Buddhism is blended with spirit worship • *Mantrayana* (Himalayan area, Mongolia, Japan), in which intimate relationship with a guru and recitations of secret mantras are emphasized; belief in sexual symbolism and demons • *Ch'an* (China) *Zen* (Japan), in which self-reliance and awareness through intuitive understanding are stressed. • *Satori* (enlightenment) may come from "sudden insight" or through self-discipline, meditation, and instruction	Tripitaka (scripture) Middle Path (way of life) The Four Noble Truths Eightfold Path (guides for life) The Texts of Taoism (include the Tao Te Ching of Lao Tzu and The Writings of Chuang Tzu) Sutras (Buddhist commentaries) Sangha (Buddhist Community)	Buddhism attempts to deal with problems of human existence such as suffering and death. Life is misery, unhappiness, and suffering with no ultimate reality in the world or behind it. The cause of all human suffering and misery is desire. The "middle path" of life avoids the personal extremes of self-denial and self-indulgence. Visions can be gained through personal meditation and contemplation; good deeds and compassion also facilitate the process toward nirvana, the ultimate mode of existence. The end of suffering is the extinction of desire and emotion and ultimately the unreal self. Present behavior is a result of past deed.

Christianity

God, a unity in tripersonality; Father, Son, and Holy Ghost	Bible Teachings of Jesus through the apostles and the church fathers	God's love for all creatures is a basic belief. Salvation is gained by those who have faith and show humility toward God. Brotherly love is emphasized in acts of charity, kindness, and forgiveness.

Confucianism

No doctrine of a god or gods or life after death Individual responsibility and logical and intuitive thinking	Five Classics (Confucian thought) Analects (conversations and sayings of Confucius)	A philosophy or a system of ethics for living rather than a religion that teaches how people should act toward one another. People are born "good." Moral character is stressed through sincerity in personal and public behavior. Respect is shown for parents and figures of authority. Improvement is gained through self-responsibility, introspection, and compassion for others.

Hinduism

Brahma (the Infinite Being and Creator that pervades all reality) Other gods: Vishnu (preserver), Shiva (destroyer), Krishna (love)	Vedas (doctrine and commentaries)	All people are assigned to castes (permanent hereditary orders, each having different privileges in society; each was created from different parts of Brahma): 1. *Brahmans:* includes priests and intellectuals 2. *Kshatriyas:* includes rulers and soldiers 3. *Vaisya:* includes farmers, skilled workers, and merchants 4. *Sudras:* includes those who serve the other three castes (servants, laborers, peasants) 5. *Untouchables:* the outcasts; those not included in the other castes

Islam

Allah (the only God) Has two major sects: • *Sunni* (orthodox): traditional and simple practices are followed; human will is determined by outside forces • *Shiite*, practices are rapturous and trancelike; human beings have free will	Koran (the words of God delivered to Mohammed by the angel Gabriel) Hadith (commentaries by Mohammed) Five Pillars of Islam (religious conduct) Islam was built on Christianity and Judaism	God is just and merciful; humans are limited and sinful. God rewards the good and punishes the sinful. Mohammed, through the Koran, guides people and teaches them truth. Peace is gained through submission to Allah. The sinless go to Paradise, and the evil go to Hell. A "good" Muslim obeys the Five Pillars of Islam.

(Continued)

Table 3.1	MAJOR WORLD RELIGIONS AND BELIEF FORMS (*Continued*)	
Source of Power or Force (Deity)	Historical Sacred Texts or Beliefs	Key Beliefs or Ethical Life Philosophy
Judaism		
God	Hebrew Bible (Old Testament) Torah (first five books of Hebrew Bible) Talmud (commentaries on the Torah)	Jews have a special relationship with God: obeying God's law through ethical behavior and ritual obedience earns the mercy and justice of God. God is worshiped through love, not out of fear.
Shintoism		
Gods of nature, ancestor worship, national heroes	Tradition and custom (the way of the gods) Beliefs were influenced by Confucianism and Buddhism	Reverence for ancestors and a traditional Japanese way of life are emphasized. Loyalty to places and locations where one lives or works and purity and balance in physical and mental life are major motivators of personal conduct.
Taoism		
All the forces in nature	Tao-te-Ching ("The Way and the Power")	Quiet and happy harmony with nature is the key belief. Peace and contentment are found in the personal behaviors of optimism, passivity, humility, and internal calmness. Humility is an especially valued virtue. Conformity to the rhythm of nature and the universe leads to a simple, natural, and ideal life.
Tribal Beliefs		
Animism: Souls or spirits embodied in all beings and everything in nature (trees, rivers, mountains) *Polytheism:* Many gods, in the basic powers of nature (sun, moon, earth, water)	Passed on through ceremonies, rituals, myths, and legends Oral history, rather than written literature, is the common medium	All living things are related. Respect for powers of nature and pleasing the spirits are fundamental beliefs to meet the basic and practical needs for food, fertility, health, and interpersonal relationships and individual development. Harmonious living is comprehension and respect of natural forces.

Summary of Other Belief Forms

- *Agnosticism:* the belief that whether there is a God and a spiritual world or any ultimate reality is unknown and probably unknowable
- *Atheism:* the belief that no God exists because "God" is defined in any current existing culture of society
- *Maoism:* the faith that is centered in the leadership of the Communist Party and all the people; the major belief goal is to move away from individual personal desires and ambitions toward viewing and serving all people as a whole
- *Scientism:* the belief that values and guidance for living come from scientific knowledge, principles, and practices; systematic study and analysis of life, rather than superstition, lead to true understanding and practice of life

Adapted from Axelson, J. A., & McGrath, P. (1998, 1993, 1985). *Counseling and development in a multicultural society.* Pacific Grove, CA: Brooks/Cole Publishing Company, a division of International Thomson Publishing Inc. Used with permission of the publisher.

religious beliefs often influence approaches to mental health, it is important to understand the basis of various religions that appear to be growing in the United States. Both religion and spirituality can provide support and strength in dealing with mental illnesses and emotional problems.

People with mental illness benefit from spiritual assessment and interventions (see Chapter 10). Perception of well-being and health in persons with severe mental illness has been positively associated with spirituality and religiousness. To carry out spiritual interventions, the nurse enters a therapeutic relationship with the patient and uses the self as a therapeutic tool (Box 3.3). Examples of spiritual interventions include meditation; guided imagery; and, when appropriate, prayer to connect with inner sources of solace and hope (see Box 3.4).

BOX 3.3

Research for Best Practice: **Coping Strategies of Family Members**

Eaton, P. M., Davis, B. L., Hammond, P. V., Condon, E. H., & Zina, T. M. (2011). Coping strategies of family members of hospitalized psychiatric patients. Nursing Research and Practice. doi:10.1155./2011/392705

THE QUESTION: What are the coping strategies of family members of hospitalized patients with psychiatric disorders?

METHODS: A descriptive, correlational, mixed method research approach was guided by the Neuman Systems Model as forty-five family members of hospitalized patients with psychiatric disorders were asked to complete the Family Crisis Oriented Personal Evaluation Scale and semi-structured interviews.

FINDINGS: Family members used more emotion-coping strategies rather than problem-solving strategies. The coping strategies used included communicating with immediate family, acceptance of their situation, passive appraisal, avoidance, and spirituality.

IMPLICATIONS FOR NURSING: Families are impacted by psychiatric hospitalizations of members and need nursing support in order to have the energy to provide care and support to their family member. Spirituality is one of the coping strategies that can be supported.

SUMMARY OF KEY POINTS

- The term *culture* is defined as a way of life that manifests the learned beliefs, values, and accepted behaviors that are transmitted socially within a specific group.

- Everyone has a cultural identity, which helps define expected behavior.

- Cultural and linguistic competence is based on a set of skills that allows individuals to increase their understanding and appreciation of cultural differences and similarities within, among, and between groups. Cultural competence is demonstrated by valuing the culture beliefs, bridging any language gap, and considering the patient's literacy level when planning and implementing care.

- Mental illnesses are stigmatized in many cultural groups. A variety of cultural and religious beliefs underlie the stigmatization.

- Access to mental health treatment is particularly limited for those living in rural areas or those who live in poverty.

- Spirituality can be a source of strength and support for both the patient with mental illness and the nurse providing the care.

- Religious beliefs are closely intertwined with beliefs about health and mental illness.

Box 3.4

Using Reflection

FACILITATING SPIRITUAL CONNECTIONS

INCIDENT • A young man with severe depression, psychosis, and HIV was shunned by his family and church. He is homeless and sleeps at a shelter each night, roaming the streets during the day. As a veteran, he seeks health services at a local Veterans Administration. He is reluctant to seek out mental health care. In an interview, he asks the nurse if God is punishing him for his actions in Afghanistan.

REFLECTION • The nurse's immediate thought was to assure him that he was not being punished. As the nurse reflected on the situation, she realized that he might be asking for help in understanding the meaning of his situation and how he could understand his connection to his God. She initiated a therapeutic relationship with him and then conducted a spiritual assessment.

CRITICAL THINKING CHALLENGES

1. Assess your cultural competence with groups that have the following heritage: African, Asian, Hispanic, and Native American.

2. Compare beliefs about mental illnesses within African and Asian American groups.

3. Compare the access to mental health services in your state or county in rural areas versus urban areas.

4. Discuss the differences between spirituality and religiousness. Is it possible that someone can be spiritual and not religious?

5. Identify the religious groups that are associated with the following sacred texts: Bible, Koran, Vedas, Texts of Taoism, Talmud.

House of Sand and Fog: (2003). Colonel Massoud Amir Behrani, an Iranian immigrant played by Ben Kingsley, has spent most of his savings trying to enhance his daughter's chances of a good marriage. The rest of his funds were spent at an auction on a repossessed house owned by Kathy Nicoli (Jennifer Connelly), an emotionally unstable, depressed young woman who failed to pay property taxes. The struggle for the house ensues with tragic results.

VIEWING POINTS: Identify the cultural differences between the Behrani and Nicoli families. Are any cultural stereotypes depicted in the film? Discuss the role of prejudice and discrimination in the outcome of the movie. How did Kathy's mental illness and relationship with the police officer influence the negotiation for the house?

References

American Psychiatric Association. (2013). *Diagnostic and statistical manual of mental disorders, DSM-5* (5th ed). Arlington, VA: American Psychiatric Association.

Appel, H.B., Huang, B., Ai, A. L. & Lin, C. J. (2011). Physical, behavioral, and mental health issues in Asian American women: Results from the national Latino Asian American study. *Journal of Women's Health (2002), 20*(11), 1703–1711.

DeNavas-Walt, C., Proctor, B. D., & Smith, J. C. (2013). *Income, Poverty, and Health Insurance Coverage in the United States: 2012. U.S. Census Bureau Current population reports* (pp. 60–245). Washington, DC: U.S. Government Printing Office.

Eack, S. M., Bahorik, A. L., Newhill, C. E., Neighbors, H. W., & Davis, L. E. (2012). Interviewer-perceived honesty as a mediator of racial disparities in the diagnosis of schizophrenia. *Psychiatric services (Washington, D.C.), 63*(9), 875–880.

Eaton, P. M., Davis, B. L., Hammond, P. V., Condon, E. H., & McGee, Z. T. (2011). Coping strategies of family members of hospitalized psychiatric patients. *Nursing Research and Practice.* doi:10.1155/2011/392705

Goode, T. D., & Jones, W. (2009). Linguistic Competence. National Center for Cultural Competence, Georgetown University Center for Child and Human Development. Washington, DC. http://nccc.georgetown.edu/documents/Definition%2520of%2520Linguistic%2520Competence.pdf

Kaltman, S., de Mendoza, A. H., Gonzales, F. A., & Serrano, A. (2013). Preferences for trauma-related mental health services among Latina immigrants from Central America, South America, and Mexico. *Psychological Trauma: Theory, Research, Practice, and Policy.* doi:10.1037/a0031539

Lee, J., Min, S. K., Kim, K. H., Kim, B., Cho, S. J., Lee, S. H., et al. (2012). Differences in temperament and character dimensions of personality between patients with Hwa-byung, an anger syndrome, and patients with major depressive disorder. *Journal of Affective Disorders, 138*(1–2), 110–116.

Lee, S. L., Juon, H. S., Martinez, G, Hsu, C. E., Robinson, E. S., Bawa J, et al. (2009). Model minority at risk: Expressed needs of mental health by Asian American young adults. *Journal of Community Health, 34*(2), 144–152.

Lee, S., Laiewski, L., & Choi, S. (2014). Racial-ethnic variation in U.S. mental health service use among Latino and Asian non-U.S. citizens. *Psychiatric Services, 65*(1), 68–74.

Searles, V. B., Valley, M. A., Hedegaard, H., Betz, M. E. (2013). Suicides in urban and rural counties in the United States, 2006-2008. *Crisis: The Journal of Crisis Intervention and Suicide Prevention,* 1–9. doi:10,1027/0227-5910/a000224

Suicide Prevention Resource Center. (2013). *Suicide among racial/ethnic populations in the U.S. Asians, Pacific Islander, and Native Hawaiians. Fact sheet.* Suicide Prevention Action Network USA. Retrieved December 4, 2010, from http://www.spanusa.org

U.S. Census Bureau. (2013). U.S. Census Bureau. Statistical Abstract of the United States: 2012 (131st ed) Washington, DC, 2011. http://www.census.gov/compendia/statab/

U.S. Census Bureau. (2014). State and County Quick Facts. Data derived from Population Estimates, American Community Survey, Census of Population and Housing, State and County Housing Unit Estimates, County Business Patterns, Nonemployer Statistics, Economic Census, Survey of Business Owners, Building Permits. http://quickfacts.census.gov/qfd/states/00000.html

U.S. Department of Health and Human Services. (2013). Cultural competency. Office of Minority Health. http://minorityhealth.hhs.gov/templates/browse.aspx?lvl=2&lvlID=11

U.S. Department of Health and Human Services. (2010). The delayed update of the HHS poverty guidelines for the remainder of 2010. *Federal Register, 75*(148), 45628.

Vachon, M., Fillion, L., & Achille, M. (2009). A conceptual analysis of spirituality at the end of life. *Journal of Palliative Medicine, 12*(1), 53–59.

Ward, E. C., Wiltshire, J. C., Detry, M. A. & Brown, R. L. (2013). African American men and women's attitude toward mental illness, perceptions of stigma, and preferred coping behaviors. *Nursing Research, 62*(3), 185–194.

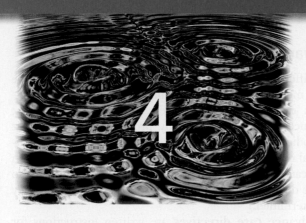

4

Patient Rights and Legal Issues

Mary Ann Boyd

KEY CONCEPT

• self-determinism

LEARNING OBJECTIVES

After studying this chapter, you will be able to:

1. Define *self-determinism* and its implications in mental health care.

2. Discuss the legal protection of the rights of people with mental disorders.

3. Discuss the legal determination of competency.

4. Delineate the differences between voluntary and involuntary treatment.

5. Discuss the difference between privacy and confidentiality.

6. Discuss HIPAA and mandates to inform and their implications in psychiatric–mental health care.

7. Identify the importance of accurate, quality documentation in electronic and non-electronic patient records.

KEY TERMS

• accreditation • advance care directives • assault • breach of confidentiality • competence • confidentiality • external advocacy system • incompetent • informed consent • internal rights protection system • involuntary commitment • least restrictive environment • living will • medical battery • negligence • power of attorney • privacy • voluntary admission • voluntary commitment

Because individuals with mental disorders are often vulnerable to mistreatment and abuse, their legal rights and the ethical health care practices of mental health providers are ongoing concerns for psychiatric–mental health nurses. For example, can a person be forced into a hospital if his or her behavior is bizarre but harmless? What human rights can be denied to a person who has a mental disorder and under what circumstances? These questions are not easily answered. This chapter summarizes some of the key patient rights and legal issues that underlie psychiatric–mental health nursing practice across the continuum of care. Discussion of the care of people with mental illness in forensic settings is found in Chapter 41.

SELF-DETERMINISM: A FUNDAMENTAL RIGHT AND NEED

At the foundation of many questions related to the rights of mental health patients is the issue of self-determinism and preservation of this right.

> **KEYCONCEPT** **Self-determinism** promotes growth and well-being toward human potential through having basic psychological needs met including autonomy (initiation and control of one's actions), competence (perceived effectiveness in social interactions), and relatedness (connections and belongingness with others) (Deci & Ryan, 2012).

A self-determined individual is internally motivated to make choices based on personal goals, not to please others or to be rewarded. That is, a person engages in activities that are interesting, challenging, pleasing, exciting, or fun, requiring no rewards other than the positive feelings that accompany them because of inner goals, needs, drives or preferences. Personal autonomy and avoidance of dependence on others are key values of self-determinism, which is integral to the recovery process (see Chapter 2).

In mental health care, self-determinism is the right to choose one's own health-related behaviors, which at times differ from those recommended by health professionals. A patient's right to refuse treatment, to choose the second or third best health care recommendation rather than the first, and to seek a second opinion are all self-deterministic acts. In mental health care, adhering to treatment regimens may be at odds with the self-deterministic views of an individual. Supporting a person's ability to choose treatment becomes complex because of related issues of competency, informed consent, voluntary and involuntary commitment, and public safety; these issues are discussed later in this chapter.

PROTECTION OF PATIENT RIGHTS

Because people with psychiatric problems are vulnerable to mistreatment and abuse, laws have been passed that guarantee them legal protection. These laws offer protection of self-determinism, protection against discrimination in employment, and protection against mistreatment in health care settings.

Self-Determination Act

The *Patient Self-Determination Act* (PSDA) was implemented on December 1, 1991, as a part of the Omnibus Budget Reconciliation Act of 1990 and requires hospitals, health maintenance organizations, skilled nursing facilities, home health agencies, and hospices receiving Medicare and Medicaid reimbursement to inform patients at the time of admission of their right to be a central part of any and all health care decisions made about them or for them. Patients have the following rights:

- Be provided with information regarding advance care documents.
- Be asked at admission or enrollment whether they have an advance care document and that this fact be recorded in the medical record.
- Be provided with information on their rights to complete advance care documents and refuse medical care (Omnibus Budget Reconciliation Act, 1990).

The Act also requires health care institutions receiving Medicare and Medicaid reimbursement to educate health care personnel and the local community about advance care planning.

Advance Care Directives in Mental Health

At different times during the course of an illness, people with mental disorders may be unable to make sound decisions regarding their treatment and care. Fortunately, advance care directives legally protect them from their periodic poor decision-making abilities. A competent individual can make a decision about a treatment—a decision that can be honored even if the person is no longer able to make decisions. (See later discussion for how competency is determined.)

Advance care directives are written instructions for health care when individuals are incapacitated. Living wills and appointment directives, often referred to as power of attorney or health proxies, are recognized under state laws and their courts. A **living will** states what treatment should be omitted or refused in the event that a person is unable to make those decisions. A durable **power of attorney** for health care appoints a proxy, usually a relative or trusted friend, to make health care decisions on an individual's behalf if that person is incapacitated.

An advance directive does not need to be written, reviewed, or signed by an attorney. It must be witnessed by two people and notarized and applies only if the individual is unable to make his or her own decisions as a result of being incapacitated or if, in the opinion of two physicians, the person is otherwise unable to make decisions for him- or herself.

Psychiatric advance directives (PADs) are relatively new legal instruments and allow patients, while competent, to document their choices of treatment and care. This declaration must be made in advance and signed by the patient and two witnesses. Through the use of a PAD, individuals are empowered to direct their treatment such as choice of medication and hospitalization. Although a physician can override this declaration during times when the patient's decision-making capacity is clearly distorted because of mental illness, the patient must be informed first and the order made by the court. During periods of competency, the PAD can be revoked.

Bill of Rights for Mental Health Patients

Rights of people with mental disorders receive additional protection beyond that afforded to patients in other health care areas (Box 4.1). The *Mental Health Systems Act* [42 U.S.C. 9501 et seq.] of 1980 requires that each state review and revise, if necessary, its laws to ensure that mental health patients receive these human rights protections and services that they require.

Americans With Disabilities Act and Job Discrimination

The *Americans With Disabilities Act* of 1990 (ADA) ensures that people with disabilities, such as severe mental

BOX 4.1

Bill of Rights for Persons Receiving Mental Health Services

- The right to treatment and services under conditions that support the person's personal liberty and restrict such liberty only as necessary to comply with treatment needs, laws, and judicial orders.
- The right to an individualized, written, treatment or service plan (to be developed promptly after admission), treatment based on the plan, periodic review and reassessment of needs and appropriate revisions of the plan, including a description of services that may be needed after discharge.
- The right to ongoing participation in the planning of services to be provided and in the development and periodic revision of the treatment plan, and the right to be provided with a reasonable explanation of all aspects of one's own condition and treatment.
- The right to refuse treatment, except during an emergency situation, or as permitted under law in the case of a person committed by a court for treatment.
- The right not to participate in experimentation in the absence of the patient's informed, voluntary, written consent, the right to appropriate protections associated with such participation, the right to an opportunity to revoke such consent.
- The right to freedom from restraints or seclusion, other than during an emergency situation.

- The right to a humane treatment environment that affords reasonable protection from harm and appropriate privacy.
- The right to confidentiality of records.
- The right to access, upon request, one's own mental health care records.
- The right (in residential or inpatient care) to converse with others privately and to have access to the telephone and mails unless denial of access is documented as necessary for treatment.
- The right to be informed promptly, in appropriate language and terms, of the rights described in this section.
- The right to assert grievances with respect to infringement of the Bill of Rights, including the right to have such grievances considered in a fair, timely, and impartial procedure.
- The right of access to protection, service, and a qualified advocate in order to understand, exercise, and protect one's rights.
- The right to exercise the rights described in this section without reprisal, including reprisal in the form of denial of any appropriate, available treatment.
- The right to referral as appropriate to other providers of mental health services upon discharge.

From Title V of the Mental Health Systems Act [42 U.S.C. 9501 et seq.]. Retrieved from http://www4.law.cornell.edu/uscode/42/10841.html.

FAME & FORTUNE

Elizabeth Parsons Ware Packard (1816–1895)
Author and Social Reformer

PUBLIC PERSONA

Elizabeth Packard, social reformer in the latter half of the 19th century, lived in Chicago and later in Springfield, Illinois. She supported herself and her six children through her writings and books that exposed the abuse of patients committed to insane asylums of the day. After her children were grown, Elizabeth Packard lobbied legislators in the Illinois state capital on behalf of her reforms.

PERSONAL REALITIES

In 1864, Elizabeth Packard was committed to the Illinois State Hospital for the Insane based solely on her husband's assertion that her religious views were different from his. In reality, she was not sufficiently subordinate to her husband. Illinois law at the time permitted any married man to consign his wife to the asylum with no requirement other than consent of the asylum superintendent. Elizabeth Packard was incarcerated in the hospital for 3 years, during which time she rejected any treatment offered.

Source: Lightner, D. L. (1999). *Asylum, prison, and poorhouse: The writings and reform work of Dorothea Dix in Illinois*. Carbondale and Edwardsville, IL: Southern Illinois University Press.

---

disorders, have legal protection against discrimination in the workplace, housing, public programs, transportation, and telecommunications. An employer is free to select the most qualified applicant available, but if the most qualified person has a mental disorder, this law mandates that reasonable accommodations need to be made for that individual. Accommodations are any adjustments to a job or work environment, such as restructuring a job, modifying work schedules, and acquiring or modifying equipment (U.S. Equal Employment Opportunity Commission, 2013).

Internal Rights Protection Systems

Mental health care systems have **internal rights protection systems,** or mechanisms to combat any violation of their patients' rights. *Public Law 99-319, the Protection and Advocacy for Mentally Ill Individuals Act of 1986,* requires each state mental health provider to establish and operate a system that protects and advocates for the rights of individuals with mental illnesses and investigates any incidents of abuse and neglect.

External Advocacy Systems

Health organizations such as the American Hospital Association, American Healthcare Association, and the

American Public Health Association serve as advocates for the rights and treatment of mental health patients and are a part of an **external advocacy system**. They are financially and administratively independent from the mental health agencies. These groups advocate through negotiation and recommendations but have no legal authority. They can resort to litigation that leads to lawsuits and consent decrees (legal mandates that are monitored by the U.S. Department of Justice) or, in some instances, a denial of accreditation to the health care institution by their certifying body.

Accreditation of Mental Health Care Delivery Systems

Patient rights are also assured of protection by an agency's **accreditation**, the recognition or approval of an institution according to the accrediting body's criteria. Accrediting bodies such as The Joint Commission require patient rights standards. The Centers for Medicare and Medicaid Services (CMS) sets patient rights standards for institutions seeking Medicare and Medicaid funding. Community mental health centers are not accredited by either the Joint Commission or CMS but by another agency, the Commission on Accreditation of Rehabilitation Facilities.

TREATMENT AND PATIENT RIGHTS

In caring for patients receiving mental health services or treatment, it is important for nurses to understand several issues related to the patient's rights to determine choices about his or her own treatment. These issues are related to competency, informed consent, least restrictive environment, and voluntary and involuntary treatment.

Competency

One of the most important concepts underlying the legal rights of individuals is competency to consent to or to refuse treatment. Although competency is a legal determination, it is not clearly defined across the states. It is generally agreed that **competence**, or the degree to which the patient can understand and appreciate the information given during the consent process, refers to a patient's cognitive ability to process information at a specific time. A patient may be competent to make a treatment decision at one time and not be competent at another time. Competence is also decision specific, so that a patient may be competent to decide on a simple treatment with a relatively clear consequence but may not be competent to decide about a treatment with a complex set of outcomes. A competent patient can refuse any aspect of the treatment plan.

Competency is different from rationality, which is a characteristic of a patient's decision, not of the patient's ability to make a decision. An irrational decision is one that involves hurting oneself pointlessly, such as stopping recommended treatment even though symptoms return. A person who is competent may make what appears to be an irrational decision, and it cannot be overruled by health care providers; however, if a person is judged **incompetent** (i.e., unable to understand and appreciate the information given during the consent process), it is possible to force treatment on the individual. Strong arguments are, however, made against forced treatment under these circumstances. Forced treatment denigrates individuals, and according to self-determinism theory and recovery concepts, individuals are not as likely to experience treatment success if it is externally imposed.

How is it determined that a patient is competent? Mental health legal experts generally agree that four areas should be directly assessed (Applebaum, 2007). Table 4.1 outlines these assessment areas. A patient who is competent to give informed consent should be able to achieve the following:

- Communicate choices.
- Understand relevant information.
- Appreciate the situation and its consequences.

Table 4.1	**DETERMINATION OF COMPETENCY**	
Assessment Area	**Definition**	**Patient Attributes**
Communicate choices	Ability to express choices	Patient should be able to repeat what he or she has heard
Understand relevant information	Capacity to comprehend the meaning of the information given about treatment	Patient should be able to paraphrase understanding of treatment
Appreciate the situation and its consequence	Capacity to grasp what the information means specifically to the patient	Patient should be able to discuss the disorder, the need for treatment, the likely outcomes, and the reason the treatment is being suggested
Use a logical thought process to compare the risks and benefits of treatment options	Capacity to reach a logical conclusion consistent with the starting premise	Patient should be able to discuss logical reasons for the choice of treatment

Adapted from Applebaum, P. (2007). Assessment of patients' competence to consent to treatment. *New England Journal of Medicine, 357*(18), 1834–1840.

- Use a logical thought process to compare the risks and benefits of treatment options.

Informed Consent

Individuals seeking mental health care must provide **informed consent**, a legal procedure to ensure that the patient knows the benefits and costs of treatment. To provide informed consent for care, the patient must be given adequate information upon which to base decisions and actively participate in the decision-making process. Informed consent is not an option but is mandated by state laws. In most states, the law mandates that a mental health provider must inform a patient in such a way that an average reasonable person would be able to make an educated decision about the interventions.

Informed consent is complicated in mental health treatment. A patient must be competent to give consent, but the individual's decision-making ability often is compromised by the mental illness. This dilemma might be illustrated by a situation in which a person who is informed of medication side effects refuses treatment, not because of the potential negative impact of the medication but because he or she denies the illness outright. The health care provider knows that when the person begins taking the medication, the symptoms of the illness will subside, and the decision-making ability will return.

Most institutions have policies that outline the nursing responsibilities within the informed consent process. The nurse has a key role in the process of informed consent, from structuring the written informed consent document to educating the patient about a particular procedure. The nurse makes sure that consent has been obtained before any treatment is given. Informed consent is especially important in research projects involving experimental drugs or therapies.

Least Restrictive Environment

The right to refuse treatment is related to a larger concept—the right to be treated in the **least restrictive environment**, which means that an individual cannot be restricted to an institution when he or she can be successfully treated in the community. In 1975, the courts ruled that a person committed to psychiatric treatment had a right to be treated in the least restrictive environment (Dixon v. Weinberger, 1975). Medication cannot be given unnecessarily. An individual cannot be restrained or locked in a room unless all other "less restrictive" interventions are tried first.

Voluntary and Involuntary Treatment

Accessing the mental health delivery system is similar to seeking any other type of health care. Whether in a public or private system, the treatment setting is usually outpatient. Treatment strategies (e.g., medication, psychotherapy) are recommended and agreed on by both the provider and the individual. Arrangements for treatment and follow up are then made. The patient leaves the outpatient setting and is responsible for following the plan.

Inpatient treatment is generally reserved for patients who are acutely ill or have a forensic commitment (see Chapter 41). If hospitalization is required, the person enters the treatment facility, participates in the treatment planning process, and follows through with the treatment. The individual maintains all civil rights and is free to leave at any time even if it is against medical advice. In most settings, this type of admission is called a **voluntary admission**. If an individual is admitted to a public facility, the state statute may refer to the process as **voluntary commitment** rather than admission; however, in both instances, full legal rights are retained.

Involuntary commitment is the confined hospitalization of a person without the person's consent but with a court order. There are also legal provisions for people to be involuntarily committed to outpatient mental health facilities through state civil laws. Because involuntary commitment is a prerogative of the state agency, each state and the District of Columbia have separate commitment statutes; however, three common elements are found in most of these statutes. The individual must be (1) mentally disordered, (2) dangerous to self or others, or (3) unable to provide for basic needs (i.e., "gravely disabled").

Patients who are involuntarily committed have the right to receive treatment, but they also may have the right to refuse it. Arguments over the rights of civilly committed patients to refuse treatment first surfaced in 1975 when a federal district court judge issued a temporary restraining order prohibiting the use of psychotropic medication against the patient's will at a state hospital in Boston. Today, laws about commitment and refusal of medication vary from state to state. Many states recognize the rights of involuntarily committed patients to refuse medication (National Mental Health Information Center, 2007). The state trend is to grant patients the right to refuse treatment whether they are competent or incompetent.

Commitment procedures vary considerably among the states. Most have provisions for an emergency short-term hospitalization of 48 to 92 hours authorized by a certified mental health provider without court approval. At the end of that period, the individual either agrees to voluntary treatment or extended commitment procedures are begun. The judge must order the commitment, and the individual is afforded several legal rights, including notice of the proceedings, a full hearing (jury trial if requested) in which the government must prove the grounds for commitment, and the right to legal counsel at state expense.

PRIVACY AND CONFIDENTIALITY

In addition to issues related to self-determinism, privacy and confidentiality are rights that need to be protected for mental health patients. **Privacy** refers to that part of an individual's personal life that is not governed by society's laws and government intrusion. Protecting an individual from intrusion is a responsibility of health care providers. **Confidentiality** can be defined as an ethical duty of nondisclosure. Providers who receive confidential information must protect that information from being accessed by others and resist disclosing it. Confidentiality involves two people: the individual who discloses and the person with whom the information is shared. If confidentiality is broken, a person's privacy is also violated; however, a person's privacy can be violated but confidentiality maintained. For example, if a nurse observes an adult patient reading pornography alone in his or her room, the patient's privacy has been violated. If the patient asks the nurse not to tell anyone and the request is honored, confidentiality is maintained.

A **breach of confidentiality** is the release of patient information without the patient's consent in the absence of legal compulsion or authorization to release information (Wettstein, 1994). For example, discussing a patient's problem with one of his or her relatives without the patient's consent is a breach of confidentiality. Even sharing patient information with another professional who is not involved in the patient's care is a breach of confidentiality because the individual has not given permission for the information to be shared. Maintaining confidentiality is not as easy as it first appears. For example, family members are legally excluded from receiving any information about an adult member without consent even if that member is receiving care from the family. Ideally, a patient gives consent for information to be shared with the family or has psychiatric advance care directive.

HIPAA and Protection of Health Information

The Health Insurance Portability and Accountability Act of 1996 (HIPAA) provides legal protection in several areas of health care, including privacy and confidentiality.

This act protects working Americans from losing existing health care coverage when changing jobs and increases opportunities for purchasing health care. It regulates the use and release of patient information, especially electronic transfer of health information. Effective April 2003, HIPAA regulations require patient authorization for the release of information with the exception of that required for treatment, payment, and health care administrative operations. The release of information related to psychotherapy requires patient permission. The underlying intent is to prevent the release of information to agencies not related to health care, such as employers, without the patient's consent. When information is released, the patient must agree to the exact information that is being disclosed, the purpose of disclosure, the recipient of the information, and an expiration date for the disclosure of information (U.S. Department of Health and Human Services, 2002).

The American Recovery and Reinvestment Act of 2009 includes several provisions affecting the management of health information. For the most part, this law focuses on maintaining privacy of electronic transfer and storage of health information and communication. In the clinical area, one way of maintaining privacy is by restricting access to records by staff members unless there is a specific reason such as caring for a patient.

Mandates to Inform

At certain times, health care professionals are legally obligated to breach confidentiality. When there is a judgment that the patient has harmed any person or is about to injure someone, professionals are mandated by law to report it to authorities. The legal "duty to warn" was a result of the 1976 decision of *Tarasoff v. Regents of the University of California*. In this case, a 26-year-old graduate student told university psychologists about his obsession with another student, Tatiana Tarasoff, whom he subsequently killed. Tatiana Tarasoff's parents initiated a separate civil action and brought suit against the therapist, the university, and the campus police, claiming that Tatiana's death was a result of negligence on the part of the defendants.

The plaintiffs claimed that the therapists should have warned Ms. Tarasoff that the graduate student presented a danger to her and that he should have been confined to a hospital. Both claims were originally dismissed in the lower courts, but in 1974, the California Supreme Court reversed the lower courts' decisions and said that Ms. Tarasoff should have been warned. The high court said that psychotherapists have a duty to warn the foreseeable victims of their patients' violent actions. Because of the outcry from professional mental health organizations, the court agreed to review the case, and in 1976, the original decision was revised by the ruling that psychotherapists have a duty to exercise reasonable care in protecting the foreseeable victims of their patients' violent actions. The results of this case have had far-reaching consequences and have influenced many decisions in the United States. Although many lawsuits have been based on the Tarasoff case, most have failed. Usually, if there are clear threats of violence toward others, the therapist is mandated to warn potential victims.

> **NCLEXNOTE**   What guides the intervention for a patient who tells the nurse that he (she) wants to hurt a family member: mandate to inform or HIPAA?
>
> Answer: Mandate to inform. Rationale: Because others are at risk for injury, the Tarasoff decision will prevail.

ACCOUNTABILITY FOR NURSES AND OTHER MENTAL HEALTH CARE PROFESSIONALS

Nurses and other health care professionals are accountable for the care they provide in mental health as well as any other practice area.

Legal Liability in Psychiatric Nursing Practice

Malpractice is based on a set of torts (a civil wrong not based on contract committed by one person that causes injury to another). An **assault** is the threat of unlawful force to inflict bodily injury upon another. An assault must be imminent and cause reasonable apprehension in the individual. Battery is the intentional and unpermitted contact with another. **Medical battery**, intentional and unauthorized harmful or offensive contact, occurs when a patient is treated without informed consent. For example, a clinician who fails to obtain consent before performing a procedure is subject to being accused of medical battery. Also, failure to respect a patient's advance directives is considered medical battery. False imprisonment is the detention or imprisonment contrary to provision of the law. Facilities that do not discharge voluntarily committed patients upon request can be subject to this type of litigation.

   Negligence is a breach of duty of reasonable care for a patient for whom a nurse is responsible that results in personal injuries. A clinician who does get consent but does not disclose the nature of the procedure and the risks involved is subject to a negligence claim. Five elements are required to prove negligence: duty (accepting assignment to care for patient), breach of duty (failure to practice according to acceptable standards of care), cause in fact (the injury would not have happened if the standards had been followed), cause in proximity (harm actually occurred within the scope of foreseeable consequence), and damages (physical or emotional injury caused by breach of standard of care). Simple mistakes are not negligent acts.

Lawsuits in Psychiatric Mental Health Care

Few lawsuits are filed against mental health clinicians and facilities compared with other health care areas. If psychiatric nurses are included in lawsuits, they are usually included in the lawsuit filed against agency. Common areas of litigation surround the nursing care of patients who are suicidal or violent. Maintaining and documenting an appropriate standard of care (see Chapter 6) can protect nurses from complicated legal proceedings. The following can help prevent negative outcomes of malpractice litigations:

* Evaluate risks, especially when privileges broaden or care is transferred.
* Document decisional processes and reasons for choices among alternatives.
* Involve family in important decisions.
* Make decisions within team model and document this shared responsibility.
* Adhere to agency's policy and procedures.
* Seek consultation and record input.

Nursing Documentation

Careful documentation is important both to help ensure protection of patient rights and for nurse accountability. Documentation can be handwritten or electronic. It is very common in psychiatric facilities that all disciplines record one progress note. Nursing documentation is based on nursing standards (see Chapter 6) and the policies of the particular facility. Many documentation styles are problem focused. That is, documentation is structured to address specific problems that are identified on the nursing care plan or interdisciplinary treatment plan. No matter the setting or structure of the documentation, nurses are responsible for documenting the following:

* Observations of the patient's subjective and objective physical, psychological, and social responses to mental disorders and emotional problems
* Interventions implemented and the patient's response
* Observations of therapeutic and side effects of medications
* Evaluation of outcomes of interventions

   Particular attention should be paid to the reason the patient is admitted for care. If the person's initial problem was suicide or homicidal ideation, the patient should routinely be assessed for suicidal and homicidal thoughts even if the treatment plan does not specifically identify suicide and homicide as potential problems. Careful documentation is always needed for patients who are suicidal, homicidal, aggressive, or restrained in any way. Medications prescribed on an as-needed (PRN) basis also require a separate entry, including reason for administration, dosage, route, and response to the medication.

A patient record is the primary documentation of a patient's problems, verifies the behavior of the patient at the point of care, and describes the care provided. The patient record is considered a legal document. Courts consider acts not recorded as acts not done. Patients also have legal access to their records. For handwritten documentation, the entries should always be written in pen with no erasures. If an entry is corrected, it should be initialed by the person making the correction. All entries should be clear, well written, and void of jargon. Judgmental statements, such as "patient is manipulating staff" have no place in patients' records. Only meaningful, accurate, objective descriptions of behavior should be used. General, stereotypic statements, such as "had a good night" or "no complaints" are meaningless and should be avoided.

With the universal use of electronic records, meaningful documentation is sometimes more difficult. Many institutions require health care workers to enter observations, assessment data, and interventions into a template that requires a "click" in a box on the monitor screen. Additional narrative entries are usually required to provide quality, individualized care. Nurses are held to the same standards of practice and documentation when entering electronic data as when entering data a non-electronic record.

SUMMARY OF KEY POINTS

- The right of self-determination entitles all patients to refuse treatment, to obtain other opinions, and to choose other forms of treatment. It is one of the basic patients' rights established by Title II, Public Law 99-139, outlining the Universal Bill of Rights for Mental Health Patients.

- Laws and systems are established to protect the rights of people with mental health issues. Some of these include the Self-Determination Act, advance directives, a patient Bill of Rights, the Americans with Disabilities Act, internal rights protection systems, external advocacy systems, and accreditation of mental health care delivery systems.

- The internal rights protection system and the external advocates combat violations of human rights.

- Informed consent is another protective right that helps patients decide what can be done to their bodies and minds. It must be obtained from a competent individual before any treatment is begun to ensure that the information is not only received but understood.

- A competent person can refuse any treatment. Incompetence is determined by the court when the patient cannot understand the information.

- The right to the least restrictive environment entitles patients to be treated in the least restrictive setting and by the least restrictive interventions and protects patients from unnecessary confinement and medication.

- Involuntary commitment procedures are specified at the state level. Patients who are involuntarily committed have the right to refuse treatment and medication.

- Patient privacy is protected through HIPAA regulations related to the transfer and storage of information. A breach in confidentiality is legally mandated when there is a threat of violence toward others.

- Nursing documentation is guided by practice standards and policies of the agency. Nurses are responsible for individualized documentation in both electronic and non-electronic health records.

CRITICAL THINKING CHALLENGES

1. Consider the relationship of self-determinism to competence by differentiating patients who are competent to give consent and those who are incompetent. Discuss the steps in determining whether a patient is competent to provide informed consent for a treatment.

2. Define competency to consent to or refuse treatment and relate the definition to the Self-Determination Act.

3. A patient is involuntarily admitted to a psychiatric unit and refuses all medication. After being unable to persuade the patient to take prescribed medication, the nurse documents the patient's refusal and notifies the prescriber. Should the nurse attempt to give the medication without patient consent? Support your answer.

4. A person who is homeless with a mental illness refuses any treatment. Although he is clearly psychotic and would benefit from treatment, he is not a danger to himself or others and seems to be able to provide for his basic needs. His family is desperate for him to be treated. What are the ethical issues underlying this situation?

5. Discuss the purposes of living wills and health proxies. Discuss their use in psychiatric–mental health care.

6. Identify the legal and ethical issues underlying the Tarasoff case and mandates to inform.

7. Compare the authority and responsibilities of the internal rights protection system with those of the external advocacy system.

MOVIES *Nuts:* 1987. Starring Barbra Streisand, Richard Dreyfuss, Maureen Stapleton, Eli Wallach, and Robert Webber. A strong-willed, high-priced prostitute is accused of manslaughter. Her family and attorney want her to plead guilty by reason of insanity. The movie revolves around the family's attempt to have her declared incompetent to stand trial, which would commit her to a mental health center before she can go to trial. She insists on proving her sanity, and to discover the truth, her lawyer must battle his prejudice and her inexplicable belligerence.

VIEWING POINTS: Watch how the family members attempt to use the competency hearings for maintaining family secrets.

References

Applebaum, P. (2007). Assessment of patients' competence to consent to treatment. *New England Journal of Medicine, 357*(18), 1834–1840.

Deci, E. L. & Ryan, R. M. (2012). Self-determination theory in health care and its relations to motivational interviewing: A few comments. *The International Journal of Behavioral Nutrition and Physical Activity*, 9, 24. http://www.ijbnapa.org/content/9/1/24

Dixon *v.* Weinberger, 405 F. Supp. 974 (D. D. C. 1975).

National Mental Health Information Center. (2007). *Know your rights*. Center for Mental Health Service. Substance Abuse and Mental Health Services Administration. Retrieved March 8, 2007, from http://mentalhealth.Samhoa.gov

Omnibus Budget Reconciliation Act of 1990. Public Law No. 101–158, Paragraph 4206, 4751.

Tarasoff v. Regents of the University of California, 551P. 2d 334 (Cal. 1976).

U.S. Department of Health and Human Services. (2002). Standards for privacy of individually identifiable health information; final rule. *Federal Register, 65*, 53182–53273.

U.S. Equal Employment Opportunity Commission, Office of the Americans with Disabilities Act. (2013). *The Americans with Disabilities Act: Questions and answers*. Washington, DC: U.S. Government Printing Office. Retrieved from www.eeoc.gov.

Wettstein, R. (1994). Confidentiality. In J. Oldham & M. Riba (Eds.), *Review of psychiatry* (Vol. 13, pp. 343–364). Washington, DC: American Psychiatric Press.

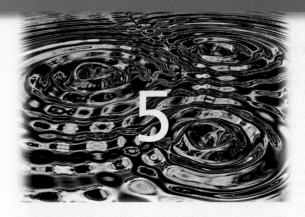

5

Mental Health Care in the Community

Peggy El-Mallakh

KEY CONCEPT

- continuum of care

LEARNING OBJECTIVES

After studying this chapter, you will be able to:

1. Define and explain the goals of the continuum of care in mental health services.

2. Identify the different mental health treatment settings and associated programs along the continuum of care.

3. Discuss the role of the psychiatric nurse at different points along the continuum of care.

4. Discuss the influence of managed care on mental health services and use of these services in the continuum of care.

5. Explain how the concept of the least restrictive environment influences the placement of patients in different mental health treatment settings.

6. Describe the nurse's role throughout the mental health continuum of care.

KEY TERMS

- assertive community treatment • board-and-care homes • case management • continuum of care • coordination of care • crisis intervention • crisis intervention teams • critical time intervention • e-mental health • in-home mental health care • intensive case management • intensive residential services • intensive outpatient program • outpatient detoxification • partial hospitalization • peer support • psychiatric rehabilitation programs • recovery centers • referral • reintegration • relapse • residential services • stabilization • therapeutic foster care • transfer • 23-hour observation

The evolution of a behavioral health care system is affected by scientific advances and social factors. Recovery from mental illness is a goal at all stages of treatment. The long-term nature of mental illnesses requires varying levels of care at different stages of the disorders as well as family and community support. Treatment costs are shared among public and private sectors. A demand exists for a comprehensive, holistic approach to care that encompasses all levels of need. Consumers, families, providers, advocacy groups, and third-party payers of mental health care no longer accept long-term institutionalization, once the hallmark of psychiatric care. Instead, they advocate for short-term treatment in an environment that promotes dignity and well-being while meeting the patient's biologic, psychological, and social needs.

Reimbursement issues have influenced health care. In the United States, health maintenance organizations

(HMOs), preferred provider organizations (PPOs), Medicaid, and Medicare have set limits on the types and lengths of treatment for which they provide reimbursement coverage, which in turn influences the kind of care the patient receives. In other countries, other regulatory bodies influence access and treatment options. Fragmentation of services is a constant threat. Today, psychiatric–mental health nurses face the challenge of providing mental health care within a complex system that is affected by financial constraints and narrowed treatment requirements.

DEFINING THE CONTINUUM OF CARE

An individual's needs for ongoing clinical treatment and care are matched with the intensity of professional health services. The continuum of care that supports recovery of mental health services can be viewed from various perspectives and ranges from intensive treatment (hospitalization) to supportive interventions (outpatient therapy).

> **KEYCONCEPT**   A **continuum of care** consists of an integrated system of settings, services, health care clinicians, and care levels, spanning illness-to-wellness states.

In a continuum, continuity of care is provided over an extended time. The appropriate medical, nursing, psychological, or social services may be delivered within one organization or across multiple organizations. The continuum facilitates the stability, continuity, and comprehensiveness of service to an individual and maximizes the coordination of care and services.

Least Restrictive Environment

The primary goal of the continuum of care is to provide treatment that allows patients to achieve the highest level of functioning in the least restrictive environment (see Chapter 4). In 1999, the U.S. Supreme Court reinforced the principle of least restrictive environment with the Olmstead decision, which states that it is a violation of the Americans with Disabilities Act to institutionalize people with severe mental illnesses when services in the community are equally effective (Seekins et al., 2011). Therefore, treatment is usually delivered in the community (as opposed to a hospital or institution) and, ideally, in an outpatient setting.

Coordination of Care

Coordination of care is the integration of appropriate services so that individualized care is provided. Appropriate services are those that are tailored to address a client's strengths and weaknesses, cultural context, service preferences, and recovery goals, including referral to community resources and liaisons with others (e.g., physician, health care organizations, community services). Several agencies could be involved, but when care is coordinated, a person's needs are met without duplication of services. Coordination of care requires collaborative and cooperative relationships among many services, including primary care, public health, mental health, social services, housing, education, and criminal justice, to name a few.

In some instances, a whole array of integrated services is needed. For example, children can benefit from treatment and specialized support at home and school. These wraparound services represent a unique set of community services and natural supports individualized for the child or adult and family to achieve a positive set of outcomes.

Case Management

Coordinated care is often accomplished through a **case management** service model in which a case manager locates services, links the patient with these services, and then monitors the patient's receipt of these services. This type of case management is referred to as the "broker" model. Case management can be provided by an individual or a team; it may include both face-to-face and telephone contact with the patient as well as contact with other service providers. **Intensive case management** is targeted for adults with serious mental illnesses and children with serious emotional disturbances. Managers of such cases have fewer caseloads and higher levels of professional training than do traditional case managers.

Case management is an integral part of mental health services and is organized around fundamental elements, including a comprehensive needs assessment, development of a plan of care to meet those needs, a method of ensuring the individual has access to care, and a method of monitoring the care provided. Case management services are most effective when a strong working alliance develops between the patient and the case manager (Kirk, Di Leo, Rehmer, Moy, & Davidson, 2013). The goal of case management is to help patients obtain access to high-quality and cost-effective mental health services (Tsai & Rosenheck, 2012). Quality is assessed by measuring patient outcomes that result from the services, such as symptom reduction, improved functioning and community integration, and patient satisfaction with the services provided (Howard, Rayens, El-Mallakh, & Clark, 2007). In addition, case managers can optimize a patient's use of resources by developing a treatment plan that closely matches the individual needs of the patient (Kirk et al., 2013) and by matching the most appropriate treatment to the patient's phase of illness.

The Nurse As Case Manager

Psychiatric nurses serve in various pivotal functions across the continuum of care. These functions can involve both direct care and coordination of the care delivered by others. The case manager role is one in which the nurse must have commanding knowledge and special training in individual and group psychotherapy, psychopharmacology, and psychosocial rehabilitation. The nurse must have expertise in psychopathology, treatment of the family as a unit, and up-to-date treatment modalities. Modalities include the therapeutic use of self, networking and social systems, crisis intervention, pharmacology, physical assessment, psychosocial and functional assessment, and psychiatric rehabilitation. The repertoire of required skills includes collaboration with members of a multidisciplinary team, teaching, management, leadership, group, and research skills. The nurse as case manager probably is the most diverse role within the psychiatric continuum.

MENTAL HEALTH SERVICES IN A CONTINUUM OF CARE

Crisis Care

An organized approach is required to treat individuals in crisis, including a mechanism for rapid access to care (within 24 hours), a referral for hospitalization, or access to outpatient services.

Crisis Intervention

Crisis intervention treatment—a specialized short-term, goal-directed therapy for those in acute distress—is brief, usually lasting fewer than 6 hours (see Chapter 20). This type of short-term care focuses on stabilization, symptom reduction, and prevention of relapse requiring inpatient services.

Crisis intervention units can be found in the emergency departments (EDs) of general and psychiatric hospitals and in crisis centers within community mental health centers. Patients in crisis demonstrate severe symptoms of acute mental illness, including labile mood swings, suicidal ideation, or self-injurious behaviors. Therefore, this treatment option commands a high degree of nursing expertise. Patients in crisis usually require medications such as anxiolytics or benzodiazepines for symptom management. Key nursing roles include assessment of short-term therapeutic interventions and medication administration. Nurses also facilitate referrals for admission to the hospital or for outpatient services.

Crisis intervention teams Behavioral problems caused by a person with acute symptoms of mental illnesses, such as schizophrenia or bipolar disorder, represent a crisis situation that can present a threat to the safety of the person and the people who live in their communities (Sands, Elsom, Gerdtz, & Khaw, 2012). Law enforcement personnel, such as police officers, are often the first responders when crises occur in the community. Police officers need to accurately assess and intervene in crisis situations and determine whether the people involved in the crisis are experiencing behavioral problems due to symptoms of mental illness. Crisis Intervention Teams (CIT) have been developed to train police officers to recognize and intervene in crisis situations in the community and determine whether emergency psychiatric services are needed. Crisis intervention by CIT-trained police officers can avoid inappropriate involvement of the patient in the criminal justice system and ensure that patients with behavioral problems due to mental illnesses receive appropriate psychiatric treatment (Canada, Angell, & Watson, 2012).

23-Hour Observation

The use of **23-hour observation** is a short-term treatment that serves the patient in immediate but short-term crisis. This type of care admits individuals to an inpatient setting for as long as 23 hours, during which time services are provided at a less-than-acute care level. The clinical problem usually is a transient disruption of baseline function, which will resolve quickly. Usually, the individual is experiencing suicidal or homicidal ideation, which presents a threat to him- or herself or others. The nurse's role in this treatment modality is assessment and monitoring. Medications also are usually administered. This treatment is used for acute trauma, such as rape and alcohol and narcotic detoxification, and for individuals with Axis II personality disorders who present with self-injurious behaviors.

Crisis Stabilization

When the immediate crisis does not resolve quickly, crisis **stabilization** is the next step. This type of care usually lasts fewer than 7 days and has a symptom-based indication for hospital admission. The primary purpose of stabilization is control of precipitating symptoms through medications, behavioral interventions, and coordination with other agencies for appropriate after-care. The major focus of nursing care in a short-term inpatient setting is symptom management. Ongoing assessment; short-term, focused interventions; and medication administration and monitoring of efficacy and side effects are major components of nursing care during stabilization. Nurses may also provide focused group psychotherapy designed to develop and strengthen the personal management strategies of patients. When treating aggressive or violent patients, the nurse monitors the appropriate use of seclusion and restraints. A physician or independent licensed practitioner is required to evaluate the patient within 1 hour after seclusion or restraints are initiated in a crisis stabilization setting (The Joint Commission, 2008).

Acute Inpatient Care

Acute inpatient hospitalization involves the most intensive treatment and is considered the most restrictive setting in the continuum. Inpatient treatment is reserved for acutely ill patients who, because of a mental illness, meet one or more of three criteria: high risk for harming themselves, high risk for harming others, or unable to care for their basic needs. Delivery of inpatient care can occur in a psychiatric hospital, psychiatric unit within a general hospital, or state-operated mental hospital.

Admission to inpatient environments can be voluntary or involuntary (see Chapter 4). The average length of stay for an involuntary admission ranges between 24 hours and several days, depending on the state or province laws; the length of stay for a voluntary admission depends on the acuity of symptoms and the patient's ability to pay the costs of treatment. It is unconstitutional in the United States to confine a nondangerous mentally ill person with an involuntary hospitalization when the patient can survive independently with the help of willing and responsible family or friends (Large, Nielssen, Ryan, & Hayes, 2008). Nevertheless, the interdisciplinary treatment team determines that the patient is no longer at risk to him- or herself or others before discharge can occur.

Both the number of available beds in psychiatric hospitals in the United States and length of inpatient stay have continually decreased since the 1980s, a trend attributed to managed care and expansion of multidisciplinary, intensive community-based services, such as assertive community treatment (ACT). Additional contributors to decreased length of stay include strict admission criteria and regulations that determine the need for continued hospitalization. Currently, admission to a hospital is determined based on medical necessity, such as dangerousness or the need for crisis stabilization. Patients are discharged when these criteria no longer apply, regardless of long-term social issues that the patient may be experiencing, such as homelessness, lack of family support, or low functioning (Sharfstein & Dickerson, 2009).

Critical Time Intervention

Many mental health consumers who receive treatment in inpatient settings are at risk for lack of engagement in outpatient treatment following discharge from the hospital, which can result in re-emergence of acute symptoms and rehospitalization (Kreyenbuhl, Nossel, & Dixon, 2009). The critical time intervention (CTI) was developed to help mental health consumers connect with outpatient care following discharge from inpatient treatment. The CTI creates a "bridge" between inpatient and outpatient treatment by coordinating care between staff in these settings. Effective care coordination is facilitated by communication about discharge plans, patient attendance at outpatient programs prior to discharge from the hospital, and family involvement in the discharge planning process (Dixon et al., 2009). CTI programs have been found to improve patient attendance at outpatient appointments (Dixon et al., 2009) and reduce homelessness following discharge from inpatient hospitalization (Herman, Conover, Gorroochurn, Hinterland, Hoepner, & Susser, 2011).

Partial Hospitalization

Partial hospitalization programs (PHPs) were developed to complement inpatient mental health care and outpatient services and provide treatment to patients with acute psychiatric symptoms who are experiencing a decline in social or occupational functioning, who cannot function autonomously on a daily basis, or who do not pose imminent danger to themselves or others. It is a time-limited, ambulatory, active treatment program that offers therapeutically intensive, coordinated, and structured clinical services within a stable milieu. The aim of PHPs is patient stabilization without hospitalization or reduced length of inpatient care. An alternative to inpatient treatment, PHP usually provides the resources to support therapeutic activities both for full-day and half-day programs. This level of care does not include overnight hospital care; however, the patient can be admitted for inpatient care within 24 hours.

In partial hospitalization, the interdisciplinary treatment team devises and executes a comprehensive plan of care encompassing behavioral therapy, social skills training, basic living skills training, education regarding illness and symptom identification and relapse prevention, community survival skills training, relaxation training, nutrition and exercise counseling, and other forms of expressive therapy. Group-based services such as wellness education and counseling for comorbid serious mental illnesses and substance abuse are also provided (Yanos, Vreeland, Minsky, Fuller, & Roe, 2009). Compared with other outpatient programs, PHPs offer more intensive nursing care.

Residential Services

Residential services provide a place for people to reside during a 24-hour period or any portion of the day on an ongoing basis. A residential facility can be publicly or privately owned. **Intensive residential services** are intensively staffed for patient treatment. These services may include medical, nursing, psychosocial, vocational, recreational, or other support services. Combining residential care and mental health services, this treatment form offers rehabilitation and therapy to people with serious and persistent mental illnesses, including chronic schizophrenia, bipolar disorder, and unrelenting depression. These services may provide short-term treatment for stays from 24 hours to 3 or 6 months or long-term treatment for several months to years.

As a result of deinstitutionalization, many patients who were unable to live independently were discharged from state hospitals to intermediate- or skilled-care nursing facilities. The use of nursing homes for residential care is controversial because many of these facilities lack mental health services. Residential care in nursing homes varies from state to state. If a facility serves a primarily geriatric population, placement of younger persons there can be problematic. If a facility with more than 16 beds is engaged primarily in providing diagnosis, treatment, or care of persons with mental disorders (including medical attention, nursing care, and related services), it is designated by the federal government as an institution for mental disease (IMD).

A Medicare-certified facility having more than 16 beds and at least 50% of residents with a mental disorder is also considered an IMD. An IMD does not qualify for matching federal Medicaid dollars, which mean that the state has principal responsibility for funding inpatient psychiatric services (Sharfstein & Dickerson, 2009).

Nursing plays an important role in the care of people who have severe and persistent mental illnesses and who require long-term stays at residential treatment facilities. Nurses provide basic psychiatric nursing care with a focus on psychoeducation, basic social skills training, aggression management, activities of daily living (ADLs) training, and group living. Education on symptom management, understanding mental illnesses, and medication is essential to recovery. The *Psychiatric-Mental Health Nursing: Scope and Standards of Practice* guide the nurse in delivering patient care (American Nurses Association, American Psychiatric Nurses Association, & International Society of Psychiatric-Mental Health Nurses, 2014) (see Chapter 6).

Respite Residential Care

Sometimes the family of a person with mental illness who lives at home may be unable to provide care continuously. In such cases, respite residential care can provide short-term necessary housing for the patient and periodic relief for the caregivers.

In-Home Mental Health Care

If at all possible, people with mental illnesses live at home, not in a residential treatment setting. The goals are choices, not placement; physical and social integration, not segregated and congregate grouping by disability; and individualized flexible services and support, not standardized levels of service. When a person can live at home but outpatient care does not meet the treatment needs, **in-home mental health care** may be provided. Home care emphasizes the personal autonomy of the patient and the need for a trusting, collaborative relationship between the nurse and the patient (Roldán-Merino, García, Ramos-Pichardo, Foix-Sanjuan, Quilez-Jover, Montserrat-Martinez, 2013). In this setting, direct patient care and case management skills are used to decrease hospital stays and increase the functionality of the patient within the home. Individuals who most benefit from in-home mental health care include patients with chronic, persistent mental illness or patients with mental illness and comorbid medical conditions that require ongoing monitoring.

In-home mental health care services rely on the skills of the mental health nurse in providing ongoing assessment and implementing a comprehensive, individualized treatment plan of care. Components of the care plan and the ongoing assessment include data on mental health status, the environment, medication compliance, family

dynamics and home safety, supportive psychotherapy, psychoeducation, coordination of services delivered by other home care staff, and communication of clinical issues to the patient's psychiatrist. In addition, the plan should address care related to collecting laboratory specimens (blood tests) and crisis intervention to reduce rehospitalization (Box 5.1).

Outpatient Care

Outpatient care is a level of care that occurs outside of a hospital or institution. Outpatient services usually are less intensive and are provided to patients who do not require inpatient, residential, or home care environments. Many patients enroll in outpatient services immediately upon discharge from an inpatient setting. Outpatient treatment can include ongoing medication management, skills training, supportive group therapy, substance abuse counseling, social support services, and case management (Johansson & Jansson, 2010). People with severe mental illnesses have high rates of comorbid medical illnesses (Howard, El-Mallakh, Rayens, & Clark, 2007), and many outpatient mental health clinics have developed integrated mental health–primary care treatment models to address the

---

BOX 5.1

Research for Best Practice: **Integrating Mental and Physical Health Care in a Community Setting**

Teachout, A., Kaiser, S. M., Wilkniss, S. M., & Moore, H. (2011). Paxton House: Integrating mental health and diabetes care for people with serious mental illnesses in a residential setting. Psychiatric Rehabilitation Journal, 34, 324–327.

THE QUESTION: This study asked whether a nurse-delivered diabetes care program would improve diabetes outcomes for people with serious mental illnesses and diabetes who live in a supported housing residence.

METHODS: Thirteen people with serious mental illnesses and diabetes participated in the program. All participants received comprehensive mental health and residential care. Clinical staff at Paxton House partnered with nurse practitioners to provide diabetes education, nutritional counseling, and exercise instruction. Clinical staff also helped program participants with healthy meal planning, shopping, and food preparation. Residents kept track of their exercise using pedometers and self-monitored daily blood glucose readings, weight, and pedometer readings.

RESULTS: All 13 participants lost weight from baseline. Weight loss averaged 20.35 pounds within 6 months of participation in the program. In addition, 40% of participants' fasting blood glucose levels were within the recommended range of 90–110 mg/dL after 6 months of participation in the program.

IMPLICATIONS: This research supports the effectiveness of a community-based program that integrates mental and physical health care for people with serious mental illnesses.

physical health needs of those with mental illnesses (Goodrich, Kilbouorne, Nord, & Bauer, 2013). These varying services promote community **reintegration** (return and acceptance of a person as a fully participating member of a community), symptom management, and optimal patient functioning. Outpatient services are provided by private practices, clinics, and community mental health centers.

Intensive Outpatient Programs

The primary focus of **intensive outpatient programs** is on stabilization and relapse prevention for highly vulnerable individuals who function autonomously on a daily basis. People who meet these criteria have returned to their previous lifestyles (e.g., interacting with family, resuming work, returning to school). Attendance in this type of program benefits individuals who still require frequent monitoring and support within a therapeutic milieu that enables them to remain connected to the community. The duration of treatment and level of services rendered are based on the patient's immediate needs. The treatment duration usually is time limited, with sessions offered 3 to 4 hours per day and 2 to 3 days per week. The treatment activities of the intensive outpatient program are similar to those offered in PHPs, but whereas PHPs emphasize social skills training, intensive outpatient programs teach patients about stress management, illness, medication, and relapse prevention.

Other Services Integrated into a Continuum of Care

Within the continuum of care, other outpatient services may be received separately or simultaneously within various settings. They involve discrete services and patient variables. Table 5.1 on page 42 defines the six levels of service variables along the continuum. Table 5.2 on page 43 outlines the patient variables.

Outpatient Detoxification

There is an increasing shift toward providing alcohol and drug detoxification in an outpatient setting. The decision to use **outpatient detoxification** depends on symptom severity and types of drugs the patient uses. Patients with alcohol dependence who show signs of tolerance and withdrawal can undergo detoxification in an outpatient setting. However, patients who undergo ambulatory detoxification must have reliable family members who are available to provide monitoring. Outpatient detoxification is not suitable for situations involving severe or complicated withdrawal, especially with delirium. In addition, patients who are pregnant or have a history of a seizure disorder are hospitalized for detoxification.

Outpatient detoxification is a specialized form of partial hospitalization for patients requiring medical supervision. During the initial withdrawal phase, use of a 23-hour bed may be a treatment option, depending on the stage of withdrawal and the type of addictive substance used. Or the patient may be required to attend a detoxification program 4 to 5 days per week until symptoms resolve. The length of participation depends on the severity of addiction.

Outpatient detoxification includes the 12-step recovery model, such as Alcoholics Anonymous (AA) and Narcotics Anonymous (NA), which provides outpatient involvement with professionals experienced in addiction counseling. It encourages abstinence and provides training in stress management and relapse prevention. Al-Anon and Alateen rely on 12-step support for families, who are usually included in the treatment program.

In-Home Detoxification

Detoxification from alcohol may be done in the home. For home detoxification to be safe and effective, symptoms of withdrawal must be mild, and a family member must be present at all times. The nurse is required to visit the patient daily for medication monitoring during the patient's first week of sobriety. Daily visits are necessary until the patient is in medically stable condition. Referrals may come from primary care physicians, court mandates, or employee assistance programs.

Assertive Community Treatment

The **assertive community treatment** (ACT) model is a multidisciplinary clinical team approach providing 24-hour, intensive community-based services. ACT typically includes low staff-to-patient ratios, but this may not be possible in rural areas with shortages of qualified mental health professionals and few services (Hilgeman et al., 2014). The ACT model helps individuals with serious mental illness live in the community (Young, Barrett, Engelhardt, & Moore, 2014). ACT provides a comprehensive range of treatment, rehabilitation, and supportive services to help patients meet the requirements of community living. Concentration of services for high-risk patients within a single multiservice team enhances continuity and coordination of care, which improves the quality of care. ACT reduces use of hospital and ED services, which reduces the cost of mental health treatment for patients with serious mental illnesses (Young et al., 2014). Initially, patients receive frequent direct assistance while reintegrating into the community. Emergency telephone numbers, or crisis numbers, are shared with patients and their families in the event that immediate assistance is needed. The ACT program is staffed 24 hours a day for emergency referral. Mobile treatment teams often are a part of the ACT model and provide assertive outreach,

Table 5.1	THE CONTINUUM OF AMBULATORY BEHAVIORAL HEALTH CARE SERVICES: SERVICE VARIABLES			
Service Variable	**Definition**	**Ambulatory Level One**	**Ambulatory Level Two**	**Ambulatory Level Three**
Service function	Specific patient care mission of the services	Crisis stabilization and acute symptoms reduction; serves as alternative to and prevention of hospitalization	Stabilization, symptom reduction, and prevention of relapse	Coordinated treatment for prevention of decline in functioning where outpatient services cannot adequately meet patient need
Scheduled programming	Planned hours of treatment	Minimum of 4 hours per day scheduled and intensive treatment over 4–7 days	Minimum of 3–4 hours per day, at least 2–3 days per week	A minimum of 4 hours per week
Crisis backup availability	Crisis intervention and emergency services or protective services during nontreatment hours	An organized and integrated system of 24-hour crisis backup with immediate access to current clinical and treatment information	A 24-hour crisis and consultation service	A 24-hour crisis and consultation service
Medical involvement	Degree of responsibility and participation assumed by medical and nursing personnel	Medical supervision	Medical consultation	Medical consultation available
Accessibility	Mechanisms by which new patient makes contact and is able to begin treatment; intake and admission procedures	Capable of admitting within 24 hours	Capable of admitting within 48 hours	Capable of admitting within 72 hours
Milieu	Cohesive, consistent, therapeutic environment	Preplanned, consistent and therapeutic; primarily within treatment setting	Active therapeutic within both treatment setting and home and community	Active therapeutic; primarily within home and community
Structure	Routines, scheduled activities, expectations, and special treatment procedures integral to non–hospital-based services	High degree of of structure and scheduling	Regularly scheduled, individualized	Individualized and coordinated
Responsibility and control	Role of treating professionals in providing a safety net for the patient	Staff aggressively monitors and supports patient and family	Monitoring and support shared with patient family and support system	Monitoring and support placed primarily with patient family and support system
Service examples		Partial hospitalization programs	Psychosocial rehabilitation	23-hour respite beds
		Day treatment programs	Intensive outpatient programs	Multi-modal outpatient services
		Intensive in-home crisis intervention	Behavioral aides	Aftercare
		Outpatient detoxification services	Assertive community treatment	Clubhouse programs
			23-hour observation beds	In-home services

From Kiser, L. J., Lefkovitz, P. M., Kennedy, L. L., & Knight, M. A. (2010). *Continuum of ambulatory behavioral health services: A position paper from the Association for Ambulatory Behavioral Healthcare.* Association for Ambulatory Behavioral Healthcare. Retrieved April 16, 2011, from www.aabh.org/content/continuum-ambulatory-behavioral-health-services.

crisis intervention, and independent-living assistance with linkage to necessary support services.

Recovery-Oriented Practice in Psychiatric Rehabilitation Settings

Psychiatric rehabilitation programs, also termed *psychosocial rehabilitation*, focus on the reintegration of people with psychiatric disabilities into the community through work, education, and social avenues while addressing their medical and residential needs. The goal is to empower patients to achieve the highest level of functioning possible. Therapeutic activities or interventions are provided individually or in groups. They may include development and maintenance of daily and community-living skills, such as communication (basic language), vocational,

Table 5.2	THE CONTINUUM OF AMBULATORY BEHAVIORAL HEALTH CARE SERVICES: PATIENT VARIABLES			
Patient Variable	Definition	Ambulatory Level One	Ambulatory Level Two	Ambulatory Level Three
Level of functioning	Ability to perform various tasks of daily living	Severe impairment in multiple areas of daily life	Marked impairment in at least one area of daily life	Moderate impairment in at least one area of daily life
Psychiatric signs and symptoms	Presenting problems and requisite assessment of suicidal, homicidal tendencies, thought processes, and orientation	Severe to disabling symptoms related to an acute condition or exacerbation of a severe or persistent disorder	Moderate to severe symptoms related to an acute condition or exacerbation of a severe or persistent disorder	Moderate symptoms related to an acute condition or exacerbation of a severe or persistent disorder
Risk or dangerousness	Degree of jeopardy present secondary to a psychiatric illnesses, including dangerousness to self and others, need for confinement, and potential for escalation of symptoms	Marked instability or dangerousness with a high risk of confinement	Moderate instability or dangerousness with some risk of confinement	Mild instability with limited dangerousness and low risk for confinement
Commitment to treatment or follow-through	Ability to comprehend and accomplish the tasks necessary to benefit from treatment at a specified level of care	Inability to form more than initial treatment contract requires close monitoring and support	Limited ability to form extended treatment contract requires frequent monitoring and support	Ability to sustain treatment contract with intermittent monitoring and support
Social support system	Ability to ask for, use, and accept assistance provided by family members or community supports	Impaired ability to access or use caretaker, family, or community support	Limited ability to form relationships or seek support	Ability to form and maintain relationships outside of treatment

From Kiser, L. J., Lefkovitz, P. M., Kennedy, L. L., & Knight, M. A. (2010). *Continuum of ambulatory behavioral health services: A position paper from the Association for Ambulatory Behavioral Healthcare*. Association for Ambulatory Behavioral Healthcare. Retrieved April 16, 2011, from www.aabh.org/content/continuum-ambulatory-behavioral-health-services.

self-care (grooming, bodily care, feeding), and social skills that help patients function in the community. These programs promote increased functioning with the least necessary ongoing professional intervention. Psychiatric rehabilitation provides a highly structured environment, similar to a PHP, in a variety of settings, such as office buildings, hospital outpatient units, and freestanding structures.

The mental health nurse's role continues to focus on the consumer's recovery goals in all treatment settings. As behavioral health care delivery occurs more in outpatient settings, so does the work of nurses. Most rehabilitation programs have a full-time nurse who functions as part of the multidisciplinary team.

Psychiatric–rehabilitation nurses are concerned with the recovery-oriented, holistic evaluation of the person and with assessing and educating the patient on compliance issues, necessary laboratory work, and environmental and lifestyle issues. This evaluation assesses the five dimensions of a person—physical, emotional, intellectual, social, and spiritual—and emphasizes recovery. Issues of psychotropic medication—evaluation of response, monitoring of side effects, and connection with pharmacy services—also fall to the nurse.

Recovery Centers

Recovery is an important goal for mental health consumers with serious mental illnesses because it emphasizes the importance of several factors that move a person from illness to wellness, such as self-direction, empowerment, a focus on strengths, peer support, respect, personal responsibility, and hope (see Chapter 2). Recovery outcomes most valued by mental health consumers include employment, education, stable housing, a social network, and participation in recreation (Whitley, Stickler, & Drake, 2012). Recovery centers assist in the mental health consumer's journey towards recovery by offering self-help groups and training in daily living. In addition, recovery centers offer illness self-management interventions, such as Wellness Recovery Action Planning (WRAP) (Wilson, Hutson, & Holston, 2013). The WRAP intervention helps consumers develop individualized plans for achieving symptom stabilization and improved quality of life (Cook et al., 2012). The recovery center also provides informal social support, in which mental health consumers experience peer acceptance in a nonstigmatizing environment.

Peer Support Services

Peer support services are provided by mental health consumers who have experienced symptom remission and are actively involved in their own recovery from mental illness. Peer support specialists typically work in outpatient settings, such as community mental health centers, therapeutic rehabilitation centers, and recovery centers. The peer support specialist works with other mental health consumers who are in the process of moving towards recovery goals. The relationship between peer specialists and mental health consumers offers an opportunity for offering mutual support for coping with mental illness and reciprocal sharing of personal experiences in the process of recovery (Grant, Reinhart, Wituk, & Meissen, 2012; Repper & Carter, 2011). Peer support specialists assist consumers with self-determination and personal responsibility for recovery. They can also teach mental health consumers effective self-management skills and self-advocacy, and encourage participation in wellness and recovery activities (Jonikas et al., 2013). Recipients of peer support services gain a sense of hope when they observe other mental health consumers who have successfully addressed the challenges of living with mental illness. In addition, mental health consumers who use peer support services have been shown to experience fewer psychiatric symptoms, increased involvement in work and education, and greater income compared to those who did not use peer services (Biegel, Pernice-Duca, Chang, & D'Angelo, 2013).

Self-Help Groups

Self-help groups are available in the community. These include AA, NA, and related 12-step programs. AA and NA use peer support as a strategy for helping people who are attempting to abstain from alcohol or drug use. Counseling, mentoring, and support are provided by individuals with alcohol or drug dependence who successfully abstain from substance use. In many cases, people with comorbid substance abuse and psychiatric diagnoses, such as schizophrenia and bipolar disorder, are unable to benefit from traditional AA self-help groups because of their psychiatric symptoms. People diagnosed with serious mental illnesses may have difficulty with feeling accepted and understood by nonmentally ill people in self-help groups, which can lead to high dropout rates (Rosenblum et al., 2014). For this reason, AA groups are available to meet the needs of individuals with comorbid psychiatric and substance abuse issues. Nurses may be asked to serve as consultants to these groups.

Relapse Prevention After-Care Programs

Relapse of mental illness symptoms and substance abuse is the major reason for rehospitalization in the United States. **Relapse** is the recurrence or marked increase in severity of the symptoms of a disease, especially after a period of apparent improvement or stability. Many issues affect a person's well-being. First and foremost, patients must believe that their lives are meaningful and worthwhile. Homelessness and unemployment create tremendous threats to a person's identity and feelings of wellness.

Much work has gone into relapse-prevention programs for the major mental illnesses and addiction disorders. Relapse prevention programs involve both patients and families and seek to (1) educate them about the illness, (2) enable them to cope with the chronic nature of the illness, (3) teach them to recognize early warning signs of relapse, (4) educate them about prescribed medications and the need for compliance, and (5) inform them about other disease management strategies (i.e., stress management, exercise) in preventing relapse.

Nurses become involved in relapse prevention programs in several different ways. They can act as referral sources for the programs, trainers or leaders of the programs, or after-care sources for patients when the programs are completed. In addition, mental health nurses can help patients and family members by promoting optimism, sticking to goals and aspirations, and focusing on individual strengths.

Supported Employment

The ability to work in a competitive job is important in recovery from severe mental illness (Baksheev, Allott, Jackson, McGorry, & Killackey, 2012). Supported employment services assist individuals to find work; assess individuals' skills, attitudes, behaviors, and interest relevant to work; offer vocational rehabilitation or other training; and provide work opportunities. Consumers receive onsite support and job-coaching services on a one-to-one basis. They occur in real work settings and are used for patients with severe mental illnesses. The primary focus is to maintain attachment between the mentally ill person and the work force.

Technology-Based Care

Access to mental health services is frequently inadequate in rural communities because of clinician shortages, lack of public transportation, and poverty. Rural communities are addressing barriers to care by creating alternative, technology-based ways to connect nurses with their patients. Telephone contact with patients after discharge from the hospital allows nurses to assess psychiatric symptoms, check on medication adherence, discuss approaches to solving problems associated with community living, and provide emotional support (Pratt et al., 2013). Patients who receive telephone contacts from nurses after discharge are more comfortable talking on the phone if the nurse meets with the patient before discharge to establish rapport. Telemedicine uses video teleconferencing equipment to link health care professionals with patients in remote rural areas. Providers of specialty psychiatric services in university settings can use telemedicine to conduct psychiatric assessments, diagnose, provide education, and consult with local providers in the care of community-based patients who need special individualized care (Hilty, Ferrer, Parish, Johnston, Callahan, & Yellowlees, 2013).

E-Mental Health

The use of electronics and the Internet is a defining feature of contemporary life in the United States. Internet users can instantaneously gain access to web-based resources for health and wellness, including mental health. E-mental health is a convenient, flexible, and cost-effective community-based resource that can communicate information about mental illnesses, facilitate self-help, reduce the stigma of seeking mental health care, and provide a forum for social support (van der Kriek, Wunderink, Emerencia, de Jonge, & Sytema, 2014). In addition, e-mental health interventions have been developed for people diagnosed with psychotic disorders; these interventions focus on self-monitoring and management of illness, medications, lifestyle, and daily living activities (van der Kriek et al., 2014). E-mental health services can be delivered in a variety of locations, such as schools, places of employment, and clinics (Lal & Adair, 2014).

Although the use of e-mental health applications is increasing, concerns have been expressed about using the Internet for the delivery of mental health care. Difficulties may occur in developing a therapeutic patient–provider relationship via the Internet. There are concerns about the ability to ensure the quality of online mental health interventions. Online treatment of certain diagnoses, such as those with severe depression, can be challenging if a depressed patient in a virtual community experiences a suicidal crisis that requires a practitioner to intervene quickly. Patient privacy and confidentiality may be compromised in a web-based e-mental health application. In addition, the Internet is often not available to subpopulations of patients with chronic and severe mental illnesses who require high-intensity services, such as those diagnosed with schizophrenia. However, the use of e-mental health applications will likely grow in the future, and psychiatric nurses are encouraged to participate in the development of high-quality e-mental health services for people diagnosed with psychiatric disorders.

Alternative Housing Arrangements

Housing is an important factor in successful community transition. Patients with psychiatric disabilities who are homeless are a vulnerable population. More than 40% of people who are homeless have a serious mental illness, which increases their risk for substance abuse, inability to access health care, assaults, incarceration, and physical health problems (National Alliance to End Homelessness, 2014). Therefore, one of the largest hurdles to overcome in treating the severely mentally ill patient is finding

appropriate housing that will meet the patient's immediate social, financial, and safety needs. Caring for people with severe mental illnesses in the home can be very stressful for family members because of the person's symptom severity and unpredictable behaviors. Many individuals with a mental illness live in some form of supervised or supported community living situation, which ranges from highly supervised congregate settings to independent apartments (Tsemberis, Kent, & Respress, 2012). The following discussion focuses on four models of alternative housing and the role of the nurse. These include personal care homes, board-and-care homes, therapeutic foster care, and supervised apartments.

Personal Care Homes

Personal care homes operate within houses in the community. Usually, six to 10 people live in one house with a health care attendant providing 24-hour supervision to assist with medication monitoring or other minor activities, including transportation to appointments, meals, and self-care skills. The clientele generally are heterogeneous and include older adults, people with mild mental retardation, and patients with chronic and subacute mental illness. Most states require these homes to be licensed.

Board-and-Care Homes

Board-and-care homes provide 24-hour supervision and assistance with medications, meals, and some self-care skills. Individualized attention to self-care skills and other ADLs generally is not available. These homes are licensed to house 50 to 150 people in one location. Rooms are shared, with two to four occupants per bedroom.

Therapeutic Foster Care

Therapeutic foster care is indicated for patients in need of a family-like environment and a high level of support. Therapeutic foster care is available for child, adolescent, and adult populations. This level of care actually places patients in residences of families specially trained to handle individuals with mental illnesses. The training usually consists of crisis management, medication education, and illness education. The family provides supervision, structure, and support for the individual living with them. The person who receives these services shares the responsibility of completing household chores and may be required to attend an outpatient program during the day.

Supervised Apartments

In a supervised apartment setting, individuals live in their own apartments, usually alone or with one roommate, and are responsible for all household chores and self-care. A staff member or "supervisor" stops by each apartment routinely to evaluate how well the patients are doing, make sure they are taking their medications, and ensure that the household is being maintained. The supervisor may also be required to mediate disagreements between roommates.

Role of Nurses in Alternative Housing

Professional registered nurses typically are not employed in alternative housing settings. However, nurses play a pivotal role in the successful reintegration of patients from more restrictive inpatient settings into society. Nurses are employed in PHPs and inpatient units and as case managers. Therefore, nurses act as liaisons for the residential placement of patients. Nurses are employed directly as consultants or provide consultation to treatment teams during discharge planning in determining appropriate outpatient settings, evaluating medication follow-up needs, and making recommendations for necessary medical care for existing physical conditions. Feedback from the residential care providers and follow-up by the treatment team regarding the patient's response to treatment interventions are essential. Rehospitalization

can be curtailed if the residential care operators identify and forward specific problems to the treatment teams. Patient interventions can be modified in an outpatient setting.

INTEGRATED PRIMARY CARE AND MENTAL HEALTH

The concept of managed care emerged in efforts to coordinate patient care efficiently and cost effectively. **Managed care organizations** provide services through HMOs or PPOs. Purchasers of health care, such as employers and government health agencies, contract with managed care organizations to provide mental health services. Traditionally, these services were separated from general medical care packages and reimbursed differently than other health care services. With the passage of the *Affordable Care Act* (see Chapter 1), the mental health services are supposed to be reimbursed at the same level as other health care problems. The recent trend is integration of many mental health services within a primary care setting. The goals of this approach to care are to increase access to care and to provide the most appropriate level of services in the least restrictive setting. Efforts focus on providing more outpatient and alternative treatment programs and avoiding costly inpatient hospitalizations. When properly conducted and administered, an integrated primary care allows patients better access to quality services while using health care dollars wisely. However, many primary care practices do not yet provide integrated services (Auxier, Miller & Rogers, 2013).

Today, managed behavioral health care has succeeded in standardizing admissions criteria, reducing length of patient stay, and directing patients to the proper level of care—inpatient and outpatient—all while attempting to control the costs. Across the continuum of care, nurses encounter integrated or collaborative organizations, and they must be familiar with the policies, procedures, and clinical criteria established by managed care organizations. As the delivery of mental health care, services become more integrated into primary care, and growing numbers of patients with mental illnesses reach older age, increasing demands are placed on the health and mental health care systems to accommodate the needs of this population. Rates of comorbid medical illnesses are high in older adults with severe mental illnesses, and the need is great for services that provide adequate psychiatric and medical care for this population, ideally in the same treatment setting (Auxier et al., 2012). Many older adults with mental illness currently receive no community services other than medication monitoring. Increasing home health care services for people with mental illness is an important alternative to institutionalization.

The Nurse's Role in Negotiating the Mental Health Delivery Systems

Because of shorter inpatient stays, inpatient psychiatric–mental health nurses maximize the short time they have by educating patients about their illness, available community resources, and medications to minimize the potential for relapse. These nurses focus on teaching social skills and self-reliance and creating empowering environments that in turn build self-confidence and help the patient move towards recovery.

The interface of psychiatric–mental health nurses with other nurses in managed care organizations and integrated primary care systems is primarily in the form of communicating the progress of individual patients to the nurses (mental health and nonmental health) and other health care workers who maintain a long-term relationship with the patient and family.

Public and Private Collaboration

Today, there are many public–private sector collaborations. The need for public–private collaboration prompted the National Association of State Mental Health Program Directors (NASMHPD), an organization representing the 55 state and territorial public mental health systems, and the American Managed Behavioral Healthcare Association (AMBHA), an organization representing private managed behavioral health care firms, to work. Nurses can expect to see more strategic alliances and joint ventures between the public and private sectors.

NURSING PRACTICE IN THE CONTINUUM OF CARE

Throughout this chapter, nurses' roles in different settings have been explained. Regardless of the situation or setting, nurses conduct assessments at the point of first patient contact. The individual's needs are then matched with the most appropriate setting, service, or program that will meet those needs. If a patient is admitted for services, the nurse also begins discharge planning upon first admission.

Assessment and Identification of Services

Choosing the level of care begins with an initial assessment to determine the need for care, the type of care to be provided, and the need for additional assessment. The nurse must discuss with the patient suicidal and homicidal thoughts. Nurses also need to consider financial issues because funding considerations may play a part in placement options. Other factors affecting the selection of care include the type of treatment the individual seeks, his or her current physical condition and ability to consent to treatment, and the organization's ability to provide direct care or to deflect care to another service provider.

Based on the results of the initial assessment, the nurse may admit the patient into services provided at that agency or initiate a referral or transfer to provide the intensity and scope of treatment required by the individual at that point in time (Figure 5.1). **Referral** involves sending an individual from one clinician to another or from one service setting to another for care or consultation. **Transfer** involves formally shifting responsibility for the care of an individual from one clinician to another or from one care unit to another. The processes of referral and transfer to other levels of care are integral for effective use of services along the continuum. These processes are based on the individual's assessed needs and the organization's capability to provide the care. Figure 5.1 depicts the process of assessment, treatment, transfer, and referral when considering appropriate levels of care.

Discharge Planning

Discharge planning begins upon admission of the individual to any level of health care. Most facilities have a written procedure for discharge planning. This procedure often provides for a transfer of clinical care information when a person is referred, transferred, or discharged to another facility or level of care. All discharge planning activities should be documented in the clinical record, including the patient's response to proposed after-care treatment, follow-up for psychiatric and physical health problems, and discharge instructions. Medication education, food–drug interactions, drug–drug interactions, and special diet instructions (if applicable) are extremely important in ensuring patient safety. Discharge planning is an integral part of psychiatric nursing care and should be considered a part of the psychiatric rehabilitation process. In addressing an individual's needs, one can coordinate after-care and discharge interventions for optimal outcomes. The overall goal of discharge planning is to provide the patient with all of the resources he or she needs to function as independently as possible in the least restrictive environment and to avoid rehospitalization.

The nurse can optimize discharge plan compliance by partnering with the patient from the first encounter. Because patients with mental illnesses may have limited cognitive abilities and residual motivational and anxiety problems, the nurse should explain in detail all after-care plans and instructions to the patient. It is helpful also to schedule all after-care appointments before the patient leaves the facility. The nurse should then give the patient written instructions about where and when to go for the appointment and a contact person's name and telephone number at the after-care placement. Finally, the nurse should review emergency telephone numbers and contacts and medication instructions with the patient.

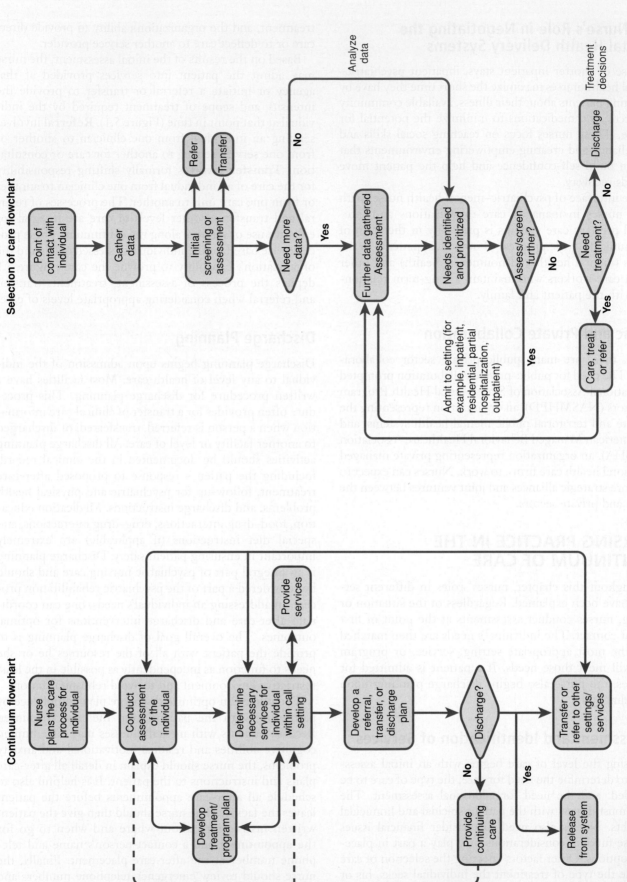

FIGURE 5.1 Flowcharts illustrating nursing care in the mental health care continuum and selection of care.

Selection of care flowchart

Point of contact with individual → Gather data → Initial screening or assessment → Need more data?

Need more data? → Yes → Further data gathered Assessment

Initial screening or assessment → Refer / Transfer

Need more data? → No → Analyze data

Further data gathered Assessment → Needs identified and prioritized → Assess/screen further?

Assess/screen further? → Yes → Admit to setting (for example, inpatient, residential, partial hospitalization, outpatient)

Assess/screen further? → No → Need treatment?

Need treatment? → Yes → Care, treat, or refer

Need treatment? → No → Discharge → Treatment decisions

Continuum flowchart

Nurse plans the care process for individual → Conduct assessment of the individual → Determine necessary services for individual within call setting → Develop a referral, transfer, or discharge plan → Discharge?

Conduct assessment of the individual → Develop treatment/program plan

Determine necessary services for individual within call setting → Provide services

Discharge? → No → Provide continuing care

Discharge? → Yes → Release from system

Transfer or refer to other settings/services

SUMMARY OF KEY POINTS

■ The continuum of care is a comprehensive system of services and programs designed to match the needs of the individual with the appropriate treatment in settings that vary according to levels of service, structure, and intensity of care.

■ Psychiatric–mental health nurses' specific responsibilities vary according to the setting. In most settings, nurses function as members of a multidisciplinary team and assume responsibility for assessment and selection of level of care, education, evaluation of response to treatment, referral or transfer to a more appropriate level of care, and discharge planning. Discharge planning provides patients with all the resources they need to function effectively in the community and avoid rehospitalization.

■ Mental health care can be given within an integrated primary care setting or a separate system. The nurse's role will vary depending upon the setting and the needs of the patient.

CRITICAL THINKING CHALLENGES

1. Define the continuum of care in mental health care and discuss the importance of the least restrictive environment.

2. Differentiate the role of the nurse in each of the following continuum settings:
   a. Crisis stabilization
   b. In-home detoxification
   c. Partial hospitalization
   d. Assertive community treatment

3. Compare alternative housing arrangements, including personal care homes, board-and-care homes, therapeutic foster care, and supervised apartments.

4. Envision using more than one service at a time. What combinations of services could benefit patients and families?

5. Identify the specific community mental health service needs of patients across the lifespan. Include the unique needs of children, adolescents, adults, and older patients. How do community mental health services meet these needs?

References

American Nurses Association, American Psychiatric Nurses Association. (2014). *Psychiatric-mental health nursing: scope and standards of practice, 2nd edition.* Silver Spring, MD: Nursesbooks.org.

Auxier, A., Miller, B. F., & Rogers, J. (2013). Integrated behavioral health and the patient-centered medical home. In: M. R. Talen & A.B. Valeras (eds.). *Integrated behavioral health in primary care.* Pg. 33–52. New York: Springer.

Auxier, A., Runyan, C., Mullin, D., Mendenhall, T., Young, J., & Kessler, R. (2012). Behavioral health referrals and treatment initiation rates in integrated primary care: A collaborative care research network study. *Translational Behavioral Medicine, 2*(3), 337–344.

Baksheev, G. N., Allot, K., Jackson, H. J., McGorry, P. D. & Killackey, E. (2012). Predictors of vocational recovery among young people with first-episode psychosis: Findings from a randomized controlled trial. *Psychiatric Rehabilitation Journal, 35*(6), 421–427.

Biegel, D. E., Pernice-Duca, F., Chang, C. W., & D'Angelo. (2013). Correlates of peer support in a clubhouse setting. *Community Mental Health Journal, 49,* 249–259.

Canada, K. E., Angell, B., & Watson, A. C. (2012). Intervening at the entry point: Differences in how CIT trained and non-CIT trained officers describe responding to mental health-related calls. *Community Mental Health Journal, 48,* 746–755.

Cook, J. A., Copeland, M. E., Jonikas, J. A., Hamilton, M. M., Razzano, L. A., Grey, D. D, et al. (2012). Results of a randomized controlled trial of mental illness self-management using Wellness Recovery Action Planning. *Schizophrenia Bulletin, 38,* 881–891.

Dixon, L. 1., Goldberg, R., Iannone, V., Lucksted, A., Brown, C., Kreyenbuhl, J., et al. (2009). Use of a critical time intervention to promote continuity of care after psychiatric inpatient hospitalization. *Psychiatric Services, 60,* 451–458.

Goodrich, D. E., Kilbourne, A. M., Nord, K. M., & Bauer, M. S. (2013). Mental health collaborative care and its role in primary care settings. *Current Psychiatry Reports, 15*(8), 383. doi: 10.1007/s11920-013-0383-2

Grant, E. A., Reinhart, C., Wituk, S., & Meissen, G. (2012). An examination of the integration of certified peer specialists into community mental health centers. *Community Mental Health Journal, 48,* 477–481.

Herman, D. B., Conover, S., Gorroochurn, P., Hinterland, K., Hoepner, L., & Susser, E. S. (2011). Randomized trial of critical time intervention to prevent homelessness after hospital discharge. *Psychiatric Services, 62,* 713–719.

Hilgeman, M. M., Mahaney-Price, A. F., Stanton, M. P., McNeal, S. F., Pettey, K. M., Tabb, K. D., et al. (2014). AlabamaVeterans Rural Health Initiative: A pilot study of enhanced community outreach in rural areas. *The Journal of Rural Health, 30*(2), 153–163. doi:10.1111/jrh.12054.

Hilty, D. M., Ferrer, D. C., Parish, M. B., Johnston, B., Callahan, E. J., & Yellowlees, P. M. (2013). The effectiveness of telemental health: A 2013 review. *Telemedicine Journal and E-Health, 19*(6), 444–454.

Howard, P. B., El-Mallakh, P., Rayens, M. K., & Clark, J. J. (2007). Comorbid medical illnesses and perceived general health among adult recipients of Medicaid mental health services. *Issues in Mental Health Nursing, 28,* 255–274.

Howard, P. B., Rayens, M. K., El-Mallakh, P. & Clark, J.J. (2007). Predictors of satisfaction among adult recipients of Medicaid mental health services. *Archives of Psychiatric Nursing, 21*(5), 257–269.

Johansson, H. & Jansson, J. A. (2010). Therapeutic alliance and outcome in routine psychiatric out-patient treatment: Patient factors and outcome. *Psychology and Psychotherapy, 83*(2), 193–206.

Jonikas, J. A., Grey, D. D., Copeland, M. E., Razzano, L. A., Hamilton, M. M., Floyd, C. B., et al. (2013). Improving propensity for patient self-advocacy through wellness recovery action planning: Results of a randomized controlled trial. *Community Mental Health Journal, 49,* 260–269.

Kirk, T. A., Di Leo, P., Rehmer, P., Moy, S. & Davidson, L. (2013). A case and care management program to reduce use of acute care by clients with substance use disorders. *Psychiatric Services, 64*(5), 491–493.

Kreyenbuhl, J., Nossel, I. R., & Dixon, L. B. (2009). Disengagement from mental health treatment among individuals with schizophrenia and strategies for facilitating connections to care: A review of the literature. *Schizophrenia Bulletin, 35,* 696–703.

Lal, S. & Adair, C. E. (2014). E-mental health: A rapid review of the literature. *Psychiatric Services, 65*(1), 24–32. doi:10.1176/appi.ps.201300009

Large, M. M., Nielssen, O., Ryan, C. J., & Hayes, R. (2008). Mental health laws that require dangerousness for involuntary admission may delay the initial treatment of schizophrenia. *Social Psychiatry and Psychiatric Epidemiology, 43*(3), 251–256.

National Alliance to End Homelessness. (2014). Issues: Health care. Retrieved June 20, 2014, from *http://www.endhomelessness.org/pages/mental_physical_health.*

Pratt, S. I., Bartels, S. J., Mueser, K. T., Naslund, J. A., Wolfe, R., Pixley, J. S., et al. (2013). Feasibility and effectiveness of an automated telehealth intervention to improve illness self-management in people with serious psychiatric and medical disorders. *Psychiatric Rehabilitation Journal, 36*(4), 297–305.

Repper, J. & Carter, T. (2011). A review of the literature on peer support in mental health services. *Journal of Mental Health, 20*, 392–411.

Roldán-Merino, J., García, I. C., Ramos-Pichardo, J. D., Foix-Sanjuan, A., Quílez-Jover, J., Montserrat-Martinez, M. (2013). Impact of personalized in-home nursing care plans on dependence in ADLs/IADLs and on family burden among adults diagnosed with schizophrenia: A randomized controlled study. *Perspectives in Psychiatric Care, 49*(3), 171–178.

Rosenblum, A., Matusow, H., Fong, C., Vogel, H., Uttaro, T., Moore, T. L., et al. (2014). Efficacy of dual focus mutual aid for persons with mental illness and substance misuse. *Drug and Alcohol Dependence, 135*, 78–87. doi:10.1016/j.drugalcdep.2013.11.012

Sands, N., Elsom, S., Gerdtz, M., & Khaw, D. (2012). Mental health-related risk factors for violence: Using the evidence to guide mental health triage decision making. *Journal of Psychiatric and Mental Health Nursing, 19*(8), 690–701.

Seekins, T., Ravesloot, C., Katz, M., Liston, B, Oxford, M., Altom, B., et al. (2011). Nursing home emancipation: A preliminary study of efforts by centers for independent living in urban and rural areas. *Disability and Health Journal, 4*(4), 245–253.

Sharfstein, S. S., & Dickerson, F. B. (2009). Hospital psychiatry for the 21st century. *Health Affairs, 28*(3), 685–688.

The Joint Commission. (2008). *Provision of care, treatment and services: Restraint and seclusion.* Retrieved May 25, 2009, from http://www.jointcommission.org/AccreditationPrograms/BehavioralHealthCare/Standards/09_FAQs/PC/Restraint+_Seclusion.htm.

Tsai, J. & Rosenheck, R. A. (2012). Outcomes of a group intensive peer-support model of case management for support housing. *Psychiatric Services, 63*(12), 1186–1194.

Teachout, A, Kaiser, S. M., Wilkniss, S. M., & Moore, H. (2011). Paxton House: Integrating mental health and diabetes care for people with serious mental illnesses in a residential setting. *Psychiatric Rehabilitation Journal, 34*, 324–327.

Tsemberis, S., Kent, D. & Respress, C. (2012). Housing stability and recovery among chronically homeless persons with co-occuring disorders in Washington, DC. *American Journal of Public Health, 102*(1), 13–16.

van der Krieke L., Wunderink L., Emerencia A. C., de Jonge P., & Sytema S. (2014). E-mental health self-management for psychotic disorders: State of the art and future perspectives. *Psychiatric Services, 65*(1), 33–49. doi:10.1176/appi.ps.201300050

Whitley, R., Strickler, D., & Drake, R. E. (2012). Recovery centers for people with severe mental illness: A survey of programs. *Community Mental Health Journal, 48*, 547–556.

Wilson, J. M., Hutson, S. P., & Holston, E. C. (2013). Participant satisfaction with Wellness Recovery Action Plan (WRAP). *Issues in Mental Health Nursing, 34*(12), 846–854.

Yanos, P. T., Vreeland, B., Minsky, S., Fuller, R. B., & Roe, D. (2009). Partial hospitalization: Compatible with evidence-based and recovery-oriented treatment? *Journal of Psychosocial Nursing and Mental Health Services, 47*(2), 41–47.

Young, M. S., Barrett, B., Engelhardt, M. A., & Moore, K. A. (2014). Six-month outcomes of an integrated assertive community treatment team serving adults with complex behavioral health and housing needs. *Community Mental Health Journal, 50*(4), 474–479. doi:10.1007/s10597-013-9692-5

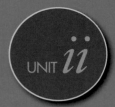
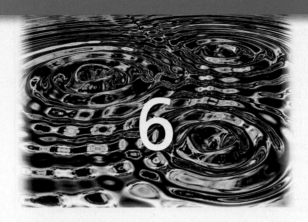

6

Ethics, Standards, and Nursing Frameworks

Mary Ann Boyd

KEY CONCEPTS

- autonomy
- beneficence
- biopsychosocial framework
- standardized nursing language

LEARNING OBJECTIVES

After studying this chapter, you will be able to:

1. Identify ethical frameworks used in psychiatric nursing practice.

2. Delineate the scope and standards of psychiatric–mental health nursing practice.

3. Discuss the impact of psychiatric–mental health nursing professional organizations on practice.

4. Integrate the biopsychosocial framework within the wellness and recovery models.

5. Discuss the basic tools of psychiatric nursing.

6. Discuss selected challenges of psychiatric–mental health nursing.

KEY TERMS

- advanced practice psychiatric–mental health registered nurse • clinical reasoning • fidelity • justice
- nonmaleficence • nursing process • paternalism • psychiatric–mental health registered nurse • reflection
- scope and standards of practice • veracity

This chapter opens with a discussion of the ethical concepts psychiatric nurses use on a daily basis. Integral to the understanding of the day-to-day practice of psychiatric–mental health nursing, the scope and standards of practice are then highlighted. This chapter integrates the biopsychosocial framework into the recovery and wellness models. The discussion of the challenges of psychiatric nursing sets the stage for the rest of the text through an overview of the dynamic nature of this specialty.

ETHICS OF PSYCHIATRIC NURSING

Psychiatric–mental health nursing actions are guided by the *Guide to the Code of Ethics for Nurses* (Box 6.1) (Fowler, 2008). The *Code* serves to inform both nurses and society of the profession's ethical expectations and requirements and provides a framework within which nurses can make ethical decisions. Psychiatric nurses face ethical problematic situations daily. To determine

---

BOX 6.1

Code of Ethics for Nurses

1. The nurse, in all professional relationships, practices with compassion and respect for the inherent dignity, worth, and uniqueness of every individual, unrestricted by considerations of social or economic status, personal attributes, or the nature of health problems.
2. The nurse's primary commitment is to the patient, whether an individual, family, group, or community.
3. The nurse promotes, advocates for, and strives to protect the health, safety, and rights of the patients.
4. The nurse is responsible and accountable for individual nursing practice and determines the appropriate delegation of tasks consistent with the nurse's obligation to provide optimum patient care.
5. The nurse owes the same duties to self as to others, including the responsibility to preserve integrity and safety, to maintain competence, and to continue personal and professional growth.
6. The nurse participates in establishing, maintaining, and improving health care environments and conditions of employment conducive to the provision of quality health care and consistent with the values of the profession through individual and collective action.
7. The nurse participates in the advancement of the profession through contributions to practice, education, administration, and knowledge development.
8. The nurse collaborates with other health professionals and the public in promoting community, national, and international efforts to meet health needs.
9. The profession of nursing, as represented by associations and their members, is responsible for articulation of nursing values, for maintaining the integrity of the profession and its practice, and for shaping social policy.

---

the best ethical action, the nurse can reflect on a series of questions, outlined in Box 6.2.

Autonomy and beneficence are fundamental ethical concepts.

> **KEYCONCEPTS** According to the principle of **autonomy,** each person has the fundamental right of self-determination. According to the principle of **beneficence,** the health care provider uses knowledge of science and incorporates the art of caring to develop an environment in which individuals achieve their maximal health care potential.

These principles can conflict when the patient is being guided by the principle of autonomy and the nurse by the

---

BOX 6.2

Basic Questions for Ethical Decision Making

- What do I know about this patient situation?
- What do I know about the patient's values and moral preferences?
- What assumptions as I making that need more data to clarify?
- What are my own feelings (and values) about the situation, and how might they be influencing how I view and respond to this situation?
- Are my own values in conflict with those of the patient?
- What else do I need to know about this case, and where can I obtain this information?
- What can I never know about this case?
- Given my primary obligation to the patient, what should I do to be ethical?

---

principle of beneficence. For example, a patient wants to stop taking medication (autonomy), and the nurse urges the patient to continue (beneficence).

> **NCLEXNOTE** Be prepared to think in terms of patient scenarios that depict the principles of beneficence versus autonomy and identify differences between views of the patient and nurse.

Other ethical principles that guide mental health care include justice, nonmaleficence, paternalism, veracity, and fidelity. **Justice** is the duty to treat all fairly, distributing the risks and benefits equally. Justice becomes an issue in mental health when a segment of a population does not have access to health care. Basic goods should be distributed, so that the least advantaged members of society are benefited. **Nonmaleficence** is the duty to cause no harm, both individual and for all. **Paternalism** is the belief that knowledge and education authorize professionals to make decisions for the good of the patient. Mandatory use of seat belts and motorcycle helmets is an example of paternalism. This principle can be in direct conflict with the mental health recovery belief of self-determinism (see Chapter 2). **Veracity** is the duty to tell the truth. This is easier said than done. Patients may ask questions when the truth is unknown. For example, if I take my medication, will the voices go away? **Fidelity** is faithfulness to obligations and duties. It is keeping promises. Fidelity is important in establishing trusting relationships.

> **NCLEXNOTE** Tracking ethical decisions that the psychiatric nurse encounters in the inpatient versus outpatient setting may be a topic for examination.

SCOPE AND STANDARDS OF PRACTICE

The practice of psychiatric nursing is regulated by law but guided by **scope and standards of practice**. The legal authority to practice nursing is granted by the states and provinces, but scope and standards of practice are defined by the profession of nursing. The ANA and the psychiatric nursing organizations (discussed later in this chapter) collaborate in defining the boundaries of psychiatric-mental health nursing and informing society about the parameters of practice. The standards are authoritative statements that describe the responsibilities for which the practitioners are accountable.

Scope of Psychiatric–Mental Health Nursing Areas of Concern

The areas of concern for the psychiatric–mental health nurse include a wide range of actual and potential mental health problems or psychiatric disorders, such as emotional stress or crisis, self-concept changes, developmental issues, physical symptoms that occur with psychological changes, and symptom management of patients with mental disorders. To understand the problem and select an appropriate intervention, integration of knowledge from the biologic, psychological, and social domains is necessary. Refer to Chapter 1, Box 1.1, for details on the actual and potential mental health problems of patients to whom psychiatric nurses attend.

Standards of Practice

Six standards of practice are organized according to the nursing process and include: assessment, diagnosis, outcome identification, planning, implementation, and evaluation (Box 6.3). The **nursing process** serves as the foundation for clinical decision making and provides a framework for nursing practice.

Each of these six standards includes competencies for which **Psychiatric-Mental Health Registered Nurse (PMH-RN)** and **Advanced Practice Psychiatric-Mental Health Registered Nurses (PMH-APRN)** are accountable. The fifth standard, implementation, has several subcategories that define standards for specific interventions. These standards of practice define the parameters of psychiatric-mental health nursing practice.

BOX 6.3

Standards of Practice

STANDARD 1. ASSESSMENT
The PMH registered nurse collects and synthesizes comprehensive health data that are pertinent to the healthcare consumer's health and/or situation.

STANDARD 2. DIAGNOSIS
The PMH registered nurse analyzes the assessment data to determine diagnoses, problems, and areas of focus for care and treatment, including level of risk.

STANDARD 3. OUTCOMES IDENTIFICATION
The PMH registered nurse identifies expected outcomes and the healthcare consumer's goals for a plan individualized to the healthcare consumer or to the situation.

STANDARD 4. PLANNING
The PMH registered nurse develops a plan that prescribes strategies and alternatives to assist the healthcare consumer in attainment of expected outcomes.

STANDARD 5. IMPLEMENTATION
The PMH registered nurse implements the specified plan.

Standard 5A Coordination of Care
The PMH registered nurse coordinates care delivery.

Standard 5B Health Teaching and Health Promotion
The PMH registered nurse employs strategies to promote health and a safe environment.

Standard 5C Consultation
The PMH advanced practice registered nurse provides consultation to influence the identified plan, enhance the abilities of other clinicians to provide services for healthcare consumers, and effect change.

Standard 5D Prescriptive Authority and Treatment
The PMH advanced practice registered nurse uses prescriptive authority, procedures, referrals, treatments, and therapies in accordance with state and federal laws and regulations.

Standard 5E Pharmacological, Biological, and Integrative Therapies
The PMH advanced practice registered nurse incorporates knowledge of pharmacological, biological, and complementary interventions with applied clinical skills to restore the healthcare consumer's health and prevent further disability.

Standard 5F Milieu Therapy
The PMH advanced practice registered nurse provides, structures, and maintains a safe, therapeutic, recovery-oriented environment in collaboration with healthcare consumers, families, and other healthcare clinicians.

Standard 5G Therapeutic Relationship and Counseling
The PMH registered nurse uses the therapeutic relationship and counseling interventions to assist healthcare consumers in their individual recovery journeys by improving and regaining their previous coping abilities, fostering mental health, and preventing mental disorder and disability.

Standard 5H Psychotherapy
The PMH advanced practice registered nurse conducts individual, couples, group, and family psychotherapy using evidence-based psychotherapeutic frameworks and the nurse–client therapeutic relationship.

STANDARD 6. EVALUATION
The PMH registered nurse evaluates progress toward attainment of expected outcomes.

From American Nurses Association, American Psychiatric Nurses Association & International Society of Psychiatric–Mental Health Nurses (2014). *Psychiatric–Mental Health Nursing: Scope and Standards of Practice,* 2nd Edition. Silver Spring, MD: Nursesbooks.org.

Table 6.1	STANDARDS OF PROFESSIONAL PERFORMANCE	
Standard	**Area of Performance**	**Description**
Standard 7	Ethics	Integrates ethical provisions in all areas of practice.
Standard 8	Education	Attains knowledge and competency that reflect current nursing practice.
Standard 9	Evidence-Based Practice & Research	Integrates evidence and research findings into practice.
Standard 10	Quality of Practice	Systematically enhances the quality and effectiveness of nursing practice.
Standard 11	Communication	Communicates effectively in a variety of formats in all areas of practice.
Standard 12	Leadership	Provides leadership in the professional practice setting and the profession.
Standard 13	Collaboration	Collaborates with the healthcare consumer, family, interprofessional health team, and others in the conduct of nursing practice.
Standard 14	Professional Practice Evaluation	Evaluates one's own practice in relation to the professional practice standards and guidelines, relevant statutes, rules, and regulations.
Standard 15	Resource Utilization	Considers factors related to safety, effectiveness, cost, and impact on practice in the planning and delivery of nursing services.
Standard 16	Environmental Health	Practices in an environmentally safe and healthy manner.

From American Nurses Association, American Psychiatric Nurses Association & International Society of Psychiatric–Mental Health Nurses (2014). *Psychiatric–Mental Health Nursing: Scope and Standards of Practice,* 2nd Edition. Silver Spring, MD: Nursesbooks.org.

It is important that nurses are prepared to practice according to these standards. Nurses ultimately are held accountable by society for practicing according to their standards.

Standards of Professional Performance

Ten standards of professional performance for psychiatric-mental health nurses follow the six standards of practice. These standards define and inform society about the professional role of psychiatric-mental health nurses and include ethics, education, evidence-based practice and research, quality of practice, communication, leadership, collaboration, professional practice evaluation, resource utilization, and environmental health. Each standard of performance includes expected competencies (ANA et al., 2014) (Table 6.1).

Levels of Practice

There are two levels of psychiatric-mental health nursing practice. The first level is the PMH-RN with educational preparation within a bachelor's degree, associate's degree, or a diploma program. The next level is the PMH-APRN with educational preparation within a master's degree or doctoral degree program. At the PMH-APRN level, two sub-categories exist including the mental health clinical specialist (PMHCNS) and psychiatric-mental health nurse practitioner (PMHMP) (Box 6.4).

Psychiatric–Mental Health Nursing Practice

According to *the Psychiatric–Mental Health Nursing: Scope and Standards of Practice*, the **psychiatric–mental health nurse** is a registered nurse who demonstrates specialized competence and knowledge, skills, and abilities in caring for persons with mental health issues and problems and

psychiatric disorders. Competency is obtained through both education and experience. The preferred educational preparation is at the baccalaureate level with credentialing by the American Nurses Credentialing Center (ANCC) or a recognized certification organization. (ANA et al., 2014).

Nursing practice at this level is "characterized by the use of the nursing process to treat people with actual or potential mental health problems, psychiatric disorders and co-occurring psychiatric and substance use disorders (ANA 2014, pg. 25). By using the nursing process, the PMH-RN promotes and fosters health and safety, assesses dysfunction and areas of strength, and assists individuals in achieving personal recovery goals. The nurse performs a wide range of interventions, including health promotion and health

---

BOX 6.4

Clinical Activities of Psychiatric–Mental Health Nurses

PSYCHIATRIC–MENTAL HEALTH REGISTERED NURSE
Health promotion and health maintenance
Intake screening, evaluation, and triage
Case management
Provision of therapeutic and safe environments
Milieu therapy
Promotion of self-care activities
Administration of psychobiologic treatment and monitoring responses
Complementary interventions
Crisis intervention and stabilization
Psychiatric rehabilitation

ADVANCED PRACTICE REGISTERED NURSE
Psychopharmacological interventions
Psychotherapy
Community interventions
Case management
Program development and management
Clinical supervision
Consultation and liaison

maintenance strategies, intake screening and evaluation and triage, case management, milieu therapy, promotion of self-care activities, psychobiologic inter-ventions, complementary interventions, health teaching, counseling, crisis care, and psychiatric rehabilitation. An overview of psychiatric nursing interventions is presented in Unit 3.

Advanced Practice

The PMH-APRN is also a licensed registered nurse but is educationally prepared at the master's level and is nationally certified as a clinical nurse specialist or a psychiatric nurse practitioner by the ANCC. The DNP (doctorate in nursing practice) requires advanced education in systems function, analysis, health policy, and advocacy may be at the PMH-RN level (RN administrators or educators) or at the APRN level (ANA et al., 2014). Researchers are prepared at the highest education level preparation with a doctorate in nursing science (DNS, DNSc) or a doctor of philosophy (PhD) degree.

Psychiatric–Mental Health Nursing Organizations

Whereas the establishment and reinforcement of standards go a long way toward legitimizing psychiatric–mental health nursing, professional organizations provide leadership in shaping mental health care. They do so by providing a strong voice for meaningful legislation that promotes quality patient care and advocates for maximal use of nursing skills.

The ANA is one such organization. Although its focus is on addressing the emergent needs of nursing in general, the ANA supports psychiatric–mental health nursing practice through liaison activities, such as advocating for psychiatric–mental health nursing at the national and state levels and working closely with psychiatric–mental health nursing organizations.

The APNA and the ISPN are two organizations for psychiatric nurses that focus on mental health care. The APNA is the largest psychiatric–mental health nursing organization, with the primary mission of advancing psychiatric–mental health nursing practice; improving mental health care for culturally diverse individuals, families, groups, and communities; and shaping health policy for the delivery of mental health services. The ISPN consists of four specialist divisions: the Association of Child and Adolescent Psychiatric Nurses, International Society of Psychiatric Consultation Liaison Nurses, Society for Education and Research in Psychiatric–Mental Health Nursing, and Adult and Geropsychiatric-Mental Health Nurses. The purpose of ISPN is to unite and strengthen the presence and the voice of psychiatric–mental health nurses and to promote quality care for individuals and families with mental health problems. The International Nurses Society on Addictions (INTNSA) is committed to the prevention, intervention, treatment, and management of addictive disorders. These organizations have annual meetings at which new research is presented. Student memberships are available.

THE BIOPSYCHOSOCIAL FRAMEWORK

The holistic, biopsychosocial model (Fig. 6.1) is well recognized as an organizing framework for understanding the interactive domains of an individual's mental health and matching appropriate interventions with patient's needs. This model is easily integrated with the recovery and wellness models and guides recovery-oriented care (see Chapter 2). The biopsychosocial framework is useful in standardized nursing languages such as NANDA International/Nursing Interventions Classification (NIC)/Nursing Outcomes Classification (NOC), Clinical Care Classification, and the Omaha system (Martin, 2005; Saba, 2012; Schwirian, 2013).

> **KEYCONCEPT** The **biopsychosocial framework** consists of three separate but interdependent domains: biologic, psychological, and social. Each domain has an independent knowledge and treatment focus but interacts and is mutually interdependent with the other domains.

Biologic Domain

The *biologic* domain consists of the biologic theories related to mental disorders and problems as well as *all* of the biologic activity related to other health problems. Biologic theories and concepts also relate to functional health patterns such as exercise, sleep, and adequate nutrition to mental health conditions. In addition, the neurobiologic theories also serve as a basis for understanding

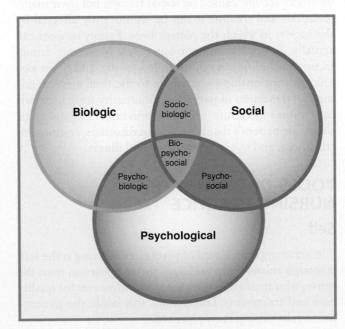

FIGURE 6.1 The biopsychosocial model.

and administering pharmacologic agents (see Chapters 8 and 11).

Psychological Domain

The *psychological* domain contains the theoretical basis of the psychological processes—thoughts, feelings, and behavior (intrapersonal dynamics) that influence one's emotion, cognition, and behavior. The psychological and nursing sciences generate theories and research that are critical in understanding patients' symptoms and responses to mental disorders. Although there are neurobiologic changes in mental disorders, symptoms are psychological. For example, even though manic behavior is caused by dysfunction in the brain, there are no laboratory tests to confirm a diagnosis, only a pattern of behavior.

Many psychiatric nursing interventions are behavioral, such as cognitive approaches, behavior therapy, and patient education. Therapeutic communication techniques require nurses to develop awareness of their own, as well as their patients', internal feelings and behavior. For mental health nurses, understanding their own and their patients' intrapersonal dynamics and motivation is critical in developing a therapeutic relationship (see Chapter 9).

Social Domain

The *social* domain includes theories that account for the influence of social forces encompassing the patient, family, and community within cultural settings. Social and nursing sciences explain the connections within the family and communities that affect the mental health, treatment, and recovery of people with mental disorders. Psychiatric disorders are not caused by social factors, but their manifestations and treatment can be significantly affected by the society in which the patient lives. Family support can actually improve treatment outcomes. Moreover, family factors, including origin, extended family, and other significant relationships, contribute to the total understanding and treatment of patients. Community forces, including cultural and ethnic groups within larger communities, shape the patient's manifestation of disorders, response to treatment, and overall view of mental illness.

TOOLS OF PSYCHIATRIC NURSING PRACTICE

Self

The most important tool of psychiatric nursing is the self. Through relationship building, patients learn to trust the nurse, who then guides, teaches, and advocates for quality care and treatment. Throughout this book, the patient–nurse relationship is emphasized.

Clinical Reasoning and Reflection

Sound **clinical reasoning** depends on the critical thinking skills and reflection. During critical thinking activities, such as problem solving and decision making, nurses analyze evaluate, explain, infer, and interpret biopsychosocial data. Some critical thinking activities, such as nursing assessments, take time, but many decisions are moment-to-moment, such as deciding whether a patient can leave a unit or whether a patient should receive a medication.

Reflection involves continual self-evaluation through observing, monitoring, and judging nursing behaviors with the goal of providing ideal interventions. Reflection skills are used in all aspects of psychiatric nursing practice, from enhancing of self awareness and examining nurse–patient interactions to evaluation of the system of care.

Interdisciplinary Care

The psychiatric–mental health nurse can expect to collaborate with other professionals and the patient in all settings. In the hospital, a patient may see a psychiatrist or psychiatric nurse practitioner who treats the symptoms and prescribes the medication; a case manager who coordinates care; a psychiatric social worker for individual psychotherapy; a psychiatric nurse for management of responses related to the mental disorder, administration of medication, and monitoring side effects; and an occupational therapist for transition into the workplace. In the community clinic, a patient may meet weekly with a therapist, monthly with a mental health provider who prescribes medication, and twice a week with a group leader in a day treatment program. All of these professionals bring a specialized skill to the patient's care.

Plan of Care

Just like patients in medical–surgical settings, patients receiving psychiatric mental health services have written plans of care. The patient and family (if appropriate) should be a participant in the development of the plan. If only nursing care is being provided, such as in-home care, a nursing care plan may be used. If other disciplines are providing services to the same patient, which often occurs in a hospital, an interdisciplinary treatment plan may be used with or instead of a traditional nursing care plan. When an interdisciplinary plan is used, components of the nursing care plan should always be easily identified. The nurse provides the care that is judged to be within the scope of practice of the psychiatric–mental health nurse. Thus, the traditional nursing care plan may or may not be used, depending on institutional policies.

Whether a nursing care plan or an interdisciplinary treatment plan is used, these plans are important because they are individualized to a patient's needs. They are sometimes approved by third-party payers who reimburse the cost of the service. In this text, the emphasis is on developing nursing care plans because they serve as a basis of practice and can be included in a multidisciplinary or interdisciplinary individual treatment plan.

CHALLENGES OF PSYCHIATRIC NURSING

The challenges of psychiatric nursing are increasing. New knowledge is being generated, technology is shaping health care into new dimensions, and nursing practice is becoming more specialized and autonomous. This section discusses a few of the challenges.

Knowledge Development, Dissemination, and Application

Knowledge is rapidly expanding in the psychiatric–mental health field. Genetic research has opened a new area of investigation into the etiology of several disorders such as schizophrenia, bipolar disorders, dementia, and autism. Psychoneuroimmunology is investigating the role of the immune system in the development of mental disorders. The presence of comorbid medical disorders gains increasing importance in the treatment of mental disorders. For example, hypertension, hypothyroidism, hyperthyroidism, and diabetes mellitus all affect the treatment of psychiatric disorders. The challenge for psychiatric nurses today is to stay abreast of the advances in total health care in order to provide safe, competent care to individuals with mental disorders.

Additional challenges for psychiatric nurses include updating their knowledge, so that significant results of studies can be applied to the care of patients. Accessing new information through journals, electronic databases, and continuing education programs takes time and vigilance but provides a sound basis for application of new knowledge.

Overcoming Stigma

Nurses can play an important role in dispelling myths of mental illnesses. Stigma often prevents individuals from seeking help for mental health problems (see Chapter 2). Reducing stigma is every nurse's responsibility, whether or not the nurse practices psychiatric nursing. To reduce the burden of mental illness and improve access to care, nurses can educate all of their patients about the etiology, symptoms, and treatment of mental illnesses.

Integration of Mental Health Care and Medical Care

There was a time when psychiatric nursing care was viewed as being separate from medical nursing. This is no longer true. Even though the focus is on mental health issues, the psychiatric nurse practices from a holistic perspective and considers the medical needs of the patient and their impact on the individual's mental health. The practice of psychiatric nursing is even more challenging as mental health promotion approaches include wellness concepts and approaches.

Health Care Delivery System Challenges

Additional continuing challenges for psychiatric nurses include providing nursing care within integrated community-based services where culturally competent, high-quality nursing care is needed to meet the emerging mental health care needs of patients. In caring for patients who require support from the social welfare system in the form of housing, job opportunities, welfare, and transportation, nurses need to be knowledgable about these systems. Moreover, in some settings, the nurse may be the only one who has a background in medical disorders, such as human immunodeficiency virus, acquired immunodeficiency syndrome, and other somatic health problems. Assertive community treatment reduces inpatient service use, promotes continuity of outpatient care, and increases the stability of people with serious mental illnesses (see Chapter 5). The nurse is involved in moving the currently fragmented health care system toward one focusing on consumer needs.

Impact of Technology and Electronic Health Records

Technologic advances have an unprecedented impact on the delivery of psychiatric nursing care and present new challenges. With the use of electronic health records, protection of patient confidentiality is more difficult in some ways. Patient records, once stored in remote areas and rarely viewed, are now readily available and easily accessed. Nurses need to be vigilant in maintaining privacy and confidentiality.

Electronic documentation enables nursing terminologies to be standardized and readily available to the nurse. The advantage of a standardized nursing language is improved patient care through better communication among nurses and other disciplines, increased visibility of nursing interventions, enhanced data collection, useful outcome evaluations, and greater adherence to standards of care (Schwirian, 2013).

> **KEYCONCEPT** A **standardized nursing language** is readily understood by all nurses to describe care. It provides a common means of communication.

Table 6.2	EXAMPLES OF THE RELATIONSHIP OF THE BIOPSYCHOSOCIAL MODEL TO STRUCTURED NURSING LANGUAGES		
Nursing Language	**Interventions**		
	Biologic	*Psychological*	*Social*
NANDA International, NIC, and NOC *Diagnosis:* Insomnia	Encourage use of sleep medications that do not contain REM sleep suppressors.	Assist to eliminate bedtime stressors.	Regulate environmental stimuli.
Clinical Care Classification (CCC) *Diagnosis:* Sleep Pattern Disturbance	Care related to improving pattern of sleep.	Teach sleep pattern control.	Manage sleep pattern control.
Omaha System *Diagnosis:* Insomnia	Take medication therapy as prescribed.	Establish routine. Use guided imagery.	Use community resources.

Saba, V. K. (2007). *Clinical care classification (CCC) system. A guide to nursing documentation.* New York: Springer Publishing Company.
Smith, K. J. & Craft-Rosenberg, M. (2010). Using NANDA, NIC, NOC in an undergraduate nursing practicum. *Nurse Educator, 35*(4), 162–166
Martin, K. S. (2005). *The Omaha system: A key to practice, documentation, and information management* (2nd ed). St. Louis: Elsevier Saunders.

There are several terminology sets being evaluated for use in electronic records (Schwirian, 2013). Table 6.2 provides an example of how some of these standardized languages relate to the biopsychosocial framework. These terminologies vary in their scope of practice and their applicability to psychiatric nursing practice. For example, NANDA International/NIC/NOC is more inclusive of mental health phenomena than the Perioperative Nursing Data Set (PNDS). To be useful in psychiatric nursing, standardized languages must specifically address responses to mental disorders and emotional problems.

Telemedicine is a reality and takes many forms, from communicating with remote sites to completing educational programs. It is important that patients have the opportunity to use technology to learn about their disorders and treatment. Because many of the disorders can affect cognitive functioning, it is also important that software programs be developed that can be used by these individuals to facilitate cognitive functioning.

SUMMARY OF KEY POINTS

- Standards for ethical behaviors for professional nurses are set by national professional organizations such as the ANA.

- There are several ethical principles to consider when providing psychiatric nursing care, including autonomy, beneficence, justice, nonmaleficence, paternalism, veracity, and fidelity.

- *Psyciatric-Mental Health Nursing: Scope and Standards of Practice, published in 2014*, establishes the areas of concern, standards of practice according to the nursing process, and standards of professional performance and differentiates between the functions of the basic and advanced practice nurse.

- Several professional nursing organizations provide leadership in shaping mental health care, including the ANA, the APNA, ISPN, and INTNSA.

- The biopsychosocial framework focuses on the three separate but interdependent dimensions of biologic, psychological, and social factors in the assessment and treatment of mental disorders. This comprehensive and holistic approach to mental disorders is the foundation for effective psychiatric–mental health nursing practice is integrated into recovery and wellness models.

- Nursing care plans and interdisciplinary treatment plans are written plans of care that are developed for each patient. Clinical reasoning skills are needed for developing and revising these tools.

- The psychiatric–mental health nurse interacts with other disciplines and many times acts as a coordinator in the delivery of care. There is always a plan of care for a patient, but it may be a nursing care plan or an individualized treatment plan that includes other disciplines.

- New challenges facing psychiatric nurses are emerging. Interpretation of research findings will assume new importance in the care of individuals with psychiatric disorders. The roles of nurses are expanding as nursing care becomes an established part of the community-based health care delivery system.

CRITICAL THINKING CHALLENGES

1. A 19-year-old patient with schizophrenia announces that he and a 47-year-old patient with bipolar disorder will be married the following week. They ask the

nurse to witness the wedding. Discuss which ethical principles may be in conflict.

2. Compare the ethical concepts of *autonomy* and *beneficence*. Focus on the difference between legal consequences and ethical dilemmas.

3. Compare the variety of patients for whom psychiatric–mental health nurses care. Factors to be considered are age, health problems, and social aspects.

4. Visit the ANA's website for a description of the psychiatric–mental health nurse's certification credentials. Compare the basic level functions of a psychiatric nurse with those of the advanced practice psychiatric nurse.

5. Explain the biopsychosocial framework and apply it to the following three clinical examples:
   a. A first-time father is extremely depressed after the birth of his child, who is perfectly healthy.
   b. A child is unable to sleep at night because of terrifying nightmares.
   c. An older woman is resentful of moving into a senior citizens residence even though the decision was hers.

6. Discuss the purposes of the following organizations in promoting quality mental health care and supporting nursing practice. Visit the organizations' websites for more information.
   a. American Nurses Association
   b. American Psychiatric Nurses Association
   c. International Society of Psychiatric–Mental Health Nurses
   d. International Nurses Society on Addictions

References

American Nurses Association, American Psychiatric Nurses Association & International Society of Psychiatric–Mental Health Nurses (2014). *Psychiatric–Mental Health Nursing: Scope and Standards of Practice, 2nd. Edition.* Silver Spring, MD: Nursesbooks.org.

Davis, A. (2008). Provision two. In M. Fowler (Ed.): *Guide to the code of ethics for nurses: Interpretation and Application* (p. 18). Washington, DC: Nursebooks.org.

Martin, K. S. (2005). *The Omaha system: A key to practice, documentation, and information management* (2nd ed). St. Louis: Elsevier Saunders.

Saba, V. K. (2012). Clinical care classification system. *Sabacare.* http://www.sabacare.com/About/?PHPSESSID=b9e97459af41b2c80d194d7434aa7800

Schwirian, P. M. (2013). Informatics and the future of nursing: Harnessing the power of standardized nursing terminology. *Bulletin of the Association for Information Science and Technology, 39*(5), 20–24.

Smith, K. J. & Craft-Rosenberg, M. (2010). Using NANDA, NIC, NOC in an undergraduate nursing practicum. *Nurse Educator, 35*(4), 162–66.

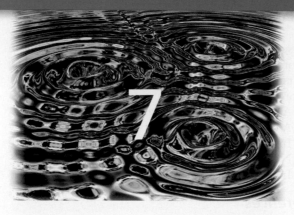

7 Psychosocial Theoretic Basis of Psychiatric Nursing

Mary Ann Boyd

KEY CONCEPTS

- anxiety
- empathic linkage

LEARNING OBJECTIVES

After studying this chapter, you will be able to:

1. Discuss psychosocial theories that support psychiatric nursing practice.

2. Identify the underlying theories that contribute to the understanding of human beings and behavior.

3. Compare the key elements of each theory that provides a basis for psychiatric–mental health nursing practice.

4. Identify common nursing theoretic models used in psychiatric–mental health nursing.

KEY TERMS

- behaviorism • classical conditioning • cognitions • cognitive theory • connections • countertransference • defense mechanisms • disconnections • empathy • family dynamics • formal support systems • informal support systems • interpersonal relations • libido • modeling • object relations • operant behavior • psychoanalysis • self-efficacy • self-system • social distance • transaction • transference • unconditional positive regard

---

This chapter presents an overview of selected psychodynamic, cognitive-behavioral, developmental, social, and nursing theories that serve as the knowledge base for psychiatric–mental health nursing practice. Many of these theories are covered in more depth in other chapters. Biologic theories are discussed in Chapters 8, 11, and 18.

PSYCHODYNAMIC THEORIES

Psychodynamic theories explain the development of mental or emotional processes and their effects on behavior and relationships. Many of the psychodynamic concepts and models that are important in psychiatric nursing began with the Austrian physician Sigmund Freud (1856–1939). Since his time, Freud's theories have been enhanced by interpersonal and humanist models. These theories

proved to be especially important in the development of therapeutic relationships, techniques, and interventions (Table 7.1).

Psychoanalytic Theory

In Freud's psychoanalytic model, the human mind is conceptualized in terms of conscious mental processes (an awareness of events, thoughts, and feelings with the ability to recall them) and unconscious mental processes (thoughts and feelings that are outside awareness and are not remembered).

Study of the Unconscious

Freud believed that the unconscious part of the human mind is only rarely recognized by the conscious, as in

Table 7.1	PSYCHODYNAMIC MODELS		
Theorist	**Overview**	**Major Concepts**	**Applicability**
Psychoanalytic Models			
Sigmund Freud (1856–1939)	Founder of psychoanalysis Believed that the unconscious could be accessed through dreams and free association Developed a personality theory and theory of infantile sexuality	Id, ego, superego Consciousness Unconscious mental processes Libido Object relations Anxiety and defense mechanisms Free associations, transference, and countertransference	Individual therapy approach used for enhancement of personal maturity and personal growth
Anna Freud (1895–1982)	Application of ego psychology to psychoanalytic treatment and child analysis with emphasis on the adaptive function of defense mechanisms	Refinement of concepts of anxiety, defense mechanisms	Individual therapy, childhood psychoanalysis
Neo-Freudian Models			
Alfred Adler (1870–1937)	First defected from Freud Founded the school of individual psychology	Inferiority	Added to the understanding of human motivation
Carl Gustav Jung (1875–1961)	After separating from Freud, founded the school of psychoanalytic psychology Developed new therapeutic approaches	Redefined libido Introversion Extroversion Persona	Personalities are often assessed on the introversion and extroversion dimensions
Otto Rank (1884–1939)	Introduced idea of primary trauma of birth Active technique of therapy, including more nurturing than Freud Emphasized feeling aspect of analytic process	Birth trauma Will	Recognized the importance of feelings within psychoanalysis
Erich Fromm (1900–1980)	Emphasized the relationship of the individual to society	Society and individual are not separate	Individual desires are formed by society
Melanie Klein (1882–1960)	Devised play therapy techniques Believed that complex unconscious fantasies existed in children younger than 6 months of age Principal source of anxiety arose from the threat to existence posed by the death instinct	Pioneer in object relations Identification	Developed different ways of applying psychoanalysis to children; influenced present-day English and American schools of child psychiatry
Karen Horney (1885–1952)	Opposed Freud's theory of castration complex in women and his emphasis on the oedipal complex Argued that neurosis was influenced by the society in which one lived	Situational neurosis Character	Beginning of feminist analysis of psychoanalytic thought
Interpersonal Relations			
Harry Stack Sullivan (1892–1949)	Impulses and striving need to be understood in terms of interpersonal situations	Participant observer Parataxic distortion Consensual validation	Provided the framework for the introduction of the interpersonal theories in nursing
Humanist Theories			
Abraham Maslow (1921–1970)	Concerned himself with healthy rather than sick people Approached individuals from a holistic-dynamic viewpoint	Needs Motivation	Used as a model to understand how people are motivated and needs that should be met
Frederick S. Perls (1893–1970)	Awareness of emotion, physical state, and repressed needs would enhance the ability to deal with emotional problems	Reality Here-and-now	Used as a therapeutic approach to resolve current life problems that are influenced by old, unresolved emotional problems
Carl Rogers (1902–1987)	Based theory on the view of human potential for goodness Used the term *client* rather than *patient* Stressed the relationship between therapist and client	Empathy Positive regard	Individual therapy approach that involves never giving advice and always clarifying client's feelings

remembered dreams (see Movies at the end of this chapter). The term *preconscious* is used to describe unconscious material that is capable of entering consciousness.

Personality and Its Development

Freud's personality structure consists of three parts: the id, ego, and superego (Freud, 1927). The *id* is formed by unconscious desires, primitive instincts, and unstructured drives, including sexual and aggressive tendencies that arise from the body. The *ego* consists of the sum of certain mental mechanisms, such as perception, memory, and motor control, as well as specific defense mechanisms (discussed below). The ego controls movement, perception, and contact with reality. The capacity to form mutually satisfying relationships is a fundamental function of the ego, which is not present at birth but is formed throughout the child's development. The *superego* is that part of the personality structure associated with ethics, standards, and self-criticism. A child's identification with important and esteemed people in early life, particularly parents, helps form the superego.

Object Relations and Identification

Freud introduced the concept of **object relations**, the psychological attachment to another person or object. He believed that the choice of a sexual partner in adulthood and the nature of that relationship depended on the quality of the child's object relationships during the early formative years.

The child's first love object is the mother, who is the source of nourishment and the provider of pleasure. Gradually, as the child separates from the mother, the nature of this initial attachment influences future relationships. The development of the child's capacity for relationships with others progresses from a state of narcissism to social relationships, first within the family and then within the larger community. Although the concept of object relations is fairly abstract, it can be understood in terms of a child who imitates her mother and then becomes like her mother in adulthood. This child incorporates her mother as a love object, identifies with her, and grows up to become like her. This process is especially important in understanding an abused child who, under certain circumstances, becomes an adult abuser.

Anxiety and Defense Mechanisms

For Freud, anxiety is the reaction to danger and is experienced as a specific state of physical unpleasantness. **Defense mechanisms** are coping styles that protect a person from unwanted anxiety. Although they are defined differently than in Freud's day, defense mechanisms still play an explanatory role in contemporary psychiatric–mental health practice. Defense mechanisms are discussed in the chapter on Communication and the Therapeutic Relationship (Chapter 9).

Sexuality

The energy or psychic drive associated with the sexual instinct, or **libido**, literally translated from Latin to mean "pleasure" or "lust," resides in the id. When sexual desire is controlled and not expressed, tension results and is transformed into anxiety (Freud, 1905). Freud believed that adult sexuality is an end product of a complex process of development that begins in early childhood and involves a variety of body functions or areas (oral, anal, and genital zones) that correspond to stages of relationships, especially with parents.

Psychoanalysis

Freud developed **psychoanalysis**, a therapeutic process of accessing the unconscious conflicts that originate in childhood and then resolving the issues with a mature adult mind. As a system of psychotherapy, psychoanalysis attempts to reconstruct the personality by examining free associations (spontaneous, uncensored verbalizations of whatever comes to mind) and the interpretation of dreams. Therapeutic relationships had their beginnings within the psychoanalytic framework.

Transference and Countertransference

Transference is the displacement of thoughts, feelings, and behaviors originally associated with significant others from childhood onto a person in a current therapeutic relationship (Moore & Fine, 1990). For example, a woman's feelings toward her parents as a child may be directed toward the therapist. If a woman were unconsciously angry with her parents, she may feel unexplainable anger and hostility toward her therapist. In psychoanalysis, the therapist uses transference as a therapeutic tool to help the patient understand emotional problems and their origin.

Countertransference, on the other hand, is defined as the direction of all of the therapist's feelings and attitudes toward the patient. Countertransference becomes a problem when these feelings and perceptions are based on other interpersonal experiences. For example, a patient may remind a nurse of a beloved grandmother. Instead of therapeutically interacting with the patient from an objective perspective, the nurse feels an unexplained attachment to her and treats the patient as if she were the nurse's grandmother. The nurse misses important assessment and intervention data.

Neo-Freudian Models

Many of Freud's followers ultimately broke away, establishing their own forms of psychoanalysis. Freud did not receive criticism well. The rejection of some of his basic tenets often cost his friendship as well. Various psychoanalytic schools have adopted other names because their doctrines deviated from Freudian theory.

Adler's Foundation for Individual Psychology

Alfred Adler (1870–1937), a Viennese psychiatrist and founder of the school of individual psychology, was a student of Freud's who believed that the motivating force in human life is an intolerable sense of inferiority. Some people try to avoid these feelings by developing an unreasonable desire for power and dominance. This compensatory mechanism can get out of hand, and these individuals become self-centered and neurotic, overcompensate, and retreat from the real world and its problems.

Today, Adler's theories and principles are adapted and applied to both psychotherapy and education. Adlerian theory is based on principles of mutual respect, choice, responsibility, consequences, and belonging.

Jung's Analytical Psychology

One of Freud's earliest students, Carl Gustav Jung (1875–1961), a Swiss psychoanalyst, created a model called analytical psychology. Jung believed in the existence of two basically different types of personalities: extroverted and introverted. Whereas extroverted people tend to be generally interested in other people and objects of the external world, introverted people are more interested in themselves and their internal environment. According to Jung, both extroverted and introverted tendencies exist in everyone, but the libido usually channels itself mainly in one direction or the other. He also developed the concept of *persona*—what a person appears to be to others in contrast to who he or she really is (Jung, 1966).

Horney's Feminine Psychology

Karen Horney (1885–1952), a German American psychiatrist, challenged many of Freud's basic concepts and introduced principles of feminine psychology. Recognizing a male bias in psychoanalysis, Horney was the first to challenge the traditional psychoanalytic belief that women felt disadvantaged because of their genital organs. Freud believed that women felt inferior to men because their bodies were less completely equipped, a theory he described as "penis envy." Horney rejected this concept, as well as the oedipal complex, arguing that there are significant cultural reasons why women may strive to obtain qualities or privileges that are defined by a society as being masculine. For example, in Horney's time, most women did not have access to a university education, the right to vote, or economic independence. She argued that women truly were at a disadvantage because of the paternalistic culture in which they lived (Horney, 1939).

Other Neo-Freudian Theories

Otto Rank: Birth Trauma

Otto Rank (1884–1939), an Austrian psychologist and psychotherapist, was also one of Freud's students. He attributed all neurotic disturbances to the primary trauma of birth. For Rank, human development is a progression from complete dependence on the mother and family to physical independence coupled with intellectual dependence on society and finally to complete intellectual and psychological emancipation. A person's will guides and organizes the integration of self.

Erich Fromm: Societal Needs

Erich Fromm (1900–1980), an American psychoanalyst, focused on the relationship of society and the individual. He argued that individual and societal needs are not separate and opposing forces; their relationship is determined by the historic background of the culture. Fromm also believed that the needs and desires of individuals are largely formed by their society. For Fromm, the fundamental purpose of psychoanalysis and psychology is to bring harmony and understanding between the individual and society (Fromm-Rieichmann, 1950).

Melanie Klein: Play Therapy

Melanie Klein (1882–1960), an Austrian psychoanalyst, devised play therapy techniques to demonstrate how a child's interaction with toys reveals earlier infantile fantasies and anxieties. She believed that complex, unconscious fantasies exist in children younger than 6 months of age. She is generally acknowledged as a pioneer in presenting an object relations viewpoint to the psychodynamic field, introducing the idea of early identification, a defense mechanism by which one patterns oneself after another person, such as a parent (Klein, 1963).

Harry Stack Sullivan: Interpersonal Forces

Interpersonal theories stress the importance of human relationships; instincts and drives are less important. Harry Stack Sullivan (1892–1949), an American psychiatrist, viewed **interpersonal relations** as a basis of human development and behavior. He believed that the health or sickness of one's personality is determined by the characteristic patterns in which one deals with other people. For example, one man is passive aggressive to everyone who contradicts him. This maladaptive behavior began when he was unable to express his disagreement to his parents. Health depends managing the constantly changing physical, social, and interpersonal environment as well as past and current life experiences (Sullivan, 1953).

Humanistic Theories

Humanistic theories are based on the belief that all human beings have the potential for goodness. Humanist therapists focus on patients' ability to learn about and accept themselves. They do not investigate repressed memories. Through therapy, patients explore personal capabilities in order to develop self-worth. They learn to experience the world in a different way.

Rogers' Client-Centered Therapy

Carl Rogers (1902–1987), an American psychologist, introduced client-centered therapy. **Empathy**, the capacity to assume the internal reference of the client in order to perceive the world in the same way as the client, is used in the therapeutic process (Rogers, 1980). The counselor is genuine but nondirect and also uses **unconditional positive regard**, a nonjudgmental caring for the client. In this therapy, the counselor's attitude and nonverbal communication are crucial. The therapist's emotional investment (i.e., true caring) in the client is essential in the therapeutic process (Rogers, 1980).

Gestalt Therapy

Another humanistic approach is Gestalt therapy, developed by Frederick S. (Fritz) Perls (1893–1970), a German-born former psychoanalyst who immigrated to the United States. Perls believed the root of human anxiety is frustration with inability to express natural biologic and psychological desires in modern civilization. The repression of these basic desires causes anxiety. In Gestalt therapy, these unmet needs are brought into awareness through individual and group exercises (Perls, 1969).

Abraham Maslow's Hierarchy of Needs

Abraham Maslow's (1921–1970) hierarchy of needs is fixture in social science and nursing (Maslow, 1970) (Figure 7.1). In nursing, Maslow's model is used to prioritize care. Basic needs (food, shelter) should be met before higher level needs (self-esteem) can be met.

Applicability of Psychodynamic Theories to Psychiatric–Mental Health Nursing

Several psychodynamic concepts are important in the practice of psychiatric–mental health nursing, such as interpersonal relationships, defense mechanisms, trans-

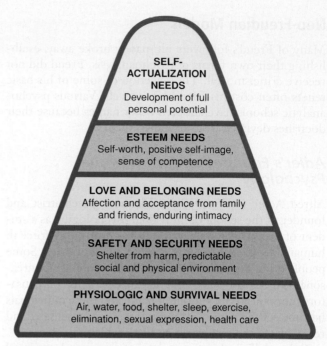

FIGURE 7.1 Maslow's hierarchy of needs.

ference, countertransference, and internal objects. In particular, a therapeutic interpersonal relationship is a core of psychiatric–mental health nursing intervention (see Chapter 10 for nursing interventions). Even though there is general consensus that most of these theories are useful, the nurse should continue to critically analyze them for utility and relevance. For example, Maslow's theory may be useful when a person with mental illness is homeless and wants food and shelter. But, another person in a similar situation may reject food and shelter because self-esteem is associated with being free to reject the confines of an institution. In this case, self-esteem need is more important than food or shelter.

Recently, there is renewed interest in psychodynamic treatment for depression. Psychodynamic therapists have a strong emphasis on affect and emotional expression, examination of topics that the patient avoids, recurring patterns of behaviors, feelings, experiences, and relationship, the past and its influence on the present, interpersonal relationships, and exploration of wishes, dreams, and fantasies (Luyten & Blatt, 2012).

COGNITIVE-BEHAVIORAL THEORIES

Behavioral Theories

Behavioral theories attempt to explain how people learn and act. Behavioral theories never attempt to explain the cause of mental disorders; instead, they focus on normal human behavior. Research results are then applied to the clinical situation. Two areas of behavioral theories relevant

Table 7.2	BEHAVIORAL THEORISTS		
Theorist	Overview	Major Concepts	Applicability
Stimulus–Response			
Edwin R. Guthrie (1886–1959)	Continued with understanding conditioning as being important in learning	Recurrence of responses tends to follow a specific stimulus	Important in analyzing habitual behavior
Ivan P. Pavlov (1849–1936)	Classical conditioning	Unconditioned stimuli Unconditioned response Conditioned stimuli	Important in understanding learning of automatic responses such as habitual behaviors
John B. Watson (1878–1958)	Introduced behaviorism Believed that learning was classical conditioning called *reflexes* Rejected distinction between mind and body	Principle of frequency Principle of recency	Focuses on the relationship between the mind and body
Reinforcement Theories			
B. F. Skinner (1904–1990)	Developed an understanding of the importance of reinforcement and differentiated types and schedules	Operant behavior Respondent behavior Continuous reinforcement Intermittent reinforcement	Important in behavior modification
Edward L. Thorndike (1874–1949)	Believed in the importance of effects that followed behavior	Reinforcement	Important in behavior modification programs

to psychiatric–nursing practice are stimulus–response theories and reinforcement theories (Table 7.2).

Early Stimulus–Response Theories

Pavlovian Theory

One of the earliest behavioral theorists was Ivan P. Pavlov (1849–1936), who noticed that stomach secretions of dogs were stimulated by triggers other than food reaching the stomach. He found that the sight and smell of food triggered stomach secretions, and he became interested in this anticipatory secretion. Through his experiments, he was able to stimulate secretions with a variety of other laboratory nonphysiologic stimuli. Thus, a clear connection was made between thought processes and physiologic responses.

In Pavlov's model, there is an unconditioned stimulus (not dependent on previous training) that elicits an unconditioned (i.e., specific) response. In his experiments, meat is the unconditioned stimulus, and salivation is the unconditioned response. Pavlov taught the dog to associate a bell (conditioned stimulus) with the meat (unconditioned stimulus) by repeatedly ringing the bell before presenting the meat. Eventually, the dog salivated when he heard the bell. This phenomenon is called **classical conditioning** (or pavlovian conditioning) (Pavlov, 1927/1960).

John B. Watson and the Behaviorist Revolution

At about the same time Pavlov was working in Russia, **behaviorism**, a learning theory that only focuses on objectively observable behaviors and discounts any independent activities of the mind, was introduced in the United States by John B. Watson (1878–1958). He rejected the distinction between body and mind and emphasized the study of objective behavior (Watson & Rayner, 1920). He developed two principles: frequency and recency. The *principle of frequency* states that the more often a response is made to a stimulus, the more likely the response to that stimulus will be repeated. The *principle of recency* states that the closer in time a response is to a particular stimulus, the more likely the response will be repeated.

Reinforcement Theories

Edward L. Thorndike

A pioneer in experimental animal psychology, Edwin L. Thorndike (1874–1949) studied the problem-solving behavior of cats to determine whether animals solved problems by reasoning or instinct. He found that neither choice was completely correct; animals gradually learn the correct response by "stamping in" the stimulus–response connection. The major difference between Thorndike and behaviorists such as Watson was that Thorndike believed that reinforcement of positive behavior was important in learning. He was the first reinforcement theorist, and his view of learning became the dominant view in American learning theory (Thorndike, 1916).

B. F. Skinner

One of the most influential behaviorists, B. F. Skinner (1904–1990), studied **operant behavior** or conditioning.

Table 7.3	COGNITIVE THEORISTS		
Theorist	Overview	Major Concepts	Applicability
Aaron Beck (b. 1921)	Conceptualized distorted cognitions as a basis for depression	Cognitions Beliefs	Important in cognitive therapy
Kurt Lewin (1890–1947)	Developed field theory, a system for understanding learning, motivation, personality, and social behavior	Life space Positive valences	Important in understanding motivation for changing behavior
Edward Chace Tolman (1886–1959)	Introduced the concept of cognitions: believed that human beings act on beliefs and attitudes and strive toward goals	Negative valences Cognition	Important in identifying person's beliefs

In this type of learning, the focus is on the consequence of the behavioral response, not a specific stimulus. If a behavior is reinforced or rewarded with success, praise, money, and so on, the behavior will probably be repeated. For example, if a child climbs on a chair, reaches the faucet, and is able to get a drink of water successfully, it is more likely that the child will repeat the behavior (Skinner, 1935). If a behavior does not have a positive outcome, it is less likely that the behavior will be repeated. Nurses use this knowledge to create behavior management plans to reinforce healthy, positive behaviors.

Cognitive Theories

The initial behavioral studies focused on human actions without much attention to the internal thinking process. When complex behaviors could not be accounted for by strictly behavioral explanations, thought processes became new subjects for study. **Cognitive theory**, an outgrowth of different theoretic perspectives, including the behavioral and the psychodynamic, attempted to link internal thought processes with human behavior (Table 7.3).

Albert Bandura's Social Cognitive Theory

Learning by watching others is the basis of Albert Bandura's (b. 1925) social cognitive theory. He developed his ideas after being concerned about television violence contributing to aggression in children. He showed learning occurs by internalizing behaviors of others through a process of **modeling** called pervasive imitation, or one person trying to be like another. The model does not have to be a real person but could be a character in history or generalized to an ideal person (Bandura, 1977, 1986).

An important concept of Bandura's is **self-efficacy**, a person's sense of his or her ability to deal effectively with the environment (Bandura, 1993). Efficacy beliefs influence how people feel, think, motivate themselves, and behave. The stronger the self-efficacy, the higher the goals people set for themselves and the firmer their commitment to them (McIntosh, 2003; Shin, Yun, Pender, & Jang, 2005).

One of Bandura's recent contributions is showing that intentions and self-motivation play roles in determining behavior, significantly expanding the reinforcement model. He believes that the human mind is not only reactive to a stimulus but is also creative, proactive, and reflective (Bandura, 2001).

Aaron Beck: Thinking and Feeling

American psychiatrist Aaron T. Beck (b. 1921) of the University of Pennsylvania devoted his career to understanding the relationship between cognition and mental health. For Beck, **cognitions** are verbal or pictorial events in the stream of consciousness. He realized the importance of cognitions when treating people with depression. He found that depression improved when patients began viewing themselves and situations in a positive light.

He believes that people with depression have faulty information-processing systems that lead to biased cognitions. These faulty beliefs cause errors in judgment that become habitual errors in thinking. These individuals incorrectly interpret life situations, judge themselves too harshly, and jump to inaccurate negative conclusions. A person may truly believe that he or she has no friends, and therefore no one cares. On examination, the evidence for the beliefs is based on the fact that there has been no contact with anyone because of moving from one city to another. Thus, a distorted belief is the basis of the cognition. Beck and his colleagues continue to develop cognitive therapy, a successful approach for the treatment of depression (Beck, 2005). Recent research supports the variability of beliefs between different generations within the same culture indicating the importance of understanding underlying beliefs (Box 7.1).

Applicability of Cognitive-Behavioral Theories to Psychiatric–Mental Health Nursing

Basing interventions on behavioral theories is widespread in psychiatric nursing. For example, patient education interventions are usually derived from the behavioral theories.

BOX 7.1

Research for Best Practice: **Differences in Beliefs in First- and Second-Generation Mothers**

Mamisachvili, L., Ardiles, P., Mancewicz, G., Thompson, S., Rabin, K., & Ross, L. E. (2013). Culture and postpartum mood problems: Similarities and differences in the experiences of first- and second-generation Canadian women. Journal of Transcultural Nursing, 24(2), 162–170.

THE QUESTION: Are there similarities and differences in experiences of postpartum mood problems (PPMP) between first- and second-generation Canadian women?

METHODS: In this exploratory qualitative study, the researchers interviewed nine first-generation and eight second-generation women to explore potential role of cultural values, beliefs, and immigration experiences in postpartum mood problems.

FINDINGS: While both generations experienced conflicts with their parents or in-laws regarding child rearing and the negative effects of PPMP stigma, the second-generation women were surprised that they needed support and experienced a loss of self. In these women, their PPMP is also related to not meeting their own and societal expectations of maternal roll fulfillment.

IMPLICATION FOR NURSING: There is variation in the beliefs associated with the state of depression. Understanding underlying belief systems is critical for providing the appropriate interventions.

Teaching patients new coping skills for their symptoms of mental illnesses is another example. Changing an entrenched habit involves helping patients identify what motivates them and how these new lifestyle habits can become permanent. In psychiatric units, behavioral interventions include the privilege systems and token economies. Behavioral approaches are discussed throughout this text. Cognitive approaches are further explained in Chapters 12 and 24.

DEVELOPMENTAL THEORIES

Developmental theories explain normal human growth and development over time. Many developmental theories are presented in terms of stages based on the assumption that normal development proceeds longitudinally from the beginning to the ending stage.

Erik Erikson: Psychosocial Development

Freud and Sullivan both published treatises on stages of human development, but Erik Erikson (1902–1994) outlined the psychosocial developmental model that is most often used in nursing. Erikson's model is an expansion of Freud's psychosexual development theory. Whereas Freud's model emphasizes intrapsychic experiences, Erikson's recognizes the role of the psychosocial environment. For example, parental divorce disrupts the family interaction pattern, and the financial and housing environment impact the development of the children.

Each of Erikson's eight stages are organized by age and developmental conflicts: basic trust versus mistrust, autonomy versus shame and doubt, initiative versus guilt, industry versus inferiority, identity versus role diffusion, intimacy versus isolation, generativity versus stagnation, and ego integrity versus despair. Successful resolution of a conflict or crisis leads to essential strength and virtues (Table 7.4). For example, a positive outcome of the trust versus mistrust crisis is the development of a basic sense of trust. If the crisis is unsuccessfully resolved, the infant moves into the next stage without a sense of trust. According to this model, a child who is mistrustful will have difficulty completing the next crisis successfully and, instead of developing a sense of autonomy, will more likely be full of shame and doubt (Erikson, 1963).

Identity and Adolescence

One of Erikson's major contributions is the recognition of the turbulence of adolescence and identity formation. When adolescence begins, childhood ways are given up,

Table 7.4	**ERIKSON'S EIGHT AGES OF MAN**	
Approximate Chronologic Age	**Developmental Conflict***	**Long-Term Outcome of Successful Resolution**
Infant	Basic trust vs. mistrust	Drive and hope
Toddler	Autonomy vs. shame and doubt	Self-control and willpower
Preschool-aged child	Initiative vs. guilt	Direction and purpose
School-aged child	Industry vs. inferiority	Method and competence
Adolescence	Identity vs. role diffusion	Devotion and fidelity
Young adult	Intimacy vs. isolation	Affiliation and love
Adulthood	Generativity vs. stagnation	Production and care
Maturity	Ego integrity vs. despair	Renunciation and wisdom

*Successful outcome is evidenced by the development of the characteristic listed first.
Adapted from Erikson, E. (1963). *Childhood and society* (pp. 273–274). New York: Norton.

and bodily changes occur. An identity is formed. Trying to reconcile a personal view of self with society's perception can be overwhelming and lead to role confusion and alienation (Erikson, 1968).

Research Evidence for Erikson's Models

Evidence is mixed that every person follows the eight stages of development as outlined by Erikson. In an early study, male college students who measured low on identity also scored low on intimacy ratings (Orlofsky, Marcia, & Lesser, 1973). These results lend support to the idea that identity precedes intimacy. In another study, intimacy was found to begin developing early in adolescence before the development of identity (Ochse & Plug, 1986). Studying fathers with young children, Christiansen and Palkovitz (1998) found that *generativity* (defined as the need or drive to produce, create, or effect a change) was associated with a paternal identity, psychosocial identity, and psychosocial intimacy. In addition, fathers who had a religious identification also had higher generativity scores than did others.

A longitudinal study of 86 men beginning at age 21 years with reassessment 32 years later at age 53 years supports Erikson's psychosocial eight-stage model (Westermeyer, 2004). In this study, 48 men (56%) achieved generativity at follow-up. Successful young adults as predicted by Erikson's model at midlife lived within a warm family environment; had an absence of troubled parental discipline; experienced a mentor relationship; and, most importantly, had favorable peer group relationships.

Erikson's model may apply differently to men and women. In one study, generativity is associated with well-being in both men and women, but in men, generativity is related to the urge for self-protection, self-assertion, self-expansion, and mastery. In women, the antecedents may be the desire for contact, connection, and union (Ackerman, Zuroff, & Moskowitz, 2000).

Studies show that generativity is significantly associated with successful marriage, work achievements, close friendships, altruistic behaviors, and overall mental health. Generativity is also associated with optimism and forgiveness in dealing with grandparenting problems within the family (Ehlman & Ligon, 2012; Pratt, Norris, Cressman, Lawford, & Hebblethwaite, 2008).

Jean Piaget: Learning in Children

One of the most influential people in child psychology is Jean Piaget (1896–1980), who contributed more than 40 books and 100 articles on child psychology alone. Piaget's theory views intelligence as an adaptation to the environment. He proposes that cognitive growth is like embryologic growth: an organized structure becomes more and more differentiated over time. Piaget's system explains how knowledge develops and changes (Table 7.5).

Each stage of cognitive development represents a particular structure with major characteristics. Piaget's theory

Table 7.5	PIAGET'S PERIODS OF INTELLECTUAL DEVELOPMENT			
Age (years)	**Period**	**Cognitive Developmental Characteristics**	**Description**	
Birth to 2	Sensorimotor	Divided into six stages, characterized by (1) inborn motor and sensory reflexes, (2) primary circular reaction and first habit, (3) secondary circular reaction, (4) use of familiar means to obtain ends, (5) tertiary circular reaction and discovery through active experimentation, and (6) insight and object permanence	The infant understands the world in terms of overt, physical action on that world. The infant moves from simple reflexes through several steps to an organized set of schemes. Significant concepts are developed, including space, time, and causality. Above all, during this period, the child develops the scheme of the permanent object.	
2–7	Preoperational	Deferred imitation; symbolic play, graphic imagery (drawing); mental imagery; and language. Egocentrism, rigidity of thought, semilogical reasoning, and limited social cognition	Child no longer only makes perceptual and motor adjustment to objects and events. Child can now use symbols (mental images, words, gestures) to represent these objects and events; uses these symbols in an increasingly organized and logical fashion.	
7–11	Concrete operations	Conservation of quantity, weight, volume, length, and time based on reversibility by inversion or reciprocity; operations: class inclusion and seriation	Conservation is the understanding of what values remain the same. For example, if liquid is poured from a short, wide glass into a tall, narrow one, the preoperational child thinks that the quantity has changed. For the concrete operation child, the amount stays the same.	
11 through the end of adolescence	Formal operations	Combination system whereby variables are isolated and all possible combinations are examined; hypothetical-deductive thinking	Mental operations are applied to objects and events. The child classifies, orders, and reverses them. Hypotheses can be generated from these concrete operations.	

was developed through observation of his own children and therefore never received formal testing.

The major strength of his model is its recognition of the central role of cognition in development and the discovery of surprising features of young children's thinking. For example, children in middle childhood become capable of considering more than one aspect of an object or situation at a time. Their thinking becomes more complex. They can understand that the area of a rectangle is determined by the length *and* width. For psychiatric–mental health nurses, Piaget's model provides a framework to recognize different levels of thinking in the assessment and intervention processes. For example, the assessment of concrete thinking is typical of some people with schizophrenia who are unable to perform abstract thinking.

Carol Gilligan: Gender Differentiation in Moral Development

Carol Gilligan (b. 1936) argues that most development models are male centered and therefore inappropriate for girls and women. She challenges Erik Erikson (psychosocial development) and Kohlberg's (moral) theories as being biased against women because they are based on primarily privileged, white men and boys. For Gilligan, attachment within relationships is the important factor for successful development. After comparing male and female personality development, she highlights differences (Gilligan, 2004). In developing identity, boys separate from their mothers, and girls attach. Girls probably learn to value relationships and become interdependent at an earlier age. They learn to value the ideal of care, begin to respond to human need, and want to take care of the world by sustaining attachments so no one is left alone. Her model of moral development, *Ethic of Care*, is divided into three stages beginning with *preconventional* or selfishness (what is best for me) to *conventional* or responsibility to others (self-sacrifice is goodness) to *postconventional* or do not hurt others or self (she is a person too) (Gilligan, 2011).

Gilligan's conclusion that female development depends on relationships has implications for everyone who provides care to women. Traditional models that advocate separation as the primary goal of human development immediately place women at a disadvantage. By negating the value and importance of attachments within relationships, the natural development of women is impaired. If Erikson's model is applied to women, their failure to separate then becomes defined as a developmental failure (Gilligan, 1982).

Jean Baker Miller: A Sense of Connection

Jean Baker Miller (1927–2006) conceptualized female development within the context of experiences and relationships. Consistent with the thinking of Carol Gilligan,

the Miller relational model views the central organizing feature of women's development as a sense of connection to others. The goal of development is to increase a woman's ability to build and enlarge mutually enhancing relationships (Miller, 1994). **Connections** (mutually responsive and enhancing relationships) lead to mutual engagement (attention), empathy, and empowerment. In relationships in which everyone interacts beneficially, mutual psychological development can occur. **Disconnections** (lack of mutually responsive and enhancing relationships) occur when a child or adult expresses a feeling or explains an experience and does not receive any response from others. The most serious types of disconnection arise from the lack of response that occurs after abuse or attacks. The theory is currently evolving and serves as a model for psychotherapy and nursing practice on psychiatric units (Riggs & Bright, 1997; Walker & Rosen, 2004).

Applicability of Developmental Theories to Psychiatric–Mental Health Nursing

Developmental theories are used in understanding childhood and adolescent experiences and their manifestations as adult problems. When working with children, nurses can use developmental models to help gauge development and mood. However, because most of the models are based on the assumptions of the linear progression of stages and have not been adequately tested, applicability has limitations. Most do not account for gender differences and diversity in lifestyles and cultures.

SOCIAL THEORIES

Numerous social theories underlie psychiatric–mental health nursing practice. Chapter 3 presents some of the sociocultural issues and discusses various social groups. This section represents a sampling of important social theories that a nurse uses. This discussion is not exhaustive and should be viewed by the student as including a few of the important social theoretic perspectives.

Family Dynamics

Family dynamics are the patterned interpersonal and social interactions that occur within the family structure over the life of a family. Family dynamics models are based on systems theory in which the change of one part affects the total functioning of the system. The family is viewed organizationally as an open system in which one member's actions influence the functioning of the total system. Family theories that are important in psychiatric–mental health nursing are based on systems models but have rarely been tested for wide-range validity. Specific family theories are discussed in depth in Chapter 14: Family Assessment and Interventions.

Family theories are especially useful to nurses who are assessing family dynamics and planning interventions. Family systems models are used to help nurses form collaborative relationships with patients and families dealing with health problems. Generalist psychiatric–mental health nurses will not be engaged in family therapy. However, they will be caring for individuals and families. Understanding family dynamics is important in every nurse's practice. Many family interventions are consistent with these theories (see Chapter 14). Many of the symptoms of mental disorders, such as hallucinations or delusions, have implications for the total family and affect interactions.

Formal and Informal Social Support

Assisting patients in the recovery process means helping patients identify supportive family and community systems. **Formal support systems** are large organizations, such as hospitals and nursing homes that provide care to individuals. **Informal support systems** are family, friends, and neighbors. Individuals with strong informal support networks actually live longer than those without this type of support. Adolescents who are survivors of sexual assault are more likely to seek support from informal support systems than formal supports (Fehler-Cabral & Campbell, 2013). In addition, classic studies showed that those without informal support have significantly higher mortality rates when the causes of death are accidents (e.g., smoking in bed) or suicides (Litwak, 1985).

An important concept is **social distance**, the degree to which the values of the formal organization and primary group members differ. In the United States, the most closely located, accessible, and available family member is expected to provide the care to a family member. Spouses are the first choice, then children, other family members, friends, and finally formal support. On the other, care-related stress can result in the informal caregiver changing the balance by placing a family member in an institution (Friedemann, Newman, Buckwalter, & Montgomery, 2014).

Formal and informal support systems are balanced when they are at a midpoint of social distance, that is, close enough to communicate but not so close to destroy each other—neither enmeshment nor isolation (Litwak, Messeri, & Silverstein, 1990; Messeri, Silverstein, & Litwak, 1993). Conflicts arise when the relationship becomes unbalanced. For example, if the primary group and the formal care system begin performing similar caregiving services, there may be disagreements. Balance is reestablished when the formal system increases the social distance by developing relationships and providing support to the caregiver and reducing contact with the patient. Thus, a balance is maintained between the two systems. In another instance, when a patient relies only

BOX 7.2

Research for Best Practice: **Formal and Informal Services**

McPherson, K. M., Kayes, N. K., Moloczij, N., & Cummins. C. (2013). *Improving the interface between informal carers and formal health and social services: A qualitative study.* International Journal of Nursing Studies, 51(3), 418–429. doi:10.1016/j.inurstu.2013.07.006

THE QUESTION: Is there a connection between informal and formal care givers? How can positive connections or interface be developed and maintained between them?

METHODS: Qualitative interviewing of formal and informal care givers (*n* = 70) using focus groups and individual interviews.

FINDINGS: Four themes emerged including (1) quality of care for the patient, (2) knowledge exchange (valuing each other's perspectives), (3) need for flexibility services, and (4) reducing the caregiver burden.

IMPLICATIONS FOR NURSING: Positive interface of formal and informal caregiver can ensure quality care for individuals.

on the health care provider for care and support (e.g., calls the nurse every day, visits the physician weekly, refuses any help from family), balance can be reestablished by linking the patient to an informal support system for help with some of the caregiving tasks.

By applying frameworks of formal and informal support systems to their patients, psychiatric nurses can understand the complex social forces that patient's with mental disorders and their caregivers experience (McPherson, Kayes, Moloczij, & Cummins, 2013) (Box 7.2). Nurses can help adjust the social distance between the formal and informal systems by identifying communication barriers and helping the two groups work together. For example, a patient misses an appointment because of a lack of transportation. The case manager helps the patient communicate the problem to the system to obtain another appointment. Informal caregivers are valued by the case manager, who recognizes the important services performed by family and friends. Thus, linkages between mental health providers (formal support) and the consumer network (informal support) are reinforced.

Role Theories

A role is a person's social position and function within an environment. Anthropologic theories explain members' roles that relate to a specific society. For example, the universal roles of healer may be assumed by a nurse in one culture and a spiritual leader in another. Societal expectations, social status, and rights are attached to these roles. Psychological theories, which are concerned about roles from a different perspective, focus on the relationship of an individual's role: the self. The responsibilities of a parent are often in conflict with the personal needs for time alone. All of the neo-Freudian and humanist models that have been discussed focus on reciprocal social relationships or interactions that determine how the mind develops.

Role theories emphasize the importance of social interaction in either the individual's choice of a particular role or society's recognition of it. Psychiatric–mental health nursing uses role concepts in understanding group interaction and the role of the patient in the family and community (see Chapters 12 and 13). In addition, milieu therapy approaches discussed in later chapters are based on the patient's assumption of a role within the psychiatric environment.

Sociocultural Perspectives

Margaret Mead: Culture and Gender

American anthropologist Margaret Mead (1901–1978) is widely known for her studies of primitive societies and her contributions to social anthropology. She conducted studies in New Guinea, Samoa, and Bali and devoted much of her studies to the patterns of child rearing in various cultures. She was particularly interested in the cultural influences determining male and female behavior (Mead, 1970). Influenced by Carl Jung and Erik Erikson, she had a vision of unity and diversity of the psychosocial development of a single human species (Sullivan, 2004). Although her research is often criticized as not having scientific rigor and being filled with misinterpretations, it is accepted as a classic in the field of anthropology (Sullivan, 2004). She established the importance of culture in determining human behavior.

Madeleine Leininger: Transcultural Health Care

Concern about the impact of culture on the treatment of children with psychiatric and emotional problems led Madeleine Leininger (1924–2012) to develop a new field, transcultural nursing, directed toward holistic, congruent, and beneficent care. Leininger developed the *Theory of Culture Care Diversity and Universality*, which explains diverse and universal dimensions of human caring (Figure 7.2). Nursing care in one culture is different from another because definitions of health, illness, and care are culturally defined (Leininger & McFarland, 2006). The goal of Leininger's theory is to discover culturally based care (Leininger, 2007).

Applicability of Social Theories to Psychiatric–Mental Health Nursing

The use of social and sociocultural theories is especially important for psychiatric–mental health nurses. In any individual or family assessment, the sociocultural aspect is integral to mental health. It would be impossible to complete an adequate assessment without considering the role of the individual within the family and society. Interventions are based on the understanding and significance of family and cultural norms. It would be impossible to interact with the family in a meaningful way without an understanding of the family's cultural values. In the inpatient setting, the nurse is responsible for designing the social environment of the unit as well as ensuring that the patient is safe from harm. To accomplish this complex task, an understanding of the unit as a small social community helps the nurse use the environment in patient treatment (see Chapter 10). In addition, many group interventions are based on sociocultural theories (see Chapter 13).

NURSING THEORIES

Nursing theories are useful to psychiatric–mental health nursing in conceptualizing the individual, family, or community and in planning nursing interventions (see Chapter 10). The use of a specific theory depends on the patient situation. For example, in people with schizophrenia who have problems related to maintaining self-care, Dorothea Orem's theory of self-care is useful. By contrast, Hildegarde Peplau's theories are appropriate when a nurse is developing a relationship with a patient. Because of the wide range of possible problems requiring different approaches, familiarity with several nursing theories is essential.

Interpersonal Relations Models

Hildegarde Peplau: The Power of Empathy

Hildegarde Peplau (1909–1999) introduced the first systematic theoretic framework for psychiatric nursing and focused on the nurse–patient relationship in her book *Inter-personal Relations in Nursing* in 1952 (Peplau, 1952). She led psychiatric–mental health nursing out of the confinement of custodial care into a theory-driven professional practice. One of her major contributions was the introduction of the nurse–patient relationship (see Chapter 9).

Peplau believed in the importance of the environment, defined as external factors considered essential to human development (Peplau, 1992): cultural forces, presence of adults, secure economic status of the family, and a healthy prenatal environment. Peplau emphasized the importance of empathic linkage.

> **KEYCONCEPT** **Empathic linkage** is the ability to feel in oneself the feelings experience by another person.

The interpersonal transmission of anxiety or panic is the most common empathic linkage. According to Peplau,

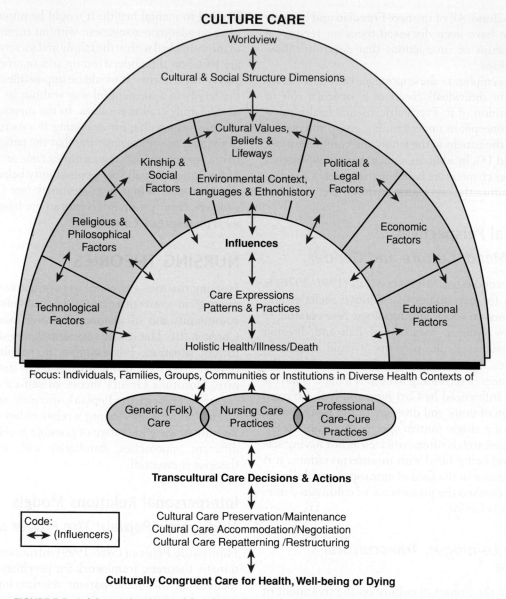

FIGURE 7.2 Leininger's Sunrise Model to depict theory of cultural care diversity and universality.

other feelings, such as anger, disgust, and envy, can also be communicated nonverbally by way of empathic transmission to others. Although the process is not yet understood, she explains that empathic communication occurs. She believes that if nurses pay attention to what they feel during a relationship with a patient, they can gain invaluable observations of feelings a patient is experiencing and has not yet noticed or talked about.

Anxiety is a key concept for Peplau, who contends that professional practice is unsafe if this concept is not understood.

> **KEYCONCEPT** **Anxiety**, according to Peplau, is an energy that arises when expectations that are present are not met.

If anxiety is not recognized, it continues to rise and escalates toward panic. There are various levels of anxiety, each having its observable behavioral cues (Box 7.3). These cues are sometimes called *defensive*, but Peplau argues that they are often "relief behaviors." For example, some people may relieve their anxiety by yelling and swearing; others seek relief by withdrawing. In both instances, anxiety was generated by an unmet security need.

BOX 7.3
Levels of Anxiety
Mild: awareness heightens **Moderate:** awareness narrows **Severe:** focused narrow awareness **Panic:** unable to function

NCLEXNOTE Peplau's model of anxiety continues to be an important concept in psychiatric nursing. Severe anxiety interferes with learning. Mild anxiety is useful for learning.

The **self-system** is another important concept in Peplau's model. Drawing from Sullivan, Peplau defined the self as an "anti-anxiety system" and a product of socialization. The self proceeds through personal development that is always open to revision but tends toward stability. For example, in parent–child relationships, patterns of approval, disapproval, and indifference are used by children to define themselves. If the verbal and nonverbal messages have been derogatory, children incorporate these messages and also view themselves negatively.

The concept of need is important to Peplau's model. Needs are primarily of biologic origin but need to be met within a sociocultural environment. When a biologic need is present, it gives rise to tension that is reduced and relieved by behaviors meeting that need. According to Peplau, nurses should recognize and support the patients' patterns and style of meeting their health care needs.

Ida Jean Orlando

In 1954, Ida Jean Orlando (1926–2007) studied the factors that enhanced or impeded the integration of mental health principles in the basic nursing curriculum. From this study, she published *The Dynamic Nurse–Patient Relationship* to offer nursing students a theory of effective nursing practice. She studied nursing care of patients on medical–surgical units, not people with psychiatric problems in mental hospitals. Orlando identified three areas of nursing concern: the nurse–patient relationship, the nurse's professional role, and the identity and development of knowledge that is distinctly nursing (Orlando, 1961). A nursing situation involves the behavior of the patient, the reaction of the nurse, and anything that does not relieve the distress of the patient. Patient distress is related to the inability of the individual to meet or communicate his or her own needs (Orlando, 1961, 1972).

Orlando helped nurses focus on the whole patient rather than on the disease or institutional demands. Her ideas continue to be useful today, and current research supports her model (Olson & Hanchett, 1997). A small nursing study investigated whether Orlando's nursing theory–based practice had a measurable impact on patients' immediate distress when compared with nonspecified nursing interventions Orlando's approach consisted of the nurse validating the patient's distress before taking any action to reduce it. Patients being cared for by the Orlando group experienced significantly less stress than those receiving traditional nursing care (Potter & Bockenhauer, 2000).

Existential and Humanistic Theoretical Perspectives

Rosemarie Rizzo Parse

The *Humanbecoming Theory* views humans as indivisible, unpredictable, ever-changing coauthors and experts about their lives (Parse, 1998, 2007). Three major themes underlie this theory: meaning (personal meaning to the situation), rhythmicity (the paradoxical patterning of the human-universe mutual processes—the ups and downs of life), and transcendence (power and originating of transforming) (Parse, 1996, 1998, 2008). The postulates involved in living a human life are *illuminating* (unbound knowing extended to infinity), *paradox* (intricate rhythm expressed as a pattern preference), *freedom* (liberation), and *mystery* (unexplainable) (Parse, 2007).

As one of the more abstract nursing theories, *humanbecoming* can used in understanding patients' life experiences and connecting psychologically with a patient. This theory has been widely studied in nursing and adds qualitative dimension to understanding the patient's human experience. For example, one of the studies addressed the positive effects of feeling strong within a community (Doucet, 2012).

Jean Watson

The theory of transpersonal caring was initiated by Jean Watson (b. 1940). Watson believes that caring is the foundation of nursing and recommends that specific theories of caring be developed in relation to specific human conditions and health and illness experiences (Watson, 2005). Her conceptualizations transcend conventional views of illness and focus on the meaning of health and quality of life (Watson, 2007). There are three foundational concepts of her theory:

- Transpersonal Caring–Healing Relations: a relational process related to philosophic, moral, and spiritual foundation
- 10 Caritas Process: the original 10 Carative Factors have evolved into the 10 Caritas Processes (Box 7.4)
- Caritas Field: a field of consciousness created when the nurse focuses on love and caring as his or her way of being and consciously manifests a healing presence with others.

Watson's theory is especially applicable to the care of those who seek help for mental illness. This model emphasizes the importance of sensitivity to self and others; the development of helping and trusting relations; the promotion of interpersonal teaching and learning; and provision for a supportive, protective, and corrective mental, physical, sociocultural, and spiritual environment. A transpersonal caring intervention guide offers protocols to assist nurses in using caring intentionally and effectively in

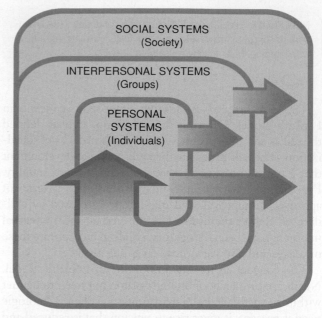

FIGURE 7.3 Imogene King's conceptual framework for nursing: dynamic interacting systems.

BOX 7.4

Nursing: Human Science and Human Care Assumptions, and Factors in Care

ASSUMPTIONS

1. Caring can be effectively demonstrated and practiced only interpersonally.
2. Caring consists of factors that result in the satisfaction of certain human needs.
3. Effective caring promotes health and individual or family growth.
4. Caring responses accept a person not only as he or she is now but also as what he or she may become.
5. A caring environment offers the development of potential while allowing the person to choose the best action for him- or herself at a given point in time.
6. Caring is more "healthogenic" than is curing. It integrates biophysical knowledge with knowledge of human behavior to generate or promote health and provide ministrations to those who are ill. A science of caring is complementary to the science of curing.
7. The practice of caring is central to nursing.

10 CARITAS PROCESSES™

1. Embrace altruistic values and practice loving kindness with self and others.
2. Instill faith, hope, and honor in others.
3. Be sensitive to self and others by nurturing individual beliefs and practices.
4. Develop helping–trusting–caring relationships.
5. Promote and accept positive and negative feelings as you authentically listen to another's story.
6. Use creative scientific problem-solving methods for caring decision making.
7. Share teaching and learning that addresses the individual needs and comprehension styles.
8. Create a healing environment for the physical and spiritual self that respects human dignity.
9. Assist with basic physical, emotional, and spiritual human needs.
10. Be open to mystery and allow miracles to enter.

From Watson Caring Science Institute, International Caritas Consortium. (2010). *Dr. Jean Watson's Human Caring Theory: Ten caritas processes.* http://www.watsoncaringscience.org/about-us/caring-science-definitions-processes-theory/

---

practice (Gallagher-Lepak & Kubsch, 2009). Watson's model is a model in the acute health care settings to guide the establishment of genuine therapeutic relationships (Hogan, 2013).

Systems Models

Imogene M. King

The theory of goal attainment developed by Imogene King (1923–2007) is based on a systems model that includes three interacting systems: personal, interpersonal, and social. In this model, human beings interact with the environment, and the individual's perceptions influence reactions and interactions (Figure 7.3). Nursing involves caring for the human being, with the goal of health defined as adjusting to the stressors in both internal and external environments (King, 2007). She defines nursing as a "process of human interactions between nurse and patient whereby each perceives the other and the situation; and through communication, they set goals, explore means, and agree on means to achieve goals" (King, 1981, p. 144). This model focuses on the process that occurs between a nurse and a patient. The process is initiated to help the patient cope with a health problem that compromises his or her ability to maintain social roles, functions, and activities of daily living (King, 1992).

In this model, the person is goal oriented and purposeful, reacting to stressors, and is viewed as an open system interacting with the environment. The variables in nursing situations are as follows:

- Geographic place of the transacting system, such as the hospital
- Perceptions of the nurse and patient
- Communications of the nurse and patient
- Expectations of the nurse and patient
- Mutual goals of the nurse and patient
- The nurse and patient as a system of interdependent roles in a nursing situation (King, 1981, p. 88)

The quality of nurse–patient interactions may have positive or negative influences on the promotion of health in any nursing situation. It is within this interpersonal system of nurse and patient that the healing process is performed. Interaction is depicted in which the outcome is a **transaction**, defined as the transfer of value between two or more people. This behavior is unique, based on experience, and is goal directed.

King's work reflects her understanding of the systematic process of theory development. Her model continues to be developed and applied in national and international settings, including psychiatric–mental health care (Shanta & Connolly, 2013).

Betty Neuman

Betty Neuman (b. 1924) uses a systems approach as a model of nursing care. Neuman wants to extend care beyond an illness model, incorporating concepts of problem finding and prevention and the newer behavioral science concepts and environmental approaches to wellness. Neuman developed her framework in the late 1960s as chairwoman of the University of California at Los Angeles graduate nursing program. The key components of the model are a client system (physiological, psychological, sociocultural, developmental, spiritual) interacting with the environment. The wholistic model can be applied to prevention and treatment.

Neuman was one of the first psychiatric nurses to include the concept of stressors in understanding nursing care. The Neuman systems model is applied to a practice and educational setting, including community health, family therapy, renal nursing, perinatal nursing, and mental health nursing of older adults (Neuman & Fawcett, 2011; Beckman, Boxley-Harges, & Kaskel, 2012). This model has been applied to the practice and educational setting including international programs (Merks, Verberk, de Kuiper, & Lowry, 2012).

Dorothea Orem

Self-care is the focus of the general theory of nursing initiated by Dorothea Orem (1914–2007) in the early 1960s. The Self-Care Deficit Nursing Theory consists of three separate parts: a theory of self-care, theory of self-care deficit, and theory of nursing systems (Biggs, 2008; Orem & Taylor, 2011; Orem, 2001). The theory of self-care defines the term as activities performed independently by an individual to promote and maintain personal well-being throughout life. The central focus of Orem's theory is the self-care deficit theory, which describes how people can be helped by nursing. Nurses can help meet self-care requisites through five approaches: acting or doing for, guiding, teaching, supporting, and providing an environment to promote the patient's ability to meet current or future demands. The nursing systems theory refers to a series of actions a nurse takes to meet the patient's self-care requisites. This system varies from the patient being totally dependent on the nurse for care to needing only some education and support.

Orem's model is used in psychiatric–mental health nursing because of its emphasis on promoting independence of the individual and on self-care activities (Burdette, 2012; Seed & Torkelson, 2012). Although

---

BOX 7.5

Research for Best Practice: Keys to Successful Self-Management of Medications

Swanlund, S. L., Scherck, K. A., Metcalfe, S. A., & Jesek-Hale, S. R. (2008). Keys to successful self-management of medications. Nursing Science Quarterly, 21(3), 238–246.

QUESTION: How do community-dwelling older adults manage their medications?

METHODS: Guided by Orem's Self-Care Deficit Nursing Theory, 19 older adults were interviewed about their medication self-management practices.

FINDINGS: Three themes emerged: successful self-management of medications, living orderly, and aging well. The clear message of this study is that self-management of medication is successful when habits are established and the use of medications is integrated into the person's lifestyle.

IMPLICATIONS FOR NURSING: Many persons with mental disorders must take medications to control symptoms. Adherence to a medication regime is problematic, and there are high noncompliance rates. The results of this study suggest the strategies should be designed to reinforce the importance of routines and building medication use into the person's normal daily lifestyle.

---

many psychiatric disorders have an underlying problem, such as motivation, these problems are generally manifested as difficulties conducting ordinary self-care activities (e.g., personal hygiene) or developing independent thinking skills. See Box 7.5 for an example.

Other Nursing Theories

Other nursing models are applied in psychiatric settings. Martha Rogers' model of unitary human beings and Calista Roy's adaptation model have been the basis of many psychiatric nursing approaches.

SUMMARY OF KEY POINTS

- The traditional psychodynamic framework helped form the basis of early nursing interpersonal interventions, including the development of therapeutic relationships and the use of such concepts as transference, countertransference, empathy, and object relations.

- The behavioral theories are often used in strategies that help patients change behavior and thinking.

- Sociocultural theories remain important in understanding and interacting with patients as members of families and cultures.

- Nursing theories form the conceptual basis for nursing practice and are useful in a variety of psychiatric–mental health settings.

CRITICAL THINKING CHALLENGES

1. Discuss the similarities and differences among Freud's ideas and those of the neo-Freudians, including Jung, Adler, Horney, and Sullivan.

2. Compare and contrast the basic ideas of psychodynamic and behavioral theories.

3. Compare and differentiate classic conditioning from operant conditioning.

4. Define the following terms and discuss their applicability to psychiatric–mental health nursing: classical conditioning, operant conditioning, positive reinforcement, and negative reinforcement.

5. List the major developmental theorists and their main ideas.

6. Discuss the cognitive therapy approaches to mental disorders and how they can be used in psychiatric–mental health nursing practice.

7. Define formal and informal support systems. How does the concept of social distance relate to these two systems?

8. Compare and contrast the basic ideas of the nursing theorists.

MOVIES

Freud: 1962. This film depicts Sigmund Freud as a young physician, focusing on his early psychiatric theories and treatments. His struggles for acceptance of his ideas among the Viennese medical community are depicted. This fascinating film is well done and gives an interesting overview of the impact of psychoanalysis.

VIEWING POINTS: Watch for the impact on political thinking during the gradual acceptance of Freud's ideas. Discuss the "dream sequence" and its impact on the development of psychoanalysis as a therapeutic technique.

An Angel at My Table: 1989, New Zealand. This three-part television miniseries tells the story of Janet Frame, New Zealand's premiere novelist and poet. Based on her autobiography, the film portrays Frame as a shy, awkward child who experiences a family tragedy that alienates her socially. She studies in England to be a teacher, but her shyness and social ineptness cause extreme anxiety. Seeking mental health care, she receives a misdiagnosis of schizophrenia and spends 8 years in a mental institution. She barely escapes a lobotomy when she is notified of a literary award. She then begins to develop friendships and a new life.

VIEWING POINTS: Observe Janet Frame's childhood development. Does she "fit" any of the models that are discussed in this chapter? Consider her life in light of Gilligan and Miller's theories that it is important for women to have a sense of connection.

References

Ackerman, S., Zuroff, D. C., & Moskowitz, D. S. (2000). Generativity in midlife and young adults: Links to agency, communion, and subjective well-being. *International Journal of Aging and Human Development, 5*(1), 17–41.

Bandura, A. (1977). *Social learning theory.* Englewood Cliffs, NJ: Prentice-Hall.

Bandura, A. (1986). *Social Foundations of thought and action: A social-cognitive theory.* Englewood Cliffs, NJ: Prentice Hall.

Bandura, A. (1993). Perceived self-efficacy in cognitive development and function. American Educational Research Association Annual Meeting. *Educational Psychologist, 28*(2), 117–148.

Bandura, A. (2001). Social cognitive theory: An agentic perspective. *Annual Review of Psychology, 52,* 1–26.

Beck, A. T. (2005). The current state of cognitive therapy: A 40-year retrospective. *Archives of General Psychiatry, 62*(9), 953–959.

Beckman, S.J., Boxley-Harges, S.L. & Kaskel, B.L. (2012). Experience informs: Spanning three decades with the Neuman Systems Model. *Nursing Science Quarterly, 25*(4), 341–346.

Biggs, A. (2008). Orem's Self-Care Deficit Nursing Theory: Update on the state of the art and science. *Nursing Science Quarterly, 21*(3), 200–206.

Burdette, L. (2012). Relationship between self-care agency, self-care practices and obesity among rural midlife women. *Self-Care, Dependent-Care & Nursing, 19*(1), 5–14.

Christiansen, S. L., & Palkovitz, R. (1998). Exploring Erikson's psychosocial theory and development: Generativity and its relationship to paternal identity, intimacy, and involvement in childcare. *The Journal of Men's Studies, 7*(1), 133–156.

Doucet, T.J. (2012). Feeling strong: A Parse research method study. *Nursing Science Quarterly, 25*(1), 62–71.

Ehlman, K. & Ligon, M. (2012). The application of a generativity model for the older adults. *International Journal of Aging and Human Development, 74*(4), 331–344.

Erikson, E. (1963). *Childhood and society* (2nd ed). New York: Norton.

Erikson, E. (1968). *Identity: Youth and crisis.* New York: Norton.

Fehler-Cabral, F. & Campbell, R. (2013). Adolescent sexual assault disclosure: The impact of peers, families, and schools. *American Journal of Community Psychology, 52*(1–2), 73–83.

Freud, S. (1905). Three essays on the theory of sexuality. In J. Strachey, A. Freud, A. Strachey, & A. Tyson (Eds.). (1953). *The standard edition of the complete psychological works of Sigmund Freud* (pp. 135–248). London: Hogarth Press.

Freud, S. (1927). The ego and the id. In E. Jones (Ed.): (1957). *The international psychoanalytical library* (No. 12). London: Hogarth Press.

Friedemann, M., Newman, F. L., Buckwalter, K. C., & Montgomery R. J. (2014). Resource need and use of multiethnic caregivers of elders in their homes. *Journal of Advanced Nursing, 70*(3), 662–673.

Fromm-Rieichmann, F. (1950). *Principles of intensive psychotherapy.* Chicago: University of Chicago Press.

Gallagher-Lepak, S., & Kubsch, S. (2009). Transpersonal caring: A nursing practice guideline. *Holistic Nursing Practice, 23*(3), 171–182.

Gilligan, C. (1982). *In a different voice.* Cambridge, MA: Harvard University Press.

Gilligan, C. (2004). Recovering psyche: Reflections on life-history and history. *Annual of Psychoanalysis, 32,* 131–147.

Gilligan, C. (2011). *Joining the resistance.* Malden, MA: Polity Press.

Hogan, B. K. (2013). Caring as a scripted discourse versus caring as an expression of an authentic relationship between self and other. *Issues in Mental Health Nursing, 34*(5), 375–379.

Horney, K. (1939). *New ways in psychoanalysis.* New York: Norton.

Jung, C. (1966). On the psychology of the unconscious. The personal and the collective unconscious. In Jung, C (Ed.), *Collected works of C. G. Jung* (2nd ed, Vol. 7, pp. 64–79). Princeton, NJ: Princeton University Press.

King, I. (1981). *A theory for nursing: Systems, concepts, process.* New York: Wiley.

King, I. (1992). King's theory of goal attainment. *Nursing Science Quarterly, 5*(1), 19–26.

King, I. (2007). King's conceptual system, theory of goal attainment, and transaction process in the 21st century. *Nursing Science Quarterly, 20*(2), 109–116.

Klein, M. (1963). *Our adult world and other essays.* London: Heinemann Medical Books.

Leininger, M. (2007). Theoretical questions and concerns: Response from the Theory of Culture Care Diversity and Universality perspective. *Nursing Science Quarterly, 20,* 9–13.

Leininger, M., & McFarland, M. (2006). *Cultural care diversity and universality theory. A theory of nursing* (2nd ed). Seaburg, MA: Jones & Bartlett Publishers.

Litwak, E. (1985). Complementary roles for formal and informal support groups: A study of nursing homes and mortality rates. *Journal of Applied Behavioral Science, 21*(4), 407–425.

Litwak, E., Messeri, P., & Silverstein, M. (1990). The role of formal and informal groups in providing help to older people. *Marriage and Family Review, 15*(1–2), 171–193.

Luyten, P. & Blatt, S. J. (2012). Psychodynamic treatment of depression. *Psychiatric Clinics of North America, 35*(1), 111–129.

Maslow, A. (1970). *Motivation and personality* (rev. ed). New York: Harper & Brothers.

McIntosh, D. (2003). *Testing an intervention to increase self-efficacy of staff in managing clients perceived as violent.* University of Cincinnati, PhD dissertation. Retrieved March 7, 2007, from http://etd.iohiolink.edu/view.cgi?acc_num=ucin1069786693

McPherson, K. M., Kayes, N. K., Moloczij, N., & Cummins C. (2013). Improving the interface between informal carers and formal health and social services: A qualitative study. *International Journal of Nursing Studies, 51*(3), 418–429. doi:10.1016/j.ijnurstu.2013.07.006

Mead, M. (1970). *Culture and commitment: A study of the generation gap.* Garden City, NY: Natural History Press/Doubleday & Co.

Merks, A., Verberk, F., de Kuiper, M., Lowry, L. W. (2012). Neuman systems model in holland: An update. *Nursing Science Quarterly, 25*(4), 364–368.

Messeri, P., Silverstein, M., & Litwak, E. (1993). Choosing optimal support groups: A review and reformulation. *Journal of Health and Social Behavior, 34*(6), 122–137.

Miller, J. (1994). Women's psychological development. Connections, disconnections, and violations. In M. Berger (Ed.): *Women beyond Freud: New concepts of feminine psychology* (pp. 79–97). New York: Brunner Mazel.

Moore, B., & Fine, B. (Eds.). (1990). *Psychoanalytic terms and concepts.* New Haven, CT: The American Psychoanalytic Association and Yale University Press.

Neuman, B., & Fawcett, J. (Eds.). (2011). *The Neuman systems model* (5th ed). Upper Saddle River, NJ: Prentice Hall.

Ochse, R., & Plug, C. (1986). Cross-cultural investigation of the validity of Erikson's theory of personality development. *Journal of Personality and Social Psychology, 50*(6), 1240–1252.

Olson, J., & Hanchett, E. (1997). Nurse-expressed empathy, patient outcomes, and the development of a middle-range theory. *Image: The Journal of Nursing Scholarship, 29*(1), 71–76.

Orem, D. (2001). *Nursing concepts of practice* (6th ed). St. Louis: Mosby.

Orem, D. E. & Taylor, S. G. (2011). Reflections on nursing practice science: The nature, the structure, and the foundation of nursing sciences. *Nursing Science Quarterly, 24*(1), 35–41.

Orlando, I. J. (1961). *The dynamic nurse–patient relationship.* New York: G. P. Putnam's Sons.

Orlando, I. J. (1972). *The discipline and teaching of nursing process.* New York: G. P. Putnam's Sons.

Orlofsky, J., Marcia, J., & Lesser, I. (1973). Ego identity status and the intimacy versus isolation crisis of young adulthood. *Journal of Personality and Social Psychology, 27*(2), 211–219.

Parse, R. R. (1996). Reality: A seamless symphony of becoming. *Nursing Science Quarterly, 9*, 181–184.

Parse, R. R. (1998). *The human becoming school of thoughts: A perspective for nurses and other health professionals.* London: Sage.

Parse, R. R. (2007). The human becoming school of thought in 2050. *Nursing Science Quarterly, 20*, 308–311.

Parse, R. R. (2008). The humanbecoming leading-following model. *Nursing Science Quarterly, 21*, 369–375.

Pavlov, I. P. (1927/1960). *Conditioned reflexes.* New York: Dover Publications.

Peplau, H. (1952). *Interpersonal relations in nursing.* New York: G. Putnam & Sons.

Peplau, H. (1992). Interpersonal relations: A theoretical framework for application in nursing practice. *Nursing Science Quarterly, 5*(1), 13–18.

Perls, F. (1969). *In and out of the garbage pail.* Lafayette, CA: Real People Press.

Potter, M. L., & Bockenhauer, B. J. (2000). Implementing Orlando's nursing theory. *Journal of Psychosocial Nursing and Mental Health Services, 38*(13), 14–21.

Pratt, M. W., Norris, J. E., Cressman, K., Lawford, H., & Hebblethwaite, S. (2008). Parents' stories of grandparenting concerns in the three-generational family: Generativity, optimism, and forgiveness. *Journal of Personality, 76*(3), 581–604.

Riggs, S. R., & Bright, M. S. (1997). Dissociative identity disorder: A feminist approach to inpatient treatment using Jean Baker Miller's relational model. *Archives of Psychiatric Nursing, 11*(4), 218–224.

Rogers, C. (1980). *A way of being.* Boston: Houghton Mifflin.

Seed, M. S. & Torkelson, D. J. (2012). Beginning the recovery journey in acute psychiatric care: Using concepts from Orem's self-care deficit nursing theory. *Issues in Mental Health Nursing, 33*(6), 394–398.

Shanta, L. L. & Connolly, M. (2013). Using King's interacting systems theory to link emotional intelligence and nursing practice. *Journal of Professional Nursing, 29*(3), 174–180.

Shin, Y., Yun, S., Pender, N. J., & Jang, H. (2005). Test of the health promotion model as a causal model of commitment to a plan for exercise among Korean adults with chronic disease. *Research in Nursing & Health, 28*(2), 117–125.

Skinner, B. F. (1935). The generic nature of the concepts of stimulus and response. *Journal of General Psychology, 12*, 40–65.

Sullivan, G. (2004). A four-fold humanity: Margaret Mead and psychological types. *Journal of the History of the Behavioral Sciences, 40*(2), 183–206.

Sullivan, H. (1953). *The interpersonal theory of psychiatry.* New York: Norton.

Thorndike, E. L. (1906). *The principles of teaching, based on psychology.* New York: A.G. Seiler.

Walker, M., & Rosen, W. B. (2004). *How connections heal: Stories from relational-cultural therapy.* New York: Guilford Press.

Watson, J. (2005). *Caring science as sacred science.* Philadelphia: F. A. Davis.

Watson, J. (2007). Theoretical questions and concerns: Response from a Caring Science Framework. *Nursing Science Quarterly, 20*, 13–15.

Watson, J. B., & Rayner, R. (1920). Conditioned emotional reactions. *Journal of Experimental Psychology, 3*, 1–14.

Westermeyer, J. F. (2004). Predictors and characteristics of Erikson's life cycle model among men: A 32-year longitudinal study. *International Journal of Aging & Human Development, 58*(1), 29–48.

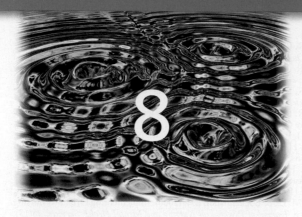

8

Biologic Foundations of Psychiatric Nursing

Mary Ann Boyd

KEY CONCEPTS

- neuroplasticity
- neurotransmitters

LEARNING OBJECTIVES

After studying this chapter, you will be able to:

1. Describe the association between biologic functioning and symptoms of psychiatric disorders.

2. Locate brain structures primarily involved in psychiatric disorders and describe the primary functions of these structures.

3. Describe basic mechanisms of neuronal transmission.

4. Identify the location and function of neurotransmitters significant to hypotheses regarding major mental disorders.

5. Discuss the role of genetics in the development of psychiatric disorders.

6. Discuss the basic utilization of new knowledge gained from fields of study, including psychoneuroimmunology and chronobiology.

KEY TERMS

- acetylcholine • amino acids • autonomic nervous system • basal ganglia • biogenic amines • biologic markers
- brain stem • cerebellum • chronobiology • circadian cycle • cortex • dopamine • extrapyramidal motor system • frontal, parietal, temporal, and occipital lobes • functional imaging • GABA • genetic susceptibility
- glutamate • hippocampus • histamine • limbic system • locus ceruleus • neurocircuitry • neurohormones
- neurons • neuromodulators • neuropeptides • norepinephrine • phenotype • pineal body • population genetics • proband • psychoneuroimmunology • receptor • serotonin • structural imaging • synaptic cleft
- working memory • zeitgebers

All behavior recognized as human results from actions that originate in the brain and its amazing interconnection of neural networks. Modern research has increased understanding of how the complex circuitry of the brain interacts with the external environment, memories, and experiences. Through the spinal column and peripheral nerves, along with other systems, such as the endocrine and immune systems, the brain constantly receives and processes information. As the brain shifts and sorts through the amazing amount of information it processes every hour, it decides on actions and initiates behaviors, allowing each person to act in entirely unique and very human ways.

Mental disorders cannot be traced to specific physiological problems but rather are complex syndromes consisting of biopsychosocial symptoms that more or less cluster together. Therefore, it is important for the nurse to understand basic nervous system functioning, as well as some of the research that is exploring the biologic basis of mental disorders.

This chapter reviews the basic information necessary for understanding neuroscience as it relates to the role of the psychiatric–mental health nurse. It reviews basic central nervous system (CNS) structures and functions, the peripheral nervous system (PNS), general functions of the major neurotransmitters and receptors, basic principles of neurotransmission, genetic models, circadian rhythms, and biologic tests. The chapter assumes that the reader has a basic knowledge of human biology, anatomy, and pathophysiology. It is not intended as a full presentation of neuroanatomy and physiology but rather as an overview of the structures and functions most critical to understanding the role of the psychiatric–mental health nurse. Psychiatric–mental health nurses must be able to make the connection between (1) patients' psychiatric symptoms, (2) the probable alterations in brain functioning linked to those symptoms, and (3) the rationale for treatment and care practices.

NEUROANATOMY OF THE CENTRAL NERVOUS SYSTEM

Although this section discusses functioning areas of the brain separately, each area is intricately connected with the others, and each functions interactively. The CNS contains the brain, brain stem, and spinal cord, and the PNS consists of the neurons that connect the CNS to the muscles, organs, and other systems in the periphery of the body. Whatever affects the CNS may also affect the PNS and vice versa.

Cerebrum

The largest region of the human brain, the cerebrum fills the entire upper portion of the cranium. The **cortex**, or outermost surface of the cerebrum, makes up about 80% of the human brain. The cortex is four to six cellular layers thick, and each layer is composed of cell bodies mixed with capillary blood vessels. This mixture makes the cortex gray brown (thus the term *gray matter*). The cortex consists of numerous bumps and grooves in a fully developed adult brain, as shown in Figure 8.1. This "wrinkling" allows for a large amount of surface area to be confined in the limited space of the skull. The increased surface area allows for more potential connections among cells within the cortex. The grooves are called *fissures* if they extend deep into the brain and *sulci* if they are shallower. The bumps or convolutions are called *gyri*. Together, they provide many of the landmarks for the subdivisions of the cortex. The longest and deepest groove, the longitudinal fissure, separates the cerebrum into left and right hemispheres. Although these two divisions are nearly symmetric, there is some variation in the location and size of the sulci and gyri in each hemisphere. Substantial variation in these convolutions is found in the cortex of different individuals.

Left and Right Hemispheres

The cerebrum can be roughly divided into two halves, or hemispheres. The left hemisphere is dominant in about 95% of people, but about 5% of individuals have mixed dominance. Each hemisphere controls functioning mainly on the opposite side of the body. Aside from controlling activities on the left side of the body, the right hemisphere

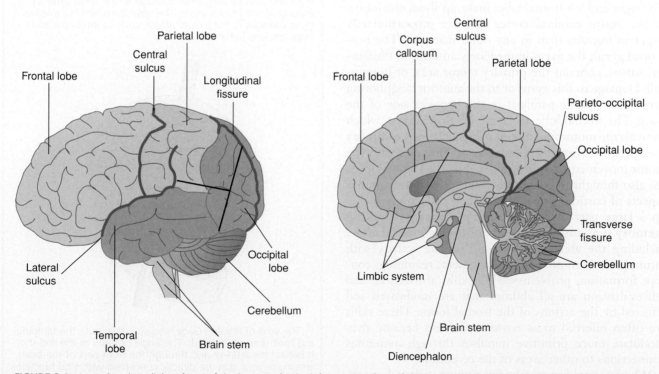

FIGURE 8.1 Lateral and medial surfaces of the brain. *Left*, The left lateral surface of the brain. *Right*, The medial surface of the right half of a sagittally hemisected brain.

also provides input into receptive nonverbal communication, spatial orientation and recognition, intonation of speech and aspects of music, facial recognition and facial expression of emotion, and nonverbal learning and memory. In general, the left hemisphere is more involved with verbal language function, including areas for both receptive and expressive speech control, and provides strong contributions to temporal order and sequencing, numeric symbols, and verbal learning and memory.

The two hemispheres are connected by the corpus callosum, a bundle of neuronal tissue that allows information to be exchanged quickly between the right and left hemispheres. An intact corpus callosum is required for the hemispheres to function in a smooth and coordinated manner.

Lobes of the Brain

The lateral surface of each hemisphere is further divided into four lobes: the **frontal, parietal, temporal, and occipital lobes** (see Figure 8.1). The lobes work in coordinated ways, but each is responsible for specific functions. An understanding of these unique functions is helpful in understanding how damage to these areas produces the symptoms of mental illness and how medications that affect the functioning of these lobes can produce certain effects.

Frontal Lobes

The right and left frontal lobes make up about one fourth of the entire cerebral cortex and are proportionately larger in humans than in any other mammal. The precentral gyrus, the gyrus immediately anterior to the central sulcus, contains the primary motor area, or homunculi. Damage to this gyrus or to the anterior neighboring gyri causes spastic paralysis in the opposite side of the body. The frontal lobe also contains Broca's area, which controls the motor function of speech. Damage to Broca's area produces expressive aphasia, or difficulty with the motor movements required for speech. The frontal lobes are also thought to contain the highest or most complex aspects of cortical functioning, which collectively makes up a large part of what we call personality. **Working memory** is an important aspect of frontal lobe function, including the ability to plan and initiate activity with future goals in mind. Insight, judgment, reasoning, concept formation, problem-solving skills, abstraction, and self-evaluation are all abilities that are modulated and affected by the actions of the frontal lobes. These skills are often referred to as *executive functions* because they modulate more primitive impulses through numerous connections to other areas of the cerebrum.

When normal frontal lobe functioning is altered, executive functioning is decreased, and modulation of impulses

can be lost, leading to changes in mood and personality. The importance of the frontal lobe and its role in the development of symptoms common to psychiatric disorders are emphasized in later chapters that discuss disorders such as schizophrenia, attention deficit hyperactivity disorder (ADHD), and dementia. Box 8.1 describes how altered frontal lobe function can affect mood and personality.

Parietal Lobes

The postcentral gyrus, immediately behind the central sulcus, contains the primary somatosensory area. Damage to this area and neighboring gyri results in deficits in discriminative sensory function but not in the ability to perceive sensory input. The posterior areas of the parietal lobe appear to coordinate visual and somatosensory

---

BOX 8.1

Frontal Lobe Syndrome

In the 1860s, Phineas Gage became a famous example of frontal lobe dysfunction. Mr. Gage was a New England railroad worker who had a thick iron-tamping rod propelled through his frontal lobes by an explosion. He survived, but suffered significant changes in his personality. Mr. Gage, who had previously been a capable and calm supervisor, began to show impatience, labile mood, disrespect for others, and frequent use of profanity after his injury (Harlow, 1868). Similar conditions are often called *frontal lobe syndrome*. Symptoms vary widely from individual to individual. In general, after damage to the dorsolateral (upper and outer) areas of the frontal lobes, the symptoms include a lack of drive and spontaneity. With damage to the most anterior aspects of the frontal lobes, the symptoms tend to involve more changes in mood and affect, such as impulsive and inappropriate behavior.

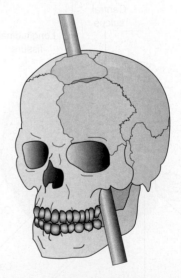

The skull of Phineas Gage, showing the route the tamping rod took through his skull. The angle of entry of the rod shot it behind the left eye and through the front part of the brain, sparing regions that are directly concerned with vital functions like breathing and heartbeat.

information. Damage to this area produces complex sensory deficits, including neglect of contralateral sensory stimuli and spatial relationships. The parietal lobes contribute to the ability to recognize objects by touch, calculate, write, recognize fingers of the opposite hands, draw, and organize spatial directions (e.g., how to travel to familiar places).

Temporal Lobes

The temporal lobes contain the primary auditory and olfactory areas. Wernicke's area, located at the posterior aspect of the superior temporal gyrus, is primarily responsible for receptive speech. The temporal lobes also integrate sensory and visual information involved in control of written and verbal language skills as well as visual recognition. The hippocampus, an important structure discussed later, lies in the internal aspects of each temporal lobe and contributes to memory. Other internal structures of this lobe are involved in the modulation of mood and emotion.

Occipital Lobes

The primary visual area is located in the most posterior aspect of the occipital lobes. Damage to this area results in a condition called *cortical blindness*. In other words, the retina and optic nerve remain intact, but the individual cannot see. The occipital lobes are involved in many aspects of visual integration of information, including color vision, object and facial recognition, and the ability to perceive objects in motion.

Association Cortex

Although not a lobe, the association cortex is an important area that allows the lobes to work in an integrated manner. Areas of one lobe of the cortex often share functions with an area of the adjacent lobe. When these neighboring nerve fibers are related to the same sensory modality, they are often referred to as *association areas*. For example, an area in the inferior parietal, posterior temporal, and anterior occipital lobes integrates visual, somatosensory, and auditory information to provide the abilities required for basic academic skills. These areas, along with numerous connections beneath the cortex, are part of the mechanisms that allow the human brain to work as an integrated whole.

Subcortical Structures

Beneath the cortex are layers of tissue composed of the axons of cell bodies. The axonal tissue forms pathways that are surrounded by glia, a fatty or lipid substance, which has a white appearance and give these layers of neuron axons their name—white matter. Structures inside the hemispheres, beneath the cortex, are considered subcortical. Many of these structures, essential in the regulation of emotions and behaviors, play important roles in our understanding of mental disorders. Figure 8.2 provides a coronal section view of the gray matter, white matter, and important subcortical structures.

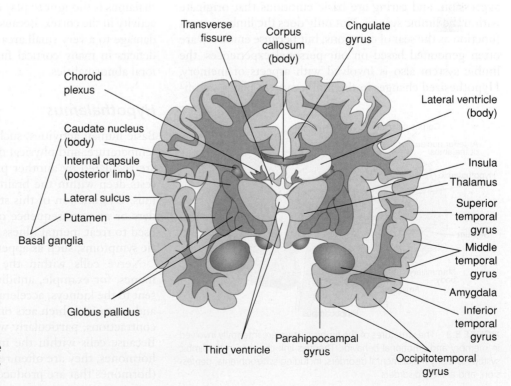

FIGURE 8.2 Coronal section of the brain, illustrating the corpus callosum, basal ganglia, and lateral ventricles.

The **basal ganglia** are subcortical gray matter areas in both the right and the left hemisphere that contain many cell bodies or nuclei. The primary subdivisions of the basal ganglia are the putamen, globus pallidus, and caudate. The basal ganglia are involved with motor functions and association in both the learning and the programming of behavior or activities that are repetitive and, done over time, become automatic. The basal ganglia have many connections with the cerebral cortex, thalamus, midbrain structures, and spinal cord. Damage to portions of these nuclei may produce changes in posture or muscle tone. In addition, damage may produce abnormal movements, such as twitches or tremors. The basal ganglia can be adversely affected by some of the medications used to treat psychiatric disorders, leading to side effects and other motor-related problems.

Limbic System

The **limbic system** is essential to understanding the many hypotheses related to psychiatric disorders and emotional behavior in general. The limbic system is called a "system" because it comprises several small structures that work in a highly organized way. These structures include the hippocampus, thalamus, hypothalamus, amygdala, and limbic midbrain nuclei. See Figure 8.3 for identification and location of the structures within the limbic system and their relationships to other common CNS structures.

Basic emotions, needs, drives, and instinct begin and are modulated in the limbic system. Hate, love, anger, aggression, and caring are basic emotions that originate within the limbic system. Not only does the limbic system function as the seat of emotions, but because emotions are often generated based on our personal experiences, the limbic system also is involved with aspects of memory. Hypothesized changes in the limbic system play a signifi-

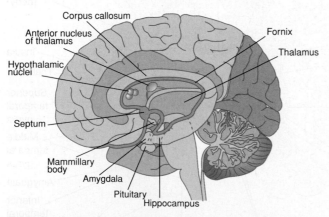

FIGURE 8.3 The structures of the limbic system are integrally involved in memory and emotional behavior. Theories link changes in the limbic system to many major mental disorders, including schizophrenia, depression, and anxiety disorders.

cant role in many theories of major mental disorders, including schizophrenia, depression, and anxiety disorders (discussed in later chapters).

Hippocampus

The **hippocampus** is involved in storing information, especially the emotions attached to a memory. Our emotional responses to memories and our associations with other related memories are functions of how information is stored within the hippocampus. Although memory storage is not limited to one area of the brain, destruction of the left hippocampus impairs verbal memory, and damage to the right hippocampus results in difficulty with recognition and recall of complex visual and auditory patterns. Deterioration of the nerves of the hippocampus and other related temporal lobe structures found in Alzheimer's disease produces the disorder's hallmark symptoms of memory dysfunction.

Thalamus

Sometimes called the "relay-switching center of the brain," the thalamus functions as a regulatory structure to relay all sensory information, except smell, sent to the CNS from the PNS. From the thalamus, the sensory information is relayed mostly to the cerebral cortex. The thalamus relays and regulates by filtering incoming information and determining what to pass on or not pass on to the cortex. In this fashion, the thalamus prevents the cortex from becoming overloaded with sensory stimulus. The thalamus is thought to play a part in controlling electrical activity in the cortex. Because of its primary relay function, damage to a very small area of the thalamus may produce deficits in many cortical functions, thus, causing behavioral abnormalities.

Hypothalamus

Basic human activities, such as sleep–rest patterns, body temperature, and physical drives such as hunger and sex, are regulated by another part of the limbic system that rests deep within the brain and is called the hypothalamus. Dysfunction of this structure, whether from disorders or as a consequence of the adverse effect of drugs used to treat mental illness, produces common psychiatric symptoms, such as appetite and sleep problems.

Nerve cells within the hypothalamus secrete hormones, for example, antidiuretic hormone, which when sent to the kidneys, accelerates the reabsorption of water; and oxytocin, which acts on smooth muscles to promote contractions, particularly within the walls of the uterus. Because cells within the nervous system produce these hormones, they are often referred to as **neurohormones** (hormones that are produced by cells within the nervous system) and form a communication mechanism through the bloodstream to control organs that are not directly connected to nervous system structures.

The pituitary gland, often called the *master gland*, is directly connected by thousands of neurons that attach it to the ventral aspects of the hypothalamus. Together with the pituitary gland, the hypothalamus functions as one of the primary regulators of many aspects of the endocrine system. Its functions are involved in control of visceral activities, such as body temperature, arterial blood pressure, hunger, thirst, fluid balance, gastric motility, and gastric secretions. Deregulation of the hypothalamus can be manifested in symptoms of certain psychiatric disorders. For example, in schizophrenia, patients often wear heavy coats during the hot summer months and do not appear hot. Before the role of the hypothalamus in schizophrenia was understood, psychological reasons were used to explain such symptoms. Now it is increasingly clear that such a symptom relates to deregulation of the hypothalamus's normal role in temperature regulation and is a biologically based symptom (Kreuzer et al., 2012).

Amygdala

The amygdala is directly connected to more primitive centers of the brain involving the sense of smell. It has numerous connections to the hypothalamus and lies adjacent to the hippocampus. The amygdala provides an emotional component to memory and is involved in modulating aggression and sexuality. Impulsive acts of aggression and violence have been linked to dysregulation of the amygdala, and erratic firing of the nerve cells in the amygdala is a focus of investigation in bipolar mood disorders (see Chapter 25).

Limbic Midbrain Nuclei

The limbic midbrain nuclei are a collection of neurons (including the ventral tegmental area and the locus ceruleus) that appear to play a role in the biologic basis of addiction. Sometimes referred to as the pleasure center or reward center of the brain, the limbic midbrain nuclei function to chemically reinforce certain behaviors, ensuring their repetition. Emotions such as feeling satisfied with good food, the pleasure of nurturing young, and the enjoyment of sexual activity originate in the limbic midbrain nuclei. The reinforcement of activities such as nutrition, procreation, and nurturing young are all primitive aspects of ensuring the survival of a species. When functioning in abnormal ways, the limbic midbrain nuclei can begin to reinforce unhealthy or risky behaviors, such as drug abuse. Exploration of this area of the brain is in its infancy but offers potential insight into addictions and their treatment.

Other Central Nervous System Structures

The **extrapyramidal motor system** is a bundle of nerve fibers connecting the thalamus to the basal ganglia and cerebral cortex. Muscle tone, common reflexes, and automatic voluntary motor functioning (e.g., walking) are controlled by this nerve track. Dysfunction of this motor track can produce hypertonicity in muscle groups. In Parkinson's disease, the cells that compose the extrapyramidal motor system are severely affected, producing many involuntary motor movements. A number of medications, which are discussed in Chapter 11, also affect this system.

The **pineal body** is located above and medial to the thalamus. Because the pineal gland easily calcifies, it can be visualized by neuroimaging and often is a medial landmark. Its functions remain somewhat of a mystery despite long knowledge of its existence. It contains secretory cells that emit the neurohormone melatonin and other substances. These hormones are thought to have a number of regulatory functions within the endocrine system. Information received from light–dark sources controls release of melatonin, which has been associated with sleep and emotional disorders. In addition, a modulation of immune function has been postulated for melatonin from the pineal gland.

The **locus ceruleus** is a tiny cluster of neurons that fan out and innervate almost every part of the brain, including most of the cortex, the thalamus and hypothalamus, the cerebellum, and the spinal cord. Just one neuron from the ceruleus can connect to more than 250,000 other neurons. Despite its small size, the wide-ranging neuronal connections allow this tiny structure to influence the regulation of attention, time perception, sleep–rest cycles, arousal, learning, pain, and mood. It also plays a role in information processing of new, unexpected, and novel experiences. Some think its function or dysfunction may explain why individuals become addicted to substances and seek out risky behaviors despite awareness of negative consequences.

The **brain stem**, which is located beneath the thalamus and composed of the midbrain, pons, and medulla, has important life-sustaining functions. Nuclei of numerous neural pathways to the cerebrum are located in the brain stem. They are significantly involved in mediating symptoms of emotional dysfunction. These nuclei are also the primary source of several neurochemicals, such as serotonin, that are commonly associated with psychiatric disorders.

The **cerebellum** is in the posterior aspect of the skull beneath the cerebral hemispheres. This large structure controls movements and postural adjustments. To regulate postural balance and positioning, the cerebellum receives information from all parts of the body, including the muscles, joints, skin, and visceral organs, as well as from many parts of the CNS.

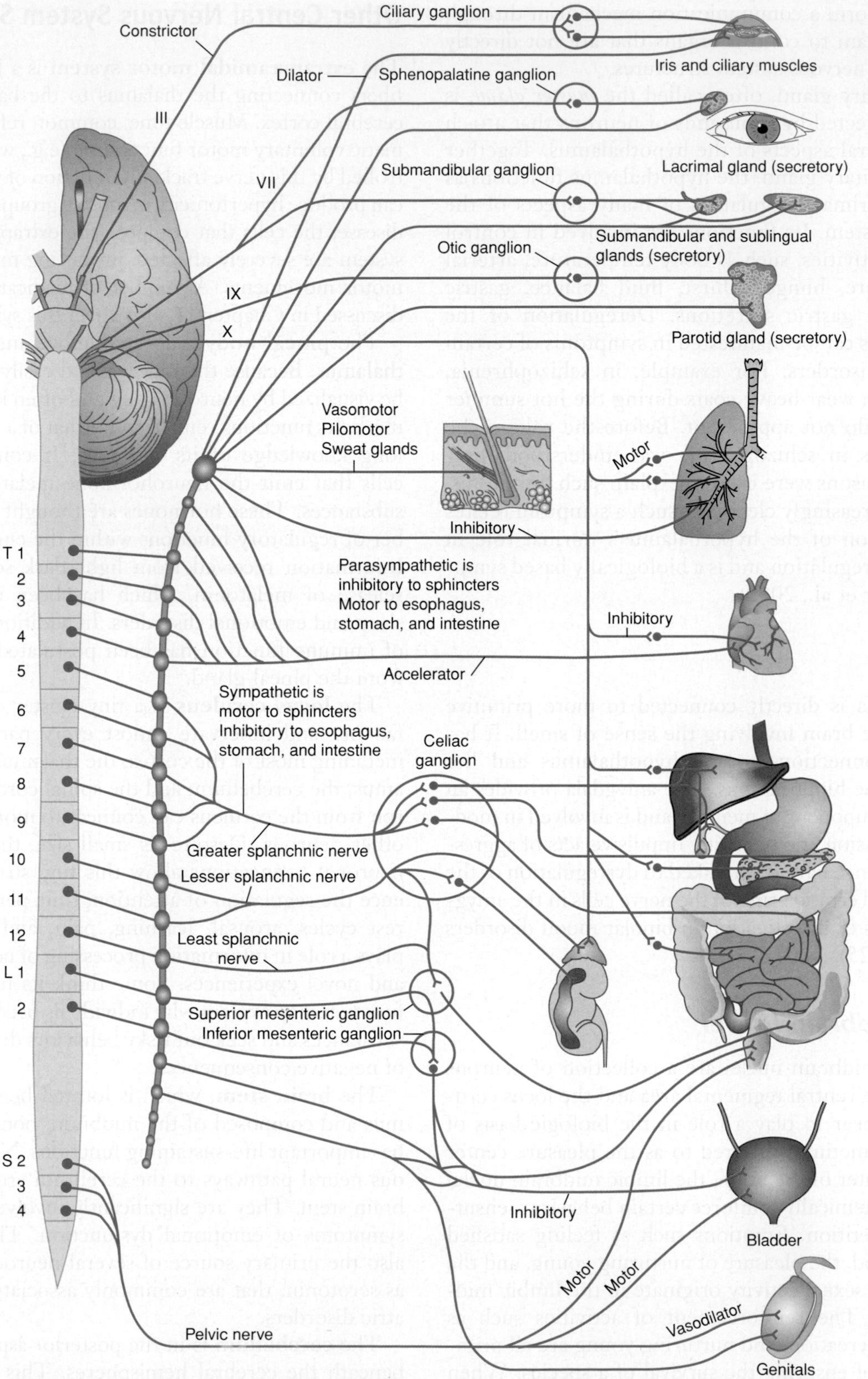

FIGURE 8.4 Diagram of the autonomic nervous system. Note that many organs are innervated by both sympathetic and parasympathetic nerves. (Adapted from Schaffe, E. E., & Lytle, I. M. [1980]. *Basic physiology and anatomy*. Philadelphia: J. B. Lippincott.)

Autonomic Nervous System

Closely associated with the spinal cord but not lying entirely within its column is the **autonomic nervous system**, a subdivision of the PNS. It was originally given this name for being independent of conscious thought, that is, automatic. However, it does not necessarily function as autonomously as the name indicates. This system contains efferent (nerves moving away from the CNS), or motor system neurons, which affect target tissues such as cardiac muscle, smooth muscle, and the glands. It also contains afferent nerves, which are sensory and conduct information from these organs back to the CNS.

The autonomic nervous system is further divided into the sympathetic and parasympathetic nervous systems. These systems, although peripheral, are included here because they are involved in the emergency, or "fight-or-flight," response as well as the peripheral actions of many

medications (see Chapter 11). Figure 8.4 illustrates the innervations of various target organs by the autonomic nervous system. Table 8.1 identifies the actions of the sympathetic and parasympathetic nervous systems on various target organs.

NEUROPHYSIOLOGY OF THE CENTRAL NERVOUS SYSTEM

At their most basic level, the human brain and connecting nervous system are composed of billions of cells. Most are connective and supportive glial cells with ancillary functions in the nervous system.

> **KEYCONCEPT** **Neuroplasticity** is a continuous process of modulation of neuronal structure and function in response to the changing environment.

Table 8.1	PERIPHERAL ORGAN RESPONSE IN THE AUTONOMIC NERVOUS SYSTEM	
Effector Organ	**Sympathetic Response (Mostly Norepinephrine)**	**Parasympathetic Response (Acetylcholine)**
Eye		
• Iris sphincter muscle	Dilation	Constriction
• Ciliary muscle	Relaxation	Accommodation for near vision
Heart		
• Sinoatrial node	Increased rate	Decrease is rare
• Atria	Increased contractility	Decrease in contractility
• Atrioventricular node	Increased contractility	Decrease in conduction velocity
Blood vessels	Constriction	Dilation
Lungs		
• Bronchial muscles	Relaxation	Bronchoconstriction
• Bronchial glands		Secretion
Gastrointestinal Tract		
• Motility and tone	Relaxation	Increased
• Sphincters	Contraction	Relaxation
• Secretion		Stimulation
Urinary Bladder		
• Detrusor muscle	Relaxation	Contraction
• Trigone and sphincter	Contraction	Relaxation
Uterus	Contraction (pregnant) Relaxation (nonpregnant)	Variable
Skin		
• Pilomotor muscles	Contraction	No effect
• Sweat glands	Increased secretion	No effect
Glands		
• Salivary, lachrymal		Increased secretion
• Sweat		Increased secretion

The changes in neural environment can come from internal sources, such as a change in electrolytes, or from external sources, such as a virus or toxin. Because of neuroplasticity, nerve signals may be rerouted, cells may learn new functions, the sensitivity or number of cells may increase or decrease, and some nerve tissue may undergo limited regeneration. Brains are most plastic during infancy and young childhood, when large adaptive learning tasks should normally occur. With age, brains become less plastic, which explains why it is easier to learn a second language at the age of 5 years than 55 years. Neuroplasticity contributes to understanding how function may be restored over time after brain damage occurs, or how an individual may react over time to continuous pharmacotherapy regimens.

Neurons and Nerve Impulses

In the human body, approximately 10 billion nerve cells, or **neurons**, function to receive, organize, and transmit information (Figure 8.5). Each neuron has a cell body, or soma, which holds the nucleus containing most of the cell's genetic information. The soma also includes other organelles, such as ribosomes and endoplasmic reticulum, which carry out protein synthesis; the Golgi apparatus, which contains enzymes to modify the proteins for specific functions; vesicles, which transport and store proteins; and lysosomes, which are responsible for degradation of these proteins. Located throughout the neurons, mitochondria, containing enzymes and often called the "powerhouse" are the sites of many energy-producing chemical reactions. These cell structures provide the basis for secreting numerous chemicals by which neurons communicate.

It is not just the vast number of neurons that accounts for the complexities of the brain but also the enormous number of neurochemical interconnections and interactions among neurons. A single motor neuron in the spinal cord may receive signals from more than 10,000 sources of interconnections with other nerves. Although most neurons have only one axon, which varies in length and conducts impulses away from the soma, each has numerous dendrites, receiving signals from other neurons. Because

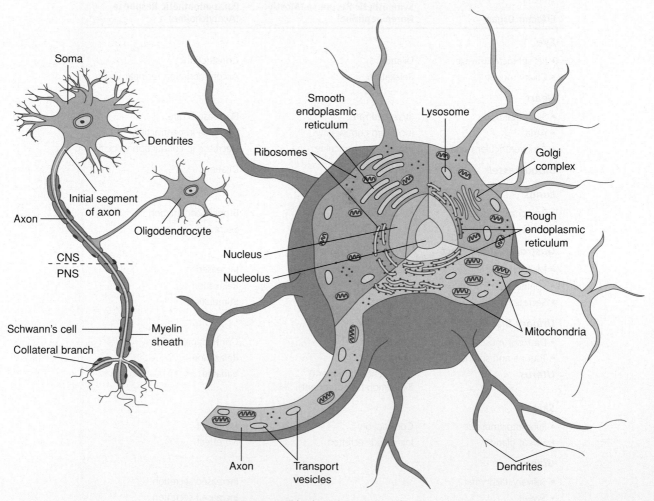

FIGURE 8.5 Cell body and organelles of neuron.

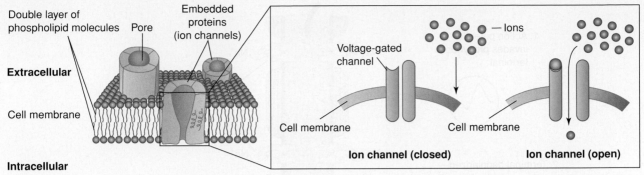

FIGURE 8.6 Initiation of a nerve impulse. The initiation of an action potential, or nerve impulse, involves the opening and closing of the voltage-gated channels on the cell membrane and the passage of ions into the cell. The resulting electrical activity sends communication impulses from the dendrites or axon into the body.

axons may branch as they terminate, they also have multiple contacts with other neurons.

Nerve signals are prompted to fire by a variety of chemical or physical stimuli. This firing produces an electrical impulse. The cell's membrane is a double layer of phospholipid molecules with embedded proteins. Some of these proteins provide water-filled channels through which inorganic ions may pass (Figure 8.6). Each of the common ions—sodium, potassium, calcium, and chloride—has its own specific molecular channel. Many of these channels are voltage gated and thus open or close in response to changes in the electrical potential across the membrane. At rest, the cell membrane is polarized with a positive charge on the outside and about a 270-millivolt charge on the inside, owing to the resting distribution of sodium and potassium ions. As potassium passively diffuses across the membrane, the sodium pump uses energy to move sodium from the inside of the cell against a concentration gradient to maintain this distribution. An action potential, or *nerve impulse*, is generated as the membrane is depolarized and a threshold value is reached, which triggers the opening of the voltage-gated sodium channels, allowing sodium to surge into the cell. The inside of the cell briefly becomes positively charged and the outside negatively charged. Once initiated, the action potential becomes self-propagating, opening nearby sodium channels. This electrical communication moves into the soma from the dendrites or down the axon by this mechanism.

Synaptic Transmission

For one neuron to communicate with another, the electrical process described must change to a chemical communication. The **synaptic cleft**, a junction between one nerve and another, is the space where the electrical intracellular signal becomes a chemical extracellular signal. Various substances are recognized as the chemical messengers among neurons.

As the electrical action potential reaches the ends of the axons, called *terminals*, calcium ion channels are opened, allowing an influx of Ca++ ions into the neuron. This increase in calcium stimulates the release of neurotransmitters into the synapse. Rapid signaling among neurons requires a ready supply of neurotransmitter. These neurotransmitters are stored in small vesicles grouped near the cell membrane at the end of the axon. When stimulated, the vesicles containing the neurotransmitter fuse with the cell membrane, and the neurotransmitter is released into the synapse (Figure 8.7). The neurotransmitter then crosses the synaptic cleft to a receptor site on the postsynaptic neuron and stimulates adjacent neurons. This is the process of neuronal communication.

When the neurotransmitter has completed its interaction with the postsynaptic receptor and stimulated that cell, its work is done, and it needs to be removed. It can be removed by natural diffusion away from the area of high neurotransmitter concentration at the receptors by being broken down by enzymes in the synaptic cleft or through reuptake through highly specific mechanisms into the presynaptic terminal. The primary steps in synaptic transmission are summarized in Figure 8.7.

Neurotransmitters

As described in the overview above, neurotransmitters are key in the process of synaptic transmission. Neurotransmitters are small molecules that directly and indirectly control the opening or closing of ion channels. **Neuromodulators** are chemical messengers that make the target cell membrane or postsynaptic membrane more or less susceptible to the effects of the primary neurotransmitter.

> **KEYCONCEPT** **Neurotransmitters** are small molecules that directly and indirectly control the opening or closing of ion channels.

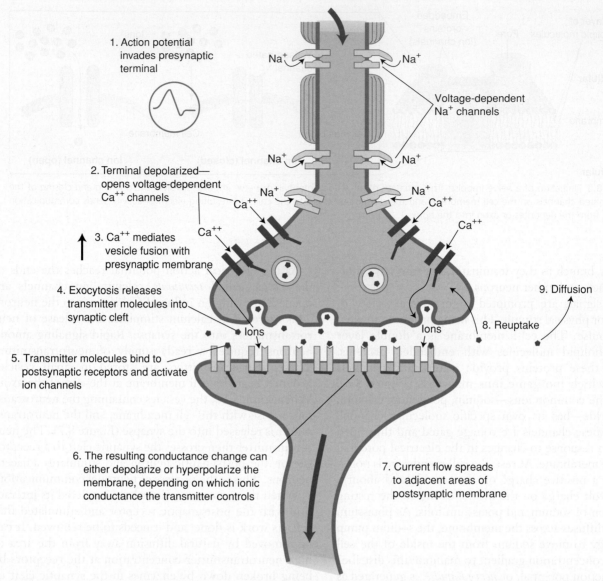

1. Action potential invades presynaptic terminal

Na⁺ ← → Na⁺

Voltage-dependent Na⁺ channels

Na⁺ Na⁺

2. Terminal depolarized— opens voltage-dependent Ca⁺⁺ channels

Na⁺ Na⁺

Ca⁺⁺ Ca⁺⁺

Ca⁺⁺ Ca⁺⁺

3. Ca⁺⁺ mediates vesicle fusion with presynaptic membrane

4. Exocytosis releases transmitter molecules into synaptic cleft

9. Diffusion

8. Reuptake

Ions Ions

5. Transmitter molecules bind to postsynaptic receptors and activate ion channels

6. The resulting conductance change can either depolarize or hyperpolarize the membrane, depending on which ionic conductance the transmitter controls

7. Current flow spreads to adjacent areas of postsynaptic membrane

FIGURE 8.7 Synaptic transmission. The most significant events that occur during synaptic transmission: (1) the action potential reaches the presynaptic terminal; (2) membrane depolarization causes Ca⁺⁺ terminals to open; (3) Ca⁺⁺ mediates fusion of the vesicles with the presynaptic membrane; (4) transmitter molecules are released into the synaptic cleft by exocytosis; (5) transmitter molecules bind to postsynaptic receptors and activate ion channels; (6) conductance changes cause an excitatory or inhibitory postsynaptic potential, depending on the specific transmitter; (7) current flow spreads along the postsynaptic membrane; (8) transmitter remaining in the synaptic cleft returns to the presynaptic terminal by reuptake; and (9) diffuses into the extracellular fluid. (Adapted from Schauf, C., Moffett, D., & Moffett, S. [1990]. *Human physiology.* St. Louis: Times Mirror/Mosby.)

Excitatory neurotransmitters reduce the membrane potential and enhance the transmission of the signal between neurons. *Inhibitory neurotransmitters* have the opposite effect and slow down nerve impulses. Although some are synthesized from dietary precursors, such as tyrosine or tryptophan, most synthesis occurs in the terminals or the neuron itself. Neurotransmitters are commonly classified as the following: cholinergic, biogenic amine (monoamines or bioamines), amino acid, and neuropeptides. Table 8.2 summarizes some of the key neurotransmitters and their proposed functions.

Acetylcholine

Acetylcholine (ACh) is the primary cholinergic neurotransmitter. Found in the greatest concentration in the PNS, ACh provides the basic synaptic communication for the parasympathetic neurons and part of the sympathetic neurons, which send information to the CNS.

Table 8.2	CLASSIC AND PUTATIVE NEUROTRANSMITTERS: THEIR DISTRIBUTION AND PROPOSED FUNCTIONS		
Neurotransmitter	**Cell Bodies**	**Projections**	**Proposed Function**
Acetylcholine			
Dietary precursor: choline	Basal forebrain Pons Other areas	Diffuse throughout the cortex, hippocampus PNS	Important role in learning and memory Some role in wakefulness and basic attention Peripherally activates muscles and is the major neurochemical in the autonomic system
Monoamines			
Dopamine (dietary precursor: tyrosine)	Substantia nigra Ventral tegmental area Arcuate nucleus Retina olfactory bulb	Striatum (basal ganglia) Limbic system and cerebral cortex Pituitary	Involved in involuntary motor movements Some role in mood states, pleasure components in reward systems, and complex behavior (e.g., judgment, reasoning, insight)
Norepinephrine (dietary precursor: tyrosine)	Locus ceruleus Lateral tegmental area and others throughout the pons and medulla	Very widespread throughout the cortex, thalamus, cerebellum, brain stem, and spinal cord Basal forebrain, thalamus, hypothalamus, brain stem, and spinal cord	Proposed role in learning and memory, attributing value in reward systems, fluctuates in sleep and wakefulness Major component of the sympathetic nervous system responses, including "fight or flight"
Serotonin (dietary precursor: tryptophan)	Raphe nuclei Others in the pons and medulla	Very widespread throughout the cortex, thalamus, cerebellum, brain stem, and spinal cord	Proposed role in the control of appetite, sleep, mood states, hallucinations, pain perception, and vomiting
Histamine (precursor: histidine)	Hypothalamus	Cerebral cortex Limbic system Hypothalamus Found in all mast cells	Control of gastric secretions, smooth muscle control, cardiac stimulation, stimulation of sensory nerve endings, and alertness
Amino Acids			
GABA	Derived from glutamate without localized cell bodies	Found in cells and projections throughout the CNS, especially in intrinsic feedback loops and interneurons of the cerebrum Also in the extrapyramidal motor system and cerebellum	Fast inhibitory response postsynaptically, inhibits the excitability of the neurons and therefore contributes to seizure, agitation, and anxiety control
Glycine	Primarily the spinal cord and brain stem	Limited projection, but especially in the auditory system and olfactory bulb Also found in the spinal cord, medulla, midbrain, cerebellum, and cortex	Inhibitory Decreases the excitability of spinal motor neurons but not cortical
Glutamate	Diffuse	Diffuse, but especially in the sensory organs	Excitatory Responsible for the bulk of information flow
Neuropeptides			
Endogenous opioids (i.e., endorphins, enkephalins)	A large family of neuropeptides that has three distinct subgroups, all of which are manufactured widely throughout the CNS	Widely distributed within and outside of the CNS	Suppress pain, modulate mood and stress Likely involvement in reward systems and addiction Also may regulate pituitary hormone release Implicated in the pathophysiology of diseases of the basal ganglia
Melatonin (one of its precursors: serotonin)	Pineal body	Widely distributed within and outside of the CNS	Secreted in dark and suppressed in light, helps regulate the sleep–wake cycle as well as other biologic rhythms
Substance P	Widespread, significant in the raphe system and spinal cord	Spinal cord, cortex, brain stem, and especially sensory neurons associated with pain perception	Involved in pain transmission, movement, and mood regulation
Cholecystokinin	Predominates in the ventral tegmental area of the midbrain	Frontal cortex, where it is often colocalized with dopamine Widely distributed within and outside of the CNS	Primary intestinal hormone involved in satiety; also has some involvement in the control of anxiety and panic

CNS, central nervous system; GABA, gamma-aminobutyric acid; PNS, peripheral nervous system.

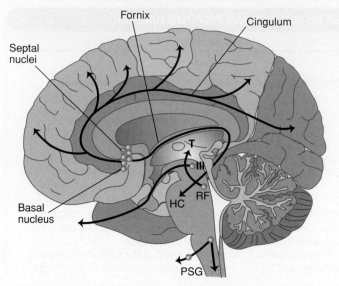

FIGURE 8.8 Cholinergic pathways. HC, hippocampal formation; PSG, parasympathetic ganglion cell; RF, reticular formation; T, thalamus. (Adapted from Nolte, J., & Angevine, J. [1995]. *The human brain: In photographs and diagrams.* St. Louis: Mosby.)

ACh is an excitatory neurotransmitter that is found throughout the cerebral cortex and limbic system. It arises primarily from cell bodies in the basal forebrain constellation, which provides innervations to the cerebral cortex, amygdala, hippocampus, and thalamus as well as from the dorsolateral tegmentum of the pons that projects to the basal ganglia, thalamus, hypothalamus, medullary reticular formation, and deep cerebellar nuclei (Siegel & Sapru, 2010) (Figure 8.8). These connections suggest that ACh is involved in higher intellectual functioning and memory. Individuals who have Alzheimer's disease or Down syndrome often exhibit patterns of cholinergic neuron loss in regions innervated by these pathways (e.g., the hippocampus), which may contribute to their memory difficulties and other cognitive deficits. Some cholinergic neurons are afferent to these areas bringing information from the limbic system, highlighting the role that ACh plays in communicating one's emotional state to the cerebral cortex.

Biogenic Amines

The **biogenic amines** (bioamines) consist of small molecules manufactured in the neuron that contain an amine group, thus the name. The catecholamines (amine attached to a catechol group) include dopamine, norepinephrine, and epinephrine, which are all synthesized from the amino acid tyrosine. Another monoamine, serotonin, is synthesized from tryptophan. Melatonin is derived from serotonin. All of these neurotransmitters are critical in many of the mental disorders.

Dopamine

Dopamine is an excitatory neurotransmitter found in distinct regions of the CNS and is involved in cognition, motor, and neuroendocrine functions. Dopamine is the neurotransmitter that stimulates the body's natural "feel good' reward pathways, producing pleasant euphoric sensation under certain conditions. It is involved in the regulation of action, emotion, motivation, and attention. Dopamine levels are decreased in Parkinson's disease, and abnormally high activity of dopamine has been associated with schizophrenia (discussed in more detail in Chapter 22). Abnormalities of dopamine activity within the reward system pathways are suspected to be a critical aspect of the development of drug and other addictions. The dopamine pathways are distinct neuronal areas within the CNS in which the neurotransmitter dopamine predominates. Three major dopaminergic pathways have been identified.

The *mesocortical* and *mesolimbic pathways* originate in the ventral tegmental area and project into the medial aspects of the cortex (mesocortical) and the limbic system inside the temporal lobes, including the hippocampus and amygdala (mesolimbic). Sometimes they are considered to be one pathway and at other times two separate pathways. The mesocortical pathway has major effects on cognition, including such functions as judgment, reasoning, insight, social conscience, motivation, the ability to generalize learning, and reward systems in the human brain. It contributes to some of the highest seats of cortical functioning. The mesolimbic pathway also strongly influences emotions and has projections that affect memory and auditory reception. Abnormalities in these pathways have been associated with schizophrenia.

Another major dopaminergic pathway begins in the substantia nigra and projects into the basal ganglia, parts of which are known as the *striatum*. Therefore, this pathway is called the *nigrostriatal pathway*. This influences the extrapyramidal motor system, which serves the voluntary motor system and allows involuntary motor movements. Destruction of dopaminergic neurons in this pathway has been associated with Parkinson's disease.

The final dopamine pathway originates from projections of the mesolimbic pathway and continues into the hypothalamus, which then projects into the pituitary gland. Therefore, this pathway, called the *tuberoinfundibular pathway*, has an impact on endocrine function and other functions, such as metabolism, hunger, thirst, sexual function, circadian rhythms, digestion, and temperature control. Figure 8.9 illustrates the dopaminergic pathways.

Norepinephrine

Norepinephrine is an excitatory neurochemical that plays a major role in generating and maintaining mood

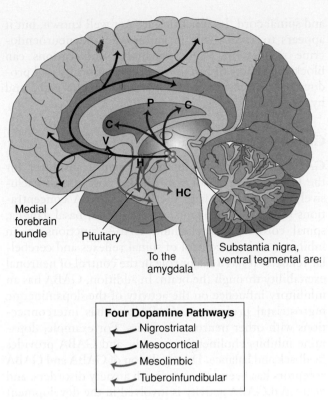

Four Dopamine Pathways
- Nigrostriatal
- Mesocortical
- Mesolimbic
- Tuberoinfundibular

FIGURE 8.9 Dopaminergic pathways. C, caudate nucleus; H, hypothalamus; HC, hippocampal formation; P, putamen; S, striatum; V, ventral striatum. (Adapted from Nolte, J., & Angevine, J. [1995]. *The human brain: In photographs and diagrams.* St. Louis: Mosby.)

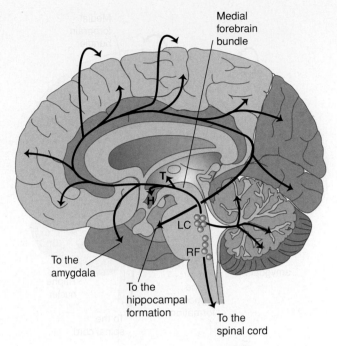

FIGURE 8.10 Noradrenergic pathways. H, hypothalamus; LC, locus ceruleus; RF, reticular formation; T, thalamus. (Adapted from Nolte, J., & Angevine, J. [1995]. *The human brain: In photographs and diagrams.* St. Louis: Mosby.)

states. Decreased norepinephrine has been associated with depression, and excessive norepinephrine has been associated with manic symptoms (Blier & El Mansari, 2013). Because norepinephrine is so heavily concentrated in the terminal sites of sympathetic nerves, it can be released quickly to ready the individual for a fight-or-flight response to threats in the environment. For this reason, norepinephrine is thought to play a role in the physical symptoms of anxiety.

Nerve tracts and pathways containing predominantly norepinephrine are called *noradrenergic* and are less clearly delineated than the dopamine pathways. In the CNS, noradrenergic neurons originate in the locus ceruleus, where more than half of the noradrenergic cell bodies are located. Because the locus ceruleus is one of the major timekeepers of the human body, norepinephrine is involved in sleep and wakefulness. From the locus ceruleus, noradrenergic pathways ascend into the neocortex, spread diffusely (Figure 8.10), and enhance the ability of neurons to respond to whatever input they may be receiving. In addition, norepinephrine appears to be involved in the process of reinforcement, which facilitates learning. Noradrenergic pathways innervate the hypothalamus and thus are involved to some degree in endocrine function. Anxiety disorders and depression are examples

of psychiatric illnesses in which dysfunction of the noradrenergic neurons may be involved. (Refer to Table 8.1 for the effects of ACh on various organs in the parasympathetic system.)

Serotonin

Serotonin (also called 5-hydroxytryptamine or 5-HT) is primarily an excitatory neurotransmitter that is diffusely distributed within the cerebral cortex, limbic system, and basal ganglia of the CNS. Serotonergic neurons also project into the hypothalamus and cerebellum. Figure 8.11 illustrates serotonergic pathways. Serotonin plays a role in emotions, cognition, sensory perceptions, and essential biologic functions, such as sleep and appetite. During the rapid eye movement (REM) phase of sleep, or the dream state, serotonin concentrations decrease, and muscles subsequently relax. Serotonin is also involved in the control of food intake, hormone secretion, sexual behavior, thermoregulation, and cardiovascular regulation. Some serotonergic fibers reach the cranial blood vessels within the brain and the *pia mater* where they have a vasoconstrictive effect. The potency of some new medications for migraine headaches is related to their ability to block serotonin transmission in the cranial blood vessels. Descending serotonergic pathways are important in central pain control. Whereas depression and insomnia have been associated with decreased levels of 5-HT, mania has been associated

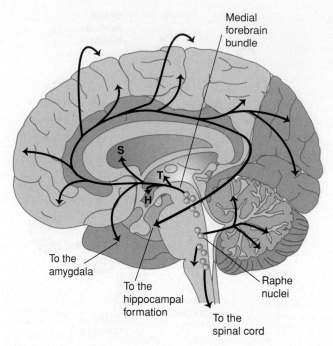

FIGURE 8.11 Serotonergic pathways. H, hypothalamus; S, septal nuclei; T, thalamus. (Adapted from Nolte, J., & Angevine, J. [1995]. *The human brain: In photographs and diagrams.* St. Louis: Mosby.)

with increased 5-HT. Some of the most well-known antidepressant medications, such as Prozac and Zoloft, which are discussed in more depth in Chapter 11, function by raising serotonin levels within certain areas of the CNS. Melatonin, which is derived from serotonin, is produced by the pineal gland and plays a role in sleep, aging, and mood changes.

Amino Acids

Amino acids, the building blocks of proteins, have many roles in intraneuronal metabolism. In addition, amino acids can function as neurotransmitters in as many as 60% to 70% of the synaptic sites in the brain. Amino acids are the most prevalent neurotransmitters. Virtually all of the neurons in the CNS are activated by excitatory amino acids, such as glutamate, and inhibited by inhibitory amino acids, such as gamma-aminobutyric acid (GABA) and glycine. Many of these amino acids coexist with other neurotransmitters.

Histamine

Histamine, derived from the amino acid histidine, has been identified as a neurotransmitter. Its cell bodies originate predominantly in the hypothalamus and project to all major structures in the cerebrum, brain stem,

and spinal cord. Its functions are not well known, but it appears to have a role in autonomic and neuroendocrine regulation. Many psychiatric medications can block the effects of histamine postsynaptically and produce side effects such as sedation, weight gain, and hypotension.

Gamma-Aminobutyric Acid

GABA is the primary inhibitory neurotransmitter for the CNS. The pathways of GABA exist almost exclusively in the CNS, with the largest GABA concentrations in the hypothalamus, hippocampus, basal ganglia, spinal cord, and cerebellum. GABA functions in an inhibitory role in control of spinal reflexes and cerebellar reflexes. It has a major role in the control of neuronal excitability through the brain. In addition, GABA has an inhibitory influence on the activity of the dopaminergic nigrostriatal projections. GABA also has interconnections with other neurotransmitters. For example, dopamine inhibits cholinergic neurons, and GABA provides feedback and balance. Dysregulation of GABA and GABA receptors has been associated with anxiety disorders, and decreased GABA activity is involved in the development of seizure disorders.

Glutamate

Glutamate, the most widely distributed excitatory neurotransmitter, is the main transmitter in the associational areas of the cortex. Glutamate can be found in a number of pathways from the cortex to the thalamus, pons, striatum, and spinal cord. In addition, glutamate pathways have a number of connections with the hippocampus. Some glutamate receptors may play a role in the long-lasting enhancement of synaptic activity. In turn, in the hippocampus, this enhancement may have a role in learning and memory. Too much glutamate is harmful to neurons, and considerable interest has emerged regarding its neurotoxic effects.

Conditions that produce an excess of endogenous glutamate can cause neurotoxicity by overexcitation of neuronal tissue. This process, called excitotoxicity, increases the sensitivity of glutamate receptors, produces overactivation of the receptors, and is increasingly being understood as a critical piece of the cascade of events involved in physical symptoms of alcohol withdrawal in dependent individuals. Excitotoxicity is also believed to be part of the pathology of conditions such as ischemia, hypoxia, hypoglycemia, and hepatic failure. Damage to the CNS from chronic malfunctioning of the glutamate system may be involved in the psychiatric symptoms seen in neurodegenerative diseases such as Huntington's, Parkinson's, and Alzheimer's diseases; vascular dementia; amyotrophic lateral sclerosis;

and acquired immune deficiency syndrome (AIDS)–related dementia. Degeneration of glutamate neurons is implicated in the development of schizophrenia.

Neuropeptides

Neuropeptides, short chains of amino acids, exist in the CNS and have a number of important roles as neurotransmitters, neuromodulators, or neurohormones. Neuropeptides were first thought to be pituitary hormones, such as adrenocorticotropin, oxytocin, and vasopressin, or hypothalamic-releasing hormones (e.g., corticotropin-releasing hormone and thyrotropin-releasing hormone [TRH]). However, when an endogenous morphine-like substance was discovered in the 1970s, the term *endorphin*, or endogenous morphine, was introduced. Although the amino acids and monoamine neurotransmitters can be produced directly from dietary precursors in any part of the neuron, neuropeptides are, almost without exception, synthesized from messenger RNA in the cell body. Currently, two types of neuropeptides have been identified. Opioid neuropeptides, such as endorphins, enkephalins, and dynorphins, function in endocrine functioning and pain suppression. The nonopioid neuropeptides, such as substance P and somatostatin, play roles in pain transmission and endocrine functioning, respectively.

There are considerable variations in the distribution of individual neuropeptides, but some areas are especially rich in cell bodies containing neuropeptides. These areas include the amygdala, striatum, hypothalamus, raphe nuclei, brain stem, and spinal cord. Many of the interneurons of the cerebral cortex contain neuropeptides, but there are considerably fewer in the thalamus and almost none in the cerebellum.

Receptors

Embedded in the postsynaptic membrane are a number of proteins that act as receptors for the released neurotransmitters. Each neurotransmitter has a specific **receptor**, or protein, for which it and only it will fit.

Lock and Key

The "lock-and-key" analogy has often been used to describe the fit of a given neurotransmitter to its receptor site. The target cell, when stimulated by the neurotransmitter, will then respond by evoking its own action potential and either producing some action common to that cell or acting as a relay to keep the messages moving throughout the CNS. This pattern of the electrical signal from one neuron, converted to chemical signal at the synaptic cleft, picked up by an adjacent neuron, again converted to an electrical action potential, and then to a chemical signal, occurs billions of times a day in billions of different neurons. This electrical–chemical communication process allows the structures of the brain to function together in a coordinated and organized manner.

Receptor Sensitivity

Both presynaptic and postsynaptic receptors have the capacity to change, developing either a greater-than-usual response to the neurotransmitter, known as supersensitivity, or a less-than-usual response, called subsensitivity. These changes represent the concept of neuroplasticity of brain tissue discussed earlier in the chapter. The change in sensitivity of the receptor is most commonly caused by the effect of a drug on a receptor site or by disease that affects the normal functioning of a receptor site. Drugs can affect the sensitivity of the receptor by altering the strength of attraction or affinity of a receptor for the neurotransmitter, by changing the efficiency with which the receptor activity translates the message inside the receiving cell, or by decreasing over time the number of receptors.

These mechanisms may account for the long-term, sometimes severely adverse, effects of psychopharmacologic drugs, the loss of effectiveness of a given medication, or the loss of effectiveness of a medication after repeated use in treating recurring episodes of a psychiatric disorder. Disease may cause a change in the normal number or function of receptors, thereby altering their sensitivity. For example, depression is associated with a reduction in the normal number of certain receptors, leading to an abnormality in their sensitivity to neurotransmitters such as serotonin and norepinephrine (Bewernick & Schlaepfer, 2013). A decreased response to continued stimulation of these receptors is usually referred to as *desensitization* or *refractoriness*. This suspected subsensitivity is referred to as *downregulation* of the receptors.

Receptor Subtypes

The nervous system uses many different neurochemicals for communication, and each specific chemical messenger requires a specific receptor on which the chemical can act. More than 100 different chemical messengers have been identified, with new ones being uncovered. In addition to the sheer number of receptors needed to accommodate these chemicals, the neurotransmitters may produce different effects at different synaptic sites.

Each major neurotransmitter has several different subtypes of receptors, allowing the neurotransmitter to have different effects in different areas of the brain. The receptors usually have the same name as the neurotransmitter, but the classification of the subtypes varies. For example, dopamine receptors are named D1, D2, D3, and so on. Serotonin receptors are grouped in families such at 5HT 1a, 5HT 1b, and so on. The receptors for Ach have completely different names: muscarinic and nicotinic. Two specific subtype receptors have been identified for GABA: A and B.

Neurocircuitry

Brain structures such as the prefrontal cortex, striatum, hippocampus, and amygdala are linked through complex neural functional networks (Haber & Rauch, 2010; Sequira, Martin, & Vawter, 2012). Recent research indicates that a dysfunctional **neurocircuitry** underlies most psychiatric disorders (Figure 8.12). Various neurocircuits are the focus of study of different illness. For example, the cingulo-frontal-parietal network is associated with attention-deficit disorder, and the amygdalo-cortical circuitry is the focus in psychosis and schizophrenia.

STUDIES OF THE BIOLOGIC BASIS OF MENTAL DISORDERS

As described earlier, mental disorders are complex syndromes consisting of clusters of biopsychosocial symptoms. These syndromes are not specific physiological disorders, and research efforts are focused on piecing the puzzle together. One important area of study is genetics; it is well established that genetic factors play an important role in the development of mental disorders. In addition, as the complexity of the nervous system and its interrelationship with other body systems and the environment has become more fully understood, new fields of study have emerged. One field worth noting is **psychoneuroimmunology** (PNI). Although it has long been observed that individuals under stress have compromised immune systems and are more likely to acquire common diseases, only recently have changes in the immune system been noted as widespread in some psychiatric illnesses. Another

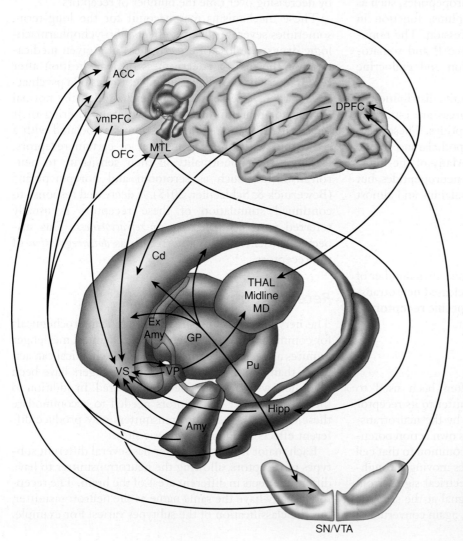

FIGURE 8.12 Key structures and pathways involved in neuropsychiatric disorders. *Arrows* illustrate projections. ACC, anterior cingulate cortex; Amy, amygdala; Cd, caudate nucleus; DPFC, dorsal prefrontal cortex; GP, globus pallidus; Ex Amy, extended amygdala; Hipp, hippocampus; MD, medial dorsal nucleus of the thalamus; MTL, medial temporal lobe; OFC, orbital frontal cortex; Pu, Putamen; SN, substantia nigra; Thal, thalamus; vmPFC, ventral medial prefrontal cortex; VP, ventral pallidum; VS, ventral striatum; VTA, ventral tegmental area. (Redrawn with permission from Haber, S. N., & Rauch, S. L. [2010]. Neurocircuitry: A window into the networks underlying neuropsychiatric disease. *Neuropsychopharmacology Reviews, 35*[1], 1–3.)

field, chronobiology, has provided new information suggesting that dysfunction of biologic rhythms may not only result from a psychiatric illness but also contribute to its development.

Genetics

The sequence of the human genome is the beginning of our understanding of complex genetic connections that leads to a **phenotype** or observable characteristics or expressions of a specific trait. The genome provides researchers with a road map of the exact sequence of the three billion nucleotide bases that make up human organisms. Many thought that after the human genome was mapped, it would be easy to determine the genes responsible for mental disorders. Unfortunately, it is not that simple. Knowing the location of the gene and its sequence are just pieces of the complex puzzle. The location of the genes does not tell us which genes are responsible for a mental illness or how mutations occur.

Population Genetics

Inheritance of mental disorders is studied by using epidemiologic methods that identifies risks and patterns of illness or traits from generation to generation. Beginning with a **proband**, a person who has the disorder or trait, **population genetics** relies on the following principle epidemiologic methods:

- **Family studies** analyze the occurrence of a disorder in first-degree relatives (biologic parents, siblings, and children), second-degree relatives (grandparents, uncles, aunts, nieces, nephews, and grandchildren), and so on.
- **Twin studies** analyze the presence or absence of the disorder in pairs of twins. The *concordance rate* is the measure of similarity of occurrence in individuals with a similar genetic makeup.
- **Adoption studies** compare the risk for the illness developing in offspring raised in different environments. The strongest inferences may be drawn from studies that involve children separated from their parents at birth.

Mental disorders and their symptoms are not an expression of a single gene. The transmission pattern does not follow classic Mendelian genetics in which the dominant allele (variant) on only one chromosome or recessive alleles on both chromosomes are responsible for manifestation of a disorder. Monozygotic (identical) twins do not manifest the same mental disorder with 100% concordance rate, but they have a higher rate of a disorder than dizygotic (fraternal) twins, who share roughly the same proportion of genes that ordinary siblings do (50%). Internal and external environmental events influence the development of a disorder with a genetic contribution. This interaction between the environment and a genetic predisposition underlies several mental disorders such as schizophrenia, autism, and ADHD.

Molecular Genetics

A gene comprises short segments of DNA and is packed with the instructions for making proteins that have a specific function. When genes are absent or malfunction, protein production is altered, and bodily functions are disrupted. In this fashion, genes play a role in cancer, heart disease, diabetes, and many psychiatric disorders. Although no conclusive evidence exists for a complete genetic cause of most psychiatric disorders, significant evidence suggests that strong genetic contributions exist for most (Sullivan, Daly, & O'Donovan, 2012).

Intracellular genes direct protein production responsible for genetic expression. Individual nerve cells outside

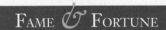

FAME & FORTUNE

King George III (1739–1830)

Bipolar Illness Misdiagnosed

PUBLIC PERSONA

Crowned King of England at age 22 years, George III headed the most influential colonial power in the world at that time. England thrived in the peacetime after the Seven Years' War with France but simultaneously taxed its American colonies so heavily and resolutely that the colonies rebelled. Could the American Revolution be blamed on King George III's state of mind?

PERSONAL REALITIES

At age 50 years, the king first experienced abdominal pain and constipation followed by weak limbs, fever, tachycardia, hoarseness, and dark red urine. Later, he experienced confusion, racing thoughts, visual problems, restlessness, delirium, convulsions, and stupor. His strange behavior included ripping off his wig and running about naked. Although he recovered and did not have a relapse for 13 years, he was considered to be mad. Relapses after the first relapse became more frequent, and the king was eventually dethroned by the Prince of Wales.

Was George's madness in reality a genetically transmitted blood disease that caused thought disturbances, delirium, and stupor? The genetic disease porphyria is caused by defects in the body's ability to make haem. The diseases are generally inherited in an autosomal dominant fashion. The retrospective diagnosis was not made until 1966 (Macalpine & Hunter, 1966). Before that, it was believed that he had bipolar disorder.

Other members of the royal family who had this hereditary disease were Queen Anne of Great Britain; Frederic the Great of Germany; George IV of Great Britain (son of George III); and George IV's daughter, Princess Charlotte, who died during childbirth from complications of the disease.

Source: Macalpine, I. & Hunter, R. (1966). The "insanity" of King George 3d: A classic case of porphyria. *British Medical Journal, 1*(5479), 65–71.

of the cell respond to these changes, modifying proteins to adapt to the new environment. This dynamic nature of gene function highlights the manner in which the body and the environment interact and in how environmental factors influence gene expression.

The study of molecular genetics in psychiatric disorders is in its infancy. It is likely that psychiatric disorders are polygenic. This means that psychiatric disorders develop when genes interact with each other and with environmental factors such as stress, infections, poor nutrition, catastrophic loss, complications during pregnancy, and exposure to toxins. Thus, genetic makeup conveys vulnerability, or a risk for the illness, but the right set of environmental factors must be present for the disorder to develop in an at-risk individual (Sequeira, Martin, & Vawter, 2012).

Genetic Susceptibility

The concept of **genetic susceptibility** suggests that an individual may be at increased risk for a psychiatric disorder. Specific risk factors for psychiatric disorders are just beginning to be understood, and environmental influences are examples of risk factors. In the absence of one specific gene for the major psychiatric disorders, risk factor assessment is a logical alternative for predicting who is more likely to experience psychiatric disorders or certain conditions, such as aggression or suicidality (Wasserman, Terenius, Wasserman, & Sokolowski, 2010).

When considering information regarding risks for genetic transmission of psychiatric disorders, there are several key points to remember:

- Psychiatric disorders have been described and labeled quite differently across generations, and errors in diagnosis may occur.
- Similar psychiatric symptoms may have considerably different causes, just as symptoms such as chest pain may occur in relation to many different causes.
- Genes that are present may not always cause the appearance of the trait.
- Several genes work together in an individual to produce a given trait or disorder.
- A biologic cause is not necessarily solely genetic in origin. Environmental influences alter the body's functioning and often mediate or worsen genetic risk factors.

Psychoneuroimmunology

PNI examines the relationships among the immune system, nervous system, and endocrine system and our behaviors, thoughts, and feelings. The immune system is composed of the thymus, spleen, lymph nodes, lymphatic vessels, tonsils, adenoids, and bone marrow, which manufactures all the cells that eventually develop into T cells, B cells, phagocytes, macrophages, and natural killer (NK)

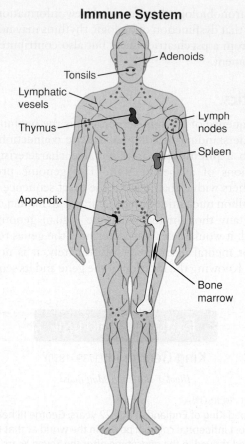

FIGURE 8.13 The immune system.

cells (Figure 8.13). Many contemporary stress research studies are examining the role of the NK cells in the early recognition of foreign bodies. Lower NK cell function is related to increased disease susceptibility. NK cell function is affected by stress-induced physiologic arousal in humans. NK cell activity has been shown to vary in response to many emotional, cognitive, and physiologic stressors, including anxiety, depression, perceived lack of personal control, bereavement, pain, and surgery (Pace & Heim, 2011).

Overactivity of the immune system can occur in autoimmune diseases such as systemic lupus erythematosus (SLE), allergies, and anaphylaxis. Evidence suggests that the nervous system regulates many aspects of immune function. Specific immune system dysfunctions may result from damage to the hypothalamus, hippocampus, or pituitary and may produce symptoms of psychiatric disorders. Figure 8.14 illustrates the interaction between stress and the immune system. This figure also demonstrates the true biopsychosocial nature of the complex interrelationship of the nervous system, the endocrine system, the immune system, and environmental or emotional stress.

Immune dysregulation may also be involved in the development of psychiatric disorders. This can occur

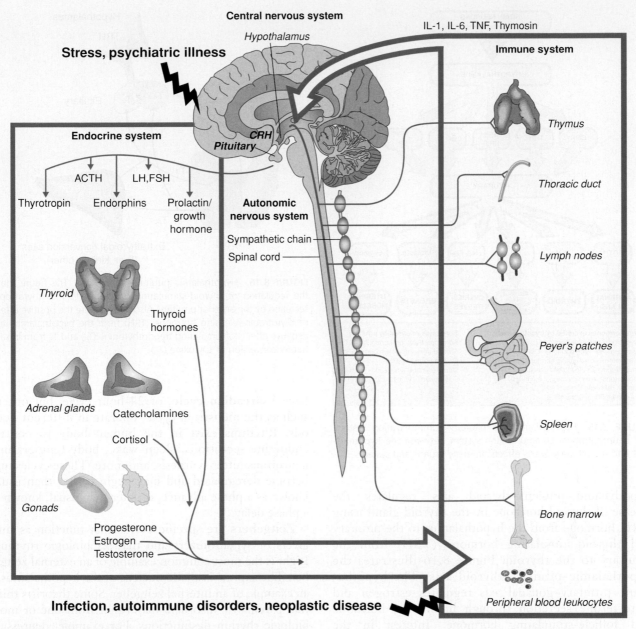

FIGURE 8.14   Examples of the interaction between stress or psychiatric illness and the immune system through the endocrine system. ACTH, adrenocorticotropic hormone; CRH, corticotropin-releasing hormone; FSH, follicle-stimulating hormone; IL, interleukin; LH, luteinizing hormone; TNF, tumor necrosis factor.

by allowing neurotoxins to affect the brain, damaging neuroendocrine tissue, or damaging tissues in the brain at locations such as the receptor sites. Some antidepressants have been thought to have antiviral effects. Symptoms of diseases such as depression may occur after an occurrence of serious infection, and prenatal exposure to infectious organisms has been associated with the development of schizophrenia. Stress and conditioning have specific effects on the suppression of immune function (Pace & Heim, 2011).

Normal functioning of the endocrine system is often disturbed in people with psychiatric disorders. For exam-

ple, thyroid functioning is often low in those with bipolar disorder, and people with schizophrenia have a higher incidence of diabetes (see Unit VI). The hypothalamus sends and receives information through the pituitary, which then communicates with structures in the peripheral aspects of the body. Figure 8.15 presents an example of the communication of the anterior pituitary with a number of organs and structures.

Axes, the structures within which the neurohormones are providing messages, are the most often studied aspect of the neuroendocrine system. These axes always involve a feedback mechanism. For example, the

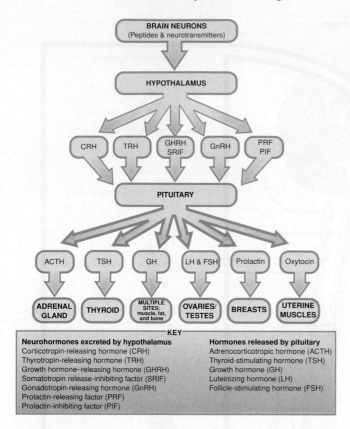

FIGURE 8.15 Hypothalamic and pituitary communication system. The neurohormonal communication system between the hypothalamus and the pituitary exerts effects on many organs and systems.

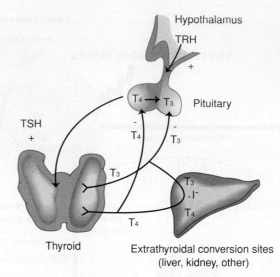

FIGURE 8.16 Hypothalamic–pituitary–thyroid axis. This figure shows the regulation of thyroid-stimulating hormone (TSH or thyrotropin) secretion by the anterior pituitary. Also depicted are the positive effects of thyrotropin-releasing hormone (TRH) from the hypothalamus and negative effects of circulating triiodothyronine (T_3) and T_3 from intrapituitary conversion of thyroxine (T_4).

hypothalamus–pituitary–thyroid axis regulates the release of thyroid hormone by the thyroid gland using TRH hormone from the hypothalamus to the pituitary and thyroid-stimulating hormone (TSH) from the pituitary to the thyroid. Figure 8.16 illustrates the hypothalamic–pituitary–thyroid axis. The hypothalamic–pituitary–gonadal axis regulates estrogen and testosterone secretion through luteinizing hormone and follicle-stimulating hormone. Interest in the endocrine system is heightened by various endocrine disorders that produce psychiatric symptoms. Addison's disease (hypoadrenalism) produces depression, apathy, fatigue, and occasionally psychosis. Hypothyroidism produces depression and some anxiety. Administration of steroids can cause depression, hypomania, irritability, and in some cases, psychosis. Some psychiatric disorders have been associated with endocrine system dysfunction. For example, some individuals with mood disorders show evidence of dysregulation in adrenal, thyroid, and growth hormone axes (see Chapter 25).

Chronobiology

Chronobiology involves the study and measure of time structures or biologic rhythms. Some rhythms

have a **circadian cycle**, or 24-hour cycle, but others, such as the menstrual cycle, operate in different periods. Rhythms exist in the human body to control endocrine secretions, sleep–wake, body temperature, neurotransmitter synthesis, and more. These cycles may become deregulated and may begin earlier than usual, known as a phase advance, or later than usual, known as a phase delay.

Zeitgebers are specific events that function as time givers or synchronizers and that set biologic rhythms. Light is the most common example of an external zeitgeber. The suprachiasmatic nucleus of the hypothalamus is an example of an internal zeitgeber. Some theorists think that psychiatric disorders may result from one or more biologic rhythm dysfunctions. For example, depression may be, in part, a phase advance disorder, including early morning awakening and decreased time of onset of REM sleep. Seasonal affective disorder may be the result of shortened exposure to light during the winter months. Exposure to specific artificial light often relieves symptoms of fatigue, overeating, hypersomnia, and depression (see Chapters 11, 24, and 32).

DIAGNOSTIC APPROACHES

Although no commonly used laboratory tests exist that directly confirm a mental disorder, they are still used as part of the diagnosis of these illnesses. **Biologic markers** are diagnostic test findings that occur only in the presence of the psychiatric disorder and include such findings as laboratory and other diagnostic test results and neuropathologic changes noticeable in assessment. These markers increase diagnostic certainty and reliability and may have predictive value, allowing for the possibility of preventive interventions to forestall or avoid the onset of illness. In addition, biologic markers could assist in developing evidence-based care practices. If markers are used reliably, it is much easier to identify the most effective treatments and to determine the expected prognoses for given conditions. The psychiatric–mental health nurse should be aware of the most current information on biologic markers so that information, limitations, and results can be discussed knowledgeably with the patient.

Laboratory Tests

For many years, laboratory tests have attempted to measure levels of neurotransmitters and other CNS substances in the bloodstream. Many of the metabolites of neurotransmitters can be found in the urine and cerebrospinal fluid (CSF) as well. However, these measures have had only limited utility in elucidating what is happening in the brain. Levels of neurotransmitters and metabolites in the bloodstream or urine do not necessarily equate with levels in the CNS. In addition, availability of the neurotransmitter or metabolite does not predict the availability of the neurotransmitter in the synapse, where it must act, or directly relate to the receptor sensitivity. Nonetheless, numerous research studies have focused on changes in neurotransmitters and metabolites in blood, urine, and CSF. These studies have provided clues but remain without conclusive predictive value and therefore are not routinely used.

Another laboratory approach to the study of some of the psychiatric disorders is the challenge test. A challenge test has been most often used in the study of panic disorders. These tests are usually conducted by intravenously administering a chemical known to produce a specific set of psychiatric symptoms. For example, lactate or caffeine may be used to induce the symptoms of panic in a person who has panic disorder. The biologic response of the individual is then monitored.

Beyond their role in helping to diagnose mental disorders, laboratory tests are also an active part of the normal care and assessment of patients with psychiatric disorders. Many physical conditions mimic the symptoms of mental illness, and many of the medications used to treat psychiatric illness can produce health problems. For these reasons, the routine care of patients with psychiatric disorders includes the use of laboratory tests such as complete blood counts, thyroid studies, electrolytes, hepatic enzymes, and other evaluative tests. Psychiatric–mental health nurses need to be familiar with these procedures and assist patients in understanding the use and implications of such tests.

Neurophysiologic Procedures

Several neurophysiological procedures are used in mental health for diagnostic purposes.

Electroencephalography

Electroencephalography (EEG) is a tried and true method for investigating what is happening inside the living brain. Developed in the 1920s, EEG measures electrical activity in the uppermost nerve layers of the cortex. Usually, 16 electrodes are placed on the patient's scalp. The EEG machine, equipped with graph paper and recording pens, is turned on, and the pens then trace the electrical impulses generated over each electrode. Until the use of computed tomography (CT) in the 1970s, the EEG was the only method for identifying brain abnormalities. It remains the simplest and most noninvasive method for identifying some disorders. It is increasingly being used to identify individual neuronal differences.

An EEG may be used in psychiatry to differentiate possible causes of the patient's symptoms. For example, some types of seizure disorders, such as temporal lobe epilepsy, head injuries, or tumors, may present with predominantly psychiatric symptoms. In addition, metabolic dysfunction, delirium, dementia, altered levels of consciousness, hallucinations, and dissociative states may require EEG evaluation.

Spikes and wave-pattern changes are indications of brain abnormalities. Spikes may be the focal point from which a seizure occurs. However, abnormal activity often is not discovered on a routine EEG while the individual is awake. For this reason, additional methods are sometimes used. Nasopharyngeal leads may be used to get physically closer to the limbic regions. The patient may be exposed to a flashing strobe light while the examiner looks for activity that is not in phase with the flashing light or the patient may be asked to hyperventilate for 3 minutes to induce abnormal activity if it exists. Sleep deprivation may also be used. This involves keeping the patient awake throughout the night before the EEG evaluation. The patient may then be drowsy and fall asleep during the procedure. Abnormalities are more likely to occur when the patient is asleep. Sleep may also be induced using medication; however, many medications change the wave patterns on an EEG. For example, the benzodiazepine class of drugs increases the rapid and fast beta activity. Many other prescribed and illicit drugs, such as lithium, which increases theta activity, can cause EEG alterations.

In addition to reassuring, preparing, and educating the patient for the examination, the nurse should carefully assess the history of substance use and report this information to the examiner. If a sleep-deprivation EEG is to be done, caffeine or other stimulants that might assist the patient in staying awake should be withheld because they may change the EEG patterns.

Polysomnography

Polysomnography is a special procedure that involves recording the EEG throughout a night of sleep. This test is usually conducted in a sleep laboratory. Other tests are usually performed at the same time, including electrocardiography and electromyography. Blood oxygenation, body movement, body temperature, and other data may be collected as well, especially in research settings. This procedure is usually conducted for evaluating sleep disorders, such as sleep apnea, enuresis, or somnambulism. However, sleep pattern changes are frequently researched in mental disorders as well.

Researchers have found that normal sleep divisions and stages are affected by many factors, including drugs, alcohol, general medical conditions, and psychiatric disorders. For example, REM latency, the length of time it takes an individual to enter the first REM episode, is shortened in depression. Reduced delta sleep is also observed. These findings have been replicated so frequently that some researchers consider them biologic markers for depression.

Structural and Functional Imaging

Neuroimaging of the brain involves **structural imaging**, which visualizes the structure of brain and allows diagnosis of gross intracranial disease and injury, and **functional imaging**, which visualizes processing of information. One of the most well-known examples of structural imaging is magnetic resonance imaging (MRI), which produces two- or three-dimensional images of brain structures without the use of X-rays or radioactive tracers. An MRI creates a magnetic field around the patient's head through which radio waves are sent. A functional MRI (fMRI) that creates functional images relies on the properties of oxygenated and deoxygenated hemoglobin to see images of changes in blood flow. The advantage of fMRI is that it is possible to see how the brain works when different stimuli are presented and problems that exist, such as a stroke. The fMRI has replaced most use of positron emission tomography (PET), which measures blood flow and oxygen and glucose metabolism. The emissions from the injected radioactive tracers are rapidly decayed and limit the monitoring of PET to short tasks.

Neuroimaging has limited clinical use in mental health, with the exception of the diagnosis of some of the dementias, particularly Alzheimer's (Frisoni, Fox, Jack, Scheltens, & Thompson, 2010). Neuroimaging has promising potential for unlocking the pathophysiology of several mental disorders. With the introduction of the fMRI, it is now possible to study the circuitry and pinpoint genetic-based predisposing factors. An MRI technique, diffusion tensor imaging, allows for viewing macroscopic changes that occur at the axon level (Radanovic et al., 2013).

Other Neurophysiologic Methods

Evoked potentials (EPs), also called event-related potentials, use the same basic principles as an EEG. They measure changes in electrical activity of the brain in specific regions as a response to a given stimulus. Electrodes placed on the scalp measure a large waveform that stands out after the administration of repetitive stimuli, such as a click or flash of light. There are several different types of EPs to be measured, depending on the sensory area affected by the stimulus, the cognitive task required, or the region monitored, any of which can change the length of time until the wave occurrence. EPs are used extensively in psychiatric research. In clinical practice, EPs are used primarily in the assessment of demyelinating disorders, such as multiple sclerosis.

However, brain electrical activity mapping studies, which involve a 20-electrode EEG that generates computerized maps of the brain's electrical activity, have found a slowing of electrical activity in the frontal lobes of individuals who have schizophrenia.

SUMMARY OF KEY POINTS

- Neuroscientists now view behavior and cognitive function as a result of complex interactions within the CNS and its plasticity, or its ability to adapt and change in both structure and function.

- Each hemisphere of the brain is divided into four lobes: the frontal lobe, which controls motor speech function, personality, and working memory—often called the executive functions that govern one's ability to plan and initiate action; the parietal lobe, which controls the sensory functions; the temporal lobe, which contains the primary auditory and olfactory areas; and the occipital lobe, which controls visual integration of information.

- The structures of the limbic system are integrally involved in memory and emotional behavior. Dysfunction of the limbic system has been linked with major mental disorders, including schizophrenia, depression, and anxiety disorders.

- Neurons communicate with each other through synaptic transmission. Neurotransmitters excite or inhibit a response at the receptor sites and have been linked to certain mental disorders. These neurotransmitters include Ach, dopamine, norepinephrine, serotonin, GABA, and glutamate.

- Although no one gene has been found to produce any psychiatric disorder, significant evidence indicates there most psychiatric disorders have a genetic predisposition or susceptibility. For individuals who have such genetic susceptibility, the identification of risk factors is crucial in helping to plan interventions to prevent development of that disorder or to prevent certain behavior patterns, such as aggression or suicide.

- PNI examines the relationship among the immune system; the nervous system; the endocrine system; and thoughts, emotions, and behavior.

- Chronobiology focuses on the study and measure of time structures or biologic rhythms occurring in the body and associates dysregulation of these cycles as contributing factors to the development of psychiatric disorders.

- Biologic markers are physical indicators of disturbances within the CNS that differentiate one disease process from another, such as biochemical changes or neuropathologic changes. These biologic markers can be measured by several methods of testing, including challenge tests, EEG, polysomnography, EPs, CT scanning, MRI, PET, and single-photon emission computed tomography; the psychiatric nurse must be familiar with all of these methods.

CRITICAL THINKING CHALLENGES

1. A woman who has experienced a "ministroke" continues to regain lost cognitive function months after the stroke. Her husband takes this as evidence that she never had a stroke. How would you approach patient teaching and counseling for this couple to help them understand this occurrence if the stroke did damage to her brain?

2. Your patient has "impaired executive functioning." Consider what would be a reasonable follow-up schedule for this patient for counseling sessions. Would it be reasonable to schedule visits at 1:00 PM weekly? Is the patient able to keep to this schedule? Why or why not? What would be the best schedule?

3. Mr. S. is unable to sleep after watching an upsetting documentary. Identify the neurotransmitter activity that may be interfering with sleep. (Hint: Fight or flight.)

4. Describe what behavioral symptoms or problems may be present in a patient with dysfunction of the following brain area:
   a. Basal ganglia
   b. Hippocampus
   c. Limbic system
   d. Thalamus
   e. Hypothalamus
   f. Frontal lobe

5. Compare and contrast the functions of the sympathetic and parasympathetic nervous systems.

6. Discuss the steps in synaptic transmission, beginning with the action potential and ending with how the neurotransmitter no longer communicates its message to the receiving neuron.

7. Examine how a receptor's usual response to a neurotransmitter might change.

8. Compare the roles of dopamine and Ach in the CNS.

9. Explain how dopamine, norepinephrine, and serotonin all contribute to endocrine system regulation. Suggest some other transmitters that may affect endocrine function.

10. Discuss how the fields of psychoneuroimmunology and chronobiology overlap.

11. Compare the methods used to find biologic markers of psychiatric disorders reviewed in this chapter. Consider the potential risks and benefits to the patient.

References

Bewernick, B. H., & Schlaepfer, T. E. (2013). Chronic depression as a model disease for cerebral aging. (Review). *Dialogues in Neuroscience, 15*(1), 77–85.

Blier, P., & El Mansari, M. (2013). Serotonin and beyond: Therapeutics for major depression. *Philosophical Transactions of the Royal Society of London. Series B, Biological Sciences, 368*(1615), 20120536. doi:10.1098/rstb.2012.0536

Frisoni, G. B., Fox, N. C., Jack, C. R., Scheltens, P., & Thompson, P. M. (2010). The clinical use of structural MRI in Alzheimer Disease. *Nature Reviews Neurology, 6*(2), 67–77.

Haber, S. N., & Rauch, S. L. (2010). Neurocircuitry: A window into the networks underlying neuropsychiatric disease. *Neuropsychopharmacology Reviews, 35*(1), 1–3.

Harlow, J. M. (1868). Recovery after severe injury to the head. *Publication of the Massachusetts Medical Society, 2,* 327.

Kreuzer, P., Landgrebe, M., Wittmann, M., Schecklmann, M., Poeppl, T. B., Hajak, G., et al. (2012). Hypothermia associated with antipsychotic drug use: A clinical case series and review of current literature. *Journal of Clinical Pharmacology, 52*(7), 1090–1097.

Macalpine, I., & Hunter, R. (1966). The "insanity" of King George 3d: A classic case of porphyria. *British Medical Journal, 1*(5479), 65–71.

Nolte, J., & Angevine, J. (1995). *The human brain: In photographs and diagrams.* St. Louis: Mosby.

Pace, T. W. & Heim, C. M. (2011). A short review on the psychoneuroim-munology of posttraumatic stress disorder: From risk factors to medical comorbidities. (Review). *Brain, Behavior, and Immunity, 25*(1), 6–13.

Radanovic, M., Pereira, F. R., Stella, F., Aprahamian, I., Ferreira, L. K., Forlenza, O. V., et al. (2013). White matter abnormalities associated with Alzheimer's disease and mild cognitive impairment: A critical review of MRI studies. (Review). *Expert Review of Neurotherapeutics, 13*(5), 483–493.

Sequeira, P. A., Martin, M. V., & Vawter, M. P. (2012). The first decade and beyond of transcriptional profiling in schizophrenia. (Review). *Neurobiology of Disease, 45*(1), 23–26.

Siegel, A., & Sapru, H. N. (2010). *Essential neuroscience* (2nd ed). Philadelphia: Lippincott Williams & Wilkins.

Sullivan, P. F., Daly, M. F., & O'Donovan, M. (2012). Genetic architectures of psychiatric disorders: The emerging picture and its implications. (Review). *Nature Reviews Genetics. 13*(8), 537–551.

Wasserman, D., Terenius, L., Wasserman, J., & Sokolowski, M. (2010). The 2009 Nobel conference on the role of genetics in promoting suicide prevention and the mental health of the population. *Molecular Psychiatry, 15*(1), 12–17.

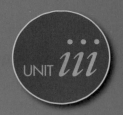

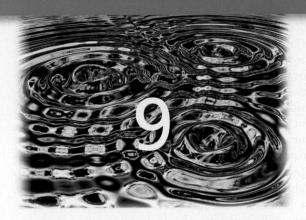

9

Communication and the Therapeutic Relationship

Cheryl Forchuk and Mary Ann Boyd

KEY CONCEPTS

- nurse–patient relationship
- self-awareness
- therapeutic communication

LEARNING OBJECTIVES

After studying this chapter, you will be able to:

1. Identify the importance of self-awareness in nursing practice.

2. Develop a repertoire of verbal and nonverbal communication skills.

3. Develop a process for selecting effective communication techniques.

4. Explain how the nurse can establish a therapeutic relationship with patients by using rapport and empathy.

5. Explain the physical, emotional, and social boundaries of the nurse–patient relationship.

6. Discuss the significance of defense mechanisms.

7. Explain what occurs in each of the three phases of the nurse–patient relationship: orientation, working, and resolution.

8. Describe what characterizes a nontherapeutic or deteriorating nurse–patient relationship.

KEY TERMS

- active listening • boundaries • communication blocks • content themes • countertransference • defense mechanisms • deteriorating relationship • empathy • empathic linkages • introspective • nontherapeutic relationship • nonverbal communication • orientation phase • passive listening • process recording • rapport • resolution • self-disclosure • symbolism • transference • verbal communication • working phase

Patients with psychiatric disorders have special communication needs that require advanced therapeutic communication skills. In psychiatric nursing, the nurse–patient relationship is an important tool used to reach treatment goals. The purposes of this chapter are to (1) help the nurse develop self-awareness and communication techniques needed for a therapeutic nurse–patient relationship, (2) examine the specific stages or steps involved in establishing the relationship, (3) explore the specific factors that make a nurse–patient relationship successful and therapeutic, and (4) differentiate therapeutic from nontherapeutic relationships.

SELF-AWARENESS

Self-awareness is the process of understanding one's own beliefs, thoughts, motivations, biases, and limitations and recognizing how they affect others. Without self-awareness, nurses will find it impossible to establish and maintain therapeutic relationships with patients. "Know thyself" is a basic tenet of psychiatric–mental health nursing (Box 9.1).

A well-developed sense of self-awareness can only come after nurses carry out self-examination. This process can provoke anxiety and is rarely comfortable, either when done alone or with help from others. Self-examination involves reflecting on the personal meaning of the current nursing situation. This reflection can relate to similar past situations and issues related to one's own personal values. Self-examination without the benefit of another's perspective can lead to a biased view of self. Conducting self-examinations with a trusted individual who can give objective but realistic feedback is best. The development of self-awareness requires a willingness to be **introspective** and to examine personal beliefs, attitudes, and motivations.

> **KEYCONCEPT** **Self-awareness** is the process of understanding one's own beliefs, thoughts, motivations, biases, and limitations, and recognizing how they affect others.

The Biopsychosocial Self

Each nurse brings a biopsychosocial self to nursing practice. The patient perceives the biologic dimension of the nurse in terms of physical characteristics: age, gender, body weight, height, ethnic or racial background, and any other observed physical characteristics. Additionally, the nurse can have a certain genetic composition, illness, or an unobservable physical disability that may influence the quality or delivery of nursing care. The nurse's psychological state also influences how he or she analyzes patient information and selects treatment interventions. An emotional state or behavior can inadvertently influence

---

the therapeutic relationship. For example, a nurse who has just learned that her child is using illegal drugs and who has a patient with a history of drug use may inadvertently project a judgmental attitude toward her patient, which would interfere with the formation of a therapeutic relationship. The nurse needs to examine underlying emotions, motivations, and beliefs and determine how these factors shape behavior.

The nurse's social biases can be particularly problematic for the nurse–patient relationship. Although the nurse may not verbalize these values to patients, some are readily evident in the nurse's behavior and appearance. A patient may perceive biases in the nurse as a result of how the nurse acts or appears at work. Other sociocultural values may not be immediately obvious to the patient; for example, the nurse's religious or spiritual beliefs or feelings about death, divorce, abortion, or homosexuality. These beliefs and thoughts can influence how the nurse interacts with a patient who is dealing with such issues. Similarly, cultural beliefs and patterns of communicating may influence the emerging relationship by each partner's behaviors conforming to or confronting cultural norms.

Understanding Personal Feelings and Beliefs and Changing Behavior

Nurses must understand their own personal feelings and beliefs and try to avoid projecting them onto patients. The development of self-awareness will enhance the nurse's objectivity and foster a nonjudgmental attitude, which is so important for building and maintaining trust throughout the nurse–patient relationship. Soliciting feedback from colleagues and supervisors about how personal beliefs or thoughts are being projected onto others is a useful self-assessment technique. One of the reasons that ongoing clinical supervision is so important is that the supervisor really knows the nurse and can continually observe for inappropriate communication and question assumptions that the nurse may hold. Clinical supervision is different from administrative supervision in that the focus is on the therapeutic development of the helper and it does not generally involve an administrative or reporting relationship.

After a nurse has identified and analyzed his or her personal beliefs and attitudes, behaviors that were driven by prejudicial ideas may change. The change process requires introspective analysis that may result in viewing the world differently. Through self-awareness and conscious effort, the nurse can change learned behaviors to engage effectively in therapeutic relationships with patients. Nevertheless, sometimes a nurse realizes that some attitudes are too ingrained to support a therapeutic relationship with a patient with different beliefs. In such cases, the nurse should refer the patient to someone with whom the patient is more likely to develop a successful therapeutic relationship.

BOX 9.1

"Know Thyself"

- What physical problems or illnesses have you experienced?
- What significant traumatic life events (e.g., divorce, death of significant person, abuse, disaster) have you experienced?
- What prejudiced or embarrassing beliefs and attitudes about groups different from yours can you identify from your family, significant others, and yourself?
- Which sociocultural factors in your background could contribute to being rejected by members of other cultures?
- How would the above experiences affect your ability to care for patients?

COMMUNICATION TYPES AND TECHNIQUES

Effective communication skills, including verbal and non-verbal techniques, are the building blocks for all successful relationships. The nurse–patient relationship is built on therapeutic communication, the ongoing process of interaction through which meaning emerges (Box 9.2). **Verbal communication**, which is principally achieved by spoken words, includes the underlying emotion, context, and connotation of what is actually said. **Nonverbal communication** includes gestures, expressions, and body language. Both the patient and the nurse use verbal and nonverbal communication. To respond therapeutically in a nurse–patient relationship, the nurse is responsible for assessing and interpreting all forms of patient communication.

> **NCLEXNOTE**   In analyzing patient–nurse communication, nonverbal behaviors and gestures are communicated first. If a patient's verbal and nonverbal communications are contradictory, priority should be given to the nonverbal behavior and gestures.

> **KEYCONCEPT**   **Therapeutic communication** is the ongoing process of interaction through which meaning emerges.

Therapeutic and social relationships are very different. In a therapeutic relationship, the nurse focuses on the patient and patient-related issues even when engaging in social activities with that patient. For example, a nurse may take a patient shopping and out for lunch. Even though the nurse is engaged in a social activity, the trip should

---

BOX 9.2

Principles of Therapeutic Communication

- The patient should be the primary focus of the interaction.
- A professional attitude sets the tone of the therapeutic relationship.
- Use self-disclosure cautiously and only when the disclosure has a therapeutic purpose.
- Avoid social relationships with patients.
- Maintain patient confidentiality.
- Assess the patient's intellectual competence to determine the level of understanding.
- Implement interventions from a theoretic base.
- Maintain a nonjudgmental attitude. Avoid making judgments about the patient's behavior.
- Avoid giving advice. By the time the patient sees the nurse, he or she has had plenty of advice.
- Guide the patient to reinterpret his or her experiences rationally.
- Track the patient's verbal interaction through the use of clarifying statements.
- Avoid changing the subject unless the content change is in the patient's best interest.

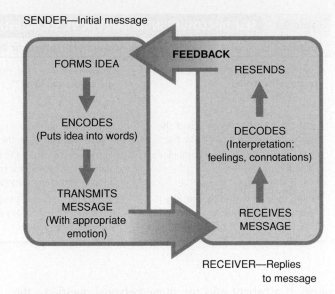

FIGURE 9.1   The communication process. (Adapted from Boyd, M. [1995]. Communication with patients, families, healthcare providers, and diverse cultures. In Strader, M. K., & Decker, P. J. [Eds.]. *Role transition to patient care management* [p. 431]. Norwalk, CT: Appleton & Lange.)

have a definite purpose, and conversation should focus only on the patient. The nurse must not attempt to meet his or her own social or other needs during the activity.

Verbal Communication

The process of verbal communication involves a sender, a message, and a receiver. The patient is often the sender, and the nurse is often the receiver, but communication is always two-way (Figure 9.1). The patient formulates an idea, encodes that message (puts ideas into words), and then transmits the message with emotion. The patient's words and their underlying emotional tone and connotation communicate the individual's needs and emotional problems. The nurse receives the message, decodes it (interprets the message, including its feelings, connotation, and context), and then responds to the patient.

On the surface, this interaction is deceptively simple; unseen complexities lie beneath. Is the message the nurse receives consistent with the patient's original idea? Did the nurse interpret the message as the patient intended? Is the verbal message consistent with the nonverbal flourishes that accompany it? Validation is essential to ensure that the nurse has received the information accurately.

Limiting Self-Disclosure

One of the most important principles of therapeutic communication for the nurse to follow is to focus the interaction on the patient's concerns. **Self-disclosure**, telling the patient personal information, generally is not a good idea. The conversation should focus on the patient, not the

Table 9.1	SELF-DISCLOSURE IN THERAPEUTIC VS. SOCIAL RELATIONSHIPS	
Situation	**Appropriate Therapeutic Response**	**Inappropriate Social Response with Rationale**
A patient asks the nurse if she had fun over the weekend.	"The weekend was fine. How did you spend your weekend?"	"It was great. My boyfriend and I went to dinner and a movie." *(This self-disclosure has no therapeutic purpose. The response focuses the conversation on the nurse, not the patient.)*
A patient asks a student nurse if she has ever been to a particular bar.	"Many people go there. I'm wondering if you have ever been there?"	"Oh yes—all the time. It's a lot of fun." *(Sharing information about outside activities is inappropriate.)*
A patient asks a nurse if mental illness is in the nurse's family.	"Mental illnesses do run in families. I've had a lot of experience caring for people with mental illnesses."	"My sister is being treated for depression." *(This self-disclosure has no purpose, and the nurse is missing the meaning of the question.)*
While shopping with a patient, the nurse sees a friend, who approaches them.	To her friend: "I know it looks like I'm not working, but I really am. I'll see you later."	"Hi, Bob. This is Jane Doe, a patient." *(Introducing the patient to the friend is very inappropriate and violates patient confidentiality.)*

nurse. If a patient asks the nurse personal questions, the nurse should elicit the underlying reason for the request. The nurse can then determine how much personal information to disclose, if any. In revealing personal information, the nurse should be purposeful and have identified therapeutic outcomes. For example, a male patient who was struggling with the implications of marriage and fidelity asked a male nurse if he had ever had an extramarital affair. The nurse interpreted the patient's statement as seeking role-modeling behavior for an adult man and judged self-disclosure in this instance to be therapeutic. He honestly responded that he did not engage in affairs and redirected the discussion back to the patient's concerns.

Nurses sometimes may feel uncomfortable avoiding patients' questions for fear of seeming rude. As a result, they might sometimes disclose too much personal information because they are trying to be "nice." However, being nice is not necessarily therapeutic. As appropriate, redirecting the patient, giving a neutral or vague answer, or saying, "Let's talk about you," may be all that is necessary to limit self-disclosure. In some instances, nurses may need to tell the patient directly that the nurse will not share personal information (Table 9.1).

Using Verbal Communication Techniques

Psychiatric nurses use many verbal techniques in establishing relationships and helping patients focus on their problems. Asking a question, restating, and reflecting are examples of such techniques. These techniques may at first seem artificial, but with practice, they can be useful. Table 9.2 lists some techniques along with examples.

Silence and Listening

One of the most difficult but often most effective communication techniques is the use of silence during verbal interactions. By maintaining silence, the nurse allows the

patient to gather thoughts and to proceed at his or her own pace. It is important that the nurse not interrupt silences because of his or her own anxiety or concern of "not doing anything" if sitting quietly with a patient.

Listening is another valuable tool. Silence and listening differ in that silence consists of deliberate pauses to

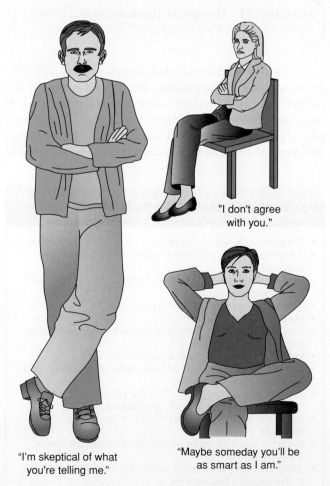

"I don't agree with you."

"I'm skeptical of what you're telling me."

"Maybe someday you'll be as smart as I am."

FIGURE 9.2 Negative body language.

encourage the patient to reflect and eventually respond. Listening is an ongoing activity by which the nurse attends to the patient's verbal and nonverbal communication. The art of listening is developed through careful attention to the content and meaning of the patient's speech. There are two types of listening: passive and active. **Passive listening** involves sitting quietly and letting the patient talk. A passive listener allows the patient to ramble and does not focus or guide the thought process. This form of listening does not foster a therapeutic relationship. Body language during passive listening usually communicates boredom, indifference, or hostility (Figure 9.2).

Through **active listening**, the nurse focuses on what the patient is saying to interpret and respond to the message objectively. While listening, the nurse concentrates only on what the patient says and the underlying meaning. The nurse's verbal and nonverbal behaviors indicate active listening. The nurse usually responds indirectly using techniques such as open-ended statements, reflection (see Table 9.2), and questions that elicit additional responses from the patient. In active listening, the nurse should avoid changing the subject and instead follow the patient's lead. At times, however, it is necessary to respond directly to help a patient focus on a specific topic or to clarify his or her thoughts or beliefs about that topic.

Table 9.2	VERBAL COMMUNICATION TECHNIQUES		
Technique	**Definition**	**Example**	**Use**
Acceptance	Encouraging and receiving information in a nonjudgmental and interested manner	*Patient:* I have done something terrible. *Nurse:* I would like to hear about it. It's OK to discuss it with me.	Used in establishing trust and developing empathy
Confrontation	Presenting the patient with a different reality of the situation	*Patient:* My best friend never calls me. She hates me. *Nurse:* I was in the room yesterday when she called.	Used cautiously to immediately redefine the patient's reality. However, it can alienate the patient if used inappropriately. A nonjudgmental attitude is critical for confrontation to be effective.
Doubt	Expressing or voicing doubt when a patient relates a situation.	*Patient:* My best friend hates me. She never calls me. *Nurse:* From what you have told me, that does not sound like her. When did she call you last?	Used carefully and only when the nurse feels confident about the details. It is used when the nurse wants to guide the patient toward other explanations.
Interpretation	Putting into words what the patient is implying or feeling	*Patient:* I could not sleep because someone would come in my room and rape me. *Nurse:* It sounds like you were scared last night.	Used in helping the patient identify underlying thoughts or feelings
Observation	Stating to the patient what the nurse is observing	*Nurse:* You are trembling and perspiring. When did this start?	Used when a patient's behaviors (verbal or nonverbal) are obvious and unusual for that patient
Open-ended statements	Introducing an idea and letting the patient respond	*Nurse:* Trust means… *Patient:* That someone will keep you safe.	Used when helping patient explore feelings or gain insight
Reflection	Redirecting the idea back to the patient for classification of important emotional overtones, feelings, and experiences; it gives patients permission to have feelings they may not realize they have	*Patient:* Should I go home for the weekend? *Nurse:* Should you go home for the weekend?	Used when patient is asking for the nurse's approval or judgment; use of reflection helps nurse maintain a nonjudgmental approach
Restatement	Repeating the main idea expressed; lets patient know what was heard	*Patient:* I hate this place. I don't belong here. *Nurse:* You don't want to be here.	Used when trying to clarify what the patient has said
Silence	Remaining quiet but nonverbally expressing interest during an interaction	*Patient:* I am angry! *Nurse:* (Silence) *Patient:* My wife had an affair.	Used when patient needs to express ideas but may not know quite how to do it; with silence, the patient can focus on putting thoughts together
Validation	Clarifying the nurse's understanding of the situation	*Nurse:* Let me see if I understand.	Used when nurse is trying to understand a situation the patient is trying to describe

NCLEXNOTE Self-disclosure can be used in very specific situations, but self-disclosure is not the first intervention to consider. In prioritizing interventions, active listening is one of the first to use.

Validation

Another important technique is *validation*, which means explicitly checking one's own thoughts or feelings with another person. To do so, the nurse must own his or her own thoughts or feelings by using "I" statements (Orlando, 1961). The validation generally refers to observation, thoughts, or feelings and seeks explicit feedback. For example, a nurse who sees a patient pacing the hallway before a planned family visit may conclude that the patient is anxious. Validation may occur with a statement such as, "I notice you pacing the hallway. I wonder if you are feeling anxious about the family visit?" The patient may agree, "Yes. I keep worrying about what is going to happen!" or disagree, "No. I have been trying to get into the bathroom for the last 30 minutes, but my roommate is still in there!"

Avoiding Blocks to Communication

Some verbal techniques block interactions and inhibit therapeutic communication (Table 9.3). One of the biggest blocks to communication is giving advice, particularly when others have already given the same advice. Giving advice is different from supporting a patient through decision making. The therapeutic dialogue presented in Box 9.3 differentiates between advice (telling the patient what to do or how to act) from therapeutic communication, through which the nurse and patient explore alternative ways of viewing the patient's world. The patient can then reach his or her own conclusions about the best approaches to use.

Nonverbal Communication

Gestures, facial expressions, and body language actually communicate more than verbal messages. Under the best circumstances, body language mirrors or enhances what is verbally communicated. However, if verbal and nonverbal messages conflict, the listener will believe the nonverbal message. For example, if a patient says that he feels fine but has a sad facial expression and is slumped in a chair away from others, the message of sadness and depression, rather than the patient's words, will be accepted. The same is true of a nurse's behavior. For example, if a nurse tells a patient, "I am happy to see you," but the nurse's facial expression communicates indifference, the patient will receive the message that the nurse is bored.

People with psychiatric problems often have difficulty verbally expressing themselves and interpreting the emotions of others. Because of this, nurses need to continually assess the nonverbal communication needs of patients. Eye contact (or lack thereof), posture, movement (shifting in chair, pacing), facial expressions, and gestures are nonverbal behaviors that communicate thoughts and feelings. For example, a patient who is pacing and restless may be upset or having a reaction to medication. A clenched fist usually indicates that a person feels angry or hostile.

Nonverbal behavior varies from culture to culture. The nurse must, therefore, be careful to understand his or her own cultural context as well as that of the patient. For example, in some cultures, it is considered disrespectful to look a person straight in the eye. In other cultures, not looking a person in the eye may be interpreted as "hiding something" or as having low self-esteem. Whether one points with the finger, nose, or eyes and how much hand gesturing to use are other examples of nonverbal communication that may vary considerably among cultures.

Table 9.3	**TECHNIQUES THAT INHIBIT COMMUNICATION**		
Technique	**Definition**	**Example**	**Problem**
Advice	Telling a patient what to do	*Patient:* I can't sleep. It is too noisy. *Nurse:* Turn off the light and shut your door.	The nurse solves the patient's problem, which may not be the appropriate solution and encourages dependency on the nurse.
Agreement	Agreeing with a particular viewpoint of a patient	*Patient:* Abortions are sinful. *Nurse:* I agree.	The patient is denied the opportunity to change his or her view now that the nurse agrees.
Challenges	Disputing the patient's beliefs with arguments, logical thinking, or direct order	*Patient:* I'm a cowboy. *Nurse:* If you are a cowboy, what are you doing in the hospital?	The nurse belittles the patient and decreases the patient's self-esteem. The patient will avoid relating to the nurse who challenges.
Reassurance	Telling a patient that everything will be OK	*Patient:* Everyone thinks I'm bad. *Nurse:* You are a good person.	The nurse makes a statement that may not be true. The patient is blocked from exploring his or her feelings.
Disapproval	Judging the patient's situation and behavior	*Patient:* I'm so sorry. I did not mean to kill my mother. *Nurse:* You should be. How could anyone kill their mother?	The nurse belittles the patient. The patient will avoid the nurse.

BOX 9.3 • THERAPEUTIC DIALOGUE • Giving Advice versus Recommendations

Ms. J has just received a diagnosis of phobic disorder and has been given a prescription for fluoxetine (Prozac). She was referred to the home health agency because she does not want to take her medication. She is fearful of becoming suicidal. Two approaches are given below.

INEFFECTIVE COMMUNICATION (ADVICE)

Nurse: Ms. J, the doctor has ordered the medication because it will help with your anxiety.

Ms. J: Yes, but I don't want to take the medication. I'm afraid it will make me suicidal. Some psychiatric medication does that. I haven't had any attacks for 2 weeks, and it seems too risky since I'm doing better. I'm scared of the side effects.

Nurse: This medication has rarely had that side effect. You should try it and see if you have any suicidal thoughts.

Ms. J: [Remains silent for a while, crosses her legs, and looks away from the nurse and down at her feet] . . . okay.

(The nurse leaves, and Ms. J decides not take the medication. Within 1 week, Ms. J is taken to the emergency room with a panic attack.)

EFFECTIVE COMMUNICATION

Nurse: Ms. J, how have you been doing?

Ms. J: So far, so good. I haven't had any attacks for 2 weeks.

Nurse: I understand that the doctor gave you a prescription for medication that may help with the panic attacks.

Ms. J: Yes, but I don't want to take it. I'm afraid of becoming suicidal. Some of this psychiatric medication does that. I don't really want to take a needless risk since I've been feeling better.

Nurse: Those worries are understandable. Have you ever had feelings of hurting yourself?

Ms. J: Not yet.

Nurse: If you took the medication and had thoughts like that, what would you do?

Ms. J: I don't know, that's why I'm scared.

Nurse: I think I see your dilemma. This medication may help your panic attacks, but if the medication produces suicidal thoughts then it might compromise your progress and that's a pretty serious risk. Is that correct?

Ms. J: Yeah, that's it.

Nurse: What are the circumstances under which you would feel more comfortable trying the medication?

Ms. J: If I knew that I would not have suicidal thoughts. If I could be assured of that.

Nurse: I can't guarantee that, but perhaps we could create an environment in which you would feel safe. I could call you every few days to see if you are having any of these thoughts and, if so, I could help you deal with them and make sure you see the doctor to review the medication.

Ms. J: Oh, that helps. If you do that, then I think that I will be alright.

(Ms. J successfully takes the medication.)

CRITICAL THINKING CHALLENGE

- Contrast the communication in the first scenario with that in the second.
- What therapeutic communication techniques did the second nurse use that may have contributed to a better outcome?
- Are there any cues in the first scenario that indicate that the patient will not follow the nurse's advice? Explain.

The nurse needs to be aware of cultural differences in communication in the context of each relationship and may need to consult with a cultural interpreter or use other learning opportunities to ensure that his or her communication is culturally congruent.

Nurses should use positive body language, such as sitting at the same eye level as the patient with a relaxed posture that projects interest and attention. Leaning slightly forward helps engage the patient. Generally, the nurse should not cross his or her arms or legs during therapeutic communication because such postures erect barriers to interaction. Uncrossed arms and legs project openness and a willingness to engage in conversation (Figure 9.3). Any verbal response should be consistent with nonverbal messages.

Selection of Communication Techniques

In successful therapeutic communication, the nurse chooses the best words to say and uses nonverbal behaviors that are consistent with these words. If a patient is angry and upset, should the nurse invite the patient to sit

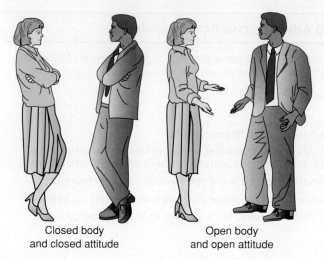

Closed body
and closed attitude

Open body
and open attitude

FIGURE 9.3 Open and closed body language.

down and discuss the problem, walk quietly with the patient, or simply observe the patient from a distance and not initiate conversation? Choosing the best response begins with assessing and interpreting the meaning of the patient's communication—both verbal and nonverbal.

Nurses should not necessarily take verbal messages literally, especially when a patient is upset or angry. For example, one nurse walked into the room of a newly admitted patient who accused, "You locked me up and threw away the key." The nurse could have responded defensively that she had nothing to do with the patient being admitted; however, that response could have ended in an argument, and communication would have been blocked. Fortunately, the nurse recognized that the patient was communicating frustration at being in a locked psychiatric unit and did not take the accusation personally.

The next step is identifying the desired patient outcome. To do so, the nurse should engage the patient with eye contact and quietly try to interpret the patient's feelings. In this example, the desired outcome was for the patient to clarify the hospitalization experience. The nurse responded, "It must be frustrating to feel locked up." The nurse focused on the patient's feelings rather than the accusations, which reflected an understanding of the patient's feelings. The patient knew that the nurse accepted these feelings, which led to further discussion. It may seem impossible to plan reactions for each situation, but with practice, the nurse will begin to respond automatically in a therapeutic way.

CONSIDERATIONS FOR EFFECTIVE COMMUNICATION AND RELATIONSHIPS

When the nurse is interacting with patients, additional considerations can enhance the quality of communica-

tion. This section describes the importance of rapport, empathy, recognition of empathic linkages, the role of boundaries and body space, and recognition of defense mechanisms in nurse–patient interactions.

Rapport

Rapport, interpersonal harmony characterized by understanding and respect, is important in developing a trusting, therapeutic relationship. Nurses establish rapport through interpersonal warmth, a nonjudgmental attitude, and a demonstration of understanding. A skilled nurse will establish rapport that will alleviate the patient's anxiety in discussing personal problems.

People with psychiatric problems often feel alone and isolated. Establishing rapport helps lessen feelings of being alone. When rapport develops, a patient feels comfortable with the nurse and finds self-disclosure easier. The nurse also feels comfortable and recognizes that an interpersonal bond or alliance is developing. All of these factors—comfort, sense of sharing, and decreased anxiety—are important in establishing and building the nurse–patient relationship.

Empathy

The use of empathy in a therapeutic relationship is central to psychiatric–mental health nursing. Empathy is sometimes confused with sympathy, which is the expression of compassion and kindness. **Empathy** is the ability to experience, in the present, a situation as another did at some time in the past. It is the ability to put oneself in another person's circumstances and to imagine what it would be like to share their feelings. The nurse does not actually have to have had the experience but has to be able to imagine the feelings associated with it. For empathy to develop, there must be a giving of self to the other individual and a reciprocal desire to know each other personally. The process involves the nurse receiving information from the patient with open, nonjudgmental acceptance and communicating this understanding of the experience and feelings so the patient feels understood.

Recognition of Empathic Linkages

While empathy is essential, it is important for the nurse to be aware of **empathic linkages**, the direct communication of feelings (Peplau, 1952). This commonly occurs with anxiety. For example, a nurse may be speaking with a patient who is highly anxious, and the nurse may notice his or her own speech becoming more rapid in tandem with the patient's. The nurse may also become aware of subjective feelings of anxiety. It may be difficult for the nurse to determine if the anxiety was communicated interpersonally or if the nurse is personally reacting to some of the content of what the patient is communicating. However, being aware of one's own feelings and analyzing them is crucial to determining the source of the feeling and addressing associated problems.

Biopsychosocial Boundaries and Body Space Zones

Boundaries are the defining limits of individuals, objects, or relationships. Boundaries mark territory, distinguishing what is "mine" from "not mine." Human beings have many different types of boundaries. Material boundaries, such as fences around property, artificially imposed state lines, and bodies of water, define territory as well as provide security and order. Personal boundaries can be conceptualized within the biopsychosocial model as including physical, psychological, and social dimensions. Physical boundaries are those established in terms of physical closeness to others—who we allow to touch us or how close we want others to stand near us.

Psychological boundaries are established in terms of emotional distance from others—how much of our innermost feelings and thoughts we want to share. Social boundaries, such as norms, customs, and roles, help us establish our closeness and place within the family, culture, and community. Boundaries are not fixed but dynamic. When boundaries are involuntarily transgressed, the individual feels threatened and responds to the perceived threat. The nurse must elicit permission before implementing interventions that invade the patient's personal space.

Personal Boundaries

Every individual is surrounded by four different body zones that provide varying degrees of protection against unwanted physical closeness during interactions. These were identified by Hall (1990) as the intimate zone (e.g., for whispering and embracing), the personal zone (e.g., for close friends), the social zone (e.g., for acquaintances), and the public zone (usually for interacting with strangers) (Figure 9.4). The actual sizes of the different zones vary according to culture. Some cultures define the intimate zone narrowly and the personal zones widely. Thus, friends in these cultures stand and sit close while interacting. People of other cultures define the intimate zone widely and are uncomfortable when others stand close to them.

The variability of intimate and personal zones has implications for nursing. For a patient to be comfortable with a nurse, the nurse needs to protect the intimate zone of that individual. The patient usually will allow the nurse to enter the personal zone but will express discomfort if the nurse breaches the intimate zone. For the nurse, the difficulty lies in differentiating the personal zone from the intimate zone for each patient.

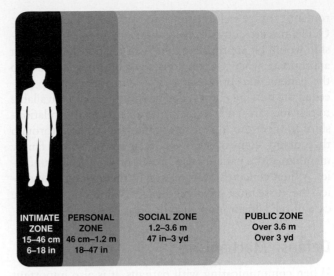

FIGURE 9.4 Body space zones.

The nurse's awareness of his or her own need for intimate and personal space is another prerequisite for therapeutic interaction with the patient. It is important that a nurse feels comfortable while interacting with patients. Establishing a comfort zone may well entail fine-tuning the size of body zones. Recognizing this will help the nurse understand occasional inexplicable reactions to the proximity of patients.

Professional Boundaries and Ethics

For nurses, professional boundaries are also essential to consider in the context of the nurse–patient relationship. Patients often enter such relationships at a very vulnerable point, and nurses need to be aware of professional boundaries to avoid exploitation of the patient. For example, in a friendship, there is a two-way sharing of personal information and feelings, but as mentioned previously, in a nurse–patient relationship, the focus is on the patient's needs, and the nurse generally does not share personal information or attempt to meet his or her own needs through the relationship. The patient may seek a friendship or sexual relationship with the nurse (or vice versa), but this would be inconsistent with the professional role and is usually considered unethical.

Indicators that the relationship may be moving outside the professional boundaries are gift giving on either party's part, spending more time than usual with a particular patient, strenuously defending or explaining the patient's behavior in team meetings, the nurse feeling that he or she is the only one who truly understands the patient, keeping secrets, or frequently thinking about the patient outside of the work situation (Forchuk et al., 2006). State or provincial regulatory bodies will have either guidelines or firm rules regarding any legal or professional restrictions about the amount of time that must pass prior to engaging in a romantic or sexual relationship with a former patient. Guidelines are comparatively vague about when a friendship would be appropriate, but such relationships are not appropriate when the nurse is actively providing care to the patient. Exceptions may be when a relationship preceded the nursing context and another nurse is unavailable to provide care, such as in a rural area. Similarly, relationships to meet the nurse's needs that are acquired through the nursing context, such as a relationship with a family member of the patient, also breach professional boundaries. When concerns arise related to therapeutic boundaries, the nurse must seek clinical supervision or transfer the care of the patient immediately.

Defense Mechanisms

When communicating with patients, it is also important for the nurse to be aware of the defense mechanisms patients may use. The concept of "defense mechanisms" is an old one, originating in Freud's theory of psychoanalysis. While defense mechanisms might seem to indicate the existence of problematic mental state, this is not true. Healthy individuals in many different contexts use defense mechanisms. **Defense mechanisms**, (also known as coping styles), are psychological mechanisms that help an individual respond to and cope with difficult situations, emotional conflicts and external stressors. Some defense mechanisms (e.g., projection, splitting, acting out) are mostly maladaptive. Others (e.g., suppression, denial) may be either maladaptive or adaptive depending on the context in which they occur. The use of defense mechanisms becomes maladaptive when its persistent use interferes with the person's ability to function and quality of life (see Table 9.4).

For example, responding to a difficult life event altruistically is very often a healthy way to recover. On the other hand, defense mechanisms such as acting out, autistic fantasies, projection, and splitting are rarely adaptive. A defense mechanism such as repression can be a natural way to react to a traumatic experience, specifically when used in appropriate moderation. However, the unchecked repression of difficult thoughts or feelings can keep someone from coming to terms with their experiences. In developing a successful therapeutic relationship, and in establishing open communication, such knowledge of defense mechanisms will prove itself invaluable.

As nurses develop therapeutic relationships, they will recognize their patients using defense mechanisms. With experience, the nurse will evaluate the purpose of a defense mechanism and then determine whether or not it should be discussed with the patient. For example, if a patient is using humor to alleviate an emotionally intense situation, that may be very appropriate. On the other hand, if someone continually rationalizes antisocial behavior, the use of the defense mechanism should be discussed.

> **NCLEXNOTE** When studying defense mechanisms, focus on mechanisms and coping styles that are similar. For example, displacement versus devaluation versus projection should be differentiated. Identify these mechanisms in your process recordings.

COMMUNICATION CONSIDERATIONS FOR PATIENTS WITH MENTAL HEALTH CHALLENGES

For patients with specific, known mental health problems or illnesses, the nurse must consider how these issues may impact communication and be prepared to analyze the content of nurse–patient interactions.

Considering Specific Mental Health Issues

It is important to consider the individual's specific mental health challenges when selecting specific communication strategies. For example, patients may frequently be experiencing increased levels of anxiety. The nurse who understands that focal attention decreases as anxiety increases will use shorter and simpler statements or questions when the patient exhibits higher levels of anxiety.

Patients who are experiencing depression may have difficulty articulating their feelings or their thinking and responses may be slowed. The nurse will frequently use silence and empathic techniques throughout this interaction. The person who is depressed may also use communication styles such as overgeneralizing ("This always happens to me . . . everything always turns out for the worse. . . ."). The nurse can assist the patient to be more specific (e.g., asking about a specific time or a specific exception).

When patients are experiencing schizophrenia, they may have hallmark symptoms such as hallucinations or delusions. If a person is having auditory hallucinations (hearing sounds that are imagined), the nurse's voice may be one of several the patient is hearing. Clear, short sentences may assist in getting the patient's attention on the nurse's voice. A person experiencing delusions may use pronouns vaguely ("they" did it) or other forms of vague or unclear communication. Clarifying and assisting the patient to be more specific may assist the patient's thinking as well as communication.

As you read through the chapters on various mental challenges, consider how the signs and symptoms of each illness could have an impact on communication and the evolving therapeutic relationship.

Table 9.4	SPECIFIC DEFENSE MECHANISMS AND COPING STYLES	

The following defense mechanisms and coping styles are commonly used when the individual deals with emotional conflict or stressors (either internal or external).

Defense Mechanism	Definition	Example
Acting out	Using actions rather than reflections or feelings during periods of emotional conflict	A teenager gets mad at his parents and begins staying out late at night.
Affiliation	Turning to others for help or support (sharing problems with others without implying that someone else is responsible for them)	An individual has a fight with her spouse and turns to her best friend for emotional support.
Altruism	Dedicating life to meeting the needs of others (receives gratification either vicariously or from the response of others)	After being rejected by her boyfriend, a young girl joins the Peace Corps.
Anticipation	Experiencing emotional reactions in advance or anticipating consequences of possible future events and considering realistic, alternative responses or solutions	A parent cries for 3 weeks before her last child leaves for college. On the day of the separation, the parent spends the day with friends.
Autistic fantasy	Excessive daydreaming as a substitute for human relationships, more effective action, or problem solving	A young man sits in his room all day and dreams about being a rock star instead of attending a baseball game with a friend.
Denial	Refusing to acknowledge some painful aspect of external reality or subjective experience that would be apparent to others (*psychotic denial* used when there is gross impairment in reality testing)	A teenager's best friend moves away, but the adolescent says he does not feel sad.
Devaluation	Attributing exaggerated negative qualities to self or others	A boy has been rejected by his long-time girlfriend. He tells his friends that he realizes that she is stupid and ugly.
Displacement	Transferring a feeling about, or a response to, one object onto another (usually less threatening), substitute object	A child is mad at her mother for leaving for the day but says she is really mad at the sitter for serving her food she does not like.
Dissociation	Experiencing a breakdown in the usually integrated functions of consciousness, memory, perception of self or the environment, or sensory and motor behavior	An adult relates severe sexual abuse experienced as a child but does it without feeling. She says that the experience was as if she were outside her body watching the abuse.
Help-rejecting complaining	Complaining or making repetitious requests for help that disguise covert feelings of hostility or reproach toward others, which are then expressed by rejecting the suggestions, advice, or help that others offer (complaints or requests may involve physical or psychological symptoms or life problems)	A college student asks a teacher for help after receiving a bad grade on a test. Every suggestion the teacher has is rejected by the student.
Humor	Emphasizing the amusing or ironic aspects of the conflict or stressor	A person makes a joke right after experiencing an embarrassing situation.
Idealization	Attributing exaggerated positive qualities to others	An adult falls in love and fails to see the negative qualities in the other person.
Intellectualization	Excessive use of abstract thinking or the making of generalizations to control or minimize disturbing feelings	After rejection in a romantic relationship, the rejected explains the relationship dynamics to a friend.
Isolation of affect	Separation of ideas from the feelings originally associated with them	The individual loses touch with the feelings associated with a rape while remaining aware of the details.
Omnipotence	Feeling or acting as if one possesses special powers or abilities and is superior to others	An individual tells a friend about personal expertise in the stock market and the ability to predict the best stocks.
Passive aggression	Indirectly and unassertively expressing aggression toward others. There is a facade of overt compliance masking covert resistance, resentment, or hostility.	One employee doesn't like another, so he secretly steals her milk from the office refrigerator. She is unaware of his hostile feelings.
Projection	Falsely attributing to another one's own unacceptable feelings, impulses, or thoughts	A child is very angry at a parent but accuses the parent of being angry.

(Continued)

Table 9.4	SPECIFIC DEFENSE MECHANISMS AND COPING STYLES (*Continued*)	
Defense Mechanism	**Definition**	**Example**
Projective identification	Falsely attributing to another one's own unacceptable feelings, impulses, or thoughts. Unlike simple projection, the individual does not fully disavow what is projected. Instead, the individual remains aware of his or her own affect or impulses but misattributes them as justifiable reactions to the other person. Frequently, the individual induces the very feelings in others that were first mistakenly believed to be there, making it difficult to clarify who did what to whom first.	A child is mad at a parent, who in turn becomes angry at the child but may be unsure of why. The child then feels justified at being angry with the parent.
Rationalization	Concealing the true motivations for one's own thoughts, actions, or feelings through the elaboration of reassuring or self-serving but incorrect explanations	A man is rejected by his girlfriend but explains to his friends that her leaving was best because she was beneath him socially and would not be liked by his family.
Reaction formation	Substituting behavior, thoughts, or feelings that are diametrically opposed to one's own unacceptable thoughts or feelings (this usually occurs in conjunction with their repression)	A wife finds out about her husband's extramarital affairs and tells her friends that she thinks his affairs are perfectly appropriate. She truly does not feel, on a conscious level, any anger or hurt.
Repression	Expelling disturbing wishes, thoughts, or experiences from conscious awareness (the feeling component may remain conscious, detached from its associated ideas)	A woman does not remember the experience of being raped in the basement but does feel anxious when going into that house.
Self-assertion	Expressing feelings and thoughts directly in a way that is not coercive or manipulative	An individual reaffirms that going to a ball game is not what she wants to do.
Self-observation	Reflecting feelings, thoughts, motivation, and behavior and responding to them appropriately	An individual notices an irritation at his friend's late arrival and decides to tell the friend of the irritation.
Splitting	Compartmentalizing opposite affect states and failing to integrate the positive and negative qualities of the self or others into cohesive images	Self and object images tend to alternate between polar opposites: exclusively loving, powerful, worthy, nurturing, and kind or exclusively bad, hateful, angry, destructive, rejecting, or worthless. One friend is wonderful and another former friend, who was at one time viewed as being perfect, is now believed to be an evil person.
Sublimation	Channeling potentially maladaptive feelings or impulses into socially acceptable behavior	An adolescent boy is very angry with his parents. On the football field, he tackles someone very forcefully.
Suppression	Intentionally avoiding thinking about disturbing problems, wishes, feelings, or experiences	A student is anxiously awaiting test results but goes to a movie to stop thinking about it.
Undoing	Words or behavior designed to negate or to make amends symbolically for unacceptable thoughts, feelings, or actions	A man has sexual fantasies about his wife's sister. He takes his wife away for a romantic weekend.

Analyzing Interactions

Many patients with psychiatric disorders have difficulty communicating. For example, perceptual, cognitive, and information-processing deficits, which are typical of people with schizophrenia, can interfere with the patient's ability to express ideas, understand concepts, and accurately perceive the environment. Because of the complexity of communication, mental health professionals monitor their interactions with patients using various methods, including audio recording; video recording; and **process recording**, which entails writing a verbatim transcript of the interaction. A video or audio recording of an interaction provides the most accurate monitoring but is cumbersome to use. Process recording, one of the easiest methods to use, is adequate in most situations. Nurses should use it when first learning therapeutic communication and during times when communication becomes a problem. In a process recording, the nurse records, from memory, the verbatim interaction immediately after the communication (Table 9.5).

The nurse then analyzes the content of the interaction in terms of the words and their meaning for both the patient and the nurse. The analysis is especially important

Table 9.5	**PROCESS RECORDING**	

Setting: The living room of Mr. S's home. Mr. S is 23 years old and was hospitalized for 2 weeks. His diagnosis is a bipolar mood disorder, and he is recovering from a depressive episode. His parents are in the room but cannot hear the conversation. Mr. S is sitting on the couch, and the nurse is sitting on a chair. This is the nurse's first visit after Mr. S's discharge from the hospital.

Patient	Nurse	Interpretation/Analysis
	How are you doing, Mr. S? (smiles and offers hand to shake)	*Plan:* Initially develop a sense of trust and initiate a therapeutic relationship.
I'm fine. It's good to be home (looking at floor, takes nurse's hand to briefly shake). I really don't like the hospital. (shakes his head while still looking at floor).	You didn't like the hospital?	Interpretation: Validating assumption that Mr. S does not want to return to hospital. Nonverbal communication may indicate sadness or low self-esteem. This needs further exploration.
No. The nurses lock you up (maintains eye contact with nurse, frowning, arms crossed). Are you a nurse?		Patient validates assumption regarding hospital, but nonverbal behavior indicates there may be further concerns.
	I'm a nurse. I'm wondering if you think that I will lock you up (maintains eye contact and open posture)?	Interpretation: Mr. S may be wondering what my role is and whether I will put him back in the hospital. This assumption needs to be validated, and my role needs clarification.
You could tell my mom to put me back in the hospital (maintains eye contact with nurse).	Any treatment that I recommend will be thoroughly discussed with you first. I am here to help you stay out of the hospital. I will not discuss anything with your mother unless you give me permission to do so (nurse maintains eye contact and open posture).	Use interpretation to clarify Mr. S's thinking. Mr. S is wondering about my relationship with his mother. Explain my role and confidentiality.
(Patient maintains eye contact and uncrosses arms.)		Patient's nonverbal communication appears to indicate he is more comfortable with this clarification.

because the ability to communicate verbally is often compromised in people with mental disorders. Because words may not have the same meaning for the patient as they do for the nurse, clarification of meaning becomes especially important. The analysis can identify symbolic meanings, themes, and blocks in communication.

Symbolism

Symbolism, the use of a word or phrase to represent an object, event, or feeling, is used universally. For example, automobiles are named for wild animals that represent speed, prowess, and beauty. In people with mental disorders, the use of words to symbolize events, objects, or feelings is often idiosyncratic, and they cannot explain their choices. For example, a person who is feeling scared and anxious may tell the nurse that bombs and guns are exploding. It is up to the nurse to make the connection between the bombs and guns and the patient's feelings and then validate this with the patient. Because of the patient's cognitive limitations, the individual may express feelings only symbolically. Another example is found in Table 9.6.

Some patients, for example, some with developmental disabilities or organic brain difficulties, may have difficulty with abstract thinking and symbolism. Conversations may be interpreted literally. For example, in response to the question: "What brings you to the hospital?" a patient might reply, "The ambulance." In these situations, the nurse must be cautious to avoid using symbols or metaphors. Concrete language, that is, language reflecting what can be observed through the senses, will be more easily understood.

Content Themes

Verbal behavior is also interpreted by analyzing **content themes**. Patients often express concerns or feelings repeatedly in several different ways. After a few sessions, a common theme emerges. Themes may emerge symbolically, as in the case with the patient who constantly talks about the "guns and bombs." Alternatively, a theme may simply be identified as a recurrent thread of a story that a patient retells at each session. For example, one patient often discussed his early abandonment by his family. This led the nurse to hypothesize that he had an underlying fear of rejection. The nurse was then able to test whether there was an underlying fear and to develop strategies to help the patient explore the fear (Box 9.4). It is important to involve patients in analyzing themes so they may learn this skill. Within the therapeutic relationship, the person who does the work is the one who

Table 9.6	USE OF SYMBOLISM	

Setting: Mr. A has been diagnosed with schizophrenia and expresses himself through the use of television characters. A nurse observed another patient shoving him against the wall. As the nurse approached the two patients, the other patient ran, leaving Mr. A noticeably shaking. The nurse checked to see if Mr. A was all right.

Patient	Nurse	Interpretation/Analysis
	Mr. A, are you OK? (approaches patient)	
Robin Hood saved the day. (trembling, arms crossed)		Mr. A could not say, "Thank you for helping me." Instead, he could only describe a fictional character's response.
	You feel that you are saved?	The nurse focused on what Mr. A must be feeling if he felt that he had been rescued.
It's a glorious day in Sherwood Forest! (trembling decreases; smiles at nurse)		He seems to be happy now.
	Mr. A, are you hurting anywhere? (eyes scan over patient, using concerned tone of voice)	The nurse wanted to check whether the patient had been hurt when pushed against the wall.
The angel of mercy put out the fire. (continues to smile and extends hand to shake hands with nurse)		The patient is apparently not hurting now.

develops the competencies, so the nurse must be careful to share this opportunity with the patient (Peplau, 1952, 1992).

Communication Blocks

Communication blocks are identified by topic changes that either the nurse or the patient makes. Topics are changed for various reasons. A patient may change the topic from one that does not interest him to one that he finds more meaningful. However, an individual usually changes the topic because he or she is uncomfortable with a particular subject. When a topic change is identified, the nurse or patient hypothesizes the reason for it. If the nurse changes the topic, he or she needs to determine why. The nurse may find that he or she is uncomfortable with the topic or may not be listening to the patient. Novice mental health nurses who are uncomfortable with silences or trying to elicit specific information from the patient often change topics.

The nurse must also record and interpret the patient's nonverbal behavior in light of the verbal behavior. Is the

---

BOX 9.4

Themes and Interactions

Session 1: Patient discusses the death of his mother at a young age.
Session 2: Patient explains that his sister is now married and never visits him.
Session 3: Patient says that his best friend in the hospital was discharged and he really misses her.
Session 4: Patient cries about a lost kitten.
Interpretation: Theme of loss is pervasive in several sessions.

---

patient saying one thing verbally and another nonverbally? The nurse must consider the patient's cultural background. Is the behavior consistent with cultural norms? For example, if a patient denies any problems but is affectionate and physically demonstrative (which is antithetical to her naturally stoic cultural beliefs and behaviors), the nonverbal behavior is inconsistent with what is normal behavior for that person. Further exploration is needed to determine the meaning of the culturally atypical behavior.

THE NURSE–PATIENT RELATIONSHIP

The nurse–patient relationship is a dynamic process that changes with time. It can be viewed in steps or phases with characteristic behaviors for both patient and nurse. This text uses an adaptation of Hildegarde Peplau's model, which she introduced in her seminal work, *Interpersonal Relations in Nursing* (1952, 1992). Emerging evidence suggests that a well-developed nurse–patient relationship positively affects patient care.

Phases

The nurse–patient relationship is conceptualized in three overlapping phases that evolve with time: orientation phase, working phase, and resolution phase. The **orientation phase** is the phase during which the nurse and patient get to know each other. During this phase, which can last from a few minutes to several months, the patient develops a sense of trust in the nurse. The second is the **working phase**, in which the patient uses the relationship to examine specific problems and learn new ways of approaching them. The final stage, **resolution phase**, is

Table 9.7	PHASES OF THE NURSE–PATIENT RELATIONSHIP		
	Orientation	**Working**	**Resolution**
Patient	Seeks assistance Identifies needs Commits to a therapeutic relationship During the later part, begins to test relationship	Discusses problems and underlying needs Uses emotional safety of relationship to examine personal issues Tests new ways of solving problems Feels comfortable with nurse May use transference	May express ambivalence about the relationship and its termination Uses personal style to say "good-bye"
Nurse	Actively listens Establishes boundaries of the relationship Clarifies expectations Identifies countertransference issues Uses empathy Establishes rapport	Supports development of healthy problem solving Encourages patient to prepare for the future	Avoids returning to patient's initial problems Encourages independence Promotes positive family interactions

the termination stage of the relationship and lasts from the time the problems are actually resolved to the close of the relationship. The relationship does not evolve as a simple linear relationship. Instead, the relationship may be predominantly in one phase, but reflections of all phases can be seen in each interaction (Table 9.7).

> **KEYCONCEPT** The **nurse–patient relationship** is a dynamic process that changes with time. It can be viewed in steps or phases with characteristic behaviors for both the patient and the nurse.

Orientation Phase

The orientation phase begins when the nurse and patient meet and ends when the patient begins to identify problems to be examined. During the orientation phase, the nurse discusses the patient's expectations, explains the purpose of the relationship and its boundaries, and facilitates the development of the relationship. It is natural for the nurse to be nervous during the first few sessions. The goal of the orientation phase is to develop trust and security within the nurse–patient relationship. During this initial phase, the nurse listens intently to the patient's history and perception of problems and begins to understand the patient and identify themes. The use of empathy facilitates the development of a positive therapeutic relationship.

First Meeting

During the first meeting, outlining both nursing and patient responsibilities is important. The nurse is responsible for providing guidance throughout the therapeutic relationship, protecting confidential information, and maintaining professional boundaries. The patient is responsible for attending agreed-upon sessions, interacting during the sessions, and participating in the nurse–patient relationship. The nurse should also explain clearly to the patient meeting times, handling of missed sessions, and the estimated length of the relationship. Issues related to recording information and how the nurse will work within the interdisciplinary team should also be made explicit.

Usually, both the nurse and the patient feel anxious at the first meeting. The nurse should recognize the anxieties and attempt to alleviate them before the meeting. The patient's behavior during this first meeting may indicate to the nurse some of the patient's problems in interpersonal relationships. For example, a patient may talk nonstop for 15 minutes or may brag of sexual conquests. What the patient chooses to tell or not to tell is significant. What a patient first does or says may not accurately indicate his or her true feelings or the situation. In the beginning, patients may deny problems or employ various forms of defense mechanisms or prevent the nurse from getting to know them. The patient is usually nervous and insecure during the first few sessions and may exhibit behavior reflective of these emotions, such as rambling. Typically, by the third session, the patient can focus on a topic.

Confidentiality in Treatment

Ideally, nurses include people who are important to the patient in planning and implementing care. The nurse and patient should discuss the issue of confidentiality in the first session. The nurse should be clear about any information that is to be shared with anyone else. The nurse shares significant assessment data and patient progress with a supervisor, team members, and a physician. Most patients expect the nurse to communicate with other mental health professionals and are comfortable with this arrangement. Restrictions regarding what can be shared and with whom are also covered by state or provincial mental health acts and health information acts.

Testing the Relationship

This first part of the orientation phase, called the "honeymoon phase," is usually pleasant. However, the therapeutic team typically hits rough spots before completing this phase. The patient begins to test the relationship to become convinced that the nurse will really accept him or her. Typical "testing behaviors" include forgetting a scheduled session or being late. Patients may also express anger at something a nurse says or accuse the nurse of breaking confidentiality. Another common pattern is for the patient to first introduce a relatively superficial issue as if it is the major problem. The nurse must recognize that these behaviors are designed to test the relationship and establish its parameters, not to express rejection or dissatisfaction with the nurse. The student nurse often feels personally rejected during the patient's testing and may even become angry with the patient. If the nurse simply accepts the behavior and continues to be available and consistent to the patient, these behaviors usually subside. Testing needs to be understood as a normal way that human beings develop trust.

Working Phase

When the patient begins identifying problems to work on, the working phase of the relationship has started. Problem identification can yield a wide range of issues, such as managing symptoms of a mental disorder, coping with chronic pain, examining issues related to sexual abuse, or dealing with problematic interpersonal relationships. Through the relationship, the patient begins to explore the identified problems and develop strategies to resolve them. By the time the working phase is reached, the patient has developed enough trust that he or she can examine the identified problems within the security of the therapeutic relationship. In the working phase, the nurse can use various verbal and nonverbal techniques to help the patient examine problems and to support the patient through the healing process.

Transference (unconscious assignment to others of the feelings and attitudes that the patient originally associated with important figures) and **countertransference** (the provider's emotional reaction to the patient based on personal unconscious needs and conflicts) become important issues in the working phase. For example, a patient could be hostile to a nurse because of underlying resentment of authority figures; the nurse, in turn, could respond defensively because of earlier experiences of anger. The patient uses transference to examine problems. During this phase, the patient is psychologically vulnerable and emotionally dependent on the nurse. The nurse needs to recognize countertransference and prevent it from eroding professional boundaries.

Many times, nurses are eager to implement rehabilitation plans. However, this cannot be done until the patient trusts the nurse and identifies what issues he or she wishes to work on in the context of the relationship.

Resolution Phase

The final stage of the nurse–patient relationship is resolution, which begins when the actual problems are resolved and ends with the termination of the relationship. During this phase, the patient is redirected toward a life without this specific therapeutic relationship. The patient connects with community resources, solidifies a newly found understanding, and practices new behaviors. The patient takes responsibility for follow-up appointments and interacts with significant others in new ways. New problems are not addressed during this phase except in terms of what was learned during the working stage. The nurse assists the client in strengthening relationships, making referrals, and recognizing and understanding signs of future relapse.

Termination begins on the first day of the relationship when the nurse explains that this relationship is time limited and was established to resolve the patient's problems and help him or her handle them. Because a therapeutic relationship is dependent, the nurse must constantly evaluate the patient's level of dependence and continually support the patient's move toward independence. Termination is usually stressful for the patient, who must sever ties with the nurse who has shared thoughts and feelings and given guidance and support over many sessions.

Depending on previous experiences with terminating relationships, some patients may not handle their emotions well during termination. Some may not show up for the last session at all to avoid their feelings of sadness and separation. Many patients display anger about the relationship's ending. Patients may express anger toward the nurse or displace it onto others. For example, a patient may shout obscenities at another patient after being told that his therapeutic relationship with the nurse would end in a few weeks. One of the best ways to handle the anger is to help the patient acknowledge it, to explain that anger is a normal emotion when a relationship is ending, and to reassure the patient that it is acceptable to feel angry. The nurse should also reassure the patient that anger subsides after the relationship is over.

Another typical termination behavior is raising old problems that have already been resolved. The nurse may feel frustrated if patients in the termination phase present resolved problems as if they were new. The nurse may feel that the sessions were unsuccessful. In reality, patients are attempting to prolong the relationship and avoid its ending. Nurses should avoid addressing these problems. Instead, they should reassure patients that they already covered those issues and learned methods to control them. They should explain that the patient may be feeling anxious about the relationship's ending and redirect the

BOX 9.5 • THERAPEUTIC DIALOGUE • The Last Meeting

INEFFECTIVE APPROACH

Ms. J: Why did the other nurses bring you flowers and cards today?

Nurse: Well, that's because today is my last day, I'm transfering to the new hospital, across town.

Ms. J: Oh, um. I was just thinking, I need to talk to you about something important.

Nurse: What is it?

Ms. J: I have been worrying about my medication again.

Nurse: Oh, have you had any side effects?

Ms. J: No, but I might.

Nurse: I think you should tell the new nurse.

Ms. J: She is too new. She won't understand and you helped me last time. I feel so worried about your leaving. Is there any way you can stay? You said that you would check in, remember?

Nurse: Well, I could check on you tomorrow?

Ms. J: Oh, would you? I would really appreciate it if you would give me your new telephone number that way I can tell you if anything happens.

Nurse: I don't know what the number will be, but you might be able to find it online.

EFFECTIVE APPROACH

Ms. J: Why did the other nurses bring you flowers and cards today?

Nurse: Oh, hello Ms. J. Do you remember? Today is my last day.

Ms. J: Oh, yes. Well, I need to talk to you about something important.

Nurse: We talked about that. Anything "important" needs to be shared with the new nurse.

Ms. J: But I want to tell *you*. You really made me feel better last time.

Nurse: Thank you, but remember that you improved a lot because you know what to do in order to continue progressing. Saying good-bye can be very hard.

Ms. J: I'll miss you.

Nurse: Your feelings are very normal when relationships are ending. I will remember you in a very special way.

Ms. J: Can I please have your telephone number in case I need to talk to you?

Nurse: No, I can't give that to you. It is important that we say good-bye today. And, remember, you can always talk to the new nurse about your concerns.

Ms. J: Okay, I know. Good-bye. Good luck.

Nurse: Good-bye.

CRITICAL THINKING CHALLENGE

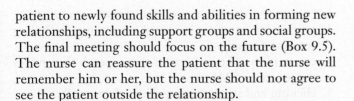

- What were some of the mistakes the nurse in the first scenario made?
- In the second scenario, how does therapeutic communication in the termination phase differ from effective communication in the working phase?

---

patient to newly found skills and abilities in forming new relationships, including support groups and social groups. The final meeting should focus on the future (Box 9.5). The nurse can reassure the patient that the nurse will remember him or her, but the nurse should not agree to see the patient outside the relationship.

Nontherapeutic Relationships

Although it is hoped that all nurse–patient relationships will go through the phases of the relationship described earlier, this is not always the case. In a **nontherapeutic relationship**, the nurse and patient both feel very frustrated and keep varying their approach with each other in an attempt to establish a meaningful relationship. This is different from a prolonged orientation phase in that the efforts are not sustained; rather, they vary constantly.

The nurse may try longer meetings, shorter meetings, being more or less directive, and varying the therapeutic stance from warm and friendly to aloof. Patients in this phase may try to talk about the past but then change to discussions of the "here and now." They will try talking about their family and in the next meeting talk about their work goals. Both *grapple and struggle* to come to a common ground, and both become increasingly frustrated with each other.

Eventually, the frustration becomes so great that the pair gives up on each other and moves to a phase of *mutual withdrawal*. The nurse may schedule seeing this patient at the end of the shift and "run out of time" so the meeting never happens. The patient will leave the unit or otherwise be unavailable during scheduled meeting times. If a meeting does occur, the nurse will try to keep it short, thinking, "What's the point—we just cover the same old ground anyway." The patient will attempt to keep it superficial and stay on safe topics ("You can always ask about your medications—nurses love to health teach, you know").

A **deteriorating relationship** is also nontherapeutic and has been shown to have predictable phases (Coatsworth-Puspoky, Forchuk, & Ward-Griffin, 2006). This relationship starts in the *withholding* phase during which the nurse is perceived as "withholding" nursing support. The nurse fails to recognize that the patient is a person with an illness or health needs. The patient feels uncomfortable, anxious, frustrated, and guilty about being ill and does not develop a sense of trust. A barrier exists between the patient and nurse.

The middle phase of a deteriorating relationship consists of two subphases: *avoiding* and *ignoring*. The patient begins to avoid the nurse and perceives that the nurse is avoiding him or her. The patient abides by the rules and because he or she does not want to cause problems. The nurse is perceived as rude and condescending. The nurse ignores and avoids the patient's requests for help; in turn, the patient becomes more anxious, frustrated, and fearful. Patients experiencing this phase report feelings of wanting to give up, being rejected, not being cared for, and not being listened to.

The end phase is named *struggling with and making sense of*. In the final phase of a nontherapeutic, deteriorating relationship, the patient struggles with and tries to understand the unsatisfactory relationship. The patient feels hopeless and frustrated as a result of the lack of support received by the nurse. In a deteriorating relationship, the patient and nurse begin as strangers and end as enemies.

Obviously, no therapeutic progress can be made in a nontherapeutic or deteriorating relationship. The nurse may be hesitant to ask for a therapeutic transfer, assuming that a relationship would similarly fail with another nurse. However, each relationship is unique, and difficulties in one relationship do not predict difficulties in the next. Clinical supervision early on may assist the development of the relationship, but often a therapeutic transfer to another nurse is required.

EXAMPLES OF STRATEGIES RELATED TO THERAPEUTIC RELATIONSHIPS

Motivational Interviewing

Motivational interviewing (MI) is a clinical method intended to engage a patient's own decision-making ability. By focusing and reinforcing the client's own arguments for change, MI can be used to achieve positive outcomes. This is an inherently collaborative process; through directed counseling, and focused discussions between the care provider and the patient. As a result, MI is inherently exploratory and adaptive.

There is a lot of evidence to suggest that MI produces positive health outcomes; however, evidence also suggests that external factors can influence the success of long-term outcomes. These external factors are often interpersonal and social (Berg, Ross, & Tikkanen, 2011). Because much of the success of MI depends on the quality of interaction between the care provider and the patient, good communication practices are essential for effective implementation of MI. Many of these problems are the result of the assumption that high-risk behaviors are entirely or mostly under the control of the individual (Berg et al., 2011). Careful attention to the effects of this assumption can make clear where MI may or may not be an ideal treatment option.

Because the success of MI is, in part, dependent on contingent factors, care providers require frequent instruction and feedback. Strong communication in the context of therapeutic relationships as discussed in this chapter, especially self-awareness, empathetic linkages, active listening, and the avoidance of unhelpful varieties of defense mechanisms, require on-going training and will affect therapeutic outcomes. While challenging to successfully implement, MI has produced positive health outcomes in many different settings (Barnett, Sussman, Smith, Rohrbach, & Spruijt-Metz, 2012; Barwick, Bennett, Johnson, McGowan, & Moore, 2012; Chen, Creedy, Lin, & Wollin, 2012; Cronk, Russell, Knowles, Matteson, Peace, & Ponferrada, 2012; Day, 2013). Every particular use of MI is likely to vary according to patient needs; Miller and Moyers (2006) have identified eight features of MI that should appear in every application of this technique:

1. "openness to collaboration with clients' own expertise,
2. proficiency in client centered counseling, including accurate empathy,
3. recognition of key aspects of client speech that guides the practice of MI,
4. eliciting and strengthening client change talk,
5. rolling with resistance,
6. negotiating change plans,
7. consolidating client commitment, and
8. switching flexibly between MI and other intervention styles." (pg. 3)

Transitional Relationship Model (TRM)/Transitional Discharge Model (TDM)

The Transitional Relationship Model (TRM) is theoretically grounded in the work of Hildegard Peplau; healing occurs in relationships. Therapeutic relationships can be formed with either professionals or peer supporters. The TRM was first developed to ease the transition from hospital to community, but its use has now been expanded in a variety of transitional care processes. There are two essential components of the TRM:

1. the therapeutic relationship should be extended until a new relationship with another care provider is established (continuing relationships formed in the hospital until new therapeutic relationships in the community are formed) and,
2. trained peer support (often through a consumer survivor group) from a psychiatric survivor who has now successfully transitioned to the community.

BOX 9.6

Research for Best Practice: **Transitional Relationship Model**

Forchuk, C., Martin, M. L., Jensen, E., Ouseley, S., Sealy, P., Beal, G., et al. (2013), Integrating an evidence-based intervention into clinical practice: 'Transitional relationship model'. Journal of Psychiatric and Mental Health Nursing, 20(7), 584–594. doi:10.1111/j.1365–2850.2012.01956.x

THE QUESTION: The Transitional Relationship Model (TRM) facilitates an effective discharge from the hospital to the community. Given this, what is the most effective way of implementing this model? What might facilitate the successful implementation of the TRM? What are the barriers to successful implementation?

METHODS: This study implemented the TRM in three waves, across six wards using a delayed implementation control group design to study how the addition of new information changed the implementation of the TRM. Following the experiences of the wards in which the TRM was initially implemented, recommendations for successful implementation of the model were developed for the subsequent waves of wards. Recommendations were developed using a combination of qualitative methods: monthly summaries, progress reports, meeting minutes, and focus groups.

FINDINGS: The results of this study can be divided into two categories: facilitators and barriers. The successful implementation of the TRM was aided by the use of educational modules (for both staff and peer training), on-site champions, and supportive documentation systems. Barriers included: feeling swamped or overwhelmed, "death by process," preexisting conflicts within teams, and changes in champions.

IMPLICATIONS FOR NURSING: The positive health outcomes associated with the TRM require careful preparation and constant attention to education, communication, and the effectiveness of the support given to caregivers.

In addition to producing positive therapeutic outcomes, the TRM also reduces time spent in hospital and readmissions (Reynolds, Lauder, Sharkey, Macivier, Veitch, & Cameron, 2004). See Box 9.6.

Technology and the Therapeutic Relationship

As technology develops and becomes increasingly accessible, traditional face-to-face communication can be replaced with technological interactions. Below are some of the most common forms of this communication:

Phone and video conferencing: this method is becoming increasingly popular, especially in remote areas where the land or the isolation of the clinic constitutes barriers to the development of a therapeutic relationship. However, three important criteria must be conceded prior to the use of this technology:

- Nonverbal communication is more difficult to detect and access
- The patient must have reliable access to the technology
- An appropriate method of documentation much still be used

Internet communication: Above all else, any communication over the internet must be secure to maintain confidentiality. Hospital firewalls can be useful in establishing such connections (Forchuk et al., 2012). One must always be aware of a hospital's or research site's policies and best practices regarding communication online. Some commonly used platforms for online communication, such as Facebook, cannot meet the standards discussed above and so ought not to be used in communication with patients. However, the internet is an invaluable resource for educational and research purposes.

SUMMARY OF KEY POINTS

- To deal therapeutically with the emotions, feelings, and problems of patients, nurses must understand their own cultural values and beliefs and interpersonal strengths and limitations.

- The nurse–patient relationship is built on therapeutic communication, including verbal and nonverbal interactions between the nurse and the patient. Some communication skills include active listening, positive body language, appropriate verbal responses, and the ability of the nurse to interpret appropriately and analyze the patient's verbal and nonverbal behaviors.

- Two of the most important communication concepts are empathy and rapport.

- In the nurse–patient relationship, as in all types of relationships, certain physical, emotional, and social boundaries and limitations need to be observed.

- The therapeutic nurse–patient relationship consists of three major and overlapping stages or phases: the orientation phase, in which the patient and nurse meet and establish the parameters of the relationship; the working phase, in which the patient identifies and explores problems; and the resolution phase, in which the patient learns to manage the problems and the relationship is terminated.

- The nontherapeutic relationship consists of three major and overlapping phases: the orientation phase, the grappling and struggling phase, and the phase of mutual withdrawal. A deteriorating relationship begins with a withholding phase, continues through the phases of avoiding and ignoring, and finally ends unsatisfactorily with a phase named "struggling with and making sense of."

CRITICAL THINKING CHALLENGES

1. Describe how you would do a suicide assessment on a distraught patient who comes to the physician's office expressing concerns about her ability to cope with her current situation. Describe how you would approach this patient if you determined she was suicidal. How might this assessment look different depending on the phase of the therapeutic relationship?

2. Describe how you would communicate with a patient who is concerned that the diagnosis of bipolar disorder will negatively affect his or her social and work relationships.

3. Your depressed patient does not seem inclined to talk about the depression. Describe the measures you would take to initiate a therapeutic relationship with him or her.

4. Think of a time that you worked with a patient you did not like. What was behind the dislike? How did you handle the therapeutic relationship? What could you do differently?

MOVIES *Good Will Hunting:* 1997. Robin Williams plays therapist, Dr. Sean Maguire. His patient, Will Hunting (Matt Damon), is a janitor at MIT who is also a troubled genius. Through a strong relationship, Will begins to realize his potential. This film deals with intense blocks to communication, as well as issues around justice system use and class.

VIEWING POINTS: Watch closely how the relationship develops between the characters played by Williams and Damon. How does the relationship change as the characters move through different stages of their relationship? Do you think that the level of self-disclosure depicted is therapeutic?

Analyze That: 2002. In this comedy sequel to *Analyze This* (1999), Billy Crystal plays psychiatrist Dr. Ben Sobel. The patient is Paul Vitti (Robert De Niro), a mobster who has been sent to prison. Vitti is either having a psychotic break or is faking one, and his former psychiatrist is called back to assess the situation. Vitti is sent to Sobel's home for treatment. Both the psychiatrist and patient have unresolved feelings related to the deaths of their fathers.

VIEWING POINTS: The issue of therapeutic boundaries is a source of comedy in this film. What normal therapeutic boundaries are being violated? Whose needs are being met throughout the film? What would be appropriate if a patient evoked personal unresolved issues for the therapist?

In Treatment: 2008. This television show is about a Washington-based psychotherapist, Paul Weston (Gabriel Byrne). The series runs throughout the week. From Monday to Thursday, Dr. Weston meets with patients and on Friday, he visits his own therapist. (Being analyzed yourself is an expectation for psychoanalysts.)

VIEWING POINTS: What aspects of therapeutic relationships can you identify in Dr. Weston's session? Look for ways in which transference and countertransference are portrayed. How is self-awareness developed for Dr. Weston?

Silver Linings Playbook: 2012. This film portrays one man's struggle to return to society after he is released from a psychiatric inpatient hospital. Patrick, (Bradley Cooper) who is trying to reconnect with his ex-wife and manage bipolar disorder, meets Tiffany (Jennifer Lawrence), who is struggling with depression following the death of her husband. Throughout the film, issues relating to stigma, establishing a therapeutic relationship, and how individuals suffering from mental illness may mutually support each other are dealt with.

VIEWING POINTS: As part of Patrick's release, he is mandated to continue meeting with a therapist. Think of this in relation to the TDM model discussed above. How is it similar and how is it different? Others often stigmatize Patrick and Tiffany. Can you identify where this happens and how such treatment might be avoided? Reflect on the fact that many other characters seem to have undiagnosed mental illnesses (such as OCD and anxiety). How do the characters help and hurt each other as they deal with the challenges of mental illness?

References

Barnett, E., Sussman, S., Smith, C., Rohrbach, L. A., & Spruijt-Metz, D. (2012). Motivational interviewing for adolescent substance use: A review of the literature. *Addictive Behaviors, 37*(12), 1325–1334. doi:10.1016/j.addbeh.2012.07.001

Barwick, M. A., Bennett, L. M., Johnson, S. N., McGowan, J., & Moore, J. E. (2012). Training health and mental health professionals in motivational interviewing: A systematic review. *Children and Youth Services Review, 34*(9), 1786–1795. doi:10.1016/j.childyouth.2012.05.012

Berg, R. C., Ross, M. W., & Tikkanen, R. (2011). The effectiveness of MI4MSM: How useful is motivational interviewing as an HIV risk prevention program for men who have sex with men? A systematic review. *AIDS Education and Prevention, 23*(6), 533–549. doi:10.1521/aeap.2011.23.6.533

Boyd, M. (1995). Communication with patients, families, healthcare providers, and diverse cultures. In M. Strader & P. Decker (Eds.). *Role transition to patient care management* (pp. 431). Norwalk, CT: Appleton & Lange.

Chen, S. M., Creedy, D., Lin, H. S., & Wollin, J. (2012). Effects of motivational interviewing intervention on self-management, psychological and glycemic outcomes in type 2 diabetes: A randomized controlled trial. *International Journal of Nursing Studies, 49*(6), 637–644. doi:10.1016/j.ijnurstu.2011.11.011

Coatsworth-Puspoky, R., Forchuk, C., & Ward-Griffin, C. (2006). "Nurse–client processes in mental health: Recipient's perspectives." *Journal of Psychiatric and Mental Health Nursing, 13*(3), 347–355.

Cronk, N. J., Russell, C. L., Knowles, N., Matteson, M., Peace, L., & Ponferrada, L. (2012). Acceptability of motivational interviewing among hemodialysis clinic staff: A pilot study. *Nephrology Nursing Journal, 39*(5), 385–391.

Day, P. (2013). Using motivational interviewing with young people: A case study. *British Journal of School Nursing, 8*(2), 97–99.

Forchuk, C., Carmichael, C., Golea, G., Johnston, N., Martin, M. L., Patterson, P., et al. (2006). *Nursing best practice guideline: Establishing therapeutic relationships (revision)*. Toronto, Canada: Registered Nurses Association of Ontario.

Forchuk, C., Martin, M. L. Jensen, E., Ouseley, S., Sealy, P., Beal, G. et al. (2012). Integrating the transitional relationship model into clinical practice. *Archives of Psychiatric Nursing, 26*(5), 374–381.

Forchuk, C., Martin, M. L., Jensen, E., Ouseley, S., Sealy, P., Beal, G., et al. (2013). Integrating an evidence-based intervention into clinical practice: 'Transitional relationship model'. *Journal of Psychiatric and Mental Health Nursing, 20*(7), 584–594. doi:10.1111/j.1365-2850.2012.01956.x

Hall, E. T. (1990). *The hidden dimension*. New York: Anchor Books.

Miller, W. R., & Moyers, T. B. (2006). Eight Stages in Learning Motivational Interviewing. *Journal of Teaching in the Addictions, 5*(1), 3–17. doi:10.1300/J188v05n01_02

Orlando, I. (1961). *Orlando's dynamic nurse-patient relationship: Function, process and principles*. New York: G.P. Putman's Sons.

Peplau, H. E. (1952, 1992). *Interpersonal relations in nursing*. New York: J. P. Putnam's Sons.

Reynolds, W., Lauder, W., Sharkey, S., Maciver, S., Veitch, T., & Cameron, D. (2004). The effects of transitional discharge model for psychiatric patients. *Journal of Psychiatric and Mental Health Nursing, 11*, 82–88.

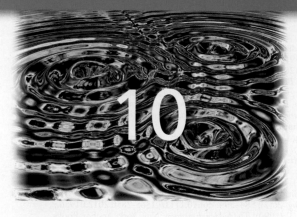

10

The Psychiatric Nursing Process

Mary Ann Boyd

KEY CONCEPTS

- assessment
- mental status examination
- nursing diagnosis
- outcomes
- nursing interventions

LEARNING OBJECTIVES

After studying this chapter, you will be able to:

1. Define the nursing process in psychiatric–mental health nursing.

2. Conduct a biopsychosocial psychiatric nursing assessment.

3. Develop nursing diagnoses following a psychiatric nursing assessment.

4. Develop patient outcomes from a nursing diagnosis.

5. Apply psychiatric nursing interventions for persons with mental health problems and mental disorders.

6. Explain how patient outcomes are evaluated in psychiatric nursing.

KEY TERMS

- affect • behavior modification • behavior therapy • bibliotherapy • body image • chemical restraint • cognition
- conflict resolution • containment • counseling • cultural brokering • de-escalation • distraction • dysphoric
- euphoric • euthymic • guided imagery • home visits • insight • judgment • labile • milieu therapy • mood
- open communication • patient observation • personal identity • psychoeducation • reminiscence • restraint
- risk factors • seclusion • self-care • self-concept • self-esteem • simple relaxation techniques • spiritual
support • structured interaction • token economy • validation • webotherapy

The nursing process is the model of care used in psychiatric nursing. In this text, the nursing process is organized around the areas of assessment, diagnosis and outcome development, intervention, and evaluation. Within this framework, this chapter delineates general areas of practice and is an introduction to some, but not all, of the commonly used interventions. Application of the nursing process to patients with specific psychiatric disorders and emotional problems are discussed in other chapters.

BIOPSYCHOSOCIAL PSYCHIATRIC NURSING ASSESSMENT

Assessment is the collection and interpretation of biopsychosocial information to determine health, functional status, and human responses to mental health problems. These responses are expressed through biologic, psychological, and social manifestations (Figure 10.1).

Assessment is not an isolated activity. Rather, it is a systematic and ongoing process that occurs throughout the

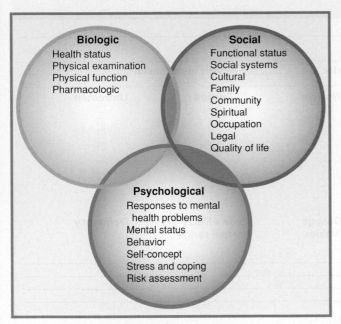

Biologic
Health status
Physical examination
Physical function
Pharmacologic

Social
Functional status
Social systems
Cultural
Family
Community
Spiritual
Occupation
Legal
Quality of life

Psychological
Responses to mental
  health problems
Mental status
Behavior
Self-concept
Stress and coping
Risk assessment

FIGURE 10.1 Biopsychosocial nursing assessment.

nurse's care of the patient. The Biopsychosocial Psychiatric Nursing Assessment (Box 10.1) is a basic guide to collecting assessment data. Assessment information is entered into the patient's written or computerized record, which may be presented in several different formats, including forms, checklists, narratives, and problem-oriented notes.

> **KEYCONCEPT   Assessment** is the deliberate and systematic collection and interpretation of biopsychosocial information or data to determine current and past health, functional status, and mental health problems, both actual and potential.

Assessment begins with the first contact with the patient and is based on the establishment of rapport with the patient (see Chapter 9). Legal consent must be given by the patient, and the nurse must follow the Health Insurance Portability and Accountability Act of 1996 (HIPAA) guidelines (see Chapter 4). The patient must develop a sense of trust before he or she will be comfortable revealing intimate life details. It is of paramount importance that the nurse has a healthy knowledge of him- or herself as well (Box 10.2). The nurse's own biases and values, which may be different from those of the patient, can influence the nurse's interpretation of assessment data. A careful self-assessment helps the nurse interpret the data objectively.

Patient Interviews

An assessment interview usually involves direct questions to obtain facts, clarify perceptions, validate observations, interpret the meanings of groups of facts, or compare information. The specific questions may take different forms. The nurse must clearly state the purpose of the interview and, if necessary, modify the interview process, so that both the patient and nurse agree on its purpose. The nurse may choose to use open- or closed-ended questions. Open-ended questions are most helpful when beginning the interview because they allow the nurse to observe how the patient responds verbally and nonverbally. They also convey caring and interest in the person's well-being, which helps to establish rapport. Nurses should use closed-ended questions when they need specific information. For example, "How old are you?" asks for specific information about the patient's age. These types of questions limit the individual's response but often serve as good follow-up questions for clarification of thoughts or feelings expressed.

Questions such as "How did you come to this clinic today?" allow patients to describe their experience in their own way. Some patients may answer this question concretely by saying, "I took a taxi" or "I came by car." Others may address this question by responding, "My family thought I should come, so they brought me" or "Well, I got up this morning . . . I took a shower, got dressed . . . and then, well you know, it's difficult sometimes to decide." Each of these answers helps the nurse assess the patient's thinking process as well as evaluate the content of the response.

Clarification is extremely important during the assessment process. Words do not have the same meaning to all people. Education, language, culture, history, and experience may influence the meaning of words. Sometimes simple and direct questioning provides clarification. In other situations, the nurse may clarify by providing a specific example for a more global thought the patient is trying to express. For example, a patient may say, "Things have been so strange since the children left." The nurse may respond with, "Sometimes, parents feel sad and empty when their children leave home. They don't know what to do with their time." Frequently summarizing what has been said allows the patient the opportunity to correct the nurse's interpretation. For example, verbalizing a sequence of events that the patient has reported may help to identify omissions or inconsistencies. Restating information or reflecting feelings that the patient has described also allows opportunity for clarification. It is essential that nurses understand exactly what patients are attempting to communicate before beginning to intervene. Box 10.3 provides a summary of other behaviors that enhance the effectiveness of an assessment interview.

Many psychiatric symptoms are beyond a patient's awareness. Family members, friends, and other health care professionals are important sources of information. Before seeking information from others, the nurse must obtain permission from the patient. The nurse needs to

BOX 10.1

Biopsychosocial Psychiatric Nursing Assessment

I. **Major reason for seeking help** _____

II. **Initial information**
   Name _____
   Age _____ Marital status _____ Gender _____ Ethnic identification _____

III. **Present and past health status** _____

	Normal	Treated	Untreated
Physical functions: System review	☐	☐	☐
Elimination	☐	☐	☐
Activity/exercise	☐	☐	☐
Sleep	☐	☐	☐
Appetite and nutrition	☐	☐	☐
Hydration	☐	☐	☐
Sexuality	☐	☐	☐
Self-care	☐	☐	☐
Existing physical illnesses	☐	☐	☐
Medications (prescription and over-the-counter)	Dosage	Side effects	Frequency
Significant laboratory tests	Values	Normal range	

IV. **Mental health problems**
   Major concerns regarding mental health problem _____
   Major loss/change in past year: No _____ Yes _____
   Fear of violence: No _____ Yes _____
   Strategies for managing problems/disorder _____

V. **Mental status examination**
   General observations (appearance, psychomotor activity, attitude) _____
   Orientation (time, place, person) _____
   Mood, affect, emotions _____
   Speech (verbal ability, speed, use of words correctly) _____
   Thought processes (tangential, logic, repetition, rhyming of words, loose connections, disorganized) _____
   Cognition and intellectual performance _____
   Attention and concentration _____
   Abstract reasoning and comprehension _____
   Memory (recall, short-term, recent, and remote) _____
   Judgment and insight _____

VI. **Significant behaviors (psychomotor, agitation, aggression, withdrawn)** _____

VII. **Self-concept (body image, self-esteem, personal identity)** _____

VIII. **Stress and coping patterns** _____

IX. **Risk assessment** _____
   Suicide: High _____ Low _____ Assault/homicide: High _____ Low _____
   Suicide thoughts or ideation: No _____ Yes _____
   Current thoughts of harming self _____
   Plan _____
   Means _____
   Means available _____
   Assault/homicide thoughts: No _____ Yes _____
   What do you do when angry with a stranger? _____
   What do you do when angry with family or partner? _____
   Have you ever hit or pushed anyone? No _____ Yes _____
   Have you ever been arrested for assault? No _____ Yes _____
   Current thoughts of harming others _____

X. **Functional status**
   Changes in functioning (work, school, home) _____

XI. **Social systems**
   Cultural assessment
      Cultural group _____
      Cultural group's view of health and mental illness _____
      What cultural rules do you try to live by? _____
      Important cultural foods _____
   Family assessment
      Family members _____
      Members important to patient _____
      Decision makers, family roles, supportive members _____
   Community resources _____

XII. **Spiritual assessment**

XIII. **Economic status**

XIV. **Legal status**

XV. **Quality of life**

Summary of significant data that can be used in formulating a nursing diagnosis

SIGNATURE/TITLE _____ Date _____

BOX 10.2

Self-Concept Awareness

Self-awareness is important in any interaction. To understand a patient's self-concept, the nurse must be aware of his or her own self-concept. By answering these questions, nurses can evaluate self-concept components and increase their self-understanding. The more comfortable the nurse is with him- or herself, the more effective the nurse can be in each and every patient interaction.

BODY IMAGE
- How do I feel about my body?
- How important is my physical appearance?
- How does my body measure up to my ideal body? (How would I like to appear?)
- What is positive about my body?
- What would I like to change about my body?
- How does my body image affect my self-esteem?

SELF-ESTEEM
- When do I feel confident and good about myself?
- When do I feel unimportant?
- What do I do when I feel good about myself? (Call friends, socialize?)
- What do I do when I have negative feelings about myself? (Withdraw, dress poorly?)
- When do I make negative statements?
- Am I able to correct my negative self-statements?

PERSONAL IDENTITY
- How do I describe myself?
- What three adjectives describe who I am?
- Do I identify with a particular cultural group, family role, or place of residence?
- What would I like to have on my tombstone?

BOX 10.3

Assessment Interview Behaviors

The following behaviors carried out by the nurse will enhance the effectiveness of the assessment interview:

- *Exhibiting empathy*—to show empathy to the patient, the nurse uses phrases such as, "That must have been upsetting for you" or "I can understand your hurt feelings."
- *Giving recognition*—the nurse gives recognition by listening actively: verbally encouraging the patient to continue, and nonverbally presenting an open, interested demeanor.
- *Demonstrating acceptance*—note that acceptance does not mean agreement or nonagreement with the patient but is a neutral stance that allows the patient to continue.
- *Restating*—the nurse tries to clarify what the patient is trying to say by restating it.
- *Reflecting*—the nurse presents the patient's last statement as a question. This gives the patient a chance to expand on the information.
- *Focusing*—the nurse attempts to bring the conversation back to the questions at hand when the patient goes off on a tangent.
- *Using open-ended questions*—general questions give the patient a chance to speak freely.
- *Presenting reality*—the nurse presents reality when the patient makes unrealistic or exaggerated statements.
- *Making observations*—the nurse says aloud what patient behaviors are observed to give the patient a chance to speak to those behaviors. For example, the nurse may say, "I notice you are twisting your fingers; are you nervous about something?"

---

provide the patient with a clear explanation of why the information is needed and how it will be used.

Assessment of the Biologic Domain

Many psychiatric disorders produce physical symptoms, such as the lack of appetite and weight loss associated with depression. A person's physical condition may also affect mental health, producing a recurrence or increase in symptoms. Many physical disorders may present first with symptoms considered to be psychiatric. For example, hypothyroidism often presents with feelings of lethargy, decreased concentration, and depressed mood. For these reasons, biologic information about the patient is always considered.

Current and Past Health Status

Beginning with a history of the patient's general medical condition, the nurse should consider the following:

- Availability of, frequency of, and most recent medical evaluation, including test results
- Past hospitalizations and surgical procedures
- Vision and hearing impairments

- Cardiac problems, including cerebrovascular accidents (strokes), myocardial infarctions (heart attacks), and childhood illnesses
- Respiratory problems, particularly those that result in a lack of oxygen to the brain
- Neurologic problems, particularly head injuries, seizure disorders, or any losses of consciousness
- Endocrine disorders, particularly unstable diabetes or thyroid or adrenal dysfunction
- Immune disorders, particularly human immunodeficiency virus (HIV) and autoimmune disorders
- Use, exposure, abuse, or dependence on substances, including alcohol, tobacco, prescription drugs, illicit drugs, and herbal preparations.

Physical Examination

Body Systems Review

After the nurse obtains historical information, he or she should examine physiologic systems to evaluate the patient's current physical condition. The psychiatric nurse should pay special attention to various systems that treatment may affect. For example, if a patient is being treated with antihypertensive medication, the dosage may need to be adjusted if an antipsychotic medication is prescribed. If a patient is overweight or has diabetes, some psychiatric medications can affect these conditions. Patients with compromised immune function (HIV, cancer) may experience mood alterations.

Neurologic Status

Particular attention is paid to recent head trauma; episodes of hypertension; and changes in personality, speech, or the ability to handle activities of daily living (ADLs). Cranial nerve dysfunction, reflexes, muscle strength, and balance are included in a thorough assessment. The nurse routinely assesses and documents movement disorders through the use of such tools as the Abnormal Involuntary Movement Scales (see Chapter 22).

Laboratory Results

The nurse reviews and documents any available laboratory data, especially any abnormalities. Hepatic, renal, or urinary abnormalities are particularly important to document because these systems metabolize or excrete many psychiatric medications. In addition, the nurse notes abnormal white blood cell and electrolyte levels. Laboratory data are especially important, particularly if the nurse is the only person in the mental health team who has a "medical" background (Table 10.1).

Physical Functions

Elimination

The nurse should inquire about and document the patient's daily urinary and bowel habits. Various medications can affect bladder and bowel functioning, so a baseline must be noted. For example, diarrhea and frequency of urination can occur with the use of lithium carbonate. Anticholinergic effects of antipsychotic medication can cause constipation and urinary hesitancy or retention.

Activity and Exercise

The patient's daily methods and levels of activity and exercise must be queried and documented. Activities are important interventions, and baseline information is needed to determine what the patient already enjoys or dislikes and whether he or she is getting sufficient exercise or adequate recreation. A patient may have altered activity or exercise in response to medication or therapies. In addition, many psychiatric medications cause weight gain, and nurses need to develop interventions that assist the patient to increase activities to counteract the weight gain.

Sleep

Changes in sleep patterns often reflect changes in a patient's emotions and are symptoms of disorders. If the patient responds positively to a question about changes in sleep patterns, it is important to clarify just what those changes are. For example, "difficulty falling asleep" means different things to different people. For a person who usually falls right to sleep, it could mean that it takes 10 extra minutes to fall asleep. For a person who normally takes 35 minutes to fall asleep, it could mean that it takes 90 minutes to do so.

Appetite and Nutrition

Changes in appetite and nutritional intake are assessed and documented because they can indicate changes in moods or relapse. For example, a patient who is depressed may not notice hunger or even that he or she does not have the energy to prepare food. Others may handle stressful emotions through eating more than usual. This information also provides valuable clues to possible eating disorders and problems with body image.

Obesity is one of the major health problems of many Americans, but it is particularly problematic for persons with psychiatric disorders. Many of the medications are associated with weight gain. A baseline body mass index (BMI) should be determined as treatment is initiated.

Hydration

Gaining perspective on how much fluid patients normally drink and how much they are drinking now provides important data. Some medications can cause retention of fluids, and others can cause diuresis; thus, the patient's current fluid status must be understood.

Sexuality

Questioning a patient on issues involving sexuality requires comfort with one's own sexuality. Changes in sexual activity as well as comfort with sexual orientation are important to assess. Issues involving sexual orientation that are unsettled in a patient or between a patient and family member may cause anxiety, shame, or discomfort. It is necessary to explore how comfortable the patient is with his or her sexuality and sexual functioning. These questions should be asked in a matter-of-fact but gentle and nonjudgmental manner. Initiating the topic of sexuality may begin with a question such as "Are you sexually active?" Birth control medications may also alter mood.

Self-Care

Self-care is the ability to perform ADLs successfully. Often, a patient's ability to care for him- or herself or carry out ADLs, such as washing and dressing, are indicative of his or her psychological state. For example, a depressed patient may not have the energy change into

Table 10.1	SELECTED HEMATOLOGIC MEASURES AND THEIR RELEVANCE TO PSYCHIATRIC DISORDERS	
Test	**Possible Results**	**Possible Cause or Meaning**
Complete Blood Count (CBC)		
Leukocyte (white blood cell [WBC]) count	Leukopenia—decrease in leukocytes (white blood cells) Agranulocytosis—decrease in number of granulocytic leukocytes Leukocytosis—increase in leukocyte count above normal limits	May be produced by: phenothiazines clozapine carbamazepine Lithium causes a benign mild to moderate increase (11,000–17,000/mcL). Neuroleptic malignant syndrome (NMS) can be associated with increases of 15,000 to 30,000/mm^3 in about 40% of cases.
WBC differential	"Shift to the left"—from segmented neutrophils to band forms	Shift often suggests a bacterial infection but has been reported in about 40% of cases of NMS.
Red blood cell (RBC) count	Polycythemia—increased RBCs	Primary form—true polycythemia caused by several disease states Secondary form—compensation for decreased oxygenation, such as in chronic pulmonary disease Blood is more viscous, and the patient should not become dehydrated.
	Decreased RBCs	Decrease may be related to some types of anemia, which requires further evaluation.
Hematocrit (Hct)	Elevations	Elevation may be caused by dehydration.
	Decreased Hct	Anemia may be associated with a wide range of mental status changes, including asthenia, depression, and psychosis. 20% of women of childbearing age in the United States have iron-deficiency anemia.
Hemoglobin (Hb)	Decreased	Another indicator of anemia; further evaluation of source requires review of erythrocyte indices.
Erythrocyte indices, such as red cell distribution width (RDW)	Elevated RDW	Finding suggests a combined anemia as in that from chronic alcoholism, resulting from both vitamin B$_{12}$ and folate acid deficiencies and iron deficiency Oral contraceptives also decrease vitamin B$_{12}$.
Other Hematologic Measures		
Vitamin B$_{12}$	Deficiency	Neuropsychiatric symptoms, such as psychosis, paranoia, fatigue, agitation, marked personality change, dementia, and delirium, may develop.
Folate	Deficiency	The use of alcohol, phenytoin, oral contraceptives, and estrogens may be responsible.
Platelet count	Thrombocytopenia—decreased platelet count	Some psychiatric medications, such as carbamazepine, phenothiazines, or clozapine, or other nonpsychiatric medications, may cause thrombocytopenia. Several medical conditions are other causes.
Serum Electrolytes		
Sodium	Hyponatremia—low serum sodium	Significant mental status changes may ensue. Condition is associated with Addison's disease, the syndrome of inappropriate secretion of antidiuretic hormone (SIADH), and polydipsia (water intoxication) as well as carbamazepine use.
Potassium	Hypokalemia—low serum potassium	Produces weakness, fatigue, electrocardiogram (ECG) changes; paralytic ileus and muscle paresis may develop. Common in individuals with bulimic behavior or psychogenic vomiting and use or abuse of diuretics; laxative abuse may contribute; can be life threatening.
Chloride	Elevation	Chloride tends to increase to compensate for lower bicarbonate.
	Decrease	Binging–purging behavior and repeated vomiting may be causes.
Bicarbonate	Elevation	Causes may be binging and purging in eating disorders, excessive use of laxatives, or psychogenic vomiting.
	Decrease	Decrease may develop in some patients with hyperventilation syndrome and panic disorder.

(Continued)

Table 10.1	SELECTED HEMATOLOGIC MEASURES AND THEIR RELEVANCE TO PSYCHIATRIC DISORDERS (*Continued*)	
Test	**Possible Results**	**Possible Cause or Meaning**
Renal Function Tests		
Blood urea nitrogen (BUN)	Elevation	Increase is associated with mental status changes, lethargy, and delirium. Cause may be dehydration. Potential toxicity of medications cleared via the kidney, such as lithium and amantadine, may increase.
Serum creatinine	Elevation	Level usually does not become elevated until about 50% of nephrons in the kidney are damaged.
Serum Enzymes		
Amylase	Elevation	Level appears to increase after binging and purging behavior in eating disorders and declines when these behaviors stop.
Alanine aminotransferase (ALT)—formerly serum glutamic pyruvic transaminase (SGPT)	ALT > AST	Disparity is common in acute forms of viral and drug-induced hepatic dysfunction.
	Elevation	Mild elevations are common with use of sodium valproate.
Aspartate aminotransferase (AST)—formerly serum glutamic oxaloacetic transaminase (SGOT)	AST > ALT	Severe elevations in chronic forms of liver disease and postmyocardial infarction may develop.
Creatine phospho-kinase (CPK)	Elevations of the isoenzyme related to muscle tissue	Muscle tissue injury is the cause. Level is elevated in neuroleptic malignant syndrome (NMS). Level is also elevated by repeated intramuscular injections (e.g., antipsychotics).
Thyroid Function		
Serum triiodothyronine (T_3)	Decrease	Hypothyroidism and nonthyroid illness cause decrease. Individuals with depression may convert less T_4 to T_3 peripherally but not out of the normal range. Medications such as lithium and sodium valproate may suppress thyroid function, but clinical significance is unknown.
	Elevations	Hyperthyroidism, T_3, toxicosis, may produce mood changes, anxiety, and symptoms of mania
Serum thyroxine (T_4)	Elevations	Hyperthyroidism is a cause.
Thyroid stimulating hormone (TSH or thyrotropin)	Elevations	Hypothyroidism—symptoms may appear very much like depression except for additional physical signs of cold intolerance, dry skin, hair loss, bradycardia, and so on. Lithium—may also cause elevations.
	Decrease	Considered nondiagnostic—may be hyperthyroidism, pituitary hypothyroidism, or even euthyroid status.

clean clothes. This information may also help the nurse to determine actual or potential obstacles to a patient's compliance with a treatment plan.

Pharmacologic Assessment

The review of systems serves as a baseline from which the nurse may judge whether the initiation of a medication exacerbates symptoms or causes new ones to develop. It is important to determine which medications the patient takes now or has taken in the past. These include over-the-counter, herbal or nonprescription medications as well as prescribed medications. This assessment is important for reasons other than serving as a baseline. It helps

target possible drug interactions, determines whether the patient has already used medications that are being considered, and identifies whether medications may be causing psychiatric symptoms.

Assessment of the Psychological Domain

The psychological domain is the traditional focus of the psychiatric nursing assessment. By definition, psychiatric disorders and emotional problems are manifested through psychological symptoms related to mental status, moods, thoughts, behaviors, and interpersonal relationships. This domain includes psychological growth and development.

Assessing this domain is important in developing a comprehensive picture of the patient.

Responses to Mental Health Problems

Individual concerns regarding a mental health problem or its consequences are included in the mental health assessment. A mental disorder, like any other illness, affects patients and families in many different ways. It is safe to say that a mental illness changes a person's life, and the nurse should identify what the changes are and their meaning to the patient and family members. Many patients experience specific fears, such as losing their job, family, or safety. Included in this part of the assessment is identifying current strategies or behaviors the patient uses in dealing with the consequences of disorder. A simple question such as "How do you deal with your voices when you are with other people?" may initiate a discussion about responses to the mental disorder or emotional problem.

Mental Status Examination

The mental status examination establishes a baseline, provides a snapshot of where the patient is at a particular moment, and creates a written record. Areas of assessment include general observations, orientation, mood and affect, speech, thought processes, and cognition. Box 10.4 provides a narrative note of the results from a patient's mental status examination.

> **KEYCONCEPT** The **mental status examination** is an organized systematic approach to assessment of an individual's current psychiatric condition.

General Observations

At the beginning of the interview, the nurse should record his or her initial impressions of the patient. These general observations include the patient's appearance, affect,

BOX 10.4
Narrative Mental Status Examination Note

The patient is a 65-year-old widowed man who is slightly disheveled. He is cooperative with the interviewer and judged to be an adequate historian. His mood and affect are depressed and anxious. He becomes tearful throughout the interview when speaking about his wife. His flow of thought is hesitant but coherent when he is speaking about his wife. He is oriented to time, place, and person. He shows good recent and remote memory. He is able to recall several items given him by the interviewer. The patient shows poor insight and judgment regarding his sadness since the loss of his wife. He repeatedly says, "Mary wouldn't want me to be sad. She would want me to continue with my life."

psychomotor activity, and overall behavior. How is the patient dressed? Is the dress appropriate for weather and setting? What is the patient's affect (emotional expression)? What behaviors is the patient displaying? For example, the same nurse assessed two male patients with depression. At the beginning of the mental status examination, the differences between these two men were very clear. The nurse described the first patient as "a large, well-dressed man who is agitated and appears angry, shifts in his seat, and does not maintain eye contact. He interrupts often in the initial explanation of mental status." The nurse described the other patient as a "small, unshaven, disheveled man with a strong body odor who appears withdrawn. He shuffles as he walks, speaks very softly, appears sad, and avoids direct eye contact."

Orientation

The nurse can determine the patient's orientation by asking the date, time, and current location of the interview setting. If a patient knows the year but not the exact date, the interviewer can ask the season. A person's orientation tells the nurse the extent of confusion. If a patient does not know the year or the place of the interview, he or she is exhibiting considerable confusion.

Mood and Affect

Mood refers to the prominent, sustained, overall emotions that the person expresses and exhibits. Mood may be sustained for days or weeks, or it may fluctuate during the course of a day. For example, some patients with depression have a diurnal variation in their mood. They experience their lowest mood in the morning, but as the day progresses, their depressed mood lifts and they feel somewhat better in the evening. Terms used to describe mood include **euthymic** (normal), **euphoric** (elated), **labile** (changeable), and **dysphoric** (depressed, disquieted, restless).

Affect refers to the person's capacity to vary outward emotional expression. Affect fluctuates with thought content and can be observed in facial expressions, vocal fluctuations, and gestures. During the assessment, the patient may exhibit anger, frustration, irritation, apathy, and helplessness while his or her overall mood remains unchanged.

Affect can be described in terms of range, intensity, appropriateness, and stability. Range can be full or restricted. An individual who expresses several different emotions consistent with the stated feelings and content being expressed is described as having a *full range* of affect that is congruent with the situation. An individual who expresses few emotions has a restricted affect. For example, a patient could be describing the recent tragic death of a loved one in a monotone with little expression.

In determining whether this response is normal, the nurse compares the patient's emotional response with the cultural norm for that particular response. *Intensity* can be increased, flat, or blunted. The nurse determines whether the emotional response is *appropriate* for the situation. For example, an inappropriate response is shown by a patient who has an extreme reaction to the death of the victims of the September 11 tragedy as if the victims were personal friends. Another patient said that his life stopped when the World Trade Center towers came down. He could not eat or sleep for weeks afterward. *Stability* can be mobile (normal) or labile. If a patient reports feeling happy one minute and reduced to tears the next, the person probably has an unstable mood. During the interview, the nurse should look for rapid mood changes that indicate lability of mood. A patient who exhibits intense, frequently shifting emotional extremes has a labile affect.

Speech

Speech provides clues about thoughts, emotional patterns, and cognitive organization. Speech may be pressured, fast, slow, or fragmented. Speech patterns reflect the patient's thought patterns, which can be logical or illogical. To check the patient's comprehension, the nurse can show a patient an object (e.g., pen, watch) and ask the person to name them. During conversation, the nurse assesses the fluency and quality of the patient's speech. The nurse listens for repetition or rhyming of words.

Thought Processes

The nurse assesses the patient for rapid change of ideas; inability or taking a long time to get to the point; loose or no connections among ideas or words; rhyming or repetition of words, questions, or phrases; or use of unheard of words. Any of these observations indicates abnormal thought patterns. The content of what the patient says is also important. What thought is the patient expressing? The nurse listens for unusual and unlikely stories, fears or behaviors; for example, "The FBI is tracking me" or "I am afraid to leave my house."

Cognition and Intellectual Performance

To assess the patient's **cognition**, that is, the ability to think and know, the nurse uses memory, calculation, and reasoning tests to identify specific areas of impairment. The cognitive areas include (1) attention and concentration, (2) abstract reasoning and comprehension, (3) memory, and (4) insight and judgment.

Attention and Concentration

To test attention and concentration, the nurse asks the patient, without pencil or paper, to start with 100 and subtract 7 until reaching 65 or to start with 20 and subtract 3. The nurse must decide which is most appropriate for the patient considering education and understanding. Subtracting 3 from 20 is the easier of the two tasks. Asking a patient to spell "world" backward is also useful in determining attention and concentration.

Abstract Reasoning and Comprehension

To test abstract reasoning and comprehension, the nurse gives the patient a proverb to interpret. Examples include "People in glass houses shouldn't throw stones," "A rolling stone gathers no moss," and "A penny saved is a penny earned."

Recall, Short-Term, Recent, and Remote Memory

There are four spheres of memory to check: recall, or immediate, memory; short-term memory; recent memory; and long-term, or remote, memory. To check immediate and short-term memory, the nurse gives the patient three unrelated words to remember and asks him or her to recite them right after telling them and at 5-minute and 15-minute intervals during the interview. To test recent memory, the nurse may question about a holiday or world event within the past few months. The nurse tests long-term or remote memory by asking about events years ago. If they are personal events and the answers seem incorrect, the nurse may check them with a family member.

Insight and Judgment

Insight and judgment are related concepts that involve the ability to examine thoughts, conceptualize facts, solve problems, think abstractly, and possess self-awareness. **Insight** is a person's awareness of his or her own thoughts and feelings and ability to compare them with the thoughts and feelings of others. It involves an awareness of how others view one's behavior and its meaning. For example, many patients do not believe that they have mental illness. They may have delusions and hallucinations or be hospitalized for bizarre and sometimes dangerous behavior, but they are completely unaware that their behavior is unusual or abnormal. During an interview, a patient may adamantly proclaim that nothing is wrong or that he or she does not have a mental illness. Even if a problem is recognized, the patient may lack insight regarding issues related to care.

Judgment is the ability to reach a logical decision about a situation and to choose a course of action after examining and analyzing various possibilities. Throughout the interview, the nurse evaluates the patient's ability to make logical decisions. For example, some patients may continually choose partners who are abusive. The nurse could logically conclude that these patients have poor judgment in selecting partners. Another way to examine a patient's judgment is to give a simple scenario and ask the person to identify the best response. An example of such a scenario is asking, "What would you do if you found a bag of money outside a bank on a busy street?" If the patient responds, "Run with it," his or her judgment is questionable.

Behavior

Throughout the assessment, the nurse observes any behavior that may have significance in understanding the patient's response or symptoms of the mental disorder or emotional problem. For example, a depressed patient may be tearful throughout the session, whereas an anxious patient may twist or pull his or her hair, shift in the chair, or be unable to maintain eye contact. The nurse may find that whenever a particular topic is addressed, the patient's behavior changes. The nurse needs to relate patterned behaviors to significant events by connecting behaviors with the assessment data. For example, a patient may change jobs frequently, causing family distress and financial problems. Exploration of the events leading up to job changes may elicit important information regarding the patient's ability to solve problems.

Self-Concept

Self-concept, which develops over a lifetime, represents the total beliefs about three interrelated dimensions of the self: body image, self-esteem, and personal identity. The importance of each of these dimensions varies among individuals. For some, beliefs about themselves are strongly tied to body image; for others, personal identity is most important. Still others develop personal identity from what others have told them over the years. The nurse carrying out an assessment must keep in mind that self-concept and its components are dynamic and variable. For example, a woman may have a consistent self-concept until her first pregnancy. At that time, the many physiologic changes of pregnancy may cause her body image to change. She may be comfortable and enjoy the "glow of pregnancy," or she may feel like a "bloated cow." Suddenly, her body image is the most important part of her self-concept, and how she handles it can increase or decrease her self-esteem or sense of personal identity. Thus, all of the components are tied together, and each one affects the others.

Self-concept is assessed through eliciting patients' thoughts about themselves, their ability to navigate in the world, and their nonverbal behaviors. A disheveled sloppy physical appearance outside cultural norms is an indication of poor self-concept. Negative self-statements, such as, "I could never do that," "I have no control over my life," and "I'm so stupid" reveal poor views of self.

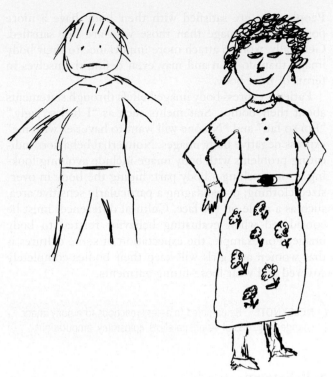

FIGURE 10.2 *Left:* Self-portrait of a 52-year-old woman at first group session following discharge from hospital for treatment of depression. *Right:* Self-portrait after 3 months of weekly group interventions.

The nurse's own self-concept can shape the nurse's view of the patient. For example, a nurse who is self-confident and feels inwardly scornful of a patient who lacks such confidence may intimidate the patient through unconscious, judgmental behaviors or inconsiderate comments.

A useful approach to measuring self-concept is asking the patient to draw a self-portrait. For many patients, drawing is much easier than writing and serves as an excellent technique for monitoring changes. Interpretation of self-concept from drawings focuses on size, color, level of detail, pressure, line quality, symmetry, and placement. Low self-esteem is expressed by small size, lack of color variation, and sparse details in the drawing. Powerlessness and feelings of inadequacy are expressed through a lack of a head, a mouth, arms, feet, or in the drawing. A lack of symmetry (placement of figure parts or entire drawings off center) represents feelings of insecurity and inadequacy. As self-esteem builds, size increases, color tends to become more varied and brighter, and more detail appears. Figure 10.2 shows a self-portrait of a patient at the beginning of treatment for depression and another drawn 3 months later.

Body Image

Body image represents a person's beliefs and attitudes about his or her body and includes such dimensions as size (large or small) and attractiveness (pretty or ugly).

People who are satisfied with their body have a more positive body image than those who are not satisfied. Generally, women attach more importance to their body image than do men and may even define themselves in terms of their body.

Patients express body image beliefs through statements about their bodies. Statements such as "I feel so ugly," "I'm so fat," and "No one will want to have sex with me" express negative body images. Nonverbal behaviors indicating problems with body image include avoiding looking at or touching a body part; hiding the body in oversized clothing; or bandaging a particularly sensitive area, such as a mole on the face. Cultural differences must be considered when evaluating behavior related to body image. For example, the expectation of some cultures is that women and girls will keep their bodies completely covered and wear loose-fitting garments.

> **NCLEXNOTE** Be prepared to assess reactions to a body image change (e.g., loss of vision, paralysis, colostomy, amputation).

Self-Esteem

Self-esteem is the person's attitude about the self. Self-esteem differs from body image because it concerns satisfaction with one's overall self. People who feel good about themselves are more likely to have the confidence to try new health behaviors. They are also less likely to be depressed. Negative self-esteem statements include "I'm a worthless person" and "I never do anything right."

Personal Identity

Personal identity is knowing "who I am." Every life experience and interaction contributes to knowing oneself better. Personal identity allows people to establish boundaries and understand personal strengths and limitations. In some psychiatric disorders, individuals cannot separate themselves from others, which shows that their personal identity is not strongly developed. A problem with personal identity is difficult to assess. Statements such as, "I'm just like my mother, and she was always in trouble," "I become whatever my current boyfriend wants me to be," and "I can't make a decision unless I check it out first" are all statements that require further exploration into the person's view of self.

Stress and Coping Patterns

Everyone has stress (see Chapter 18). Sometimes the experience of stress contributes to the development of mental disorders. Identification of major stresses in a patient's life helps the nurse understand the person and support the use of successful coping behaviors in the future. The nurse should explore how the patient deals with stress and identify successful coping mechanisms in order to encourage their use.

> **NCLEXNOTE** Every assessment should focus on stress and coping patterns. Identifying how a patient copes with stress can be used as a basis of care in all nursing situations. Include content from Chapter 18 when studying these concepts.

Risk Assessment

Risk factors are characteristics, conditions, situations, or events that increase the patient's vulnerability to threats to safety or well-being. Throughout this text, the sections concerning risk factors focus on the following:

- Risks to the patient's safety
- Risks for developing psychiatric disorders
- Risks for increasing, or exacerbating, symptoms and impairment in an individual who already has a psychiatric disorder.

Consideration of risk factors involving patient safety should be included in each assessment. Examples of these risks include the risk for suicide and violence toward others or the risk for events, such as falling, seizures, allergic reactions, or elopement (unauthorized absence from health care facility). Nurses assess factors on a priority basis. For example, threats of violence or suicide take priority.

Suicidal Ideation

During the assessment, the nurse needs to listen closely to whether the patient describes or mentions thinking about self-harm. If the patient does not openly express ideas of self-harm, it is necessary to ask in a straightforward and gentle manner, "Have you ever thought about injuring or killing yourself?" If the patient answers, "Yes, I am thinking about it right now," the nurse knows not to leave the patient unobserved and to institute suicide precautions as indicated by the facility protocols. General questions to ask to ascertain suicidal ideation follow:

- Have you ever tried to harm or kill yourself?
- Do you have thoughts of suicide at this time? If yes, do you have a plan? If yes, can you tell me the details of the plan?
- Do you have the means to carry out this plan? (If the plan requires a weapon, does the patient have it available?)
- Have you made preparations for your death (e.g., writing a note to loved ones, putting finances in order, giving away possessions)?
- Has a significant episode in your life caused you to think this way (e.g., recent loss of spouse or job)?

If any of these responses are "yes," the nurse should explore the issue in detail, notify the supervisor, and clearly document the patient responses and nursing follow-up. The nurse is expected follow the agency policies.

Assaultive or Homicidal Ideation

When assessing a patient, the nurse also needs to listen carefully to any delusions or hallucinations that the patient shares. If the patient gives any indication that he or she must or is being told to harm someone, the nurse must first think of self-safety and institute assaultive precautions as indicated by the facility protocols. General questions to ascertain assaultive or homicidal ideation follow:

- Do you intend to harm someone? If yes, who?
- Do you have a plan? If yes, what are the details of the plan?
- Do you have the means to carry out the plan? (If the plan requires a weapon, is it readily available?)

Assessment of the Social Domain

The assessment continues with examination of the patient's social domain. The nurse inquires about interactions with others in the family and community (work, church, or other organizations); the patient's parents and their marital relationship; the patient's place in birth order; names and ages of any siblings; and relationships with spouse, siblings, and children. The nurse also assesses work and education history and community activities. The nurse observes how the patient relates to any family or friends who may be in attendance. This component of the assessment helps the nurse anticipate how the patient may get along with other patients in an inpatient setting. It also allows the nurse to plan for any anticipated difficulties.

Functional Status

An important aspect of the assessment is determining the functioning of the patient (i.e., is an adult working and living independently? is a student attending classes?). How the patient copes with strangers and those with whom he or she does not get along is also important information.

Social Systems

A significant component of the patient's life involves the social systems in which he or she may be enmeshed. The social systems to examine include the family, the culture to which the patient belongs, and the community in which he or she lives.

Family Assessment

How the patient fits in with and relates to his or her family is important to know. See Chapter 14 for a discussion of a comprehensive family assessment. General questions to ask include the following:

- Who do you consider family?
- How important to you is your family?
- How does your family make decisions?
- What are the roles in your family, and who fills them?
- Where do you fit in your family?
- With whom in your family do you get along best?
- With whom in your family do you have the most conflict?
- Who in your family is supportive of you?

Cultural Assessment

Culture can profoundly affect a person's world view (see Chapter 3). Culture helps a person frame beliefs about life, death, health and illness, and roles and relationships. During cultural assessment, the nurse must consider factors that influence the manifestations of the current mental disorder. For example, a patient mentions "speaking in tongues." The nurse may identify this experience as a hallucination when, in fact, the patient was having a religious experience common within some branches of Christianity. In this instance, knowing and understanding such religious practices will prevent a misinterpretation of the symptoms.

The nurse can elicit important cultural information by asking the following questions:

- To what cultural group do you belong?
- Were you raised in an ethnic community?
- How do you define health?
- How do you define illness?
- How do you define good and evil?
- What do you do to get better when you are physically ill? Mentally ill?
- Whom do you see for help when you are physically ill? Mentally ill?
- By what cultural rules or taboos do you try to live?
- Do you eat special foods?

Community Support and Resources

Many patients are connected to community resources, and the nurse needs to assess what they are and the patterns of usage. For example, a patient who is homeless may know of a church where he or she can sleep but may go there only on cold nights. Or a patient may go to the community center daily for lunch to be with other people.

Spiritual Assessment

Among the many definitions of spirituality is one offered by Burkhardt and Nagai-Jacobson (1997). Spirituality is

> the unifying force of a person; the essence of being that shapes, gives meaning to, and is aware of one's self-becoming. Spirituality permeates all of life and is manifested in one's being, knowing, and doing. It is expressed and experienced uniquely by each individual through and within connection to God, Life Force, the Absolute, the environment, nature, other people, and the self (Burkhardt & Nagai-Jacobson, 1997, p. 42).

Nurses must be clear about their own spirituality to be sure it does not interfere with assessment of the patient's spirituality. General questions to ask include the following:

- What gives your life meaning?
- What is the purpose of your life?
- What do you do to bring joy into your life?
- What life goals have you set for yourself?
- Do you think that stress in any way has caused your illness?
- Can you forgive others?
- Can you forgive yourself?
- Is your faith helpful to you in stressful situations?
- Is worship important to you?
- Do you participate in any religious activities?
- Do any religious beliefs control your life?
- Do you believe in God or a higher power?
- Do you pray?
- Do you meditate?
- Do you feel connected with the world?

NCLEXNOTE Identify emotional problems that are related to religion or spiritual beliefs such as conflicts between recommended treatments and beliefs.

Occupational Status

The nurse should document the occupation the patient is now in as well as a history of jobs. If the patient has changed jobs frequently, the nurse should ask about the reasons. Perhaps the patient has faced such problems as an inability to focus on the job at hand or to get along with others. If so, such issues require further exploration.

Economic Status

Finances are very private for many people; thus, the nurse must ask questions about economic status carefully. What the nurse needs to ascertain is not specific dollar amounts but whether the patient feels stressed by finances and has enough for basic needs.

Legal Status

Because of laws governing mentally ill people, ascertaining the patient's correct age, marital status, and any legal guardianship is important. The nurse may need to check the patient's medical records for this information.

Quality of Life

The patient's perspective on quality of life means how the patient rates his or her life. Does a patient feel his life is poor because he cannot purchase everything he wants? Does another patient feel blessed because the sun is shining today? Listening carefully to the patient's discussion of his or her life and how he or she measures the quality of that life provides important information about self-concept, coping skills, desires, and dreams.

NURSING DIAGNOSIS

After completing an assessment of the patient, the nurse generates nursing diagnoses based on the assessment data. With experience, the nurse can easily cluster the assessment data to support one nursing diagnosis over another. Nursing diagnoses are universally used in nursing practice and education. In this text, primarily NANDA diagnoses are used. See Box 10.5 for more information. For each disorder, data are presented to support related nursing diagnoses.

KEYCONCEPT A **nursing diagnosis** is a clinical judgment about an identified problem or need that requires nursing interventions and nursing management. It is based on data generated from a nursing assessment (Carpenito-Moyet, 2014).

DEVELOPING PATIENT OUTCOMES

Mutually agreed-upon goals flow from the nursing diagnoses and provide guidance in determining appropriate interventions. Initial outcomes are determined and then are monitored and evaluated throughout the care process. Measuring outcomes not only demonstrates clinical effectiveness but also helps to promote rational clinical decision making and is reflective of the nursing interventions.

KEYCONCEPT **Outcomes** are the changes—favorable or unfavorable—in a patient's health status that can be attributed to nursing care at a given point in time (Moorhead, Johnson, Maas, & Swanson, 2008). An outcome is concise, stated in few words and in neutral terms. Outcomes describe a patient's state, behavior, or perception. Outcomes are variable and can be measured (Table 10.2, p. 138).

BOX 10.5

NANDA International Nursing Diagnoses (2012–2014)

HEALTH PROMOTION
Deficient Diversional Activity
Sedentary Lifestyle
Deficient Community Health
Risk-Prone Health Behavior
Ineffective Health Maintenance
Readiness for Enhanced Immunization Status
Ineffective Protection
Ineffective Self-Health Management
Readiness for Enhanced Self-Health Management
Ineffective Family Therapeutic Regimen Management

NUTRITION
Insufficient Breast Milk
Ineffective Infant Feeding Pattern
Imbalanced Nutrition: Less Than Body Requirements
Imbalanced Nutrition: More Than Body Requirements
Readiness for Enhanced Nutrition
Risk for Imbalanced Nutrition: More Than Body Requirements
Impaired Swallowing
Risk for Unstable Blood Glucose Level
Neonatal Jaundice
Risk for Neonatal Jaundice
Risk for Impaired Liver Function
Risk for Electrolyte Imbalance
Readiness for Enhanced Fluid Balance
Deficient Fluid Volume
Excess Fluid Volume
Risk for Deficient Fluid Volume
Risk for Imbalanced Fluid Volume

ELIMINATION AND EXCHANGE
Functional Urinary Incontinence
Overflow Urinary Incontinence
Reflex Urinary Incontinence
Stress Urinary Incontinence
Urge Urinary Incontinence
Risk for Urge Urinary Incontinence
Impaired Urinary Elimination
Readiness for Enhanced Urinary Elimination
Urinary Retention
Constipation
Perceived Constipation
Risk for Constipation
Diarrhea
Dysfunctional Gastrointestinal Motility
Risk for Dysfunctional Gastrointestinal Motility
Bowel Incontinence
Impaired Gas Exchange

ACTIVITY/REST
Insomnia
Sleep Deprivation
Readiness for Enhanced Sleep
Disturbed Sleep Pattern
Risk for Disuse Syndrome
Impaired Bed Mobility
Impaired Physical Mobility
Impaired Wheelchair Mobility
Impaired Transfer Ability
Impaired Walking
Disturbed Energy Field
Fatigue
Wandering
Activity Intolerance
Risk for Activity Intolerance
Ineffective Breathing Pattern
Decreased Cardiac Output
Risk for Ineffective Gastrointestinal Perfusion
Risk for Ineffective Renal Perfusion
Impaired Spontaneous Ventilation
Ineffective Peripheral Tissue Perfusion
Risk for Decreased Cardiac Tissue Perfusion
Risk for Ineffective Cerebral Tissue Perfusion

Risk for Ineffective Peripheral Tissue Perfusion
Dysfunctional Ventilatory Weaning Response
Impaired Home Maintenance
Readiness for Enhanced Self-Care
Bathing Self-Care Deficit
Dressing Self-Care Deficit
Feeding Self-Care Deficit
Toileting Self-Care Deficit
Self-Neglect

PERCEPTION/COGNITION
Unilateral Neglect
Impaired Environmental Interpretation Syndrome
Acute Confusion
Chronic Confusion
Risk for Acute Confusion
Ineffective Impulse Control
Deficient Knowledge
Readiness for Enhanced Knowledge
Impaired Memory
Readiness for Enhanced Communication
Impaired Verbal Communication

SELF-PERCEPTION
Hopelessness
Risk for Compromised Human Dignity
Risk for Loneliness
Disturbed Personal Identity
Risk for Disturbed Personal Identity
Readiness for Enhanced Self-Control
Chronic Low Self-Esteem
Situational Low Self-Esteem
Risk for Chronic Low Self-Esteem
Risk for Situational Low Self-Esteem
Disturbed Body Image

ROLE RELATIONSHIPS
Ineffective Breastfeeding
Interrupted Breastfeeding
Readiness for Enhanced Breastfeeding
Caregiver Role Strain
Risk for Caregiver Role Strain
Impaired Parenting
Readiness for Enhanced Parenting
Risk for Impaired Parenting
Risk for Impaired Attachment
Dysfunctional Family Processes
Interrupted Family Processes
Readiness for Enhanced Family Processes
Ineffective Relationship
Readiness for Enhanced Relationship
Risk for Ineffective Relationship
Parental Role Conflict
Ineffective Role Performance
Impaired Social Interaction

SEXUALITY
Sexual Dysfunction
Ineffective Sexuality Pattern
Ineffective Childbearing Process
Readiness for Enhanced Childbearing Process
Risk for Ineffective Childbearing Process
Risk for Disturbed Maternal–Fetal Dyad

COPING/STRESS TOLERANCE
Post-Trauma Syndrome
Risk for Post-Trauma Syndrome
Rape Trauma Syndrome
Relocation Stress Syndrome
Risk for Relocation Stress Syndrome
Ineffective Activity Planning
Risk for Ineffective Activity Planning
Anxiety
Defensive Coping
Ineffective Coping

(Continued)

BOX 10.5

NANDA International Nursing Diagnoses (2012–2014) *(Continued)*

Readiness for Enhanced Coping
Ineffective Community Coping
Readiness for Enhanced Community Coping
Compromised Family Coping
Disabled Family Coping
Readiness for Enhanced Family Coping
Death Anxiety
Ineffective Denial
Adult Failure To Thrive
Fear
Grieving
Complicated Grieving
Risk for Complicated Grieving
Readiness for Enhanced Power
Powerlessness
Risk for Powerlessness
Impaired Individual Resilience
Readiness for Enhanced Resilience
Risk for Compromised Resilience
Chronic Sorrow
Stress Overload
Autonomic Dysreflexia
Risk for Autonomic Dysreflexia
Disorganized Infant Behavior
Readiness for Enhanced Organized Infant Behavior
Risk for Disorganized Infant Behavior
Decreased Intracranial Adaptive Capacity

LIFE PRINCIPLES
Readiness for Enhanced Hope
Readiness for Enhanced Spiritual Well Being
Readiness for Enhanced Decision Making
Decisional Conflict
Moral Distress
Noncompliance
Impaired Religiosity
Readiness for Enhanced Religiosity
Risk for Impaired Religiosity
Spiritual Distress
Risk for Spiritual Distress

SAFETY/PROTECTION
Risk for Infection
Ineffective Airway Clearance
Risk for Aspiration
Risk for Bleeding

Impaired Dentition
Risk for Dry Eye
Risk for Falls
Risk for Injury
Impaired Oral Mucous Membrane
Risk for Perioperative Positioning Injury
Risk for Peripheral Neurovascular Dysfunction
Risk for Shock
Impaired Skin Integrity
Risk for Impaired Skin Integrity
Risk for Sudden Infant Death Syndrome
Risk for Suffocation
Delayed Surgical Recovery
Risk for Thermal Injury
Impaired Tissue Integrity
Risk for Trauma
Risk for Vascular Trauma
Risk for Other Directed Violence
Risk for Self-Directed Violence
Self-Mutilation
Risk for Self-Mutilation
Risk for Suicide
Contamination
Risk for Contamination
Risk for Poisoning
Risk for Adverse Reaction to Iodinated Contrast Media
Latex Allergy Response
Risk for Allergy Response
Risk for Latex Allergy Response
Risk for Imbalanced Body Temperature
Hyperthermia
Hypothermia
Ineffective Thermoregulation

COMFORT
Impaired Comfort
Readiness for Enhanced Comfort
Nausea
Acute Pain
Chronic Pain
Social Isolation

GROWTH/DEVELOPMENT
Risk for Disproportionate Growth
Delayed Growth And Development
Risk for Delayed Development

From *Nursing Diagnoses: Definitions and Classification 2012–2014.* © 2012, 2009, 2007, 2005, 2003, 2001, 1998, 1996, 1994 NANDA International. Used by arrangement with Wiley-Blackwell Publishing. In order to make safe and effective judgments using NANDA-I nursing diagnoses, it is essential that nurses refer to the definitions and defining characteristics of the diagnoses listed in this work.

Outcomes focus on the individual recipient of care (patient or family caregivers) and include patient statements, behaviors, or perceptions that are sensitive to or influenced by nursing interventions (Moorhead et al., 2008). Nurses are accountable for documenting patient

Table 10.2	EXAMPLE OF OUTCOMES	
Diagnosis	**Outcome**	**Intervention**
Impaired social interaction (isolates self from others)	Social involvement Indicators: 1. Interact with other patients. 2. Attend group meetings.	Using a contract format, explain role and responsibility of patients

outcomes; nursing interventions; and any changes in diagnosis, care plan, or both. Outcomes can be expressed in terms of the patient's actual responses (no longer reports hearing voices) or the status of a nursing diagnosis at a point in time after implementation of nursing interventions, such as Caregiver Role Strain resolved. This documentation is important for further research, cost, and continuity and quality of care studies.

NURSING INTERVENTIONS

Interventions can be either nurse-initiated treatment, which is an autonomous action in response to a nursing diagnosis, or physician-initiated treatment with an order written in the patient's record.

> KEYCONCEPT   **Nursing interventions** are nursing actions or treatment, selected based on clinical judgment, that are designed to achieve patient, family, or community outcomes. Interventions can be direct or indirect.

There are several nursing interventions systems, including the Nursing Interventions Classification (NIC), the Clinical Care Classification system, and the Omaha nursing model. All of these systems are recognized by the American Nurses Association (ANA) (Bulechek, Butcher, Dochterman, & Wagner, 2013; Martin, 2005; Saba, 2012). See Chapter 6. In this text, the *Psychiatric-Mental Health Nursing: Scope and Standards of Practice* guides the use of interventions (ANA, APNA, & ISPN, 2014). Some are adapted from classification systems and others from the psychiatric mental health nursing literature.

Interventions for the Biologic Domain

Biologic interventions focus on physical functioning and are directed toward the patient's self-care, activities and exercise, sleep, nutrition, relaxation, hydration, and thermoregulation as well as pain management and medication management.

Promotion of Self-Care Activities

Many patients with psychiatric–mental health problems can manage ADLs or self-care activities such as bathing, dressing appropriately, selecting adequate nutrition, and sleeping regularly. Others cannot manage such self-care activities, either because of their symptoms or as a result of the side effects of medications.

In the inpatient setting, the psychiatric nurse structures the patient's activities, so that basic self-care activities are completed. During acute phases of psychiatric disorders, the inability to attend to basic self-care tasks, such as getting dressed, is very common. Thus, the ability to complete personal hygiene activities (e.g., dental care, grooming) is monitored, and patients are assisted in completing such activities. In a psychiatric facility, patients are encouraged and expected to develop independence in completing these basic self-care activities. In the community, monitoring these basic self-care activities is always a part of the nursing visit or clinic appointment.

Activity and Exercise Interventions

In some psychiatric disorders (e.g., schizophrenia), people become sedentary and appear to lack the motivation to complete ADLs. This lack of motivation is part of the disorder and requires nursing intervention. In addition, side effects of medication often include sedation and lethargy. Encouraging regular activity and exercise can improve general well-being and physical health. In some instances, exercise behavior becomes an abnormal focus of attention, as may be observed in some patients with anorexia nervosa.

When assuming the responsibility of direct care provider, the nurse can help patients identify realistic activities and exercise goals. As leader or manager of a psychiatric unit, the nurse can influence ward routine. Alternatively, the nurse can delegate activity and exercise interventions to nurses' aides. Some institutions have other professionals (e.g., recreational therapists) available for the implementation of exercise programs. As a case manager, the nurse should consider the activity needs of individuals when coordinating care.

Sleep Interventions

Many psychiatric disorders and medications are associated with sleep disturbances. Sleep is also disrupted in patients with dementia; such patients may have difficulty falling asleep or may frequently awaken during the night. In dementia of the Alzheimer's type, individuals may reverse their sleeping patterns by napping during the day and staying awake at night.

Nonpharmacologic interventions are always used first because of the side-effect risks associated with the use of sedatives and hypnotics (see Chapter 11). Sleep interventions to communicate to patients include the following:

- Go to bed only when tired or sleepy.
- Establish a consistent bedtime routine.
- Avoid stimulating foods, beverages, or medications.
- Avoid naps in the late afternoon or evening.
- Eat lightly before retiring and limit fluid intake.
- Use your bed only for sleep or intimacy.
- Avoid emotional stimulation before bedtime.
- Use behavioral and relaxation techniques.
- Limit distractions.

Nutrition Interventions

Psychiatric disorders and medication side effects can affect eating behaviors. For varying reasons, some patients eat too little, but others eat too much. For instance, homeless patients with mental illnesses have difficulty maintaining adequate nutrition because of their deprived lifestyle. Substance abuse also interferes with maintaining adequate nutrition, either through stimulation or suppression of appetite or neglecting nutrition because of drug-seeking behavior. Thus, nutrition interventions should be specific and relevant to the individual's circumstances and mental health. In addition, recommended daily nutritional allowances are important in the promotion of physical and mental health, and nurses should consider them when planning care.

BOX 10.6

Relaxation Techniques: Descriptions and Implementation

SIMPLE RELAXATION TECHNIQUES
- Create a quiet, nondisrupting environment with dim lights and a comfortable temperature.
- Instruct the patient to assume a relaxed position, wearing loose and comfortable clothing.
- Instruct the patient to relax and to let the sensations happen.
- Use a low tone of voice with a slow, rhythmic pace of words.
- Instruct the patient to take an initial slow, deep breath (abdominal breathing) while thinking about pleasant events.
- Use soothing music (without words) to enhance relaxation.
- Reinforce the use of relaxation by praising efforts and helping the patient to schedule time regularly for it.
- Evaluate and document the patient's response to relaxation.

DISTRACTION
- Distraction techniques include music, counting, television, reading, play, and exercise. Help the patient choose a technique that will work for him or her.
- Advise the patient to practice the distraction technique before he or she will need to use it.
- Have the patient develop a specific plan for how and when he or she will use distraction.
- Evaluate and document the patient's response to distraction.

GUIDED IMAGERY
- Help the patient choose a particular guided imagery technique (alone or with others).

- Discuss an image the patient has experienced as pleasurable and relaxing, such as lying on a beach, watching snow fall, floating on a raft, or watching the sun set.
- Individualize the images chosen, considering religious or spiritual beliefs, artistic interests, or other individual preferences.
- Make suggestions to induce relaxation (e.g., peaceful images, pleasant sensations, or rhythmic breathing).
- Use modulated voice when guiding the imagery experience.
- Have the patient travel mentally to the scene, and assist in describing the setting in detail.
- Use permissive directions and suggestions when leading the imagery, such as "perhaps," "if you wish," or "you might like."
- Have the patient slowly experience the scene. How does it look? smell? sound? feel? taste?
- Use words or phrases that convey pleasurable images, such as floating, melting, and releasing.
- Develop cleansing or clearing portion of imagery (e.g., all pain appears as red dust and washes downstream in a creek as you enter).
- Assist the patient in developing a method of ending the imagery technique, such as counting slowly while breathing deeply.
- Encourage expression of thoughts and feelings regarding the experience.
- Prepare the patient for unexpected (but often therapeutic) experiences, such as crying.
- Evaluate and document the patient's response.

Adapted from Bulechek et al. (2013).

Some psychiatric symptoms involve changes in perceptions of food, appetite, and eating habits. If a patient believes that food is poisonous, he or she may eat sparingly or not at all. Interventions are then necessary to address the suspiciousness as well as to encourage adequate intake of recommended daily allowances. Allowing patients to examine foods, participate in preparations, and test the safety of the meal by eating slowly or after everyone else may be necessary. For patients who are paranoid, it is sometimes helpful to serve prepackaged foods.

Relaxation Interventions

Relaxation promotes comfort, reduces anxiety, alleviates stress, eases pain, and prevents aggression. It can diminish the effects of hallucinations and delusions. The many different relaxation techniques used as mental health interventions range from simple deep breathing to biofeedback to hypnosis. Although some techniques, such as biofeedback, require additional training and, in some instances, certification, nurses can easily apply simple relaxation, distraction, and imagery techniques. **Simple relaxation techniques** encourage and elicit relaxation to decrease undesirable signs and symptoms. **Distraction** is the purposeful focusing of attention away from undesirable sensations, and **guided imagery** is the

purposeful use of imagination to achieve relaxation or direct attention away from undesirable sensations (Box 10.6). These interventions are helpful for people experiencing anxiety; guided imagery is especially useful in stress management.

Relaxation techniques that involve physical touch (e.g., back rubs) usually are not used for people with mental disorders. Touching and massaging usually are not appropriate, especially for those who have a history of physical or sexual abuse. Such patients may find touching too stimulating or misinterpret it as being sexual or aggressive.

Hydration Interventions

Assessing fluid status and monitoring fluid intake and output are often important interventions. Overhydration or underhydration can be a symptom of a disorder. For example, some patients with psychotic disorders experience chronic fluid imbalance. Many psychiatric medications affect fluid and electrolyte balance (see Chapter 11). For example, when taking lithium carbonate, patients must have adequate fluid intake and pay special attention to testing serum sodium levels. Interventions that help patients understand the relationship of medications to fluid and electrolyte balance are important in their overall care.

Thermoregulation Interventions

Many psychiatric disorders can disturb the body's normal temperature regulation. Thus, patients cannot sense temperature increases or decreases and consequently cannot protect themselves from extremes of hot or cold. This problem is especially difficult for people who are homeless or live outside the protected environments of institutions and boarding homes. In addition, many psychiatric medications affect the ability to regulate body temperature.

Interventions include educating patients about the problem of thermoregulation, identifying potential extremes in temperatures, and developing strategies to protect the patient from the adverse effects of temperature changes. For example, reminding patients to wear coats and sweaters in the winter or to wear loose, lightweight garments in the summer may prevent frostbite or heat exhaustion, respectively.

Pain Management

Psychiatric nurses are more likely to provide care to patients experiencing chronic pain than acute pain. However, a single intervention is seldom successful for relieving chronic pain. In some instances, pain is managed by medication; in other instances, nonpharmacologic strategies, such as simple relaxation techniques, distraction, or imagery, are used. Indeed, relaxation is one of the most widely used cognitive and behavioral approaches to pain. Education, stress management techniques, hypnosis, and biofeedback are also used in pain management. Physical agents include heat and cold therapy, exercise, and transcutaneous nerve stimulation.

The key to managing pain is identifying how it disrupts the patient's personal, social, professional, and family life. Education focusing on the pain, use of medications for treatment, and development of cognitive skills are important pain management components. In some cases, redefining treatment success as improvement in functioning, rather than alleviation of pain, may be necessary. The interaction between stress and pain is important; that is, increased stress leads to increased pain. Patients can better manage their pain when stress is reduced.

Medication Management

The psychiatric–mental health nurse uses many medication management interventions to help patients maintain therapeutic regimens. Medication management involves more than the actual administration of medications. Nurses also assess medication effectiveness and side effects and consider drug–drug interactions. Monitoring the amount of lethal prescription medication is particularly important. For example, check if patients have old prescriptions of tricyclic antidepressants in their medicine cabinets. Treatment with psychopharmacologic agents can be lengthy because of the chronic nature of many disorders; many patients remain on medication regimens for years, never becoming free of medication. Thus, medication education is an ongoing intervention that requires careful documentation. Medication follow-up may include home visits as well as telephone calls.

Interventions for the Psychological Domain

A major emphasis in psychiatric–mental health nursing is on the psychological domain: emotion, behavior, and cognition. The nurse–patient relationship serves as the basis for interventions directed toward the psychological domain. Because the therapeutic relationship was extensively discussed in Chapter 9, it is not covered in this chapter. This section does cover counseling, conflict resolution, bibliotherapy and webotherapy, reminiscence, behavior therapy, psychoeducation, health teaching, and spiritual interventions. Cognitive interventions are presented in Chapter 12. Chapter 7 presents the theoretic basis for many of these interventions.

Counseling Interventions

Counseling interventions are specific, time-limited interactions between a nurse and a patient, family, or group experiencing immediate or ongoing difficulties related to their health or well-being. Counseling is usually short term and focuses on improving coping abilities, reinforcing healthy behaviors, fostering positive interactions, or preventing illness and disability. Counseling strategies are discussed throughout the text. Psychotherapy, which differs from counseling, is generally a long-term approach aimed at improving or helping patients regain previous health status and functional abilities. Mental health specialists, such as advanced practice nurses, use psychotherapy.

Conflict Resolution and Cultural Brokering

Conflict resolution is a specific type of intervention through which the nurse helps patients resolve disagreements or disputes with family, friends, or other patients. Conflict can be positive if individuals see the problem as solvable and providing an opportunity for growth and interpersonal understanding. The nurse may be in the position of actually resolving a family conflict or teaching family members how to resolve their own conflicts positively. In addition, because nurses are in positions of leadership, they often need conflict resolution skills to settle employee conflicts.

At times, patients who are politically and economically powerless find themselves in conflict with the health care system. Differences in cultural values and languages among patients and health care organizations contribute to feelings of powerlessness. For example, migrant farm workers, people who are homeless, and people who need to make informed decisions under stressful conditions may be unable to navigate the health care system. The nurse can help to resolve such conflicts through **cultural brokering**, the act of bridging, linking, or mediating messages, instructions, and belief systems between groups of people of differing cultural systems to reduce conflict or produce change (Esperat, Inouye, Gonzalez, Owen, & Feng, 2004).

For the "nurse as broker" to be effective, he or she establishes and maintains a sense of connectedness or relationship with the patient. In turn, the nurse also establishes and cultivates networks with other health care facilities and resources. Cultural sensitivity enables the nurse to be aware of and sensitive to the needs of patients from a variety of cultures. Cultural competence is necessary for the brokering process to be effective.

Bibliotherapy and Internet Use

Bibliotherapy, sometimes referred to as bibliocounseling, is the reading of selected written materials to express feelings or gain insight under the guidance of a health care provider. The provider assigns and discusses with the patient a book, story, or article. The provider makes the assignment because he or she believes that the patient can receive therapeutic benefit from the reading. (It is assumed that the provider who assigned the reading has also read it.) The provider needs to consider the patient's reading level before making an assignment. If a patient has limited reading ability, the provider should not use bibliotherapy.

Literary works serve as a projective screen through which people see themselves in the story. Literature can help patients identify with characters and vicariously experience their reality. It can also expose patients to situations that they have not personally experienced—the vicarious experience allows growth in self-knowledge and compassion (Macdonald, Vallance, & McGrath, 2013). Through reading, patients can enrich their lives in the following ways:

• *Catharsis:* expression of feelings stimulated by parallel experiences
• *Problem solving:* development of solutions to problems in the literature from practical ideas about problem solving
• *Insight:* increased self-awareness and understanding as the reader explores personal meaning from what is read
• *Anxiety reduction:* self-help written materials can reduce concerns about a diagnosed problem and treatment.

Using the internet can be helpful to patients, but it also has drawbacks. Some web sites can help patients gain insight into their problems through acquiring new knowledge and interacting with others in the privacy of their own surroundings. Web materials and chat groups are variable in quality and accuracy. Nurses should carefully evaluate the quality of the website when patients are engaging in webotherapy.

Reminiscence

Reminiscence, the thinking about or relating of past experiences, is used as a nursing intervention to enhance life review in older patients. Reminiscence encourages patients, either in individual or group settings, to discuss their past and review their lives. Through reminiscence, individuals can identify past coping strategies that can support them in current stressful situations. Patients can also use reminiscence to maintain self-esteem, stimulate thinking, and support the natural healing process of life review. Activities that facilitate reminiscence include writing an account of past events, making a tape recording and playing it back, explaining pictures in old family albums, drawing a family tree, and writing to old friends (Box 10.7).

Behavior Therapy

Behavior therapy interventions focus on reinforcing or promoting desirable behaviors or altering undesirable ones. The basic premise is that because most behaviors are learned, new functional behaviors can also be learned. Behaviors—not internal psychic processes—are the targets

---

BOX 10.7

Research for Best Practice: Reminiscence Treatment in Older Adults with Dementia

Huang, S., Li., C., Yang, C., & Chen, J. J. (2009). Application of reminiscence treatment on older people with dementia: A case study in Pingtung, Taiwan. Journal of Nursing Research, 17(2), 112–119.

THE QUESTION: Does cognition improve and depression decrease following participation in an eight-week reminiscence social group organized around cooking?

METHODS: A social work group of 10 older adult female residents of a nursing home completed eight sessions of reminiscence cooking lessons consisting of preparing traditional foods. Changes in memory, cognition, brain functioning, and personal interaction were measured pre- and post-session by the mental health status, depression scale, EEG, and feeling of participation scale.

FINDINGS: There were positive changes in all of the measures, but none of these changes were significant.

IMPLICATIONS FOR NURSING: This small study is clinically interesting because the intervention, cooking food as an activity for reminiscence therapy, is unique and rarely reported. The problem with the study is the small sample. The lack of significant findings is predictable with this small group. However, the intervention is logical and deserves further study.

of the interventions. The models of behavioral theorists serve as a basis for these interventions (see Chapter 7).

Behavior Modification

Behavior modification is a specific, systematized behavior therapy technique that can be applied to individuals, groups, or systems. The aim of behavior modification is to reinforce desired behaviors and extinguish undesired ones. Desired behavior is rewarded to increase the likelihood that patients will repeat it, and over time, replace the problematic behavior with it. Behavior modification is used for various problematic behaviors, such as dysfunctional eating, addictions, anger management, and impulse control and often is used in the care of children and adolescents.

Token Economy

Used in inpatient settings and in group homes, a **token economy** applies behavior modification techniques to multiple behaviors. In a token economy, patients are rewarded with tokens for selected desired behaviors. They can use these tokens to purchase meals, leave the unit, watch television, or wear street clothes. In less restrictive environments, patients use tokens to purchase additional privileges, such as attending social events. Token economy systems have been especially effective in reinforcing positive behaviors in people who are developmentally disabled or have severe and persistent mental illnesses. The strategy has been expanded to rehabilitation programs for children (Jones, Webb, Estes, & Dawson, 2013), and cocaine addiction (Farronato, Dursteler-Macfarland, Wiesbeck, & Petitjean, et al., 2013).

> NCLEXNOTE Focus on helping patient achieve and maintain self-control of behavior (e.g., contract, behavior modification).

Psychoeducation

Psychoeducation uses educational strategies to teach patients the skills they lack because of a psychiatric disorder. The goal of psychoeducation is a change in knowledge and behavior. Nurses use psychoeducation to meet the educational needs of patients by adapting teaching strategies to their disorder-related deficits (Box 10.8). As patients gain skills, functioning improves. Some patients may need to learn how to maintain their morning hygiene. Others may need to understand their illness and cope with hearing voices that others do not hear.

Specific psychoeducation techniques are based on adult learning principles, such as beginning at the point where the learner is currently and building on his or her current experiences. Thus, the nurse assesses the patient's current skills and readiness to learn. From there, the

---

BOX 10.8

Research for Best Practices: Educational and Self-Management Interventions

Coster, S & Norman, I. (2009). Cochrane reviews of educational and self-management interventions to guide nursing practice: A review. International Journal of Nursing Studies, 46, 508–528.

THE QUESTION: What interventions improve patients' knowledge and skills to manage chronic disease?

METHODS: Thirty Cochrane systematic reviews were identified. Data were extracted and summarized.

FINDINGS: Most of the studies provided inadequate evidence (n = 18, 60%), but of those studies with adequate evidence, mental health is one of the chronic disease states for which patient education makes a difference.

IMPLICATIONS FOR NURSING: Education can be effective in the area of mental health and is a key intervention for patients with emotional problems and mental disorders.

---

nurse individualizes a teaching plan for each patient. He or she can conduct such teaching in a one-to-one situation or a group format.

Psychoeducation is a continuous process of assessing, setting goals, developing learning activities, and evaluating for changes in knowledge and behavior. Nurses use it with individuals, groups, families, and communities. Psychoeducation serves as a basis for psychosocial rehabilitation, a service-delivery approach for those with severe and persistent mental illness (see Chapter 22).

> NCLEXNOTE Apply knowledge from social sciences to help patients manage responses to psychiatric disorders and emotional problems.

Health Teaching

Health teaching is one of the standards of care for the psychiatric nurse. Teaching methods should be appropriate to the patient's development level, learning needs, readiness, ability to learn, language preference, and culture. Based on principles of learning, health teaching involves transmitting new information to the patient and providing constructive feedback and positive rewards, practice sessions, homework, and experimental learning. Health teaching is the integration of principles of teaching and learning with the knowledge of health and illness (Figure 10.3).

Thus, in health teaching, the psychiatric nurse attends to potential health care problems other than mental disorders and emotional problems. For example, if a person has diabetes mellitus and is taking insulin, the nurse provides health care teaching related to diabetes and the interaction of this problem with the mental disorder.

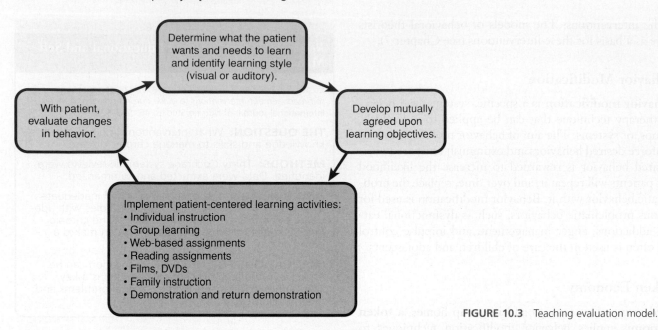

FIGURE 10.3 Teaching evaluation model.

Spiritual Interventions

Spiritual care is based on an assessment of the patient's spiritual needs. A nonjudgmental relationship and just "being with" (not doing for) the patient are key to providing spiritual intervention. In some instances, patients ask to see a religious leader. Nurses should always respect and never deny these requests. To assist people in spiritual distress, the nurse should know and understand the beliefs and practices of various spiritual groups. **Spiritual support**, assisting patients to feel balance and connection within their relationships, involves listening to expressions of loneliness, using empathy, and providing patients with desired spiritual articles.

Interventions for the Social Domain

The social domain includes the individual's environment and its effect on his or her responses to mental disorders and distress. Interventions within the social domain are geared toward couples, families, friends, and large and small social groups, with special attention given to ethnicity and community interactions. In some instances, nurses design interventions that affect a patient's environment, such as helping a family member decide to admit a loved one to a long-term care facility. In other instances, the nurse actually modifies the environment to promote positive behaviors. Group and family interventions are discussed in Chapters 13 and 14, respectively.

Social Behavior and Privilege Systems in Inpatient Units

In psychiatric units, unrelated strangers who have problems interacting live together in close quarters, sometimes with two to four people sharing bedrooms and bathrooms. For this reason, most psychiatric units develop a list of behavioral expectations called unit rules that staff members post and explain to patients upon admittance. Their purpose is to facilitate a comfortable and safe environment; they have little to do with the patients' reasons for admission. Getting up at certain times, showering before breakfast, making the bed, and not visiting in others' rooms are typical expectations. It is usually the nurse manager who oversees the operation of the unit and implementation of privilege systems.

Most psychiatric facilities use a privilege system to protect patients and to reinforce unit rules and other appropriate behavior (also see the previous section discussing a token economies). The more appropriate the behavior, the more privileges of freedom the person has. Privileges are based on the assessment of a patient's risk to harm himself or herself or others and ability to follow treatment regimens. For example, a patient with few privileges may be required to stay on the unit and eat only with other patients. A patient with full privileges may have freedom to leave the unit and go outside the hospital and into the community for short periods.

Milieu Therapy

Milieu therapy provides a stable and coherent social organization to facilitate an individual's treatment. (The terms *milieu therapy* and *therapeutic environment* are often used interchangeably.) In milieu therapy, the design of the physical surroundings, structure of patient activities, and promotion of a stable social structure and cultural setting enhance the setting's therapeutic potential. A therapeutic milieu facilitates patient interactions and promotes personal growth. Milieu therapy is the responsibility of the nurse in collaboration with the patient and other health care providers. The key concepts of milieu therapy include containment, validation, structured interaction, and open communication.

Containment

Containment is the process of providing safety and security and involves the patient's access to food and shelter. In a well-contained milieu, patients feel safe from their illnesses and protected against social stigma. The physical surroundings are also important in this process and should be clean and comfortable, with special attention paid to promoting a noninstitutionalized environment. Pictures on walls, comfortable furniture, and soothing colors help patients relax. Most facilities encourage patients and nursing staff to wear street clothes, which help decrease the formalized nature of hospital settings and promotes nurse–patient relationships.

Therapeutic milieus emphasize patient involvement in treatment decisions and operation of the unit; nurses should encourage freedom of movement within the contained environment. Patients participate in maintaining the quality of the physical surroundings, assuming responsibility for making their own beds, attending to their own belongings, and keeping an acceptable living area. Families are viewed as a part of the patient's life, and ties are maintained. In most inpatient settings, specific times are set for family interaction, education, and treatment. Family involvement is often a criterion for admission for treatment, and the involvement may include regular family attendance at therapy sessions.

Validation

In a therapeutic environment, **validation** is another process that affirms patient individuality. Staff–patient interactions should constantly reaffirm the patient's humanity and human rights. All interaction a staff member initiates with a patient should reflect his or her respect for that patient. Patients must believe that staff members truly like and respect them.

Structured Interaction

One of the most interesting milieu concepts is **structured interaction**, which is purposeful interaction that allows patients to interact with others in a useful way. For instance, the daily community meeting provides structure to explain unit rules and consequences of violations. Ideally, patients who are either elected or volunteer for the responsibility assume leadership for these meetings. In the meeting, the group discusses behavioral expectations, such as making beds daily, appropriate dress, and

rules for leaving the unit. Usually, there are other rules, such as no fighting or name calling.

In some instances, the treatment team assigns structured interactions to specific patients as part of their treatment. Specific attitudes or approaches are directed toward individual patients who benefit from a particular type of interaction. Nurses consistently assume indulgence, flexibility, passive or active friendliness, matter-of-fact attitude, casualness, watchfulness, or kind firmness when interacting with specific patients. For example, if a patient is known to overreact and dramatize events, the staff may provide a matter-of-fact attitude when the patient engages in dramatic behavior.

Open Communication

In **open communication**, the staff and patient willingly share information. Staff members invite patient self-disclosure within the support of a nurse–patient relationship. In addition, they provide a model of effective communication when interacting with one another as well as with patients. They arrange an environment to facilitate optimal interaction and resocialization. Support, attention, praise, and reassurance given to patients improve self-esteem and increase confidence. Patient education is also a part of this support, as are directions to foster coping skills.

Milieu Therapy in Different Settings

Milieu therapy is applied in various settings. In long-term care settings, the therapeutic milieu becomes essential because patients may reside there for months or years. These patients typically have schizophrenia or developmental disabilities. Structure in daily living is important to the successful functioning of the individuals and the overall group but must be applied within the context of individual needs. For example, if a patient cannot get up one morning in time to complete assigned tasks (e.g., showering or making a bed) because of a personal crisis the night before, the nurse should consider the situation compassionately and flexibly, not applying the "consequences" rule or taking away the patient's privileges. In turn, the nurse must weigh individual needs against the collective needs of all the patients. For a patient who is consistently late for treatment activities, the nurse should apply the rules of the unit even if it means taking away privileges.

Recently, concepts of milieu therapy have been applied to short-term inpatient and community settings. In acute-care inpatient settings, nursing actions provide limits to and controls on patient behavior and provide structure and safety for the patients. Milieu treatments are based on the individual needs of the patients and include relaxation groups, discussion groups, and medication groups. Spontaneous and planned activities are possible on a short-term unit as well as in a long-term setting. In the community, it is possible to apply milieu therapy approaches in day treatment centers, group homes, and single dwellings.

Promotion of Patient Safety

Although the use of social rules of conduct and privilege systems can enhance smooth operation of a unit, some potentially serious problems can be associated with these practices. A most critical aspect of psychiatric–mental health nursing is the promotion of patient safety, especially in inpatient units.

Observation

Patient observation is the ongoing assessment of the patient's mental status to identify and subvert any potential problem. An important process in all nursing practice, observation is particularly important in psychiatric nursing. In psychiatric settings, patients are ambulatory and thus more susceptible to environmental hazards. In addition, judgment and cognition impairment are symptoms of many psychiatric disorders. Often, patients are admitted because they pose a danger to themselves or others. In psychiatric nursing, observation is more than just "seeing" patients. It means continually monitoring them for any indication of harm to themselves or others.

All patients who are hospitalized for psychiatric reasons are continually monitored. The intensity of the observation depends on their risk to themselves and others. Some patients are merely asked to "check in" at different times of the day, but others have a staff member assigned to only them, such as in instances of potential suicide. Often "sharps," such as razors, are locked up and given to patients at specified times. Mental health facilities and units all have policies that specify levels of observation for patients of varying degrees of risk.

De-escalation

De-escalation is an interactive process of calming and redirecting a patient who has an immediate potential for violence directed toward self or others. This intervention involves assessing the situation and preventing it from escalating to one in which injury occurs to the patient, staff, or other patients. After the nurse has assessed the situation, he or she calmly calls to the patient and asks the individual to leave the situation. The nurse must avoid rushing toward the patient or giving orders (see Chapter 19). Nurses can use various interventions in this situation, including distraction, conflict resolution, and cognitive interventions.

Seclusion

Seclusion is the involuntary confinement of a person in a room or an area where the person is physically prevented from leaving (Centers for Medicare & Medicaid Services [CMS], 2012). A patient is placed in seclusion for purposes of safety or behavioral management. The seclusion room has no furniture except a mattress and a blanket. The walls usually are padded. The room is environmentally safe, with no hanging devices, electrical outlets, or windows from which the patient could jump. When a patient is placed in seclusion, he or she is observed at all times.

There are several types of seclusion arrangements. Some facilities place seclusion rooms next to the nurses' stations. These seclusion rooms have an observation window. Other facilities use a modified patient room and assign a staff member to view the patient at all times. Seclusion is an extremely negative patient experience; consequently, its use is seriously questioned, and many facilities have completely abandoned its practice (Box 10.9). Patient outcomes may actually be worse if seclusion is used.

Restraints

The most restrictive safety intervention is the use of **restraint**, any manual method, physical or mechanical, that immobilizes or reduces the ability of the patient to move. Tucking a patient's sheet in so tightly that the

---

BOX 10.9

Research for Best Practice: **Evidence for Seclusion and Restraint Use**

Sailas, E., & Fenton, M. (2012). Seclusion and restraint for people with serious mental illnesses. The Cochrane Library (Oxford) (ID 00075320-100000000-00215.

THE QUESTION: How effective are seclusion, restraint, or alternative controls for people with serious mental illness?

METHODS: A meta-analysis of the effectiveness of seclusion and restraint compared with the alternatives for persons with serious mental illnesses was conducted. Randomized controlled trials were included if they focused on the use of restraint or seclusion or strategies designed to reduce the need for restraint or seclusion in the treatment of serious mental illness. The search yielded 2,155 citations. Of these, 35 studies were obtained.

FINDINGS: No controlled studies exist that evaluate the value of seclusion or restraint in those with serious mental illness. There are reports of serious adverse effects for these techniques in qualitative reviews.

IMPLICATIONS FOR NURSING: Alternative ways of dealing with unwanted or harmful behaviors need to be developed. Continuing use of seclusion or restraint must, therefore, be questioned.

person cannot move is considered a restraint as is the use of leather restraints. **Chemical restraint** is the use of medications for restricting patients' behavior or their freedom of movement. These chemical restraints include drugs that are not a part of their standard psychiatric treatment or that are an inappropriate dosage of their standard medication. If hospitals choose to use any type of restraints for behavioral control, the restraints are applied only after every other intervention is used and the patient continues to be a danger to self or others. Documentation must reflect a careful assessment of the patient that indicates the need for an intervention to protect the patient from harm (CMS, 2012).

The least restrictive type of restraint is selected to keep a patient safe. Wrist restraints restrict arm movement. Walking restraints or ankle restraints are used if a patient cannot resist the impulse to run from a facility but is safe to go outside and to activities. Three- and four-point restraints are applied to the wrist and ankles in bed. When five-point restraints are used, all extremities are secured, and another restraint is placed across the chest.

The use of both seclusion and restraints must follow the Medicare regulations contained in the *Patients' Rights Condition of Participation* (CMS, 2012). Agencies that do not follow the regulations may lose their Medicare and Medicaid certification and, consequently, their funding. The application of physical restraints should also follow hospital policies. Nurses should document all the previously tried de-escalation interventions before the application of restraints. They should limit use of restraints to times when an individual is judged to be a danger to self or others; they should apply restraints only until the patient regains control over his or her behavior. When a patient is in physical restraints, the nurse should closely observe the patient and protect him or her from self-injury. See Box 10.9.

Home Visits

Patients usually have been hospitalized or have received treatment for acute psychiatric symptoms before being referred to psychiatric home service. The goal of **home visits**, the delivery of nursing care in the patient's living environment, is to maximize the patient's functional ability within the nurse–patient relationship and with the family or partner as appropriate. The psychiatric nurse who makes home visits needs to be able to work independently, is skilled in teaching patients and families, can administer and monitor medications, and uses community resources for the patient's needs.

Home visits are especially useful in certain situations, including helping reluctant patients enter therapy, conducting a comprehensive assessment, strengthening a support network, and maintaining patients in the community when their condition deteriorates. Home visits are also useful in helping individuals comply with taking medication. The home visit process consists of three steps: the previsit phase, the home visit, and the postvisit phase. During previsit planning, the nurse sets goals for the home visit based on data received from other health care providers or the patient. In addition, the nurse and patient agree on the time of the visit. As the nurse travels to the home, he or she should assess the neighborhood for access to services, socioeconomic factors, and safety.

The actual visit can be divided into four parts. The first is the greeting phase, in which the nurse establishes rapport with family members. Greetings, which are usually brief, establish the communication process and the atmosphere for the visit. Greetings should be friendly but professional. In cultures that consider greetings important, this phase may involve more formal interactions, such as eating food or drinking tea with family members. The next phase establishes the focus of the visit. Sometimes the purpose of the visit is medication administration, health teaching, or counseling. The patient and family must be clear regarding the purpose. The implementation of the service is the next phase and should use most of the visit time. If the purpose of the visit is problem solving or decision making, the family's cultural values may determine the types of interaction and decision-making approaches. Closure is the last phase, the end of the home visit. It is a time to summarize and clarify important points. The nurse should also schedule any additional visits and reiterate patient expectations between visits. Usually, the nurse is the only provider to see the patient regularly. The nurse should acknowledge family members on leaving if they were not a part of the visit.

The postvisit phase includes documentation, reporting, and follow-up planning. This is also when the nurse meets with the supervisor and presents data from the home visit at the team meeting.

Community Action

Nurses have a unique opportunity to promote mental health awareness and support humane treatment for people with mental disorders. Activities range from being an advisor to support groups to participating in the political process through lobbying efforts and serving on community mental health boards. These unpaid activities are usually outside the realm of a particular job. However, an important role of professionals is to provide community service in addition to service through income-generating positions.

EVALUATING OUTCOMES

Evaluation of patient outcomes involves answering the following questions:

- What is the cost effectiveness of the intervention?
- What benefits did the patient receive?

- What was the patient's level of satisfaction?
- Was the outcome diagnosis specific or nonspecific?

Outcomes can be measured immediately after the nursing intervention or after time passes. For example, a patient may be able to resolve the acute depression and demonstrate confidence and improved self-esteem during a hospital stay. In various cases, it may be several months before the person can engage in positive interpersonal relationships.

SUMMARY OF KEY POINTS

- Assessment is the deliberate and systematic collection of biopsychosocial information or data to determine current and past health and functional status and to evaluate present and past coping patterns.

- The biologic assessment includes current and past health status, physical examination with review of body systems, review of physical functions, and pharmacologic assessment.

- The psychological assessment includes the mental status examination, behavioral responses, and risk factor assessment.

  - The mental status examination includes general observation of appearance, psychomotor activity, and attitude; orientations; mood; affect; emotions; speech; and thought processes.

  - Behavioral responses are assessed as are self-concept and current and past coping patterns.

  - Risk factor assessment includes ascertaining whether the patient has any suicidal, assaultive, or homicidal ideation.

- The social assessment includes functional status; social systems; spirituality; occupational, economic, and legal status; and quality of life.

- The biopsychosocial assessment provides the data for nursing diagnoses and planning patient outcomes. Anticipated patient outcomes are the basis for psychiatric–mental health nursing interventions.

- Nursing interventions are implemented for each domain include biologic (self-care, activity and exercise, sleep, nutrition, thermoregulation, and pain and medication management); psychological (counseling, conflict resolution, bibliotherapy and webotherapy, reminiscence, behavior therapy, psychoeducation, health teaching, and spiritual interventions); and social (behavior therapy and modification, milieu therapy, and various home and community interventions).

- Evaluation of patient outcomes involves assessing cost effectiveness of the interventions, benefits to the patient, and the patient's level of satisfaction. Outcomes should be measurable, either immediately after intervention or after some time passes.

CRITICAL THINKING CHALLENGES

1. A 23-year-old white woman is admitted to an acute psychiatric setting for depression and suicidal gestures. This admission is her first, but she has experienced bouts of depression since early adolescence. She and her fiancé have just broken their engagement and moved into separate apartments. She has not yet told anyone that she is pregnant. She said that her mother had told her that she was "living in sin" and that she would "pay for it." The patient wants to "end it all!" From this scenario, develop three assessment questions for each domain: biologic, psychological, and social.

2. Identify normal laboratory values for sodium, blood urea nitrogen, liver enzymes, leukocyte count and differential, and thyroid functioning. Why are these values important to know?

3. Write a paragraph on your self-concept, including all three components: body image, self-esteem, and personal identity. Explore the type of patient situations in which your self-concept can help your interactions with patients. Explore the types of patient situations in which your self-concept can hinder your interactions with patients.

4. Tom, a 25-year-old man with schizophrenia, lives with his parents, who want to retire to Florida. Tom goes to work each day but relies on his mother for meals, laundry, and reminders to take his medication. Tom believes that he can manage the home, but his mother is concerned. She asks the nurse for advice about leaving her son to manage on his own. Generate a nursing diagnosis, outcomes, and interventions that would meet some of Tom's potential responses to his changing lifestyle.

5. Joan, a 35-year-old married woman, is admitted to an acute psychiatric unit for stabilization of her mood disorder. She is extremely depressed but refuses to consider a recommended medication change. She asks the nurse what to do. Using a nursing intervention, explain how you would approach Joan's problem.

6. A nurse reports to work for the evening shift. The unit is chaotic. The television in the day room is loud; two patients are arguing about the program. Visitors are mingling in patients' rooms. The temperature of the unit is hot. One patient is running up and down the hall yelling, "Help me, help me." Using a milieu therapy approach, what would you do to calm the unit?

References

American Nurses Association, American Psychiatric Nurses Association and International Society of Psychiatric-Mental Health Nurses. (2014). *Psychiatric-Mental Health Nursing: Scope and Standards of Practice, 2nd Edition.* Silver spring, MD: Nursebooks.org.

Bulechek, G. M., Butcher, H. K., Dochterman, J., & Wagner, C. (Eds.). (2013). *Nursing interventions classification (NIC)* (6th ed.). St. Louis, MO: Elsevier.

Burkhardt, M. A., & Nagai-Jacobson, M. G. (1997). Spirituality and healing. In B. M. Dossey (Ed.). *Core curriculum for holistic nursing* (pp 42–51). Gaithersburg, MD: Aspen.

Carpenito-Moyet, L. J. (2014). *Nursing diagnosis: Application to clinical practice* (14th ed.). Philadelphia: Wolters Kluwer | Lippincott Williams & Wilkins.

Centers for Medicare & Medicaid Services. (2012). *Interpretive guidelines for hospital CoP for patient rights. Quality of care information, quality standards 482.13.* Retrieved May 14, 2014, www.cms.hhs.gov/manuals.

Esperat, M. C., Inouye, J., Gonzalez, E. W., Owen, D. C., & Feng, D. (2004). Health disparities among Asian Americans and Pacific Islanders. *Annual Review of Nursing Research, 22,* 135–159.

Farronato, N. S., Dursteler-Macfarland, K. M., Wiesbeck, G. A., & Petitjean, S. A. (2013). A systematic review comparing cognitive-behavioral therapy and contingency management for cocaine dependence (Review). *Journal of Addictive Diseases, 32*(3), 274–287.

Jones, E. J., Webb, S. J., Estes, A., & Dawson, G. (2013). Rule learning in autism: the role of reward type and social context. *Developmental Neuropsychology, 38*(1), 58–77.

Macdonald, J., Vallance, D., & McGrath, M. (2013). An evaluation of a collaborative bibliotherapy scheme delivered via a library service. *Journal of Psychiatric & Mental Health Nursing, 20*(10), 857–865.

Martin, K. S. (2005). *The Omaha system: A key to practice, documentation, and information management.* (2nd ed). St. Louis: Elsevier Saunders.

Moorhead, S., Johnson, M., Maas, M. L., & Swanson, E. (2008). *Nursing outcomes classification (NOC)* (4th ed). St. Louis: Mosby.

Saba, V. K. (2012). *Clinical care classification (CCC) system (Version 2.1) (User's Guide)* (2nd ed). New York: Springer Publishing Company, LLC.

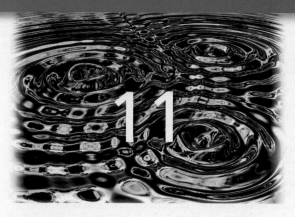

11

Psychopharmacology, Dietary Supplements, and Biologic Interventions

Mary Ann Boyd

KEY CONCEPTS

- agonists
- antagonists
- pharmacokinetics
- pharmacodynamics

LEARNING OBJECTIVES

After studying this chapter, you will be able to:

1. Differentiate target symptoms from side effects.

2. Identify nursing interventions for common side effects of psychiatric medications.

3. Explain the role of the governmental regulatory process in the approval of medication and the use of other biologic interventions.

4. Discuss the pharmacodynamics of psychiatric medications.

5. Discuss the pharmacokinetics of psychiatric medications.

6. Explain the major classifications of psychiatric medications.

7. Identify typical nursing interventions related to the administration of psychiatric medications.

8. Analyze the potential benefits of other forms of somatic treatments, including herbal supplements, nutrition therapies, electroconvulsive therapy, light therapy, transcranial magnetic stimulation, and vagus nerve stimulation.

9. Evaluate the significance of non-adherence and discuss strategies supportive of medication adherence.

KEY TERMS

- absorption • adherence • adverse reactions • affinity • agonists • akathisia • antagonists • atypical antipsychotics • augmentation • bioavailability • biotransformation • boxed warning • carrier protein • chronic syndromes • clearance • compliance • conventional antipsychotics • cytochrome P450 (CYP450) system • desensitization • distribution • dosing • drug–drug interaction • dystonia • efficacy • enzymes • ethnopsychopharmacology • excretion • extrapyramidal symptoms (EPS) • first-pass effect • half-life • hypnotics • inducer • inhibitor • intrinsic activity • metabolism • metabolites • off-label • package insert • partial agonists • pharmacogenomics • phototherapy • polypharmacy • potency • protein binding • pseudoparkinsonism • relapse • repetitive transcranial magnetic stimulation • sedative–hypnotics • sedatives • selectivity • serotonin syndrome • side effects • solubility • steady state • substrate • tardive dyskinesia • target symptoms • therapeutic index • tolerance • toxicity • uptake receptors

Recent scientific and technologic developments have opened the door for the development of new medications that treat mental disorders. Although nurses administer these medications, monitor their effectiveness, and manage side effects, they also have an important role in educating patients about their medications. Advanced practice nurses also prescribe medications. Psychiatric medications are increasingly prescribed in primary care settings, and nurses practicing in nonpsychiatric settings now need an in-depth knowledge of them.

This chapter focuses on the pharmacodynamics and pharmacokinetics of psychiatric medications. Included in this chapter is an overview of the major classes of psychopharmacologic drugs used in treating patients with mental disorders and the role of herbal supplements and nutritional therapies. In addition, other biologic treatments are discussed, including electroconvulsive therapy (ECT), light therapy, repetitive transcranial magnetic stimulation (rTMS), and vagus nerve stimulation.

CONSIDERATIONS IN USING PSYCHIATRIC MEDICATIONS

As with any drug, psychiatric medications are designated for use in certain conditions for specific symptoms. The nurse quickly realizes that these symptoms are present in several conditions, leading to medications being prescribed off-label or for other conditions other than those that are approved. Because medications can have both desirable and undesirable effects, it is important for the nurse to consider these factors to help ensure patient safety.

Target Symptoms and Side Effects

Psychiatric medications and other biologic interventions are indicated for **target symptoms**, which are specific measurable symptoms expected to improve with treatment. Standards of care guide nurses in monitoring and documenting the effects of medications and other biologic treatments on target symptoms.

As yet, no drug has been developed that is so specific it affects only its target symptoms; instead, drugs typically act on a number of other organs and sites within the body. Even drugs with a high affinity and selectivity for a specific neurotransmitter will cause some responses in the body that are not related to the target symptoms. These unwanted effects of medications are called **side effects**. If unwanted effects have serious physiologic consequences, they are considered **adverse reactions**. The nurse monitors, documents, and reports the appearance of side effects and adverse reactions and implements nursing interventions for relief of medication side effects (Table 11.1).

Drug Regulation and Use

The U.S. Food and Drug Administration (FDA) is responsible for ensuring the safety, efficacy, and security of human and veterinary drugs, biologic products, medical devices, our nation's food supply, cosmetics, and products that emit radiation (www.FDA.gov). The FDA approves the labeling of medications and other biologic treatments after a thorough review of efficacy and safety data (Box 11.1). Nurses administering medications are responsible for knowing the labeling content, which is found in each medication's **package insert** (PI) or pre-

scribing information and includes approved indications for the medication, side effects, adverse reactions, contraindications, and other important information. If a medication is ordered and administered for a condition that is not approved by the FDA, it is considered **off-label** use. In psychiatric care, many medications are safely used off-label. Although their use is supported by evidence-based studies, the use of drugs for off-label purposes increases risk for the patient and liability for the nurse. If the FDA identifies serious adverse reactions that can occur with the use of a specific medication, it may issue a warning found in a **boxed warning** in the PI. The nurse should be aware of these boxed warnings and monitor for the appearance of the adverse reactions. If a PI is not readily available, the labeling information is easily found on the FDA's website and in most pharmacy departments.

PSYCHOPHARMACOLOGY

A comparatively small amount of medication can have a significant and large impact on cell function and resulting behavior. When tiny molecules of medication are compared with the vast amount of cell surface in the human body, the fraction seems disproportionate. Yet the drugs used to treat mental disorders often have profound effects on behavior. To understand how this occurs, one needs to understand both where and how drugs work. The following discussion highlights important concepts relevant to psychiatric medications.

Pharmacodynamics: Where Drugs Act

Drug molecules act at specific sites, not on the entire cell surface. Psychiatric medications primarily target the central nervous system (CNS) at the cellular, synaptic level at four sites: receptors, ion channels, enzymes, and carrier proteins.

> **KEYCONCEPT** **Pharmacodynamics** is the action or effects of drugs on living organisms.

Receptors

Receptors are specific proteins intended to respond to a chemical (i.e., neurotransmitter) normally present in blood or tissues (see Chapter 8). Receptors also respond to drugs with similar chemical structures. When drugs attach to a receptor, they can act as **agonists**—substances that initiate the same response as the chemical normally present in the body—or as **antagonists**—substances that block the response of a given receptor. Figure 11.1 illustrates the action of an agonist and an antagonist drug at a receptor site. A drug's ability to interact with a given receptor type may be judged by three properties: selectivity, affinity, and intrinsic activity.

Table 11.1	MANAGING COMMON SIDE EFFECTS OF PSYCHIATRIC MEDICATIONS
Side Effect or Discomfort	**Intervention**
Blurred vision	Reassurance (generally subsides in 2 to 6 wk)
Dry eyes	Artificial tears may be required; increased use of wetting solutions for those wearing contact lens Alert ophthalmologist; no eye examination for new glasses for at least 3 wk after a stable dose
Dry mouth and lips	Frequent rinsing of mouth, good oral hygiene, sucking sugarless candies or lozenges, lip balm, lemon juice, and glycerin mouth swabs
Constipation	High-fiber diet; encourage bran, fresh fruits, and vegetables Metamucil (must consume at least 16 oz of fluid with dose) Increase hydration Exercise; increase fluids Mild laxative
Urinary hesitancy or retention	Monitor frequently for difficulty with urination, including changes in starting or stopping stream Notify prescriber if difficulty develops A cholinergic agonist, such as bethanechol, may be required
Nasal congestion	Nose drops, moisturizer, *not* nasal spray
Sinus tachycardia	Assess for infections Monitor pulse for rate and irregularities Withhold medication and notify prescriber if resting rate exceeds 120 bpm
Decreased libido, anorgasmia, ejaculatory inhibition	Reassurance (reversible); change to another medication
Postural hypotension	Frequent monitoring of lying-to-standing blood pressure during dosage adjustment period, immediate changes and accommodation, measure pulse in both positions; consider change to less anti-adrenergic drug Advise patient to get up slowly, sit for at least 1 min before standing (dangling legs over side of bed), and stand for 1 min before walking or until lightheadedness subsides Increase hydration, avoid caffeine Elastic stockings if necessary Notify prescriber if symptoms persist or significant blood pressure changes are present; medication may have to be changed if patient does not have impulse control to get up slowly
Photosensitivity	Protective clothing Dark glasses Use of sun block; remember to cover all exposed areas
Dermatitis	Stop medication usage Consider medication change; may require a systemic antihistamine Initiate comfort measures to decrease itching
Impaired psychomotor functions	Advise patient to avoid dangerous tasks, such as driving Avoid alcohol, which increases this impairment
Drowsiness or sedation	Encourage activity during the day to increase accommodation Avoid tasks that require mental alertness, such as driving May need to adjust dosing schedule or, if possible, give a single daily dose at bedtime May need a cholinergic medication if sedation is the problem Avoid driving or operating potentially dangerous equipment May need change to less-sedating medication Provide quiet and decreased stimulation when sedation is the desired effect
Weight gain and metabolic changes	Exercise and diet teaching Caloric control
Edema	Check fluid retention Reassurance May need a diuretic
Irregular menstruation or amenorrhea	Reassurance (reversible) May need to change class of drug Reassurance and counseling (does not indicate lack of ovulation) Instruct patient to continue birth control measures
Vaginal dryness	Instruct in use of lubricants

KEYCONCEPT *Agonists* (mimic the neurotransmitter) have all three properties: selectivity, affinity, and intrinsic activity. *Antagonists* (block the receptor) have only selectivity and affinity properties; they do not have intrinsic activity because they produce no biologic response by attaching to the receptor.

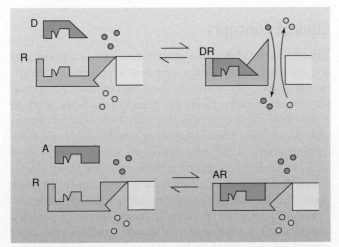

FIGURE 11.1 Agonist and antagonist drug actions at a receptor site. This schematic drawing represents drug–receptor interactions. At the *top*, drug D has the correct shape to fit receptor R, forming a drug–receptor complex, which results in a conformational change in the receptor and the opening of a pore in the adjacent membrane. Drug D is an agonist. At the *bottom*, drug A also has the correct shape to fit the receptor, forming a drug–receptor complex, but in this case, there is no conformational change and therefore no response. Drug A is, therefore, an antagonist.

Some drugs are referred to as **partial agonists** because they have some intrinsic activity (although weak). Because there are no "pure" drugs affecting only one neurotransmitter, most drugs have multiple effects. A drug may act as an agonist for one neurotransmitter and an antagonist for another. Medications that have both agonist and antagonist effects are called *mixed agonist–antagonists.*

Selectivity

Selectivity is the ability of a drug to be specific for a particular receptor. If a drug is highly selective, it will interact only with its specific receptors in the areas of the body where these receptors occur and therefore not affect tissues and organs where its receptors do not occur. Using a "lock-and-key" analogy, only a specific, highly selective key will fit a given lock. The more selective or structurally specific a drug is, the more likely it will affect only the specific receptor for which it is meant. The less selective the drug, the more receptors are affected and the more likely there will be unintended effects or side effects.

Affinity

Affinity is the degree of attraction or strength of the bond between the drug and its biologic target. Affinity is strengthened when a drug has more than one type of chemical bond with its target. If a cell membrane contains several receptors to which a drug will adhere, the affinity is increased. The weaker the chemical bond, the more likely a drug's effects are reversible. Most drugs used in psychiatry adhere to receptors through weak chemical bonds, but some drugs, specifically the monoamine oxidase inhibitors (MAOIs; discussed later), have a different type of bond, called a covalent bond. A covalent bond is formed when two atoms share a pair of electrons. This type of bond is stronger and irreversible at normal temperatures. The effects of the drugs that form covalent bonds are often called "irreversible" because they are long lasting, taking several weeks to resolve. Knowledge of a medication's affinity for receptors and subtypes of receptors may give some indication of the likelihood that specific target symptoms might improve and what side effects might be predicted.

Intrinsic Activity

A drug's ability to interact with a given receptor is its **intrinsic activity**, or the ability to produce a response after it becomes attached to the receptor. Some drugs have selectivity and affinity but produce no response. An important measure of a drug is whether it produces a change in the cell containing the receptor.

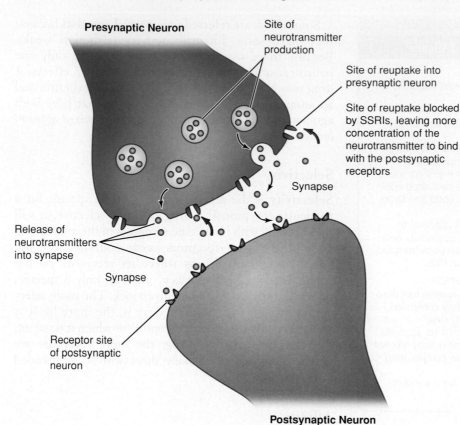

Presynaptic Neuron

Site of neurotransmitter production

Site of reuptake into presynaptic neuron

Site of reuptake blocked by SSRIs, leaving more concentration of the neurotransmitter to bind with the postsynaptic receptors

Synapse

Release of neurotransmitters into synapse

Synapse

Receptor site of postsynaptic neuron

Postsynaptic Neuron

FIGURE 11.2 Reuptake blockade of a carrier molecule for serotonin by a selective serotonin reuptake inhibitor.

Ion Channels

Some drugs directly block the ion channels of the nerve cell membrane. For example, the antianxiety benzodiazepine drugs, such as diazepam (Valium), bind to a region of the gamma-aminobutyric acid (GABA)–receptor chloride channel complex, which helps to open the chloride ion channel. In turn, the activity of GABA is enhanced.

Enzymes

Enzymes are usually proteins that act as catalysts for physiologic reactions and can be targets for drugs. For example, monoamine oxidase is an enzyme required to break down neurotransmitters associated with depression (norepinephrine, serotonin, and dopamine). The MAOI antidepressants inhibit this enzyme, resulting in more neurotransmitter activity.

Carrier Proteins: Uptake Receptors

A **carrier protein** is a membrane protein that transports a specific molecule across the cell membrane. Carrier proteins (also referred to as **uptake receptors**) recognize sites specific for the type of molecule to be transported. When a neurotransmitter is removed from the synapse, specific carrier molecules return it to the presynaptic nerve where

most of it is stored to be used again. Medications specific for this site block or inhibit this transport and therefore increase the activity of the neurotransmitter in the synapse. Figure 11.2 illustrates the reuptake blockade.

Clinical Concepts

Efficacy is the ability of a drug to produce a response and is considered when a drug is selected. The degree of receptor occupancy contributes to the drug's efficacy, but a drug may occupy a large number of receptors and not produce a response. Table 11.2 provides a brief summation of possible physiologic effects from drug actions on specific neurotransmitters. This information should serve only as a guide in predicting side effects because many physical outcomes or behaviors resulting from neural transmission are controlled by multiple receptors and neurotransmitters.

Potency refers to the dose of drug required to produce a specific effect. One drug may be able to achieve the same clinical effect as another drug but at a lower dose, making it more potent. Although the drug given at the lower dose is more potent because both drugs achieve similar effects, they may be considered to have equal efficacy.

In some instances, the effects of medications diminish with time, especially when they are given repeatedly, as in the treatment of chronic psychiatric disorders. This loss of effect is most often a form of physiologic adaptation that

Table 11.2	DRUG ACTIONS ON NEUROTRANSMITTERS	
Action by Drug on Neurotransmitter	**Physiologic Effects**	**Example of Drugs**
Reuptake Inhibition		
Norepinephrine reuptake inhibition	Antidepressant action Potentiation of pressor effects of norepinephrine Interaction with guanethidine Side effects: tachycardia, tremors, insomnia, erectile and ejaculation dysfunction	Desipramine Venlafaxine
Serotonin reuptake inhibition	Antidepressant action Anti-obsessional effect Increase or decrease in anxiety (dose dependent) Side effects: gastrointestinal distress; nausea; headache; nervousness; motor restlessness; and sexual side effects, including anorgasmia	Fluoxetine Fluvoxamine
Dopamine reuptake inhibition	Antidepressant action Antiparkinsonian effect Side effects: increase in psychomotor activity, aggravation of psychosis	Bupropion
Receptor Blockade		
Histamine receptor blockade (H₁)	Side effects: sedation, drowsiness, hypotension, and weight gain	Quetiapine Imipramine Clozapine Olanzapine
Acetylcholine receptor blockade (muscarinic)	Side effects: anticholinergic (dry mouth, blurred vision, constipation, urinary hesitancy and retention, memory dysfunction) and sinus tachycardia	Imipramine Amitriptyline Thioridazine Clozapine
Norepinephrine receptor blockade (α₁ receptor)	Potentiation of antihypertensive effect of prazosin and terazosin Side effects: postural hypotension, dizziness, reflex tachycardia, sedation	Amitriptyline Clomipramine Clozapine
Norepinephrine receptor blockade (α₂ receptor)	Increased sexual desire (yohimbine) Interactions with antihypertensive medications, blockade of the antihypertensive effects of clonidine Side effect: priapism	Amitriptyline Clomipramine Clozapine Trazodone Yohimbine
Norepinephrine receptor blockade (β₁ receptor)	Antihypertensive action (propranolol) Side effects: orthostatic hypotension, sedation, depression, sexual dysfunction (including impotence and decreased ejaculation)	Propranolol
Serotonin receptor blockade (5-HT₁ₐ)	Antidepressant action Antianxiety effect Possible control of aggression	Trazodone Risperidone Ziprasidone
Serotonin receptor blockade (5-HT₂)	Antipsychotic action Some antimigraine effect Decreased rhinitis Side effects: hypotension, ejaculatory problems	Risperidone Clozapine Olanzapine Ziprasidone
Dopamine receptor blockade (D₂)	Antipsychotic action Side effects: extrapyramidal symptoms, such as tremor, rigidity (especially acute dystonia and parkinsonism); endocrine changes, including elevated prolactin levels	Haloperidol Ziprasidone

may develop as the cell attempts to regain homeostatic control to counteract the effects of the drug. There are many reasons for decreased drug effectiveness (Box 11.2).

Desensitization is a rapid decrease in drug effects that may develop in a few minutes of exposure to a drug. This reaction is rare with most psychiatric medications but can occur with some medications used to treat serious side effects (e.g., physostigmine, sometimes used to relieve severe anticholinergic side effects). A rapid decrease can also occur with some drugs because of immediate transformation of the receptor when the drug molecule binds to the receptor. Other drugs cause a decrease in the number of receptors or exhaust the mediators of neurotransmission.

Tolerance is a gradual decrease in the action of a drug at a given dose or concentration in the blood. This decrease may take days or weeks to develop and results in

---

BOX 11.2

Mechanisms Causing Decreases in Medication Effects

- Change in receptors
- Loss of receptors
- Exhaustion of neurotransmitter supply
- Increased metabolism of the drug
- Physiologic adaptation

---

loss of therapeutic effect of a drug. For therapeutic drugs, this loss of effect is often called *treatment refractoriness*. In the abuse of substances such as alcohol or cocaine, tolerance is a part of the addiction (see Chapter 31).

Toxicity generally refers to the point at which concentrations of the drug in the bloodstream are high enough to become harmful or poisonous to the body. Individuals vary widely in their responses to medications. Some patients experience adverse reactions more easily than others. The **therapeutic index** is the ratio of the maximum nontoxic dose to the minimum effective dose. A high therapeutic index means that there is a large range between the dose at which the drug begins to take effect and a dose that would be toxic to the body. Drugs with a low therapeutic index have a narrow range.

This concept of toxicity has some limitations. The range can be affected by drug tolerance. For example, when tolerance develops, the person increases the dosage, which makes him or her more susceptible to an accidental suicide. The therapeutic index of a medication also may be greatly changed by the coadministration of other medications or drugs. For example, alcohol consumed with most CNS-depressant drugs will have added depressant effects, greatly increasing the likelihood of toxicity or death.

Pharmacokinetics: How the Body Acts on the Drugs

The field of pharmacokinetics studies the process of how drugs are acted on by the body through absorption, distribution, metabolism (biotransformation), and excretion. Pharmacokinetics for specific medications are always explained in a drug's PI. Together with the principles of pharmacodynamics, this information is helpful in monitoring drug effects and predicting behavioral response.

> **KEYCONCEPT** **Pharmacokinetics** is the process by which a drug is absorbed, distributed, metabolized and eliminated by the body.

Absorption and Routes of Administration

The first phase of **absorption** is the movement of the drug from the site of administration into the plasma. The typical routes of administration of psychiatric medications include oral (tablet, capsule, and liquid), deltoid and gluteal intramuscular (IM; short- and long-acting agents), and intravenous (IV; rarely used for treatment of the primary psychiatric disorder but instead for rapid treatment of adverse reactions). A transdermal patch antidepressant and oral inhalation are also available. The advantages and disadvantages of each route and the subsequent effects on absorption are listed in Table 11.3.

Drugs taken orally are usually the most convenient for the patient; however, this route is also the most variable because absorption can be slowed or enhanced by a number of factors. Taking certain drugs orally with food or antacids may slow the rate of absorption or change the amount of the drug absorbed. For example, antacids containing aluminum salts decrease the absorption of most antipsychotic drugs; thus, antacids must be given at least 1 hour before administration or 2 hours after.

Oral preparations are absorbed from the gastrointestinal tract into the bloodstream through the portal vein and then to the liver. They may be metabolized within the gastrointestinal wall or liver before reaching the rest of the body. This is called the **first-pass effect**. The consequence of first-pass effect is that only a fraction of the drug reaches systemic circulation. Oral dosages are adjusted for the first-pass effect. That is, the dose of the oral form is significantly higher than the IM or IV formulations.

Bioavailability describes the amount of the drug that actually reaches systemic circulation unchanged. The route by which a drug is administered significantly affects bioavailability. With some oral drugs, the amount of drug entering the bloodstream is decreased by first-pass metabolism, and bioavailability is lower. On the other hand, some rapidly dissolving oral medications have increased bioavailability.

Distribution

Distribution of a drug is the amount of the drug found in various tissues, particularly the target organ at the site of drug action. Factors that affect distribution include the size of the organ; amount of blood flow or perfusion within the organ; solubility of the drug; plasma **protein binding** (the degree to which the drug binds to plasma proteins); and anatomic barriers, such as the blood–brain barrier, that the drug must cross. A psychiatric drug may have rapid absorption and high bioavailability, but if it does not cross the blood–brain barrier to reach the CNS, it is of little use. Table 11.4 provides a summary of how some significant factors affect distribution. Two of these factors, **solubility** (ability of a drug to dissolve) and protein binding, warrant additional discussion with regard to how they relate to psychiatric medications.

Table 11.3	SELECTED FORMS AND ROUTES OF PSYCHIATRIC MEDICATIONS		
Preparation and Route	**Examples**	**Advantages**	**Disadvantages**
Oral tablet	Basic preparation for most psychopharmacologic agents, including antidepressants, antipsychotics, mood stabilizers, anxiolytics, and so on	Usually most convenient	Variable rate and extent of absorption, depending on the drug May be affected by the contents of the intestines May show first-pass metabolism effects May not be easily swallowed by some individuals
Oral liquid	Also known as concentrates Many antipsychotics, such as haloperidol, chlorpromazine, thioridazine, risperidone The antidepressant fluoxetine Antihistamines, such as diphenhydramine Mood stabilizers, such as lithium citrate	Ease of incremental dosing Easily swallowed In some cases, more quickly absorbed	More difficult to measure accurately Depending on drug: • Possible interactions with other liquids such as juice, forming precipitants • Possible irritation to mucosal lining of mouth if not properly diluted
Rapidly dissolving tablet	Atypical antipsychotics, such as olanzapine, risperidone, asenapine	Dissolves almost instantaneously in mouth	Patient needs to remember to have completely dry hands and to place tablet in mouth immediately Tablet should not linger in the hand Handy for people who have trouble swallowing or for patients who let medication linger in the cheek for later expectoration Can be taken when water or other liquid is unavailable
Intramuscular	Some antipsychotics, such as ziprasidone, haloperidol, and chlorpromazine Anxiolytics, such as lorazepam Anticholinergics, such as benztropine mesylate No antidepressants No mood stabilizers	More rapid acting than oral preparations No first-pass metabolism	Injection-site pain and irritation Some medications may have erratic absorption if heavy muscle tissue at the site of injection is not in use
Intramuscular depot (or long acting)	Risperidone (Risperdal Consta), paliperidone palmitate (Invega Sustenna), olanzapine (Zyprexa Relprevv) haloperidol decanoate, fluphenazine decanoate	May be more convenient for some individuals who have difficulty following medication regimens	Pain at injection site
Intravenous	Anticholinergics, such as diphenhydramine, benztropine mesylate Anxiolytics, such as diazepam, lorazepam, and chlordiazepoxide	Rapid and complete availability to systemic circulation	Inflammation of tissue surrounding site Often inconvenient for patient and uncomfortable Continuous dosage requires use of a constant-rate IV infusion
Transdermal patch	Antidepressant, selegiline	Avoid daily oral ingestion of medication	Skin irritation
Oral inhalation	Conventional antipsychotic, loxapine	Rapidly absorbed to treat psychomotor agitation	Bronchospasm

IV, intravenous.

Solubility

Substances may cross a membrane in a number of ways, but passive diffusion is by far the simplest. To do this, the drug must dissolve in the structure of the cell membrane. Therefore, the solubility of a drug is an important characteristic. Being soluble in lipids allows a drug to cross most of the membranes in the body, and the tissues of the CNS are less permeable to water-soluble drugs than are other areas of the body. Most psychopharmacologic agents are lipid soluble and easily cross the blood–brain barrier. However, this characteristic means that psychopharmacologic agents also cross the placenta; consequently, most are contraindicated during pregnancy.

Protein Binding

Of considerable importance is the degree to which a drug binds to plasma proteins. Only unbound or "free" drugs act at the receptor sites. High protein binding reduces the concentration of the drug at the receptor sites.

Table 11.4	FACTORS AFFECTING DISTRIBUTION OF A DRUG
Factor	**Effect on Drug Distribution**
Size of the organ	Larger organs require more drug to reach a concentration level equivalent to other organs and tissues.
Blood flow to the organ	The more blood flow to and within an organ (perfusion), the greater the drug concentration. The brain has high perfusion.
Solubility of the drug	The greater the solubility of a drug within a tissue, the greater its concentration.
Plasma protein binding	If a drug binds well to plasma proteins, particularly to albumin, it will stay in the body longer but have a slower distribution.
Anatomic barriers	Both the gastrointestinal tract and the brain are surrounded by layers of cells that control the passage or uptake of substances. Lipid-soluble substances are usually readily absorbed and pass the blood–brain barrier.

However, because the binding is reversible, as the unbound drug is metabolized, more drug is released from the protein bonds. Drugs are also released from storage in the fat depots. These processes can prolong the duration of action of the drug. When patients stop taking their medication, they often do not experience an immediate return of symptoms because they continue to receive the drug as it is released from storage sites in the body.

Metabolism

Metabolism, also called **biotransformation**, is the process by which a drug is altered and broken down into smaller substances, known as **metabolites**. Most metabolism occurs in the liver, but it can also occur in the kidneys, lungs, and intestines. Biotransformation in the liver occurs in phases. Phase I includes oxidation, hydrolysis, and reduction reactions. In most cases, metabolites are inactive, but in some psychiatric drugs, such as norfluoxetine (metabolite of fluoxetine [Prozac]), they are also active. Phase II reactions or conjugation combines a drug or metabolite with other chemicals. Through the phases of biotransformation, lipid-soluble drugs eventually become more water soluble, so they may be readily excreted.

Phase I oxidation reactions are carried out by the **cytochrome P450 (CYP450) system**, a set of microsomal enzymes (usually hepatic) referred to as CYP1, CYP2, and CYP3. Within each CYP family, there are enzyme subgroups identified by a number–letter sequence (i.e., 1A2 or 3A4). There are more than 50 enzymes, but most of the metabolism occurs in only a few of them. A **substrate** is the drug or compound that is identified as a target of an enzyme. For example, clozapine is the substrate for the CYP1A2 enzyme.

The functioning of these enzymes is influenced by drugs and other chemical substances. An **inhibitor** of a CYP enzyme slows down metabolism, which in turn decreases the clearance of the substrate and elevates its plasma level. An **inducer** speeds up metabolism, which in turn increases the clearance of the substrate and decreases its plasma level. For example, cigarette smoke is a potent inducer of CYP1A2, which in turn speeds up the clearance of clozapine and decreases its plasma level. A smoker will clear clozapine faster than a nonsmoker even though both take the same dose.

A **drug–drug interaction** can occur if one substance inhibits an enzyme system. For example, nortriptyline (an antidepressant with a narrow therapeutic index) is the substrate of the CYP2D6 enzyme. By adding paroxetine (a selective serotonin reuptake inhibitor [SSRI] antidepressant and an inhibitor of the CYP2D6 enzyme), the 2D6 enzyme is inhibited, and nortriptyline's blood level increases. Toxicity can easily develop because of a low therapeutic index.

Each human CYP450 enzyme is an expression of a unique gene. The science of **pharmacogenomics** blends pharmacology with genetic knowledge and is concerned with understanding and determining an individual's specific CYP450 makeup and then individualizing medications to match the person's CYP450 profile. Genetically (inherited as an autosomal recessive trait), some individuals are poor metabolizers, and others may be rapid metabolizers. Whereas poor metabolizers are more likely to have adverse reactions, rapid metabolizers may not allow certain drugs to reach therapeutic levels. Research has suggested that there are variations among ethnic groups with poor metabolizers accounting for up to 7% of whites for CYP2D6 and up to 25% of East Asians for CYP2C19.

Knowing whether patients are poor or rapid metabolizers is important because most psychiatric medications are metabolized by these enzymes. DNA laboratory tests are available for patients who have a personal or family history of adverse drug reactions to medications metabolized by 2D6 and 2D19 to confirm the presence of genotypes that affect metabolism. Enzyme CYP2D6 is important in the metabolism of many antidepressants and antipsychotics, and CYP2C19 is important for some antidepressant metabolism (Preskorn et al., 2013; Teh & Bertilsson, 2012).

Excretion

Excretion refers to the removal of drugs from the body either unchanged or as metabolites. **Clearance** refers to the total volume of blood, serum, or plasma from which a drug is completely removed per unit of time to account for the excretion. The **half-life** of a drug provides a measure of the expected rate of clearance. Half-life refers to the time required for plasma concentrations of the drug to be reduced by 50%. For most drugs, the rate of excretion slows, but the half-life remains unchanged. It usually takes four half-lives or more of a drug in total time for more than 90% of a drug to be eliminated.

Drugs bound to plasma proteins do not cross the glomerular filter freely. These lipid-soluble drugs are passively reabsorbed by diffusion across the renal tubule and thus are not rapidly excreted in the urine. Because many psychiatric medications are protein bound and lipid soluble, most of their excretion occurs through the liver where they are excreted in the bile and delivered into the intestine. Lithium and gabapentin, mood stabilizers, are notable examples of renal excretion. Any impairment in renal function or renal disease may lead to toxic symptoms.

Dosing refers to the administration of medication over time, so that therapeutic levels may be achieved or maintained without reaching toxic levels. In general, it is necessary to give a drug at intervals no greater than the half-life of the medication to avoid excessive fluctuation of concentration in the plasma between doses. With repeated dosing, a certain amount of the drug is accumulated in the body.

Steady-state plasma concentration, or simply **steady state**, occurs when absorption equals excretion and the therapeutic level plateaus. The rate of accumulation is determined by the half-life of the drug. Drugs generally reach steady state in four to five times the elimination half-life. However, because elimination or excretion rates may vary significantly in any individual, fluctuations may still occur, and dose schedules may need to be modified.

Individual Variations in Drug Effects

Many factors affect drug absorption, distribution, metabolism, and excretion. These factors may vary among individuals, depending on their age, genetics, and ethnicity.

Age

Pharmacokinetics are significantly altered at the extremes of the life cycle. Gastric absorption changes as individuals age. Gastric pH increases, and gastric emptying decreases. Gastric motility slows and splanchnic circulation is reduced. Normally, these changes do not significantly impair oral absorption of a medication, but addition of common conditions, such as diarrhea, may significantly alter and reduce absorption. Malnutrition, cancer, and liver disease decrease the production of the primary protein albumin. More free drug is acting in the system, producing higher blood levels of the medication and potentially toxic effects. The activity of hepatic enzymes also slows with age. As a result, the ability of the liver to metabolize medications may slow as much as a fourfold decrease between the ages of 20 and 70 years. Production of albumin by the liver generally declines with age. Changes in the parasympathetic nervous system produce

a greater sensitivity in older adults to anticholinergic side effects, which are more severe with this age group.

Renal function also declines with age. Creatinine clearance in a young adult is normally 100 to 120 mL/min, but after age 40 years, this rate declines by about 10% per decade (Glassock, 2009). Medical illnesses, such as diabetes and hypertension, may further the loss of renal function. When creatinine clearance falls below 30 mL/min, the excretion of drugs by the kidneys is significantly impaired, and potentially toxic levels may accumulate.

Ethnopsychopharmacology

Ethnopsychopharmacology investigates cultural variations and differences that influence the effectiveness of pharmacotherapies used in mental health. These differences include genetics and psychosocial factors. Studies of identical and nonidentical twins show that much of the individual variability in elimination half-life of a given drug is genetically determined. For example, some individuals of Asian descent produce higher concentrations of

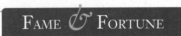

FAME & FORTUNE

Abraham Lincoln (1809–1865)
Civil War President

PUBLIC PERSONA

The 16th president of the United States led a nation through turbulent times during a civil war. Ultimately, his leadership preserved the United States as the republic we know today despite periods of "melancholy" or depression throughout his life. At times, he had strong thoughts of committing suicide. Yet he had an enormous ability to cope with depression, especially in later life. He generally coped with the depression through his work, humor, fatalistic resignation, and even religious feelings. He generally did not let his depression interfere with his work as president. In 1841, he wrote of his ongoing depression, "A tendency to melancholy. . . let it be observed, is a misfortune, not a fault" (letter to Mary Speed, September 27, 1841).

PERSONAL REALITIES

Lincoln's depression began in early childhood and can be traced to multiple causes. There is evidence that there was a genetic basis because both of his parents had depression. Lincoln was partially isolated from his peers because of his unique interests in politics and reading. Additionally, he suffered through the deaths of his younger brother, mother, and older sister. There is speculation that Lincoln's depression may have dated to Thomas Lincoln's cold treatment of his son. There is also evidence that Abraham Lincoln took a commonly prescribed medication called *blue mass*, which contained mercury. Consequently, some speculate that he had mercury poisoning.

SOURCE: Hirschhorn, N., Feldman, R. G., & Greaves, I. A. (2001). Abraham Lincoln's blue pills: Did our 16th president suffer from mercury poisoning? *Perspectives in Biology and Medicine, 44*(3), 315–322.

acetaldehyde with alcohol use than do those of European descent, resulting in a higher incidence of adverse reactions such as flushing and palpitations. Asians often require one half to one third the dose of antipsychotic medications and lower doses of antidepressants than whites require (Silva, 2013). Although many of these variations may be related to the CYP450 genetic differences discussed earlier, more research is needed to understand fully the underlying mechanisms and to identify groups that may require different approaches to medication treatment.

PHASES OF DRUG TREATMENT AND THE NURSE'S ROLE

Phases of drug treatment include initiation, stabilization, maintenance, and discontinuation of the medication. The following explains the role of the nurse in these phases.

Initiation Phase

Before the initiation of medications, patients must undergo several assessments.

- A psychiatric evaluation to determine the diagnosis and target symptoms
- A nursing assessment that includes cultural beliefs and practices (see Chapter 10)
- Physical examination and indicated laboratory tests, often including baseline determinations such as a complete blood count (CBC), liver and kidney function tests, electrolyte levels, urinalysis, and possibly thyroid function tests and electrocardiography (ECG), to determine whether a physical condition may be causing the symptoms and to establish that it is safe to initiate use of a particular medication.

During the initiation of medication, the nurse assesses, observes, and monitors the patient's response to the medication; teaches the patient about the action, dosage, frequency of administration, and side effects; and develops a plan for ongoing contact with clinicians. The first medication dose should be treated as if it were a "test" dose. Patients should be monitored for adverse reactions such as changes in blood pressure, pulse, or temperature; changes in mental status; allergic reactions; dizziness; ataxia; or gastric distress. If any of these symptoms develop, they should be reported to the prescriber.

Stabilization Phase

During stabilization, the prescriber adjusts or titrates the medication dosage to achieve the maximum amount of improvement with a minimum of side effects. Psychiatric–mental health nurses assess for improvements in the target symptoms and for the appearance of side effects. If medications are being increased rapidly, such as in a hospital

setting, nurses must closely monitor temperature, blood pressure, pulse, mental status, common side effects, and unusual adverse reactions.

In the outpatient setting, nurses focus on patient education, emphasizing the importance of taking the medication, expected outcomes, and potential side effects. Patients need to know how and when to take their medications, how to minimize any side effects, and which side effects require immediate attention. A plan should be developed for patients and their families to clearly identify what to do if adverse reactions develop. The plan, which should include emergency telephone numbers or available emergency treatment, should be reviewed frequently.

Therapeutic drug monitoring is most important in this phase of treatment. Many medications used in psychiatry improve target symptoms only when a therapeutic level of medication has been obtained in the individual's blood. Some medications, such as lithium, have a narrow therapeutic range and must be monitored frequently and accurately. Nurses must be aware of when and how these levels are to be determined and assist patients in learning these procedures. Because of protein binding and lipid solubility, most medications do not have obtainable plasma levels that are clinically relevant. However, plasma levels of these medications may still be requested to evaluate further such issues as absorption and adverse reactions.

Sometimes the first medication chosen does not adequately improve the patient's target symptoms. In such cases, use of the medication will be discontinued, and treatment with a new medication will be started. Medications may also be changed when adverse reactions or seriously uncomfortable side effects occur or these effects substantially interfere with the individual's quality of life. Nurses should be familiar with the pharmacokinetics of both drugs to be able to monitor side effects and possible drug–drug interactions during this change.

At times, an individual may show only partial improvement from a medication, and the prescriber may try an **augmentation** strategy by adding another medication. For example, a prescriber may add a mood stabilizer, such as lithium, to an antidepressant to improve the effects of the antidepressant. **Polypharmacy**, using more than one group from a class of medications, is increasingly being used as an acceptable strategy with most psychopharmacologic agents to match the drug action to the neurochemical needs of the patient. Nurses must be familiar with the potential effects, side effects, drug interactions, and rationale for the treatment regimen.

Maintenance Phase

After the individual's target symptoms have improved, medications are usually continued to prevent **relapse** or return of the symptoms. In some cases, this may occur despite the patient's continued use of the medication. Patients must be educated about their target symptoms and have a plan of action if the symptoms return. In other cases, the patient may experience medication side effects. The psychiatric–mental health nurse has a central role in assisting individuals to monitor their own symptoms, identify emerging side effects, manage psychosocial stressors, and avoid other factors that may cause the medications to lose effect.

Discontinuation Phase

Some psychiatric medications will be discontinued; others will not. Some require a tapered discontinuation, which involves slowly reducing dosage while monitoring closely for reemergence of the symptoms. Some psychiatric disorders, such as mild depression, respond to treatment and do not recur. Other disorders, such as schizophrenia, usually require lifetime medication. Discontinuance of some medications, such as controlled substances, produces withdrawal symptoms; discontinuance of others does not.

MAJOR PSYCHOPHARMACOLOGIC DRUG CLASSES

Major classes of psychiatric drugs include antipsychotics, mood stabilizers, antidepressants, antianxiety and sedative–hypnotic medications, and stimulants.

Antipsychotic Medications

Antipsychotic medications can be thought of as "newer" and "older" medications. Newer or **atypical antipsychotics** appear to be equally or more effective but have fewer side effects than the traditional older agents. The term *typical* or **conventional antipsychotics** identifies the older antipsychotic drugs. Table 11.5 provides a list of selected antipsychotics.

Table 11.5	ANTIPSYCHOTIC MEDICATIONS			
Generic (Trade) Drug Name	Usual Dosage Range	Half-Life	Therapeutic Blood Level	Approximate Equivalent Dosage (mg)
Atypical Antipsychotics				
Aripiprazole (Abilify)	5–30 mg/d	75–94 h	Not available	Not available
Aripiprazole (Maintena)	200–400 mg	30–47 days	Not available	Not available
Clozapine (Clozaril)	300–900 mg/d	4–12 h	141–204 ng/mL	50
Risperidone (Risperdal) Oral	2–8 mg/d	20 h	Not available	1
Risperdal Consta	25–50 mg every 2 weeks		Not available	
Olanzapine (Zyprexa)	5–15 mg/d 2.5–10 mg/d IM	21–54 h	Not available	Not available
Olanzapine (Relprevv)	150–300 mg every 2–4 weeks	30 days	Not available	Not available
Paliperidone (Invega Extended Release)	3–12 mg once daily in AM	23 h	Not available	Not available
Paliperidone (Invega Sustenna)	117 mg monthly	29–49 days	Not available	Not available
Quetiapine fumarate (Seroquel)	150–750 mg/d	7 h	Not available	Not available
Ziprasidone HCl (Geodon)	40–160 mg/d 10–20 mg/d IM	7 h	Not available	Not available
Iloperidone (Fanapt)	6–12 mg BID	18–33 h	Not available	Not available
Asenapine (Saphris)	5–10 mg BID, (sublingual)	24 h	Not available	Not available
Lurasidone HCL (Latuda)	40–80 mg	18 h	Not available	Not available
Conventional (Typical) Antipsychotics				
Chlorpromazine	50–1200 mg/d	2–30 h	30–100 mg/mL	100
Fluphenazine	2–20 mg/d	4.5–15.3 h	0.2–0.3 ng/mL	2
Perphenazine	12–64 mg/d	Unknown	0.8–12.0 ng/mL	10
Trifluoperazine (Stelazine)	5–40 mg/d	47–100 h	1–2.3 ng/mL	5
Thiothixene (Navane)	5–60 mg/d	34 h	2–20 ng/mL	4
Loxapine (Adasuve)	10 mg/d (inhalation)	7 h	Not available	
Haloperidol (Haldol)	2–60 mg/d	21–24 h	5–15 ng/mL	2

BID, twice a day; IM, intramuscular.

Indications and Mechanism of Action

Antipsychotic medications are indicated for schizophrenia, mania, and autism and to treat the symptoms of psychosis, such as hallucinations, delusions, bizarre behavior, disorganized thinking, and agitation. (These symptoms are described more fully in later chapters.) Off-label uses of these drugs are quite common. These medications also reduce aggressiveness and inappropriate behavior associated with psychosis. Within the typical antipsychotics, haloperidol and pimozide are approved for treating patients with Tourette's syndrome, reducing the frequency and severity of vocal tics. Some of the typical antipsychotics, particularly chlorpromazine, are used as antiemetics or for postoperative intractable hiccoughs.

The atypical antipsychotic medications differ from the typical antipsychotics in that they block serotonin receptors more potently than the dopamine receptors. The differences between the mechanism of action of the typical and atypical antipsychotic helps to explain their differences in terms of effect on target symptoms and in the degree of side effects they produce.

Pharmacokinetics

Antipsychotic medications administered orally have a variable rate of absorption complicated by the presence of food, antacids, and smoking and even the coadministration of anticholinergics, which slow gastric motility. Clinical effects begin to appear in about 30 to 60 minutes. Absorption after IM administration is less variable because this method avoids the first-pass effects. Therefore, IM administration produces greater bioavailability. It is important to remember that IM medications are absorbed more slowly when patients are immobile because erratic absorption may occur when muscles are not in use, which is especially important to remember when administering IM antipsychotic medication to patients who are restrained. For example, a patient's arm may be more mobile than the buttocks. The deltoid has better blood perfusion, and the medication will be more readily absorbed, especially with use.

Metabolism of these drugs occurs almost entirely in the liver with the exception of paliperidone (Invega Sustenna), which is not extensively metabolized by the liver but is excreted largely unchanged through the kidney and lurasidone (Latuda), which is excreted through the urine and feces. These medications are subject to the effects of other drugs that induce or inhibit the CYP450 system described earlier (Table 11.6). Careful observance of concurrent medication use, including prescribed, over-the-counter, and substances of abuse, is required to avoid drug–drug interactions. Atypical antipsychotic concentrations may be affected by CYP450-inhibiting drugs such as paroxetine and fluoxetine.

Excretion of these substances tends to be slow. Most antipsychotics have a half-life of 24 hours or longer, but many also have active metabolites with longer half-lives. These two effects make it difficult to predict elimination time, and metabolites of some of these agents may be found in the urine months later. When a medication is discontinued, the adverse reactions may not immediately subside. The patient may continue to experience and sometimes need treatment for the adverse reactions for several days. Similarly, patients who discontinue their antipsychotic drugs may still derive therapeutic benefit for several days to weeks after drug discontinuation.

High lipid solubility, accumulation in the body, and other factors have also made it difficult to correlate blood levels with therapeutic effects. Table 11.5 shows the therapeutic ranges available for some of the antipsychotic

Table 11.6	CYP450 METABOLISM OF COMMONLY USED ANTIPSYCHOTICS		
Drug	How Metabolized	Induces	Inhibits
Aripiprazole	2D6, 3A4	None	None
Clozapine	1A2, 2C19, 2D6, 3A4	None	None
Haloperidol	1A2, 2D6, 3A4	None	2D6
Iloperidone	3A4, 2D6	None	3A
Lurasidone	3A4 Eliminated in urine and feces	None	None
Olanzapine	1A2, 2D6	None	None
Paliperidone	<10% 2D6, 3A4; primarily renal elimination	None	None
Quetiapine	3A4	None	None
Risperidone	2D6	None	Mild 2D6
Ziprasidone	1A2, 3A4	None	None

Information based on Prescribing 2013 Information of each medication.

medications. The potency of the antipsychotics also varies widely and is of specific concern when considering typical antipsychotic drugs. As Table 11.5 (on page 161) indicates, 50 mg of clozapine is roughly equivalent to 1 mg of risperidone and 5 mg of trifluoperazine.

Long-Acting Preparations

Currently, in the United States, atypical and conventional antipsychotics are available in long-acting forms. These antipsychotics are administered by injection once every 2 to 4 weeks. Whereas the long-acting injectable atypical antipsychotics (risperidone, paliperidone, olanzapine, and aripiprazole) are water-based suspensions, the conventional antipsychotics are oil-based solutions. Long-acting injectable medications maintain a fairly constant blood level between injections. Because they bypass problems with gastrointestinal absorption and first-pass metabolism, this method may enhance therapeutic outcomes for the patient. The use of these medications increases the likelihood of adhering to a prescribed medication regimen.

Nurses should be aware that the injection site may become sore and inflamed if certain precautions are not taken. The oil-based injections (fluphenazine and haloperidol) are viscous liquids. For these injections, a large-gauge needle (at least 21 gauge) should be used. Because the medication is meant to remain in the injection site, the needle should be dry, and a deep IM injection should be given by the Z-track method. (Note: Do not massage the injection site. Rotate sites and document in the patient's record.) Manufacturer recommendations should be followed.

Side Effects, Adverse Reactions, and Toxicity

Various side effects and interactions can occur with antipsychotics, with the conventional (typical) antipsychotics producing different side effects than the atypical antipsychotics. The side effects vary largely based on their degree of attraction to different neurotransmitter receptors and their subtypes. See Box 11.3 for assessments that should be completed before starting an antipsychotic to reduce the risk of adverse reactions.

Cardiovascular Side Effects

Cardiovascular side effects include orthostatic hypotension and prolongation of the QTc interval. Orthostatic hypotension is very common and depends on the degree of blockade of α-adrenergic receptors. Typical and atypical antipsychotics have been associated with prolonged QTc intervals and should be used cautiously in patients who have increased QTc intervals or are taking other medications that may prolong the QTc interval (Beach,

---

BOX 11.3

Recommended Assessments Before and During Antipsychotic Therapy

- Weigh all patients and track BMI during treatment
  - Determine if overweight (BMI 25–29.9) or obese (BMI ≥30)
  - Monitor BMI monthly for first 3 months; then quarterly
- Obtain baseline personal and family history of diabetes, obesity, dyslipidemia, hypertension, and cardiovascular disease
- Get waist circumference (at umbilicus)
  - Men: >40 inches (102 cm)
  - Women: >35 inches (88)
- Monitor BP, fasting plasma glucose, and fasting lipid profile within 3 months and then annually (more frequently for patients with diabetes or have gained >5% of initial weight)
  - Prediabetes (fasting plasma glucose 100–125 mg/dL)
  - Diabetes (fasting plasma glucose >126 mg/dL)
  - Hypertension (BP >140/90 mm Hg)
  - Dyslipidemia (increased total cholesterol [>200 mg], decreased HDL, and increased LDL)

BMI, body mass index; BP, blood pressure; HDL, high-density lipoprotein; LDL, low-density lipoprotein.

Celano, Noseworthy, Januzzi, & Huffman, 2013). Other cardiovascular side effects from typical antipsychotics have been rare, but occasionally they cause ECG changes that have a benign or undetermined clinical effect.

Anticholinergic Side Effects

Anticholinergic side effects resulting from blockade of acetylcholine are another common side effect associated with antipsychotic drugs. Dry mouth, slowed gastric motility, constipation, urinary hesitancy or retention, vaginal dryness, blurred vision, dry eyes, nasal congestion, and confusion or decreased memory are examples of these side effects. Interventions for decreasing the impact of these side effects are outlined in Table 11.1 on page 152.

This group of side effects occurs with many of the medications used for psychiatric treatment. Using more than one medication with anticholinergic effects often increases the symptoms. Older patients are often most susceptible to a potential toxicity that results from high blockade of acetylcholine. This toxicity is called an *anticholinergic crisis* and is described more fully, along with its treatment, in Chapter 22.

Weight Gain

Weight gain is a common side effect of the atypical antipsychotics, particularly clozapine and olanzapine (Zyprexa), which can cause a weight gain of up to 20 lb within 1 year. Ziprasidone (Geodon), aripiprazole (Abilify), and lurasidone (Latuda) are associated with little to no weight gain. If a patient becomes overweight or obese, switching to another antipsychotic should be considered and weight control interventions implemented.

Diabetes

One of the more serious side effects is the risk of type II diabetes. The FDA has determined that all atypical antipsychotics increase the risk for type II diabetes. Nurses should routinely assess for emerging symptoms of diabetes and alert the prescriber of these symptoms (see Box 11.3).

Sexual Side Effects

Sexual side effects result primarily from the blockade of dopamine in the tuberoinfundibular pathways of the hypothalamus. As a result, blood levels of prolactin may increase, particularly with risperidone and the typical antipsychotics. Increased prolactin causes breast enlargement and rare but potential galactorrhea (milk production and flow), decreased sexual drive, amenorrhea, menstrual irregularities, and increased risk for growth in preexisting breast cancers. Other sexual side effects include retrograde ejaculation (backward flow of semen), erectile dysfunction, and anorgasmia.

Blood Disorders

Blood dyscrasias are rare but have received renewed attention since the introduction of clozapine. Agranulocytosis is an acute reaction that causes the individual's white blood cell count to drop to very low levels, and concurrent neutropenia, a drop in neutrophils in the blood, develops. In the case of the antipsychotics, the medication suppresses the bone marrow precursors to blood factors. The exact mechanism by which the drugs produce this effect is unknown. The most notable symptoms of this disorder include high fever, sore throat, and mouth sores. Although benign elevations in temperature have been reported in individuals taking clozapine, no fever should go uninvestigated. Untreated agranulocytosis can be life threatening. Although agranulocytosis can occur with any of the antipsychotics, the risk with clozapine is greater than with the other antipsychotics. Therefore, prescription of clozapine requires weekly blood samples for the first 6 months of treatment and then every 2 weeks after that for as long as the drug is taken. Drawing of these samples must continue for 4 weeks after clozapine use has been discontinued. If sore throat or fever develops, medications should be withheld until a leukocyte count can be obtained. Hospitalization, including reverse isolation to prevent infections, is usually required. Agranulocytosis is more likely to develop during the first 18 weeks of treatment. Some research indicates that it is more common in women (Novartis, 2013).

Neuroleptic Malignant Syndrome

Neuroleptic malignant syndrome (NMS) is a serious complication that may result from antipsychotic medications. Characterized by rigidity and high fever, NMS is a rare condition that may occur abruptly with even one dose of medication. Temperature must always be monitored when administering antipsychotics, especially high-potency medications. This condition is discussed more fully in Chapter 22.

Other Side Effects

Photosensitivity reactions to antipsychotics, including severe sunburns or rash, most commonly develop with the use of low-potency typical medications. Sun block must be worn on all areas of exposed skin when taking these drugs. In addition, sun exposure may cause pigmentary deposits to develop, resulting in discoloration of exposed areas, especially the neck and face. This discoloration may progress from a deep orange color to a blue gray. Skin exposure should be limited and skin tone changes reported to the prescriber. Pigmentary deposits, retinitis pigmentosa, may also develop on the retina of the eye.

Antipsychotics may also lower the seizure threshold. Patients with an undetected seizure disorder may experience seizures early in treatment. Those who have a preexisting condition should be monitored closely.

Medication-Related Movement Disorders

Medication-related movement disorders are side effects or adverse reactions that are commonly caused by typical antipsychotic medications but less commonly with atypical antipsychotic drugs. These disorders of abnormal motor movements can be divided into two groups: acute **extrapyramidal symptoms (EPS)**, which develop early in the course of treatment (sometimes after just one dose), and chronic syndromes, which develop from longer exposure to antipsychotic drugs.

Acute Extrapyramidal Symptoms

Acute EPS are acute abnormal movements that include dystonia, pseudoparkinsonism, and akathisia. They develop early in treatment, sometimes from as little as one dose. Although the abnormal movements are treatable, they are at times dramatic and frightening, causing physical and emotional impairments that often prompt patients to stop taking their medication. EPS occurs when there is an imbalance of acetylcholine, dopamine, and gamma-aminobutyric acid (GABA) in the basal ganglia as a result of blocking dopamine.

Dystonia, sometimes referred to as an *acute dystonic reaction*, is impaired muscle tone that generally is the first EPS to occur, usually within a few days of initiating use of an antipsychotic. Acetylcholine is overactive because one of its modulators, dopamine, is blocked. Dystonia is characterized by involuntary muscle spasms that lead to abnormal postures, especially of the head and neck muscles. Acute dystonia occurs most often in young men, adolescents, and children. Patients usually first report a thick tongue, tight jaw, or stiff neck. Dystonia can progress to a protruding tongue, oculogyric crisis (eyes rolled up in the head), torticollis (muscle stiffness in the neck, which draws the head to one side with the chin pointing to the other), and laryngopharyngeal constriction. Abnormal postures of the upper limbs and torso may be held briefly or sustained. In severe cases, the spasms may progress to the intercostal muscles, producing more significant breathing difficulty for patients who already have respiratory impairment from asthma or emphysema. The treatment is the administration of a medication such as the anticholinergic agents that inhibit acetylcholine and thereby restore the balance of neurotransmitters (Table 11.7).

Drug-induced parkinsonism is sometimes referred to as **pseudoparkinsonism** because its presentation is identical to Parkinson's disease. The difference is that the activity of dopamine is blocked in pseudoparkinsonism, and in Parkinson's disease, the cells of the basal ganglia are destroyed. Older patients are at the greatest risk for experiencing pseudoparkinsonism (Lopez et al., 2013). Symptoms include the classic triad of rigidity, slowed movements (akinesia), and tremor. The rigid muscle stiffness is usually seen in the arms. Akinesia can be observed by the loss of spontaneous movements, such as the absence of the usual relaxed swing of the arms while walking. In addition, masklike facies or loss of facial expression and a decrease in the ability to initiate movements also are present. Usually, tremor is more pronounced at rest, but it can also be observed with intentional movements, such as eating. If the tremor becomes severe, it may interfere with the patient's ability to eat or

Table 11.7	DRUG THERAPIES FOR ACUTE MEDICATION-RELATED MOVEMENT DISORDERS		
Agents	**Typical Dosage Ranges**	**Routes Available**	**Common Side Effects**
Anticholinergics			
Benztropine (Cogentin)	2–6 mg/d	PO, IM, IV	Dry mouth, blurred vision, slowed gastric motility causing constipation, urinary retention, increased intraocular pressure; overdose produces toxic psychosis
Trihexyphenidyl	4–15 mg/d	PO	Same as benztropine, plus gastrointestinal distress Older adults are most prone to mental confusion and delirium
Biperiden (Akineton)	2–8 mg/d	PO	Fewer peripheral anticholinergic effects Euphoria and increased tremor may occur
Antihistamines			
Diphenhydramine	25–50 mg QID to 400 mg daily	PO, IM, IV	Sedation and confusion, especially in older adults
Dopamine Agonists			
Amantadine	100–400 mg daily	PO	Indigestion, decreased concentration, dizziness, anxiety, ataxia, insomnia, lethargy, tremors, and slurred speech may occur with higher doses Tolerance may develop on fixed dose
β-Blockers			
Propranolol (Inderal)	10 mg TID to 120 mg daily	PO	Hypotension and bradycardia Must monitor pulse and blood pressure Do not stop abruptly because doing so may cause rebound tachycardia
Benzodiazepines			
Lorazepam (Ativan)	1–2 mg IM 0.5–2 mg PO	PO, IM	All may cause drowsiness, lethargy, and general sedation or paradoxical agitation Confusion and disorientation in older adults
Diazepam (Valium)	2–5 mg tid	PO, IV	Most side effects are rare and will disappear if dose is decreased
Clonazepam (Klonopin)	1–4 mg/d	PO	Tolerance and withdrawal are potential problems

IM, intramuscular; IV, intravenous; PO, oral; QID, four times a day; TID, three times a day.

maintain adequate fluid intake. Hypersalivation is possible as well. Pseudoparkinsonism symptoms may occur on one or both sides of the body and develop abruptly or subtly but usually within the first 30 days of treatment. The treatment is the reduction in dosage or a change of antipsychotic that has less affinity for the dopamine receptor. Anticholinergic medication is sometimes given.

Akathisia is characterized by an inability to sit still or restlessness and is more common in middle-aged patients. The person will pace, rock while sitting or standing, march in place, or cross and uncross the legs. All of these repetitive motions have an intensity that is frequently beyond the explanation of the individual. In addition, akathisia may be present as a primarily subjective experience without obvious motor behavior. This subjective experience includes feelings of anxiety, jitteriness, or the inability to relax, which the individual may or may not be able to communicate. It is extremely uncomfortable for a person experiencing akathisia to be forced to sit still or be confined. These symptoms are sometimes misdiagnosed as agitation or an increase in psychotic symptoms. If an antipsychotic medication is given, the symptoms will not abate and will often worsen. Differentiating akathisia from agitation may be aided by knowing the person's symptoms before the introduction of medication. Whereas psychotic agitation does not usually begin abruptly after antipsychotic medication use has been started, akathisia may occur after administration. In addition, the nurse may ask the patient if the experience is felt primarily in the muscles (akathisia) or in the mind or emotions (agitation).

Akathisia is the most difficult acute medication-related movement disorder to relieve. It does not usually respond well to anticholinergic medications. The pathology of akathisia may involve more than just the extrapyramidal motor system. It may include serotonin changes that also affect the dopamine system. The usual approach to treatment is to change or reduce the antipsychotic. A number of medications are used to reduce symptoms, including β-adrenergic blockers, anticholinergics, antihistamines, and low-dose antianxiety agents (Laoutidis & Luckhaus, 2014). The β-adrenergic blockers, such as propranolol (Inderal), given in doses of 30 to 120 mg/d, are the most successful.

A number of nursing interventions reduce the impact of these syndromes. Individuals with acute EPS need frequent reassurance that this is not a worsening of their psychiatric condition but instead is a treatable side effect of the medication. They also need validation that what they are experiencing is real and that the nurse is concerned and will be responsive to changes in these symptoms. Physical and psychological stress appears to increase the symptoms and further frighten the patient; therefore, decreasing stressful situations becomes important. These symptoms are often physically exhausting for the patient, and the nurse should ensure that the patient receives adequate rest and hydration. Because tremors, muscle rigidity, and motor restlessness may interfere with the individual's ability to eat, the nurse may need to assist the patient with eating and drinking fluids to maintain nutrition and hydration.

Risk factors for acute EPS include previous episodes of EPS. The nurse should listen closely when patients say they are "allergic" or have had "bad reactions" to antipsychotic medications. Often, they are describing one of the medication-related movement disorders, particularly dystonia, rather than a rash or other allergic symptoms.

Chronic Syndromes: Tardive Dyskinesia

Chronic syndromes develop from long-term use of antipsychotics. They are serious and affect about 20% of the patients who receive typical antipsychotics for an extended period. These conditions are typically irreversible and cause significant impairment in self-image, social interactions, and occupational functioning. Early symptoms and mild forms may go unnoticed by the person experiencing them.

Tardive dyskinesia, the most well-known of the chronic syndromes, involves irregular, repetitive involuntary movements of the mouth, face, and tongue, including chewing, tongue protrusion, lip smacking, puckering of the lips, and rapid eye blinking. Abnormal finger movements are common as well. In some individuals, the trunk and extremities are also involved, and in rare cases, irregular breathing and swallowing lead to belching and grunting noises. These symptoms usually begin no earlier than after 6 months of treatment or when the medication is reduced or withdrawn. Once thought to be irreversible, considerable controversy now exists as to whether this is true.

Part of the difficulty in determining the irreversibility of tardive dyskinesia is that any movement disorder that persists after discontinuation of antipsychotic medication has been described as tardive dyskinesia. Atypical forms are now receiving more attention because some researchers believe they may have different underlying mechanisms of causation. Some of these forms of the disorder appear to remit spontaneously. Symptoms of what is now called *withdrawal tardive dyskinesia* appear when use of an antipsychotic medication is reduced or discontinued and remit spontaneously in 1 to 3 months. Tardive dystonia and tardive akathisia have also been described. Both appear in a manner similar to the acute syndromes but continue after the antipsychotic medication has been withdrawn. More research is needed to determine whether these syndromes are distinctly different in origin and outcome.

The risk for experiencing tardive dyskinesia increases with age. Although the prevalence of tardive dyskinesia averages 15% to 20%, the rate rises to 50% to 70% in older patients receiving antipsychotic medications; in addition, cumulative incidence of tardive dyskinesia appears to

- Age older than 50 years
- Female
- Affective disorders, particularly depression
- Brain damage or dysfunction
- Increased duration of treatment
- Standard antipsychotic medication
- Possible—higher doses of antipsychotic medication

increase 5% per year of continued exposure to antipsychotic medications (Woods et al., 2010). Women are at higher risk than men. Anyone receiving antipsychotic medication can develop tardive dyskinesia. Risk factors are summarized in Box 11.4. The causes of tardive dyskinesia remain unclear. No one medication relieves the symptoms. Dopamine agonists, such as bromocriptine, and many other drugs have been tried with little success. Dietary precursors of acetylcholine, such as lecithin and vitamin E supplements, may prove to be beneficial.

The best approach to treatment remains avoiding the development of the chronic syndromes. Preventive measures include use of atypical antipsychotics, using the lowest possible dose of typical medication, minimizing use of as-needed (PRN) medication, and closely monitoring individuals in high-risk groups for development of the symptoms of tardive dyskinesia. All members of the mental health treatment team who have contact with individuals taking antipsychotics for longer than 3 months must be alert to the risk factors and earliest possible signs of chronic medication-related movement disorders.

Monitoring tools, such as the Abnormal Involuntary Movement Scale (AIMS) (see Appendix B), should be used routinely to standardize assessment and provide the earliest possible recognition of the symptoms. Standardized assessments should be performed at a minimum of 3- to 6-month intervals. The earlier the symptoms are recognized, the more likely they will resolve if the medication can be changed or its use discontinued. Newer, atypical antipsychotic medications have a much lower risk of causing tardive dyskinesia and are increasingly being considered first-line medications for treating patients with schizophrenia. Other medications are under development to provide alternatives that limit the risk for tardive dyskinesia.

Mood Stabilizers (Antimania Medications)

Mood stabilizers, or antimania medications, are psychopharmacologic agents used primarily for stabilizing mood swings, particularly those of mania in bipolar disorders. Lithium, the oldest, is the gold standard of treatment for acute mania and maintenance of bipolar disorders. Not all respond to lithium, and increasingly, other drugs are being used as first-line agents. Anticonvulsants, calcium channel blockers, adrenergic blocking agents, and atypical antipsychotics are used for mood stabilization.

Lithium

Lithium, a naturally occurring element, is effective in only about 40% of patients with bipolar disorder. Although lithium is not a perfect drug, a great deal is known regarding its use—it is inexpensive, it has restored stability to the lives of thousands of people, and it remains the gold standard of bipolar pharmacologic treatment.

Indications and Mechanisms of Action

Lithium is indicated for symptoms of mania characterized by rapid speech, flight of ideas (jumping from topic to topic), irritability, grandiose thinking, impulsiveness, and agitation. Because it has mild antidepressant effects, lithium is used in treating depressive episodes of bipolar illness. It is also used as augmentation in patients experiencing major depression that has only partially responded to antidepressants alone. Lithium also has been shown to be helpful in reducing impulsivity and aggression in certain psychiatric patients.

The exact action by which lithium improves the symptoms of mania is unknown, but it is thought to exert multiple neurotransmitter effects, including enhancing serotonergic transmission, increasing synthesis of norepinephrine, and blocking postsynaptic dopamine. Lithium is actively transported across cell membranes, altering sodium transport in both nerve and muscle cells. It replaces sodium in the sodium–potassium pump and is retained more readily than sodium inside the cells. Conditions that alter sodium content in the body, such as vomiting, diuresis, and diaphoresis, also alter lithium retention. The results of lithium influx into the nerve cell lead to increased storage of catecholamines within the cell, reduced dopamine neurotransmission, increased norepinephrine reuptake, increased GABA activity, and increased serotonin receptor sensitivity. Lithium also alters the distribution of calcium and magnesium ions and inhibits second messenger systems within the neuron. The mechanisms by which lithium improves the symptoms of mania are complex and interrelated, involving the sum of all or part of these actions and more (Malhi, Tanious, Das, Coulston, & Berk, 2013).

Pharmacokinetics

Lithium carbonate is available orally in capsule, tablet, and liquid forms. Slow-release preparations are also available. Lithium is readily absorbed in the gastric system and may be taken with food, which does not impair absorption. Peak blood levels are reached in 1 to 4 hours, and the medication is usually completely absorbed in

8 hours. Slow-release preparations are absorbed at a slower, more variable rate.

Lithium is not protein bound, and its distribution into the CNS across the blood–brain barrier is slow. The onset of action is usually 5 to 7 days and may take as long as 2 weeks. The elimination half-life is 8 to 12 hours and is 18 to 36 hours in individuals whose blood levels have reached steady state and whose symptoms are stable. Lithium is almost entirely excreted by the kidneys but is present in all body fluids. Conditions of renal impairment or decreased renal function in older patients decrease lithium clearance and may lead to toxicity. Several medications affect renal function and therefore change lithium clearance. See Chapter 25 for a list of these and other medication interactions with lithium. About 80% of lithium is reabsorbed in the proximal tubule of the kidney along with water and sodium. In conditions that cause sodium depletion, such as dehydration caused by fever, strenuous exercise, hot weather, increased perspiration, and vomiting, the kidneys attempts to conserve sodium. Because lithium is a salt, the kidneys retain lithium as well, leading to increased blood levels and potential toxicity. Significantly increasing sodium intake causes lithium levels to fall.

Lithium is usually administered in doses of 300 mg two to three times daily. Because it is a drug with a narrow therapeutic range or index, blood levels are monitored frequently during acute mania, and the dosage is increased every 3 to 5 days. These increases may be slower in older adult patients or patients who experience uncomfortable side effects. Blood levels should be monitored 12 hours after the last dose of medication. In the hospital setting, nurses should withhold the morning dose of lithium until the serum sample is drawn to avoid falsely elevated levels. Individuals who are at home should be instructed to have their blood drawn in the morning about 12 hours after their last dose and before they take their first dose of medication. During the acute phases of mania, blood levels of 0.8 to 1.4 mEq/L are usually attained and maintained until symptoms are under control. The therapeutic range for lithium is narrow, and patients in the higher end of that range usually experience more uncomfortable side effects. During maintenance, the dosage is reduced, and dosages are adjusted to maintain blood levels of 0.4 to 1 mEq/L.

Lithium clears the body relatively quickly after discontinuation of its use. Withdrawal symptoms are rare, but occasional anxiety and emotional lability have been reported. It is important to remember that almost half of the individuals who discontinue lithium treatment abruptly experience a relapse of symptoms within a few weeks. Some research suggests that discontinuation of the use of lithium for individuals whose symptoms have been stable may lead to lithium's losing its effectiveness when use of the medication is restarted. Patients should be warned of the risks in abruptly discontinuing their medication and should be advised to consider the options carefully in consultation with their prescriber.

Side Effects, Adverse Reactions, and Toxicity

At lower therapeutic blood levels, side effects from lithium are relatively mild. These reactions correspond with peaks in plasma concentrations of the medication after administration, and most subside during the first few weeks of therapy. Frequently, individuals taking lithium complain of excessive thirst and an unpleasant metallic-like taste. Sugarless throat lozenges may be useful in minimizing this side effect. Other common side effects include increased frequency of urination, fine head tremor, drowsiness, and mild diarrhea. Weight gain occurs in about 20% of the individuals taking lithium. Nausea may be minimized by taking the medication with food or by use of a slow-release preparation. However, slow-release forms of lithium increase diarrhea. Muscle weakness, restlessness, headache, acne, rashes, and exacerbation of psoriasis have also been reported. See Chapter 25 for a summary of selected nursing interventions to minimize the impact of common side effects associated with lithium treatment. Patients most frequently discontinued their own medication use because of concerns with mental slowness, poor concentration, and memory problems.

As blood levels of lithium increase, the side effects of lithium become more numerous and severe. Early signs of lithium toxicity include severe diarrhea, vomiting, drowsiness, muscular weakness, and lack of coordination. Lithium should be withheld and the prescriber consulted if these symptoms develop. Lithium toxicity can easily be resolved in 24 to 48 hours by discontinuing the medication, but hemodialysis may be required in severe situations. See Chapter 25 for a summary of the side effects and symptoms of toxicity associated with various blood levels of lithium.

Monitoring of creatinine concentration, thyroid hormones, and CBC every 6 months during maintenance therapy helps to assess the occurrence of other potential adverse reactions. Kidney damage is considered an uncommon but potentially serious risk of long-term lithium treatment. This damage is usually reversible after discontinuation of the lithium use. A gradual rise in serum creatinine and decline in creatinine clearance indicate the development of renal dysfunction. Individuals with preexisting kidney dysfunction are susceptible to lithium toxicity.

Lithium may alter thyroid function, usually after 6 to 18 months of treatment. About 30% of the individuals taking lithium exhibit elevations in thyroid-stimulating hormone (TSH), but most do not show suppression of circulating thyroid hormone. Thyroid dysfunction from lithium treatment is more common in women, and some individuals require the addition of thyroxine to their care. During maintenance, TSH levels may be monitored. Nurses should observe for dry skin, constipation, bradycardia, hair loss, cold intolerance, and other symptoms of hypothyroidism. Other endocrine system effects result from hypoparathyroidism, which increases parathyroid hormone levels and calcium. Clinically, this change is not significant, but elevated calcium levels may cause mood changes, anxiety, lethargy, and sleep disturbances. These symptoms may erroneously be attributed to depression if hypercalcemia is not investigated.

Lithium use must be avoided during pregnancy because it has been associated with birth defects, especially when administered during the first trimester. If lithium is given during the third trimester, toxicity may develop in a newborn, producing signs of hypotonia, cyanosis, bradykinesia, cardiac changes, gastrointestinal bleeding, and shock. Diabetes insipidus may persist for months. Lithium is also present in breast milk, and women should not breastfeed while taking lithium. Women expecting to become pregnant should be advised to consult with a physician before discontinuing use of birth control methods.

Anticonvulsants

In the psychiatric mental health area, anticonvulsants are commonly used to treat patients with bipolar disorder and are considered mood stabilizers. The following discussion highlights the use of anticonvulsants as mood stabilizers in the treatment of bipolar disorder.

Indications and Mechanisms of Action

Valproate (valproic acid; Depakote), carbamazepine (Tegretol), and lamotrigine (Lamictal) have FDA approval for the treatment of bipolar disorder, mania, or mixed episodes (see Chapter 25). Other anticonvulsants, such as topiramate (Topamax), oxcarbazepine (Trileptal), and gabapentin (Neurontin) are used off-label as adjunctive treatments. In general, the anticonvulsant mood stabilizers have many actions, but their effects on ion channels, reducing repetitive firing of action potentials in the nerves, most directly decrease manic symptoms. In addition, carbamazepine affects the release and reuptake of several neurotransmitters, including norepinephrine, GABA, dopamine, and glutamate. It also changes several second messenger systems. No one action has successfully accounted for the anticonvulsants' ability to stabilize mood (Bialer, 2012).

Pharmacokinetics

Valproic acid is rapidly absorbed, but the enteric coating of divalproex sodium adds a delay of as long as 1 hour. Peak serum levels occur in about 1 to 4 hours. The liquid form (sodium valproate) is absorbed more rapidly and peaks in 15 minutes to 2 hours. Food appears to slow absorption but does not lower bioavailability of the drug.

Carbamazepine is absorbed in a somewhat variable manner. The liquid suspension is absorbed more quickly than the tablet form, but food does not appear to interfere with absorption. Peak plasma levels occur in 2 to 6 hours. Because high doses influence peak plasma levels and increase the risk for side effects, carbamazepine should be given in divided doses two or three times a day. The suspension, which has higher peak plasma levels and lower trough levels, must be given more frequently than the tablet form.

These medications cross easily into the CNS, move into the placenta as well, and are associated with an increased risk for birth defects. Carbamazepine, valproic acid, and lamotrigine are metabolized by the CYP450 system. However, one of the metabolites of carbamazepine is potentially toxic. If other concurrent medications inhibit the enzymes that break down this toxic metabolite, severe adverse reactions are often the result. Medications that inhibit this breakdown include erythromycin, verapamil, and cimetidine (now available in nonprescription form).

Teaching Points

Nurses need to educate patients about potential drug interactions, especially with nonprescription medications. Nurses can also inform other health care practitioners who may be prescribing medication that these patients are taking carbamazepine. It is important to note that oral contraceptives may become ineffective, and female patients should be advised to use other methods of birth control.

Side Effects, Adverse Reactions, and Toxicity of Anticonvulsants

The most common side effects of carbamazepine are dizziness, drowsiness, tremor, visual disturbance, nausea, and vomiting. These side effects may be minimized by initiating treatment in low doses. Patients should be advised that these symptoms will diminish, but care should be taken when changing positions or performing tasks that require visual alertness. Giving the drug with food may diminish nausea. Adverse reactions include rare aplastic anemia, agranulocytosis, severe rash, rare cardiac problems, and SIADH (syndrome of inappropriate secretion of the diuretic hormone) caused by hyponatremia.

Valproic acid also causes gastrointestinal disturbances, tremor, and lethargy. In addition, it can produce weight gain and alopecia (hair loss). These symptoms are transient and should diminish with the course of treatment. Dietary supplements of zinc and selenium may be helpful to patients experiencing hair loss. Constipation and urinary retention occur in some individuals. Nurses should monitor urinary output and assist patients to increase fluid consumption to decrease constipation.

Benign skin rash, sedation, blurred or double vision, dizziness, nausea, vomiting, and other gastrointestinal symptoms are side effects of lamotrigine. In rare cases, lamotrigine (Lamictal) produces severe, life-threatening rashes that usually occur within 2 to 8 weeks of treatment. This risk is highest in children. Use of lamotrigine should be immediately discontinued if a rash is noted.

Transient elevations in liver enzymes occur with both carbamazepine and valproic acid but symptoms of hepatic injury rarely occur. If the patient reports abnormal pain or shows signs of jaundice, the prescriber should be notified immediately. Several blood dyscrasias are associated with carbamazepine, including aplastic anemia, agranulocytosis, and leukopenia. Patients should be advised to report fever, sore throat, rash, petechiae, or bruising immediately. In addition, advise patients of the importance of completing routine blood tests throughout treatment. The increased risks for aplastic anemia and agranulocytosis with carbamazepine use still require close monitoring of CBCs during treatment. Valproate and its derivatives have had a similar course of development.

Off-label mood stabilizer, gabapentin (Neurontin) has relatively few side effects. Topamax (Topiramate) carries an increased risk of kidney stone formation. It can also cause a decrease in serum digoxin levels and may decrease effectiveness of oral birth control agents. In addition, ongoing ophthalmologic monitoring is required because of reports of acute myopia with secondary glaucoma. Trileptal (oxcarbazepine) has the potential for causing hyponatremia and may also decrease the effectiveness of oral birth control agents. Because of the potentially significant adverse reactions that the anticonvulsants can produce, careful patient teaching and monitoring are required.

Antidepressant Medications

Medications classified as antidepressants are used not only for the treatment of depression but also in the treatment of anxiety disorders, eating disorders, and other mental health states (Table 11.8). They are used very cautiously in persons with bipolar disorder because of the possibility of precipitating a manic episode. The exact neuromechanism for the antidepressant effect is unknown in all of them. The onset of action also varies considerably and appears to depend on factors outside of steady-state plasma levels. Initial improvement with some antidepressants, such as the SSRIs, may appear within 7 days, but complete relief of symptoms may take several weeks. Antidepressants should not be discontinued abruptly because of uncomfortable symptoms that result. Discontinuance of use of these medications

requires slow tapering. Individuals taking these medications should be cautioned not to abruptly stop using them without consulting their prescriber. Antidepressant medications are well absorbed from the gastrointestinal system; however, some individual variations exist. Most of the antidepressants are metabolized by the CYP450 enzyme system, so that drugs that activate this system tend to decrease blood levels of the antidepressants, and inhibitors of this system increase antidepressant blood levels (Table 11.9). All of these medications have a "boxed warning" for increased risk of suicidal behavior in children and adolescents compared with placebo.

Serotonin syndrome, or serotonin intoxication syndrome, can occur if there is an overactivity of serotonin or an impairment of the serotonin metabolism. Concomitant medications such as triptans used to treat migraines also can increase the serotonergic activity. With the advent of widely used antidepressants targeting the serotonergic systems, symptoms of this serious side effect should be assessed. Symptoms include mental status changes (hallucinations, agitation, coma), autonomic instability (tachycardia, hyperthermia, changes in blood pressure), neuromuscular problems (hyperreflexia, incoordination), and gastrointestinal disturbance (nausea, vomiting, diarrhea). Serotonin syndrome can be life threatening. The treatment for serotonin syndrome is discontinuation of the medication and symptom management.

Selective Serotonin Reuptake Inhibitors

The serotonergic system is associated with mood, emotion, sleep, and appetite and is implicated in the control of numerous emotional, physical, and behavioral functions (see Chapter 8). Decreased serotonergic neurotransmission has been proposed to play a key role in depression. In 1988, fluoxetine (Prozac) was the first of a class of drugs that acted "selectively" on serotonin, one group of neurotransmitters associated with depression. Other similarly selective medications, sertraline (Zoloft), paroxetine (Paxil), and fluvoxamine (Luvox), soon followed. The newest SSRI is escitalopram oxalate (Lexapro).

All of the SSRIs inhibit the reuptake of serotonin by blocking its transport into the presynaptic neuron, which in turn increases the concentration of synaptic serotonin. The concentration of synaptic serotonin is controlled directly by its reuptake; thus, drugs blocking serotonin transport have been successfully used for the treatment of depression and other conditions associated with serotonergic activity.

The SSRIs also have other properties that account for the common side effects, which include headache, anxiety, insomnia, transient nausea, vomiting, and diarrhea. Sedation may also occur, especially with paroxetine. Most often, these medications are given in the morning, but if daytime sedation occurs, they may be given in the evening. Higher

Table 11.8 ANTIDEPRESSANT MEDICATIONS			
Generic (Trade) Drug Name	Usual Dosage Range (mg/d)	Half-Life (h)	Therapeutic Blood Level (ng/mL)
Selective Serotonin Reuptake Inhibitors			
Citalopram (Celexa)	20–50	35	Not available
Escitalopram (Lexapro)	10–20	27–32	Not available
Fluoxetine (Prozac)	20–80	2–9 days	72–300
Fluvoxamine (Luvox)	50–300	17–22	Not available
Paroxetine (Paxil)	10–50	10–24	Not available
Sertraline (Zoloft)	50–200	24	Not available
Serotonin Norepinephrine Reuptake Inhibitors			
Desvenlafaxine (Pristiq Extended Release)	50	11	Not available
Duloxetine (Cymbalta)	40–60	8–17	Not available
Levomilnacipran (Fetzima)	40–120	12	Not available
Nefazodone (Serzone)	100–600	2–4	Not available
Venlafaxine (Effexor)	75–375	5–11	100–500
Norepinephrine Dopamine Reuptake Inhibitor			
Bupropion (Wellbutrin)	200–450	8–24	10–29
α_2 Antagonist			
Mirtazapine (Remeron)	15–45	20–40	Not available
Others			
Trazodone	150–600	4–9	650–1,600
Vilazodone (Viibryd)	10–40	25	Not available
Vortioxetine (Brintellix)	5–20	66	Not available
Tricyclic Antidepressants			
Amitriptyline (Elavil)	50–300	31–46	110–250
Amoxapine	50–600	8	200–500
Clomipramine (Anafranil)	25–250	19–37	80–100
Imipramine (Tofranil)	30–300	11–25	200–350
Desipramine (Norpramin)	25–300	12–24	125–300
Doxepin	25–300	8–24	100–200
Nortriptyline (Aventyl, Pamelor)	30–100	18–44	50–150
Protriptyline (Vivactil)	15–60	67–89	100–200
Tetracyclic			
Maprotiline (Ludiomil)	50–225	21–25	200–300
Monoamine Oxidase Inhibitors			
Isocarboxazid (Marplan)	20–60	Not available	Not available
Phenelzine (Nardil)	15–90	24 (effect lasts 3–4 d)	Not available
Tranylcypromine (Parnate)	10–60	24 (effect lasts 3–10 d)	Not available
Selegiline (Emsam)	6–12 mg/ 24 h	25%–50% delivered in 24 h	Not available

doses, especially of fluoxetine, are more likely to produce sedation. Tolerance develops to the common side effects of nausea and dizziness. These symptoms, along with sexual dysfunction, sedation, diastolic hypertension, and increased perspiration, tend to be dose dependent, occurring more frequently at higher doses. Other common side effects include insomnia, constipation, dry mouth, tremors, blurred vision, and asthenia or muscle weakness.

Sexual dysfunction is a relatively common side effect with most antidepressants. Erectile and ejaculation disturbances occur in men and anorgasmia in women. This side effect is often difficult to assess if the nurse has not obtained a sexual history before initiation of use of the medication. Anorgasmia is particularly common with the SSRIs and often goes unreported, frequently because nurses and other health care providers do not ask.

Table 11.9	CYP450 METABOLISM OF COMMON ANTIDEPRESSANTS		
Drug	How Metabolized	Induces	Inhibits
Bupropion	2B6	None	2D6
Citalopram	2C19, 2D6, 3A4	None	Mild 2D6
Desvenlafaxine	3A4	None	Mild 2D6
Duloxetine	1A2, 2D6	None	2D6
Escitalopram	2C19, 2D6, 3A4	None	Mild 2D6
Fluoxetine	2C9, 2C19, 2D6, 3A4	None	2C19, 2D6 3A4, norfluoxetine
Fluvoxamine	1A2, 2D6	None	1A2, 2C9, 2C19, 3A4
Mirtazapine	1A2, 2D6, 3A4	None	None
Nefazodone	2D6, 3A4	None	3A4
Paroxetine	2D6	None	2D6, 2B6
Selegiline	2A6, 2C9, 3A4/5	None	2D6, 3A4/5
Sertraline	2B6, 2C9, 2D6, 3A4	None	2B6, 2C9, 2C19, 2D6, 3A4 (dosage >200 mg)
St. John's Wort*	3A4	3A4	None
Trazodone	2D6, 3A4	None	None
Tricyclic antidepressants	2D6, others depending on drug	None	Mild 2D6
Venlafaxine	2D6	None	Mild 2D6
Vilazodone	3A4, 2C19, 2D6	None	2C8
Vortioxetine	2D6, 3A4/5, 2C9, 2A6, 2C8, 2B6	None	None

*Not a U. S. Food and Drug Administration–approved antidepressant.
Information from the Prescribing Information of each medication.

Serotonin Norepinephrine Reuptake Inhibitors

Decreased activity of the neurotransmitter norepinephrine is also associated with depression and anxiety disorders. Venlafaxine (Effexor), nefazodone (Serzone), duloxetine (Cymbalta), and desvenlafaxine (Pristiq) prevent the reuptake of both serotonin and norepinephrine at the presynaptic site and are classified as serotonin norepinephrine reuptake inhibitors (SNRIs). Desipramine (Norpramin) is technically a tricyclic antidepressant (TCA) and is usually categorized as such. It works, however, on both serotonin and norepinephrine, so it can also be considered an SNRI.

The side effects are similar to those of the SSRIs; there is also a risk for an associated increase in blood pressure. Elevations in blood pressure have been described, and nurses should monitor blood pressure, especially in patients who have a history of hypertension. Venlafaxine (Effexor) has little effect on acetylcholine and histamine; thus, it creates only mild sedation and anticholinergic symptoms. This medication is often used if a depressed patient is sleeping excessively and reports little energy. The most common side effects of nefazodone (Serzone) include dry mouth, nausea, dizziness, muscle weakness, constipation, and tremor. It is unlikely to cause sexual disturbance. Nefazodone also has a "boxed warning" for hepatic failure and should not be used in those with acute liver disease.

Norepinephrine Dopamine Reuptake Inhibitors

Bupropion (Wellbutrin, Zyban) inhibits reuptake of norepinephrine, serotonin, and dopamine. Wellbutrin is indicated for depression and Zyban for nicotine addiction. The smoking cessation medication, Zyban, is given at a lower dose than Wellbutrin. Patients should not take Zyban if they are taking Wellbutrin. Bupropion has a chemical structure unlike any of the other antidepressants and somewhat resembles a few of the psychostimulants. Bupropion's activating effects may be experienced as agitation or anxiety by some patients. Others also experience insomnia and appetite suppression. For a few individuals, bupropion has produced psychosis, including hallucinations and delusions. Most likely, this is secondary to overstimulation of the dopamine system. Bupropion is contraindicated for people with seizure disorders and those at risk for seizures. The rate of seizures is similar to that with the SSRIs and mirtazapine but is lower than the rate associated with the older antidepressants. Most important, bupropion has a lower incidence of sexual dysfunction and often is used in individuals who are experiencing these side effects with other antidepressants (GlaxoSmithKline, 2013).

α₂ Antagonist

Mirtazapine (Remeron) boosts norepinephrine or nor-adrenaline and serotonin by blocking α_2 adrenergic pre-synaptic receptors on a serotonin receptor ($5HT_{2A}$; $5HT_{2C}$, $5HT_3$). This is a different action than the other antidepressants. A histamine receptor, which is also blocked, may explain its sedative side effect. Mirtazapine is indicated for depression. Side effects include sedation (at lower doses), dizziness, weight gain, dry mouth, constipation, and change in urinary functioning.

Other Antidepressants

Trazodone blocks serotonin 2A receptor potently and blocks the serotonin reuptake pump less potently. It is indicated for depression but is often used off-label for insomnia and anxiety. Sedation is a very common side effect. Other side effects include weight gain, nausea, vomiting, constipation, dizziness, fatigue, incoordination, and tremor.

Other newly FDA approved antidepressants target other receptor sites. For example, vilazodone (Viibryd) is a serotonin reuptake inhibitor and a partial agonist of $5\text{-}HT_{1A}$; vortioxetine (Brintellix) inhibits reuptake of serotonin and norepinephrine but is also a partial agonist to $5\text{-}HT_{1A}$. These subtle differences translate into subtle clinical effects.

Tricyclic Antidepressants

The TCAs were once the primary medication used for treating depression. With the introduction of the SSRIs and other previously discussed antidepressants, the use of TCAs has significantly declined. In most cases, these medications are as effective as the other drugs, but they have more serious side effects and a higher lethal potential (see Table 11.8, p. 171). The TCAs act on a variety of neurotransmitter systems, including the norepinephrine and serotonin reuptake systems.

Pharmacokinetics

The TCAs are highly bound to plasma proteins, which make the association between blood levels and therapeutic clinical effects difficult. However, some plasma ranges have been established (see Table 11.8). Most of the TCAs have active metabolites that act in much the same manner as the parent drug. Most of these antidepressants may be given in a once-daily single dose. If the medication causes sedation, this dose should be given at bedtime.

Side Effects, Adverse Reactions, and Toxicity

Because the TCAs act on several neurotransmitters in addition to serotonin and norepinephrine, these drugs have many unwanted effects. With the TCAs, sedation, orthostatic hypotension, and anticholinergic side effects are the most common sources of discomfort for patients receiving these medications. Other side effects of the TCAs include tremors, restlessness, insomnia, nausea and vomiting, confusion, pedal edema, headache, and seizures. Blood dyscrasias may also occur, and any fever, sore throat, malaise, or rash should be reported to the prescriber. Interventions to assist in minimizing these side effects are listed in Table 11.1 on page 152.

The TCAs have the potential for cardiotoxicity. Symptoms include prolongation of cardiac conduction that may worsen preexisting cardiac conduction problems. The TCAs are contraindicated with second-degree atrioventricular block and should be used cautiously in patients who have other cardiac problems. Occasionally, they may precipitate heart failure, myocardial infarction, arrhythmias, and stroke.

Antidepressants that block the dopamine (D_2) receptor, such as amoxapine, have produced symptoms of NMS. Mild forms of EPS and endocrine changes, including galactorrhea and amenorrhea, may develop.

Monoamine Oxidase Inhibitors

The MAOIs, as their name indicates, inhibit monoamine oxidase (MAO), an enzyme that breaks down the biogenic amine neurotransmitters serotonin, norepinephrine, and others. By inhibiting this enzyme, serotonin and norepinephrine activity is increased in the synapse. In the United States, there are three oral formulations: phenelzine (Nardil), tranylcypromine (Parnate), and isocarboxazid (Marplan) and one available by a transdermal patch: selegiline (Emsam). These are considered MAOIs because they form strong covalent bonds to block the enzyme monoamine oxidase. This inhibition of this enzyme increases with repeated administration of these medications and takes at least 2 weeks to resolve after discontinuation of use of the medication.

The major problem with the MAOIs is their interaction with tyramine-rich foods and certain medications that can result in a hypertensive crisis. All of the MAOIs have dietary modification except the 6 mg/24 hours dose of selegiline. The enzyme monoamine is important in the breakdown of dietary amines (e.g., tyramine). When the enzyme is inhibited, tyramine, a precursor for dopamine, increases in the nerve cells. Tyramine has a vasopressor action that induces hypertension. If the individual ingests food that contains high levels of tyramine while taking MAOIs, severe headaches, palpitation, neck stiffness and soreness, nausea, vomiting, sweating, hypertension, stroke, and, in rare instances,

Table 11.10	EXAMPLE OF A TYRAMINE-RESTRICTED DIET	
Category of Food	**Food to Avoid**	**Food Allowed**
Cheese	All matured or aged cheeses	Fresh cottage cheese, cream cheese, ricotta cheese, and processed cheese slices; all fresh milk products that have been stored properly (e.g., sour cream, yogurt, ice cream). All casseroles made with these cheeses, (e.g., pizza, lasagna) *Note:* All cheeses are considered matured or aged except those listed under "foods allowed"
Meat, fish, and poultry	• Air dried, aged, and fermented meats, sausages, and salamis • Pickled herring • Any spoiled or improperly stored meat • Spoiled or improperly stored animal liver	Fresh meat, poultry, and fish, including fresh processed meats (e.g., lunch meats, hot dogs, breakfast sausage, and cooked sliced ham)
Fruits and vegetables	Broad bean pods (Fava bean pods)	All other vegetables
Alcoholic beverages	All tap beers and other beers that have not been pasteurized	Alcohol: no more than two domestic bottled or canned beers or 4-fluid-oz glasses of red or white wine per day; this applies to nonalcoholic beer also; please note that red wine may produce a headache unrelated to an increase in blood pressure
Miscellaneous foods	Marmite concentrated yeast extract Sauerkraut Soy sauce and other soybean condiments	Other yeast extracts (e.g., brewer's yeast) Soy milk Pizzas from commercial chain restaurants prepared with cheeses low in tyramine

Source: Krishnan, K.R. (2009). Monoamine oxidase inhibitors. In A. F. Schatzberg, & C. B. Nemeroff (Eds.). *The American Psychiatric Publishing textbook of psychopharmacology* (4th ed). Arlington, VA: American Psychiatric Publishing.

death may result. Patients who are taking MAOIs are prescribed a low-tyramine diet (Table 11.10).

In addition to food restrictions, many prescription and nonprescription medications that stimulate the sympathetic nervous system (sympathomimetic) produce the same risk for hypertensive crisis as do foods containing tyramine. The nonprescription medication interactions involve primarily diet pills and cold remedies. Patients should be advised to check the labels of any nonprescription drugs carefully for a warning against use with antidepressants, especially the MAOIs, and then consult their prescriber before consuming these medications. In addition, symptoms of other serious drug–drug interactions may develop, such as coma, hypertension, and fever, which may occur when patients receive meperidine (Demerol) while taking an MAOI. Patients should notify other health care providers, including dentists, that they are taking an MAOI before being prescribed or given any other medication.

The MAOIs frequently produce dizziness, headache, insomnia, dry mouth, blurred vision, constipation, nausea, peripheral edema, urinary hesitancy, muscle weakness, forgetfulness, and weight gain. Older patients are especially sensitive to the side effect of orthostatic hypotension and require frequent assessment of lying and standing blood pressures. They may be at risk for falls and subsequent bone fractures and require assistance in changing position.

Sexual dysfunction, including decreased libido, impotence, and anorgasmia, also is common with MAOIs.

Antianxiety and Sedative–Hypnotic Medications

Sometimes called *anxiolytics*, antianxiety medications, such as buspirone (BuSpar), and sedative–hypnotic medications, such as lorazepam (Ativan), come from various pharmacologic classifications, including barbiturates, benzodiazepines, nonbenzodiazepines, and nonbarbiturate sedative–hypnotic medications, such as chloral hydrate. These drugs represent some of the most widely prescribed medications today for the short-term relief of anxiety or anxiety associated with depression.

Benzodiazepines

Commonly prescribed benzodiazepines include alprazolam (Xanax), lorazepam (Ativan), diazepam (Valium), chlordiazepoxide (Librium), flurazepam, and triazolam (Halcion). Although benzodiazepines are known to enhance the effects of the inhibitory neurotransmitter GABA, their exact mechanisms of action are not well understood. Of the various benzodiazepines in use to relieve anxiety (and treat insomnia), oxazepam (Serax) and lorazepam (Ativan) are often preferred for patients

Table 11.11	ANTIANXIETY AND SEDATIVE–HYPNOTIC MEDICATIONS		
Generic (Trade) Drug Name	Usual Dosage Range (mg/d)	Half-Life (h)	Speed of Onset After Single Dose
Benzodiazepines			
Diazepam (Valium)	4–40	30–100	Very fast
Chlordiazepoxide (Librium)	15–100	50–100	Intermediate
Clorazepate (Tranxene)	15–60	30–200	Fast
Lorazepam (Ativan)	2–8	10–20	Slow-intermediate
Oxazepam	30–120	3–21	Slow-intermediate
Alprazolam (Xanax)	0.5–10	12–15	Intermediate
Clonazepam (Klonopin)	1.5–20	18–50	Intermediate
Nonbenzodiazepine			
Buspirone	15–30	3–11	Very slow

with liver disease and for older patients because of their short half-lives.

Pharmacokinetics

The variable rate of absorption of the benzodiazepines determines the speed of onset. Table 11.11 provides relative indications of the speed of onset, from very fast to slow, for some of the commonly prescribed benzodiazepines. Whereas chlordiazepoxide (Librium) and diazepam (Valium) are slow, erratic, and sometimes incompletely absorbed when given intramuscularly, lorazepam (Ativan) is rapidly and completely absorbed when given intramuscularly.

All of the benzodiazepines are highly lipid soluble and highly protein bound. They are distributed throughout the body and enter the CNS quickly. Other drugs that compete for protein-binding sites may produce drug–drug interactions. The degree to which each of these drugs is lipid soluble affects its duration of action. Most of these drugs have active metabolites, but the degree of activity of each metabolite affects duration of action and elimination half-life. Most of these drugs vary markedly in length of half-life. Oxazepam and lorazepam have no active metabolites and thus have shorter half-lives. Elimination half-lives may also be sustained for obese patients when using diazepam, chlordiazepoxide, and halazepam (Paxipam).

Side Effects, Adverse Reactions, and Toxicity

The most commonly reported side effects of benzodiazepines result from the sedative and CNS depression effects of these medications. Drowsiness, intellectual impairment, memory impairment, ataxia, and reduced motor coordination are common adverse reactions. If used for sleep, many of these medications, especially the long-acting benzodiazepines, produce significant "hangover" effects experienced on awakening. Older patients receiving repeated doses of medications such as flurazepam (Dalmane) at bedtime may experience paradoxical confusion, agitation, and delirium, sometimes after the first dose. In addition, daytime fatigue, drowsiness, and cognitive impairments may continue while the person is awake. For most patients, the effects subside as tolerance develops; however, alcohol increases all of these symptoms and potentiates the CNS depression. Individuals using these medications should be warned to be cautious when driving or performing other tasks that require mental alertness. If these tasks are part of the person's work requirements, another medication may be chosen. Administered intravenously, benzodiazepines often cause phlebitis and thrombosis at the IV sites, which should be monitored closely and changed if redness or swelling develops.

Because tolerance develops to most of the CNS depressant effects, individuals who wish to experience the feeling of "intoxication" from these medications may be tempted to increase their own dosage. Psychological dependence is more likely to occur when using these medications for a longer period. Abrupt discontinuation of the use of benzodiazepines may result in a recurrence of the target symptoms, such as rebound insomnia or anxiety. Other withdrawal symptoms appear rapidly, including tremors, increased perspiration, palpitations, increased sensitivity to light, abdominal discomfort or pain, and elevations in systolic blood pressure. These symptoms may be more pronounced with the short-acting benzodiazepines, such as lorazepam. Gradual tapering is recommended for discontinuing use of benzodiazepines after long-term treatment. When tapering short-acting medications, the prescriber may switch the patient to a long-acting benzodiazepine before discontinuing use of the short-acting drug.

Individual reactions to the benzodiazepines appear to be associated with sensitivity to their effects. Some patients feel apathy, fatigue, tearfulness, emotional lability, irritability, and nervousness. Symptoms of depression may worsen. The psychiatric–mental health nurse should closely monitor these symptoms when individuals are receiving benzodiazepines as adjunctive treatment for anxiety that coexists with depression. Gastrointestinal disturbances, including nausea, vomiting, anorexia, dry mouth, and constipation, may develop. These medications may be taken with food to ease the gastrointestinal distress.

Older patients are particularly susceptible to incontinence, memory disturbances, dizziness, and increased risk for falls when using benzodiazepines. Pregnant patients should be aware that these medications cross the placenta and are associated with increased risk for birth defects, such as cleft palate, mental retardation, and pyloric stenosis. Infants born addicted to benzodiazepines often exhibit flaccid muscle tone, lethargy, and difficulties sucking. All of the benzodiazepines are excreted in breast milk, and breastfeeding women should avoid using these medications. Infants and children metabolize these medications more slowly; therefore, more drug accumulates in their bodies.

Toxicity develops in overdose or accumulation of the drug in the body from liver dysfunction or disease. Symptoms include worsening of the CNS depression, ataxia, confusion, delirium, agitation, hypotension, diminished reflexes, and lethargy. Rarely do the benzodiazepines cause respiratory depression or death. In overdose, these medications have a high therapeutic index and rarely result in death unless combined with another CNS depressant drug, such as alcohol.

Nonbenzodiazepines: Buspirone

Buspirone, a nonbenzodiazepine, is effective in controlling the symptoms of anxiety but has no effect on panic disorders and little effect on obsessive-compulsive disorder.

Indications and Mechanisms of Actions

Nonbenzodiazepines are effective for treating anxiety disorders without the CNS depressant effects or the potential for abuse and withdrawal syndromes. Buspirone is indicated for treating generalized anxiety disorder; therefore, its target symptoms include anxiety and related symptoms, such as difficulty concentrating, tension, insomnia, restlessness, irritability, and fatigue. Because buspirone does not add to depression symptoms, it has been tried for treating anxiety that coexists with depression. In some instances, it is thought to potentiate the antidepressant actions of other medications.

Buspirone has no effect on the benzodiazepine–GABA complex but instead appears to control anxiety by blocking the serotonin subtype of receptor, 5-HT_{1a}, at both presynaptic reuptake and postsynaptic receptor sites. It has no sedative, muscle relaxant, or anticonvulsant effects. It also lacks potential for abuse.

Pharmacokinetics

Buspirone is rapidly absorbed but undergoes extensive first-pass metabolism. Food slows absorption but appears to reduce first-pass effects, increasing the bioavailability of the medication. Buspirone is given on a continual dosing schedule of three times a day because of its short half-life of 2 to 3 hours. Clinical action depends on reaching steady-state concentrations; taking this medication with food may facilitate this process.

Buspirone is highly protein bound but does not displace most other medications. However, it does displace digoxin and may increase digoxin levels to the point of toxicity. It is metabolized in the liver and excreted predominantly by the kidneys but also via the gastrointestinal tract. Patients with liver or kidney impairment should be given this medication with caution.

Buspirone cannot be used on a PRN basis; rather, it takes 2 to 4 weeks of continual use for symptom relief to occur. It is more effective in reducing anxiety in patients who have never taken a benzodiazepine.

Buspirone does not block the withdrawal of other benzodiazepines. Therefore, a switch to buspirone must be initiated gradually to avoid withdrawal symptoms. Nurses should closely monitor patients who are undergoing this change of medication for emergence of withdrawal symptoms from the benzodiazepines and report such symptoms to the prescriber.

Side Effects, Adverse Reactions, and Toxicity

Common side effects from buspirone include dizziness, drowsiness, nausea, excitement, and headache. Most other side effects occur at an incidence of less than 1%. There have been no reports of death from an overdose of buspirone alone. Older patients, pregnant women, and children have not been adequately studied. For now, buspirone can be assumed to cross the placenta and is present in breast milk; therefore, its use should be avoided in pregnant women, and women who are taking this medication should not breastfeed.

Sedative–Hypnotics

Sedatives reduce activity, nervousness, irritability and excitability without causing sleep, but if given in large

Table 11.12 **HYPNOTICS FOR INSOMNIA**			
Generic (Trade) Drug Name	Usual Dosage Range (mg/d)	Elimination Half-Life (h)	Speed of Onset After Single Dose
Benzodiazepine Hypnotics			
Flurazepam	15–30	47–100	Fast
Temazepam (Restoril)	15–30	9.5–20	Moderately fast
Triazolam (Halcion)	0.25–0.5	1.5–5	Fast
Quazepam (Doral)	0.75–15	39	Fast
Estazolam (ProSom)	1	10–24	Fast
Nonbenzodiazepine Hypnotics			
Eszopiclone (Lunesta)	2–3	6	Fast
Zaleplon (Sonata)	10	1	Fast
Zolpidem (Ambien)	5–10	2.6	Fast
Zolpidem CR (Ambien CR)	12.5	2.6	Fast
Melatonergic Hypnotics			
Melatonin	0.1–10	0.5–0.75	Fast
Ramelteon (Rozerem)	8	1–2.6	Fast
Antihistamines			
Hydroxyzine (Vistaril)	50–100	20	Fast
Doxylamine (Unisom)	25	10	Fast

enough doses, they have a hypnotic effect. **Hypnotics** cause drowsiness and facilitate the onset and maintenance of sleep. These two classifications are usually referred to as **sedative–hypnotics**—drugs that have a calming effect or depress the CNS. These medications include (1) benzodiazepines (2) GABA enhancers, (3) melatonergic hypnotics, and (4) the antihistamines (Table 11.12). The benzodiazepines have been previously discussed. The GABA enhancers modulate GABA-A receptors. They do not cause a high degree of tolerance or dependence and are easier to discontinue than the benzodiazepines. Melatonergic hypnotics are melatonin agonists, and antihistamines are block histamines, causing sedation (Stahl, 2013). These medications are discussed thoroughly in Chapter 32.

Stimulants and Wakefulness-Promoting Agents

Amphetamines were first synthesized in the late 1800s but were not used for psychiatric disorders until the 1930s. Initially, amphetamines were prescribed for a variety of symptoms and disorders, but their high abuse potential soon became obvious.

Currently among the medications known as stimulants are methylphenidate (Ritalin, Methylin, Metadate), D-amphetamine (Dexedrine), amphetamine/dextroamphetamine (Adderall), dexmethylphenidate (Focalin), lisamphetamine (Vyvanse), and CNS stimulants. Modafinil (Provigil) and armodafinil (Nuvigil) are wakefulness-promoting agents used for narcolepsy and other sleep disorders.

Indications and Mechanisms of Action

Medical use of these stimulants is now restricted to a few disorders, including narcolepsy, attention deficit hyperactivity disorder (ADHD)—particularly in children—and obesity unresponsive to other treatments. However, stimulants are increasingly being used as an adjunctive treatment in depression and other mood disorders to address the fatigue and low energy common to these conditions.

Amphetamines indirectly stimulate the sympathetic nervous system, producing alertness, wakefulness, vasoconstriction, suppressed appetite, and hypothermia. Tolerance develops to some of these effects, such as suppression of appetite, but the CNS stimulation continues. Although the exact mechanism of action is not completely understood, stimulants cause a release of catecholamines, particularly norepinephrine and dopamine, into the synapse from the presynaptic nerve cell. They also block reuptake of these catecholamines. Methylphenidate is structurally similar to the amphetamines but produces a milder CNS stimulation. Psychostimulants should be used very cautiously in individuals who have a history of substance abuse.

Although the stimulant effects of these medications may seem logically indicated for narcolepsy, a disorder in which the individual frequently and abruptly falls asleep, the indications for childhood ADHD seem less obvious. The etiology and neurobiology of ADHD remain unclear, but psychostimulants produce a paradoxic calming of the increased motor activity characteristic of ADHD. Studies show that medication decreases disruptive activity during school hours, reduces noise and verbal activity, improves attention span and short-term memory, improves ability to follow directions, and decreases distractibility and impulsivity. Although these improvements have been well documented in the literature, the diagnosis of ADHD and subsequent use of psychostimulants with children remain matters of controversy (see Chapter 35).

Modafinil (Provigil) and armodafinil (Nuvigil), wake-promoting agents, are used for treating excessive sleepiness associated with narcolepsy, sleep apnea, and residual sleepiness for shift work sleep disorder. Armodafinil is longer acting than modafinil. The mechanism of action is unclear, but it is hypothesized that they increase glutamate and suppress GABA in the hypothalamus, hippocampus, and thalamus. There is no evidence of direct effects on dopamine, but there may be action on a dopamine transport. These drugs may increase the risk of Stevens-Johnson syndrome (Wood, Sage, Shuman, & Anagnostaras, 2013).

Pharmacokinetics

Psychostimulants are rapidly absorbed from the gastrointestinal tract and reach peak plasma levels in 1 to 3 hours. Considerable individual variations occur between the drugs in terms of their bioavailability, plasma levels, and half-lives. Table 11.13 compares the primary psychostimulants used in psychiatry. Some of these differences are age dependent because children metabolize these medications more rapidly, producing shorter elimination half-lives.

The psychostimulants appear to be unaffected by food in the stomach and should be given after meals to reduce the appetite-suppressant effects when indicated. However,

changes in urine pH may affect the rates of excretion. Excessive sodium bicarbonate alkalizes the urine and reduces amphetamine secretion. Increased vitamin C or citric acid intake may acidify the urine and increase its excretion. Starvation from appetite suppression may have a similar effect. All of these drugs are highly lipid soluble, crossing easily into the CNS and the placenta. Psychostimulants undergo metabolic changes in the liver where they may affect, or be affected by, other drugs. They are primarily excreted through the kidneys; therefore, renal dysfunction may interfere with excretion.

Psychostimulants are usually begun at a low dose and increased weekly, depending on the improvement of symptoms and occurrence of side effects. Initially, children with ADHD are given a morning dose, so their school performance may be compared from morning to afternoon. Rebound symptoms of excitability and overtalkativeness may occur when use of the medication is withdrawn or after dose reduction. These symptoms also begin about 5 hours after the last dose of medication, which may affect the dosing regimen for some individuals. The return of symptoms in the afternoon for children with ADHD may require that a second dose be given at school. Prescribers should work with parents to implement other interventions after school and on weekends when the psychostimulants are not used. The severity of symptoms may require that the medications be continued during these times, but this dosing schedule should be determined after careful evaluation on an individual basis. Use of these medications should not be stopped abruptly, especially with higher doses, because the rebound effects may last for several days.

Modafinil (Provigil) is absorbed rapidly and reaches peak plasma concentration in 2 to 4 hours. Armodafinil reaches peak plasma concentration later and is maintained for 6 to 14 hours. Absorption of both may be delayed by 1 to 2 hours if taken with food. Modafinil is eliminated via liver metabolism with subsequent excretion of metabolites through renal excretion. They may interact with drugs that inhibit, induce, or are metabolized

Table 11.13	PSYCHOSTIMULANT MEDICATIONS	
Generic (Trade) Drug Name	Usual Dosage Range (mg/d)	Elimination Half-Life
Dextroamphetamine (Dexedrine)	5–40	Highly variable depending on urine pH
Methylphenidate (Ritalin)	10–60	2.4 h (children); 2.1 h (adults)
Amphetamine/dextroamphetamine (Adderall)	2.5 mg (3–5 yr) 5 mg (6 yr) 5–60 mg for narcolepsy	9–11 h
Dexmethylphenidate extended release (Focalin XR)	5–40 mg	3 h
Lisdexamfetamine (Vyvanse)	30 mg	<1 h

by CYP450 isoenzymes, including phenytoin, diazepam, and propranolol. Concurrent use of modafinil or armodafinil and other drugs metabolized by the CYP450 isoenzyme system may lead to increased circulating blood levels of the other drugs.

Side Effects, Adverse Reactions, and Toxicity

Side effects associated with psychostimulants typically arise within 2 to 3 weeks after use of the medication begins. From most to least common, these side effects include appetite suppression, insomnia, irritability, weight loss, nausea, headache, palpitations, blurred vision, dry mouth, constipation, and dizziness. Because of the effects on the sympathetic nervous system, some individuals experience blood pressure changes (both hypertension and hypotension), tachycardia, tremors, and irregular heart rates. Blood pressure and pulse should be monitored initially and after each dosage change.

Rarely, psychostimulants suppress growth and development in children. These effects are a matter of controversy, and research has produced conflicting results. Although suppression of height seems unlikely to some researchers, others have indicated that psychostimulants may have an effect on cartilage. Height and weight should be monitored several times annually for children taking these medications and compared with prior history of growth. Weight should be monitored, especially closely during the initial phases of treatment. These effects also may be minimized by drug "holidays," such as during school vacations.

Rarely, individuals may experience mild dysphoria, social withdrawal, or mild to moderate depression. These symptoms are more common at higher doses and may require discontinuation of use of medication. Abnormal movements and motor tics may also increase in individuals who have a history of Tourette's syndrome. Psychostimulants should be avoided by patients with Tourette's symptoms or with a positive family history of the disorder. In addition, dextroamphetamine has been associated with an increased risk for congenital abnormalities. Because there is no compelling reason for a pregnant woman to continue to take these medications, patients should be informed and should advise their prescriber immediately if they plan to become pregnant or if pregnancy is a possibility.

Death is rare from overdose or toxicity of the psychostimulants, but a 10-day supply may be lethal, especially in children. Symptoms of overdose include agitation, chest pain, hallucinations, paranoia, confusion, and dysphoria. Seizures may develop, along with fever, tremor, hypertension or hypotension, aggression, headache, palpitations, rashes, difficulty breathing, leg pain, and abdominal pain. Toxic doses of dextroamphetamine are above 20 mg, with potential death resulting from a 400-mg dose. Parents should be warned regarding the

potential lethality of these medications and take preventive measures by keeping the medication in a safe place.

Side effects associated with modafinil and armodafinil include nausea, nervousness, headache, dizziness, and trouble sleeping. If the effects continue or are bothersome, patients should consult the prescriber. Modafinil and armodafinil are generally well tolerated with few clinically significant side effects. It is potentially habit forming and must be used with great caution in individuals with a history of substance abuse or dependence (Cephalon, 2013).

DIETARY SUPPLEMENTS

Herbal Supplements

Many individuals are turning to dietary herbal preparations to address psychiatric symptoms. If these supplements were classified as drugs, their efficacy and safety would have to be approved by the FDA before marketing. However, herbal supplements are regulated like foods, not medications, and thus are exempt from the FDA's efficacy and safety standards. Lack of regulation does not mean that these herbal supplements are effective and safe. These substances often have adverse reactions and interact with prescribed medications. Nurses need to include an assessment of these agents into their overall patient assessment to understand the total picture.

Herbal supplements popular for psychiatric disorders include St. John's Wort (SJW) and kava. SJW, derived from *Hypericum perforatum L.*, is used for depression, pain, anxiety, insomnia, and premenstrual syndrome. SJW is believed to modulate serotonin, dopamine, and norepinephrine. The risk of developing serotonin syndrome is increased when taken with other serotonergic drugs. It is recognized as a potent inducer of CYP3A4 (Sarris, 2013) and has the potential to interact with substrates of this enzyme. It should not be taken with prescribed antidepressants.

Kava, derived from the *Piper methysticum* plant, is used for anxiety reduction. Kava interacts with dopaminergic transmission, inhibits the MAO-B enzyme system, and modulates the GABA receptor. It may also inhibit uptake of noradrenaline. Kava is widely used by Pacific Islanders as a social and ceremonial tranquilizing drink. In 2002, the FDA issued warnings about the risk of severe liver injury associated with kava. Several countries have restricted its use. Thrombocytopenia, leukopenia, and hearing impairment have been reported with the use of kava (Bunchorntavakul & Reddy, 2013).

Valerian, (*Valeriana officinalis*) a member of the Valerianaceae family, is a perennial plant native to Europe and Asia and naturalized to North America. Valerian is a common ingredient in products promoted for insomnia and nervousness. The evidence of its effectiveness is inconclusive. The mechanism of action is unclear but appears to be relatively safe. There are some reports that suggest hepatotoxicity in humans (Modabbernia & Akhondzadeh, 2013).

Vitamin, Mineral, and Other Dietary Supplements

The neurotransmitters necessary for normal healthy functioning are produced from chemical building blocks taken in with the foods we eat. Many nutritional deficiencies may produce symptoms of psychiatric disorders. Fatigue, apathy, and depression are caused by deficiencies in iron, folic acid, pantothenic acid, magnesium, vitamin C, or biotin. Logically, treating these deficiencies with dietary supplements should improve the psychiatric symptoms. The question becomes: Can nutritional supplements improve psychiatric symptoms that are not the result of such deficiencies?

Tryptophan, the dietary precursor for serotonin, has been most extensively investigated as it relates to low serotonin levels and increased aggression. Individuals who have low tryptophan levels are prone to have lower levels of serotonin in the brain, resulting in depressed mood and aggressive behavior (Qureshi & Al-Bedah, 2013).

Dietary supplements such as melatonin, 2-dimethylaminoethanol (DMAE), and lecithin target CNS functioning. Melatonin, a naturally occurring hormone secreted from the pineal gland, is used for treatment of insomnia and prevention of "jet lag" in air travelers. DMAE is promoted for the treatment of ADHD, Alzheimer's disease, Huntington's chorea, and tardive dyskinesia (Copinschi & Caufriez, 2013). DMAE is similar to a former prescription medication removed from the market in 1983 for lack of efficacy. Lecithin, a precursor to acetylcholine, is used to improve memory and treat dementia. The extent to which the level of acetylcholine is raised by ingestion of lecithin is unknown (Tayebati & Amenta, 2013).

Medications may also influence the development of nutritional deficiencies that may worsen psychiatric symptoms. For example, drugs with strong anticholinergic activity often produce impaired or enhanced gastric motility, which may lead to generalized malabsorption of vitamins and minerals. In addition, many vitamin and mineral supplements have toxicities of their own when given in excess. For example, daily ingestion of more than 100 mg of pyridoxine (vitamin B_6) can produce neurotoxic symptoms, photosensitivity, and ataxia. More research is needed to identify the underlying mechanisms and relationships of dietary supplements and dietary precursors of the bioamines to mood and behavior and psychopharmacologic medications. For now, it is important for the psychiatric–mental health nurse to recognize that these issues may be potential factors in improvement of the patient's mental status and target symptoms.

OTHER BIOLOGIC TREATMENTS

Although the primary biologic interventions remain pharmacologic, other somatic treatments have gained acceptance, remain under investigation, or show promise for the future. These include neurosurgery, ECT, phototherapy, and (most recently) **repetitive transcranial magnetic stimulation** (rTMS) and vagus nerve stimulation (VNS). The use of neurosurgery is very limited and outside the scope of this text.

Electroconvulsive Therapy

For hundreds of years, seizures have been known to produce improvement in some psychiatric symptoms. Camphor-induced seizures were used in the 16th century to reduce psychosis and mania. With time, other substances, such as inhalants, were tried, but most were difficult to control or produced adverse reactions, sometimes even fatalities. ECT was formally introduced in Italy in 1938. It is one of the oldest medical treatments available and remains safely in use today. It is one of the most effective treatments for severe depression but has been used for other disorders, including mania and schizophrenia when other treatments have failed.

With ECT, a brief electrical current is passed through the brain to produce generalized seizures lasting 25 to 150 seconds. The patient does not feel the stimulus or recall the procedure. A short-acting anesthetic and a muscle relaxant are given before induction of the current. A brief pulse stimulus, administered unilaterally on the nondominant side of the head, is associated with less confusion after ECT. However, some individuals require bilateral treatment for effective resolution of depressive symptoms. Induction of a seizure is necessary to produce positive treatment outcomes. Because individual seizure thresholds vary, the electrical impulse and treatment method also may vary. In general, the lowest possible electrical stimulus necessary to produce seizure activity is used. Blood pressure and the ECG are monitored during the procedure. This procedure is repeated two or three times a week, usually for a total of six to 12 treatments. Because there is no particular difference in treatment efficacy and a twice-weekly regimen produces less accumulative memory loss, this treatment course is often chosen. After symptoms have improved, antidepressant medication may be used to prevent relapse. Some patients who cannot take or do not experience response to antidepressant treatment may continue to have ECT treatment. Usually, once-weekly treatments are gradually decreased in frequency to once monthly. The number and frequency vary depending on the individual's response.

Although ECT produces rapid improvement in depressive symptoms, its exact mechanism of antidepressant action remains unclear. It is known to downregulate β-adrenergic receptors in much the same way as antidepressant medications. However, unlike antidepressant therapy, ECT produces an upregulation in serotonin, especially 5-HT$_2$. ECT also has several other actions on neurochemistry, including increased influx of calcium and effects on second messenger systems.

Brief episodes of hypotension or hypertension, bradycardia or tachycardia, and minor arrhythmias are among the adverse reactions that may occur during and immediately after the procedure but usually resolve quickly. Common aftereffects from ECT include headache, nausea, and muscle pain. Memory loss is the most troublesome long-term effect of ECT. Many patients do not experience amnesia, but others report some memory loss for months or even years. Evidence is conflicting on the effects of ECT on the formation of memories after the treatments and on learning, but most patients experience no noticeable change. Memory loss occurring as part of the symptoms of untreated depression presents a confounding factor in determining the exact nature of the memory deficits from ECT. It is important to remember that patient surveys are positive, with most individuals reporting that they were helped by ECT and would have it again (Rajagopal, Chakrabarti, & Grover, 2013).

ECT is contraindicated in patients with increased intracranial pressure. Risk also increases in patients with recent myocardial infarction, recent cerebrovascular accident, retinal detachment, or pheochromocytoma (a tumor on the adrenal cortex) and in patients at high risk for complications from anesthesia. Although ECT should be considered cautiously because of its specific side effects, added risks of general anesthesia, possible contraindications, and substantial social stigma, it is a safe and effective treatment.

Psychiatric–mental health nurses are involved in many aspects of care for individuals undergoing ECT. Informed consent is required, and all treating professionals have a responsibility to ensure that the patient's and family's questions are answered completely. Available treatment options, risks, and consequences must be fully discussed. Sometimes memory difficulties associated with severe depression make it difficult for patients to retain information or ask questions. Nurses should be prepared to restate or explain the procedure as often as necessary. Whenever possible, the individual's family or other support systems should be educated and involved in the consent process. Educational videos are available, but they should not replace direct discussions. Language should be in terms the patient and family members can understand. Other nursing interventions involve preparation of the patient before treatment, monitoring immediately after treatment, and follow-up. Many of these considerations are listed in Box 11.5.

BOX 11.5

Interventions for the Patient Receiving Electroconvulsive Therapy

- Discuss treatment alternatives, procedures, risks, and benefits with patient and family. Make sure that informed consent for ECT has been given in writing.
- Provide initial and ongoing patient and family education.
- Assist and monitor the patient who must take NPO after midnight the evening before the procedure.
- Make sure that the patient wears loose, comfortable, nonrestrictive clothing to the procedure.
- If the procedure is performed on an outpatient basis, ensure that the patient has someone to accompany him or her home and stay with him or her after the procedure.
- Ensure that pretreatment laboratory tests are complete, including a CBC, serum electrolytes, urinalysis, ECG, chest radiography, and physical examination.
- Teach the patient to create memory helps, such as lists and notepads, before the ECT.
- Explain that no foreign or loose objects can be in the patient's mouth during the procedure. Dentures will be removed, and a bite block may be inserted.
- Insert an IV line and provide oxygen by nasal cannula (usually 100% oxygen at 5 L/min).
- Obtain emergency equipment and be sure it is available and ready if needed.
- Monitor vital signs frequently immediately after the procedure, as in every postanesthesia recovery period.
- When the patient is fully conscious and vital signs are stable, assist him or her to get up slowly, sitting for some time before standing.
- Monitor confusion closely; the patient may need reorientation to the bathroom and other areas.
- Maintain close supervision for at least 12 hours and continue observation for 48 hours after treatment. Advise family members to observe how the patient manages at home, provide assistance as needed, and report any problems.
- Assist the patient to keep or schedule follow-up appointments.

CBC, complete blood count; ECG, electrocardiogram; ECT, electroconvulsive therapy; IV, intravenous; NPO, nothing by mouth.

Light Therapy (Phototherapy)

Human circadian rhythms are set by time clues (*Zeitgebers*) inside and outside the body. One of the most powerful regulators of these body patterns is the cycle of daylight and darkness.

Research findings indicate that some individuals with certain types of depression may experience disturbance in these normal body patterns or of circadian rhythms, particularly those who experience a seasonal variation in their depression. These individuals are more depressed during the winter months when there is less light; they improve spontaneously in the spring (see Chapter 24). These individuals usually have symptoms that are somewhat different from classic depression, including fatigue, increased need to sleep, increased appetite and weight gain, irritability, and carbohydrate craving. Sometimes, the symptoms appear in the summer, and some individuals have only subtle changes without developing the full pattern. Administering artificial light to these patients during winter months has reduced these depressive symptoms.

Light therapy, sometimes called **phototherapy**, involves exposing the patient to an artificial light source during winter months to relieve seasonal depression. Artificial light is believed to trigger a shift in the patient's circadian rhythm to an earlier time. Research remains ongoing. The light source must be very bright, full-spectrum light, usually 2,500 lux, which is about 200 times brighter than normal indoor lighting. Harmful ultraviolet light is filtered out. Exposure to this light source has produced improvement and relief of depressive symptoms for significant numbers of seasonally depressed individuals. It produces no change for individuals who are not seasonally depressed.

Studies have shown that morning phototherapy produces a better response than either evening or morning and evening timing of the phototherapy session. Light banks with full-spectrum light may be put together by the individual or obtained from various companies now producing these light sources. Light visors (visors containing small, full-spectrum light bulbs that shine on the eyelids) have also been developed. The patient is instructed to sit in front of the lights at a distance of about 3 feet, engaging in a variety of other activities, but glancing directly into the light every few minutes. This should be done immediately on arising and is most effective before 8 AM. The duration of administration may begin with as little as 30 minutes and increase to 2 to 5 hours. One to 2 hours is usually sufficient, and the antidepressant response begins in 1 to 4 days, with the full effect usually complete after 2 weeks. Full antidepressant effect is usually maintained with daily sessions of 30 minutes (Fisher et al., 2013).

Side effects of phototherapy are rare, but eye strain, headache, and insomnia are possible. An ophthalmologist should be consulted if the patient has a preexisting eye disorder. In rare instances, phototherapy has been reported to produce an episode of mania. Irritability is a more common complaint. Follow-up visits with the prescriber or therapist are needed to help manage side effects and assess positive results. Phototherapy should be implemented only by a provider knowledgeable in its use.

Transcranial Magnetic Stimulation

Transcranial magnetic stimulation was introduced in 1985 as a noninvasive, painless method to stimulate the cerebral cortex. Undergirding this procedure is the hypothesis that a time-varying magnetic field will induce an electrical field, which, in brain tissue, activates inhibitory and excitatory neurons, thereby modulating neuroplasticity in the brain. The low-frequency electrical stimulation from rTMS triggers lasting anticonvulsant effects in rats, and the therapeutic benefits of rTMS in humans are thought to be related to an action similar to that produced by anticonvulsant medication. The rTMS has been used for both clinical and research purposes. The rTMS stimulation of the brain's prefrontal cortex may help some depressed patients in much the same way as ECT but without its side effects (Kirsch & Nichols, 2013). Thus, it has been proposed as an alternative to ECT in managing symptoms of depression. The rTMS treatment is administered daily for at least 1 week, much like ECT, except that subjects remain awake. Although proven effective for depression, rTMS does have some side effects, including mild headaches.

Vagus Nerve Stimulation

VNS sends electrical impulses to the brain to improve depression. The vagus nerve has traditionally been considered a parasympathetic efferent nerve that was responsible only for regulating autonomic functions, such as heart rate and gastric tone. However, the vagus nerve (cranial X) also carries sensory information to the brain from the head, neck, thorax, and abdomen, and research has identified that the vagus nerve has extensive projections of its sensory afferent connections to many brain areas. Although the basic mechanism of action of VNS is unknown, incoming sensory, or afferent, connections of the left vagus nerve directly project into many of the very same brain regions implicated in neuropsychiatric disorders. These help us to understand how VNS is helpful in treating psychiatric disorders. Vagus nerve stimulation connections change levels of several neurotransmitters implicated in the development of major depression, including serotonin, norepinephrine, GABA, and glutamate, in the same way that antidepressant medications produce their therapeutic effect (Wani, Trevino, Marnell, & Husain, 2013).

Approved by the FDA for the adjunctive treatment of severe depression for adults who are unresponsive to four or more adequate antidepressant treatments, VNS is a permanent implant. VNS is not a cure for depression, and patients must be seen regularly for assessment of mood states and suicidality.

THE ISSUE OF ADHERENCE

Medications and other biologic treatments work only if they are used. On the surface, **adherence**, or **compliance** to a therapeutic routine, seems amazingly simple. However, following therapeutic regimens, self-administering medications as prescribed, and keeping appointments are amazingly complex activities that often prevent successful treatment. Adherence exists on a continuum and can be conceived of as full, partial, or nil. Partial

BOX 11.6

Common Reasons for Nonadherence to Medication Regimens

- Uncomfortable side effects and those that interfere with quality of life, such as work performance or intimate relationships
- Lack of awareness of or denial of illness
- Stigma
- Feeling better
- Confusion about dosage or timing
- Difficulties in access to treatment
- Substance abuse

adherence whereby a patient either attempts to take medications but misses doses or takes more than prescribed, is by far the most common. Recent estimates indicate that on the average, 50% or more of the individuals with schizophrenia taking antipsychotic medications stop taking the medications or do not take them as prescribed. It should be remembered that problems with adherence are an issue with many chronic health states, including diabetes and arthritis, not just psychiatric disorders. Box 11.6 lists some of the common reasons for nonadherence. Psychiatric–mental health nurses should be aware that a number of factors influence individuals to stop taking their medications.

The most often cited reasons for noncompliance are related to side effects of the medication. Improved functioning may be observed by health care professionals but not felt by the patient. Side effects may interfere with work performance or other important aspects of the individual's life. For example, a construction worker cannot afford to be drowsy and sedated while operating a crane at a construction site, and a woman in an intimate relationship may find anorgasmia intolerable. Nurses need to be sensitive to the patient's ability to tolerate side effects and to the impact that side effects have on the patient's life. Medication choice, dosing schedules, and prompt treatment of side effects may be crucial factors in helping patients to continue their treatment even if the symptoms for which they initially sought help have improved.

Cognitive deficits associated with some psychiatric disorders may make it difficult for the individual to self-monitor, develop insight, make choices, remember to fill prescriptions, or keep appointments. Forgetfulness, cost, and confusion regarding dosage or timing may also contribute to noncompliance.

Family members may have similar difficulties that influence the individual not to take the medication. They may misunderstand or deny the illness, thinking, for example, "My wife's better, so she doesn't need that medicine anymore." Family members may be distressed when observable side effects occur. Adherence concerns must not be dismissed as the patient's or family's problem.

Psychiatric nurses should actively address this issue. A positive therapeutic relationship between the nurse and patient and family must provide a strong sense of trust that side effects and other difficulties in treatment will be addressed and minimized. When individuals report experiencing distressing side effects, the nurse should immediately respond with assessment and interventions to reduce these effects. It is important to assess compliance often, asking questions in a nonthreatening, nonjudgmental manner. It also may be helpful to seek information from others who are involved with the patient.

Adherence can be improved by psychoeducation. This approach is most helpful if it addresses the individual's specific symptoms and concerns. For example, if the patient is having difficulty with understanding the purpose of the medication, it may be helpful to link taking it to reduction of specific unwanted symptoms or improved functioning, such as continuing to work. Family members should also be included in these discussions.

Other factors that interfere with adherence should also be assessed and plans developed to minimize their effect. For example, an individual who is being considered for clozapine therapy may have missed a number of appointments in the past. On assessment, the nurse may discover that it takes the individual 2 hours on three different buses each way to reach the clinic. The nurse can then assist with arranging for a home health nurse to visit the patient's apartment, draw blood samples for analysis, and assess side effects, thus decreasing the number of trips the patient must make to the clinic.

SUMMARY OF KEY POINTS

- Target symptoms and side effects of medications should be clearly identified. The FDA approves the use of medications for specific disorders and symptoms.

- Psychiatric medications primarily act on CNS receptors, ion channels, enzymes, and carrier proteins. Agonists mimic the action of a specific neurotransmitter; antagonists block the response.

- A drug's ability to interact with a given receptor type depends on three qualities: selectivity—the ability to interact with specific receptors while not affecting other tissues and organs; affinity—the degree of strength of the bond between drug and receptor; and intrinsic activity—the ability to produce a certain biologic response.

- Pharmacokinetics refers to how the human body processes the drug, including absorption, distribution, metabolism, and excretion. Bioavailability describes the amount of the drug that actually reaches circulation throughout the body. The wide variations in the way each individual processes any medication often are related to physiologic differences caused by age, genetic makeup, other disease processes, and chemical interactions.

■ Antipsychotic medications are drugs used in treating patients with psychotic disorders, such as schizophrenia. They act primarily by blocking dopamine or serotonin postsynaptically. In addition, they have a number of actions on other neurotransmitters. Older typical antipsychotic drugs work on positive symptoms and are inexpensive but produce many side effects. Newer atypical antipsychotic drugs work on positive and negative symptoms and are much more expensive but have far fewer side effects and are better tolerated by patients.

■ Medication-related movement disorders are a particularly serious group of side effects that principally occur with the typical antipsychotic medications and that may be acute syndromes, such as dystonia, pseudoparkinsonism, and akathisia, or chronic syndromes, such as tardive dyskinesia.

■ The mood stabilizers, or antimania medications, are drugs used to control wide variations in mood related to mania, but these agents may also be used to treat patients with other disorders. Lithium and the anticonvulsants are chemically unrelated and act in different ways to stabilize mood.

■ Antidepressant medications are drugs used primarily for treating symptoms of depression. They act by blocking reuptake of one or more of the bioamines, especially serotonin and norepinephrine. These medications vary considerably in their structure and action. Newer antidepressants, such as the SSRIs, have fewer side effects and are less lethal in overdose than the older TCAs.

■ Antianxiety medications also include several subgroups of medications, but the benzodiazepines and nonbenzodiazepines are those principally used in psychiatry. The benzodiazepines act by enhancing the effects of GABA, and the nonbenzodiazepine buspirone acts on serotonin. Benzodiazepines can be used on a PRN basis, but buspirone, the one available nonbenzodiazepine, must be taken regularly.

■ Psychostimulants enhance neurotransmitter activity, acting at a number of sites in the nerves. These medications are most often used for treating symptoms related to ADHD and narcolepsy.

■ ECT uses the application of an electrical pulsation to induce seizures in the brain. These seizures produce a number of effects on neurotransmission that result in the rapid relief of depressive symptoms.

■ rTMS and VNS are two emerging somatic treatments for psychiatric disorders. They are both means to directly affect brain function through stimulation of the nerves that are direct extensions of the brain.

■ Phototherapy involves the application of full-spectrum light, in the morning hours, which appears to reset circadian rhythm delays related to seasonal affective disorder and other forms of depression. Nutritional therapies are in various stages of investigation.

■ Adherence refers to the ability of an individual to self-administer medications as prescribed and to follow other instructions related to medication treatment. It can be full, partial, or nil. Nonadherence is related to factors such as medication side effects, stigma, and family influences. Nurses play a key role in educating patients and helping them to improve adherence.

CRITICAL THINKING CHALLENGES

1. Discuss how you would go about identifying the target symptoms for a specific patient for the following medications: antipsychotic, antidepressant, and antianxiety drugs.

2. Track the approval process from identification of a potential substance to marketing a medication. Compare at least three psychiatric medications that are in phase III trials (hint: www.FDA.gov).

3. Obtain the PIs for the three atypical antipsychotics, two SSRIs, and one SNRI. Compare their boxed warnings, pharmacodynamics, pharmacokinetics, indications, side effects, and dosages.

4. Compare the oral and IM dose of lorazepam. Why are these doses similar?

5. Mr. J. has schizophrenia and was just prescribed an antipsychotic. His family wants to know the risk–benefits of the medication. How would you answer?

6. Identify the CYP450 enzyme that metabolizes the following medications: risperidone, olanzapine, quetiapine, clozapine, fluoxetine, venlafaxine, trazodone, nefazodone, and bupropion.

7. Find the four medications or substances that induce or inhibit the following CYP450 enzymes: 2D6, 2C19, 3A4, and 1A2.

8. Obtain the PI for clozapine, risperidone, quetiapine, and Risperdal Consta. Compare the half-lives of each drug. Discuss the relationship of the drug's half-life to the dosing schedule. When is steady state reached in each of these medications?

9. Explain the health problems associated with anticholinergic side effects of the antipsychotic medications.

10. Compare the type of movements that characterize tardive dyskinesia with those that characterize akathisia and dystonia and explore which one is easier for a patient to experience.

11. One patient is prescribed the MAOI Emsam, 6 mg per day, and another is taking another MAOI, Nardil, 15 mg per day. Are the dietary restrictions different?

12. A patient who is taking an MAOI asks you to explain what will happen if she eats pizza. Prepare a short teaching intervention beginning with the action of the medication and its consequences.

13. Explain how your nursing care would be different for a male patient taking lithium carbonate than for a female patient.

14. Patient A is taking valproic acid (Depakote) for mood stabilization, and patient B is taking lamotrigine (Lamictal). After comparing notes with each other, they ask you why patient A has to have drug blood levels and patient B does not. How are these two drugs alike? How are they different?

15. Two patients are getting their blood drawn. One patient is getting lithium and the other clozapine. What laboratory tests are being ordered?

16. A patient who is depressed has been started on sertraline. During the assessment, she tells you that she is also taking SJW, lecithin, and a multiple vitamin. What is your next step?

17. Compare different approaches that you might use with a patient with schizophrenia who has decided to stop taking his or her medication because of intolerance to side effects.

References

Beach, S. R., Celano, C. M., Noseworthy, P. A., Januzzi, J. L., & Huffman, J. C. (2013). QTc prolongation, torsades de pointes, and psychotropic medications. (Review). *Psychosomatics, 54*(1), 1–13.

Bialer, M. (2012). Why are antiepileptic drugs used for nonepileptic conditions? *Epilepsia,* 53(suppl 7), 26–33.

Bunchorntavakul, C., & Reddy, K. R. (2013). Review article: Herbal and dietary supplement hepatotoxicity. *Alimentary Pharmacology & Therapeutics, 37*(1), 3–17.

Cephalon. (2013). *Nuvigil (armodafinil) tablets.* Retrieved from http://www.nuvigil.com/PDF/Full_Prescribing_Information.pdf

Copinschi, G., & Caufriez, A. (2013). Sleep and hormonal changes in aging. (Review). *Endocrinology and Metabolism Clinics of North America, 42*(2), 371–389.

Fisher, P. M., Madsen, M. K., Mc Mahon, B., Holst, K. K., Andersen, S. B., Laursen, H. R., et al. (2013). Three-Week Bright-Light Intervention Has Dose-Related Effects on Threat-Related Corticolimbic Reactivity and Functional Coupling. *Biological Psychiatry, 19* pii: S0006–3223(13)01102–01105. doi:10.1016/j.biopsych.2013.11.031

Glassock, R. J. (2009). The GFR decline with aging: A sign of normal senescence, not disease. *Nephrology Times, 9*(2), 6–8.

GlaxoSmithKline. (2013). Wellbutrin Prescribing Information. www.wellbutrin.com

Kirsch, D. L., & Nichols, F. (2013). Cranial electrotherapy stimulation for treatment of anxiety, depression, and insomnia. *Psychiatric Clinics of North America, 36*(1), 169–176.

Laoutidis, Z. G., & Luckhaus, C. (2014). 5-HT2A receptor antagonists for the treatment of neuroleptic-induced akathisia: A systematic review and meta-analysis. *International Journal of Neuropsychopharmacology, 17*(5), 823–832.

Lopez, O. L., Becker, J. T., Chang, Y. F., Sweet, R. A., Aizenstein, H., Snitz, B., et al. (2013). The long-term effects of conventional and atypical antipsychotics in patients with probable Alzheimer's Disease. *The American Journal of Psychiatry, 170*(9), 1051–1058.

Malhi, G. S., Tanious, M., Das, P., Coulston, C. M., & Berk, M. (2013). Potential mechanisms of action of lithium in bipolar disorder. Current understanding. *CNS Drugs, 27*(2), 135–153.

Modabbernia, A., & Akhondzadeh, S. (2013). Saffron, passionflower, valerian and sage for mental health. *The Psychiatric Clinics of North America, 36*(1), 85–91.

Novartis. (2013). *Clozaril (prescribing information).* Retrieved from http://www.clozaril.com.

Preskorn, S. H., Kane, C. P., Lobello, K., Nichols, A. L., Fayyad, R., Buckley, G., et al. (2013). Cytochrome P450 2D6 phenoconversion is common in patients being treated for depression: Implications for personalized medicine. *The Journal of Clinical Psychiatry, 74*(6), 614–621.

Qureshi, M. A., & Al-Bedah, A. M. (2013). Mood disorders and complementary and alternative medicine: A literature review. *Neuropsychiatric Disease and Treatment, 9,* 639–658. doi:10.2147/NDT.S43419

Rajagopal, R., Chakrabarti, S., & Grover, S. (2013). Satisfaction with electroconvulsive therapy among patients and their relatives. *The Journal of ECT, 29*(4), 283–290.

Sarris, J. (2013). St. John's wort for the treatment of psychiatric disorders. *The Psychiatric Clinics of North America, 36*(1), 65–72.

Silva, H. (2013). Ethnopsychopharmacology and pharmacogenomics. *Advances in Psychosomatic Medicine, 33,* 88–96.

Stahl, S. M. (2013). *Stahl's essential psychopharmacology* (4th ed.). New York: Cambridge University Press.

Tayebati, S. K., & Amenta, F. (2013). Choline-containing phospholipids: Relevance to brain functional pathways. (Review). *Clinical Chemistry and Laboratory Medicine, 51*(3), 513–521.

Teh, L. K., & Bertilsson, L. (2012). Pharmacogenomics of CYP2D6: Molecular genetics, interethnic differences and clinical importance. A review. *Drug, Metabolism and Pharmacokinetics, 27*(1), 55–67.

Wani, A., Trevino, K., Marnell, P., & Husain, M. M. (2013). Advances in brain stimulation for depression. *Annals of Clinical Psychiatry, 25*(3), 217–224.

Wood, S., Sage, J. R., Shuman, T., & Anagnostaras, S. G. (2013). Psychostimulants and cognition: A continuum of behavioral and cognitive activation. *Pharmacological Reviews, 66*(1), 193–221.

Woods, S. W., Morgenstern, H., Saksa, J. R., Walsh, B. C., Sullivan, M. C., Money, R., et al. (2010). Incidence of tardive dyskinesia with atypical versus conventional antipsychotic medications: A prospective cohort study. *The Journal of Clinical Psychiatry, 71*(4), 463–474.

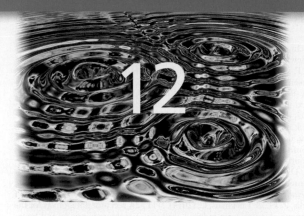

12

Cognitive Interventions

Jeanne A. Clement

KEY CONCEPTS

- cognitive behavioral therapy
- rational emotive behavior therapy
- solution-focused therapy

LEARNING OBJECTIVES

After studying this chapter, you will be able to:

1. Discuss the history of cognitively based therapeutic interventions.
2. Identify the concepts underlying cognitive interventions.
3. Discuss three forms of cognitively based therapies.
4. Apply cognitive interventions in a clinical setting.
5. Describe the contexts in which psychiatric nurses use cognitive interventions.

KEY TERMS

- ABCDE • activating event • belief system • cognitions • cognitive interventions • cognitive triad
- cognitive distortions • compliments • dysfunctional consequences • exception questions
- functional consequences • miracle questions • relationship questions • scaling questions • schema

Psychiatric nurses use evidence-based cognitive interventions in a variety of practice settings (inpatient and outpatient). The knowledge and skills inherent in cognitively based interventions have been extensively studied and their effectiveness has been demonstrated for a variety of psychiatric disorders, especially depression (see Chapter 24) and anxiety disorders (see Chapter 26). **Cognitive interventions** are based on the concept of cognition. **Cognition** can be defined as an internal process of perception, memory, and judgment through which an understanding of self and the world is developed. Cognitive interventions aim to change or reframe an individual's automatic thought patterns that have developed over time and which interfere with the individual's ability to function optimally. The skills and techniques that were developed on the basis of cognitive theory result in a new view of self and the environment.

Cognitive interventions had their beginnings in the long-term inpatient environment, but today they are a mainstay of psychiatric care in all settings and are used by all disciplines and at all levels of practice. Evidence from a number of studies, reinforced by meta-analysis of groups in the past decade, supports the use of cognitive therapies with a wide variety of psychological and psychiatric conditions, and it has been shown to be effective with diverse individuals in diverse settings (Hopper et al., 2013; Hunot et al., 2013). Cognitive therapies are incorporating additional therapeutic modalities such as mindfulness and targeting for persons with anxiety and depressive disorders (Hofman, Asmundson, & Beck, 2013). The current chapter explains the theoretical perspectives and application of cognitive interventions.

DEVELOPMENT OF COGNITIVE THERAPIES

Cognitive therapy was first developed and implemented in the 1950s by Albert Ellis (1913–2007), a psychologist, who was uncomfortable with the nondirective Freudian and neo-Freudian approaches. According to Ellis, cognition, emotions, and behavior are integrated and holistic. From the 1950s until his death, Ellis continued to develop and refine his theory and therapeutic approach into what he calls rational emotive behavior therapy (Ellis, Abrams, & Abrams, 2008).

Beginning in the 1960s, other cognitively based theories and therapeutic approaches were developed, the most prominent being cognitive behavioral therapy (CBT) by Aaron Beck (see Chapter 7) (Beck, 2008). Steven de Shazer (1940–2005) and Insoo Kim Berg (1934–1997) developed solution-focused brief therapy (SFBT), an approach that is useful with persons who have diagnoses such as depression, obsessive–compulsive disorder (OCD), schizophrenia, and other psychiatric disorders (de Shazer, Dolan, Korman, Trepper, McCollum, & Berg, 2007; Laaksonen, Knekt, Sares-Jaske, & Lindfors, 2013). All of these models will be discussed in the current chapter.

COGNITIVE THERAPY MODELS

Psychiatric nurses have found that cognitive approaches are congruent with the standards of practice and are particularly effective in challenging care environments. Brief cognitive therapies offer approaches that can be applied within the therapeutic patient–nurse relationship and the nursing process. Patients undergoing cognitively based psychotherapy are frequently treated by an interdisciplinary team that supports this approach.

Cognitive Behavioral Therapy

> **KEYCONCEPT** Cognitive behavioral therapy (CBT) is a highly structured psychotherapeutic method used to alter distorted beliefs and problem behaviors by identifying and replacing negative inaccurate thoughts and changing the rewards for behaviors.

In CBT, the relationship between thoughts, feelings, and behavior are examined and identified. CBT operates on the following assumptions:

- People are disturbed not by an event but by the perception of that event.
- Whenever and however a belief develops, the individual believes it.
- Work and practice can modify beliefs that create difficulties in living.

Figure 12.1 depicts the interaction of individual experiences, perception of these experiences, and the unique thoughts attached to these experiences that influence the development of beliefs (functional or dysfunctional). The person develops an explanation of their relationship to their environment and to other people from these beliefs. Dysfunctional thinking develops from a variety of human experiences and can become the predominant way the

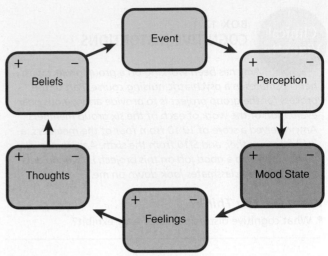

FIGURE 12.1 Model of perception, thoughts, and mood states: the cycle of cognition.

world is viewed. To quote from Shakespeare's *Hamlet,* "For there is nothing either good or bad but thinking makes it so."

Thoughts have a powerful effect on emotion and behavior. By changing dysfunctional thinking, a person can alter their emotional reaction to a situation and reinterpret the meaning of an event. That is, by identifying, analyzing, and changing thoughts and behaviors that are counterproductive, feelings such as helplessness, anxiety, and depression can be reduced. The goal of CBT is to restructure how a person perceives events in his or her life to facilitate behavioral and emotional change.

Cognitive Processes

Three cognitive processes are involved in the development of common mental disorders such as depression. These processes include the cognitive triad, cognitive distortions, and schema.

The **cognitive triad** includes thoughts about oneself, the world, and the future. Accumulation of thoughts about oneself is reflected in spoken and unspoken beliefs and moods that grow out of these beliefs. Emotions and behavior reflect the strength of the accumulated beliefs. Dysfunctional thoughts about the self are usually overly negative or overly positive whereas functional thoughts more closely reflect the reality of the perceived situation. For example, one student has the belief that learning is very difficult for him and that he will fail the examination no matter how hard he studies. He does not study for the examination because he believes that he will fail anyway. A second student believes that she is very bright, understands the material, and does not need to study. She attends a concert the night before the test. A third student believes that he has a grasp of the material to be

Clinical Vignette

BOX 12.1
COGNITIVE DISTORTIONS

Amy has been working on a group project with her classmates in a psychiatric nursing course. Part of the process for the group project is to provide anonymous peer evaluation of the work of each of the six group members. Amy received a score of 10/10 from four of the members, a 7/10 from another, and 5/10 from the sixth. Amy thinks, "I guess I didn't do a good job on this project. I never do anything right. My classmates look down on me."

What Do You Think?
• What cognitive distortions does Amy exhibit?

covered on the test but ensures this by studying notes and the text before the examination. The first two students fail the examination. Failure for the first student reinforces the dysfunctional belief that no matter what, he will fail. The second student argues that the test was unfair, which also reinforces her dysfunctional belief that she is bright and understands the material. The third student earned a good grade. His functional thoughts and behaviors are also reinforced.

Students one and two above both hold distinctive views that are not supported by empirical evidence but are generated automatically in response to a given situation. These automatic thoughts are called **cognitive distortions** and are generated by organizing distorted information and/or inaccurate interpretation of a situation. Cognitive distortions or "twisted thinking" occur in a variety of ways; however, there are some common distortions (Burns, 2008) (see Box 12.1).

Schema are the individual's life rules that act as a sieve or filter. They allow only information compatible with the internal picture of self and the world to be brought to the person's awareness. Schema develop in early childhood and become relatively fixed by middle childhood. They are the accumulation of both learning and experience from the individual's genetic makeup, family and school environments, peer relationships, and society as a whole. Ethnicity, culture, gender, and religious affiliation influence schema development. In addition, the age of the individual at the time a given event occurs, the persons or circumstances involved influence how that event is perceived and the relative strength of that influence. In the example, student number one believes that he is not intelligent. This belief could have initiated in early childhood if the student was constantly unfavorably compared with an older sibling. This schema increases vulnerability in a host of interpersonal situations, particularly those that relate to scholarly endeavors. Student number two was overly praised by parents and other relatives and developed a schema of being more accomplished than most.

Implementing Cognitive Behavioral Therapy

The use of CBT is based on a collaborative therapeutic relationship in which a mutual trust develops through promoting patients' strengths and control over their own lives. CBT assumes that individuals have the innate ability to solve their own problems; thus, the overarching treatment goal is for the patient to be able to engage in self-care, independent of professional assistance.

In CBT, goals are developed in partnership and supply a forward-looking focus for what "can be" in the future as opposed to "what happened" in the past. The present serves as a platform from which current perceptions of earlier events can be reexamined. Movement toward goals is facilitated by strategies designed to engage the patient in the service of their own mental health. Strategies emerge when nurse and patient develop a working conceptualization of the issue or problem as the patient sees it. The nurse educates the patient about the therapeutic approach. An agenda is mutually established for each therapeutic interaction. Techniques that focus on both cognition and behavior are used to promote patient growth.

Engagement and Assessment

The first step in CBT is engagement and assessment. In this phase, the therapist establishes rapport with the patient and develops the theme that problems are manageable. The patient's definition of the problem that brought him or her into treatment is explored through a series of open-ended questions. A problem list is developed and reframed into manageable goals that are prioritized. The prioritized list forms the agenda for the treatment plan and structures the content of each individual session. A contract is developed for a number of sessions (frequently 10 to 12). The therapist seeks information about the patient's strengths and successes on which to base re-examination and reframing of negative beliefs and to design interventions. During all sessions the therapist summarizes issues identified and develops homework assignments that enhance and expand the work done during the sessions.

Intervention Framework

Specific interventions used with CBT, in addition to the interaction that takes place in the therapy sessions, revolve around carefully crafted homework assignments that the patient works on in the time between sessions. Subsequently, sessions may be scheduled regularly once or twice a month. Typical homework assignments include evaluating the accuracy of automatic thoughts and beliefs.

It is important for the therapist to realize that the thoughts a person has about a problem are not beliefs. In CBT the therapist helps the patient identify the underlying belief, and then they

- explore the evidence that supports or refutes the belief about the event;
- identify alterative explanations for the event;
- examine the real implications if the belief is true (e.g., "What is the worst thing that could happen?").

In the sessions, the therapist challenges negative beliefs and helps the patient examine the "self-talk" that helps to sustain these beliefs. Cognitive techniques focus on the patient's patterns of automatic thinking, first identifying what they are by examining the patient's recurrent patterns in everyday life and then testing the validity of these automatic thoughts.

Other tools that are used to help change the patient's self-perception include bibliotherapy (the use of books that offer alternative thoughts and responses), journaling, and keeping a diary focused on emotional and behavioral responses to upsetting situations that documents small changes that might otherwise go unnoticed. The patient is also encouraged to make note of positive events and positive thoughts about themselves and their ability to cope with negative events. These positive thoughts and effective coping responses are reinforced in interactions with the therapist. As goals are developed at the beginning of each therapy session, the last few minutes are spent reviewing the progress toward the goals for that day.

Evaluation and Termination

Evaluation and termination begins with the original contract when patient and therapist determined the number of sessions. The patient's progress toward treatment goals is continually evaluated, and the patient is urged to become more self-reliant and independent. As progress is never a continuous upward process, therapists prepare the patient for setbacks by acknowledging that setbacks are normal and expected and crafting ways in which the patient can deal with them. It is not uncommon for the time between sessions to lengthen as the final session approaches. At the final session, the use of "booster" sessions is discussed, and frequently a session is scheduled in 6 months to do a quick "check-up" and review continuing progress.

Strengths and Limitations of Cognitive Behavioral Therapy

One of the strengths of CBT lies in the body of empirical evidence supporting the effectiveness of these interventions (Antoniades, Mazza, & Brijnath, 2014; Nordgren

et al., 2014). Many studies show positive, sustained improvement in people treated with this form of intervention. Critics, however, identify some limitations. Chief among the limitations identified is the concern that the therapeutic relationship, long believed to be the main factor in patient improvement, may be forgotten in the rigid adherence to specific techniques. Others believe that change is dependent on the patient developing a clear understanding of their belief system and the origin of that system; thus, CBT is not effective with persons who have thought disorders and other issues that interfere with the ability to do so.

Rational Emotive Behavior Therapy

> **KEYCONCEPT** Rational emotive behavior therapy (REBT) is a psychotherapeutic approach that proposes that unrealistic and irrational beliefs cause many emotional problems. It is a form of CBT with a primary emphasis on changing irrational beliefs that cause emotional distress into thoughts that are more reasonable and rational.

REBT is based on the assumptions that people are born with the potential to be rational (self-constructive) and irrational (self-defeating). Ellis believes that highly cognitive, active, directive homework assignments, and structured therapies are likely to be more effective in a shorter time than other therapies. Irrational thinking, self-damaging habituations, wishful thinking, and intolerance are exacerbated by culture and family groups (Ellis et al., 2008).

Rational Emotive Behavior Therapy Framework

The basic framework for REBT uses the acronym ABCDE (see Box 12.2).

The **activating event** may be either external or internal and not necessarily an actual event, but it may also be an emotion or a thought/expectation. For example, a person who is lonely and feels isolated but is uncomfortable in interpersonal situations may see a flyer advertising a

---

BOX 12.2

The Rational Emotive Behavior Therapy Framework

A Activating event that triggers automatic thoughts and emotions
B Beliefs that underlie the thoughts and emotions
C Consequences of this automatic process
D Dispute or challenge unreasonable expectations
E Effective outlook developed by disputing or challenging negative belief systems

gathering of people who are interested in discussing solutions to global warming and would really like to attend (**A**ctivating event). However, when this person thinks about going to the gathering he imagines going into the room where he does not know anybody and someone coming up to him and trying to engage him in conversation. His imagination provides a picture of not being able to respond and leaving the room after suffering great embarrassment (**B**elief system: "I am a failure in social situations, and everybody can see what a loser I am."). Of course, he decides not to go (**C**onsequences of his belief system).

Belief systems are shaped by rationality, which is self-constructive, and irrationality, which is self-defeating. Rational beliefs are flexible and lead to reasonable evaluations of negative activating events. For example, after a low grade on an examination, instead of believing "I am stupid" or "that instructor is out to get me," student might conclude that "I earned a low grade on the test; I really need to work to develop a better understanding of the content," or "I think I need to get help with my test-taking skills." Other rational beliefs might be "I really didn't have time to study; so I can accept this grade and just move on." In other words, "I don't like it, but I can live with it." Rational beliefs accept that human beings are fallible and reject absolutes such as always and never.

Irrational beliefs promote dysfunctional negative emotions that in turn lead to psychic pain and discomfort. Behaviors directed at relief of this pain tend to be self-defeating: "I can't fight the system; I will never succeed in this class." There are five themes common in irrational beliefs:

1. A demand: "This *must* happen."
2. Absolute thinking: "All or nothing at all."
3. Catastrophizing: exaggerating negative consequences of an event.
4. Low frustration tolerance: everything should be easy.
5. Global evaluations of human worth: "People can be rated and some are better than others."

Dysfunctional consequences of the interaction between A (activating event) and B (belief system) follow from absolute, rigid, and irrational beliefs whereas **functional consequences** follow from flexible and rational beliefs. For example, demands about self based on "musts" reinforce dysfunctional beliefs such as: "I must do well and be approved by significant others, and if I'm not, then it's awful." The consequences of these beliefs are often anxiety, depression, shame, and guilt that lead to the inability to develop or achieve life's goals or to develop satisfying interpersonal relationships. Self-regard that is dependent on the approval of others demands that others "treat me fairly and considerately; it's terrible I can't bear it when you don't." Thus, when fairness and consideration is not forthcoming, passive-aggressiveness, anger, rage, and violence may erupt. Demands that the world or life be exactly as one wants can also lead to self-pity as well as problems of self-discipline and addictive behaviors.

Rational Emotive Behavior Therapy Interventions

REBT uses role-playing, assertion training, desensitization, humor, operant conditioning, suggestion, support, and other interventions. According to Ellis, there are two basic forms of REBT: general and preferential. General REBT is synonymous with CBT and teaches patients rational and healthy behavior. Preferential REBT includes general REBT but also emphasizes a profound philosophic change. It teaches patients how to dispute irrational ideas and unhealthy behaviors and to become more creative, scientific, and skeptical thinkers (Ellis et al., 2008). The therapist uses the ABCDE model in a structured manner (Box 12.2). A major challenge for the therapist is to teach the patient the difference between thoughts and beliefs. Automatic thoughts are not irrational beliefs but are inferences about the belief. The focus of interventions during the therapy sessions (frequently several weeks or months apart) is on developing rational beliefs to replace those that are irrational and interfere with the patient's quality of life. Figure 12.2 examines the sequence of treatment used in REBT.

Solution-Focused Brief Therapy

KEYCONCEPT   **Solution-focused brief therapy (SFBT)** focuses on solutions rather than problems. This approach does not challenge the existence of problems but proposes that problems are best understood in relation to their solutions. Solution-focused therapy assists the client in exploring life without the problem (Miller & Berg, 1995).

SFBT, although basically a cognitive approach, differs in philosophy and approach from other cognitively based approaches. The primary difference is the de-emphasis on the patient's "problems," or symptoms, and an emphasis on what is functional and healthful. SFBT assists the patient in exploring life without the problem, and it asserts that what is expected to happen influences what the patient does. By discovering what future the client sees as worth striving for, the present becomes important to that future. Otherwise, there is no sense in the patient doing something different or in seeing something in a different light. Empirical evidence exists that supports the use of solution-focused approaches as a best practice (Kim, 2008).

Solution-focused theory views the patient as an individual with a collection of strengths and successes as

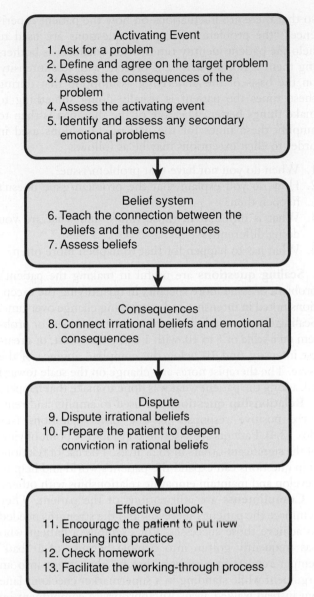

Activating Event
1. Ask for a problem
2. Define and agree on the target problem
3. Assess the consequences of the problem
4. Assess the activating event
5. Identify and assess any secondary emotional problems

Belief system
6. Teach the connection between the beliefs and the consequences
7. Assess beliefs

Consequences
8. Connect irrational beliefs and emotional consequences

Dispute
9. Dispute irrational beliefs
10. Prepare the patient to deepen conviction in rational beliefs

Effective outlook
11. Encourage the patient to put new learning into practice
12. Check homework
13. Facilitate the working-through process

FIGURE 12.2 Rational emotive behavior therapy sequence of treatment.

opposed to a diagnosis and collection of symptoms. Solution-focused approaches emphasize the uniqueness of the individual and their capacity to make changes or to deal with their day-to-day lives despite what may seem to be the predominant pathology (Iveson, 2002; Bond et al., 2014).

Solution-Focused Behavior Therapy Assumptions

SFBT assumes that change is constant and inevitable. Essentially, everyone changes constantly and is never the same from 1 minute to the next. A person interacts, if only in a minute way, with a constantly changing environment. Very small changes can lead to larger changes,

---

BOX 12.3

Solution-Focused Behavior Therapy Assumptions

1. People have the strengths and resources needed to solve their problems; therefore, the therapist's role is to recognize and emphasize these by amplifying them primarily through asking questions that enable a collaborative approach to co-constructing solutions.
2. It isn't necessary to know a lot about the complaint and its origins or functions in order to resolve it.
3. Define and dissect the "problem" from the perspective of the patient and look for exceptions to the "problem" in the patient's life.
4. Even long-standing issues can be resolved in a relatively short period of time.
5. There is no right or wrong way to see things.
6. Change is most likely to occur when the focus is on what is changeable.
7. The job of the therapist is to identify and amplify change and maintain a focus on the present and the future.
8. The therapist and patient cocreate reality, utilizing what the patient perceives is "truth," and develop small, concrete, specific, and reality-based goals that are realistic in the context of the patient's life.
9. The therapist expects change and movement and that expectation is inherent in the questions used and the attitude of the therapist.

Adapted from O'Hanlon, W. H., & Weiner-Davis, M. (1989). *In search of solutions: A new direction in psychotherapy.* New York: W. W. Norton.

---

and the stimulus to change comes from a variety of sources. Constant change and its "ripple effect" direct the strategies and interventions used by the therapist. Both assumptions and strategies point the patient toward a positive, future-oriented change. Box 12.3 lists the assumptions that underlie this approach.

Solution-Focused Behavior Therapy Interventions

In SFBT, the therapist takes a position of curiosity in learning about the patient, as opposed to an expert to whom the person has come to be helped. This curiosity is manifested in the questions and techniques that are integral to this approach and enable the development of realistic goals at each session. Questions used in eliciting the "problem" (frequently referred to as the "issue(s)" to avoid focusing on the "problem") seek very specific information. Examples of questioning in the initial session might include the following:

1. What brought you here today?
   What is going on that made you choose to seek help?
2. Give me a recent example of how that was demonstrated in your life.
3. Who was present when this happened? What did they say and do, and what did you say or do?
   And then what happened?

4. When does this kind of thing happen most often?
5. Where is it likely to occur?
6. Where is it least likely to occur?
7. Is there a particular time (of day, month, year) when this is **un**likely to happen?
8. How does this interfere with your life, your relationships, self-image, etc.?

If your spouse/significant other/coworker were here now, how would he or she say that you were trying to solve the issue or problem?

Interventions in SFBT focus on achievement of specific, concrete, and achievable goals developed in the collaboration between therapist and patient. These goals, formed using the patient's language, are specific and focus on strengths. Primary techniques used to facilitate progress toward goal attainment are skillfully crafted questions that include the use of the "miracle question," exceptions, scaling, relationship questions, as well as the use of feedback, with an emphasis on complimenting any small, goal-oriented change the patient makes. Feedback conveys to the patient that the therapist has listened carefully and recognizes that working toward a goal of change is difficult and requires hard work.

In **miracle questions**, the therapist structures a scenario that the patient is asked to think about carefully (even though it sounds strange) and to use their imagination in crafting the response, again to very specific questions (see Box 12.4 for a sample scenario and questions).

Other ways of facilitating a similar focus on what the solution would look like are to ask the patient to keep track of what goes well in their life that he or she would like to see happen again. The patient is encouraged to keep a written list of what they have noticed and bring it to the next session.

Exception questions are rooted in the belief that nothing is constantly present at the same level of intensity, so that there are fluctuations on how the patient experiences "the problem." Exception questions are used to help the patient identify times when whatever is bothering them is not present or is present with less intensity, on the basis of the underlying assumption that during these times the patient is usually doing something to make things better. The role of the therapist is then to amplify these times for the patient. Questions used in order to elicit exceptions may be as follows:

1. When do you not have that problem/issue?
2. How do you explain that the problem/issue doesn't happen then?
3. What is different in those times, and what are you doing differently?
4. What has to happen for that to happen more often?

Scaling questions are useful in making the patient's problem or issue more specific, in quantifying the exceptions noted in intensity, and in tracking change over time. Scaling questions ask the patient to rate the issue or problem on a scale of 1 to 10, with 1 being the worst, or greatest intensity, and 10 being the complete absence of the issue. The therapist notes any change on the scale toward 10, asking the patient what was done to make that happen.

Relationship questions are used to amplify and reinforce positive responses to the other questions (see Box 12.4). Patients are asked to consider the point of view of the significant others in their lives. The use of relationship questions can expand the patient's world and help to develop and maintain empathic relationships with others.

Compliments are affirmations of the patient. They reinforce the patient's successes and the strengths needed to achieve those successes. For example, a patient who has frequently gotten into trouble because of a "bad" temper reports in a session that he almost got into an argument while standing in a supermarket checkout lane but instead walked away. An appropriate compliment by the therapist might be "Wow! That's great. That must have been very difficult for you." Compliments can create hope in the patient.

> **NCLEXNOTE** Application of knowledge from the social sciences such as psychology will underlie many of the psychosocial questions. Familiarity with the basic cognitive therapy models will strengthen the application of these concepts to patient situations.

USE OF COGNITIVE THERAPIES IN PSYCHIATRIC NURSING

The context of practice has changed considerably for psychiatric nurses. Length of stay for patients in inpatient settings is becoming shorter every year. The patients admitted to inpatient settings are acutely ill and dealing

---

BOX 12.4

Miracle Questions

"I want you to pretend that tonight after you go to bed and are sound asleep a miracle occurs. The miracle is that the issues that have been bothering you and interfering in your life disappear. Since you have been asleep, you are not aware that the miracle has occurred when you wake up in the morning."

1. What would be your first clue that something was different for you?
2. How will your life be different?
3. What will you be doing instead of _____?
4. How will you be doing this?
5. Beside yourself, who will be the first to notice that there is something different about you?
6. What will that person say or do?
7. How will you respond differently than you might if the issue or problem was still present?

with more complex issues than ever before. More psychiatric care occurs in prisons than in psychiatric hospitals. More and more the focus of practice is in the community, private homes, and primary care settings rather than in specialty hospitals.

Inpatient Settings

Solution-focused therapy is one of the brief cognitive therapies used by psychiatric nurses in acute inpatient psychiatric settings. SFBT's emphasis on strengths fits well with the values of psychiatric nurses, and the techniques used are well within their scope of practice (Hagen & Mitchell, 2001). Solution-focused approaches have been effective with hospitalized people who were experiencing delusions, hallucinations, and/or loosening of associations (see Box 12.5).

Other cognitive therapeutic techniques used in inpatient settings include journaling and "homework" assignments that focus on education about diagnoses and medications, as well as on group process. These interventions seem to work well in conjunction with shortened length of stay in inpatient settings.

Community Settings

In community settings, cognitive approaches are used in combination with a broad array of interpersonal, behavioral, educational, and pharmacological interventions.

In community and clinic settings, CBT is used within a holistic evaluation of patients that includes a complete health history and physical examination and evaluation of possible co-occurring disorders such as depression and alcohol and other drug use or abuse. In particular, the use of questioning such as that integral to solution-focused approaches elicits strengths in a relatively short time and can provide a means for the nurse to support positive coping. The focus on realistic goal development provides a means of evaluation of patient progress.

Home and primary care settings are also conducive to the implementation of cognitive techniques. Small, concrete, specific goals developed in a naturalistic setting such as the home can create significant change for the whole family. CBT and SFBT approaches are very useful in primary care settings where time with patients is very short. Goal setting, use of scaling questions, and compliments can be done in the course of a 15-minute interaction.

SUMMARY OF KEY POINTS

- Cognitive therapies have a long history in mental health care and have support as evidence-based interventions effective in several mental disorders.

- Psychiatric nurses use cognitive interventions in a variety of settings. Cognitive therapies serve as the framework for psychotherapy as well as interdisciplinary treatment.

- Cognitive behavioral therapy focuses on dysfunctional thinking through the examination of the cognitive triad, cognitive distortions, and schema.

- Rational emotive behavior therapy assumes that people are born with the tendency to be rational and irrational. Using the ABCDE framework, REBT focuses on identifying and changing irrational beliefs that lead to negative consequences.

- Solution-focused brief therapy identifies the possible solutions before addressing the problem.

CRITICAL THINKING CHALLENGES

1. Compare and contrast the three cognitive therapies in terms of assumptions and interventions.
2. A patient has recently been fired from her job, which is the third job that she has had within 1 year. She is depressed but denies suicidal thoughts. She tells you that she is a failure and can never get and keep a job. Discuss how CBT, REBT, and SFBT would view and treat this patient.
3. A nurse manager plans to use CBT as a theoretical model for an inpatient unit. Discuss the interventions that should be used on an inpatient unit that applies the CBT model.

BOX 12.5

Research for Best Practice: **Might Within Madness: Solution-Focused Therapy and Disordered-Thought Clients**

Hagen, B. F., & Mitchell, D. S. (2001) Might within the madness: Solution-focused therapy and thought disordered clients. Archives of Psychiatric Nursing, 15(2), 86–93.

THE QUESTION: Is it possible to use SFBT with persons with thought disorders?

METHODS: SFBT was tested with three persons with severe thought disorders.

FINDINGS: The authors found that these three persons could identify their problems, respond to scaling questions, identify exceptions, identify strengths, and use homework. The "miracle question" did not work well. SFBT worked for these individuals.

IMPLICATIONS FOR NURSING: The results of these case studies indicate that persons with thought disorders can use elements of SFBT.

References

Antoniades, J., Mazza, D., Brijnath, B. (2014). Efficacy of depression treatments for immigrant patients: results from a systematic review. *BMC Psychiatry, 14*(1), 176.

Beck, A. T. (2008). The evolution of the cognitive model of depression and its neurobiological correlates. *American Journal of Psychiatry, 165*(8), 969–977.

Bond, C., Woods, K., Humphrey, N., Symes, W., & Green, L. (2014). Practitioner review: The effectiveness of solution focused brief therapy with children and families: a systematic and critical evaluation of the literature from 1990–2010. *Journal of Child Psychology & Psychiatry, 54*(7), 707–723.

Burns, D. D. (2008). *Feeling good: The new mood therapy.* New York: Harper Collins.

de Shazer, S., Dolan, Y., Korman, H., Trepper, T. S., McCollum, E. E., & Berg, I. K. (2007). *More than miracles: The state of the art in solution focused brief therapy.* New York: Haworth.

Ellis, A., Abrams, M. & Abrams, L. D. (2008). *Personality theories: Critical perspectives.* New York: Sage.

Hagen, B. F., & Mitchell, D. S. (2001). Might within the madness: Solution-focused therapy and thought disordered clients. *Archives of Psychiatric Nursing, 15*(2), 86–93.

Hofmann, S. G., Asmundson, G. J., & Beck, A. T. (2013). The science of cognitive therapy. *Behavior Therapy, 44*(2), 199–212.

Hopper, T., Bourgeois, M., Pimentel, J., Qualis, C. D., Hickey, E., Frymark, T., et al. (2013). An evidence-based systematic review on cognitive interventions for individuals with dementia. *American Journal of Speech-Language Pathology, 22*(1), 126–145.

Hunot, V., Moore, T. H., Caldwell, D. M., Furukawa, T. A., Davies, P., Jones, H., et al. (2013). "Third wave" cognitive and behavioural therapies versus other psychological therapies for depression (Review). *Cochrane Database of Systematic Reviews, 10,* CD008704. doi:10.1002/14651858. CD008704.pub2.

Iveson, C. (2002). Solution-focused brief therapy. *Advances in Psychiatric Treatment, 8,* 149–157.

Kim, J. S., (2008). Examining the effectiveness of solution-focused brief therapy: A meta-analysis. *Research on Social Work Practice, 1*(2), 107–116.

Laaksonen, M. A., Knekt, P., Sares-Jaske, L, & Lindfors, O. (2013). Psychological predictors on the outcome of short-term psychodynamic psychotherapy and solution-focused therapy in the treatment of mood and anxiety disorder. *European Psychiatry, 28*(2), 117–124.

Miller, S. D., & Berg, I. K. (1995). *The miracle method: A radically new approach to problem drinking.* New York: Norton.

Nordgren, L. B., Hedman, E., Etienne, J., Bodin, J, Kadowaki A., Eriksson, S, Lindkvist E., Andersson G., & Carlbring P. (2014). Effectiveness and cost-effectiveness of individually tailored Internet-delivered cognitive behavior therapy for anxiety disorders in a primary care population: a randomized controlled trial. *Behaviour Research & Therapy, 2*(59C), 1–11.

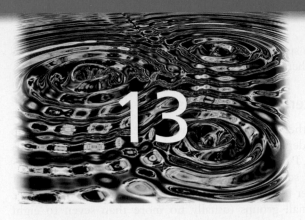

13

Group Interventions

Mary Ann Boyd

KEY CONCEPTS

- group
- group dynamics
- group process

LEARNING OBJECTIVES

After studying this chapter, you will be able to:

1. Discuss concepts used in leading groups.

2. Compare the roles that group members can assume.

3. Identify important aspects of leading a group, such as member selection, leadership skills, seating arrangements,

and ways of dealing with challenging behaviors of group members.

4. Identify types of groups: psychoeducation, supportive therapy, psychotherapy, and self-help.

5. Describe common nursing intervention groups.

KEY TERMS

- closed group • cohesion • co-leadership • communications pathways • direct leadership • dyad • formal group roles • group themes • groupthink • indirect leadership • individual roles • informal group roles • maintenance roles • open group • task roles • triad

---

Group interventions are a key nursing strategy in mental health promotion and recovery. A group experience can help an individual enhance self-understanding, conquer unwanted thoughts and feelings, and learn new behaviors. In a group, members learn from each other as well as the leader. Group interventions are efficient because several patients can participate at one time, and they can be used in most settings. Groups can vary in purpose from being a social group attending a local ball game to an intensive psychotherapy group. Although a family can also be considered a group, family interventions are discussed separately in Chapter 14.

> **KEYCONCEPT** A **group** is two or more people who develop interactive relationships and share at least one common goal or issue. *A group is more than the sum of its parts.* A group develops its own personality, patterns of interaction, and rules of behavior.

Nurses in various roles and settings may use group interventions, such as when conducting patient education or leading support groups. This chapter discusses group concepts, considerations in group leadership, and types of groups that nurses commonly lead.

PREPARING TO LEAD A GROUP

Psychiatric nurses lead a wide range of groups (see later discussion of Types of Groups). Some are structured such as a psychoeducation group, and others are unstructured (e.g., a social group). The purpose of the group will dictate the amount of structure and types of activities. In all groups, nurses maintain professional boundaries. Because some group activities are social in nature (unit parties, community trips), it is easy to forget that socialization is a treatment intervention. Nurses should avoid meeting personal social needs within this context (Box 13.1).

BOX 13.1
Using Reflection

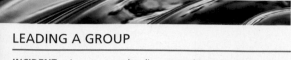

LEADING A GROUP

INCIDENT • A nurse was leading a smoking cessation group that was discussing substitute activities for smoking triggers. One of the participants asked the nurse how she spent her leisure time. The nurse described, in detail, a weekend trip to the mountains.

REFLECTION • Upon reflection, she realized that she was meeting her needs by sharing an enjoyable trip with others. She realized that she should have briefly answered the question and then redirected the discussion to the group members.

Thoughtful planning and preparation make for a successful group. The following sections discuss important considerations when planning for a group.

Selecting Members

Individuals can self-refer or be referred to a group by treatment teams or clinicians, but the leader is responsible for assessing each individual's suitability for the group. In instances when a new group is forming, the leader assesses the individual's suitability for the group based on the following criteria:

- Does the purpose of the group match the needs of the potential member?
- Does the potential member have the social skills to function comfortably in the group?
- Will the other group members accept the new group member?
- Can the potential member make a commitment to attending group meetings?

Forming an Open or Closed Group

In planning for a group, one of the early decisions is whether the group will be open or closed. In an **open group**, new members may join, and old members may leave the group at different sessions. Because length of patient hospitalization is relatively short, open groups are typical on inpatient units. For example, a newly admitted patient may join an anger management group that is part of an ongoing program in an inpatient unit.

In a **closed group**, members begin the group at one time, and no new members are admitted. If a member leaves, no replacement member joins. In a closed group, participants get to know one another very well and can develop close relationships. Closed groups are more typical of outpatient groups that have a sequential curriculum or psychotherapy groups. These groups usually meet weekly for a specified period. Outpatient smoking cessation, psychotherapy, and psychoeducation groups are examples.

Determining Composition

Another decision is the group size. The size of a group will depend on the overall group goals and patients' abilities. Patients with challenging behaviors should be carefully screened and may be able to function in smaller rather than larger groups.

Small groups (usually no more than seven to eight members) become more cohesive, are less likely to form subgroups, and can provide a richer interpersonal experience than large groups (Yalom & Leszcz, 2005). A very small group is two people (**dyad**) or three (**triad**). Small groups function nicely with one group leader although many small groups are led by two people. Even though small groups cannot easily withstand the loss of members, they are ideal for patients who are highly motivated to deal with complex emotional problems, such as sexual abuse, eating disorders, or trauma or for those who have cognitive dysfunction and require a more focused group environment with minimal distractions.

In leading a small group, the leader gets to know the members very well but maintains objectivity. The nurse observes for transference of participants toward the leader or other member. If a member becomes a "favorite patient," the leader should reflect upon any underlying personal countertransference issues (see Chapter 9).

> **NCLEXNOTE** Be prepared to select members and plan for a patient or family support group to help deal with the impact of mental illnesses on the family lifestyle.

Large groups (more than eight to 10 members) are effective for specific problems or issues, such as smoking cessation or medication information. Large groups are often used in the workplace (Cahill & Lancaster, 2014). A large group can be ongoing and open ended. Usually, transference and countertransference issues do not develop.

However, leading a large group is challenging because of the number of potential interactions and relationships that can form and the difficulty in determining the feelings and thoughts of the participants (Clark, 2009). As the size of the group increases, the level of engagement decreases and conflict increases (LoCoco, Gullo, LoVerso, & Kivlighan, 2013). It may be difficult to get everyone's attention to begin a group session. Subgroups can form, making it difficult to develop a cohesive group. If subgroups form that are detrimental to the group, the nurse can change the structure and function of communication within the subgroups by rearranging seating and encouraging the subgroup to interact with the rest of the group. Gender mix is also a consideration and can make a difference in the success of the group. For example, research shows that all-female and mixed gender groups rate their groups as more valuable and useful than did members of all-male groups. All-male groups and mixed groups are more task oriented than all-female groups. A high proportion of women in a mixed-gender group might facilitate an early development of positive group climate (LoCoco et al., 2013).

Selecting a Leadership Style

A group is led within the context of the group leader's theoretic background and the group's purpose. For example, a leader with training in cognitive-behavioral therapy may focus on treating depression by asking members to think differently about situations, which in turn lead to feeling better. A leader with a psychodynamic orientation may focus on the feelings of depression by examining situations that generate the same feelings. Whatever the leader's theoretic background, his or her leadership behavior can be viewed on a continuum of direct to indirect.

Direct leadership behavior enables the leader to control the interaction by giving directions and information and allowing little discussion. The leader literally tells the members what to do. On the other end of the continuum is **indirect leadership**, in which the leader primarily reflects the group members' discussion and offers little guidance or information to the group. Sometimes the group needs a more direct approach, such as in a psychoeducation class; other times it needs a leader who is indirect. The challenge of providing leadership is to give sufficient direction to help the group meet its goals and develop its own group process but enough freedom to allow members to make mistakes and recover from their thinking errors in a supportive, caring, learning environment.

Co-leadership, when two people share responsibility for leading the group, is useful in most groups as long as the co-leaders attend all sessions and maintain open communication. Co-leadership works well when the co-leaders plan together and meet before and after each session to discuss the group process.

Setting the Stage: Arranging Seating

Group sessions should be held in a quiet, pleasant room with adequate space and privacy. Holding a session in too large or too small a room inhibits communication. The sessions should be held in private rooms that non-members cannot access. Interruptions are distracting and can potentially compromise confidentiality. Arrangement of chairs should foster interaction and reduce communication barriers. Communication flows better when no physical barriers, such as tables, are between members. Group members should be able to see and hear each other.

BOX 13.2

Example of Group Guidelines

- Group sessions begin and end on time.
- All views are heard and respected. Cell phones are silenced; there are no side conversations.
- Only one person speaks at a time. No interrupting.
- Emotion is acceptable; aggression is not. Disagreements should be expressed calmly and objectively.
- Everyone is expected to stay for the entire meeting.
- Who we see and what is said here stay here.

Arranging a group in a circle with chairs comfortably close to one another without a table enhances group work. No one should sit outside the group. If a table is necessary, a round table is better than a rectangular one, which implicitly increases the power of those who sit at the ends.

Group members tend to sit in the same places. Those who sit close to the group leader are more likely to have more power in the group than those who sit far away.

Planning the First Meeting

The leader sets the tone of the group at the first meeting. The leader and members introduce themselves. The leader may ask participants to share some introductory information such as why they joined the group and what do they hope to gain from the experience. The leader can share name, credentials for leading group, and a brief statement about experience. The leader should avoid self-disclosing personal information.

The first session is the time to explain the structure of group, including the purpose and group rules (Box 13.2). It is important the group starts and ends at scheduled times; otherwise, members who tend to be late will not change their behavior, and those who are on time will resent waiting for the others. The leader also explains when and if new members can join the group.

During the first session, the leader begins to assess the group dynamics or interactions—both verbal and nonverbal. During the course of the group sessions, these interactions will be important in understanding the group process and may determine the success of the group.

> KEYCONCEPT   **Group dynamics** are the all the verbal and nonverbal interactions that occur in the group.

LEADING A GROUP

A group leader is responsible for monitoring and shaping the group process, as well as focusing on the group content (Puskar, Mazza, Slivka, Westcott, Campbell, & McFadden, 2012). Although models of group development differ, most follow a pattern of a beginning, middle, and ending phase (Corey, Corey, & Corey, 2010) (Table 13.1). These

Table 13.1	COMPARISON OF MODELS OF GROUP DEVELOPMENT		
Phase	Robert Bales (1955)	William Schutz (1960)	Bruce Tuckman (1965)
Beginning	• *Orientation:* What is the problem?	• *Inclusion:* Deal with issues of belonging and being in and out of the group.	• *Forming:* Get to know one another and form a group.
Middle	• *Evaluation:* How do we feel about it?	• *Control:* Deal with issues of authority (who is in charge?), dependence, and autonomy.	• *Storming:* Tension and conflict occur; subgroups form and clash with one another. • *Norming:* Develop norms of how to work together.
Ending	• *Control:* What should we do about it?	• *Affection:* Deal with issues of intimacy, closeness, and caring versus dislike and distancing.	• *Performing:* Reach consensus and develop cooperative relationships.

Sources: Bales, R. (1955). A set of categories for the analysis of small group interaction. *American Sociological Review, 15,* 257–263.
Schutz, W. (1960). *FIRO: A three-dimensional theory of interpersonal behavior.* New York: Holt, Rinehart & Winston.
Tuckman, B. (1965). Developmental sequence in small groups. *Psychological Bulletin, 63*(6), 384–399.

stages should not be viewed as a linear progression with one preceding another but as a dynamic process that is constantly revisiting and reexamining group interactions and behaviors, as well as progressing forward. The group leader needs to be aware of the group's stage of development as well as leadership responsibilities.

> KEYCONCEPT **Group process** is the development and culmination of the session-to-session interactions of the members that move the group toward its goals.

Beginning Stage: The Honeymoon

In the beginning, the group leader acknowledges each member; constructs a working environment; develops rapport with the members; begins to builds a therapeutic relationship; and clarifies outcomes, processes, and skills related to the group's purpose (Corey et al., 2010). To carry out these functions, the leader processes group interactions by staying objectives and observing members' interactions as well as participating in the group. The leader reflects on, evaluates, and responds to interactions. The use of various techniques enhances the leader's ability to lead the group effectively and to help the group meet its goals (Table 13.2).

During beginning sessions, group members get to know one another and the group leader. The length of the beginning stage depends on the purpose of the group, the number of members, and the skill of the leader. It may last for only a few sessions or several. Members often exhibit polite, congenial behavior typical of those in new social situations. They are "good patients" and often intellectualize their problems; that is, these patients deal with emotional conflict or stress by excessively using abstract thinking or generalizations to minimize disturbing feelings. Members are usually anxious and sometimes display behavior that does not truly represent their feelings.

In this phase, members begin to test whether they can trust one another and the leader. Members may come late to group or try to extend group time. Some time after the initial sessions, group members usually experience a period of conflict, either among themselves or with the leader. This conflict is a normal part of group development, and many believe that conflict is necessary to move into any working phase. Sometimes one or more group members become the scapegoat. Such situations challenge the leader to guide the group during this period by avoiding taking sides and treating all members respectfully.

Working Stage

The working stage of groups involves a real sharing of ideas and the development of closeness. A group personality may emerge that is distinct from the individual personalities of its members. The group develops norms, which are rules and standards that establish acceptable behaviors. Some norms are formalized, such as beginning group on time, but others are never really formalized, such as sitting in the same place each session. These normative standards encourage conformity and discourage behavioral deviations from the established norms. A member quickly learns the norms or is ostracized.

During this stage, the group realizes its purpose. If the purpose is education, the participants engage in learning new content or skills. If the aim of the group is to share feelings and experiences, these activities consume group meetings. During this phase, the group starts on time, and the leader often needs to remind members when it is time to stop.

Facilitating Group Communication

One of the responsibilities of the group leader is to facilitate both verbal and nonverbal communication to meet the treatment goals of the individual members and the

Table 13.2	TECHNIQUES IN LEADING GROUPS	
Technique	Purpose	Example
Support: giving feedback that provides a climate of emotional support	Helps a person or group continue with ongoing activities Informs group about what the leader thinks is important Creates a climate for expressing unpopular ideas Helps the more quiet and fearful members speak up	"We really appreciate your sharing that experience with us. It looked like it was quite painful."
Confrontation: challenging a participant (needs to be done in a supportive environment)	Helps individuals learn something about themselves Helps reduce some forms of disruptive behavior Helps members deal more openly and directly with one another	"Tom, this is the third time you have changed the subject when we have talked about spouse abuse. Is something going on?"
Advice and suggestions: sharing expertise and knowledge that the members do not have	Provides information that members can use after they have examined and evaluated it Helps focus the group's task and goals	"The medication you are taking may be causing you to be sleepy."
Summarizing: statements at the end of sessions that highlight the session's discussion, any problem resolution, and unresolved problems	Provides continuity from one session to the next Brings to focus still-unresolved issues Organizes the past in ways that clarify; brings into focus themes and patterns of interaction	"This session, we discussed Sharon's medication problems, and she will be following up with her physicians."
Clarification: restatement of an interaction	Checks on the meanings of the interaction and communication Avoids faulty communication Facilitates focus on substantive issues rather than allowing members to be sidetracked into misunderstandings	"What I heard you say was that you are feeling very sad right now. Is that correct?"
Probing and questioning: a technique for the experienced group leader that asks for more information	Helps members expand on what they were saying (when they are ready to) Gets at more extensive and wider range of information Invites members to explore their ideas in greater detail	"Could you tell us more about your relationship with your parents?"
Repeating, paraphrasing, highlighting: a simple act of repeating what was just said	Facilitates communication among group members Corrects inaccurate communication or emphasizes accurate communication	*Member:* "I forgot about my wife's birthday." *Leader:* "You forgot your wife's birthday."
Reflecting feelings: identifying feelings that are being expressed	Orients members to the feelings that may lie behind what is being said or done Helps members deal with issues they might otherwise avoid or miss	"You sound upset."
Reflecting behavior: identifying behaviors that are occurring	Gives members an opportunity to see how their behavior appears to others and to evaluate its consequences Helps members to understand others' perceptions and responses to them	"I notice that when the topic of sex is brought up, you look down and shift in your chair."

entire group. Because of the number of people involved, developing trusting relationships within groups is more complicated than is developing a single relationship with a patient. The communication techniques used in establishing and maintaining individual relationships are the same for groups, but the leader also attends to the communication patterns among the members.

Encouraging Interaction

The nurse leads the group during this phase by encouraging interaction among members and being responsive to their comments. Active listening enables the leader to process events and track interactions. The nurse can then formulate responses based on a true understanding of the discussion. A group leader who listens also models listening behavior for others, helping them improve their skills. Members may need to learn to listen to one another, track discussions without changing the subject, and not speak while others are talking. At the end of the session, the nurse summarizes the work of the session and projects the work for the next meeting.

The leader maintains a neutral, nonjudgmental style and avoids showing preference to one member over another. This may be difficult because some members may naturally seek out the leader's attention or ask for special favors. These behaviors are divisive to the group, and the leader should discourage them. Other important skills include providing everyone with an opportunity to contribute and respecting everyone's ideas. A leader who truly wants group participation and decision making does not reveal his or her beliefs.

Monitoring Verbal Communication

Group interaction can be viewed as a communication network that becomes patterned and predictable. In a group, verbal comments are linked in a chain formation. Monitoring verbal interactions and leading a group at the same time is difficult for one person. If there are two leaders, one may be the active leader of the group, and the other may sit outside the group and observe and record rather than participating. If all members agree, the leader can use an audio or video recorder for reviewing interaction after the group session.

Interesting interaction patterns can be observed and analyzed (Fig. 13.1). By analyzing the content and patterns, the leader can determine the existence of **communications pathways**—who is most liked in the group, who occupies a position of power, what subgroups have formed, and who is isolated from the group. People who sit next to each other tend to communicate among themselves. Usually, those who are well liked or display leadership abilities tend to be chosen for interactions more often than do those who are not. The leader can also determine if there is a change of subject when a sensitive topic is introduced.

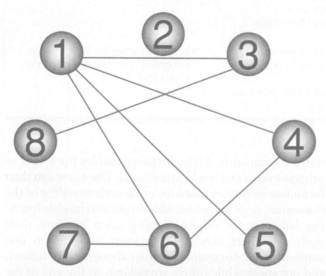

FIGURE 13.1 Sociometric analysis of group behavior. In this sociometric structure, response pattern was recorded during member interaction. Group members interacted with number 1 the most. Therefore, number 1 is the overchosen person. Numbers 5 and 7 are underchosen. Number 2 is never chosen and is determined to be the isolate.

Deciphering Content Themes

Group themes are the collective conceptual underpinnings of a group and express the members' underlying concerns or feelings regardless of the group's purpose. Themes that emerge in groups help members to understand group dynamics. Different groups have different themes. A grief group most likely would have a theme of loss or new beginnings and an adolescent group may have a theme of independence. Although some predictable themes occur in groups, the obvious or assumed themes at the beginning may actually wind up differing from reality as the process continues. In one hospice support group, the members seemed to be focusing on the memories of their loved ones. However, upon examination of the content of their interactions, discussions were revolving around financial planning for the future (Box 13.3).

Monitoring Nonverbal Communication

Observing nonverbal communication contributes to understanding the group dynamics. Members communicate nonverbally with each other, not only the group leader. Eye contact, posture, and body gestures of one member impact other members. For example, if one member is explaining a painful experience and another member looks away and tries to engage still another, the self-disclosing member may feel devalued and rejected because the disruptive behavior is interpreted as disinterest. However, if the leader interprets the disruptive behavior as anxiety over the topic,

---

BOX 13.3

Group Themes

A large symptom-management group is ongoing at a psychiatric facility. It is co-led by two nurses who are skilled in directing large groups and knowledgeable about the symptoms of mental disorders. Usually 12 people attend. The usual focus of the group is on identifying symptoms that indicate an impending reemergence of psychotic symptoms, medication side effects, and managing the numerous symptoms that medication is not controlling.

The nurses identified the appearance of the theme of powerlessness based on the following observations:

- **Session 1:** T. L. expressed his frustration at being unable to keep a job because of his symptoms. The rest of the group offered their own experiences of being unable to work.
- **Session 2:** C. R. is late to group and announces that she was late because the bus driver forgot to tell her when to get off, and she missed her stop. She is irritated with the new driver.
- **Session 3:** N. T. is out of medication and says that he cannot get more because he is out of money again. He asks the nurses to lend him some money and make arrangements to get free medication.
- **Session 4:** G. M. relies on his family for all transportation and refuses to use public transportation.

In all of these sessions, participants expressed feelings that are consistent with loss of power.

he or she may try to engage the other member in discussing the source of the anxiety.

The leaders should monitor the nonverbal behavior of group members during each session. Often, one or two people can set the overall mood of the group. Someone who comes to a session very sad or angry can set a tone of sadness or anger for the whole group. An astute group leader recognizes the effects of an individual's mood on the total group. If the purpose of the group is to deal with emotions, the group leader may choose to discuss the member's problem at the beginning of the session. The leader, thus, limits the mood to the one person experiencing it. If the group's purpose is inconsistent with self-disclosure of personal problems, the nurse should acknowledge the individual member's distress and offer a private session after the group. In this instance, the nurse would not encourage repeated episodes of self-disclosure from that member or others.

Tracking Group Communication

The leader tracks the verbal and nonverbal interactions throughout the group sessions. Depending on the group's purpose, the leader may or may not share the observations with the group. For example, if the purpose of the group is psychoeducation, the leader may incorporate the information into a lesson plan without identifying any one individual. If the purpose of the group is to improve the self-awareness and interaction skills of members, the leader may point out the observations. The leader needs to be clear about the purpose of the group and tailor leadership strategies accordingly.

Determining Roles of Group Members

There are two official or **formal group roles**, the leader and the members; however, there are also important **informal group roles** or positions with implicit rights and duties that can either help or hinder the group's process. Ideally, one or more members assume **task roles** or functions. These individuals are concerned about the purpose of the group and "keep things on task." For example, *information seeker* is the member who asks for clarification; the *coordinator* spells out relationships among ideas, and the *recorder* keeps the minutes.

Maintenance roles or functions are assumed by those who help keep the group together. Other members assume maintenance roles and make sure that the group members get along with each other and try to make peace if conflict erupts. These individuals are as interested in maintaining the group's cohesiveness as focusing on the group's tasks. The *harmonizer, compromiser,* and *standard setter* are examples of maintenance roles.

Both task and maintenance functions are needed in an effective group. In selecting members and analyzing the progress of the group, the leader pays attention to the balance between the task and maintenance functions. If too many group members assume task functions and too few assume maintenance functions, the group may have difficulty developing **cohesion**, or sticking together. If too many members assume maintenance functions, the group may never finish its work.

Individual roles are played by members to meet personal needs, such as feeling important or being an expert on a subject. These roles have nothing to do with the group's purpose or cohesion and can detract from the group's functioning (Box 13.4). If individual roles predominate, the group may be ineffective.

Dealing with Challenging Group Behaviors

Problematic behaviors occur in all groups. They can be challenging to the most experienced group leaders and frustrating to new leaders. In dealing with any problematic behavior or situation, the leader must remember to support the integrity of the individual members and the group as a whole.

Monopolizer

Some people tend to monopolize a group by constantly talking or interrupting others. This behavior is common in the beginning stages of group formation and usually represents anxiety that the member displaying such behavior is experiencing. Within a few sessions, this person usually relaxes and no longer attempts to monopolize the group. However, for some people, monopolizing discussions is part of their normal personality and will continue. Other group members usually find the behavior mildly irritating in the beginning and extremely annoying as time passes. Members may drop out of the group to avoid that person. The leader needs to decide if, how, and when to intervene. The best case scenario is when savvy group members remind the monopolizer to let others speak. The leader can then support the group in establishing rules that allow everyone the opportunity to participate. However, the group often waits for the leader to manage the situation. There are a couple of ways to deal with the situation. The leader can interrupt the monopolizer by acknowledging the member's contribution but redirecting the discussion to others, or the leader can become more directive and limit the discussion time per member.

"Yes, But . . ."

Some people have a patterned response to any suggestions from others. Initially, they agree with suggestions others offer them, but then they add "yes, but . . ." and

---

BOX 13.4

Roles and Functions of Group Members

TASK ROLES

- *Initiator-contributor* suggests or proposes new ideas or a new view of the problem or goal.
- *Information seeker* asks for clarification of the values pertinent to the group activity.
- *Information giver* offers "authoritative" facts or generalizations or gives own experiences.
- *Opinion giver* states belief or opinions with emphasis on what should be the group's values.
- *Elaborator* spells out suggestions in terms of examples, develops meanings of ideas and rationales and tries to deduce how an idea would work.
- *Coordinator* shows or clarifies the relationships among various ideas and suggestions.
- *Orienter* defines the position of the group with respect to its goals.
- *Evaluator-critic* measures the outcome of the group against some standard.
- *Energizer* attempts to stimulate the group to action or decision.
- *Procedural technician* expedites group movement by doing things for the group such as distributing copies and arranging seating.
- *Recorder* writes suggestions, keeps minutes, and serves as group memory.

MAINTENANCE ROLES

- *Encourager* praises, agrees with, and accepts the contributions of others.
- *Harmonizer* mediates differences among members and relieves tension in conflict situations.
- *Compromiser* operates from within a conflict and may yield status or admit error to maintain group harmony.

- *Gatekeeper* attempts to keep communication channels open by encouraging or facilitating the participation of others or proposes regulation of the flow of communication through limiting time.
- *Standard setter* expresses standards for the group to achieve.
- *Group observer* keeps records of various aspects of group processes and interprets data to group.
- *Follower* goes along with the movement of the group.

INDIVIDUAL ROLES

- *Aggressor* deflates the status of others; expresses disapproval of the values, acts, or feelings of others; attacks the group or problem; jokes aggressively; and tries to take credit for the work.
- *Blocker* tends to be negative and resistant, disagrees and opposes without or beyond "reason," and attempts to bring back an issue after group has rejected it.
- *Recognition seeker* calls attention to self through such activities as boasting, reporting on personal achievements, or acting in unusual ways.
- *Self-confessor* uses group setting to express personal, non–group-oriented feelings or insights.
- *Playboy* makes a display of lack of involvement in group's processes.
- *Dominator* tries to assert authority or superiority in manipulating the group or certain members of the group through flattery, being directive, or interrupting others.
- *Help-seeker* attempts to call forth sympathy from other group members through expressing insecurity, personal confusion, or depreciation of self beyond reason.
- *Special interest pleader* speaks for a special group, such as "grass roots," usually representing personal prejudices or biases.

Adapted from Benne, K., & Sheats, P. (1948). Functional roles of group members. *Journal of Social Issues, 4*(2), 41–49.

---

give several reasons why the suggestions will not work for them. Leaders and members can easily identify this patterned response. In such situations, it is best to avoid problem solving for the member and encourage the person to develop his or her own solutions. The leader can serve as a role model of the problem-solving behavior for the other members and encourage them to let the member develop a solution that would work specifically for him or her.

Disliked Member

In some groups, members clearly dislike one particular member. This situation can be challenging for the leader because it can result in considerable tension and conflict. This person could become the group's scapegoat. The group leader may have made a mistake by placing the person in this particular group, and another group may be a better match. One solution may be to move the person to a better-matched group. Whether the person stays or leaves, the group leader must stay neutral and avoid displaying negative verbal and nonverbal behaviors that

indicate that he or she too dislikes the group member or is displeased with the other members for their behavior. Often, the group leader can manage the situation by showing respect for the disliked member and acknowledging his or her contribution. In some instances, getting supervision from a more experienced group leader is useful. Defusing the situation may be possible by using conflict resolution strategies and discussing the underlying issues.

The Silent Member

The engagement of a member who does not participate in group discussion can be challenging. This member has had a lifetime of being "the quiet one" and is usually comfortable in the silent role. The leader should respect the person's silent nature. Like all the other group members, the silent member often gains a considerable amount of information and support without verbally participating. It is best for the group leader to get to know the member and understand the meaning of the silence before encouraging interaction.

Group Conflict

Most groups experience periods of conflict. The leader first needs to decide whether the conflict is a natural part of the group process or whether the group needs to address some issues. Member-to-member conflict can be handled through the previously discussed conflict resolution process (see Chapter 10). Leader-to-member conflict is more complicated because the leader has the formal position of power. In this instance, the leader can use conflict resolution strategies but should be sensitive to the power differential between the leader's role and the member's role.

Termination Stage or Saying Good-Bye

Termination can be difficult for a group, especially an effective one. During the final stages, members begin to grieve for the loss of the group's closeness and begin to reestablish themselves as individuals. Individuals terminate from groups as they do from any relationship. One person may not show up at the last session, another person may bring up issues that the group has already addressed, and others may demonstrate anger or hostility. Most members of successful groups are sad as the group terminates. During the last meetings, members may make arrangements for meeting after group. These plans rarely materialize or continue. Leaders should recognize these plans as part of the farewell process—saying good-bye to the group.

In terminating a group, the nurse discusses and summarizes the work of the group, including the accomplishments of members and their future plans. The nurse focuses on ending the group and avoids being pulled into working stage issues. For example, when a patient brings up an issue that was once resolved, the nurse reinforces the skills and then reminds the member of the actions that will be taken after the group has ended.

TYPES OF GROUPS

Psychoeducation Groups

The purposes of psychoeducation groups are to enhance knowledge, improve skills, and solve problems. The intervention strategies used in psychoeducation groups focus on transmission of information necessary for making some type of change and providing a process for making the change (Drum, Becker, & Hess, 2011). Recovery-oriented groups are psychoeducation groups that facilitate consumer involvement in the educational process and build on the recovery principles (see Chapter 2). Learning how to manage a medication regimen or control angry outbursts is an example of a recovery-oriented group.

Psychoeducation groups are formally planned, and members are purposefully selected. The group leader develops a lesson plan for each session that includes objectives, content outline, references, and evaluation tools. These groups are time limited and usually last for only a few sessions. If the group lasts longer than a few sessions, cohesiveness becomes important, especially in those that teach health maintenance behaviors such as exercise and weight control (Brown, 2011).

Task Groups

Task groups focus on completion of specific activities, such as planning a week's menu. When members are strongly committed to completing a task and the leader encourages equal participation, cohesiveness promotes satisfaction and higher performance (de Jong, Curseu, & Leenders, 2014). To complete a task, group cohesiveness is especially important. Leaders can encourage cohesiveness by placing participants in situations that promote social interaction with minimal supervision, such as refreshment periods and team-building exercises.

Without cohesiveness, the group's true existence is questionable. In cohesive groups, members are committed to the existence of the group. In large groups, cohesiveness tends to be decreased, with subsequent poorer performance among group members in completing tasks. However, cohesiveness can be a double-edged sword. In very cohesive groups, members are more likely to transgress personal boundaries. Dysfunctional relationships may develop that are destructive to the group process and ultimately not in the best interests of individual members.

Decision-Making Groups

The psychiatric nurse often leads decision-making groups that plan activities, develop unit rules, and select learning materials. The nurse who is leading a decision-making group should observe the process for any signs of **groupthink**, the tendency of group members to avoid conflict and adopt a normative pattern of thinking that is often consistent with the ideas of the group leader (Janis, 1972, 1982). Group members form opinions consistent with the group consensus rather than critically evaluation the situation. Groupthink is more likely to occur if the leader is respected or persuasive. It can also occur if a closed leadership style is used and external threat is present, particularly with time pressure (Goncalo, Polman, & Maslach, 2010). Many catastrophes, such as the *Challenger* explosion and Bay of Pigs invasion, have been attributed to groupthink.

There may be instances in which groupthink can lead to a reasonable decision: for example, a group decides to arrange a going-away party for another patient. In other situations, groupthink may inhibit individual thinking and problem solving: for example, a team is displaying groupthink if it decides that a patient should lose privileges based on the assumption that the patient is deliberately exhibiting bizarre behaviors. In this case, the team is failing to consider or examine other evidence that suggests the bizarre behavior is really an indication of psychosis.

Supportive Therapy Groups

Supportive therapy groups are usually less intense than psychotherapy groups and focus on helping individuals cope with their illnesses and problems. Implementing supportive therapy groups is one of the basic functions of the psychiatric nurse. In conducting this type of group, the nurse focuses on helping members cope with situations that are common for other group members. Counseling strategies are used. For example, a group of patients with bipolar illness whose illness is stable may discuss at a monthly meeting how to tell other people about the illness or how to cope with a family member who seems insensitive to the illness. Family caregivers of persons with mental illnesses benefit from the support of the group, as well as additional information about providing care for an ill family member.

Psychotherapy Groups

Psychotherapy groups treat individuals' emotional problems and can be implemented from various theoretic perspectives, including psychoanalytic, behavioral, and cognitive. These groups focus on examining emotions and helping individuals face their life situations. At times, these groups can be extremely intense. Psychotherapy groups provide an opportunity for patients to examine and resolve psychological and interpersonal issues within a safe environment. Mental health specialists who have a minimum of a master's degree and are trained in group psychotherapy lead such groups. Patients can be treated in psychotherapy and still be members of other nursing groups. Communication with the therapists is important for continuity of care.

One of the most respected approaches is Irvin D. Yalom's model of group psychotherapy. According to Yalom & Leszcz (2005), there are 11 primary factors through which therapeutic changes occur (Table 13.3). In this model, interpersonal relationships are very important because change occurs through a corrective emotional experience within the context of the group. The group is viewed as a social microcosm of the patients' psychosocial environment (Yalom & Leszcz, 2005).

Self-Help Groups

Self-help groups are led by people who are concerned about coping with a specific problem or life crisis. These groups do not explore psychodynamic issues in depth. Professionals usually do not attend these groups or serve as consultants. Alcoholics Anonymous, Overeaters Anonymous, and One Day at a Time (a grief group) are examples of self-help groups.

Table 13.3	YALOM'S THERAPEUTIC FACTORS
Therapeutic Factors	**Definition**
Instillation of hope	Hope is required to keep patients in therapy
Universality	Finding out that others have similar problems
Imparting information	Didactic instruction about mental health, mental illness, and so on
Altruism	Learning to give to others
Corrective recapitulation of the primary family group	Reliving and correcting early family conflicts within the group
Development of socializing techniques	Learning basic social skills
Imitative behavior	Assuming some of the behaviors and characteristics of the therapist
Interpersonal learning	Analogue of therapeutic factors in individual therapy, such as insight, working through the transference, and corrective emotional experience
Group cohesiveness	Group members' relationship to therapist and other group members
Catharsis	Open expression of affect to purge or "cleanse" self
Existential factors	Patients' ultimate concerns of existence: death, isolation, freedom, and meaninglessness

Source: Yalom, I., & Leszcz, M. (2005) *The theory and practice of group psychotherapy.* New York: Basic Books.

Age-Related Groups

Group interventions for specific age groups require attention to the developmental needs of the group members, any physical and mental impairments, social ability, and cognitive level. Children's groups should be structured to accommodate their intellectual and developmental functioning. Groups for older people should be adapted for age-related changes of the members (Box 13.5).

COMMON NURSING INTERVENTION GROUPS

Nurses lead groups of varying types that are geared toward a specific content area such as medication management, symptom management, anger management, and self-care skills. In addition, nurses groups focus on other issues such as stress management, relaxation, and women's issues. The key to being a good leader is to integrate group leadership, knowledge, and skills with nursing interventions that fit a selected group.

Working With Older People in Groups

SELF-ASSESSMENT
Because most group leaders do not have personal experience with the issues faced by older adults, the leaders should sensitize themselves to the positive and negative aspects of aging and the developmental issues facing older adults. Leaders need to be aware of their own negative reactions to aging and how this might affect their work.

COHORT EXPERIENCES
There is a wide variation in the experiences and history of older adults. Current 80- to 90-year-old adults grew up in the Great Depression of the 1930s, 65- to 80-year-old adults commonly experienced growing up during World War II, and the Baby Boomers (ages 55 to 65 years) were teenagers or young adults during the political and sexual revolution of the 1960s.

TYPICAL THEMES IN GROUP MEETINGS
- **Continuity with the past:** Older adults enjoy recalling, reliving, and reminiscing about past accomplishments.
- **Understanding the modern world:** They often use groups to understand and adapt to the modern world.
- **Independence:** They worry about becoming dependent. Physical and cognitive impairments are threats to independence. Loss of family members and friends are also threats. Leaders should be familiar with the grieving processes.
- **Changes in family relationships:** Family relationships, especially with children and grandchildren, are increasingly important as social roles change.
- **Changes in resources and environment:** Living on a fixed income focuses older people on the importance of their disposable income. They are more vulnerable to community and neighborhood changes because of their physical and financial limitations.

GROUP LEADERSHIP
- The pace of group meetings should be slowed.
- Greater emphasis should be placed on using wisdom and experience rather than learning new information.
- The group should be encouraged to use life review strategies such as autobiography and reminiscence.
- Teaching new coping skills should be placed within the context of previous attempts to resolve issues and problems (Toseland & Rizzo, 2004).

Medication Group Protocol

PURPOSE: Develop strategies that reinforce a self-medication routine.

DESCRIPTION: The medication group is an open, ongoing group that meets once a week to discuss topics germane to self-administration of medication. Members will not be asked to disclose the names of their medications.

MEMBER SELECTION: The group is open to any person taking medication for a mental illness or emotional problem who would like more information about medication, side effects, and staying on a regimen. Referrals from mental health providers are encouraged. Each person will meet with the group leader before attending the group to determine if the group will meet the individual's learning needs.

STRUCTURE: The format is a small group, with no more than eight members and one psychiatric nurse group leader facilitating a discussion about the issues. Topics are rotated.

TIME AND LOCATION: 2:00–3:00 PM, every Wednesday at the Mental Health Center

COST: No charge for attending

TOPICS
- How Do I Know If My Medications Are Working?
- Side Effect Management: Is It Worth It?
- Hints for Taking Medications Without Missing Doses!
- Health Problems That Medications Affect
- (Other topics will be developed to meet the needs of group members.)

EVALUATION: Short pretest and posttest for instructor's use only

Medication Groups

Nurse-led medication groups are common in psychiatric nursing. Not all medication groups are alike, so the nurse must be clear regarding the purpose of each specific medication group (Box 13.6). A medication group can be used primarily to transmit information about medications, such as action, dosage, and side effects, or it can focus on issues related to medications, such as compliance, management of side effects, and lifestyle adjustments. Many nurses incorporate both perspectives.

Assessing a member's medication knowledge is important before he or she joins the group to determine what the individual would like to learn. People with mental illness may have difficulty remembering new information, so assessment of cognitive abilities is important.

Assessing attention span, memory, and problem-solving skills gives valuable information that nurses can use in designing the group. The nurse should determine the members' reading and writing skills to select effective patient education materials.

An ideal group is one in which all members use the same medication. In reality, this situation is rare. Usually, the group members are using various medications. The nurse should know which medications each member is taking, but to avoid violating patient confidentiality, the nurse needs to be careful not to divulge that information to other patients. If group members choose, they can share the names of their medications with one another. A small group format works best, and the more interaction, the better. Using a lecture method of teaching is less effective than involving the members in the learning process. The nurse should expose the members to various audio and visual educational materials, including workbooks, videotapes, and handouts. The nurse should ask members to write down information to help them remember and learn through various modes. Evaluation of the learning outcomes begins with the first class.

Nurses can develop and give pre-tests and post-tests, which in combination can measure learning outcomes.

Symptom Management Groups

Nurses often lead recovery-oriented groups that focus on helping patients deal with a severe and persistent mental illness. Handling hallucinations, being socially appropriate, and staying motivated to complete activities of daily living are a few common topics. In symptom management groups, members also learn when a symptom indicates that relapse is imminent and what to do about it. Within the context of a symptom management group, patients can learn how to avoid relapse.

Anger Management Groups

Anger management is another common topic for a nurse-led group, often in the inpatient setting. The purposes of an anger management group are to discuss the concept of anger, identify antecedents to aggressive behavior, and develop new strategies to deal with anger other than verbal and physical aggression (see Chapter 19). The treatment team refers individuals with histories of being verbally and physically abusive, usually to family members, to these groups to help them better understand their emotions and behavioral responses. Impulsiveness and emotional lability are problems for many of the group members. Anger management usually includes a discussion of associated stressful situations, events that trigger anger, feelings about the situation, and unmet personal needs.

Self-Care Groups

Another common nurse-led recovery-oriented psychiatric group is a self-care group. People with psychiatric illnesses often have self-care deficits and benefit from the structure that a group provides. These groups are challenging because members usually know how to perform these daily tasks (e.g., bathing, grooming, performing personal hygiene), but their illnesses cause them to lose the motivation to complete them. The leader not only reinforces the basic self-care skills but also, more importantly, helps identify strategies that can motivate the patients and provide structure to their daily lives.

Reminiscence Groups

Reminiscence therapy has been shown to be a valuable intervention for older clients. In this type of group, members are encouraged to remember events from past years. Such a group is easily implemented. Usually, a simple question about an important family event will spark memories. Reminiscence groups are usually associated with patients who have dementia who are having difficulty with recent memory. Reminiscence groups can also be used as an intergenerational intervention with healthy older adults and children. Older adults become less lonely and experience an improved quality of life; children's attitudes toward the elderly becomes more positive (Gaggioli et al., 2014; Stinson, 2009).

SUMMARY OF KEY POINTS

- The definition of group can vary according to theoretic orientation. A general definition is that a group is two or more people who have at least one common goal or issue. Group dynamics are the interactions within a group that influence the group's development and process.

- Groups can be open, with new members joining at any time, or closed, with members admitted only once. Either small or large groups can be effective, but dynamics change in different size groups.

- The process of group development occurs in phases: beginning, middle, and termination. These stages are not fixed but dynamic. The process challenges the leader to guide the group. During the working stage, the group addresses its purpose.

- Leading a group involves many different functions, from obtaining and receiving information to testing and evaluating decisions. The leader should explain the rules of the group at the beginning of the group.

- Verbal communication includes the communication network and group themes. Nonverbal communication is more complex and involves eye contact, body posture, and the mood of the group. Decision-making groups can be victims of groupthink, which can have positive or negative outcomes. Groupthink research is ongoing.

- Seating arrangements can affect group interaction. The fewer physical barriers there are, such as tables, the better the communication. Everyone should be a part of the group, and no one should sit outside of it. In the most interactive groups, members face one another in a circle.

- Leadership skills involve listening; tracking verbal and nonverbal behaviors; and maintaining a neutral, nonjudgmental style.

- Although there are only two formal group roles, leader and member, there are many informal group roles. These roles are usually categorized according to purpose—task functions, maintenance functions, and individual roles. Members who assume task functions encourage the group members to stay focused on the group's task. Those who assume maintenance functions worry more about the group working together than the actual task itself. Individual roles can either enhance or detract from the work of the group.

■ The leader should address behaviors that challenge the leadership, group process, or other members to determine whether to intervene. In some instances, the leader redirects a monopolizing member; at other times, the leader lets the group deal with the behavior. Group conflict occurs in most groups.

■ There are many different types of groups. Psychiatric nurses lead psychoeducation and supportive therapy groups. Mental health specialists who are trained to provide intensive therapy lead psychotherapy groups. Consumers lead self-help groups, and professionals assist only as requested. Leading age-related groups requires attention to the developmental, physical, social, and intellectual abilities of the participants. Themes of older adult groups include continuity with the past, understanding the modern world, independence, and changes in family and resources. Group leadership for older adult groups builds on participants' previous experiences and coping abilities in developing new coping skills.

■ Medication, symptom management, anger management, and self-care groups are common nurse-led groups focused on specific interventions.

CRITICAL THINKING CHALLENGES

1. Group members are very polite to one another and are superficially discussing topics. You would assess the group as being in which phase? Explain your answer.

2. After three sessions of a supportive therapy group, two members begin to share their frustration with having a mental illness. The group is moving into which phase of group development? Explain your answer.

3. Define the roles of the task and maintenance functions in groups. Observe your clinical group and identify classmates who are assuming task functions and maintenance functions.

4. Observe a patient group for at least five sessions. Discuss the seating pattern that emerges. Identify the communication network and the group themes. Then identify the group's norms and standards.

5. Discuss the conditions that lead to groupthink. When is groupthink positive? When is groupthink negative? Explain.

6. List at least six behaviors that are important for a group leader, including one for age-related groups. Justify your answers.

7. During the first meeting, one member seems very anxious and tends to monopolize the conversation. Discuss how you would assess the situation and whether you would intervene.

8. At the end of the fourth meeting, one group member angrily accuses another of asking too many questions. The other members look on quietly. How would you assess the situation? Would you intervene? Explain.

MOVIES *12 Angry Men:* 1998. In this excellent film, a young man stands accused of fatally stabbing his father. A jury of his "peers" is deciding his fate. This jury is portrayed by an excellent cast, including Jack Lemmon, George C. Scott, Tony Danza, and Ossie Davis. At first, the case appears to be "open and shut." This film depicts an intense struggle to reach a verdict and is an excellent study of group process and group dynamics.

VIEWING POINTS: Identify the leaders in the group. How does leadership change throughout the film? Do you find any evidence of groupthink? How does the group handle conflict?

References

Benne, K., & Sheats, P. (1948). Functional roles of group members. *Journal of Social Issues, 4*(2), 41–49.

Brown, N. W. (2011). *Psychoeducational groups: Process and practice* (3rd ed). New York: Taylor & Frances Group.

Cahill, K., & Lancaster, T. (2014). Workplace interventions for smoking cessation. (Review). *The Cochrane Collaborative, 2* CD003440, *doi: 10.1002/14651858.CD003440.pub4*

Clark, C. C. (2009). *Group leadership skills for nurses and health professionals* (5th ed). New York: Springer.

Corey, M. S., Corey, G., & Corey, C. (2010). *Group process and practice.* New York: Brooks Cole.

de Jong, J. P., Curseu, P. L., & Leenders, R. T. (2014). When do bad apples not spoil the barrel? Negative relationships in teams, team performance, and buffering mechanism. *The Journal of Applied Psychology, 99*(3), 514–522.

Drum, D., Becker, M. S., & Hess, E. (2011). Expanding the application of group interventions: Emergence of groups in health care settings. *The Journal for Specialists in Group Work, 36*(4), 247–263.

Gaggioli, A., Morganti, L., Bonfiglio, S., Scaratti, C., Cipresso, P., Serino, S., et al. (2014). Intergenerational group reminiscence: A potentially effective intervention to enhance elderly psychosocial wellbeing and to improve children's perception of aging. *Educational Gerontology, 40*(7), 486–498.

Goncalo, J. A., Polman, E., & Maslach, C. (2010). Can confidence come too soon? collective efficaacy, conflict and group performance over time. *Organizational Behavior & Human Decision Processes, 113*(1), 13–24.

Janis, I. (1972). *Victims of groupthink.* Boston: Houghton Mifflin.

Janis, I. (1982). *Groupthink* (2nd ed). Boston: Houghton Mifflin.

Lo Coco, G., Gullo, S., Lo Verso, G., & Kivlighan, D. M. (2013). Sex composition and group climate: A group actor-partner interdependence analysis. *Group Dynamics: Theory, Research, and Practice, 17*(4), 270–280.

Puskar, K., Mazza, G., Slivka, C., Westcott, M., Campbell, F., & McFadden, T. G. (2012). Understanding content and process: Guidelines for group leaders. *Perspectives in Psychiatric care, 48*(4), 225–229.

Stinson, C. K. (2009). Structured group reminiscence: An intervention for older adults. *The Journal of Continuing Education in Nursing, 40*(11), 523–528.

Toseland, R. W., & Rizzo, V. M. (2004). What's different about working with older people in groups? *Journal of Gerontological Social Work, 44*(1/2), 5–23.

Yalom, I., & Leszcz, M. (2005). *The theory and practice of group psychotherapy.* New York: Basic Books.

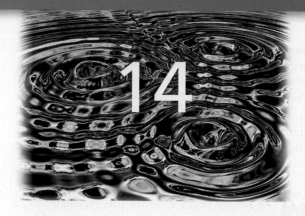

14

Family Assessment and Interventions

Mary Ann Boyd

KEY CONCEPTS

- comprehensive family assessment
- family

LEARNING OBJECTIVES

After studying this chapter, you will be able to:

1. Discuss the changing family structure and mental health implications.

2. Discuss the balance of family mental health with family dysfunction.

3. Develop a genogram that depicts the family history, relationships, and mental disorders across at least three generations.

4. Develop a plan for a comprehensive family assessment.

5. Apply family nursing diagnoses to families who need nursing care.

6. Discuss nursing interventions that are useful in caring for families.

KEY TERMS

- boundaries • differentiation of self • dysfunctional • emotional cutoff • extended family • family development • family life cycle • family projection process • family structure • genogram • multigenerational transmission process • nuclear family • nuclear family emotional process • resilience • sibling position • subsystems • transition times • triangles

A family is a group of people connected emotionally, or by blood, or in both ways that has developed patterns of interaction and relationships. Family members have a shared history and a shared future (McGoldrick, Carter, & Garcia-Preto, 2011). **A nuclear family** is two or more people living together and related by blood, marriage, or adoption. An **extended family** is several nuclear families whose members may or may not live together and function as one group. Families are unique in that, unlike all other groups, they incorporate new members only by birth, adoption, or marriage, and members can leave only by divorce or death.

KEYCONCEPT **Family** is a group of people connected by emotions, blood, or both, that has developed patterns of interaction and relationships. Family members have a shared history and a shared future (McGoldrick et al., 2011).

The psychiatric nurse interacts with families in various ways. Because of the interpersonal and chronic nature of many mental illnesses, psychiatric nurses often have frequent and long-term contact with families. Involvement may range from meeting family members only once or twice to treating the whole family as a patient. Unlike a therapeutic group (see Chapter 13), the family system has a history and continues to function when the nurse is not there. The family reacts to past, present, and anticipated future relationships within at least a three-generation family system. This chapter explains how to integrate important family concepts into the nursing process when providing psychiatric nursing care to families experiencing mental health problems.

CHANGING FAMILY STRUCTURE

Although families may be defined differently within various cultures, they all play an important role in the life of the individual and influence who and what we are. Traditionally, families are considered a source of guidance, security, love, and understanding. This is also true for people who have mental illnesses and emotional problems. It is often the family that assumes primary care for the person with mental illness and supports that individual throughout treatment. For patients, the family unit may provide their only constant support throughout their lives. Although the nuclear family remains the basic unit of social organization, its structure and size have changed drastically in recent times and so have the functions and roles of family members.

Family Size

Family size in the United States has decreased. In 1790, about one third of all households, including servants, slaves, and other people not related to the head, consisted of seven people or more. By 1960, only one household in 20 was this size. The average family household in 2013 was 2.6 people. Married couples made up most (63%) of the family groups with children under the age of 18 (Vespa, Lewis, & Keider, 2013).

Contemporary Roles

A woman's role in the family has changed drastically in the past years. Today, most women, including those who are mothers, work—both in dual-income families and in single-parent families. Women make up 47.4% of the American civilian work force. There are 161 million females and 156.1 million males in the United States as of December 2013. More than half of the female work force is married and only 24% of married mothers and 0.7% of married fathers with children are stay-at-home parents (Vespa et al., 2013).

Mobility and Relocation

Families are more mobile and may change residences more often than ever before. Leaving familiar environments and readjusting to new surroundings and lifestyles stress family members. Moreover, these moves impose separation from the extended family, which traditionally has been a stabilizing force and a much-needed support system.

Family Composition

Unmarried Couples

More unmarried couples are cohabiting before or instead of marrying. Between 1995 and 2006–2010, the percentage of women who cohabited as a first union increased for all hispanic and race groups except for Asian women. First premarital cohabitations were longest for hispanic women (33 months) and shortest for white women (19 months).

Forty percent of the cohabitations among women transitioned to marriage by 3 years, 32% remained intact, and 27% dissolved. Nearly 20% of women became pregnant in their first year of cohabitation (Copen, Daniels, & Mosher, 2013). Cohabitation among adults over 50 is rapidly rising from 1.2 million in 2000 to 2.75 million in 2010. Unlike the younger adults, the union of older adults endure an average of 8 years and appear to be an alternative to marriage (Brown, Bulanda, & Lee, 2012).

Single-Parent Families

It is estimated that 50% to 60% of all American children will reside at some point in a single-parent home. In 2012, 64% of the 74 million children in the United States were living with two married parents. Twenty-four percent of children lived with their mothers, 4% lived with their fathers, and 4% lived with neither. Seventy-four percent of white, nonhispanic, 59% of hispanic, and 33% of black children lived with two married parents in 2012. Although most children spend their childhood living with two parents, many children experience the presence of other adults within the home (Childstats, 2013).

Stepfamilies

Remarried families or stepfamilies have a unique set of challenges that are not completely understood. More than 50% of U.S. families are remarried or recoupled (U.S. Census Bureau, 2013). Many parents find that stepparenting is much more difficult than parenting a biologic child. The bonding that occurs with biologic children rarely occurs with the stepchildren, whose natural bond is with a parent not living with them. However, the stepparent often assumes a measure of financial and parental responsibility. The care and management of children often become the primary stressor to the marital partners. In addition, the children are faced with multiple sets of parents whose expectations may differ. They may also compete for the children's attention. It is not unusual for second marriages to fail because of the stressors inherent in a remarried family.

Childless Families

Couples can be involuntarily childless because of infertility or voluntarily childless by choice. Approximately 15% of all couples in the reproductive age are involuntarily childless. There is some evidence that this group experiences grief over being childless (Lechner, Bolman, & van Dalen, 2007). As the opportunities for women have increased, many people have chosen not to have children. Research on childlessness is sparse, but it appears that middle and old age childless adults are not more vulnerable to loneliness and depression than those with children (Umberson, Pudrovska, & Reczek, 2010; Vikstrom, Hammar, Marcusson, Wressle, & Sydsjo, 2011).

Same-Sex Families

Among the most stigmatized people are those who are gay or lesbian. It is estimated that most lesbian and gay populations have encountered some form of verbal harassment or violence in their lives. The exact number of people who are gay or lesbian is believed to be undercounted. In 2010, there were an estimated 581,300 same-sex couples (Lofquist & Ellis, 2011). Higher smoking and drinking rates are present in this population and may indicate higher rates of depression, stress, low self-esteem, and complications of childhood abuse (Mustanski, Garofalo, & Emerson, 2010). However, these mental health problems may improve as more states legalize same-sex marriage.

Although at one time people believed that being gay or lesbian was a result of faulty parenting or personal choice, evidence now shows that sexual orientation is determined early in life by a combination of factors, including genetic predisposition, biologic development, and environmental events (see Chapter 33). In the past, it was also believed that sexual orientation could be changed through counseling by making a concerted effort to establish new relationships. However, no evidence supports the hypothesis that changes in sexual orientation are possible.

FAMILY MENTAL HEALTH AND ILLNESS

In a mentally healthy family, members live in harmony among themselves and within society. Ideally, these families support and nurture their members throughout their lives. However, dysfunction and mental illness can affect a family's overall mental health.

Family Dysfunction

A family becomes **dysfunctional** when interactions, decisions, or behaviors interfere with the positive development of the family and its individual members. Most families have periods of dysfunction such as during a crisis or stressful situation when the coping skills are not available. Families usually adapt and regain their mentally healthy balance. A family can be mentally healthy and at the same time have a member who has a mental illness. Conversely, a family can be dysfunctional and have no member with a diagnosable mental illness.

Effects of Mental Illness on Family Functioning

Families of people with persistent mental disorders have special needs. Many mentally ill adults live with their parents well into their 30s and beyond. For these adults with persistent mental illness, the family serves several functions that those without mental illness do not need. Such functions include the following:

- *Providing support.* People with mental illness have difficulty maintaining nonfamilial support networks and may rely exclusively on their families.
- *Providing information.* Families often have complete and continuous information about care and treatment over the years.
- *Monitoring services.* Families observe the progress of their relative and report concerns to those in charge of care.
- *Advocating for services.* Family groups advocate for money for residential care services.

The stigma associated with having a family member with a psychiatric disorder underlies much of the burden and stress the caregivers experience. Families can become socially isolated and financially stressed and lose employment opportunities as they struggle to care for their loved one. Frustration, anxiety, and low-self esteem may result (Zauszniewski, Bekhet, & Suresky, 2009).

Conflicts can occur between parents and mental health workers who place a high value on independence. Members of the mental health care system may criticize families for being overly protective when, in reality, the patient with mental illness may face real barriers to independent living. Housing may be unavailable; when available, quality may be poor. The patient may fear leaving home, may be at risk for relapse if he or she does leave, or may be too comfortable at home to want to leave. When long-term caregivers, usually the parents, die, their adult children with mental illness experience housing disruptions and potentially traumatic transitions. Siblings who have other responsibilities expect to be less involved than their parents in the care and oversight of the mentally ill brother or sister. Few families actually plan for this difficult eventuality (Griffiths & Sin, 2013).

Nurses must use an objective and rational approach when discussing independence and dependence of those with mental illness who live with aging parents. Family emotions often obscure the underlying issues, but nurses can diffuse such emotions, so that everyone can explore the alternatives comfortably. Although separation must eventually occur, the timing and process vary according to each family's particular situation. Parents may be highly anxious when their adult children first leave home and need reassurance and support.

COMPREHENSIVE FAMILY ASSESSMENT

A comprehensive family assessment is the collection of all relevant data related to family health, psychological well-being, and social functioning to identify problems for which the nurse can generate nursing diagnoses. The assessment consists of a face-to-face interview with family members and can be conducted during several sessions. Nurses conduct a comprehensive family assessment

BOX 14.1

Family Mental Health Assessment

I. Family members present
Name   **Age**   **Relationship**
_____   _____   _____
_____   _____   _____
_____   _____   _____

II. Health status
Member   **Disorder and current treatment**
_____   _____
_____   _____

III. Mental health status
Member   **Disorder and current treatment**
_____   _____
_____   _____

IV. Impact of mental illness on family function
Describe the changes that occur in the family as a result of the family member's disorder:
_____
_____
_____

V. Family life cycle
Describe the family life cycle stage and any transitions that are occurring.
_____
_____

VI. Communication patterns
Describe the family communication patterns in terms of usual times of communication (morning, dinner etc.), which family members talk to each other, who communicates the family rules, who carries out discipline. Identify triangulated messages. _____
_____
_____
_____

VII. Stress and coping
Identify current family stressful events and family coping mechanisms. _____
_____
_____

VIII. Problem-solving skills
Determine who solves problems in the family. Are the problem-solving skills of the family able to manage most family problems?
_____
_____
_____

IX. Family system (from the genogram)
Family composition _____
_____

Health and illness patterns _____
_____

Relationship patterns _____
_____

(Continued)

BOX 14.1

Family Mental Health Assessment (*Continued*)

Social functioning patterns _____

_____

_____

Financial and legal status _____

_____

_____

Formal and informal network _____

_____

_____

_____

X. Nursing diagnoses

_____

_____

_____

when they care for patients and their families for an extended period. They also use them when a patient's mental health problems are so complex that family support is important for optimal care (Box 14.1).

KEYCONCEPT A **comprehensive family assessment** is the collection of all relevant data related to family health, psychological well-being, and social functioning to identify problems for which the nurse can generate nursing diagnoses.

Relationship Building

In preparing for a family assessment, nurses must concentrate on developing a relationship with the family. Although necessary when working with any family, relationship development is particularly important for families from ethnic minority cultures; because of the discrimination that they have experienced, they may be less likely to trust those from outside their family or community. Developing a relationship takes time, so the nurse may need to complete the assessment during several meetings rather than just one.

To develop a positive relationship with a family, nurses must establish credibility with the family and address its immediate intervention needs. To establish credibility, the family must see the nurse as knowledgeable and skillful. Possessing culturally competent nursing skills and projecting a professional image are crucial to establishing credibility. With regard to immediate intervention needs, a family that needs shelter or food is not ready to discuss a member's medication regimen until the first needs are met. The nurse will make considerable progress in establishing a relationship with a family when he or she helps members meet their immediate needs.

Genograms

Families possess various structural configurations (e.g., single-parent, multigenerational, same-gender relationships). The nurse can facilitate taking the family history by completing a **genogram**, which is a multigenerational schematic depiction of biological, legal, and emotional relationships from generation to generation (McGoldrick, Gerson, & Petry, 2008). The nurse can use a genogram as a framework for exploring relationships and patterns of health and illness.

Creating Genograms

A genogram includes the age, dates of marriage and death, and geographic location of each member. Symbols are used in the genogram and are defined in a legend. Squares represent men, and circles represent women; ages are listed inside the squares and circles. Horizontal lines represent marriages with dates; vertical lines connect parents and children. Genograms can be particularly useful in understanding family history, composition, relationships, and illnesses (Fig. 14.1).

Genograms vary from simple to elaborate. The patient's and family's assessment needs guide the level of detail. In a small family with limited problems, the genogram can be rather general. In a large family with multiple problems, the genogram should reflect these complexities. Thus, depending on the level of detail, nurses collect various data. They can study important events such as marriages, divorces, deaths, and geographic movements. They can include cultural or religious affiliations, education and economic levels, and the nature of the work of each family member. Psychiatric nurses should always include mental disorders and other significant health problems in the genogram.

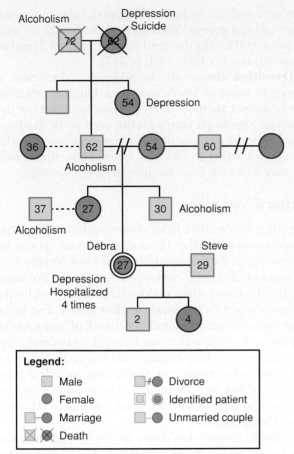

FIGURE 14.1 Analysis of genogram for Debra. Illness patterns are depression (paternal aunt, grandmother [suicide]) and alcoholism (brother, father, grandfather). Relationship patterns show that the parents are divorced and neither sibling is married.

Analyzing and Using Genograms

For a genogram to be useful in assessment, the nurse needs to analyze the data for family composition, relationship problems, and mental health patterns. Nurses can begin with composition. How large is the family? Where do family members live? A large family whose members live in the same city is more likely to have support than a family in which distance separates members. Of course, this is not always the case. Sometimes even when family members live geographically close, they are emotionally distant from one another.

The nurse should also study the genogram for relationship and illness patterns. For instance, in terms of relationship patterns, the nurse may find a history of divorces or family members who do not keep in touch with the rest of the family. The nurse can then explore the significance of these and other relationships. In terms of illness patterns, alcoholism, often seen across several generations, may be prevalent in men on one side of a family. The nurse can then hypothesize that alcoholism is one of the mental health risks for the family and design interventions to reduce the risk. Or the

nurse may find via a genogram that members of a family's previous generation were in "state hospitals" or had "nerve problems."

Family Biologic Domain

In the family biologic domain, the family assessment includes a thorough picture of physical and mental health status and how the status affects family functioning. The family with multiple health problems, both physical and mental, must try to manage these problems as well as obtain the many financial and health care resources the family members need.

Physical Health Status

The family health status includes the physical illnesses and disabilities of all members; the nurse can record such information on the genogram and also include the physical illnesses and disabilities of other generations. Illnesses of family members are an indication not only of their physical status but also of the stress currently being placed on the family and its resources. The nurse should pay particular attention to any physical problems that affect family functioning. For example, if a member requires frequent visits to a provider or hospitalizations, the whole family will feel the effects of focusing excessive time and financial resources on that member. The nurse should explore how such situations specifically affect other members.

Mental Health Status

Detecting mental disorders in families may be difficult because these disorders often are hidden or the "family secret." Very calmly, the nurse should ask family members to identify anyone who has had or has a mental illness. He or she should record the information on the genogram as well as in the narrative. If family members do not know if anyone in the family had or has a mental illness, the nurse should ask if anyone was treated for "nerves" or had a "nervous breakdown." Overall, a good family history of mental illness across multiple generations helps the nurse understand the significance of mental illness in the current generation. If one family member has a serious mental illness, the whole family will be affected. Usually, siblings of the mentally ill member receive less parental attention than the affected member.

Family's Psychological Domain

Assessment of the family's psychological domain focuses on the family's development and life cycle, communication patterns, stress and coping abilities, and problem-solving skills. One aim of the assessment is to understand the relationships within the family. Although family roles and structures are important, the true value of the family is in its relationships, which are irreplaceable. For example, if a parent leaves or dies, another person (e.g., stepparent, grandparent) can assume some parental functions but can never really replace the emotional relationship with the missing parent.

Family Development

Family development is a broad term that refers to all the processes connected with the growth of a family, including changes associated with work, geographic location, migration, acculturation, and serious illness. In optimal family development, family members are relatively differentiated (capable of autonomous functioning) from one another, anxiety is low, and the parents have good emotional relationships with their own families of origin.

Family Life Cycles

The concept of **family life cycle** refers to stages that evolve based on significant events related to the arrival and departure of members, such as birth or adoption, child rearing, departure of children from home, occupational retirement, and death. Identifying the family life cycle is helpful in assessing family relationships, roles, and stresses. The family life cycle is a process of expansion, contraction, and realignment of relationship systems to support the entry, exit, and development of family members in a functional way (McGoldrick et al., 2011) (Table 14.1). A family's life cycle is conceptualized in terms of stages throughout the years. To move from one stage to the next, the family system undergoes changes. Structural and potential structural changes within stages can usually be handled by rearranging the family system (first-order changes), but transition from one stage to the next requires changes in the system itself (second-order changes). An example of a first-order change is when all the children are finally in school and the stay-at-home parent returns to work. The system is rearranged, but the structure remains the same. In second-order changes, the family structure does change, such as when a member moves away from the family home to live independently.

> **NCLEXNOTE** Apply family life cycle stages to a specific family with a member who has a psychiatric disorder. Identify the emotional transitions and the required family changes.

The nurse should not view this model as the "normal" life cycle for every family and should limit its use to those families it clearly fits. As second marriages, career changes in midlife, and other phenomena occur with increasing frequency, this traditional model is being challenged, modified, and redesigned to address such contemporary structural and role changes. This model also may not fit many cultural groups. Variations of the family life cycle are presented for the divorced family (Table 14.2) and the remarried family (Table 14.3, p. 217).

Transition times are the addition, subtraction, or change in status of family members. During transitions, family stresses are more likely to cause symptoms or dysfunction. Significant family events, such as the death of a member or the introduction of a new member, also affect the family's ability to function. During transitions, families may seek help from the mental health system.

Cultural Variations

In caring for families from diverse cultures, the nurse should examine whether the underlying assumptions and frameworks of the dominant life-cycle models apply. Even the concept of "family" varies among cultures. For example, the dominant white middle-class culture's definition of family refers to the intact nuclear family. For Italian Americans, the entire extended network of aunts, uncles, cousins, and grandparents may be involved in family decision making and share holidays and life-cycle transitions. For African Americans, the family may include a broad network of kin and community that includes long-time friends who are considered family members (Hines & Boyd-Franklin, 2005).

Cultural groups also differ in the importance they give to certain life-cycle transitions. For example, Irish American families may emphasize the wake, viewing death as an important life-cycle transition. African American families may emphasize funerals, going to considerable expense and delaying services until all family members arrive. Italian American and Polish American families may place great emphasis on weddings (McGoldrick, Giordano, & Garcia-Preto, 2005).

The life cycle of Mexican immigrant families can be examined in the context of *familismo* (a value of close connection between immediate and extended family members), parental authority, and extended family. The impact of living in a different country, learning a different language, and lack of extended family may create family conflict as they adjust to a different cultural environment. Their children are faced with academic expectations that need parental involvement and support. Family emotional climate increases as both parents share parenting responsibilities (Sotomayor-Peterson, Figueredo, Christensen, & Taylor, 2012).

Families in Poverty

An estimated 15% of the U.S. population lives below the poverty level (U.S. Department of Commerce, 2014), and a disproportionate number of children from minority groups live in poverty. Single-sex couples are as likely to live in poverty as different-sex couples. Lesbian couples

Table 14.1	STAGES OF THE FAMILY LIFE CYCLE	
Family Life Cycle Stage	**Emotional Transition**	**Required Family Changes**
Leaving home: emerging young adults	Accepting emotional and financial responsibility for self	Differentiation of self in relation to family of origin Development of intimate peer relationships Establishment of self in respect to work and financial independence Establishment of self in community and larger society Spirituality?
Joining of families through marriage or union	Commitment to new system	Formation of partner systems Realignment of relationships with extended family, friends, and larger community to include new partners
Families with young children	Accepting new members into the system	Adjustment of couple system to make space for children Collaboration in child-rearing, financial, and housekeeping tasks Realignment of relationships with extended family to include parenting and grandparenting roles Realignment of relationships with community and larger social system to include new family structure and relationships
Families with adolescents	Increasing flexibility of family boundaries to permit children's independence and grandparents' frailties	Shift of parent–child relationships to permit adolescent to move into and out of system Refocus on midlife couple and career issues Begin shift toward caring for older generation Realignment with community and larger social system to include shifting family of emerging adolescent and parents in new formation pattern of relating
Launching children and moving on at midlife	Accepting a multitude of exits from and entries into the system	Renegotiation of couple system as a dyad Development of adult-to-adult relationships between parents and grown children Realignment of relationships to include in-laws and grandchildren Realignment of relationships with community and larger social system to include new structure and constellation of family relationships Exploration of new interests or career given the freedom from child care responsibilities Dealing with care needs, disabilities, and death of parents (grandparents)
Families in late middle age	Accepting the shifting generational roles	Maintenance of own or couple functioning and interests in face of physiologic decline: exploration of new familial and social role options Supporting more central role of middle generations Realignment of system in relation to community and larger social system to acknowledge changed pattern of family relationships of this stage Making room in the system for the wisdom and experience of elders Supporting the older generation without overfunctioning for them
Families nearing the end of life	Accepting the realities of limitations and death and the completion of one cycle of life	Dealing with loss of spouse, siblings, and other peers Making preparations for death and legacy Managing reversed roles in caretaking between middle and older generations Realignment of relationships with larger community and social system to acknowledge changing life-cycle relationships

Reprinted with modifications from McGoldrick, M., Carter, B., & Garcia-Preto, N. (2011). *The expanded family life cycle: Individual, family, and social perspectives* (4th ed, pp. 16–17). Boston, MA: Allyn & Bacon. Used with permission.

Table 14.2	FAMILY LIFE CYCLE FOR THE DIVORCING FAMILY	
Family Life Cycle Stage	Emotional Process	Developmental Issues
Divorce		
Decision to divorce	Acceptance of inability to resolve marital problems sufficiently to continue relationship	Acceptance of one's own part in the failure of the marriage
Planning the breakup of the system	Supporting viable arrangements for all parts of the system	Working cooperatively on problems of custody, visitation, and finances Dealing with extended family about the divorce
Separation	Willingness to continue cooperative co-parental relationship and joint financial support of children Working on resolution of attachment to spouse	Mourning loss of intact family Restructuring marital and parent–child relationships and finances; adaptation to living apart Realignment of relationships with extended family; staying connected with spouse's extended family
The divorce	Working on emotional divorce: overcoming hurt, anger, guilt, and so on	Mourning loss of intact family; giving up fantasies of reunion Retrieving hopes, dreams, expectations from the marriage Staying connected with extended families
Postdivorce family		
Single parent (custodial household or primary residence)	Willingness to maintain financial responsibilities, continue parental contact with ex-spouse, and support contact of children with ex-spouse and his or her family	Making flexible visitation arrangements with ex-spouse and family Rebuilding own financial resources Rebuilding own social network
Single parent (noncustodial)	Willingness to maintain financial responsibilities and parental contact with ex-spouse and to support custodial parent's relationship with children	Finding ways to continue effective parenting Maintaining financial responsibilities to ex-spouse and children Rebuilding own social network

Reprinted with modifications from McGoldrick, M., Carter, B., & Garcia-Preto, N. (2011). *The expanded family life cycle: Individual, family, and social perspectives* (4th ed, p. 320). Boston, MA: Allyn & Bacon. Used with permission.

have much higher poverty rates than either different-sex couples or gay male couples (Badget, Durso, Schneebaum, 2013; Eamon, 2013).

The family life cycle of those living in poverty may vary from those with adequate financial means. People living in poverty struggle to make ends meet, and family members may face difficulties in meeting their own or other members' basic developmental needs. To be poor does not mean that a family is automatically dysfunctional. But poverty is an important factor that can force even the healthiest families to crumble.

In studying African American families living in poverty, Hines (1999) observed a condensed life cycle during which family members leave home, mate, have children, and become grandparents at much earlier ages than their working-class and middle-class counterparts. Consequently, many individuals in such families assume new roles and responsibilities before they are developmentally capable. Education subsequently becomes a low priority, and teenagers often drop out of school. Male adolescents cannot differentiate themselves from either family or peers. They often cannot find employment except for

menial work and may assert their masculinity in transient heterosexual relationships. Adolescent females become pregnant, and older family members (usually the baby's grandmother) often become the primary sources of assistance. A woman, her children, and her daughter's children often live together without clear delineation of their respective roles. Subsequent pregnancies may increase the burden of caregiving. Despite possible poor health, older family members continue to work to support their children and grandchildren. These families experience chronic stress and untimely losses. Families living in poverty are subject to family disruption via abrupt loss of members, loss of unemployment compensation, illness, death, imprisonment, or alcohol or drug addiction. Poor families are often forced to seek public assistance, which ultimately can result in additional stress (Hines, 1999).

Communication Patterns

Family communication patterns develop over a lifetime and are important information during an assessment. Some family members communicate more openly and

Table 14.3	FAMILY LIFE CYCLE FOR THE REMARRIED FAMILY	
Family Life Cycle Stage	**Emotional Process**	**Developmental Issues**
Entering new relationship	Recovery from loss of first marriage (adequate "emotional divorce")	Recommitment to marriage and to forming a family with readiness to deal with the complexity and ambiguity
Conceptualizing and planning new marriage and family	Accepting one's own fears and those of new spouse and children about forming a new family Accepting the need for time and patience for adjustment to complexity and ambiguity of: 1. Multiple new roles 2. Boundaries: space, time, membership, and authority 3. Affective issues: guilt, loyalty conflicts, desire for mutuality, unresolvable past hurts	Working on openness in the new relationships to avoid pseudomutuality Planning for maintenance of cooperative financial and co-parental relationships with ex-spouses Planning to help children deal with fears, loyalty conflicts, and membership in two systems Realignment of relationships with extended family to include new spouse and children Plan maintenance of connections for children with extended family of ex-spouses
Remarriage and reconstruction of family	Resolution of attachment to previous spouse and ideal of "intact" family Acceptance of different model of family with permeable boundaries	Restructuring family boundaries to allow for inclusion of new spouse–stepparent Realignment of relationships and financial arrangements to permit interweaving of several systems Making room for relationships of all children with all parents, grandparents, and other extended family Sharing memories and histories to enhance stepfamily integration
Renegotiation of remarried family at all future life-cycle transitions	Accepting evolving relationships of transformed remarried family	Changes as each child graduates, marries, dies, or becomes ill Changes as each spouse forms new couple relationship, remarries, moves, becomes ill, or dies

Reprinted with modifications from McGoldrick, M., Carter, B., & Garcia-Preto, N. (2011). *The expanded family life cycle: Individual, family, and social perspectives* (4th ed, p. 321). Boston, MA: Allyn & Bacon. Used with permission.

honestly than others. In addition, family subgroups develop from communication patterns. Just as in any assessment interview, the nurse should observe the verbal and nonverbal communication of the family members. Who sits next to each other? Who talks to whom? Who answers most questions? Who volunteers information? Who changes the subject? Which subjects seem acceptable to discuss? Which topics are not discussed? Can spouses be intimate with each other? Are any family secrets revealed? Does the nonverbal communication match the verbal communication? Nurses can use all of this information to help identify family problems and communication issues.

Nurses should also assess the family for its daily communication patterns. Identifying which family members confide in one another is a place to start examining ongoing communication. Other areas include how often children talk with parents, which child talks to the parents most, and who is most likely to discipline the children. Another question considers whether family members can express positive and negative feelings. In determining how open or closed the family is, the nurse explores the type of information the family shares with nonfamily members.

For example, whereas one family may tell others about a member's mental illness, another family may not discuss any illnesses with those outside the family.

Stress and Coping Abilities

One of the most important assessment tasks is to determine how family members deal with major and minor stressful events and their available coping skills. Some families seem able to cope with overwhelming stresses, such as the death of a member, major illness, or severe conflict, but other families seem to fall apart over relatively minor events. Some family caregivers of persons with mental illness have **resilience**, the ability to ability to recover or adjust to challenges over time. For some families, they not only survive the day-to-day stresses of caring for a family member with a serious mental health problem but seem to grow stronger and healthier (Bekhet, Johnson, & Zauszniewski, 2012). It is important for the nurse to listen to which situations a family appraises as stressful and help the family identify usual coping responses. The nurse can then evaluate these responses. On the other hand, if the family's responses are maladaptive (e.g., substance abuse, physical abuse), the nurse will discuss the need to develop coping skills that lead to family well-being (see Chapter 18).

> **NCLEXNOTE**   Identifying stressful events and coping mechanisms should be a priority in a family assessment.

Problem-Solving Skills

Nurses assess family problem-solving skills by focusing on the more recent problems the family has experienced and determining the process that members used to solve them. For example, a child is sick at school and needs to go home. Does the mother, father, grandparent, or babysitter receive the call from the school? Who then cares for the child? Underlying the ability to solve problems is the decision-making process. Who makes and implements decisions? How does the family handle conflict? All of these data provide information regarding the family's problem-solving abilities. After these abilities are identified, the nurse can build on these strengths in helping families deal with additional problems.

Family Social Domain

An assessment of the family's social domain provides important data about the operation of the family as a system and its interaction within its environment. Areas of concern include the system itself, social and financial status, and formal and informal support networks.

Family Systems

Just as any group can be viewed as a system, a family can be understood as a system with interdependent members. Family system theories view the family as an open system whose members interact with their environment as well as among themselves. One family member's change in thoughts or behavior can cause a ripple effect and change everyone else's. For example, a mother who decides not to pick up her children's clothing from their bedroom floors anymore forces the children to deal with cluttered rooms and dirty clothes in a different way than before.

One common scenario in the mental health field is the effect of a patient's improvement on the family. With new medications and treatment, patients are more likely to be able to live independently, and this subsequently changes the responsibilities and activities of family caregivers. Although on the surface members may seem relieved that their caregiving burden is lifted, in reality, they must adjust their time and energies to fill the remaining void. This transition may not be easy because it is often less stressful to maintain familiar activities than to venture into uncharted territory. Families may seem as though

they want to keep an ill member dependent, but in reality, they are struggling with the change in their family system.

Several system models are used in caring for families: the Wright Leahey Calgary model (2013); Bowen's family system (1975, 1976); and Minuchin, Lee, and Simon's (1996) structural family system.

Calgary Family Model

Lorraine M. Wright and Maureen Leahey developed the Calgary Family Assessment Model (CFAM) and the Calgary Family Intervention Model (CFIM). These nursing models are based on systems, cybernetics, and communication and change theories (Wright & Leahey, 2013). Families seek help when they have family health and illness problems, difficulties, and suffering. These two models are multidimensional frameworks that conceptualize the family into structural, developmental, and functional categories. Each assessment category contains several subcategories. Structure is further categorized into internal (e.g., family, gender, sexual orientation), external (extended family and larger systems), and context (ethnicity, race, social class, religion, spirituality, environment). Family developmental assessment is organized according to stages, tasks, and attachments. Functional assessment areas include instrumental (e.g., activities of daily living) and expressive (communication, problem-solving roles, beliefs). The application of this model helps family members of individuals with eating disorders understand behaviors, concern with weight and food, and denial of the problem (Gisladottir & Svavarsdottir, 2011).

The CFAM and CFIM are built around four stages: engagement, assessment, intervention, and termination. The *engagement* stage is the initial stage in which the family is greeted and made comfortable. In the *assessment* stage, problems are identified and relationships among family members and health providers develop. During this stage, the nurse opens space for the family members to tell their story. The *intervention* stage is the core of the clinical work and involves providing a context in which the family can make changes (see Intervention section in this chapter). The *termination* phase refers to the process of ending the therapeutic relationship (Wright & Leahey, 2013).

Family Systems Therapy Model

Bowen recognized the power of a system and believed that there is a balance between the family system and the individual. Bowen developed several concepts that professionals often use today when working with families (Bowen, 1975, 1976; Knauth, Skowron, & Escobar, 2006; Prince-Embury & Saklofske, 2013; Wright, 2009).

Differentiation of self involves two processes: intrapsychic and interpersonal. Intrapsychic differentiation means separating thinking from feeling: a differentiated individual can distinguish between thoughts and feelings and can consequently think through behavior. For example, a person who has experienced intrapsychic differentiation, even though angry, will think through the underlying issue before acting. However, the feeling of the moment will drive the behavior of an undifferentiated individual. Interpersonal differentiation is the process of freeing oneself from the family's emotional chaos. That is, the individual can recognize the family turmoil but avoid reentering arguments and issues. For Bowen, the individual must resolve attachment to this chaos before he or she can differentiate into a mature, healthy personality. Nursing research is currently testing a theoretical model to explain adolescent risk behaviors (Box 14.2).

Triangles: According to Bowen, the triangle is a three-person system and the smallest stable unit in human relations. Cycles of closeness and distance characterize a two-person relationship. When anxiety is high during periods of distance, one party "triangulates" a third person or thing into the relationship. For example, two partners may have a stable relationship when anxiety is low. When anxiety and tension rise, one partner may be so uncomfortable that he or she confides in a friend instead of the other partner. In these cases, triangulating reduces the tension but freezes the conflict in place. In families, triangulating occurs when a husband and wife diffuse tension by focusing on the children. To maintain the status quo and avoid the conflict, which tends to produce symptoms in the child (e.g., bed wetting, fear of school), one of the parents develops an overly intense relationship with one of the children.

Family projection process: Through this process, the triangulated member becomes the center of the family conflicts; that is, the family projects its conflicts onto the child or other triangulated person. Projection is anxious, enmeshed concern. For example, a husband and wife are having difficulty deciding how to spend money. One of their children is having difficulty with interpersonal relationships in school. Instead of the parents resolving their differences over money, one parent focuses on the child's needs and becomes intensely involved in the child's issues. The other parent then relates coolly and distantly to the involved parent.

Nuclear family emotional process: This concept describes patterns of emotional functioning in a family in a single generation. This emotional distance is a patterned reaction in daily interactions with the spouse.

Multigenerational transmission process: Bowen believed that one generation transfers its emotional processes to the next generation. Certain basic patterns among parents and children are replicas of those of past generations, and generations to follow will repeat them as well. The child who is the most involved with the family is least able to differentiate from his or her family of origin and passes on conflicts from one generation to another. For example, a spouse may stay emotionally distant from his partner just as his father was with his mother.

Sibling position: Children develop fixed personality characteristics based on their sibling position in their families. For example, a first-born child may have more confidence and be more outgoing than the second-born child, who has grown up in the older child's shadow. Conversely, the second-born child may be more inclined to identify with the oppressed and be more open to other experiences than the first-born child. These attitudinal and behavioral patterns become fixed parts of both children's personalities. Knowledge of these general personality characteristics is helpful in predicting the family's emotional processes and patterns. These theoretical ideas of Bowen have not been supported by research, but the more general principle that a child's position in the family origin affects the child has significant empirical support (Bleske-Rechek & Kelley, 2014; Green, 2014).

Emotional cutoff: If a member cannot differentiate from his or her family, that member may just flee from the family, either by moving away or avoiding personal subjects of conversation. Yet a brief visit from parents can render these individuals helpless.

BOX 14.2

Research for Best Practice: **Psychometric Evaluation of the Differentiation of Self Inventory for Adolescents**

Knauth, D. G., Skowron, E. A., & Escobar, M. (2006). Effect of differentiation of self on adolescent risk behavior: Test of the theoretical model. Nursing Research, 55(5), 336–345.

THE QUESTION: What is the relationship between the predictor variables of differentiation of self, chronic anxiety, and social problem solving and adolescent high-risk sexual behaviors alcohol and other-drug use and academic engagement?

METHODS: Data were collected from 161 racially or ethnically diverse adolescents (14–19 years old) who completed questions for the variables including the Differentiation of Self Inventory, State-Trait Anxiety Inventory, Social Problem Solving for Adolescents, Drug Involvement Scale for Adolescents, and Sexual Behavior Questionnaire.

FINDINGS: Consistent with the model, higher levels of differentiation of self related to lower levels of chronic anxiety and higher levels of social problem solving. Findings support the theoretical model's credibility and provide evidence of the importance of differentiation of self.

IMPLICATIONS FOR NURSING: Nurses can study and understand adolescent risk behaviors from a family system perspective.

In using the family systems therapy model, the nurse can observe family interactions to determine how differentiated family members are from one another. Are members autonomous in thinking and feeling? Do triangulated relationships develop during periods of stress and tension? Are family members interacting in the same manner as their parents or grandparents? How do the personalities of older siblings compare with those of younger siblings? Who lives close to one another? Does any family member live in another city? The Bowen model can provide a way of assessing the system of family relationships.

Family Structure Model

Minuchin et al. (1996) emphasize the importance of family structure. In their model, the family consists of three essential components: structure, subsystems, and boundaries.

Family structure is the organized pattern in which family members interact. As two adult partners come together to form a family, they develop the quantity of their interactions, or how much time they spend interacting. For example, a newly married couple may establish their evening interaction pattern by talking to each other during dinner but not while watching television. The quality of the interactions also becomes patterned. Whereas some topics are appropriate for conversation during their evening walk (e.g., reciting daily events), controversial or emotionally provocative topics are relegated to other times and places.

Family rules are important influences on interaction patterns. For example, "family problems stay in the family" is a common rule. Both the number of people in the family and its development also influence the interaction pattern. For instance, the interaction between a single mother and her children changes when she remarries and introduces a stepfather. Over time, families repeat interactions, which develop into enduring patterns. For example, if a mother tells her son to straighten his room and the son refuses until his father yells at him, the family has initiated an interactional pattern. If this pattern continues, the child will come to see the father as the disciplinarian and the mother as incompetent. However, the mother will be more affectionate to her son, and the father will remain the disciplinarian on the "outside."

Subsystems develop when family members join together for various activities or functions. Minuchin et al. (1996) view each member, as well as dyads and other larger groups that form, as a subsystem. Obvious groups are parents and children. Sometimes there are "boy" and "girl" systems. Such systems become obvious in an assessment when family members talk about "the boys going fishing with dad" and "the girls going shopping with mother." Family members belong to several different subgroups. A mother may also be a wife, sister, and daughter. Sometimes these roles can conflict. It may be acceptable for a woman to be very firm as a disciplinarian in her role as mother. However, in her sister, wife, or daughter role, similar behavior would provoke anger and resentment.

Boundaries are invisible barriers with varying permeabilities that surround each subsystem. They regulate the amount of contact a person has with others and protect the autonomy of the family and its subsystems. If family members do not take telephone calls at dinner, they are protecting themselves from outside intrusion. When parents do not allow children to interrupt them, they are establishing a boundary between themselves and their children. According to Minuchin et al. (1996), the spouse subsystem must have a boundary that separates it from parents, children, and the outside world. A clear boundary between parent and child enables children to interact with their parents but excludes them from the spouse subsystem.

Boundaries vary from rigid to diffuse. If boundaries are too rigid and permit little contact from outside subsystems, disengagement results, and disengaged individuals are relatively isolated. On the other hand, rigid boundaries permit independence, growth, and mastery within the subsystem, particularly if parents do not hover over their children, telling them what to do or fighting their battles for them. Enmeshed subsystems result when boundaries are diffuse. That is, when boundaries are too relaxed, parents may become too involved with their children, and the children learn to rely on the parents to make decisions, resulting in decreased independence. According to Minuchin et al. (1996), if children see their parents as friends and treat them as they would treat their peers, then enmeshment exists.

Indeed, autonomy and interdependence are key concepts, important both to individual growth and family system maintenance. Relationship patterns are maintained by universal rules governing family organization (especially power hierarchy) and mutual behavioral expectations. In the well-functioning family, boundaries are clear, and a hierarchy exists with a strong parental subsystem. Problems result when there is a malfunctioning of the hierarchical arrangement or boundaries or a maladaptive reaction to changing developmental or environmental requirements. Minuchin et al. (1996) believe in clear, flexible boundaries by which all family members can live comfortably.

In the family structural theory, what distinguishes normal families is not the absence of problems but a functional family structure to handle them. Normal husbands and wives must learn to adjust to each other, rear their children, deal with their parents, cope with their jobs, and fit into their communities. The types of struggles change with developmental stages and situational crises. The psychiatric nurse assesses the family structure and the presence of subsystems or boundaries. He or she uses these data to determine how the subsystems and boundaries affect the family's functioning. Helping family members change a subsystem, such as including girls in the boys' activities, may improve family functioning.

Social and Financial Status

Social status is often linked directly to financial status. The nurse should assess the occupations of the family members. Who works? Who is primarily responsible for the family's financial support? Families of low social status are more likely to have limited financial resources, which can place additional stresses on the family. Nurses can use information regarding the family's financial status to determine whether to refer the family to social services.

Cultural expectations and beliefs about acceptable behaviors may cause additional stress. For example, in a qualitative study of Korean American caregivers, spouse caregivers' perceptions were compared with child caregivers'. In the Korean culture dementia is called *no-mang* and viewed as a normal consequence of aging. Caregivers are selected based on cultural belief of filial piety—the eldest son and wife provide the care. Eight female Korean American caregivers (four spouses, four adult children) were interviewed about their perceptions of caregiving for their family members. Spouse caregivers perceived their caregiving as part of their life work. Child caregivers viewed their caregiving as extra work (Lee & Smith, 2012).

Formal and Informal Support Networks

Both formal and informal networks are important in providing support to individuals and families and should be identified in the assessment. These networks are the link among the individual, families, and the community. Assessing the extent of formal support (e.g., hospitals, agencies) and informal support (e.g., extended family, friends, and neighbors) gives a clearer picture of the availability of support. In assessing formal support, the nurse should ask about the family's involvement with government institutions and self-help groups such as Alcoholics Anonymous. Assessing the informal network is particularly important in cultural groups with extended family networks or close friends because these individuals can be major sources of support to patients. If the nurse does not ask about the informal network, these important people may be missed. Nurses can inquire whether family members volunteer at schools, local hospitals, or nursing homes. They can also ask whether the family attends religious services or activities.

FAMILY NURSING DIAGNOSES

From the assessment data, nurses can choose several possible nursing diagnoses. Ineffective Family Therapeutic Regimen Management and Disabled Family Coping are possibilities. Nurses choose Interrupted Family Processes if a usually supportive family is experiencing stressful events that challenge its previously effective functioning. They choose Ineffective Family Therapeutic Regimen Management if the family is experiencing difficulty integrating into daily living a program for the treatment of illness and the sequela of illness that meets specific health goals. They select Compromised Family Coping when the primary supportive person is providing insufficient, ineffective, or compromised support, comfort, or assistance to the patient in managing or mastering adaptive tasks related to the individual's health challenge.

The assessment data may also reveal other nursing diagnoses of individual family members, such as Caregiver Role Strain, Ineffective Denial, or Complicated Grieving. If the nurse finds that any other nursing diagnosis is appropriate, the individual family member should have an opportunity to explore ways of managing the problem.

FAMILY INTERVENTIONS

Family interventions focus on supporting the biopsychosocial integrity and functioning of the family as defined by its members. Although family therapy is reserved for mental health specialists, the generalist psychiatric–mental health nurse can implement several biopsychosocial interventions, such as counseling, promotion of self-care activities, supportive therapy, education and health teaching, and the use of genograms.

In implementing any family intervention, flexibility is essential, particularly when working with culturally diverse groups. The nurse creates the context for change by making sure the interventions are possible for the family (Wright & Leahy, 2005). For example, weekly appointments may be ideal but impossible for a busy family. To implement successful, culturally competent family interventions, nurses need to be open to modifying the structure and format of the sessions. Longer sessions are often useful, especially when a translator or interpreter is used. Nurses also need to respect and work with the changing family composition of family and nonfamily participants (e.g., extended family members, intimate partners, friends and neighbors, community helpers) in sessions. Because of the stigma that some cultural groups associate with seeking help, nurses may need to hold intervention sessions in community settings (e.g., churches and schools) or at the family's home. If adequate progress is made, it is time to decrease the frequency of sessions and move toward termination. Families may move toward termination if they recognize that improvement has been made (Wright & Leahey, 2013).

Counseling

Nurses often use counseling when working with families because it is a short-term problem-solving approach that addresses current issues. The nurse should avoid taking sides by forming an alliance with one family member or subgroup (Wright & Leahy, 2013). If the assessment reveals complex, longstanding relationship problems, the nurse needs to refer the family to a family therapist. If the family is struggling with psychiatric problems of one or more family members or the family system is in a life-cycle transition, the nurse should use short-term counseling. Instead of giving advice, the counseling sessions should focus on specific issues or problems using sound group process theory. Usually, a problem-solving approach works well after an issue has been identified (see Chapter 10).

Promoting Self-Care Activities

Families often need support in changing behaviors that promote self-care activities. For example, families may inadvertently reinforce a family member's dependency out of fear of the patient's being taken advantage of in work or social situations. A nurse can help the family explore how to meet the patient's need for work and social activity and at the same time help alleviate the family's fears.

Caregiver distress or role strain can occur in families that are responsible for the care of members with long-term illness. Family interventions can help families deal with the burden of caring for members with psychiatric disorders. An analysis of 16 studies indicated that family interventions can affect relatives' burden, psychological distress, and the relationship between patient and relative and family functioning. Family intervention may decrease the frequency of relapse (in persons with schizophrenia) and encourage compliance with medication (Pharoah, Mari, Rathbone, & Wong, 2010).

Supporting Family Functioning and Resilience

Supporting family functioning involves various nursing approaches. In meeting with the family, the nurse should identify and acknowledge its values. In developing a trusting relationship with the family, the nurse should confirm that all members have a sense of self and self-worth. Encouraging positive thinking and participating in support groups will contribute to the family's well-being (Box 14.3). Supporting family subsystems (e.g., encouraging the children to play while meeting with the spouses) reinforces family boundaries. Based on assessment of the family system's operation and communication patterns, the nurse can reinforce open, honest communication.

In communicating with the family, the nurse needs to observe boundaries constantly and avoid becoming triangulated into family issues. An objective, empathic leadership style can set the tone for the family sessions.

BOX 14.3

Research for Best Practice: **Resilience and Women Family Caregivers**

Zauszniewski, J. A., Bekhet, A. K., & Suresky, M. J. (2009). Effects on resilience of women family caregivers of adults with serious mental illness: The role of positive cognitions. Archives of Psychiatric Nursing, 23(6), 412–422.

THE QUESTION: What are the risks and protective factors on resilience in women family members of adults with serious mental illness?

METHODS: This study is based on a secondary analysis using data from a larger study of resourcefulness and quality of life in women caregivers of adults with serious mental illness.

FINDINGS: Both the caregiver risk and protective factors, including eight positive cognitions, were found to predict two indicators of resilience: resourcefulness and sense of coherence.

IMPLICATIONS FOR NURSING: Enhancement of the resilience of family members by encouraging members to participate in support groups and develop skills for positive thinking will contribute to the family member's well being.

Providing Education and Health Teaching

One of the most important family interventions is education and health teaching, particularly in families with mental illness. Families have a central role in the treatment of mental illnesses. Members need to learn about mental disorders, medications, actions, side effects, and overall treatment approaches and outcomes. For example, families are often reluctant to have members take psychiatric medications because they believe the medications will "drug" the patient or become addictive. The family's beliefs about mental illnesses and treatment can affect whether patients will be able to manage their illness.

Using Genograms

Genograms not only are useful in assessment but also can be used as intervention strategies. Nurses can use genograms to help family members understand current feelings and emotions as well as the family's evolution over several generations. Genograms allow the family to examine relationships from a factual, objective perspective. Often, family members gain new insights and can begin to understand their problems within the context of their family system. For example, families may begin to view depression in an adolescent daughter with new seriousness when they see it as part of a pattern of several generations of women who have struggled with depression. A husband, raised as an only child in a small Midwestern town, may better understand his feelings of

BOX 14.4

John and Judy Jones

John and Judy Jones were married 3 years ago after their graduation from a small liberal arts college in the Midwest. Judy's career choice required that she live on the East Coast where she should be near her large family. John willingly moved with her and quickly found a satisfying position. After about 6 months of marriage, John became extremely irritable and depressed. He kept saying that his life was not his own. Judy was very concerned but could not understand his feelings of being overwhelmed. His job was going well, and they had a very busy social life, mostly revolving around her family, whom John loved. They decided to seek counseling and completed the following genogram:

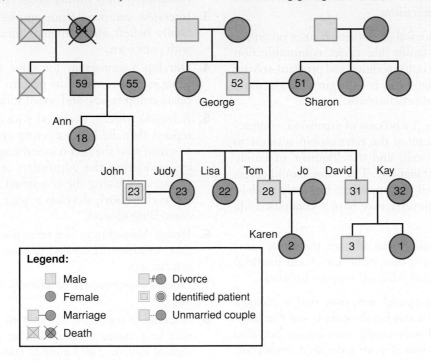

Legend:
- ☐ Male
- ● Female
- ☐● Marriage
- ⊠ ⊗ Death
- ☐#● Divorce
- ☐ ◉ Identified patient
- ☐--● Unmarried couple

After looking at the genogram, both John and Judy began to realize that part of John's discomfort had to do with the number of family members who were involved in their lives.

Judy and John began to redefine their social life, allowing more time with friends and each other.

being overwhelmed after comparing his family structure with that of his wife, who comes from a large family of several generations living together in the urban Northeast (Box 14.4).

SUMMARY OF KEY POINTS

- The family is an important societal unit that often is responsible for the care and coordination of treatment of members with mental disorders. The family structure, size, and roles are rapidly changing. Traditional health care services will have to adapt to meet the mental health care needs of these families.

- A family is a group of people who are connected emotionally, by blood, or in both ways that has developed patterns of interactions and relationships. Families come in various compositions, including nuclear, extended, multigenerational, single-parent, and same-gender families. Cultural values and beliefs define family composition and roles.

- Nurses complete a comprehensive family assessment when they care for families for extended periods or if a patient has complex mental health problems.

- In building relationships with families, nurses must establish credibility and competence with the family. Unless the nurse addresses the family's immediate needs first, the family will have difficulty engaging in the challenges of caring for someone with a mental disorder.

- The genogram is an assessment and intervention tool that is useful in understanding health problems, relationship issues, and social functioning across several generations.

- In assessing the family biologic domain, the nurse determines physical and mental health status and their effects on family functioning.

- Family members are often reluctant to discuss the mental disorders of family members because of the stigma associated with mental illness. In many instances, family members do not know whether mental illnesses were present in other generations.

- The family psychological assessment focuses on family development, the family life cycle, communication patterns, stress and coping abilities, and problem-solving skills. One assessment aim is to begin to understand family interpersonal relationships.

- The family life cycle is a process of expansion, contraction, and realignment of the relationship systems to support the entry, exit, and development of family members in a functional way. The nurse should determine whether a family fits any of the life-cycle models. Families living in poverty may have a condensed life cycle.

- In assessing the family social domain, the nurse compiles data about the system itself, social and financial status, and formal and informal support networks.

- The family system model proposes that a balance should exist between the family system and the individual. A person needs family connection but also needs to be differentiated as an individual. Important concepts include triangles, family projection process, nuclear family emotional process, multigenerational transmission, sibling position, and emotional cutoff.

- The family structure model explains patterns of family interaction. Subsystems develop that also influence interaction patterns. Boundaries can vary from rigid to relaxed. The rigidity of the boundaries affects family functioning.

- Family interventions focus on supporting the family's biopsychosocial integrity and functioning as defined by its members. Family psychiatric nursing interventions include counseling, promotion of self-care activities, supportive therapy, education and health teaching, and the use of genograms. Mental health specialists, including advanced practice nurses, conduct family therapy.

- Education of the family is one of the most useful interventions. Teaching the family about mental disorders, life cycles, family systems, and family interactions can help the family develop a new understanding of family functioning and the effects of mental disorders on the family.

CRITICAL THINKING CHALLENGES

1. Differentiate between a nuclear and extended family. How can a group of people who are unrelated by blood consider themselves a family?

2. Interview a family with a member who has a mental illness and identify who provides support to the individual and family during acute episodes of illness.

3. Interview someone from another culture regarding family beliefs about mental illness. Compare them with your own.

4. Develop a genogram for your family. Analyze the genogram in terms of its pattern of health problems, relationship issues, and social functioning.

5. A female patient, divorced with two small children, reports that she is considering getting married again to a man who she met 6 months ago. She asks for help in considering the advantages and disadvantages of remarriage. Using the remarried family formulations life-cycle model, develop a plan for structuring the counseling session.

6. Define Minuchin et al.'s term *family structure* and use that definition in observing your own family and its interaction.

7. Discuss what happens to a family that has rigid boundaries.

8. A family is finding it difficult to provide transportation to a support group for an adult member with mental illness. The family is committed to his treatment but is also experiencing severe financial stress because of another family illness. Using a problem-solving approach, outline a plan for helping the family explore solutions to the transportation problem.

Brokeback Mountain: 2005. This movie is a powerful story of two young men, a Wyoming ranch hand and a rodeo cowboy, who meet in the summer of 1963 sheepherding in the harsh, high grasslands and have an unorthodox yet lifelong bond. At the end of the summer, a love affair begins that the two of them desperately try to hide from those around them.

VIEWING POINTS: Observe your feelings as you watch this movie. Identify the cultural mores that prevent Jack and Ennis from being open about their relationship. Develop a genogram of Ennis and Jack.

My Big Fat Greek Wedding: 2002. This movie is about Fotoula "Toula" Portokalos, a Greek American woman who falls in love with a non-Greek protestant fellow, Ian Miller. Toula is the only one in her family who had not met her family expectations of marrying a Greek and having children. Whereas Toula is stuck working in the family business, a restaurant, her sister has the perfect Greek family. Toula's father is adamantly opposed to marriage to a non-Greek. A wedding is eventually planned with multiple problems throughout the year.

VIEWING POINTS: Discuss the stigma that faces Toula and Ian as they plan their life together. How would you intervene if Toula approached you for help with her family? Identify the cultural beliefs that are shaping and interfering with the wishes of the newly engaged couple.

References

Badgett, M. V. L., Durso, L. E., & Schneebaum, A. (2013). *New patterns of poverty in the Lesbian, gay, and bisexual community*. The Williams Institute, Los Angeles: University of California.

Bekhet, A. K., Johnson, J. L., & Zauszniewski, J. A. (2012). Resilience in family members of persons with autism spectrum disorder: A review of the literature. *Issues in Mental Health Nursing, 33*(10), 650–656.

Bleske-Rechek, A., & Kelley, J. A. (2014). Birth order and personality: A within-family test using independent self-reports from both firstborn and laterborn siblings. *Personality and Individual Differences, 56*(1), 15–18.

Bowen, M. (1975). Family therapy after twenty years. In S. Arieti, D. Freedman, & J. Dyrud (Eds.), *American handbook of psychiatry* (2nd ed, vol. 5, pp. 379–391). New York: Basic Books.

Bowen, M. (1976). Theory in the practice of psychotherapy. In P. Guerin (Ed.), *Family therapy: Theory and practice* (pp. 42–90). New York: Gardner Press.

Brown, S. L., Bulanda, J. R., & Lee, G. R. (2012). Transitions into and out of cohabitation in later life. *Journal of Marriage & Family, 74*(4), 774–793.

ChildStats. (2013). *America's Children: Key National Indicators of Well-Being, 2013*. Forum on Child and Family Statistics. www.childstats.gov

Copen, C. E., Daniels, K., & Mosher, W. D. (2013). First premarital cohabitation in the United States: 2006-2010 National Survey of Family Growth. *National Health Statistics Reports, 64*. National Center for Health Statistics, Center for Disease Control and Prevention.

Eamon, M. K. (2013). Employment, economic hardship and sources of assistance in low-income, single-mother families before versus during and after the Great Recession. *Journal of Poverty, 17*(2), 135–156.

Gisladottir, M. & Svavarsdottir, E. K. (2011). Educational and support intervention to help families assist in the recovery of relatives with eating disorders. *Journal of Psychiatric and Mental health Nursing, 18*(2), 122–130.

Green, B. (2014). Birth order and post-traumatic stress disorder. *Psychology, Health & Medicine, 19*(1), 24–32.

Griffiths, C. & Sin, J. (2013). Rethinking siblings and mental illness. *The Psychologist, 26*(11), 808–810.

Hines, P. M. (1999). The family life cycle of African American families living in poverty. In B. Carter & M. McGoldrick (Eds.), *The expanded family life cycle* (pp. 327–345). New York: Allyn & Bacon.

Hines, P. M., & Boyd-Franklin, N. (2005). African American families. In M. McGoldrick, J. Giordano, & N. Garcia-Preto (Eds.), *Ethnicity & family therapy* (3rd ed, pp. 87–116). New York: The Guilford Press.

Knauth, D., Skowron, E. A., & Escobar, M. (2006). Effect of differentiation of self on adolescent risk behavior: Test of the theoretical model. *Nursing Research, 55*(5), 336–345.

Lee, Y., & Smith, L. (2012). Qualitative research on Korean American dementia caregivers' perception of caregiving: Heterogeneity between spouse caregivers and child caregivers. *Journal of Human Behavior in the Social Environment, 22*(2), 115–129.

Lechner, L., Bolman, C., & van Dalen, A. (2007). Definite involuntary childlessness: associations between coping, social support and psychological distress. *Human Reproduction, 22*(1), 288–294.

Lofquist, D., & Ellis, R. (2011). Comparison of estimates of same-sex couple households from the ACS and CPS. Annual Meeting of the Population Association of America, Washington, D.S., March 31–April 2, 2011.

McGoldrick, M., Carter, B., & Garcia-Preto, N. (2011). *The expanded family life cycle: Individual, family, and social perspectives* (4th ed). Boston, MA: Allyn & Bacon.

McGoldrick, M., Gerson, R. & Petry, S. (2008). *Genograms: Assessment and intervention* (3rd ed). New York: W. W. Norton & Company.

McGoldrick, M., Giordano, F., & Garcia-Preto, N. (Eds.). (2005). *Ethnicity and family therapy*. New York: The Guilford Press.

Minuchin, S., Lee, W., & Simon, G. (1996). *Mastering family therapy: Journey of growth and transformation*. New York: John Wiley & Sons.

Mustanski, B. S., Garofalo, R., & Emerson, E. M. (2010). Mental health disorders, psychological distress, and suicidality in a diverse sample of lesbian, gay, bisexual, and transgender youths. *American Journal of Public Health, 100*(12), 2426–2432.

Pharoah, F. M., Mari, J. J., Rathbone, J., & Wong, W. (2010). Family intervention for schizophrenia. *Cochrane Database of Systematic Reviews*, (12):CD000088.

Prince-Embury, S. & Saklofske, D. H., (Eds.) (2013). *Resiliency in children, Youth and Adults: Translating Research into Practice*. New York: Springer.

Sotomayor-Peterson, M., Figueredo, A. J., Christensen, D. H., & Taylor, A. R. (2012). Couples' cultural values, shared parenting, and family emotional climate within Mexican American families. *Family Process, 51*(2), 218–233.

U.S. Census Bureau. (2013). Current population survey. *2013 Annual Social and Economic Supplement*. www.census.gov.

U.S. Department of Commerce. (2014). *American Community Survey 2008–2012*. Retrieved from http://www.census.gov/

Umberson, D., Pudrovska, T., & Reczek, C. (2010). Parenthood, childlessness, and well-being: A life course perspective. *Journal of Marriage & Family, 72*(3), 612–629.

Vespa, J., Lewis, J. M., & Kreider, R. M. (2013). *America's families and living arrangements: 2012*. U.S. Department of Commerce, U.S. Census Bureau. www.census.gov.

Vikstrom, J., Bladh, M., Hammar, M., Marcusson, J., Wressle, E., & Sydsjo, G. (2011). The influences of childlessness on the psychological well-being and social network of the oldes old. *BMC Geriatrics, 11*, 78. www.biomedcentral.com/1471-2318/11/78

Wright, J. (2009). Self-soothing-A recursive intrapsychic and relational process: The contribution of the Bowen theory to the process of self-soothing. *The Australian and New Zealand Journal of Family Therapy, 30*(1), 29–31.

Wright. L. M. & Leahey, L. M. (2005). The three most common errors in family nursing: How to avoid or sidestep. *Journal of Family Nursing, 11*(2), 90–101.

Wright, L. M., & Leahey, L. M. (2013). *Nurses and families: A guide to family assessment and intervention* (6th ed). Philadelphia: F. A. Davis Company.

Zauszniewski, J. A., Bekhet, A. K., & Suresky, M. J. (2009). Effects on resilience of women family caregivers of adults with serious mental illness: The role of positive cognitions. *Archives of Psychiatric Nursing, 23*(6), 412–422.

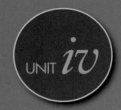

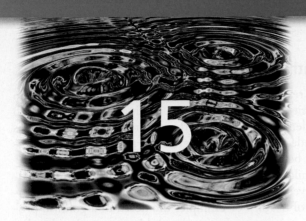

15

Mental Health Promotion for Children and Adolescents

Catherine Gray Deering

KEY CONCEPTS

- egocentric thinking
- invincibility fable

LEARNING OBJECTIVES

After studying this chapter, you will be able to:

1. Describe common problems for children and adolescents.

2. Identify risk factors for the development of psychopathology in childhood and adolescence.

3. Describe protective factors in the mental health promotion of children and adolescents.

4. Analyze the role of the nurse in mental health promotion for children and families.

KEY TERMS

- attachment • bibliotherapy • bullying • child abuse and neglect • developmental delays • early intervention programs • family preservation • fetal alcohol syndrome • formal operations • normalization • protective factors • psychoeducational programs • relational aggression • resilience • risk factors • social skills training • vulnerable child syndrome

Children and adolescents respond to the stresses of life in different ways according to their developmental levels. **Resilience** is the phenomenon by which some children at risk for psychopathology—because of genetic or experiential circumstances (or both)—attain good mental health, maintain hope, and achieve healthy outcomes (Garcia-Dia, DiNapoli, Garcia-Ona, Jakubowski, & O'Flaherty, 2013). This chapter examines specific determinants of childhood and adolescent mental health, discusses the effects of common childhood stressors, and identifies **risk factors** for psychopathology, or the characteristics that increase the

likelihood of developing a disorder. This chapter also considers **protective factors**, or the characteristics that reduce the probability that a child will develop a disorder, and provides guidelines for mental health promotion and risk reduction. Nurses are in a key position to identify and intervene with children and adolescents at risk for psychopathology by virtue of their close contact with families in health care settings and their roles as educators. Knowing the difference between typical and atypical child development is crucial in helping parents to view their children's behavior realistically and to respond appropriately.

CHILDHOOD AND ADOLESCENT MENTAL HEALTH

Supportive social networks and positive childhood and adolescent experiences maximize the mental health of children and adolescents. Children are more likely to be mentally healthy if they have good physical health, positive social development, an easy temperament (adaptable, low intensity, positive mood), and secure **attachment** through the emotional bonds formed between them and their parents at an early age. These areas are considered in the mental health assessment of children (see Chapter 34). **Developmental delays** not only slow the child's progress but also can interfere with the development of positive self-esteem. Children with an easy temperament can adapt to change without intense emotional reactions. A secure attachment helps the child test the world without fear of rejection.

> **NCLEXNOTE** Attachment and temperament are key concepts in the behavior of children and adolescents in any health care setting. Apply these concepts to any pediatric patient.

COMMON PROBLEMS IN CHILDHOOD

Children and adolescents are faced with many challenges while growing up. Loss is an inevitable part of life. All children experience significant losses, the most common being death of a grandparent, parental divorce, death of a pet, and loss of friends through moving or changing schools. Learning to mourn losses can lead to a renewed appreciation of the precious value of life and close relationships. Sibling rivalry, illness, and common adolescent risk-taking tendencies also may pose challenges for children as they grow and develop.

Death and Grief

Vast research shows that similar to adults, children who experience major losses are at risk for mental health problems, particularly if the natural grieving process is impeded. However, the grieving process differs somewhat between children and adults (Table 15.1).

Children's responses to loss reflect their developmental level. As early as age 3 years, children have some concept of death. For example, the death of a goldfish provides an opportunity for the child to grasp the idea that the fish will never swim again. However, not until about age 7 years can most children understand the permanence of death. Before this age, they may verbalize that someone has "died" but in the next sentence ask when the dead person will be "coming back." Even adolescents sometimes flirt with death by driving dangerously or engaging in other risky behaviors as if they believe they are immune to death. This phenomenon is known as the invincibility fable because adolescents view themselves in an egocentric way, as unique and invulnerable to the consequences experienced by others.

Table 15.1	GRIEVING IN CHILDHOOD, ADOLESCENCE, AND ADULTHOOD	
Children	**Adolescents**	**Adults**
• View death as reversible; do not understand that death is permanent until about age 7 years	• Understand that death is permanent but may flirt with death (e.g., reckless driving, unprotected sex) because of omnipotent feelings	• Understand that death is permanent; may struggle with spiritual beliefs about death
• Experiment with ideas about death by killing bugs, staging funerals, acting out death in play	• May be fascinated by death, enjoy morbid books and movies, listen to rock music about death and suicide	• May try not to think about death, depending on cultural background
• Mourn through activities (e.g., mock funerals, playing with things owned by the loved one); may not cry	• Mourn by talking about the loss, crying, and reflecting on it, sometimes becoming dramatic (e.g., overidentifying with the lost person, developing poetic or romantic ideas about death)	• Mourn through talking about the loss, crying, reviewing memories, and thinking privately about it
• May not discuss the loss openly but may instead express grief through regression, somatic complaints, behavior problems, or withdrawal	• Often withdraw when mourning or seek comfort through peer groups; may feel parents do not understand their feelings	• Usually discuss loss openly, depending on level of support available; may feel there is a "time limit" on how long it is socially acceptable to grieve
• Need repeated explanations to fully understand the loss; it may be helpful to read children's books that explain death	• Need permission to grieve openly because they may believe they should act strong or take care of the adults involved; need acceptance of their sometimes extreme reactions	• Need friends, family, and other supportive people to listen and allow them to mourn for however long it takes; need opportunities to review their feelings and memories

> **KEYCONCEPT**   The **invincibility fable** is an aspect of egocentric thinking in adolescence that causes teens to view themselves as immune to dangerous situations, such as unprotected sex, fast driving, and drug abuse.

If the concept of death is difficult for adults to grasp, it is particularly important to be sensitive to children's struggle to understand and cope with it. Most children closely watch their parents' response to grief and loss and use fantasy to fill the gaps in their understanding. In many cases, family members take turns grieving, with children sensing that their parents are so overwhelmed by their own emotional pain that they cannot bear the children's grief. They also see adults taking turns being strong for each other.

Loss and Preschool-Aged Children

The preschool-aged child may react more to the parents' distress about a death than to the death itself. Young children who depend totally on their parents may be frightened when they see their parents upset. Anything the parent can do to alleviate their children's anxiety, such as reassuring them that the parent will be okay and continuing the child's routine (e.g., normal bedtimes, snacks, play times) will help the child to feel secure (Worden, 2009). Because preschool-aged children have limited ability to verbalize their feelings, they may need to express them through fantasy play and activities, such as mock funerals. Books that explain death, such as *Charlotte's Web* by E. B. White, may also be helpful. Parents should take care not to use euphemisms that could fuel misconceptions of death, such as "He went to sleep" or "Jesus took him." Young children may interpret these messages literally and fear going to sleep (because they might die) or focus their natural, grief-related anger on the irrational idea that the person deliberately has not returned. The best approach is to explain honestly that the person has died and is not coming back, elicit the child's understanding and questions about what has happened, and then repeat this process continually as the child gradually begins to grasp the reality of the situation. The decision of whether to take a young child to a funeral may be particularly complex. Figure 15.1 enumerates some factors to consider.

Loss and School-Aged Children

School-aged children understand the permanence of death more clearly than do preschoolers, but they may still struggle to articulate their feelings. Children in this age group may express their grief through somatic complaints, regression, behavior problems, withdrawal, and even anger toward their parents. They may think that others expect them to cry and react with immediate emotional intensity to the death; when they do not react this way, they feel guilty.

The death of a sibling can be a particularly difficult loss for both the child and the family. Common reactions to this are for the surviving child to feel guilt because of natural sibling rivalry and for the parents to unconsciously endow the surviving child with qualities of the lost sibling as if to fill the empty space in the family (Worden, 2009). Of course, the death of a parent can be even more devastating. The functioning level of the surviving parent is the best predictor of a child's adjustment to the loss (Silverman, 2000). Parents should provide grieving children with support; nurturance; continuity; and the opportunity to remember the lost person in concrete ways through photographs, stories, and family activities that allow the child to memorialize the loved one.

Loss and Adolescents

Adolescents who are in Piaget's stage of **formal operations**, characterized by the ability to use abstract reasoning to conceptualize and solve problems, can better understand death as an abstract concept (see Chapter 7). Because adolescents tend to be idealistic and to think in extremes, they may even have poetic or romantic notions about death. Many teenagers become fascinated with morbid rock music, movies, and books. Although they may be able to express their thoughts and feelings about death more clearly than younger children, they often are reluctant to do so for fear of being viewed as childish. Some adolescents assume a parental role in the family after a death, denying their own needs. School settings may be particularly helpful in providing group and individual support for grieving adolescents; structured programs for children and adolescents can prevent complicated (pathological) bereavement (Dopp & Cain, 2012).

Separation and Divorce

Although many families adapt to separation and divorce without long-term negative effects for the children, youth often show at least temporary difficulties in dealing with this common stressor (Kelly, 2012). Parental separation and divorce change the family structure, usually resulting in a substantial reduction in the contact that children have with one of their parents. The child's response to divorce is similar to the response to death. In some ways, divorce may be harder for the child to understand because the noncustodial parent is gone but still alive, and the parents have made a conscious choice to separate. Children of divorce are at increased risk for emotional, behavioral, and academic problems. However, the response to the loss that divorce imposes varies depending on the child's temperament; the parents' interventions; and the level of stress, change, and conflict surrounding the divorce

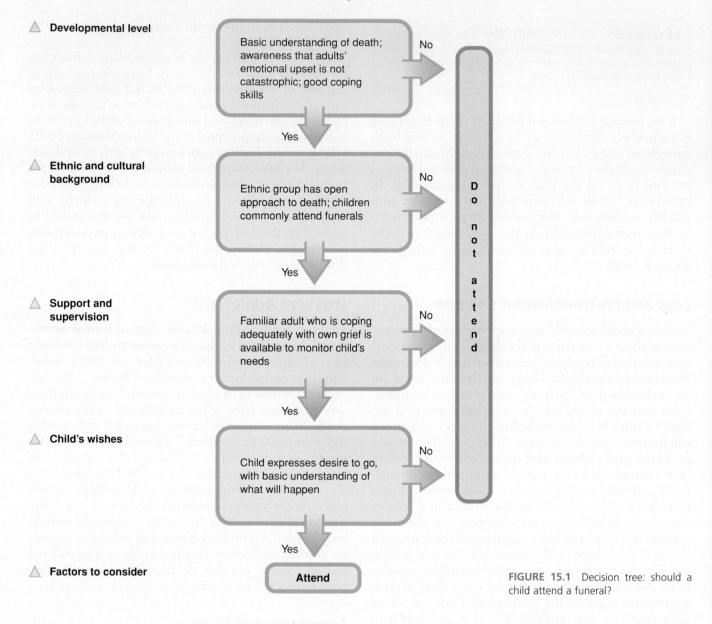

Developmental level

Basic understanding of death; awareness that adults' emotional upset is not catastrophic; good coping skills

No

Yes

Ethnic and cultural background

Ethnic group has open approach to death; children commonly attend funerals

No

Yes

Support and supervision

Familiar adult who is coping adequately with own grief is available to monitor child's needs

No

Yes

Child's wishes

Child expresses desire to go, with basic understanding of what will happen

No

Yes

Do not attend

Factors to consider

Attend

FIGURE 15.1 Decision tree: should a child attend a funeral?

(Hetherington & Kelly, 2002). A major change in socio-economic status, such as moving from dual-earner status to single-parent family status, may account for much of the variation in levels of distress among divorcing families (Ryan & Claessens, 2013).

The first 2 or 3 years after the couple's breakup tend to be the most difficult. Typical childhood reactions include confusion, guilt, depression, regression, somatic symptoms, acting-out behaviors (e.g., stealing, disobedience), fantasies that the parents will reunite, fear of losing the custodial parent, and alignment with one parent against the other. After an initial adjustment period, children usually accept the reality of the situation and begin coping adaptively. Most divorced parents eventually remarry new partners, which often imposes another period of coping difficulties for the children. Children with step-

parents and stepsiblings are at renewed risk for emotional and behavioral problems as they struggle to cope with the new relationships (Gonzales, 2009).

Protective factors against emotional problems in children of divorce and remarriage include a structured home and school environment with reasonable and consistent limit setting and a warm, supportive relationship with stepparents (Kelly, 2012). Helpful interventions for children of divorce include education regarding children's reactions; promotion of regular and predictable visitation; reduction of conflict between the parents through counseling, mediation, and clear visitation policies; continuance of usual routines; and family counseling to facilitate adjustment after remarriage (Table 15.2). It is also important to make it clear to children that the divorce was not caused by them. Egocentric thinking, which is

Table 15.2	PLAY THERAPY WITH A 4-YEAR-OLD CHILD WHOSE PARENTS ARE DIVORCING	
Patient Statement	**Nurse Response**	**Analysis and Rationale**
(Child smashes two cars together and makes loud, crashing sound.)	That's a loud crash. They really hit hard.	Child may be expressing anger and frustration nonverbally through play. Nurse attempts to establish rapport with child by relating at child's level using age-appropriate vocabulary.
Crrrash!	I know a boy who gets so mad sometimes that he feels like smashing something.	Child is engrossed in fantasy play, typical of preschoolers. Children often use toys as symbols of human figures (animism). Nurse uses indirect method of eliciting child's feelings because preschoolers often do not express feelings directly. Reference to another child's anger helps to normalize this child's feelings.
Yeah!	Sounds like you feel that way sometimes, too.	Child is beginning to relate to nurse and sense her empathy. Nurse reflects the child's feelings to facilitate further communication.
Yeah, when my mom and dad fight.	It's hard to listen to parents fighting. Sometimes it's scary. You wonder what's going to happen.	Child is experiencing frustration and helplessness related to family conflict. Nurse expresses empathy and attempts to articulate child's feelings because preschool children have a limited ability to identify and label feelings.
My mom and dad are getting a divorce.	That's too bad. What's going to happen when they get the divorce?	Child has basic awareness of the reality of parents' divorce but may not understand this concept. Nurse expresses empathy and attempts to assess the child's level of understanding of the divorce.
Dad's not going to live in our house.	Oh, I guess you'll miss having him there all the time. It would be nice if you all could live together, but I guess that's not going to happen.	Preschool child focuses on the effects the divorce will have on him (egocentrism). Child seems to have a clear understanding of the consequences of the divorce. Nurse articulates the child's perspective and reinforces the reality of the divorce to avoid fueling child's possible denial and reconciliation fantasies.
(Silently moves cars across the floor.)	What do you think is the reason your parents decided to get a divorce?	Child expresses sadness nonverbally. Nurse further attempts to assess the child's understanding of the circumstances surrounding the divorce.
Because I did it.	What do you mean—you did it?	Child provides clue that he may be feeling responsible. Nurse uses clarification to fully assess child's understanding.
I made them mad 'cause I left my bike in the driveway and Dad ran over it.	How? Do you think that's why they're getting the divorce?	Child uses egocentric thinking to draw conclusion that his actions caused the divorce. Nurse continues to clarify the child's thinking. The goal is to elicit the child's perceptions, so that misperceptions can be corrected.
Yeah, they had a big fight.	They may have been upset about the bike, but I don't think that's why they're getting a divorce.	The nurse goes on to explain why parents get divorced and to provide opportunities for the child to ask questions.
Why?	Because parents get divorced when they're upset with *each other*—when they can't get along—not when they're upset with their children.	

normal for children, may cause children to believe that they are at the root of the problem. Some evidence shows that it is not the divorce itself but rather the continuing conflict between the parents that is most damaging to children. Parents manage divorce better if they can remember that children naturally idealize and identify with both parents and need to view both of them positively. Therefore, it is helpful for parents to guard against making negative statements about each other and focus on evidence of their former partner's love and respect for the child.

> **KEYCONCEPT** In **egocentric thinking**, children naturally view themselves as the center of their own universe. Common examples of this are children looking out the car window at night and claiming that "the moon is following me" and children sitting in front of the television set, blocking the view for the parent, but believing that if they can see the television, that parent can, too. This kind of magical, self-focused thinking is charming, but it has a downside when children believe that they have caused a divorce or death in the family because of their own actions.

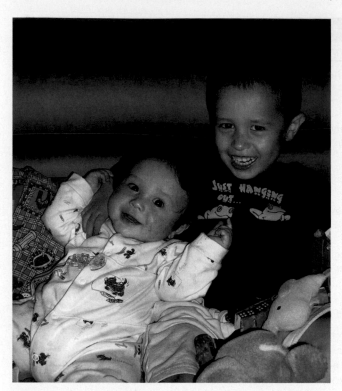

FIGURE 15.2 Sibling relationships significantly influence personality development.

Sibling Relationships

Until recently, the role of siblings in children's development was underemphasized. A growing body of research shows that sibling relationships significantly influence personality development. Positive sibling relationships can be protective factors against the development of psychopathology (Figure 15.2), particularly in troubled families in which the parents are emotionally unavailable (Kramer & Bank, 2005). Thus, nurses should emphasize to parents that minimizing sibling rivalry and maximizing cooperative behavior will benefit their children's social and emotional development throughout life.

Sibling rivalry begins with the birth of the second child. Often, this event is traumatic for the first child who, up until then, was the sole focus of the parents' attention (Kramer & Ramsburg, 2002). The older sibling usually reacts with anger and may reveal not-so-subtle fantasies of getting rid of the new sibling (e.g., "I dreamed that the new baby died"). Parents should recognize that these reactions are natural and allow the child to express feelings, both positive and negative, about the baby while reassuring the child that he or she has a very special place in the family. Allowing the older child opportunities to care for the baby and reinforcing any nurturing or affectionate behavior will promote positive bonding.

Some sibling rivalry is natural and inevitable, even into adulthood. However, intense rivalry and conflict between siblings correlates with behavior problems in children.

However, positive temperament and effective, supportive coparenting can buffer against the negative outcomes associated with sibling conflict (Kolak & Volling, 2013). One factor that can exacerbate this sibling rivalry is differential treatment of children. Although it is natural and appropriate for parents to use different methods to manage children with different personalities, parents must be sensitive to their children's perceptions of their behavior and emphasize each child's strengths. Helping each child to develop a separate identity based on unique talents and interests can minimize rivalry and perceptions of favoritism.

Children with siblings who have psychological disorders are also at increased risk for mental health problems. (Sanders & Szymanski, 2013). Nurses should be alert to behavior problems of other family members and include siblings in family interventions.

Bullying

Children have been victimized by bullies throughout history, but this problem has only recently become a topic of widespread concern for mental health professionals.

Bullying is defined as repeated, deliberate attempts to harm someone, usually unprovoked. An imbalance in strength is a part of the pattern, with most victims having difficulty defending themselves. Boys are more likely to use physical aggression, and bigger boys usually pick on smaller, weaker ones (Olweus, 2003). Girls are more likely to use **relational aggression**, which involves disrupting peer relationships by excluding or manipulating others and spreading rumors. Cyberbullying (spreading pictures, rumors, or smear campaigns via the Internet) has become an increasingly common phenomenon that can have devastating effects because of the speed and scope of its impact (Ybarra & Mitchell, 2004).

Children who have insecure attachments; who have distant or authoritarian parents; and who have been physically, sexually, or verbally abused are at risk for becoming bullies (Rodkin & Hodges, 2003; Shields & Cicchetti, 2001). On the other side, victims of bullies often suffer from low self-esteem and relationship difficulties, even into adulthood.

Nurses who work with children and adolescents should assess for the occurrence of bullying by asking direct questions because this problem is often hidden (Hensley, 2013). Immediate intervention should involve a coordinated effort by the school, parents, bullies, and victims because studies show that bullying does not occur in a vacuum. Rather, numerous "henchmen," supporters, and bystanders participate in the process (Olweus, 2003). The most effective programs involve educating and changing the climate in the whole school (not just working with the bullies) (Berger, 2007).

Physical Illness

Many children experience a major physical illness or injury at some point during development. Hospitalization and intrusive medical procedures are acutely traumatic for most children. The likelihood of lasting psychological problems resulting from physical illness depends on the child's developmental level and previous coping mechanisms, the family's level of functioning before and after the illness, and the nature and severity of the illness. As with any major stressor, the perception of the event (i.e., meaning of the illness) will influence the family's ability to cope. One possible outcome of early childhood illness or injury is the phenomenon of **vulnerable child syndrome**, in which the family perceives the child as fragile despite current good health, causing them to be overprotective (Duncan & Caughy, 2009).

Common childhood reactions to physical illness include regression (e.g., loss of previous developmental gains in toilet training, social maturity, autonomous behavior), sleep and feeding difficulties, behavior problems (negativism, withdrawal), somatic complaints that mask attempts at emotional expression (e.g., headaches, stomach aches), and depression. Infants and children younger than school age are particularly vulnerable to separation anxiety during illness and may regress to earlier levels of anxiety about strangers, becoming fearful of health care providers. Young children often have magical thinking about the illness, and their tendency to process information in concrete terms may lead to misperceptions about the illness and treatment procedures (e.g., dye = die; stretcher = stretch her) (Deering & Cody, 2002). Adolescents may be concerned about body image and maintaining their sense of independence and control.

Nurses must remember that parents are the primary resource to the child and the experts who know the child's needs and reactions. Thus, nurses must maintain a collaborative approach in working with parents of physically ill children. If the child is a sick infant, nurses should take care to allow the normal attachment process between parents and the infant to unfold despite health care professionals' efforts to assume some parenting functions.

Many parents react with guilt to their child's illness or injury, especially if the illness is genetically based or partially the result of their own behavior (e.g., drug or alcohol abuse during pregnancy). Parents may project their guilt onto each other or health care professionals, lashing out in anger and blame. Nurses should view this behavior as part of the grieving process and help parents to move forward in caring for their children and regaining competence. Teaching parents how to care for their children's medical problems and reinforcing their successes in doing so will help.

Chronic physical illness in childhood presents a unique set of challenges. Although most children with chronic illnesses and their families are remarkably resilient and adjust to the stressors and regimens involved in their care, children with chronic health conditions are three to four times more likely to experience psychiatric symptoms than are their healthy peers (LeBlanc, Goldsmith, & Patel, 2003; Lewis & Vitulano, 2003). Conditions that affect the central nervous system (CNS) (e.g., infections, metabolic diseases, CNS malformations, brain and spinal cord trauma) are particularly likely to result in psychiatric difficulties. Nurses who understand pathophysiologic processes are in a unique position to assess the interaction between biologic and psychological factors that contribute to mental health problems in chronically ill children (e.g., lethargy from high blood sugar levels or respiratory problems, mood swings from steroid use). Inactivity and lack of sensory stimulation from hospitalization or bed rest may contribute to neurologic deficits and developmental delays.

The major challenge for a chronically ill child is to remain active despite the limitations of the illness and to become fully integrated into school and social activities. Children who view themselves as different or defective will experience low self-esteem and be more at risk for depression, anxiety, and behavior problems. Studies show that parental perceptions of the child's vulnerability predict greater adjustment problems even after controlling for age and disease severity (Anthony, Gil, & Schanberg, 2003). Educating parents and helping them to foster maximum independence within the limitations of the child's health problem is the key.

Adolescent Risk-Taking Behaviors

Adolescence is a time of growing independence and, consequently, experimentation. Emotional extremes prevail. To adolescents, the world seems great one day and terrible the next; people are either for them or against them. Adolescents are struggling to consolidate their abilities to control their impulses and react to the many "crises" that may seem trivial to adults but are very important to teens. Biologic changes (e.g., onset of puberty, height and weight changes, hormonal changes), psychological changes (increased ability for abstract thinking), and social changes (dating, driving, increased autonomy) are all significant. Unevenness in adolescent brain development, specifically in the amygdala, may contribute to difficulties with impulse control or the ability to "think twice" before acting (Steinberg, 2013).

Teenagers test different roles and struggle to find a peer group that fits their unfolding self-image. During this process, many adolescents experiment with risk-taking behaviors, such as smoking, using alcohol and drugs, having unprotected sex, engaging in truancy or delinquent behaviors, and running away from home. Although most youths eventually become more responsible, some develop harmful behavior patterns and addictions that endanger their mental and physical health. One recent trend is self-mutilation or cutting by adolescents who use this as a cry for help or a tension release (Askew & Byrne, 2009;

Rissanen, Kylma, & Laukkanen, 2009). Adolescents whose psychiatric problems have already developed are particularly vulnerable to engaging in risky behaviors because they have limited coping skills, may attempt to self-medicate their symptoms, and may feel increased pressure to fit in with other teens.

Several approaches to mental health promotion with adolescents are recommended. First, intervening at the peer group level through education programs, alternative recreation activities, and peer counseling is most successful. Second, training in values clarification, problem solving, social skills, and assertiveness helps give adolescents the skills to cope with situations in which they are pressured by their peers. If just one person can find the strength to express an unpopular viewpoint in a group and decline to participate in a destructive activity, others will quickly follow. It takes enormous courage, as well as concrete knowledge and practice with assertiveness, to speak up in these situations. A third type of intervention is a program that uses team efforts by teachers, parents, community leaders, and teen role models. These programs help at-risk youth by building self-esteem, setting positive examples, and working to involve the youth in community activities.

Approaches that have not proved effective include mere education about dangerous activities without behavior training and programs that provide inadequate training for the professionals implementing them. In any intervention, it is also important to keep in mind that adolescents are skeptical of authority figures and tend to take cues from one another. Nurses working with teenagers find it helpful to use a discussion approach that encourages questioning and argument as opposed to talking down to or "talking at" teenagers (Deering & Cody, 2002).

RISK FACTORS FOR CHILDHOOD PSYCHOPATHOLOGY

Understanding the risk factors for psychopathology is vital in mental health promotion and the prevention of disorders. Any intervention must recognize and work to address these factors if it is to be successful.

Poverty and Homelessness

An estimated 15% of the U.S. population lives below the poverty level (U.S. Census Bureau, 2013), and a disproportionate number of children from minority groups live in poverty. The effects of poverty are numerous and pervasive. Lack of proper nutrition and access to prenatal and infant care place children from poor families at risk for physical and mental health problems. Adolescence may be truncated when children from impoverished families are forced into adult roles as parents work long hours to meet

basic needs (Dashiff, DiMicco, Myers, & Sheppard, 2009; see Chapter 14).

Although crime, drug abuse, gang activity, and teenage pregnancy are seen in adolescents from all socioeconomic backgrounds, children living in poverty may be more vulnerable to these problems because they may view their options as limited. Thus, they may have an increased need to maintain a tough image and struggle more for a sense of control over their environment. The obstacles inherent in overcoming the effects of poverty can seem insurmountable to young people.

A major focus of preventive nursing interventions for disadvantaged families involves simply forming an alliance that conveys respect and willingness to work as an advocate

---

BOX 15.1

Research for Best Practice: **Risk and Protective Factors for Out-of-Home Youth**

Harpin, S., Kenyon, D. B., Kools, S., Bearinger, L. H., & Ireland, M. (2013). Correlates of emotional distress in out-of-home youth. *Journal of Child and Adolescent Psychiatric Nursing. 26(3),* 110–118.

THE QUESTION: What are the major risk and protective factors for mental health outcomes among youth in out-of-home placements?

METHODS: Nurse researchers examined data from a large survey of high school students in Minnesota who reported living in out-of-home placements (*n* = 5,500) and a comparison group (*n* = 5,500). They performed regression analyses to identify risk and proctective factors for the two groups.

FINDINGS: Of the nearly 140,000 total student respondents in the survey, 5,516 (4%) reported being in out-of-home placements. Young people of color were over-represented (43.1%) in the out-of-home placement group. Youth in placements had higher suicidal risk, mental health distress, and rates of physical and sexual abuse, and fewer protective factors (feeling parents care about them, other adults care, and school connectedness) than those in the comparison group. For the youth in out-of-home placements, physical and sexual abuse and suicidality significantly predicted higher emotional distress. Conversely, the most significant protective factors for youth in placements were perceptions of parental caring and feeling connected to their schools.

IMPLICATIONS FOR NURSING PRACTICE: Nurses and other healthcare workers are often on the front lines of screening efforts and should assess risk and protective factors among youth as they enter and move between out-of-home placements. Particular attention should be paid to the history and impact of physical and sexual abuse and suicidality. Youth in out-of-home placements may continue to idealize their parents despite the trauma that they may have faced at their hands. This need to remain attached to their parents should be supported since the emotional bond and perception of parental caring may be a protective factor for their mental health. Other research has demonstrated that programs promoting school connectedness increase the mental health of youth, and the current study underscores how these programs may be of particular benefit to youth in out-of-home placements.

to help patients gain access to resources. In terms of Maslow's need hierarchy, families living in poverty may be more focused on survival needs (e.g., food, shelter) than self-actualization needs (e.g., insight-oriented psychotherapy for themselves or their children). Unless the nurse can work as a partner with the family and address the issues that are most pressing for the family with an active, problem-solving approach, other types of intervention may be fruitless. At the same time, it is inappropriate to assume that poor families will be resistant to or unable to benefit from psychotherapy or other mental health interventions.

Additional risks arise from homelessness in children and teens, which may result from loss of shelter for the entire family, running away, or being thrown out of their homes (Box 15.1; see also Chapter 38). For youths who are homeless, there is an increased risk for physical health problems (e.g., nutrition deficiencies, infections, chronic illnesses), mental health problems (particularly developmental delays in language, fine or gross motor coordination, and social development; depression; anxiety; disruptive behavior disorders), and educational under-achievement. Many homeless youth have been physically and/or sexually abused, leading to elevated rates of mental disorders (Oliveira & Burke, 2009). Adolescents who run away from an abusive home can find themselves living on the streets where staying alive and developing self-reliance are a daily struggle.

The living conditions of many shelters place children at risk for lead poisoning and communicable diseases and make the regular sleep, feeding, play, and bathing patterns important for normal development nearly impossible. Nurses working with homeless families need to be aware of the effects of this lifestyle on children because they have a limited ability to speak for themselves and because their needs are often overlooked.

Child Abuse and Neglect

Early recognition and reduction of risk factors are the keys to preventing **child abuse and neglect**, which includes any actions that endanger or impair a child's physical, psychological, or emotional health and development. Risk factors for child abuse and neglect include high levels of family stress, drug or alcohol abuse, a stepparent or parental boyfriend or girlfriend who is unstable or unloving toward the child, and lack of social support for the parents. In addition, young children (particularly those younger than 3 years) and children with a history of prematurity, medical problems, and severe emotional problems are at high risk because they place great demands on their parents. Abuse can have lifelong effects on development. Children who have been maltreated are more likely to enter aggressive relationships, abuse drugs or alcohol to numb emotions, develop eating disorders, become depressed, and engage in self-destructive behavior (Mersky, Topitzes, & Reynolds, 2013; Putnam, 2003).

Box 15.2 lists signs of physical and sexual abuse in children. Nurses are legally mandated to report any reasonable

---

BOX 15.2

Signs of Possible Child Abuse

SEXUAL ABUSE
- Bruises or bleeding on the genitals or in the rectum
- Sexually transmitted infection (e.g., HIV, gonorrhea, syphilis, herpes genitalis)
- Vaginal or penile discharge
- Sore throats
- Enuresis or encopresis
- Foreign bodies in the vagina or rectum
- Pregnancy, especially in a young adolescent
- Difficulty in walking or sitting
- Sexual acting out with siblings or peers
- Sophisticated knowledge of sexual activities
- Preoccupation with sexual ideas
- Somatic complaints, especially abdominal pain and constipation
- Sleep difficulties
- Hyperalertness to the environment
- Withdrawal
- Excessive daydreaming or seeming preoccupied
- Regressed behavior

PHYSICAL ABUSE
- Bruises or lacerations, especially in clusters on back, buttocks, thighs, or large areas of the torso*

- Fractures inconsistent with the child's history
- Old and new injuries at the same time
- Unwilling to change clothes in front of others; wears heavy clothes in warm weather
- Identifiable marks from belt buckles, electrical cords, or handprints
- Cigarette burns
- Rope burns on arms, legs, face, neck, or torso from being bound and gagged
- Adult-size bite marks
- Bald spots interspersed with normal hair
- Shrinking at the touch of an adult
- Fear of adults, especially parents
- Apprehensive when other children cry
- Scanning the environment, staying very still, failing to cry when hurt
- Aggression or withdrawal
- Indiscriminant seeking of affection
- Defensive reactions when questioned about injuries
- History of being taken to many different clinics and emergency departments for different injuries

*Note: Because many injuries do not represent child abuse, a careful history must be taken.

suspicion of abuse and neglect to the appropriate state authorities. Mandated reporting laws allow the state to investigate the possibility of abuse, provide protection to children, and link families with support and services. Nurses are immune from liability for reporting suspected abuse, but they may be held legally accountable for not reporting it. The decision to report abuse sometimes poses an ethical dilemma for nurses as they try to balance the need to maintain the family's trust against the need to protect the child. This decision is further complicated by the knowledge that if temporary out-of-home placement is necessary, the quality of the placement may not be optimum, and the child and family may suffer in the process of the separation.

To minimize damaging the nurse–family relationship, experts recommend that nurses report abuse in the presence of the parents, preferably with the parent initiating the telephone call. The professional should explain that reporting is necessary to provide safety for the child and to obtain services for the family. If the parents cannot be present when the report is made, the nurse should, at minimum, notify the family that the report was made.

Preventing child abuse and neglect occurs with any intervention that supports the parents with physical, financial, mental health, and medical resources that will reduce stress within the family system. Early intervention and family support programs are considered the cornerstone of preventive efforts. A major protective factor against psychopathology stemming from abuse and neglect is the establishment of a supportive relationship with at least one adult who can provide empathy, consistency, and possibly, a corrective experience (e.g., a foster parent or other family member) for the child (Afifi & MacMillan, 2011).

Nurses working with abused children should resist the temptation to view the child as the only victim. Remembering that most abusive parents were abused themselves as children and therefore may have limited coping mechanisms or little access to positive parental role models will help the nurse maintain empathy toward the parents. After state agencies intervene to establish the child's safety, a family systems approach that is supportive of the whole family unit is most effective.

Substance-Abusing Families

Children whose parents are substance abusing (see Chapter 31) live in an unpredictable family environment, coping with stress that may disrupt their ability to perform in school and lead to other emotional problems. The codependency movement, which emphasizes the effects of addiction on family members and groups such as Adult Children of Alcoholics (ACOA) and Al-Anon have brought increasing attention to the effects of parental substance abuse on child development.

Biologic factors affecting children of those who abuse substances include **fetal alcohol syndrome**, nutritional deficits stemming from neglect, and neuropsychiatric dysfunction. Genetic factors are at least partly responsible for the well-documented increased risk for substance abuse among children whose parents abuse substances. Recent studies are beginning to link a family history of anxiety disorders and alcoholism with genetically transmitted anxiety disorders, which may be a precursor to alcohol abuse. The precise mechanism of family transmission of alcoholism remains unknown. Recent studies suggest that children of those who abuse substances may inherit a predisposition to a nonspecific form of biologic dysregulation that may be expressed either as alcoholism or some other psychiatric disorder (e.g., hyperactivity, conduct disorder, depression), depending on the individual's developmental history.

Children of those who abuse substances are at high risk for both substance abuse and behavior disorders (Straussner & Fewell, 2011). Moreover, some evidence shows that other factors related to addiction, such as family stress, violence, divorce, dysfunction, and other concurrent parental psychiatric disorders (e.g., depression, anxiety), are as important as the substance abuse itself in increasing this risk (Ritter, Stewart, Bernet, Coe, & Brown, 2002). The experience of growing up in a substance-abusing family is marked by unpredictability, fear, and helplessness because of the cyclic nature of addictive patterns.

The literature on children of parents who have alcoholism has described several typical roles that children assume, including the "hero" (overly responsible children who may ignore their own needs to take care of parents and other children), "scapegoat" (problem children who divert attention away from the parent with alcoholism), "mascot" (family clowns who relieve tension and mask feelings through joking), and "lost child" (children who suffer in silence but may exhibit difficulties at school or in later life) (Veronie & Freuhstorfer, 2001). These roles, combined with the enabling behaviors of other family members who attempt to cover up and minimize the effects of the addiction, may become so rigid and effective in masking the problem that children of substance abusers may not come to the attention of mental health professionals until after the parent stops drinking and family roles are disrupted.

Even for children who do not experience significant psychopathology, the experience of growing up in a substance-abusing family can lead to a poor self-concept when children feel responsible for their parents' behavior, become isolated, and learn to mistrust their own perceptions because the family denies the reality of the addiction. Despite the well-documented risk for children in substance-abusing families, there is no uniform pattern of outcomes, and many children demonstrate resilience. School-based interventions with children from substance-abusing families can significantly increase resilience (Gance-Cleveland & Mays, 2008).

Out-of-Home Placement

The tendency to blame parents and view out-of-home placement as a refuge for children has sharply declined in recent years. This change in attitudes results from public awareness of the deficiencies in the foster care system, greater support for parents' rights, and increased knowledge of the biologic basis for many of the disorders of parents and children that lead to out-of-home placement.

Family preservation involves supporting and educating the family in order to secure the attachment between children and parents and to preserve the family unit and prevent the removal of children from their homes. Today children are removed from their homes only as a last resort. Family support services are designed to assist families with access to resources and education regarding child rearing, monitor and facilitate the development of the bond between child and caregiver, and increase the caregiver's confidence in his or her abilities (Turnbull et al., 2007).

However, despite recent trends toward family preservation, an increasing number of children are placed in foster homes, group homes, or residential treatment centers—in many cases for months to years (Bruskas, 2008). Factors leading to the increased number of children in out-of-home placement include increased willingness of the public and professionals to report child abuse and neglect; the epidemic proportions of substance abuse and cases of AIDS; and the increasing number of families living in poverty. Those may lead to abuse, neglect, and homelessness. About 50% of children in out-of-home placement are adolescents, but the numbers of infants and young children are growing, particularly those with serious physical and emotional problems, who pose particular challenges for placement (Scribano, 2010). Infants who are abandoned by drug-abusing parents and children with HIV whose parents are sick or deceased need permanent out-of-home placements, which are often difficult to find.

The adjustment to an out-of-home placement can be viewed through the conceptual framework of Bowlby's stages of coping with parental separation. According to Bowlby (1960), the child initially responds to separation from parents with protest (crying, kicking, screaming, pleading, and attempting to elicit the parent's return). The child then moves to a state of despair (listlessness, apathy, and withdrawal, which lead to some acceptance of caregiving by others but a reluctance to reattach fully). Finally, the child experiences detachment if the child and new parent cannot manage to form an emotional bond. Because children often experience multiple placements, the potential for a disrupted attachment may be great by the time the child faces the prospect of a permanent family. After repeatedly undergoing separation and mourning, the child learns that rejection is inevitable and may automatically maintain distance from a new caregiver.

Typical coping styles seen in children exposed to multiple placements include detachment, diffuse rage, chronic depression, antisocial behavior, low self-esteem, and chronic dependency or exaggerated demands for nurturing and support. Sometimes these symptoms develop into attachment disorders that can be difficult to treat. It takes a very committed and resilient parent to continue caring for a child who does not reinforce attempts at caregiving and who exhibits these kinds of significant emotional and behavior problems.

INTERVENTION APPROACHES

The goal of health promotion and prevention interventions is to maximize the mental health of children and adolescents. The selected interventions should allow maximal autonomy for the child and family; keep the family unit intact, if possible; and provide the appropriate level of care to meet the needs of the child and family. A view of parents as partners is important to effective interventions. Interdisciplinary approaches are ideal in which the nurse acts as coordinator, case manager, and advocate to establish linkages with physicians and nurse practitioners, teachers, speech and language specialists, social workers, and other professionals to develop and implement a

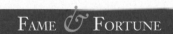

FAME & FORTUNE

Dave Pelzer (1960–)

Resilient Survivor

PUBLIC PERSONA

Dave Pelzer entered the U.S. Air Force at age 18 years and developed into a dedicated, sensitive human being who helped children when working as a juvenile hall counselor, youth service worker, and adviser to foster care and youth service boards. He also became, and still is, a noted author and lecturer. Dave has appeared on numerous television talk shows. He is especially admired for his sense of humor, intriguing outlook on life, and sense of personal responsibility.

PERSONAL REALITIES

Dave Pelzer is a survivor of extreme physical and emotional abuse by his alcoholic mother. He was rescued by teachers who reported his abuse and got him the help he needed at the age of 12 years. He chronicles his experiences of abuse and foster placements in his internationally best-selling books (best known for *A Child Called "It"*). Although Dave endured years of torture, he is a wonderful example of resilient coping.

BOX 15.3
PREVENTIVE INTERVENTIONS WITH AN ADOLESCENT IN CRISIS

Ben and Rita were just transferred to a second foster home after being removed from their mother's care when she relapsed on cocaine and left them unattended. The plan is for the two children to return to their mother's home after she completes a 30-day drug treatment program. Ben, a high school freshman, is in the school nurse's office asking for aspirin for another headache.

The nurse notices that Ben's nose looks inflamed, he is sniffling, and he seems more "hyper" than usual. In a concerned tone of voice, she asks him if he's been using cocaine, and he snaps back, "Just because my mother's a coke head doesn't give you the right to suspect me!" When the nurse gently says, "Tell me about what's been happening with your mother; I had no idea," Ben responds less defensively and explains the situation about the foster home and his mother's drug problem. He says that if it weren't for Rita, his younger sister, he would have run away by now. His foster parents are "making him" go to school, but he's going to drop out as soon as he returns to live with his mother. The only thing that he likes about school is playing basketball, and the basketball coach, who is his physical education teacher, wants him on the team.

After a lengthy talk with Ben, the nurse finishes the assessment interview and concludes that he is at risk for drug

abuse, running away, and dropping out of school. He is also showing symptoms of depression, which he may be attempting to medicate with cocaine. Protective factors for Ben include his strong attachment to his sister, his ability and willingness to express his thoughts and feelings, his interest in basketball, and a positive relationship with the basketball coach.

The nurse develops a plan with Ben to attend the weekly drug and alcohol discussion group at the school, so he can talk with other teens from substance-abusing families and learn coping skills to prevent addiction. The nurse contacts the basketball coach, who agrees to find a student mentor who can shoot hoops with Ben and help him come up with a plan to stay in school, maybe find a part-time job, and join the basketball team. Ben agrees to check in regularly with the nurse to report how the plan is working and revise it if needed. The nurse feels optimistic that with support from his peers, coach, mentor, and herself, Ben can overcome what is probably a genetically based risk for depression and addiction. Ben shows signs of resilience. He is motivated to "keep his act together for Rita," capable of forming positive attachments, and willing to seek help when he knows where to find it.

What Do You Think?
- If Ben "forgets" to check in regularly with the nurse, what would be the next course of action?

- When are the times Ben is most susceptible to change his mind about staying in school and avoiding drugs? What action should be taken to avoid these times?

---

comprehensive biopsychosocial plan of intervention (Box 15.3). Support groups are available for just about every kind of stressor that a family can experience, including substance abuse, death, divorce, and coping with a chronic illness. A continuum of modalities of care is available to children and families (Figure 15.3).

Early intervention programs offer regular home visits, support, education, and concrete services to those in need. The assumption underlying these programs is that parents are the most consistent and important figures in children's lives, and they should be afforded the opportunity to define their own needs and priorities. With support and education, parents are empowered to respond more effectively to their children. The effectiveness of these programs may be the key to preventing the placement of children outside the home (Heckman, 2013).

Psychoeducational programs designed to teach parents and children basic coping skills for dealing with various stressors are a particularly effective form of mental health intervention. By focusing on **normalization** (teaching families normal behaviors and expected responses) and providing families with information about

typical child development and expected reactions to various stressors, families feel less isolated, know what to expect, and put their reactions into perspective. For example, if families learn that anger is a natural part of grieving, they will be less likely to view it as abnormal and more likely to accept and cope with it constructively.

Social skills training is useful with youth who have low self-esteem or aggressive behavior or who are at high risk for substance abuse (Kvarme, Helseth, Sorum, Luth-Hansen, Haugland, & Nativig, 2010; Steele, Elkin, & Roberts, 2008). Social skills training involves instruction, feedback, support, and practice with learning behaviors that help children to interact more effectively with peers and adults. When combined with assertiveness training, social skills training can be particularly helpful in providing children with coping skills to resist engaging in addictive or antisocial behaviors and to prevent social withdrawal under stress. Social skills training may be particularly helpful for children who are bullies or who are rejected by their peers (Fopma-Loy, 2000).

Bibliotherapy is a particularly potent form of intervention because it empowers families to learn and develop coping mechanisms on their own (see Chapter 10). A wide

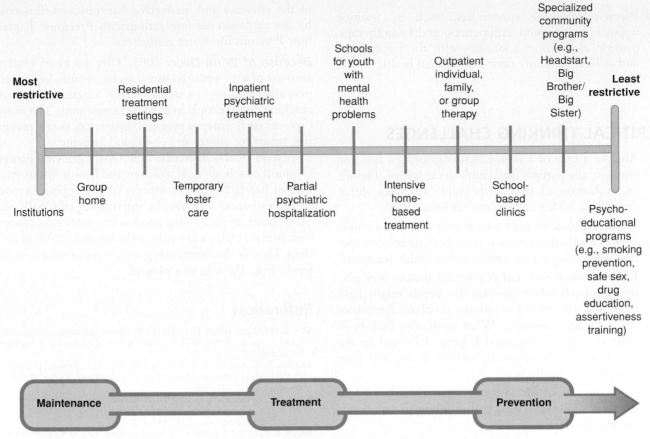

FIGURE 15.3 The continuum of mental health care for children and adolescents.

variety of books are available to help children understand issues such as death, divorce, chronic illness, stepfamilies, adoption, and birth of a sibling. In addition, many mental health organizations and public health agencies have pamphlets designed to educate parents about various physical and psychological problems. By providing concrete information and advice, these reading materials help to reduce anxiety by pointing out common reactions to the various stressors, so that families do not feel alone.

SUMMARY OF KEY POINTS

- Children who experience major losses, such as death or divorce, are at risk for developing mental health problems.

- Sibling relationships have significant effects on personality development. Positive sibling relationships can be protective factors against the development of mental health problems.

- Bullying is a serious problem that is often hidden yet can cause longstanding psychological harm; it must be addressed on a school-wide level.

- Medical problems in childhood and adolescence may cause psychological problems when illness leads to regression or lack of full participation in family, school, and social activities.

- Striving for identity and independence may lead adolescents to participate in high-risk activities (e.g., drug use, unprotected sex, smoking, delinquent behaviors) that may lead to mental health problems.

- Poverty, homelessness, abuse, neglect, and parental substance abuse all create conditions that undermine a child's ability to make normal developmental gains and contribute to vulnerability for various emotional and behavioral problems.

- Children who experience disrupted attachments because of out-of-home placements may have difficulty forming close relationships with their new parents and trusting others.

- Family support services and early intervention programs are designed to prevent removal of the child from the family as a result of abuse or neglect and to maintain a strong, nurturing family system.

■ Psychoeducational approaches, such as training opportunities, group experiences, and bibliotherapy, provide children and families with the information and skills to promote their own mental health.

CRITICAL THINKING CHALLENGES

1. Analyze a case of a family that is grieving a loss and compare the parents' and children's reactions. Include an evaluation of how each child's reactions differ, depending on his or her developmental level.

2. Watch a movie or read a book that provides a child's view of death, divorce, or some other loss and consider how adults may be insensitive to the child's reactions.

3. Examine your own developmental history and pinpoint periods when stressful life events might have increased the risk for emotional problems for you or other family members. What protective factors in your own personality and coping skills and in the environment around you helped you to maintain your good mental health?

4. What aspects of life are more stressful for children than for adults (i.e., how is it different to experience life as a child)?

5. Examine how your own social and cultural background may either facilitate or create barriers to your ability to interact with families from other ethnic groups or those who are poor or homeless.

6. Allow yourself to reflect on how your own judgmental attitudes might interfere with your ability to communicate effectively with families who have abused or neglected their children.

7. Why is the process of normalization of feelings such a powerful intervention with children and families? What kinds of mental health issues, developmental processes, or both would benefit from teaching related to normal reactions? How can nurses incorporate this kind of intervention into their practice roles?

8. How can nurses expand their roles to have maximal effects on primary, secondary, and tertiary mental health intervention with children and families?

Precious: 2009. This powerful and disturbing movie portrays the life of an African American adolescent girl who is physically, sexually, and emotionally abused by her family. It demonstrates the devastating effects of abuse, poverty, substandard schooling, and family dysfunction, at the same time conveying hope through this girl's amazing resilience.

Viewing Points: Give some examples of how Precious uses dissociation to cope with her abuse. What are some of the effective and ineffective interventions illustrated by the professionals interacting with Precious? Explain how Precious illustrates resilience.

Because of Winn Dixie: 2005. This is a heart-rending account of a 10-year-old girl who overcomes her loneliness after moving to a small town by adopting a dog and reaching out to people in her new community. The movie explores such issues as parental separation, single parenting, substance abuse, and childhood grieving.

Viewing Points: Describe how Opal's grieving process is typical of school-aged children and how it differs from that of her father. What aspects of her coping demonstrate resilience? Explain the importance of Opal's dog, Winn Dixie, in the healing process for this family. Discuss how pets may play a key role in the mental health of children. How is the relationship with a pet similar and different from the role of a sibling?

References

Afifi, T. O., & MacMillan, H. L. (2011). Resilience following child maltreatment: A review of protective factors. *The Canadian Journal of Psychiatry, 56*(5), 266–272.

Anthony, K. K., Gil, K. M., & Schanberg, L. E. (2003). Parental perceptions of child vulnerability in children with chronic illness. *Journal of Pediatric Psychology, 28*(3), 185–190.

Askew, M., & Byrne, M. W. (2009). Biopsychosocial approach to treating self-injurious behaviors: An adolescent case study. *Journal of Child and Adolescent Psychiatric Nursing, 22*(3), 115–119.

Berger, K. S. (2007). Update on bullying at school: Science forgotten? *Developmental Review, 27,* 90–126.

Bowlby, J. (1960). Grief and mourning in infancy and early childhood. *Psychoanalytic Study of the Child, 15,* 9–52.

Bruskas, D. (2008). Children in foster care: A vulnerable population at risk. *Journal of Child and Adolescent Psychiatric Nursing, 21*(2), 70–77.

Dashiff, C., DiMicco, W., Myers, B., & Sheppard, K. (2009). Poverty and adolescent mental health. *Journal of Child and Adolescent Psychiatric Nursing, 22*(1), 23–32.

Deering, C. G., & Cody, D. J. (2002). Communicating effectively with children and adolescents. *American Journal of Nursing, 102*(3), 34–42.

Dopp, A. R., & Cain, A. C. (2012). The role of peer relationships in parental bereavement during childhood and adolescence. *Death Studies, 36*(1), 41–60.

Duncan, A. F., & Caughy, M. O. (2009). Parenting style and the vulnerable child syndrome. *Journal of Child and Adolescent Psychiatric Nursing, 22*(4), 228–234.

Fopma-Loy, J. (2000). Peer rejection and neglect of latency age children: Pathways and group psychotherapy model. *Journal of Child and Adolescent Psychiatric Nursing, 13,* 29–38.

Gance-Cleveland, B., & Mays, M. Z. (2008). School-based support groups for adolescents with a substance-abusing parent. *Journal of the American Psychiatric Nurses Association, 14,* 4, 297–309.

Garcia-Dia, M. J., DiNapoli, J. M., Garcia-Ona, L., Jakubowski, R., & O'Flaherty, D. (2013). Concept analysis: Reslience. *Archives of Psychiatric Nursing, 27*(6), 264–270.

Gonzales, J. (2009). Prefamily counseling: Working with blended families. *Journal of Divorce and Remarriage, 50*(2), 148–157.

Heckman, J. J. (2013). *Giving kids a fair chance.* Boston: MIT Press.

Hensley, V. (2013). Childhood bullying: A review and implications for healthcare professionals. *Nursing Clinics of North America, 48*(2), 203–213.

Hetherington, E. M., & Kelly, J. (2002). *For better or for worse: Divorce reconsidered.* New York: W. W. Norton.

Kelly, J. (2012). Risk and protective factors associated with child and adolescent adjustment following separation and divorce: Social science applications. In K. Kuehnle & L. Drozd (Eds.) *Parenting plan evalautions: Applied research for the family court* (pp. 49–84). Oxford, New York: Oxford University Press.

Kolak, A. M., & Volling, B. L. (2013). Coparenting moderates the association between firstborn children's temperament and problem behavior across the transition to siblinghood. *Journal of Family Psychology, 27*(3), 355–364.

Kramer, L., & Bank, L. (2005). Sibling relationship contributes to individual and family well-being. *Journal of Family Psychology, 19*(4), 483–485.

Kramer, L., & Ramsburg, D. (2002). Advice given to parents on welcoming a second child: A critical review. *Family Relations: Interdisciplinary Journal of Applied Family Studies, 51*(1), 2–14.

Kvarme, L. G., Helseth, S., Sorum, R., Luth-Hansen, V., Haugland, S., & Nativig, G. K. (2010). The effect of a solution-focused approach to improve self-efficacy in socially withdrawn school children: A non-randomized controlled trial. *International Journal of Nursing Studies, 47*(11), 1389–1996.

LeBlanc, L. A., Goldsmith, T., & Patel, D. R. (2003). Behavioral aspects of chronic illness in children and adolescents. *Pediatric Clinics of North America, 50*(4), 859–878.

Lewis, M., & Vitulano, L. A. (2003). Biopsychosocial issues and risk factors in the family when the child has a chronic illness. *Child & Adolescent Psychiatric Clinics of North America, 12*(3), 389–399.

Mersky, J. P., Topitzes, J., & Reynolds, A. J. (2013). Impacts of adverse childhood experiences on health, mental health, and substance use in early adulthood: A cohort study of an urban, minority sample in the U.S. *Child Abuse and Neglect, 37*(11), 917–925.

Oliveira J. O., & Burke, P. J. (2009). Lost in the shuffle: culture of homeless adolescents. *Pediatric Nursing, 35*(3), 154–161.

Olweus, D. (2003). A profile of bullying at school. *Educational Leadership, 60*(6), 12–17.

Putnam, F. W. (2003). Ten-year research update review: Child sexual abuse. *Journal of the American Academy of Child & Adolescent Psychiatry, 42*(3), 269–278.

Rissanen, M. L., Kylma, J., & Laukkanen, E. (2009). Descriptions of help by Finnish adolescents who self-mutilate. *Journal of Child and Adolescent Psychiatric Nursing, 22*(1), 7–15.

Ritter, J., Stewart, M., Bernet, C., Coe, M., & Brown, S. A. (2002). Effects of childhood exposure to familial alcoholism and family violence on adolescent substance use, conduct problems, and self-esteem. *Journal of Traumatic Stress, 15*(2), 113–122.

Rodkin, P. C., & Hodges, E. V. (2003). Bullies and victims in the peer ecology: Four questions for psychologists and school professionals. *School Psychology Review, 32*, 384–400.

Ryan, R. M., & Claessens, A. (2013). Associations between family structure changes and children's behavior problems: The mediating effects of timing and marital birth. *Developmental Psychology, 40*(7), 1219–1231.

Sanders, A., & Szmanski, K. (2013). Siblings of people diagnosed with a mental disorder and posttraumatic growth. *Community Mental Health Journal, 49*(5), 554–559.

Scribano, P. V. (2010). Prevention strategies in child maltreatment. *Current Opinion in Pediatrics, 22*(5), 616–620.

Shields, A., & Cicchetti, D. (2001). Parental mistreatment and emotional dysregulation as risk factors for bullying and victimization in middle school children. *Journal of Clinical Child Psychology, 30*, 349–363.

Silverman, P. R. (2000). *Never too young to know: Death in children's lives.* New York: Oxford University Press.

Steele, R. G., Elkin, T. D., & Roberts, M. C. (2008). *Handbook of evidence-based therapies for children and adolescents: Bridging science and practice.* New York: Springer.

Steinberg, L. (2013). *Adolescence* (10th ed). New York: McGraw-Hill.

Straussner, S. L. A., & Fewell, C. F. (2011). *Children of substance-abusing parents: Dynamics and treatment.* New York: Springer.

Turnbull, A. P., Summers, J. A., Turnbull, R., Brotherson, M. J., Winton, P., Roberts, R., et al. (2007). Family supports and services in early intervention: A bold vision. *Journal of Early Intervention, 29*, 187–206.

U.S. Census–Bureau. (2013). *Poverty.* Retrieved from http://www.census.gov

Veronie, L., & Freuhstorfer, D. B. (2001). Gender, birth order and family role identification among children of alcoholics. *Current Psychology: Developmental, Learning, Personality, Social, 20*(1), 53–67.

Worden, J. W. (2009). Grief counseling and grief therapy: A handbook for the mental health practitioner (4th ed). New York: Springer.

Ybarra, M. L., & Mitchell, K. J. (2004). Youth engaging in online harassment: Associations with caregiver-child relationships, Internet use, and personal characteristics. *Journal of Adolescence, 27*(3), 319–336.

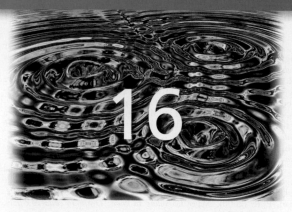

16

Mental Health Promotion for Young and Middle-Aged Adults

Richard Yakimo

KEY CONCEPTS

- middle-age adulthood
- young adulthood

LEARNING OBJECTIVES

After studying this chapter, you will be able to:

1. Describe psychosocial challenges common to young and middle-aged adults.

2. Identify risk factors related to psychopathology in young and middle-aged adults.

3. Describe protective factors in the mental health promotion of young and middle-aged adults.

4. Analyze the role of the nurse in mental health promotion for young and middle-aged adults.

KEY TERMS

- empty nest • informal caregivers • peak marriage age • protective factors • risk factors • sandwich generation

---

Concepts of young and middle-age adulthood are relatively new in American culture.

> **KEYCONCEPTS** The generally accepted age range for **young adulthood** is from 18 to 44 years. **Middle-age adulthood** spans the period from approximately 45 to 65 years.

Western families have achieved unprecedented economic stability that provides for long periods of development. Technological advances such as economic development, improved nutrition, public health control of infectious diseases, access to health care, and other modern developments have resulted in the lengthening of the lifespan chronologically in the developed world. This extended adulthood provides for an increased range of life choices, such as education; job selection; and lifestyle, including relationships, marriage, and family. Such advances do not exist worldwide because of the differences in the chronological life span in different societies. In many nondeveloped areas, the lifespan is characterized by a brief childhood followed by a mature adulthood that evolves quickly into old age.

YOUNG AND MIDDLE-AGED ADULTHOOD MENTAL HEALTH

Psychological changes in adulthood occur slowly and subtly with age and experience, not in fixed stepwise manner. Until recently, adult development was viewed as a relatively stationary plateau with the rapid and complex changes of childhood and adolescence forming one steep side and the declining changes of old age the other. Any rigid stage theory of adult life is oversimplifying young and middle-aged development. Today, young and middle-aged development is viewed as dynamic and multifaceted.

The developmental issues reported by young, middle-aged, and older adults are recurrent, taking new forms as their lives unfold. The developmental concepts of identity, intimacy, and generativity may have their initial blooming during adolescence, young adulthood, and middle age, but they continue to be renegotiated in the face of life stresses such as job loss, career change, relocation, illness, divorce, and widowhood (see Chapter 7).

Chronological age is also losing its customary social meaning, resulting in a more fluid life cycle. Traditional notions of young adulthood as a time of leaving the parental home and establishing an independent career and family life, of college education taking place during late adolescence, or of the middle-aged parents facing the **"empty nest"**—a home devoid of children and caregiving responsibilities—are being replaced with fewer age-defined life roles.

The timing of life events such as education, marriage, childrearing, career development, and retirement is becoming less regular, and more alternatives are tolerated by society. Some people never marry, and others retire very early. Many young adults now remain in their parents' homes while they pursue their professional education rather than strike out on their own as was customary in previous generations. Their middle-aged parents are often already caring for their own parents, creating the **sandwich generation**, with its responsibilities toward the elder generation above and two generations of children below them. Many women choose to marry and establish a family and then return to finish their college education when their children start school.

COMMON CHALLENGES IN ADULTHOOD

Young and middle-aged adulthood are marked by many significant life events. Among them are leaving the primary family home for the first time, getting married (or not), and taking on new caregiving responsibilities. For adults in a breadwinning role, the prospect of unemployment can also present a major life challenge that affects their ability to be effective in other life roles.

Changes in Family Structure

The young adult and middle-aged years are characterized by changes in family structures. Older adolescents finish school and often leave home, which alters the primary family structure. Marriage establishes new roles for adults who previously lived by themselves or their parents. The arrival of children changes the structure and dynamics of the newly formed family. These are all normal developmental events, but they can also lead to mental distress, physical problems, and social alienation.

Married adults are healthier than those in other nonmarried groups. See Table 16.1 for a breakdown of marital status in the U.S. adult population. Married adults are least likely to experience health problems and least likely to engage in risky health behaviors with one exception: middle-aged married men have the highest rate of overweight or obesity. Widowed, divorced, or separated adults

Table 16.1	MARITAL STATUS OF THE U.S. ADULT POPULATION OVER THE AGE OF 15 YEARS
Marital Status	**Percent of Adult Population**
Married	50.4
Widowed	5.7
Divorced	10.2
Separated	2.2
Never married	31.4

Source: U.S. Census Bureau. (2014). Families and Living Arrangements: 2013. People & Households. Washington, DC: Author. Retrieved June 27, 2014, from http://www.census.gov/hhes/families/data/cps2013FG.html.

are more likely to experience serious psychological distress than married adults. The prevalence of physical inactivity in leisure time, current cigarette smoking, and heavier drinking of alcohol are higher in those who are widowed, divorced, separated, never married, or living with a partner (Schoenborn & Adams, 2010). Rates of separation or divorce are at least twice as high for those with almost any psychiatric disorder as for those without disorder.

There appears to be a **"peak marriage age"** in the mid-twenties. People who get married between the ages of 23 and 27 years are much less likely to get divorced than those who marry as teens. Nearly half of marriages in which the woman is 18 years old or younger divorce or separate within 10 years (Schoenborn & Adams, 2010). Middle-aged adults are most likely to be married compared with younger adults and adults 65 year or older. But this group is also twice as likely as younger and older adults to be divorced or separated.

Caring for Others

In 2012, 73.7 million children (younger than the age of 18 years) resided in the United States, up from 64 million in 1990. Most of these children (64%) lived with two parents, and approximately 24% lived with only their mother, 4% lived with only their father, and another 4% lived in households with neither parent present. Within these numbers, there are further variations in ethnic groups. Seventy-four percent of white, nonhispanic, 59% of hispanic and 33% of black children lived with two married parents in 2012 (U.S. Census Bureau, 2013).

Whether functioning in a two-parent or single-parent home, parents who work out of the home must provide for the care and safety of their children during their absence. Childcare outside the home is often disproportionately expensive compared with income and often is not available for parents working evenings, nights, holidays, or weekends and during periods of illness and other crises. Federal support to single parent families is limited. Working parents could formerly rely on their own parents and other family members to assist with childcare, but today many parents have no family available locally or are also serving as caretakers to family members in addition to their children.

In fact, **informal caregivers**, unpaid individuals who provide care, are the largest source of long-term care services in the United States. It is estimated that more than 62 million people provide care for a chronically ill, disabled, or aged family member or friend during any given year. Although men are increasingly becoming more involved in caregiving, women comprise the majority and perform the more difficult tasks of caregiving. The average caregiver is age 48 years, female, married, working outside the home, and earning a median household income of $57,200. The duration of caregiving spans from less than a year to more than 40 years, with an average duration of 4 to 5 years (Family Caregiver Alliance, 2012).

Caregivers are under considerable stress and often neglect their physical and mental health needs. Caregivers also report higher levels of loneliness, anxiety and depressive symptoms, and other mental health problems than noncaregiving peers. In turn, altered physical and mental health reduces the quality, satisfaction, and ability to cope with daily stresses related to caregiving (Family Caregiver Alliance, 2012).

Unemployment

Employment is an important societal value and thus serves as a source of economic, social, and emotional stability and self-esteem. Young and middle-aged adults seek and maintain employment that maintains their lifestyle and provides for their children. In a society that is consumer driven, the ability to generate resources becomes critical. Yet shifts in the ownership and organizational structure of companies, downsizing, and the job market's ever-changing demands for workers with particular skills make employment stability questionable, both now and in the future. Career changes and the continuing necessity of training for new positions are now the norm.

In late 2007, the United States began facing an economic recession resulting in there being fewer jobs available. In mid 2010, the unemployment rate rose to 9.5%, up 4.5% from when the recession began in late 2007. In 2014, the unemployment rate is declining and is hovering around 6.3%. (U.S. Bureau of Labor Statistics, 2014).

Disparities in these unemployment rates exist by race, gender, and ethnic groups. According to recent numbers, African Americans are faring the worst. By 2013, the overall African-American unemployment rate was 13.1%. Unemployment for Hispanic populations was 9.1%, with rural Hispanic populations facing especially stretched resources and limited opportunities because of a tendency to have larger families and be significantly younger than rural white families. Generally, those with limited education and nonskilled workers remained at special risk for low wages and unemployment (U.S. Bureau of Labor Statistics, 2014).

Single mothers are another group at high risk for low wages and unemployment. The proportion of single mothers who were unemployed decreased in the mid- and late 1990s but has risen in the last few years. Education levels of single stay-at-home mothers are lower than those of single working mothers. Most stay-at-home mothers (71% in 2012) are below the poverty level, compared with a quarter of single working mothers (Cohn, Livingston, & Wang, 2014). Mothers with older children (6 to 17 years of age, none younger) were more likely to participate in the labor force than mothers with younger children (younger than 6 years of age). This is most likely because of the limited availability of safe and affordable childcare (U.S. Department of Labor, 2014).

Within the cohort of unemployed workers, there are twice as many people with mental disorders when compared with a similar group of employed persons. Many people who live with mental illness are underemployed; about 70% who hold college degrees earn less than $10 per hour (SAMSHA, 2014; NAMI, 2010). Men have traditionally gained self-esteem through their jobs, so they are particularly susceptible to the psychological strains of unemployment (Chatterji, Alegria, & Takeuchi, 2009).

MENTAL DISORDERS IN YOUNG AND MIDDLE-AGED ADULTS

The great majority of people experience their first symptoms of mental illness when they are adolescents or early in the young adult stage. By far, the highest rates of mental disorder occur among young adults. Late-life onset of mental disorder (older than age 40 years) is relatively rare, with the exception of cognitive impairment, which typically occurs past the age of 70 years. Recent research suggests that 46% of people will experience a mental disorder in their lifetime and that the average age of onset for anxiety and impulse control disorders is 8 years and substance use disorders is 16 years (Kessler et al., 2012).

Changes in the biologic, psychological, and social domains can create a matrix of stress that may foster mental disorder. The vast majority of people with mental disorders do not come to the attention of the mental health system. In fact, fewer than half of those with mental disorders receive any kind of treatment from mental health professionals (Wang, Ulbricht, & Schoenbaum, 2009).

RISK FACTORS FOR YOUNG AND MIDDLE-AGED ADULT PSYCHOPATHOLOGY

Mental health promotion and illness prevention are driven by cultivating awareness of personal risk factors for mental illness and modifying those that can be changed. Specific **risk factors**, or characteristics that increase the likelihood of developing a disorder, can contribute to poor mental health and influence the development of a mental disorder. Risk factors do not cause the disorder or problem and are not symptoms of the illness but are factors that influence the likelihood that the symptoms will appear. The existence of a risk factor does not always mean the person will get the disorder or disease; it just increases the chances. There are many different kinds of risk factors, including genetic, biologic, environmental, cultural, and occupational. Even gender is a risk factor for some disorders (e.g., more women experience depression than men) (see Chapter 24). In general, gender, age, unemployment, and lower education are risk factors associated with mental illness.

Biologic Risk Factors

The biologic functioning of young versus middle-aged adults is a contrast between optimally running physiological systems and those showing definite signs of wear and inefficiency. Of course, there are wide variations in the health of the various systems within each stage, with some young adults more physiologically and functionally compromised than their middle-aged counterparts. Most physical and mental systems have completed development by the time an individual reaches young adulthood. In general, the optimal health state of young adults begins to show changes around the age of 30 years. The perception of these physical changes often makes individuals aware of their aging process and may result in threats to bodily integrity and self-esteem. This section reviews the primary changes in the health of physiological symptoms and possible mental health implications.

Skin

The most obvious change in physical appearance starts with the skin. Although the young adult's skin is smooth and taut, by late young adulthood, the skin begins to lose moisture and tone, and wrinkles develop. Self-esteem issues can erupt as the skin ages, especially for women.

Cardiovascular and Respiratory Systems

Maximum cardiac output is reached between 20 and 30 years of age. Thereafter, blood pressure and cholesterol levels gradually increase. Although men are especially prone to cardiovascular disease in middle age because of testosterone levels, women are not exempt from risk of heart disease. In a parallel manner, respiratory function also decreases with age. After the age of 30 years, maximum breathing capacity slowly decreases and may be reduced up to 75% compared with during young

adulthood. Such changes are compounded if the individual smoked throughout adulthood. Alterations in cardiac and respiratory efficiency may result in limited energy for daily tasks and preference for lower activity levels, which makes exercise less of an enjoyable activity (Brown, Pavey, & Bauman, 2014).

Sensory Function

Sensory functions are also compromised as an individual moves from young adulthood into middle age. Although the visual sense is at its peak in early young adulthood, the lenses of the eyes gradually lose their elasticity around age 30 years, and corrective lenses may be necessary. Such changes may result in issues regarding physical appearance that may affect self-esteem. Hearing is optimal in young adulthood, but middle age brings changes in the bones of the inner ear and auditory nerve, resulting in the gradual inability to hear high-pitched tones and detect certain consonants. Such alterations in hearing may also present issues related to body integrity.

Neurologic System

In middle age, brain structural changes are minimal. Although neurons are gradually being lost, changes in cognition are not evident. There may be some slowing of speed of reflexes because of small changes in nerve conduction speed during middle age.

Basal Metabolic Rate

Basal metabolic rate is at maximum functional capacity at age 30 years and then gradually decreases at a rate of 2% per decade, related to a gradual loss in highly physiologically active muscle mass. The ratio of fat tissue to lean body mass gradually increases, which may result in weight gain if calories are not restricted. There is currently an epidemic of obesity within the Unites States because of poor nutrition and low activity levels. Weight gain also raises concerns changes about physical attractiveness, especially in women. It is also related to decreased cardiac and respiratory efficiency, which makes exercise less of a preferred activity (Brown et al., 2014).

Sexual and Reproductive Functioning

Concerns about changing physical appearance may also be tied to reactions to changes in sexual functioning. In middle-aged men, testosterone production decreases, resulting in a lower sex drive, more time needed to achieve erection, and production of fewer sperm cells. Men whose sense of self was dependent on the level of sexual functioning typical of young adulthood may experience anxiety over such changes. Diminishing estrogen levels in middle age in women result in the cessation of menses and capacity for pregnancy. The beginning of menopause may bring unpleasant symptoms such as hot flashes, night sweats, fatigue, and nausea. However, most women experience menopause as a relief from menses, fluctuating hormone levels, and the possibility of pregnancy. Women whose view of self was based on sexual characteristics may also be prone to anxiety because of these changes.

Psychosocial Risk Factors

Any of the common challenges of adulthood previously discussed such as unemployment, changing family structure, and caregiving may serve as risks factors for mental disorders. These more general problems reveal underlying risk factors that have shown to be common in the development of mental disorders. Also, risk factors rarely occur in isolation but tend to cluster because one may bring about another, and they influence each other.

Age

The majority of mental disorders occur among young adults and appear to be less common with increasing age. The first symptoms may occur in childhood but are usually evident in late adolescence and early middle adulthood. Such symptoms may be partially tied to the increasing demands for independence and social responsibility that Western society places on developing individuals. As some adults get older, they may experience decreasing stress because of learning to cope more efficiently.

Marital Status

Individuals who are happily married experience higher rates of both physical and mental health compared with those who are single, separated, or divorced. Marriage may serve as a general marker for psychological health and the ability to connect with larger social networks. However, an unhappy marriage can have negative health effects. Unmarried individuals may also experience positive physical and mental health especially if they are not isolated from others and have support from a larger social system (Prouix & Snyder-Rivas, 2013; Schoenborn & Adams, 2010).

Unemployment and Other Job Stresses

In this consumer-oriented society, economic stability is a major value. Unemployment is a larger indicator of such socioeconomically related variables such as poverty, lack of education, and the ability to obtain economic power within the larger social system. This creates an environment of stress that may contribute to the development of

mental disorder or may indicate the negative effect that mental disorder has had on obtaining the education and independence necessary for obtaining job security and advancement (Worach-Kardas & Kostrzewski, 2014).

Of course, employment has its own set of stresses. Many people with low-paying jobs work two jobs, often going directly from one job to another. Shift work causes changes in circadian rhythms and sleep patterns, leading to an increase in stress. Interpersonal problems with coworkers can lead to emotional distress. Challenges even arise related to the different learning styles and career expectations of workers of different ages and backgrounds or who are reentering the workforce (Box 16.1).

Gender

Women come to the attention of the mental health system because of their greater awareness of health issues and willingness to seek interventions. However, women also differ in the types of mental disorders that they show. Whereas women are more prone to anxiety and depression, men tend to show problems with impulse control that result in disorders such as alcohol and drug abuse.

History of Child Abuse

Being abused as a child increases the risk of a mental disorder as an adult. Data from a national survey indicated that there are long-term consequences of early childhood abuse. Reported emotional abuse was associated with lower personal control, which in turn leads to lower health ratings (Fryers & Brugha, 2013).

Prior Mental Disorder

Mental illness tends to be a chronic disorder whose symptoms manifest fairly early in life. Research has shown that mental illness arising in childhood and adolescence predicts further disorder in later years. Because most mental disorders are never cured, the existence of prior symptoms or full-blown disorder is a risk for mental illness at later periods in life. Increased stress provides the ground for the current emergence of symptoms of mental disorders that may have appeared to be in remission (Fryers & Brugha, 2013).

Coping

Although the quality of coping is important in the reduction of stress, little is known about the continuity and changes in coping styles over the lifespan. Because past behavior is the best predictor of future behavior, it would appear that coping styles used in the past would be repeated in the present time. The quality of such coping would determine how well stress is handled in the present

BOX 16.1

Research for Best Practice: **Generational Differences Among Novice Registered Nurses**

Keepnews, D. M., Kovner, C. T., & Shin, J. H. (2010). Generational differences among newly licensed registered nurses. Nursing Outlook, 58, 155–163.

THE QUESTION: Registered nurses (RNs) are entering the workforce from three generations: the Baby Boomers (born 1946–1964), Generation X (1965–1979), and Generation Y (born after 1980). Novice nurses, thus, may come from young adult and middle-age developmental groups. What are the differences in the characteristics, work-related experiences, and attitudes of newly licensed RNs across the three generations?

METHODS: A 16-page survey regarding work values and experiences was mailed to a randomly selected sample of 14,512 newly licensed RNs located across the United States. A total of 30.1% completed the survey.

FINDINGS: Baby Boomers were less likely to have had a formal orientation to their first position. They were more likely to assume head nurse positions during their first year of practice. This may reflect supervisors' expectations that Baby Boomers are less in need of formal orientation and better prepared to move rapidly into management positions. Novice Generation Y and X nurses were much more likely than Baby Boomers to work in an intensive care unit. Generation X and Y RNs may seek greater levels of stimulation in their work and may also possess greater comfort with technology. Generation X and Y nurses were also more likely than Baby Boomers to work 10- or 12-hour shifts, showing Baby Boomer preference for shorter and less taxing work times. A total of 14.5% of newly licensed Baby Boomer RNs and 9.5% of Generation X RNs were male compared with 3.4% of Generation Y. The stability and relatively high pay of RN jobs may be more attractive to Baby Boomer and X Generation men who have formerly worked in and perhaps been displaced from other professions.

IMPLICATIONS FOR NURSING: Retention of experienced RNs is important because the current recruitment rate of new RNs will not solve the nursing shortage problem. Middle-aged RNs also have developed the expertise needed to ensure quality care. Job redesign and improvements in the work environment are necessary to prevent related illnesses and injuries that may prompt nurses to leave the workforce. Recent legislation enforcing minimum staffing levels and limiting mandatory overtime may also result in improved work environments. In addition, management should recognize the generational diversity of the nursing workforce by assessing the age composition per unit, understanding differing expectations, and building on the values and strengths of different generations while emphasizing common organizational goals.

at midlife (defined as 40–60 years) with those in young and older adulthood. The results of this study suggest that coping is a process that improves in quality as life continues and is shown in increasing satisfaction with life. A longitudinal follow-up of MIDUS respondents occurred in 2002–2006. The purposes of the follow-up were to repeat the assessments obtained in the original study and to expand into other areas of biological and neurological assessments. A third phase is currently being extended to 2016.

BOX 16.2

Research for Best Practice: **The MIDUS National Survey: An Overview**

Brim, O. G., Ryff, C. D., & Kessler, R. C. (2004). The MIDUS National Survey: An overview. In O. G. Brim, C. D. Ryff, & R. C. Kessler (Eds.), How healthy are we? A national study of well-being at midlife (pp. 1–34). Chicago: University of Chicago Press.

THE QUESTION: The John D. and Catherine T. MacArthur Foundation established the Research Network on Successful Midlife Development to generate new knowledge related to the challenges faced by those in the middle years. The network created and implemented a national survey of midlife Americans to determine the well-being of those in the middle of their lives. The goals were to develop indicators (physical, psychological, social) for assessing midlife development; establish an empirical basis of what happens in midlife; and identify factors that influence midlife development, including illness, life stresses, work, and family.

METHODS: This study involved surveying more than 7,000 subjects between 25 and 74 years of age to compare those at midlife (defined as 40–60 years) with those in young and older adulthood. Demographics, psychosocial factors, mental health, physical illnesses, and health-related beliefs were surveyed.

FINDINGS: Many findings are being generated from this large data set. One set of findings suggests that coping is a process that improves in quality as life continues and is shown in increasing satisfaction with life. Initial findings of the study are that mood in midlife is more contextually determined, influenced by work and social relationships, compared with younger and older adults. Self-reported quality of life improves with age, but increases do not significantly start until middle age (around age 40 years), with the strongest predictors being the quality of the marital relationship and finances. Only a quarter of middle-aged adults report having a midlife crisis, and the majority of middle-aged Americans report that they are healthy and in control of their lives.

IMPLICATIONS FOR NURSING: From this study, nurses can appreciate that most people in midlife are able to cope as long as they have a good quality of life, including social relationships and financial security. By assessing coping skills, nurses can identify strengths that can be supported in times of emotional turmoil and exacerbation of illnesses. Because work and social relationships are very important to this group, these areas should always be assessed.

and sets the stage for continued positive outcomes or more problems in the future.

There is an absence of epidemiologic studies that directly compare adult life stages according to mental health variables such as coping. An exception is the Midlife Development in the United States (MIDUS) Study (Box 16.2). The study involved more than 7,000 subjects between 25 and 74 years of age to compare those

Sad, Blue, or Depressed Days

Although depression is a major public health problem that is related to disability and impaired quality of life, little is known about lesser symptoms of feeling sad or blue that may not meet the diagnostic criteria for a mood disorder. As part of the Behavioral Risk Factor Surveillance System, a national survey that monitors behaviors that place individuals at risk for health problems, respondents were asked how many days in the past month they experienced sad, blue, or depressed days (SBDDs). Such symptoms were common, with respondents reporting a mean of 3 days in which they experienced SBDDs within the past month. Women reported more SBDDs than men; young adults reported the highest number and older adults the fewest. The difference between men and women's SBDDs decreased with increasing age (Kobau, Safran, Zack, Moriarty, & Chapman, 2004).

The number of reported SBDDs was highly associated with problems in health maintenance. Those who reported more SBDDs also engaged in more unhealthy behaviors such smoking, binge drinking, and physical inactivity. These findings suggest the link between depressive symptoms and lack of health-promoting activities and the need for interventions that increase positive feelings, self-efficacy, and the motivation to engage in health-promoting behaviors (Kobau et al., 2004).

Lack of Health Promotion Behaviors

People with mental disorders in young adult and middle age appear to lack basic health promotion behaviors. This lack results in high rates of physical illness and premature mortality compared with the general population. This includes low levels of awareness about physical and mental health issues, smoking, poor quality diets, lack of exercise, lack of leisure activities and contact with friends, negative attitudes toward help seeking, and stigma associated with mental health problems (Aschbrenner, Mueser, Bartels, & Pratt, 2013; Cerimele, Halperin, & Saxon, 2014; Jacka, Cherbuin, Anstey, & Butterworth, 2014).

NCLEXNOTE People with mental disorders frequently neglect their physical health and have premature mortality. Assessment of physical health and health-promoting activities is important in the care of people with mental disorders because of their high rate of smoking, lack of physical activity, and resistance to seeking help for physical concerns.

Parenting Stress

Young adults often find that the addition of children to the family, particularly the birth of the second child, tends to insulate the nuclear family from larger social networks. The responsibilities and time constraints involved in rearing small children may limit the couple's worldview to the home, and definitions of self may be constricted to the activities of the nuclear family. However, as children grow and create their own lives, the social connectedness of the parents tends to expand. By middle age, couples may anticipate the emancipation of their children and may entertain more options for socializing with other people.

Factors Associated with Suicide

Suicide ideation and suicide are serious public health problems in the United States. In one large epidemiological study, the prevalence rate of suicide during the past year among younger adults (age 18 to 25), was 6.6% and 4.0% for adults 26 to 49 years. These rates were higher than that among adults aged 50 years or older (Han, McKeon, & Gfroerer, 2014). Among adults with major depression the prevalence was 37.7% and adults who received mental health treatment but perceived unmet treatment needs was 33.5%. There is no one risk factor associated with suicide, but a variety of factors include age, family stress, illness, and social circumstances. For example, during the recent recession years, the suicide rate increased as home foreclosures increased (Houle & Light, 2014). Traumatic brain injuries are associated with suicide ideation and attempts. Discrimination experienced by ethnic and sexual minorities is related to suicide (Bostwick et al., 2014; Mackelprang, Bombardier, Fann, Temkin, Barber, & Dikmen, 2014).

PROTECTIVE FACTORS

In contrast to risk factors, **protective factors** are characteristics that reduce the probability that a person will develop a mental health disorder or problem or decrease the severity of existing problems. Common protective factors exist in multiple contexts—families, communities, and society. All of these contexts should be considered when promoting mental health. For example, parental involvement can help combat drug abuse in their children, but a strong school policy is also needed. In addition, other community resources must be used to support the drug-free community environment. Targeting only one context is unlikely to make a lasting impact.

INTERVENTION APPROACHES

Many nursing interventions are effective in helping young and middle-aged adults achieve greater mental health. Whereas some are geared toward helping adults cope with the challenges typical of this period of life, others are more specifically designed toward preventing depression and suicide. Another aspect of intervention is helping adults overcome societal pressures that might prevent them from seeking care in the first place.

Mental Health Promotion

The psychiatric mental health nurse supports the young and middle-aged adult through the developmental journey of life. Stresses associated with balancing the psychosocial demands and the adjustment to changes in the biologic, psychological, and social domains can be overwhelming. Validation and education are important interventions in helping these individuals cope with these changes (see Chapter 18).

A person's mental health can be challenged by a variety of factors; biologic changes or illnesses, psychological pressures, and interpersonal tensions are only a few. Developing coping strategies to eliminate or reduce the impact of these potentially destructive factors is a part of normal growth and development. In addition, sustaining positive health behaviors such as relaxation, proper nutrition, adequate sleep, regular exercise, and forming a network of trusting relationships can support one's mental health. Mental health promotion focuses on increasing the individual's physical, mental, emotional, and social competencies to increase well-being and actualize potential.

Social Support During Life Transitions

Young and middle-aged adults are prone to many life transitions: entrance into the work force, job loss, career change, separation, divorce, the birth of children and their eventual leaving home, and changes in health status. Middle-aged adults are also subject to watching their parents age and possibly lose independence. Both young and middle adults can benefit from education about coping with the stresses involved with such transitions, linking with sources of social support, and anticipating the changes in role and adjustment (Box 16.3).

Lifestyle Support

Although health may be at its maximum during the young adult years, changes in bodily appearance and function become evident by age 30 years and become more pronounced as middle age begins. Although such changes are inevitable, their magnitude can be tempered by health promotion activities such as attention to regular exercise, good nutrition, adequate sleep, health screening, relaxation, leisure, and other forms of stress management. The young adult years are times of learning positive coping strategies for the stresses inherent to personal, marital, family, and occupational life. Such learning can be enhanced by a social support network consisting of people

BOX 16.3

Using Reflection

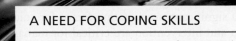

A NEED FOR COPING SKILLS

INCIDENT • The young woman kept repeating that she was scared and not ready for marriage. The elaborate wedding was the following week. The nurse assured her that everything would be fine and her concerns were normal. The following week, the local newspaper reported that this bride had run away the day of the wedding.

REFLECTION • Upon reflection, the nurse realized that the young woman had been raised by a single parent who had several short-term romantic relationships and had no exposure to a successful marriage. The young woman was clearly telling the nurse that she did not have the coping skills that are needed for marriage.

who are currently undergoing such stresses as well as older people who have the perspective and experience in handling these domains of life. These networks can be informal, such as regular contact with a circle of friends, or more formal such as support groups sponsored by social, occupational, and religious organizations. Research has consistently shown the crucial importance of the sense of belonging and availability of social support for the maintenance of health and recovery from illness of all kinds (Farber, Lamis, Shahane, & Campos, 2014).

Self-Care Enhancement

The latter part of young adulthood and middle age are times when chronic illnesses such as hypertension, heart disease, and arthritis may become evident. Symptoms of mental disorders may have arisen earlier in life but require continuous care because of their chronic and episodic nature. It is important for both young and middle-aged adults to be educated about the physiological aspects of such disorders, the advances in medications used in treating them, possible side effects, the importance of medication adherence, lifestyle changes that can be instituted to control such disorders, and the possible use of complementary healing methods (e.g., massage, meditation). Such strategies require a good relationship with a health care provider as well as initiative from individuals to contributing to their own care through seeking and evaluating information available from the press, on the Internet, or from advocacy groups.

Prevention of Depression and Suicide

Although suicide is highest among older adults and adolescents, it still poses a major mental health issue for young and middle-aged adults. Symptoms of most psychiatric disorders have made their appearance by the time an individual enters young adulthood. In particular, mood disorders may first arise during the young adult years and continue through middle age and older adulthood. Because depression is a significant precipitating factor for suicide, early detection and intervention are critical for managing mood disorders and preventing suicide. Routine screening for depression and associated substance abuse is recommended in primary care settings (U.S. Preventive Services Task Force, 2009).

Reducing the Stigma of Mental Health Treatment

Although mental disorders are common within the community and the rate of treatment has risen over the past 20 years, more than half of people do not receive mental health treatment of any kind. Part of this lack of attention is certainly because of the lack of available treatment in many communities (e.g., rural areas), but another major factor is the stigma that continues to be associated with mental illness and seeking help for mental health problems. Organizations such as the National Alliance on Mental Illness (NAMI) have spearheaded the movement toward viewing mental disorders as biologically based and devoid of moral implications, putting them on par with physical disorders. NAMI is an important organization for obtaining information, support, and referrals for treatment for individuals with mental disorders as well as their families.

The Future of Mental Health for Young and Middle-Aged Adults

The periods of adult development known as young adulthood and middle age can be some of the most productive in life. They can also be the most stressful and debilitating because of the rapid rate of social change and economic instability that society is currently experiencing. The division of adulthood into young- and middle-aged stages and the interest in adult development have paved the way for examining the challenges unique to these stages in which individuals spend the majority of their lives. More needs to be known about the stresses of these stages, the ways that individuals cope, the changes that bring about increased life satisfaction, and the ways in which nurses can support adaptation and ensure health promotion. Such health-promoting interventions may serve as the foundation for future mental health.

Although more is known about childhood and older adults because of the more dramatic and time-dependent aspects of their development, the more subtle changes of adulthood also deserve consideration. Development does not end at childhood, and more needs to be known

about the manner in which young adults progress within their lives and achieve the satisfactions reported with middle age.

Research also needs to examine the variables that promote and protect mental health as well as understanding risk factors. Researchers and clinicians often equate promotive or protective factors with the absence of risk factors. This is tantamount to equating health with the absence of illness. Models of thriving and flourishing in response to life's challenges have been proposed by theorists as a more appropriate model for mental health promotion rather than adequate functioning or the lack of criteria for a psychiatric disorder. Those who flourish do not merely lack psychiatric disorders; they also have lower risk for cardiovascular disease and other chronic physical illnesses, fewer health related limitations, lower health care utilization, fewer missed days of work, and high resilience and intimacy. The adoption of such positive models has implications not only for prevention of mental illness but also for more proactive interventions that ensure continued wellness that progresses into older adulthood.

SUMMARY OF KEY POINTS

- Western families have achieved unprecedented economic stability that provides for long periods of development and a range of choices in lifestyle.

- The periods of young and middle adulthood do not exist in less developed countries; a brief childhood progresses quickly into old age.

- Western society has recently shown greater tolerance for the timing of life events such as education, marriage, and childrearing.

- The periods of young and middle-age are characterized by changes in family structure caused by children leaving and returning home, marriage, and divorce.

- Caregiving for both children and older parents is a potential stress faced by both young and middle-aged adults.

- Unemployment is a growing common problem in adulthood, particularly for single mothers and African Americans.

- Mental disorders are most common in young adults, with the first symptoms evident in late adolescence and young adulthood, with the exception of cognitive impairment.

- As individuals progress from young to middle-aged adulthood, they experience changes from optimally running physiological systems to those showing wear and inefficiency.

- Psychosocial risk factors for mental disorder include age, marital status, unemployment and job stresses, gender, prior mental disorder, coping, SBDDs, lack of health promotion behaviors, parenting stress, and factors associated with suicide.

- Despite decreases in the efficiency of physiological functioning, young and middle-aged adults often lack health promoting behaviors, especially if they have mental disorders.

- Suicide is a growing problem in young and middle adulthood, especially in the light of recent economic downturns, and requires early detection and treatment.

- Social support and stress management are important in helping people to cope with the stresses involved in life transitions.

- Fewer than half of individuals receive treatment for their mental health issues, and stigma remains toward those experiencing problems.

- Mental health promotion in adulthood needs to embrace positive models of people who flourish in life rather than those who lack mental illness. Little is known about the factors that promote or protect mental health.

CRITICAL THINKING CHALLENGES

1. What are your assumptions about the psychosocial tasks that should be accomplished by an individual in American society who is young versus middle aged? Describe the challenges that each age group faces in terms of education, marriage, career, children, financial stability, and health and the expected outcomes for each of these challenges. Then compare your answers with another person's. In which areas do you agree and disagree? Why does the perception of the tasks of young and middle adulthood differ from person to person?

2. Describe the modifiable risk factors for mental disorders for young and middle-aged adults and suggest mental health promotion activities that can be used to address these risk factors.

3. What factors do you think are protective or promotive of mental health? How do physical and mental health overlap? What kinds of interventions may promote both physical and mental health?

 The Kids Are All Right: 2010. This is a film about a lesbian couple and their adolescent daughter and son who were both conceived from the same anonymous donor via artificial insemination.

The daughter, who is preparing to leave home for college, decides to initiate contact with her biologic father. The introduction of the father, although pleasant at first, ultimately reveals the strains in the family's relationships and functioning. This film illustrates the children negotiating the identity tasks of adolescence and ambivalently assuming initial responsibilities of young adulthood. The parents mirror their children's struggles in terms of renegotiating the roles played in their marriage, their lesbian identities, the level of independence given to their children, and acknowledging the imminent "empty nest."

VIEWING POINTS: Identify the life transitions faced by each of the family members in the film. How does each member cope with the stresses they are experiencing? How are the developmental issues the parents are facing similar to their children's? How did the entrance of the father highlight the conflicts and ultimately change the dynamics in this family?

References

Aschbrenner, K. A., Mueser, K. T., Bartels, S. J., & Pratt, S. I. (2013). Perceived social support for diet and exercise among persons with serious mental illness enrolled in a healthy lifestyle intervention. *Psychiatric Rehabilitation Journal, 36*(2), 65–71.

Bostwick, W. B., Meyer, I., Aranda, F., Russell, S., Hughes, T., Birkett, M., et al. (2014). Mental health and suicidality among racially/ethnically diverse sexual minority youths. *American Journal of Public Health, 104*(6), 1129–1136.

Brim, O. G., Ryff, C. D., & Kessler, R. C. (2004). The MIDUS National Survey: An overview. In O. G. Grim, C. D. Ryff, & R. C. Kessler (Eds.). *How healthy are we? A national study of well-being at midlife* (pp. 1–34). Chicago: University of Chicago Press.

Brown, W. J., Pavey, T., & Bauman, A. E. (2014). Comparing population attributable risks for heart disease across the adult lifespan in women. *British Journal of Sports Medicine,* doi:10.1136/bjsports-2013-093090

Chatterji, P., & Alegria, M., & Takeuchi, M. (2009). Racial/ethnic differences in the effects of psychiatric disorders on employment. *Atlantic Economic Journal, 37,* 243–257.

Cerimele, J. M., Halperin, A. C., & Saxon, A. J. (2014). Tobacco use treatment in primary care patients with psychiatric illness. *Journal of the American Board of Family Medicine, 27*(3), 399–410.

Cohn, C., Livingston, G., & Wang, W. (2014). Comparing stay-at-home and working mothers. Pew Research, Social & Demographic Trends. Pew Research Center. Retrieved June 27, 2014, from http://www.pewsocialtrends.org/2014/04/08/after-decades-of-decline-a-rise-in-stay-at-home-mothers/

Fryers, T., & Brugha, F. (2013). Childhood determinants of adult psychiatric disorder. *Clinical Practice & Epidemiology in Mental Health, 9,* 1–50. doi:10.2174/1745017901209010001

Family Caregiver Alliance. (2012). *Selected caregiver statistics.* Family Caregiver Alliance. Retrieved from http://www.caregiving.org.

Farber, E. W., Lamis, D. A., Shahane, A. A., & Campos, P. E. (2014). Personal meaning, social support, and perceived stigma in individuals receiving HIV mental health services. *Journal of Clinical Psychology in Medical Settings, 21*(2), 173–182.

Han, B., McKeon, R., & Gfroerer, J. (2014). Suicidal ideation among community-dwelling adults in the United States. *American Journal of Public Health, 104*(3), 488–497.

Houle, J. N., & Light, M. T. (2014). The home foreclosure crisis and rising suicide rates, 2005 to 2010. *American Journal of Public Health, 104*(6), 1073–1079.

Jacka, F. N., Cherbuin, N., Anstey, K. J., & Butterworth, P. (2014). Dietary patterns and depressive symptoms over time: Examining the relationships with socioeconomic position, health behaviours and cardiovascular risk. *Plos One, 9*(1), e87657. doi:10.1371/journal.pone.0087657

Kessler, R. C., Avenevoli, S., McLaughlin, K. A., Green, J. G., Lakoma, M. D., Petukhova, M., et al. (2012). Lifetime co-morbidity of DMS-IV disorders in the US National Comorbidity Survey Replication Adolescent Supplement (NCS-A). *Psychol Med*, 42(9), 1997–2010.

Kobau, R., Safran, M. A., Zack, M. M., Moriarty, D. G., & Chapman, D. (2004). Sad, blue, or depressed days, health behaviors and health-related quality of life, Behavioral Risk Factor Surveillance System, 1995–2000. *Health and Quality of Life Outcomes*, 2, 40–53.

Mackelprang, J. L., Bombardier, C. H., Fann, J. R., Temkin, N. R., Barber, J. K., & Dikmen, S. S. (2014). Rates and predictors of suicidal ideation during the first year after traumatic brain injury. *American Journal of Public Health*, 104(7), e100–e107.

NAMI. (2010). *The high costs of cutting mental health: unemployment*. National Alliance on Mental Illness: Arlington, VA.

Prouix, C. M., & Snyder-Rivas, L. A. (2013). The longitudinal associations between marital happiness, problems, and self-rated health. *Journal of Family Psychology*, 27(2), 194–202.

SAMSHA (2014). *The NSDUH Report*. Center for Behavioral Health U.S. Department of Health & Human Services. Washington, DC.

Schoenborn, C A. & Adams, P. F. (2010). Health behaviors of adults: United States, 2005–2007. National Center for Health Statistics. *Vital Health Statistics*, 10(245), 1–132.

U.S. Bureau of Labor Statistics (2014, April). Regional and State Employment and Unemployment (Monthly). Retrieved from http://www.bls.gov/home.htm.

U.S. Census Bureau. (2013). *America's families and living arrangements: 2010*. Washington D.C: Author.

U.S. Preventive Services Task Force. (2009). *Guide to clinical preventive services*. Washington, DC: Agency for Healthcare Research and Quality. Retrieved from http://www.ahrq.gov/clinic/pocketgd09/pocketgd09.pdf.

Wang, P. S., Ulbricht, C. M., & Schoenbaum, M. (2009). Improving mental health treatments through comparative effectiveness research. *Health Affairs*, 28(3), 783–791. *doi:10.1377/hlthaff.28.3.783.*

Worach-Kardas, J., & Kostrzewski, S. (2014). Quality of life and health state of long-term unemployed in older production age. *Applied Research in Quality of Life*, 9, 335–353.

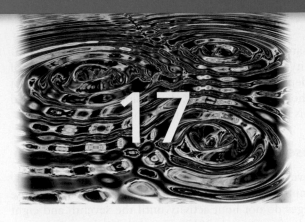

17

Mental Health Promotion for Older Adults

Georgia L. Stevens

KEY CONCEPT

- late adulthood

LEARNING OBJECTIVES

After studying this chapter, you will be able to:

1. Describe important biopsychosocial processes impacting late adulthood.

2. Identify risk factors related to geriatric psychopathology.

3. Identify protective factors in the mental health promotion of older adults.

4. Discuss mental health prevention and promotion interventions that are especially effective with older adults and the nurse's role in them.

KEY TERMS

- elder mistreatment • functional status • gerotranscendence • middle-old • old-old • resilience
- speed–accuracy shift • young-old

Older adults are at somewhat greater risk than younger age groups for the development or recurrence of mental health problems. One in four older adults has a significant mental disorder, with depression, anxiety disorders, and dementia being among the most common (U.S. Department of Health and Human Services, 2010). Yet despite the high prevalence of psychiatric disorders and mental health problems in later life, older people remain vastly underserved by the current mental health system. The future need for services will be even greater as the number of adults aged 65 years and older doubles in the next 25 years, coupled with a significant increase in older adult ethnic minorities, who tend to be even more underserved while having higher than average healthcare needs, thereby supporting the need for an improved mental health system (Canive & Escobar, 2009). This chapter explains the effects of aging on mental health and identifies risks and protective factors related to the psychopathology of older adults.

OLDER ADULT MENTAL HEALTH

Our understanding of successful aging has evolved from a view of inevitable decline based on solely objective measures to a richer and more optimistic picture based on qualitative studies. It is, therefore, critical that the study of late adulthood occurs over time through listening to the perspectives of older adults and learning from their wisdom.

Older adulthood is a gradual biopsychosocial process of change and personal development that can be conceptualized in roughly three stages: **young-old** (ages 65–74 years), **middle-old** (ages 75–84 years), and **old-old** (age 85 years and older).

> **KEYCONCEPT** **Late adulthood** can be divided into three chronological groups: young-old, middle-old, and old-old.

These changes can be negative or positive. For example, family relationships and roles change as once-dependent children grow into adulthood and become parents themselves. No longer having dependent children can be viewed positively with more time to pursue personal interest or negatively with feelings of abandonment. When older adults retire from their lifelong work, they are challenged to establish a new meaning in life. There are opportunities to do the things, such as traveling and visiting friends, that were impossible when work and family responsibilities took precedence. When losses occur, friendship relationships also change. The nurse can be instrumental in helping older adults consider the potential growth opportunities during this time.

COMMON CHALLENGES IN OLDER ADULTHOOD

Biologic Domain

Changes in vital biologic structures and processes occur gradually over decades and become evident in late adulthood. However, many older adults can integrate profound decrements in physical capacity without significantly affecting their ability to function under normal conditions. It is only when functional reserves are needed, such as during an infection, that the absence of these reserves may be observed. Changes in health status, for example, can lead to loss in physical functioning and independence, which in turn can result in an unplanned change in residence. The risk of depression is increased as functional limitation increase and perceived physical health declines (Hybels, Blazer, & Hays, 2011).

Physical Changes

Many physical changes occur in older adults. Typically, body fat increases (18%–36% in men; 33%–48% in women), total body water decreases (10%–15%), and muscle mass decreases. In the renal system, there is a predictable decline in glomerular filtration and tubular secretion. Although less efficient, the renal system without disease or injury can function adequately throughout late adulthood (Saxon, Etten, & Perkins, 2010). Liver function may be reduced because of decreases in blood flow and enzyme activity, resulting in increased blood and tissue concentrations of medications as well as half-life prolongation. Also, fat-soluble drugs may become sequestered in fatty tissue, rather than remaining in the circulating plasma increasing the risk for drug accumulation and toxicity (see Chapter 11). In the brain, healthy older adults have a reduction in gray matter volume, increase in cerebrospinal fluid, increased white matter abnormalities, and lower metabolic rates at rest (Eyler & Kovaceviv, 2010).

Any of these changes over time can compromise the physiological reserves to manage the everyday stresses of life. There has been a significant increase in use of anti-anxiety, sedative, and hypnotic medications in community-dwelling older adults as well as an increase use of antidepressants in this group. Even with a high usage of psychotropic medications, depression remains untreated in this population (Hybels et al., 2011).

Sensory Changes

All five senses gradually decline in acuity with age, usually beginning in the fourth and fifth decades of life, but these changes do not limit activity until the seventh and eight decades (Saxon et al., 2010). Visual and auditory losses can significantly impact independence and self-mastery. Taste, touch, and smell undergo a uniform dulling although the rate of decline is highly variable among individuals. Sensory decline is important to consider when assessing psychiatrically ill older adults because diminished senses may affect information processing, potentially affecting interpretation of standard mental status examinations. For example, patients who do not reveal hearing difficulty may be evaluated instead for dementia or depression.

Sexuality

Interest in and enjoyment of sexual activities can continue until one's death despite physical changes that affect sexual functioning. Health, a desire to remain sexually active, access to a partner, and a conducive environment contribute to positive sexual experiences. Physiological changes in women related to sexual functioning include decreasing estrogen levels, alterations in the structural integrity of the vagina (e.g., decreased blood flow, decreased flexibility, diminished lubrication, and diminished response during orgasm), and decreased breast engorgement during arousal (Saxon et al., 2010). Physiological changes in men include a decline in testosterone production, increased time to achieve erection, less firm erections, decreased urgency for ejaculation, decreased sperm production, and a longer refractory period (i.e., the amount of time before the man can achieve another erection). Problems with sexual performance in aging men are usually centered around erectile dysfunction, which in turn, affects self-esteem (Saxon et al., 2010).

Access to a conducive environment for sexual expression may be hindered if an older adult resides with an adult child or in a nursing home. Stigma associated with sexual activity in later life is also perpetuated by young adults' negative attitudes toward late-life sexuality and further contributes to lack of acceptance that sexual feelings and behaviors are normal at all ages (Allen, Petro, & Phillips, 2009). Lack of acceptance by others, particularly family members, and lack of privacy further contribute to a sense of isolation, loneliness, and poor social support, which are all associated with risks for depression (Hybels et al., 2011).

Psychological Domain

Cognitive Function

Many cognitive abilities (e.g., knowledge accumulated over a lifetime) are preserved or even enhanced during aging (Palmer & Dawes, 2010). Normal aging does not impair consciousness, alertness, or attention. Individual factors, including customary activity levels, socioeconomic status, education, and personality, may modify the development or expression of age-related changes in cognition.

Mental processing speed and reaction time do gradually decrease from mid to late adulthood and may affect how quickly the older adult responds to questions (Palmer & Dawes, 2010). This phenomenon has been labeled the **speed–accuracy shift**, by which the older adult focuses more on accuracy than speed in responding. Older adults are more likely to make errors of omission (leave out the answer) than errors of commission (make a guess). Hurrying older adults to answer questions may interfere with their ability to provide the correct answer (Saxon et al., 2010). Communication with older adults requires special attention to verbal interactions and environmental influences. Box 17.1 highlights many of the considerations necessary when interacting with older adults.

Memory loss is not a normal part of aging, but memory may be less efficient. Older people may well dismiss information that is not important to them. Memory problems in later life are believed to result from encoding or retrieval problems (or both). Other factors associated with memory changes include a lack of perceived relevance, sensory problems, not paying attention, a general failure to link the "to be remembered" information to existing knowledge through association, and a lack of using repetition to strengthen memory. Although a decline in memory efficiency may be frustrating for the older individual, it does not necessarily hamper his or her ability to function daily (Palmer & Dawes, 2010). Threats to memory include medications, depression (impairs concentration and attention), poor nutrition, infection, heart and lung disease (lack of oxygen), thyroid problems (can cause symptoms of depression or confusion that mimic memory loss), alcohol use, and sensory loss (interferes with perception). However, it is important not to confuse memory decline with deficits in memory storage such as those that are seen in dementias (see Chapter 37).

Intelligence and Personality

Intelligence and personality are stable across the life span in the absence of disease; however, the learning abilities of older people may be more selective, requiring motivation ("How important is this information?"), depend on meaningful content ("Why do I need to know this?"), and related to familiarity with the idea or content. Although age causes no differences in the ability to process knowledge to learn a skill, younger people are more likely to use strategies to learn tasks. Level of education needs to be considered in evaluating responses on mental status examinations because lower education may represent a deficit in early-life cognitive reserve often related to socioeconomic status (Jeste & Depp, 2010).

Development

Late-life adult developmental phenomena is not well defined (see Chapter 7). Although Erik Erikson identified "integrity versus despair" as a developmental task specific to late adulthood, recently his wife, Joan Serson, published an extension of his theory that included old age as a ninth stage, **gerotranscendence** (Erikson & Erikson, 1997). Rather than emphasizing decrements in physical capacity for function, gerotranscendence theory provides for continued growth in dimensions such as spirituality and inner strength. The concept of gerotranscendence may be used in establishing health promotion interventions. Gerotranscendence is also congruent with more recent research about mental health in late adulthood, which is more optimistic and addresses successful aging. This approach is examining constructs such as empowerment, mastery, resilience, and wisdom (López, Orrell, Morgan, & Warner, 2010; Read, Braam, Lyyra, & Deeg, 2014). See Box 17.2 for one study related to continued development in older adulthood.

BOX 17.1

Communicating with Older Adults

- Focus the person's attention on the exchange of communication; the older adult may need extra time to begin to process information.
- Face the person when speaking to him or her.
- Minimize distractions in the room, including other people, objects in your hands, noise, and other activities.
- Reduce glare from room lighting by dimming too-bright lights. Conversely, avoid sitting in shadows.
- Speak slowly and clearly. Older adults may depend on lip reading, so ensure that the individual can see you. Speak loudly but do not shout.
- Use short, simple sentences and be prepared to repeat or revise what you have said.
- Limit the number of topics discussed at one time to prevent information overload.
- Ask one question at a time to minimize confusion. Allow plenty of time for the person to answer and express ideas.
- Frequently summarize the important points of the conversation to improve understanding and comprehension.
- Avoid the urge to finish sentences.
- Consider factors such as fatigue and discomfort in structuring the communication.
- If the communication exchange is going poorly, postpone it for another time.

BOX 17.2

Research for Best Practice: **Gerotranscendence Support Group**

Wang, J. J., Lin, Y. H., & Hsieh, L. Y. (2011). Effects of gerotranscendence support group on gerotranscendence perspective, depression, and life satisfaction of institutionalized elders. Aging and Mental Health, 15(5), 580–586.

THE QUESTION: Can a gerotranscendence theory (GT) support group improve life satisfaction and reduce depression?

METHODS: Over an 8-week period, depression and life satisfaction scores of 35 residents (average age 80 years) of an assisted-living facility and one nursing home who participated in a GT support group were compared to the 41 similar residents who participated on a weekly "chat" session. The GTs session focused on topics of universe and self transcendence, saying goodbye to worries, forward life, and sharing perspectives of end-of-life.

FINDINGS: Depression and life satisfaction in the GT support improved compared to the "chat" group. A GT perspective developed in the GT support group.

IMPLICATIONS FOR NURSING: This study suggests that GT support groups can influence elder's life satisfaction and depression.

Emotional Health

Although personality is fairly stable across adulthood, emotional changes are small but generally positive. Aging adults tend to become more emotionally stable, more agreeable, and more conscientious, with a higher level of well-being. These positive changes are thought to be related to the development of better emotional regulation because of life experiences and involvement in meaningful activities, networks, and goals. Threats to emotional and physical well-being include loss of social belonging, unrelenting stressors, and neurologic dysregulation (Charles & Horwitz, 2010).

Social Domain

Functional Status

Functional status, the extent to which a person can independently carry out personal care, home management, and social functions in everyday life in a way that has meaning and purpose, often changes during the later years. Estimates of the prevalence of functional dependency vary, but in general, studies show that difficulty in performing activities of daily living (ADLs) and instrumental activities of daily living (IADLs) increase with advancing age and that cognitive impairment significantly predicts functional decline (Pirogovsky et al., 2014). It is important to remember that most older adults live in the community and perceive that they are aging well despite chronic illnesses and some physical disability

(Jeste et al., 2013). A sense of control and self-efficacy contributes to an older person's sense of self mastery despite limitations.

Retirement

Research shows an association between successful aging and a happy retirement. The ability to adapt to change and remain engaged and involved in life and social networks contributes to the successful negotiation of the retirement transition (Kahana, Bhatta, Lovegreen, Kahana, & Midlarsky, 2013). On the other hand, changing roles and circumstances can cause stress and contribute to the onset of psychiatric disorders (Virtanen et al., 2014).

Financial concerns certainly impact one's adjustment to retirement. Social security continues to provide the largest single source of income for older adults (Purcell, 2009). The traditional "three-legged stool" on which retirement rests—Social Security, pensions, and savings and investments—disproportionately excludes some groups such as people of color, gays and lesbians, women, and immigrants who have faced barriers to education, health, a stable work history, or financial stability (Badgett, Durso, & Schneebaum, 2013; Cawthorne, 2008).

The economic downturn had significant implications in terms of personal financial concerns; there is increased competition for jobs as well as a potential delay in retirement (Purcell, 2009). Although mandatory retirement is becoming a thing of the past, older workers may be overlooked for promotions and employment opportunities because of their age and likelihood of retiring. Impairment or dissatisfaction with one's social network has been associated with increased anxiety symptoms in late life (Hybels et al., 2011).

Leisure and Social Activities

As with younger populations, lifestyle is crucial in late adulthood. As age increases, participation in leisure and social activities decreases for many people. Health conditions such as depression, lung disease, and diabetes may prevent participation in home maintenance and leisure activities, especially walking, gardening, and active sports. Maintaining a positive mental attitude and participating in cognitively engaging, regularly scheduled leisure activities appears to exert a protective factor and is associated with a reduced risk of dementia even after adjusting for baseline cognitive status (Tolppanen et al., 2014). Higher education levels are also associated with increased participation in both formal and informal activities.

Family Relationship Changes

As family relationships change, interpersonal relationship strains can develop. Disappointments with the lifestyles of adult children and changes in caregiving responsibilities affect the quality of a long-term family relationship. In some instances, the young-old assume caregiving responsibilities for their old-old relatives. It is also common for grandparents to assume some caregiving responsibilities for their grandchildren. Although there are stresses associated with grandparenting, positive benefits appear to outweigh negatives. The frequency of grandparents raising grandchildren in co-parenting and custodial households has increased significantly in the past 35 years, occurring most frequently in African American families (Holt-Hill, 2009; Yancura, 2013).

Cultural Impact

With our communities increasingly becoming a reflection of multiple ethnic histories and values, the aging population is likewise becoming more diverse. It is expected that the percentage of older adult minorities in 2000 (16.4%) will rise to 22% in 2020 and to 42% in 2050 (Vincent & Velkoff, 2010). Based on the latest census, it is projected that between 1990 and 2030, the percentage of older adults will increase by 395% for Hispanics and 247% for African Americans (Salazar, 2010). Ethnic minorities face disparities in access and provision of health care at the same time that they have higher than average health care needs (D'Avolio, Strumpf, Feldman, Mitchell, & Rebholz, 2013). Cultural variations also exist in family expectations of and responsibilities for older adults. For example, some groups, such as Asian cultures, tend to highly value the experience and wisdom of their elders, and family members feel a responsibility for their care.

Community Factors

Although most older adults live in their own homes, they may find themselves living in changing or deteriorating neighborhoods with inadequate social resources, such as church, community centers, shopping, and health care. Relocating to smaller and more protective housing may be welcomed by some and fiercely resisted by others.

Residential Care

Residential care in foster care homes, family homes, personal care homes, residential care facilities, or assisted living arrangements provides the older adult with a protected environment. The quality of services and affordability of the arrangement needs to be carefully evaluated to determine whether the older adult's needs and abilities match the care provided in that facility, including staff training and staffing patterns, medication supervision, approaches to behavior management, activities provided, services available (e.g., care management, family support, counseling, day care), safety and security issues, provision of personal care with attention to dignity and privacy, health and nutrition concerns, and full disclosure of costs and funding and payment issues.

RISK FACTORS FOR OLDER ADULT PSYCHOPATHOLOGY

Chronic Illnesses

Although the frequency of acute conditions declines with advancing age, about 80% of older adults have at least one chronic health condition; 50% have at least two. Poor physical health is associated with mental disorders both as a risk factor as well as an outcome, with those with severe disabilities reporting lower levels of well-being (Jefferis et al., 2014). Common chronic conditions that cause activity limitation include arthritis, hypertension, heart disease, and respiratory disorders. Chronic illnesses can reduce physiologic capacity and consequently increase functional dependency. In addition, during acute episodes of illness, many older adults lose functional ability because they have limited reserves or cannot mobilize reserves to regain their premorbid performance levels (Sánchex, Vidán, Serra, Fernández-Avilés, & Bueno, 2011).

Alcohol and Substance Abuse

Alcohol and substance abuse are underestimated and undertreated. By 2020, the number of adults aged 50 or older needing substance abuse treatment is expected to double from 2.8 million (2002–2006 annual average) to 5.7 million (U.S. Department of Health and Human Services, 2012). Substance abuse is associated with poor health outcomes, higher health care utilization, and increased complexity of the course of the disorder. In addition, older adults with substance abuse problems have increased disability and impairment, compromised quality of life, increased caregiver stress, increased mortality, and a higher risk of suicide. The majority of older adults with substance abuse problems do not receive adequate treatment (U.S. DHHS, 2012).

Polypharmacy

Polypharmacy, the use of several medications, is often associated with chronic illness and long-term drug therapy. Older persons consume an average of two to six prescription medications and two to three over-the-counter medications. Medication misuse can easily occur and in some combinations, lead to drug abuse (National Council on Aging, 2012). The aging process affects pharmacokinetics and the strength and number of protein-binding sites (see Chapter 11). These changes place older adults at increased risk for adverse drug reactions. Difficulties in managing medications arising from memory impairment further compound the problem of medication misuse. Serious problems result when the treatment regimen and care delivery specific to prescribed medications are not coordinated. These problems are compounded when an older adult uses over-the-counter drugs, herbal remedies, and

---

BOX 17.3

Drug Therapy Interventions

- Minimize the number of drugs that the patient uses, keeping only those drugs that are essential. One third of the residents in one long-term care facility received eight to 16 drugs daily.
- Always consider alternatives among different drug classifications or dosage forms that are more suitable for older adult patients.
- Implement preventive measures to reduce the need for certain medications. Such prevention includes health promotion through proper nutrition, exercise, and stress reduction.
- Most age-dependent pharmacokinetic changes lead to potential accumulation of the drug; therefore, medication dosages should start low and go slow.
- Exercise caution when administering medication with a long half-life or in an older adult with impaired renal or liver function. Under these conditions, the time may be extended between doses.
- Be knowledgeable of each drug's properties, including such factors as half-life, excretion, and adverse effects.

(For example, venlafaxine HCl (Effexor), a structurally novel antidepressant that inhibits the reuptake of serotonin and norepinephrine, requires regular monitoring of the patient's blood pressure.)
- Assess the patient's clinical history for physical problems that may affect excretion of medications.
- Monitor laboratory values (e.g., creatinine clearance) and urinary output in patients receiving medications eliminated by the kidneys.
- Monitor plasma albumin levels in patients receiving drugs that have high binding affinity to protein.
- Regularly monitor the patient's reaction to all medications to ensure a therapeutic response.
- Look for potential drug interactions that may complicate therapy. Antacids lower gastric acidity and may decrease the rate at which other medications are dissolved and absorbed.
- Instruct patients to consult with their providers before taking any over-the-counter medications.

---

home or folk remedies without considering their potential interaction with prescribed drugs. Nurses can follow the principles delineated in Box 17.3 to improve drug therapy in the older adult population.

Bereavement and Loss

Older adults experience many losses—friends and family members die, physical health can be compromised, choices and independence may be limited, and social status may diminish. Loss of one's spouse, particularly when the relationship has been long and satisfying, constitutes a major life event. Women are more likely to lose their spouses and tend to be widowed at a younger age than are men. Consequently, women have more time to adjust and develop substitute social relationships to replace the spouse. Conversely, men tend to lose their wives at an older age, have fewer social networks to replace the spouse, and express feelings of loneliness and abandonment. Because of differences in longevity, men and women usually experience life events at different ages. Regardless of gender differences, survivors are at higher risk for depression and face financial issues after the death of a loved one. Health care professionals should work closely with grieving survivors to help them understand that their lives will be displaced for some time. Support sessions on the grief process and financial and employment planning could become a standard part of care.

Poverty

Because retirement and widowhood are common events in late life and usually involve a loss in financial resources, older adults are high risk for poverty, which contributes to higher mortality rates, poorer health, and lower

health-related quality of life. This is of particular concern now, with the economic downturn, negative impact on pension funds, and the larger numbers of older adults. There are two groups of poor older adults: those who have lived in poverty all their lives and those who became impoverished in late life.

Health care costs probably are the largest contributor to economic insecurity in older people. The aging of the population has significant implications in terms of health care costs associated with Medicare as two million "Baby Boomers" were eligible to sign up by the end of 2010. Older women are more likely to live in poverty than older men (11.5% compared with 6.6%) (U.S. Department of Commerce Economics and Statistics Administration, 2011). Older people living alone have the highest poverty rates. Older people of color live below the poverty line more than white Americans, as do older adults living in rural areas compared with their urban counterparts (U.S. Department of Commerce Economics and Statistical Administration, 2013).

Lack of Social Support and Suicide

A lack of social support and substance use are linked to the high rate of suicide in older adults. Suicide rate for men are highest for those 75 years of age and older. The rate of suicide attempts to completed suicides among adults ages 65 year and older is four to one. The rate of suicide for those 75 years of age and older is 16.3 per 100,000 (Centers for Disease Control and Prevention, 2012). Suicide rates are consistently higher among older adults than any other age group. The rate of suicide in men 65 years of age or older is seven times that of women of the same age. Rates are the highest for divorced or widowed white men (CDC, 2012). See Box 17.4 for risk factors.

BOX 17.4

Risk Factors for Suicide in Late Life (Age Older Than 65 Years)

- White and male
- Poor mental or physical health
- Depression
- Alcohol or drug abuse
- History of prior suicide attempts
- Family history of suicide
- Preoccupied with suicidal talk and plans
- Social isolation: widowed, divorced, living alone in an urban area
- History of poor interpersonal relationships
- Bereavement
- Rigid coping style
- Financial strain
- Access to firearms

Conwell, Y., & Thompson, C. (2008). Suicidal behavior in elders. *Psychiatric Clinics of North America, 31*(2), 333–356.

NCLEXNOTE Safety concerns are a priority. Review suicide risk factors. Carefully explore any suicidal ideation and develop a plan for prevention.

Shared Living Arrangements and Elder Mistreatment

Elder mistreatment can be defined as intentional actions that cause harm or create a serious risk of harm to a vulnerable older adult by a caregiver or other person who stands in a trust relationship to the individual (National Center for Elder Abuse [NCEA], 2014). Estimates of occurrence of abuse and neglect vary from 7.6% to 10%, but actual cases may actually be 12 times the number of reported cases (NCEA, 2014). Clinical and empirical evidence suggests that a shared living arrangement increases the opportunities for contact that can lead to conflict and mistreatment. Abuse of older adults tends to take place where the individuals live: most often in the home where abusers are apt to be adult children, other family members such as grandchildren, or spouses or partners of older adults. Institutional settings, especially long-term care facilities, can also be sources of abuse. The prevalence of mistreatment of the older adult appears to be related to low income, poor health, and lack of social support. Race and ethnic differences have not been shown to play a role (Alexandra Hernandez-Tejada, Amstadter, Muzzy, & Acierno, 2013).

PROTECTIVE FACTORS FOR MENTAL ILLNESS IN OLDER PERSONS

Protective factors for minimizing the occurrence of mental disorders in older adults are similar to those in younger adults. Evidence supports protective factors that include marriage, education and income level, resilience and positive outlook, healthy lifestyle, nutrition, and exercise.

The Marriage Effect

It has long been thought that married people have lower mortality rates than unmarried at all ages. Many studies have reported that being part of a couple and the quality of the relationship are positively correlated with longevity and health, including cognitive and emotional function (Hakansson et al., 2009). There are several possible explanations for the marriage advantage. For example, married people may be less likely to engage in high-risk and health-damaging behaviors. They may also be more likely to receive care and support when needed. They have shared economic resources and a social network of relatives and friends who can provide vital support at older ages. Negotiating a partner relationship which presents ongoing social and emotional challenges, may also contribute to higher functioning. However, recent studies show that cohabitation for men and women over the age of 45 also has health benefits and never being married does not negatively impact health. Only divorce marginally harms the health of younger men (Kohn & Averett, 2014) (Figure 17.1).

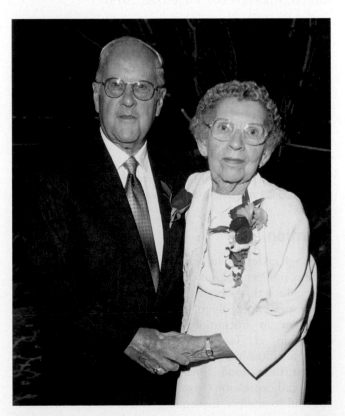

FIGURE 17.1 Lifelong marriage is associated with positive physical and mental health.

Education and Income

Education and income provide older adults with cognitive, economical, and coping reserves that support function and well-being and are related to physical activity and physical and cognitive function and disability. Those with higher education and income are more likely to engage in physical activity and have the resources to provide care when needed. Higher levels of education are associated with higher levels of cognitive function as well as a lower risk of dementia (Cabello, Bravo, Latorre, & Fernandez-Berrocal, 2014; Shpanskaya et al., 2014).

Resilience and Positive Outlook

Research has shown that those with a positive attitude toward aging age better and live longer. Although it is not known why a positive attitude increases longevity, it is thought to be linked to the will to live, **resilience** (the ability to adapt successfully to stress, trauma, or chronic adversity), and a proactive approach to health. It may also be that people with a positive attitude have lower stress (Stibich, 2009). Research has proposed that resilience enables one to adapt positively to adversity and characteristics associated with resilience include optimism, social engagement, emotional well-being, fewer cognitive complaints, and successful aging (Jeste et al., 2013; Kuwert, Knaevelsrud, & Pietrzak, 2014).

Healthy Lifestyle

A healthy lifestyle is important in preventing illness and promoting well-being at all ages, including in late adulthood. Such behaviors include not smoking; drinking alcohol in moderation; getting adequate rest and sleep; getting adequate hydration and nutrition, especially fruits and vegetables; exercising; and coping with stress (Franklin & Tate, 2009). Both a healthy diet and higher physical activity have been shown to be independently associated with reduced risk for Alzheimer's disease (Scarmeas et al., 2009).

Nutrition

Although older adults who are overweight number 14.3 million, undernutrition is a greater problem in today's older adults than obesity. The prevalence of undernutrition appears to be high in older adults, especially those living in an institutionalized setting (17% to 65%) (Bernstein, & Touhy, 2010). Factors contributing to undernutrition include living alone, poor intake of fluid and nutritious foods, medications, malignancy, bereavement, and depression (Saxon et al., 2010). Undernutrition can lead to anemia, inadequate wound healing, increased incidence of pressure sores, impaired elimination, impaired immunological functions, weakness, fatigue, and mental problems (including depression, dementia, and agitation) (Saxon et al., 2010). Adequate nutrition is an important factor in maintaining mental health.

Physical Activity

Emerging evidence suggests that physical activity is related to positive mental health and may be a protective factor. There is a moderate amount of evidence that exercise can prevent the onset or worsening of depression. Structured exercise programs enhance older persons' overall physical functioning and well-being and reduce anxiety symptoms among sedentary adults with chronic illnesses (Buman et al., 2010; Herring, O'Connor, & Dishman, 2010).

INTERVENTION APPROACHES

Reducing the Stigma of Mental Health Treatment

The stigma of mental illness continues to interfere with the willingness of older adults to seek treatment. Today's older Americans grew up during a time when institutionalization in asylums, electroconvulsive treatments, and other treatment approaches were regarded with fear. This fear can lead to denial of problems. Nurses can help reduce the stigma through educational interventions and facilitation of access to services.

Early Recognition of Depressive Symptoms and Suicide Risk

Depression is one of the most common mental disorders of older adults (see Chapter 24). Because depression can be debilitating and can lead to suicide, recognition and early intervention are the keys to avoiding ongoing depressive episodes. Depressive symptomotology among older adults is more likely to include vague somatic complaints, cognitive symptoms, hypersomnia, and appetite changes rather than complaints of depressed mood. Early indications of symptomatology can be identified in primary care settings using a screening tool such as the Geriatric Depression Scale (Yesavage et al., 1983). Several preventive interventions are helpful, such as grief counseling for widows and widowers, self-help groups, and physical and social activities.

Monitoring Medications

With the approval of new medications, older adults' health problems can be treated with pharmacologic agents that were not previously available. It is important to make sure that medications are being taken correctly as well as whether they are having the desired effects. Side effects and drug interactions should be carefully monitored to detect untoward symptoms and delirium. Dosages may need to be adjusted slowly. It is important to review all medications, including over-the-counter, natural, and alternative remedies.

Avoiding Premature Institutionalization

Although many people require nursing home care, integrated care in the community is effective and can delay nursing home placement. Home visits that focus on assessment of symptoms and coordination of health care needs can result in older adults receiving their mental health support within the community and, therefore, aging in place. Older adults and those with disabilities prefer to receive community-based care, which to be most effective must include prevention and rehabilitation services as well as acute care.

Promoting Mental Health

Social Support Transitions

Compensating for loss of family by expanding friendship networks and employment may become an important method of establishing a network in late life. Older adults can be prepared for the transition by receiving information about internal developmental processes, sources of social support, and opportunities for personal growth and role supplementation. Interventions to support successful aging promote productive and social engagement and effective coping (Reichstadt, Sengupta, Depp, Palinkas, & Jeste, 2010). Groups can be particularly effective in developing a sense of community, decreasing isolation, and strengthening a safety network.

Cognitive Engagement

Frequent engagement in cognitive activities may positively impact cognitive functioning in memory. Successful cognitive aging appears to be supported not only by cognitive reserve but also by the older adult's development and use of compensatory strategies. For example, a nursing intervention would be teaching the patient to write notes to self about upcoming events. Such compensatory strategies support cognitive functioning as well as a sense of personal control.

Lifestyle Support

Lifestyle interventions, such as exercise promotion and nutrition counseling, are particularly important in late life because a tendency to slow down and become more sedentary usually accompanies aging. For many, retirement provides an opportunity to restructure the time that was previously spent working. Developing regular exercise habits can help maintain physical and psychological well-being, especially if done with others. Self-

help programs generally include components of exercise, nutrition, health screening, and health habits. Maintaining social support is an integral part of lifestyle support.

Self-Care Enhancement

Enhancing health self-care is a major area for mental health promotion. Education of older adults and their families is crucial to ensuring adherence to agreed upon care regimens. The nurse must consider the individual's educational level, pace of learning, and visual and hearing deficits. The nurse should provide instructional aids, large-print labeling, and devices such as medication calendars that encourage adherence. Self-care enhancements assist the older adult to use compensatory strategies and aids to be as functionally independent as possible for as long as possible. Supporting a sense of control and decisional capacity is critical to self-care (O'Neal, Adams, McHugo, Van Citters, Drake, & Bartels, 2008).

Spiritual Support

Spirituality can be extremely important to older adults and can positively affect attitude, particularly as health declines. Participation in a community of faith is associated with better health outcomes, including less depression (Blazer & Meador, 2010). Supporting contact with spiritual leaders important to the patient is an ongoing mental health promotion intervention. The nurse can also support a patient's spiritual growth by exploring the meanings that a particular life change has for the patient. In late life, existential issues such as experiencing losses, redefining meanings in existence, and living in the present become the standard, replacing the performance and future orientation that characterize earlier adulthood.

Community Services

More emphasis should be placed on community care options, services that provide both sustenance and growth (Shpanskaya et al., 2014). Examples of supportive services that foster independent community living include information and referral services; transportation and nutrition services; legal and protective services; comprehensive senior centers; homemaker and handyman services; matching of older with younger individuals to share housing; and use of the supports available through churches, community groups, or mental health and other community agencies (e.g., area agencies on aging) to maintain older adults in the community for as long as possible. The availability and accessibility of these services vary greatly, and eligibility requirements may exist.

POSITIVE MENTAL AGING

At this time, there are many questions about the course of aging for future cohorts of older adults. It is probable that some of the losses and decrements associated with aging are in fact artifacts of a more sedentary, less healthy lifestyle over a lifetime. Furthermore, we must consider that positive mental aging is more than the absence of mental disorders and impairment but rather is more a reflection of resilience—the capacity to adapt, feel in control, and make decisions about care and life (Jeste & Depp, 2010). Most important is to listen to older adults themselves. Research shows that four qualities contribute to successful aging: the capacity to adapt to change; engagement and involvement in life; the importance of stability and security with reliable social support; and least importantly, physical health (Jeste et al., 2013). As nurses, it is incumbent upon us to help older adults to recognize and use their strengths to cope with and transcend losses and limitations. Recognizing and tapping into the wisdom accumulated over a lifetime may help older adults to negotiate the many challenges faced in later life.

SUMMARY OF KEY POINTS

- Changes in vital biologic structures and processes occur, but older adults can sustain some structural losses without losing function.

- All five special senses (sight, hearing, touch, taste, and smell) decline with age, which may affect information processing.

- Although older adults experience many physical changes, they can and have the desire to remain sexually active.

- Threats to cognitive function in older adults include medications, depression, poor nutrition, infection, heart and lung disease, thyroid problems, alcohol use, and sensory loss.

- Intelligence and personality are stable throughout the life span; however, reaction time slows with age.

- Major changes in social roles with aging include retirement, loss of partner, and changes in residence.

- Polypharmacy is prevalent in older adults, particularly in nursing homes. Ongoing assessment of medications is needed to prevent inappropriate medication administration.

- Older people are at higher risk for poverty and suicide.

- Mental health protective factors include marriage, education, resilience and positive outlook, and healthy lifestyle (including nutrition and exercise).

- Interventions to prevent mental illness include reducing the stigma of mental health treatment, preventing depression and suicide, monitoring medications, and preventing premature institutionalization.

- Nurses can provide a number of interventions to promote mental health, addressing social support transitions, cognitive engagement, lifestyle support, self-care enhancement, spiritual support, and community-based services.

- Positive mental aging is more than the absence of mental disorders and impairment but rather is more a reflection of resilience, which is the capacity to adapt, feel in control, and be engaged, with a positive outlook.

CRITICAL THINKING CHALLENGES

1. Compare the three late adulthood chronological groups in terms of age. Using the recommendations in Box 17.1, interview people representing each of the three chronological groups about their views of mental health.
2. Highlight normal biologic changes that occur during the aging process.
3. Hypothesize why IQ tests and personality do not change with time.
4. Explain the concept of *gerotranscendence* and use the concept to explain differences between the young-old and the old-old.
5. Identify positive and negative perspectives of retirement.
6. Explain why chronic illnesses, polypharmacy, and poverty are all risk factors for mental health problems in later life.

7. Describe mental health promotion interventions that relate to social support transitions, cognitive engagement, lifestyle support, and self-care.

8. Describe factors that contribute to successful aging.

 Driving Miss Daisy: 1989. This delightful film stars Jessica Tandy as Daisy Werthan, a cantankerous old woman. Morgan Freeman plays Hoke Colburn, Daisy's chauffeur. This beautiful story examines a relationship between two people who have more in common than just getting old. *Driving Miss Daisy* challenges some of the myths about getting old.

VIEWING POINTS: Identify the normal behaviors in the growth and development of older adults. Observe the verbal and nonverbal communication of Daisy and Hoke. How do they support each other?

References

Alexandra Hernandez-Tejada, M. A., Amstadter, A., Muzzy, W., & Acierno, R. (2013). The National Elder Mistreatment Study: Race and ethnicity findings. *Journal of Elder Abuse & Neglect, 25*(4), 281–293. doi:10.1080/08946566.2013.770305

Allen, R. S., Petro, K. N., & Phillips, L. L. (2009). Factors influencing young attitudes and knowledge of late-life sexuality among older women. *Aging & Mental Health, 13*(2), 238–245.

Badgett, M. V., Durso, L. E., & Schneebaum, A. (2013). *New patterns of poverty in the lesbian, gay, and bisexual community.* The Williams Institute. http:willamsinstitute.law.ucla.edu

Bernstein, M., & Touhy, A. S. (2010). Nutrition for the older adult. Sudbury, MD: Jones & Bartlett Publisher, LLC.

Blazer, D. G., & Meador, K. G. (2010). The role of spirituality in healthy aging. In C. A. Depp & D. V. Jeste (Eds.). *Successful cognitive and emotional aging* (pp. 73–86). Washington, DC: American Psychiatric Publishing.

Buman, M. P., Hekler, E. B., Haskell, W. L., Pruitt, L., Conway, T. L., Cain, K. L., et al. (2010). Objective light-intensity physical activity associations with rated health in older aduts. *American Journal of Epidemiology, 172*(10), 1156–1165.

Cabello, R., Navarro Bravo, B., Latorre, J. M., & Fernández-Berrocal, P. (2014). Ability of university-level education to prevent age-related decline in emotional intelligence. *Frontiers in Aging Neuroscience, 6,* 37. doi:10.3389/fnagi.2014.00037

Canive, J. M., & Escobar, J. I. (2009). New research on aging minority groups is timely and incorporates state of the art methodologies. *American Journal of Geriatriatric Psychiatry, 17*(11), 913–915.

Cawthorne A. (2008). *Elderly poverty: the challenge before us.* Center for American Progress. Retrieved from http://www.americanprogress.org/issues/2008/07/elderly_poverty.html.

Centers for Disease Control and Prevention (2012). *Suicide: Facts at a glance.* Retrieved May 20, 2014, from http://www.cdc.gov/violenceprevention/pdf/Suicide_DataSheet-a.pdf

Charles, S. T., & Horwitz, B. N. (2010). Positive emotions and health: What we know about aging. In C. A. Depp & D. V. Jeste (Eds.). *Successful cognitive and emotional aging* (pp. 55–72). Washington, DC: American Psychiatric Publishing.

Conwell, Y., & Thompson, C. (2008). Suicidal behavior in elders. *Psychiatric Clinics of North America, 31*(2), 333–356.

D'Avolio, D. A., Strumpf, N. E., Feldman, J., Mitchell, P., & Rebholz, C. M. (2013). Barriers to primary care: perceptions of older adults utilizing the ED for nonurgent visits. *Clinical Nursing Research, 22*(4), 416–431.

Erikson, E. H., & Erikson, J. M. (1997). *The lifecycle completed, extended version.* New York: WW Norton.

Eyler, L. T., & Kovaceviv, S. (2010). Neuroimaging of successful cognitive and emotional aging. In C. A. Depp & D. V. Jeste (Eds.). *Successful cognitive and emotional aging* (pp. 137–156). Washington, DC: American Psychiatric Publishing.

Franklin, N. C., & Tate, C. A. (2009). Lifestyle and successful aging: An overview. *American Journal of Lifestyle Medicine, 3*(1), 6–11.

Jefferis, B. J., Sartini, C., Lee, I. M., Choi, M., Amuzu, A., Gutierrez, C., et al. (2014). Adherence to physical activity guidelines in older adults, using obectively measured physical activity in a population-based study. *BMC Public Health, 14,* 382. www.biomedcentral.com/1471-2458/14/322

Hakansson, K., Rovio, S., Helkala, E., Vilska, A. Winblad, B., Soininen, H, et al. (2009). Association between mid-life marital status and cognitive function in later life: Population based cohort study. *BMJ, 339,* b2462.

Herring, M. P., O'Connor, P. J., & Dishman, R. K. (2010). The effect of exercise training on anxiety symptoms among patients: A systematic review. *Archives of Internal Medicine, 170*(4), 321–331.

Holt-Hill, S. A. (2009). Stress and coping among elderly African-Americans. *Journal of National Black Nurses Association, 20*(2), 1–12.

Hybels, C.F., Blazer, D. G., & Hays, J. C. (2011). Demography and epidemiology of psychiatric disorders in late life. In D. G. Blazer, & D. Steffens (Eds.). *The American Psychatric Publishing textbook of geriatric psychiatry* (4th ed). Arlington, VA: American Psychiatric Publishing, Inc. Retrieved March 6, 2011, from http://10.1176/appi.books.9781585623754.www.psychiatryonline.com/.

Jeste, D. J., & Depp, C. A. (2010). Positive mental aging. *American Journal of Geriatriatric Psychiatry, 18*(1), 1–3.

Jeste, D. V., Savla, G. N., Thompson, W. K., Vahia, I. V., Glorioso, D. K., Martin, A.S., et al. (2013). Association between older age and more successful aging: Critical role of resilience and depression. *American Journal of Psychiatry, 170*(2), 188–196.

Kahana, E., Bhatta, T., Lovegreen, L. D., Kahana, B., & Midlarsky, E. (2013). Altruism, helping, and volunteering: Pathways to well-being in late life. *Journal of Aging & Health, 25*(1), 159–187.

Kohn, J. L., & Averett, S. L. (2014). The effect of relationship status on health with dynamic health and persistent relationships. *Journal of Health Economics, 36,* 69–83. doi:10.1016/j.jhealeco.2014.03.010

Kuwert, P., Knaevelsrud, C., & Pietrzak, R. H. (2014). Loneliness among older veterans in the United States: Results from the National Health and Resilience in Veterans Study. *American Journal of Geriatric Psychiatry, 22*(6), 564–569.

López, J. E., Orrell, M., Morgan, L., & Warner, J. (2010). Empowerment in older psychiatric in-patients: Development of the EQuIP Empowerment Questionnaire for In-Patients. *American Journal of Geriatriatric Psychiatry, 18*(1), 21–32.

National Center for Elder Abuse (NCEA). (2014). Statistics/data. Administration on Aging. U.S. Department of Health & Human Services. Retrieved May 21, 2014 from http://www.ncea.aoa.gov/Library/Data/index.aspx. www.ncea.aoa.gov/Library/Data/index.aspx.

National Council on Aging. (2012). Issue Brief 5: Prescription medication misuse and abuse among older adults. *Older Americans Behavioral Health,* SAMSHA & Administration on Aging. www.ncoa.org

O'Neal, E. L., Adams, J. R., McHugo, G. J., Van Citters, A. D., Drake, R. E., & Bartels, S. J. (2008). Preferences of older and younger adults with serious mental illness for involvement in decision-making in medical and psychiatric settings. *American Journal of Geriatriatric Psychiatry, 16*(10), 826–833.

Palmer, B. P., & Dawes, S. E. (2010). Cognitive aging: From basic skills to scripts and schemata. In C. A. Depp & D. V. Jeste (Eds.). *Successful cognitive and emotional aging* (pp. 37–54). Washington, DC: American Psychiatric Publishing.

Pirogovsky, E., Schiehser, D. M., Obtera, K. M., Burke, M. M., Lessig, S. L., Song, D. D., et al. (2014). Instrumental activities of daily living are impaired in Parkinson's disease in patients with mild cognitive impairment. *Neuropsychology, 28*(2), 229–237.

Purcell, P. (2009). *Income and poverty among older Americans in 2008.* Congressional Research Service Reports for the People, October 2, 2009. Retrieved November 2, 2010, from http://www.opencrs.com

Read, S., Braam, A. W., Lyyra, T., & Deeg, D. J. (2014). Do negative life events promote gerotranscendence in the second half of life? *Aging & Mental health, 18*(1), 117–124.

Reichstadt, J., Sengupta, G., Depp, C. A., Palinkas, L. A., & Jeste, D. V. (2010). Older adults' perspectives on successful aging: Qualitative interviews. *American Journal of Geriatriatric Psychiatry, 18*(7), 567–575.

Salazar, J. C. (2010). Substance abuse and the older adult: How to offer caring, culturally competent treatment. *Aging Today, 31*(1), 1–3. Retrieved April 26, 2010, from http://www.agingtoday.org

Sánchex, E., Vidán, M. T., Serra, J. A., Fernández-Avilés, F., & Bueno, H. (2011). Prevalence of geriatric syndromes and impact on clinical and functional outcomes in older patients with acute cardiac disease. *Heart, 87*(19), 1602–1606.

Saxon, S. V., Etten, M. J., & Perkins, E. A. (2010). *Physical change and aging* (5th ed). New York: Springer.

Scarmeas, N., Luchsinger, J. A., Schupf, N., Brickman, A. M., Cosentino, S., Tang, M. X., et al. (2009). *Journal of the American Medical Association, 302*(6), 627–637.

Shpanskaya, K. S., Choudhury, K. R., Hostage, C Jr, Murphy, K. R., Petrella, J. R., Doraiswamy, P. M., et al. (2014). Educational attainment and hippocampal atrophy in the Alzheimer's disease neuroimaging initiative cohort. *Journal of Neuroradiology*. doi:10.1016/j.neurad.2013.11.004

Stibich, M. (2009). Think positive about aging and live longer. *About.com*, April 26, 2009. Retrieved April 26, 2010, from http://www.longevity.about.com.

Tolppanen, A. M., Solomon, A., Kulmala, J., Kareholt, I., Ngandu, T., Rusanen, M., et al. (2014). Leisure-time physical activity from mid- to late life, body mass index, and risk of dementia. *Alzheirmer's & Dementia*. doi: 10.1016/j.jalz.2014.01.008

U.S. Department of Commerce Economics and Statistics Administration. (2011). *Women in America: Indicators of social and economic well-being*. Revised May 12, 2014. www.esa.doc.gov.

U.S. Department of Commerce Economics and Statistical Administration. (2013). Poverty: 200e to 2012. *American Community Survey*. U.S. Census Bureau. www.census.gov.

U.S. Department of Health and Human Services. (2010). *The numbers count: Mental disorders in America. Transforming the understanding and treatment of mental illness through research*. Washington, DC: National Institute of Mental Health. Retrieved December 6, 2010, from http://www.nimh.mih.gov/health/publications.

U.S. Department of Health and Human Services. (2012). Older adult substance abuse treatment admissions have increased; Number of special treatment programs for this population has decreased. *Data Spotlight*. Center for Behavioral Health Statistics and Quality. Substance Abuse & Mental Health Services Administration. Retrieved June 27, 2014, http://www.samhsa.gov/data/spotlight/WEB_SPOT_043/WEB_SPOT_043.pdf

Vincent, G. K., & Velkoff, V. A. (2010). *The next four decades, the older population in the United States: 2010 to 2050*. Current Population Reports, P25-1138. Washington, DC: U.S. Census Bureau.

Virtanen, M., Ferrie, J. E., Batty, G. D., Elovainio, M., Jokela, M., Vahtera, J., et al. (2014). Socioeconomicand Psychosocial Adversity in Midlife and Depressive Symptoms Post Retirement: A 21-year Follow-up of the Whitehall II Study. *The American Journal of Geriatric Psychiatry*. doi:10.1016/j.jagp.2014.4.001

Watkins, T. (2010). *Aging issues can be tougher on gays*. Retrieved September 30, 2010, from http://www.cnn.com

Yancura, L. A. (2013). Justifications for caregiving in white, Asian American, and native Hawaiian grandparents raising grandchildren. *The Journal of Gerontology. Series B. Psychological Science & Social Science, 68*(1), 139–144.

Yesavage, J. A., Brink, T. L., Rose, T. L., Lum, O., Huang, V., Adey, M. B., et al. (1983). Development and validation of a geriatric depression screening scale: A preliminary report. *Journal of Psychiatric Research, 17*, 37–49.

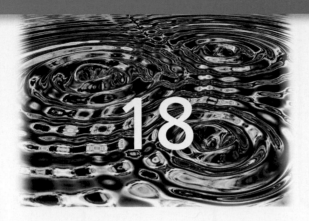

18

Stress and Mental Health

Mary Ann Boyd

KEY CONCEPTS

- allostatic load
- adaptation
- coping
- stress

LEARNING OBJECTIVES

After studying this chapter, you will be able to:

1. Discuss the concept of stress as it relates to mental health and mental illness.

2. Discuss interpersonal and psychological factors affecting the experience of stress, including the person–environment relationship and appraisal.

3. Discuss the variety of stress responses experienced by individuals.

4. Explain the role of coping and adaptation in maintaining and promoting mental health.

5. Apply critical thinking skills to the nursing management process for a person experiencing stress.

KEY TERMS

- allostasis • appraisal • constraints • demands • diathesis • emotion-focused coping • emotions • homeostasis • life events • person–environment relationship • problem-focused coping • reappraisal • social functioning • social network • social support • stress response

---

Stress is a natural part of life, yet it is one of the most complex concepts in health and nursing. Although often thought of as negative, stress can be a positive experience when an individual approaches it with successful coping skills. For example, children learn to cope with stressful situations in preparation for adulthood. During severe stress, some people draw on resources that they never realized they had and grow from those experiences. However, early childhood stress and trauma, unresolved stress, or chronic stress can have negative mental and physical health consequences.

THE ROLE OF STRESS IN MENTAL HEALTH

Stress is a transactional process arising from real or perceived internal or external environmental demands that are appraised as threatening or benign (Lazarus &

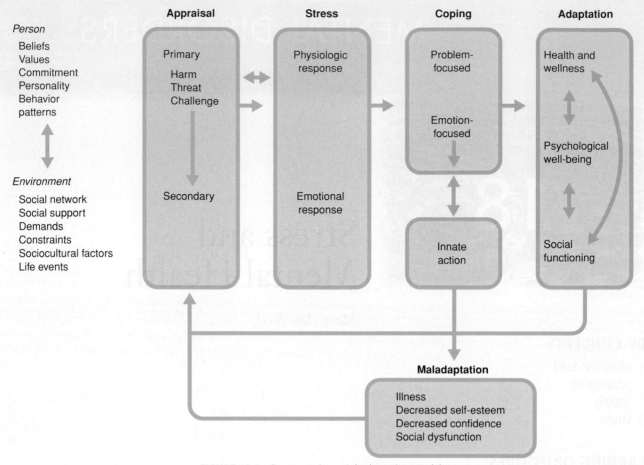

FIGURE 18.1 Stress, coping, and adaptation model.

Folkman, 1984) (Figure 18.1). No one lives in a stress-free environment, yet stress reduction leads to positive mental health. Conversely, many patients attribute their first illness episode to a stressful event such as an assault, rape, or family tragedy.

> **KEYCONCEPT** **Stress** is a transactional process arising from real or perceived internal or external environmental demands that are appraised as threatening or benign (Lazarus & Folkman, 1984).

Stress responses can be acute or chronic. Acute stress can lead to physiologic overload, which in turn can have a negative impact on a person's health. Chronic stress is clearly associated with negative health incomes. Stress is also associated with the development or exacerbation of symptoms of mental illness. For example, psychiatric disorders are prevalent in caregivers of persons with chronic illnesses. Many caregivers of family members with dementia, AIDS, and other long-term illnesses experience severe and chronic stress leading to depression as they continually monitor the family member, cope with illness-related behaviors,

and often witness deterioration of their significant other. In addition, the caregiver's own activities are curtailed (Zegwaard, Aartsen, Cuijpers, & Grypdonck, 2011).

When stress is associated with the development or exacerbation of a mental illness, the diathesis-stress model can be applied. In this model, a **diathesis** or a genetic predisposition increases susceptibility of developing a disorder. For example, in animal models, maternal separation and abandonment demonstrate that early stress experiences alter hypothalamus–pituitary–adrenal (HPA) axis response to stress (discussed later in this chapter). Impaired functioning of the stress response is central to many psychiatric, immune, and physical disorders (Kumari, Badrick, Sacker, Kirschbaum, Marmot, & Chandola, 2010). As a result, adverse events during childhood increase risk of alcohol and drug dependence, eating disorders, affective disorders, posttraumatic stress disorder (PTSD), and suicidal behavior. Another example is the story of a woman whose mother had a long history of depression (indicating a genetic predisposition to mental disorders for the daughter) and who was assaulted as she was leaving work and sustained multiple injuries. Her first manic episode occurred within 2 months (see Chapter 25).

INTERPERSONAL AND PSYCHOSOCIAL ASPECTS OF STRESS

Two important factors determine whether an individual experiences a **stress response**, which is the physiological, behavioral, and cognitive reaction to a perceived threat. They are the person–environment relationship and the person's cognitive appraisal of the risks and benefits of a given situation.

Person–Environment Relationship

The **person–environment relationship** is the interactions between an individual and the environment that change throughout a stress experience. It is based on the values and beliefs people they carry with them in life, as well as personality factors and factors related to the individual's social and physical environment.

Values and Goals

Personal values are developed throughout a lifetime and are shaped by cultural, ethnic, family, and religious beliefs. These values influence the significance of a particular event. What is important to one person may not be to another. For example, one person may value a high-paying salary and another may value the freedom to move around without the boundaries of material things.

If a goal is important, a person is more likely to do what it takes to reach the goal. The more important the goal or the more difficult the goal is to obtain, the greater the likelihood of stress. For example, students who earn mostly or all As often feel more stress about examinations than do students who earn Bs and Cs because the higher grade is more difficult to obtain.

Personality and Behavior Patterns

The association of personality types to health or illness status has been studied for over fifty years (Friedman & Rosenman, 1974). There are four general personality types. Type A personalities are characterized as competitive, aggressive, ambitious, impatient, alert, tense, and restless. They think, speak, and act at an accelerated pace and reflect an aggressive, hostile, and time-urgent style of living that is often associated with increased psychophysiologic arousal (Sogaard, Dalgard, Holme, Roysamb, & Haheim, 2008). In contrast, type B personalities do not exhibit these behaviors and generally are more relaxed, easygoing, and easily satisfied. They have an accepting attitude about trivial mistakes and use a problem-solving approach to major problems. Rarely do type B people push themselves to obtain excesses from the environment or try to accomplish too much in too little time (Tishler, Bartholomae, & Rhodes, 2005).

Type C personalities are described as having difficulty expressing emotion and are introverted, respectful, conforming, compliant, and eager to please and avoid conflict. They respond to stress with depression and hopelessness. This personality type was initially associated with the development of cancer, specifically breast cancer in women, but there has been no clear evidence that the stress associated with this personality type has a role in the etiology of cancer (Bryant-Lukosius, 2003; Lală, Bobîrnac, & Tipa, 2010). The type D (distressed) personalities experience increased negative emotion (depression) and pessimism and are unlikely to show their emotions to others. There is mixed research support for an association between a type D personality and mental health disorders and poor physical health status (Mols & Denollet, 2010; Marchesi et al., 2014; Stevenson & Williams, 2014).

However, overall, research supporting associations between personality types and health status is mixed. Personality characteristics, such as hostility and anger, associated with illnesses continue to be the focus of these studies (Rafanelli, Sirri, Grandi, & Fava, 2013; Shen, Countryman, Spiro, & Niaura, 2008).

Physical and Social Environment

A person has unique interactions daily with the physical and social environments. The external environment includes physical aspects such as air quality, cleanliness of food and water, temperature, and noise. Social aspects include living arrangements and personal contacts.

Social Networks

A **social network** consists of linkages among a defined set of people with whom an individual has personal contacts. A social identity develops within this network (Azmitia, Syed, & Radmacher, 2008). Emotional support, material aid, services, information, and new social contacts increase personal resources, enhance the ability to cope with change, and influence the course of illnesses (Li & Wu, 2010).

A social network may be large, consisting of numerous family and community contacts, or small, consisting of few. Contacts can be categorized according to three levels:

1. Level I consists of six to 12 people with whom the person has close contact.
2. Level II consists of a larger number of contacts, generally 30 to 40 people whom the person sees regularly.
3. Level III consists of the large number of people with whom a person has direct contact, such as the grocer and mail carrier, and can represent several hundred people.

Each person's social network is slightly different. Multiple contacts allow several networks to interact.

Generally, the larger the network, the more support is available. An ideal network structure is fairly dense and interconnected; people within the network are in contact with one another. Dense networks are better able to respond in times of stress and crisis and to provide emotional support to those in distress. For example, residents of a small town are more likely to provide food and shelter to fire victims than neighbors in a large urban area who have little contact with each other.

Ideally, a balance between intense and less intense relationships exists in a social network. When relationships are intense and include only one or two people, the opportunity to interact with other network members is limited. On the other hand, isolation can occur without at least a few intense relationships.

Social networks provide opportunities for give and take. Network members both provide and receive support, aid, services, and information. Reciprocity is particularly important because most friendships do not last without the give and take of support and services. A person who is always on the receiving end eventually becomes isolated from others.

Social Support

One of the important functions of the social network is to provide **social support** in the form of positive interpersonal interactions as part of a dynamic process that is in constant flux and varies with life events and health status (Whatley, Dilorio, & Yeager, 2010). Not all interpersonal interactions within a network are supportive. A person can have a large, complex social network but little social support. Some life events, such as marriage, divorce, and bereavement, actually change the level of social support by adding to or subtracting from a person's social network.

Social support serves three functions:

1. Emotional support contributes to a person's feelings of being cared for or loved.
2. Tangible support provides a person with additional resources.
3. Informational support helps a person view situations in a new light (Table 18.1).

Social support enhances health outcomes and reduces mortality by helping members make needed behavior changes and buffering stressful life events. In a supportive social environment, members feel helped, valued, and in personal control. Healthy people are likely to have strong support systems that help them cope with undesirable life events.

Demands and Constraints

Internal **demands** that pull on an individual's resources are generated by physiologic and psychological needs. External demands are imposed by the physical environment such as crowding, crime, noise, and pollution. The social environment imposes other demands, such as behavioral and role expectations. In contrast to demands, **constraints** are limitations that are both personal and environmental. Personal constraints include internalized cultural values and beliefs and psychological deficits that dictate actions or feelings. Finite resources, such as money and time, are examples of environmental constraints that many people have.

These demands and constraints vary with the individual and contribute to or initiate a stress response (Lazarus, 2001; Segerstrom, 2010). They also interact with one another; for example, work demands, such as changing shifts, may interact with physical demands, such as a need for sleep, creating a high-risk situation in which stress is likely to occur (Box 18.1).

Table 18.1   EXAMPLES OF FUNCTIONS OF SOCIAL SUPPORT

Function	Example
Emotional support	Attachment, reassurance, being able to rely on and confide in a person
Tangible support	Direct aid such as loans or gifts, services such as taking care of someone who is ill, doing a job or chore
Informational support	Providing information or advice, giving feedback about how a person is doing

From Schaefer, C., Coyne, J., & Lazarus, R. (1982). The health-related functions of social support. *Journal of Behavioral Medicine, 4*(4), 381–406.

BOX 18.1
Using Reflection

THE MEANING OF A LOSS OF JOB

INCIDENT • Two women lost their jobs at a local company. One was a single parent who was the sole supporter of two small children, and the other had no children but lived with a man who paid most of their expenses. Both women were being treated at the mental health center for depression. The single parent was devastated, but the other woman seemed almost relieved that she no longer had to work. The nurse was confused about the different reactions of the two women.

REFLECTION • Upon reflection, the nurse understood the variation in reactions to the job loss. Because the demands and constraints of the environment are different for the two women, the meaning of the job loss is different for each. Whereas the job loss significantly affects the single parent's ability to support her children, it is merely an inconvenience for the other woman because her partner helps share expenses. The economic demands on the single parent are greater, and thus she is likely to experience greater stress.

Sociocultural Factors

Cultural expectations and role strain serve as both demands and constraints in the experience of stress. If a person violates cultural group values to meet role expectations, stress occurs; for example, a person may stay in an abusive relationship to avoid the stress of violating a cultural norm that values lifelong marriage, no matter what the circumstances. The potential guilt associated with norm violation and the anticipated isolation from being ostracized seem worse than the physical and psychological pain caused by the abusive situation.

Employment is another highly valued cultural norm and provides social, psychological, and financial benefits. In all cultures, work is assigned significance beyond economic compensation. It is often the central focus of adulthood and, for many, a source of personal identity. Even if employment brings little real happiness, being employed implies financial needs are being met. Work offers status, regulates life activities, permits association with others, and provides a meaningful life experience. Although work is demanding, unemployment can actually be more stressful because of the associated isolation and loss of social status.

Gender expectations often become an additional source of demands and constraints for women, who assume multiple roles. In most cultures, women who work outside the home are expected to assume primary responsibility for care of the children and household duties. Most women are adept at separating these roles and can compartmentalize problems at work from those at home. When there is a healthy balance between work and home, women experience a low level of psychological stress. However, when the balance is disturbed, daily stress contributes to health problems (Low, Thurston, & Matthews, 2010).

Life Events

In 1967, Holmes and Rahe presented a psychosocial view of illness by pointing out the complex relationship between life changes and the development of illnesses (Holmes & Rahe, 1967). They hypothesized that people become ill after they experience major **life events**, such as marriage, divorce, and bereavement. The more frequent the changes, the greater the possibility of becoming sick. The investigators cited the events that they believed partially accounted for the onset of illnesses and began testing whether these life changes were actual precursors to illness. It soon became clear that not all events have the same effects. For example, the death of a spouse is usually much more devastating and stressful than a change in residence. From their research, the investigators were able to assign relative weights to various life events according to the degree of associated stress. Rahe devised the Recent Life Changes Questionnaire (Table 18.2) to evaluate the frequency and significance of

life change events (Rahe, 1994). Numerous research studies subsequently demonstrated the relationship between a recent life change and the severity of near-future illness (Rahe, 1994; Rahe, Taylor, Tolles, Newhall, Veach, & Bryson, 2002). Recent studies show that life changes in older adults that resulted in feeling helpless or fearing for their life reported higher body mass index and more chronic illnesses (Seib et al., 2014). If several life changes occur within a short period, the likelihood that an illness will appear is even greater (Tamers, Okechukwu, Bohl, Gueguen, Goldberg, & Zins, 2014).

Appraisal

All stress responses are affected by the personal meaning of a situation; for example, chest pain is stressful to a person not only because of the immediate pain and incapacitation it causes but also because of the fear that the chest pain may mean that the person is having a heart attack. Thus, the significance of the event actually determines the importance of the person–environment relationship (Lazarus, 2001; Moran, 2001). Stress is initiated not by a single stress but by an unfavorable person–environment relationship that is meaningful in terms of the risks or benefits to that person's well-being.

A given event or situation may be extremely stressful to one person but not to another (Box 18.2, p. 271). The more important or meaningful the outcome, the more vulnerable the person is to stress. **Appraisal** is the process where all aspects are considered—the demands, constraints, and resources are balanced with personal goals and beliefs. A critical factor is the risk involved (Aguilera, 1998; Kendall & Terry, 2009; Lazarus, 2001).

The appraisal process has two levels: primary and secondary. In a primary appraisal, a person evaluates the events occurring in his or her life as a threat, harm, or challenge. During primary appraisal of a goal, the person determines whether (1) the goal is relevant, (2) the goal is consistent with his or her values and beliefs, and (3) whether a personal commitment is present. In the vignette, Susan's commitment to the goal of doing well on the test was consistent with her valuing the content, which in turn motivated her to study regularly and prepare carefully for the examination. She believed that the test would be difficult. Joanne had a commitment to pass the test but did not value the content. Unlike Susan, Joanne believed that the test would be relatively easy because she expected the questions to be the same as those on the previous examination.

In a secondary appraisal, the person explains the outcome of events. There may be blame or credit given for the outcome. In the example, Susan was nervous but took the test. Joanne's secondary appraisal of the test-taking situation began with the realization that she might not pass the test because the questions were

Table 18.2	RECENT LIFE CHANGES QUESTIONNAIRE

Directions: Sum the life change units (LCUs) for your life change events during the past 12 months.
250 to 400 LCUs per year: Minor life crisis
Over 400 LCUs per year: Major life crisis

Life Changes	LCU Values*	Life Changes	LCU Values*
Family		Change in sleeping habits	31
Death of spouse	105	Revision of personal habits	31
Marital separation	65	Change in eating habits	29
Death of close family member	65	Change in church activities	29
Divorce	62	Vacation	29
Pregnancy	60	Change in school	28
Change in health of family member	52	Change in recreation	28
Marriage	50	Christmas	26
Gain of new family member	50	**Work**	
Marital reconciliation	42	Fired at work	64
Spouse begins or stops work	37	Retirement from work	49
Son or daughter leaves home	29	Trouble with boss	39
In-law trouble	29	Business readjustment	38
Change in number of family get-togethers	26	Change to different line of work	38
		Change in work responsibilities	33
Personal		Change in work hours or conditions	30
Jail term	56	**Financial**	
Sex difficulties	49	Foreclosure of mortgage or loan	57
Death of a close friend	46	Change in financial state	43
Personal injury or illness	42	Mortgage (e.g., home, car)	39
Change in living conditions	39	Mortgage or loan less than $10,000 (e.g., stereo)	26
Outstanding personal achievement	33		
Change in residence	33		
Minor violations of the law	32		
Begin or end school	32		

*LCU, life change unit. The number of LCUs reflects the average degree or intensity of the life change.

From Rahe, R. H. (2000). Recent Life Changes Questionnaire (RLCQ).

different. She acted impulsively by blaming the teacher for giving a different examination and by storming out of the room. She clearly did not cope effectively with a difficult situation.

RESPONSES TO STRESS

After a person–environment relationship is established and an individual appraises a situation as threatening or harmful, an internal stress response occurs. This includes simultaneous physiologic and emotional responses.

Physiologic Responses

Physiologic changes in response to stress are automatic and differ based on the type of stress, duration, and intensity, which depend on the appraised risk of the situation. The riskier the situation, the more intense is the physiologic response.

Homeostasis and the Fight or Flight Response

The concept of **homeostasis**, which is the body's tendency to resist physiologic change and hold bodily functions relatively consistent, well-coordinated, and usually stable, was introduced by Walter Cannon in the 1930s. The body's internal equilibrium is regulated by physiologic processes such as blood glucose, pH, and oxygen. Set points (normal reference ranges of physiological parameters) are maintained (Cannon, 1932).

When the brain (amygdala and hippocampus) interprets an event as a threat, the hypothalamus and autonomic nervous system are signaled to secrete adrenaline,

BOX 18.2

STRESS RESPONSES TO AN EXAMINATION

Two students are preparing for the same examination. Susan is genuinely interested in the subject, prepares by studying throughout the semester, and reviews the content two days before test day. The night before the examination, she goes to bed early, gets a good night's sleep, and wakes refreshed but is slightly nervous about the test. She wants to do well and expects a difficult test but knows that she can retake it at a later date if she does poorly.

In contrast, Joanne is not interested in the subject matter and does not study throughout the semester. She "crams" 2 days before the test date and does an "all nighter" the night before. This is the last time that Joanne can take the examination, but she believes that she will pass because she has already taken it twice and is familiar with the questions. If she does not pass, she will not be able to return to school. On entering the room, Joanne is physically tired and somewhat fearful of not passing the test. As she looks at the test, she instantly realizes that it is not the examination she expected. The questions are new. She begins hyperventilating and tremoring. After yelling obscenities at the teacher, she storms out of the room. She is very distressed and describes herself as "being in a panic."

What Do You Think?

- How are the students' experiences different? Are there any similarities?
- Are there any nursing diagnoses that apply to Joanne's situation?

cortisol, and epinephrine. These hormones activate the sympathetic nervous system, physiological stability is challenged, and a "fight or flight" response occurs. Heart rate, blood pressure, and blood sugar increase. Energy is mobilized for survival. As the sympathetic system is activated, the parasympathic is muted (Table 18.3). After there is no longer a need for more energy and the threat is over, the body returns to a state of homeostasis.

Chronic Stress and Illness

The HPA axis, introduced earlier, is another important part of the stress response. Hans Seyle, who first initiated the study of stress, defined stress as a nonspecific response to an irritant, a perceived danger, or a life threat. He called stress evoked by positive emotions or events *eustress* and stress evoked by negative feelings and events *distress*. He showed that corticosteroid secretion from the pituitary gland increased during stress and contributed to development of illnesses. Seyle described this process as general adaptation syndrome (GAS), which he defined as consisting of three stages: the alarm reaction (a threat is perceived, and the body responds physiologically), stage of resistance (coping mechanisms are used to try to reestablish homeostasis), and stage of exhaustion (occurs if homeostasis is not achieved) (Selye, 1956, 1974).

We now understand that the sympathetic nervous system activates the HPA axis. When the hypothalamus secretes corticotropin-releasing hormone (CRH), the pituitary gland increases secretion of adrenocorticotropic hormone (corticotropin), which in turn stimulates the adrenocortical secretion of cortisol.

Table 18.3	FLIGHT AND FIGHT: PHYSIOLOGICAL CHANGES		
Sympathetic Nervous System Effect		**Purpose**	**Parasympathetic Nervous System Conservation of Energy**
Increased serum glucose		Increased energy	Decreased sexual and sex hormone activity
Increased cardiac output and blood pressure (increase in renin and angiotensin)		Increased blood flow	Decreased growth, repair, and maturation
Increased oxygen tension and hematocrit		Increased supply of oxygen in blood	Decreased digestion, assimilation, and whole food distribution
Other Physiological Changes			
Effect		**Purpose**	
Increased immune responses		Reduced risk of infections	
Heightened vigilance in the brain		Increased decision-making attention and memory	
Hyperactivation of the hemostatic and coagulation system		Prevention of excessive bleeding from wounds	

Adapted from Diamond, J. W. (2009). Allostatic medicine: Bringing stress, coping, and chronic disease into focus. Part 1. *Integrative Medicine, 8*(6), 40–44.

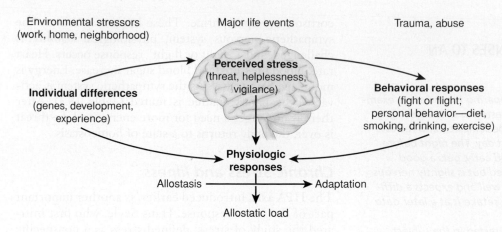

FIGURE 18.2   The development of allostatic load in response to stress. (Redrawn with permission from McEwen, B. S. [1998]. Protective and damaging effects of stress and stress mediators. *New England Journal of Medicine, 3*[38], 171–179.)

Allostasis and the Allostatic Load

Allostasis is a term used to describe the dynamic regulatory process that maintains homeostasis through a process of adaptation. Physiological stability is achieved when the autonomic nervous system; the HPA; and the cardiovascular, metabolic, and immune systems respond to internal and external stimuli (McEwen, 2005, 2010).

As wear and tear on the brain and body occur, there is a corresponding increase in the number of abnormal biologic parameters called allostatic load (AL) (Figure 18.2). AL is measured by the cumulative changes of the biologic regulatory systems as indicated by abnormal laboratory values. The greater the allostatic load, the greater the state of chronic stress and ultimately, the more negative changes in health (McEwen & Gianaros, 2010).

> **KEYCONCEPT**   **Allostatic load** is the consequence of the wear and tear on the body and brain and leads to ill health.

Paradoxically, the same systems that are protective in acute stress can damage the body when activated by chronic stress. The benefits of the increase in circulating cortisol to the human body are initially adaptive, but if it continues, it can be quite damaging to both mental (depression) and physical (immune, cardiovascular, and metabolic) health (McVicar, Ravalier, & Greenwood, 2013; Sterling, 2012).

In chronic stress, the immune system is suppressed. Cortisol is primarily immunosuppressive and contributes to reduction in lymphocyte numbers and function (primarily T-lymphocyte and monocyte subsets) and natural killer (NK) activities. The immune cells have receptors for cortisol and catecholamines that can bind with lymphatic cells and suppress the immune system. The continuous sustained activation of the sympathetic nervous system; HPA axis; cardiovascular, metabolic, and immune systems contribute to a hormonal overload, leading to

impairment in memory, immunity, cardiovascular, and metabolic function (McEwen, 2000, 2005). Over time, chronic stress compromises health and increases susceptibility to illnesses. For instance, children who have suffered psychological neglect, abuse, or parental loss are more likely to display mood or anxiety disorders during adulthood (Benjet, Borges, & Medina-Mora, 2010).

In addition, health disparities found in lower socioeconomic groups, racial and ethnic minorities, and older adults may be partly explained by the chronic stress they tend to experience. Elevated AL has been shown to exist in these groups and in relatively young women with histories of high stress and especially those with PTSD and depression (Carlson & Chamberlain, 2005; Clark, Bond, & Hecker, 2007; Glover, Stuber, & Poland, 2006; Juruena, 2013; Peek et al., 2010; Seeman, Epel, Gruenewald, Karlamangla, & McEwen, 2010). See Box 18.3.

Elevation of white blood cell counts and lower counts of T, B, and NK cells are found in those who face academic examinations, job strain, caregiving for a family member with dementia, marital conflict, and daily stress. Altered parameters of immune function are present in those with negative moods (chronic hostility, depression, and anxiety), social isolation, and marital disagreement. Antibody titers to Epstein-Barr and herpes simplex viruses are also elevated in stressed populations. If the stress is long term, the immune alteration continues (Kiecolt-Glaser et al., 2005; Segerstrom, 2010).

Emotional Responses

Emotional responses to stress depend on the significance of the event experience. The **emotions** (psychophysiological reactions that define a person's mood) are usually ones of excitement or distress marked by strong feelings and usually accompanied by an impulse toward definite action. If the emotions are intense, a disturbance in intellectual functions occurs. When the situation is viewed as a challenge, emotions are more likely to be positive. If

BOX 18.3

Research for Best Practice: **Allostatic Load**

de Castro, A. B., Voss, J. G., Ruppin, A., Dominguez, C. F., & Seixas, N. S. (2010). Stressors among Latino day laborers: A pilot study examining allostatic load. AAOHN, 58(5), 185–196.

THE QUESTION: Do participants with higher allostatic load (AL) report greater stress than those with lower AL?

METHODS: For this pilot study, 30 Latino men were recruited from a worker center. Participants completed an interview, and researchers measured six indicators of allostatic load (body mass index, waist-to-hip ration, systolic blood pressure, diastolic blood pressure, C-reactive protein, and cortisol). Percentages and mean scores were calculated for several self-reported stressors in work, economic, and social contexts. Low and high ALs were compared.

FINDINGS: Overall, participants with high ALs reported experiencing more stress than those with low ALs. Latino day laborers experience stress that places them at risk for high AL.

IMPLICATIONS FOR NURSING: Certain cultural and ethnic groups are at high risk for chronic stress. Chronic stress can be assessed by measuring changes in physiological parameters. Nurses need to recognize that the importance of a careful physical assessment as well as a psychosocial assessment.

Table 18.4 | **CORE RELATIONAL THEMES FOR EACH EMOTION**

Emotion	Relational Meaning
Anger	A demeaning offense against me and mine
Anxiety	Facing an uncertain, existential threat
Fright	Facing an immediate, concrete, and overwhelming physical danger
Guilt	Having transgressed a moral imperative
Shame	Having failed to live up to an ego ideal
Sadness	Having experienced an irrevocable loss
Envy	Wanting what someone else has
Jealousy	Resenting a third party for the loss of or a threat to another's affection
Disgust	Taking in or being too close to an indigestible object or idea (metaphorically speaking)
Happiness	Making reasonable progress toward the realization of a goal
Pride	Enhancement of one's ego identity by taking credit for a valued object or achievement, either our own or that of someone or a group with whom we identify
Relief	A distressing goal/incongruent condition that has changed for the better or gone away
Hope	Fearing the worst but yearning for better
Love	Desiring or participating in affection, usually but not necessarily reciprocated
Compassion	Being moved by another's suffering and wanting to help

Adapted from Lazarus, R. S. (1999). *Stress and emotion: A new synthesis.* New York: Springer.

the event is evaluated as threatning or harmful, negative emotions are elicited. Emotions can be categorized as follows:

- *Negative emotions* occur when there is a threat to, delay in, or thwarting of a goal or a conflict between goals: anger, fright, anxiety, guilt, shame, sadness, envy, jealousy, and disgust.
- *Positive emotions* occur when there is movement toward or attainment of a goal: happiness, pride, relief, and love.
- *Borderline emotions* are somewhat ambiguous: hope, compassion, empathy, sympathy, and contentment.
- *Nonemotions* connote emotional reactions but are too ambiguous to fit into any of the preceding categories: confidence, awe, confusion, and excitement (Lazarus, 1999).

Emotions are expressed as themes that summarize dangers or benefits of each stressful situation. For instance, physical danger provokes fear; a loss leads to feelings of sadness (Table 18.4). Emotions have their own innate responses that are automatic and unique; for example, anger may automatically provoke tremors in one person but both tremors and perspiration in another. Emotions often provoke impulsive behavior. For example, the first impulse of a young musician facing his first performance at Carnegie Hall who experiences stage fright is to run home. As he resists this impulse, he begins coping with his fears in order to perform.

COPING

Coping is a deliberate, planned, and psychological effort to manage stressful demands. The coping process may inhibit or override the innate urge to act. Positive coping leads to adaptation, which is characterized by a balance between health and illness, a sense of well-being, and maximum social functioning. When a person does not cope well, maladaptations occur that can shift the balance toward illness, a diminished self-concept, and deterioration in social functioning.

KEYCONCEPT   Coping is a deliberate, planned, and psychological effort to manage stressful demands.

There are two types of coping. In **problem-focused coping**, the person attacks the source of stress and solves the problem (eliminating it or changing its effects), which changes the person–environment relationship. In

BOX 18.4

Ways of Coping: Examples of Problem-Focused Versus Emotion-Focused Coping

PROBLEM-FOCUSED COPING
- When noise from the television interrupts a student's studying and causes the student to be stressed, the student turns off the television and eliminates the noise.
- An abused spouse is finally able to leave her husband because she realizes that the abuse will not stop even though he promises never to hit her again.

EMOTION-FOCUSED COPING
- A husband is adamantly opposed to visiting his wife's relatives because they keep dogs in their house. Even though the dogs are well cared for, their presence in the relative's home violates his need for an orderly, clean house and causes the husband sufficient stress that he copes with by refusing to visit. This becomes a source of marital conflict. One holiday, the husband is given a puppy and immediately becomes attached to the dog, who soon becomes a valued family member. The husband then begins to view his wife's relatives differently and willingly visits their house more often.
- A mother is afraid that her teenage daughter has been in an accident because she did not come home after a party. Then the woman remembers that she gave her daughter permission to stay at a friend's house. She immediately feels better.

BOX 18.5

***Research for Best Practice*: Emotion- versus Problem-Focused Coping for Health Threats**

Ahmad, M. M., Musil, C. M., Zauszniewski, J. A., & Resnick, M. I. (2005). Prostate cancer: appraisal, coping, and health status. Journal of Gerontological Nursing, 31*(10), 34–43.*

THE QUESTION: Do men use emotion- or problem-focused coping when appraising a health threat?

METHODS: A convenience sample of 131 men with prostate cancer was surveyed to identify how cognitive appraisal and types of coping affected their health status.

FINDINGS: Men who appraised more harm or loss experienced worse physical and mental health. When the men perceived their diagnosis as posing more harm or loss or greater threat, they were more likely to use emotion-focused coping. When the diagnosis was perceived as a challenge, men were more likely to use problem-focused coping.

IMPLICATIONS FOR NURSING: Patients respond differently to the same medical diagnosis depending on how they appraise the threat of the diagnosis. Problem-focused coping is more likely to be used if the diagnosis is viewed as a challenge ("I can beat it") rather than a threat ("I will die"). Assessing the coping style will provide important assessment data for planning interventions.

emotion-focused coping, the person reduces the stress by reinterpreting the situation to change its meaning (Boxes 18.4 and 18.5).

No one coping strategy is best for all situations. Coping strategies work best in particular situations. Over time, these strategies become automatic and develop into patterns for each person. Hopefully, the strategies are effective. Some situations require a combination of strategies and activities. Ideally, a stressful situation is matched with the needed resources as the events are unfolding. Social support can be critical in helping people cope with difficult situations. Successful coping with life stresses is linked to quality of life and to physical and mental health (Lazarus, 2001).

As a part of the coping process, reappraisal is important because of the changing nature of the stressful situation. **Reappraisal**, which is the same as appraisal except that it happens after coping, provides feedback about the outcomes and allows for continual adjustment to new information.

ADAPTATION

Adaptation can be conceptualized as a person's capacity to survive and flourish (Lazarus, 1999). Adaptation or lack of it affects three important areas: health, psychological well-being, and social functioning. A period of stress may compromise any or all of these areas. If a person copes successfully with stress, he or she returns to a previous level of adaptation. Successful coping results in an improvement in health, well-being, and social functioning. Unfortunately, at times, maladaptation occurs.

> **KEYCONCEPT** **Adaptation** is a person's capacity to survive and flourish. Adaptation affects three important areas: health, psychological well-being, and social functioning.

It is impossible to separate completely the adaptation areas of health, well-being, and social functioning. A maladaptation in any one area can negatively affect the others. For instance, the appearance of psychiatric symptoms can cause problems in performance in the work environment that in turn elicit a negative self-concept. Although each area will be discussed separately, the reader should realize that when one area is affected, most likely all three areas are affected (Figure 18.3).

Health

Health can be negatively affected by stress when coping is ineffective and the damaging condition or situation is not ameliorated or the emotional distress is not regulated. Examples of ineffective coping include using emotion-focused coping when a problem-focused approach is appropriate, such as if a woman reinterprets an abusive situation as her fault instead of getting help to remove

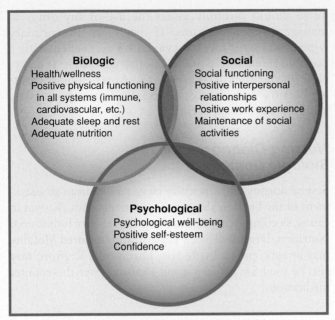

FIGURE 18.3 Biopsychosocial adaptation.

Biologic
Health/wellness
Positive physical functioning in all systems (immune, cardiovascular, etc.)
Adequate sleep and rest
Adequate nutrition

Social
Social functioning
Positive interpersonal relationships
Positive work experience
Maintenance of social activities

Psychological
Psychological well-being
Positive self-esteem
Confidence

herself from the environment. In addition, if a coping strategy violates cultural norms and lifestyle, stress is often exaggerated. Some coping strategies actually increase the risk for mortality and morbidity, such as the excessive use of alcohol, drugs, or tobacco. Many people use overeating, smoking, or drinking to reduce stress. They may feel better temporarily but are actually increasing their risk for illness. For people whose behaviors exacerbate their illnesses, learning new behaviors becomes important. Healthy coping strategies such as exercising and obtaining adequate sleep and nutrition contribute to stress reduction and the promotion of long-term health.

Psychological Well-Being

An ideal outcome to a stress response is feeling good about how stress is handled. Of course, outcome satisfaction for one person does not necessarily represent outcome satisfaction for another. For instance, suppose that two students receive the same passing score on an examination. One may feel a sense of relief, but the other may feel anxious because he appraises the score as too low. Understanding a person's emotional response to an outcome is essential to analyzing its personal meaning. People who consistently have positive outcomes from stressful experiences are more likely to have positive self-esteem and self-confidence. Unsatisfactory outcomes from stressful experiences are associated with negative mood states, such as depression, anger, guilt leading to decreased self-esteem, and feelings of helplessness. Likewise, if the situation was appraised as challenging rather than harmful or

threatening, increased self-confidence and a sense of well-being are likely to follow. If the situation was accurately appraised as harmful or threatening but viewed as manageable, the outcome may also be positive.

Social Functioning

Social functioning, the performance of daily activities within the context of interpersonal relations and family and community roles, can be seriously impaired during stressful episodes. For instance, a person who is experiencing the stress of a divorce may not be able to carry out job responsibilities satisfactorily. Social functioning continues to be impaired if the person views the outcome as unsuccessful and experiences negative emotions. If successful coping with a stressful encounter leads to a positive outcome, social functioning returns to normal or is improved.

CARE FOR THE PERSON EXPERIENCING STRESS

NURSING MANAGEMENT: Human Response to Stress

The overall goals in the nursing management of stress are to resolve the stressful person–environment situation, reduce the stress response, and develop positive coping skills. The goals for those who are at high risk for stress (experiencing recent life changes, vulnerable to stress, or have limited coping mechanisms) are to recognize the potential for stressful situations and strengthen positive coping skills through education and practice.

Stress responses vary from one person to another. Acute stress is easier to recognize than chronic stress. In many instances, living with chronic stress has become a way of life and is no longer recognized. If there are significant emotional or behavioral symptoms in response to an identifiable stressful situation, a diagnosis of adjustment disorder may be made (American Psychiatric Association, 2013). From the assessment data, the nurse can determine any illnesses, the intensity of the stress response, and the effectiveness of coping strategies. Nurses typically identify stress responses in people or family members who are receiving treatment for other health problems.

Biologic Domain

Assessment

An assessment of the biologic domain should include a careful health history, focusing on past and present illnesses and traumas. If a psychiatric disorder is present, psychiatric symptoms may spontaneously reappear even when no alteration has occurred in the patient's medication regimen. Special attention should be paid to disorders of the endocrine system, such as hypothyroidism.

Gender Differences

It is now known that people experience stress differently depending on their gender. Whereas males are more likely to respond to stress with a fight or flight response, females have less aggressive responses; they "tend and befriend." There is a difference in perception of and behavioral response to the stress, as well as a difference in the physiology of the stress response (McEwen, 2005).

Review of Systems

A systems review can elicit the person's own unique physiologic response to stress and can also provide important data on the effect of chronic illnesses. These data are useful for understanding the person–environment situation and the person's stress reactions, coping responses, and adaptation.

Physical Functioning

Physical functioning usually changes during a stress response. Typically, sleep is disturbed, appetite either increases or decreases, body weight fluctuates, and sexual activity changes. Physical appearance may be uncharacteristically disheveled—a projection of the person's feelings. Body language expresses muscle tension, which conveys a state of anxiety not usually present. Because exercise is an important strategy in stress reduction, the nurse should assess the amount of physical activity, tolerance for exercise, and usual exercise patterns. Determining the details of the person's exercise pattern and any recent changes can help in formulating reasonable interventions.

Pharmacologic Assessment

In assessing a person's coping strategies, the nurse needs to ask about the use of alcohol, tobacco, marijuana, and any other addictive substances. Many people begin or increase the frequency of using these substances as a way of coping with stress. In turn, substance abuse contributes to the stress behavior. Knowing details about the person's use of these substances (number of times a day or week, amount, circumstances, side effects) helps in determining the role these substances play in overall stress reduction or management. The more important the substances are in the person's handling of stress, the more difficult it will be to change the addictive behavior.

Stress also often prompts people to use antianxiety medication without supervision. Use of over-the-counter and herbal medications is also common. The nurse should carefully assess the use of any drugs to manage stress symptoms. If drugs are the primary coping strategy, further evaluation is needed with a possible referral to a mental health specialist. If a psychiatric disorder is present, the nurse should assess medication compliance, especially if the psychiatric symptoms are reappearing.

Nursing Diagnoses for the Biologic Domain

Several nursing diagnoses may be generated from an assessment of the biologic domain. For patients with changes in eating, sleeping, or activity, nursing diagnoses of Imbalanced Nutrition, Disturbed Sleep Pattern, and Impaired Mobility may be appropriate. Ineffective Therapeutic Regimen may also be used for patients using excessive over-the-counter medications.

Interventions for the Biologic Domain

People under stress can usually benefit from several biologic interventions. Their activities of daily living are usually interrupted, and they often feel that they have no time for themselves. The stressed patient who is normally fastidiously groomed and dressed may appear disheveled and unkempt. Simply reinstating the daily routine of shaving (for a man) or applying makeup (for a woman) can improve the person's outlook on life and ability to cope with the stress.

Stress is commonly manifested in the areas of nutrition and activity. During stressful periods, a person's eating patterns change. To cope with stress, a person may either overeat or become anorexic. Both are ineffective coping behaviors and actually contribute to stress. Educating the patient about the importance of maintaining an adequate diet during the period of stress will highlight its importance. It will also allow the nurse to help the person decide how eating behaviors can be changed.

Exercise can reduce the emotional and behavioral responses to stress. In addition to the physical benefits of exercise, a regular exercise routine can provide structure to a person's life, enhance self-confidence, and increase feelings of well-being. People who are stressed are often not receptive to the idea of exercise, particularly if it has not been a part of their routine. Exploring the patient's personal beliefs about the value of activity will help to determine whether exercise is a reasonable activity for that person.

The person under stress tends to be tense, nervous, and on edge. Simple relaxation techniques help the person relax and may improve coping skills. If these techniques do not help the patient relax, distraction or guided imagery may be taught to the patient (see Chapter 10). In some instances, spiritually oriented interventions can be used (Box 18.6). Referral to a mental health specialist for

---

BOX 18.6

Research for Best Practice: **Spiritually Based Interventions**

Bormann, J. E., Thorp, S., Wetherell, J. L., & Golshan, S. (2008). A spiritually-based group intervention for combat veterans with posttraumatic stress disorder: A feasibility study. Journal of Holistic Nursing, 29(2), 109–116.

THE QUESTION: Is it feasible to use mantram repetition—the spiritual practice of repeating a sacred word or phrase throughout the day—for managing symptoms of posttraumatic stress disorder (PTSD) in veterans?

METHODS: A two group (intervention vs. control) by two time (pre- and postintervention) experimental design was used. Veterans were randomly assigned to intervention ($n = 14$) or delayed-treatment control ($n = 15$). Measures were PTSD symptoms, psychological distress, quality of life, and patient satisfaction. Effect sizes were calculated using Cohen's d.

FINDINGS: Thirty-three male veterans were enrolled, and 29 (88%) completed the study. Large effect sizes were found for reducing PTSD symptom severity ($d = -.72$), psychological distress ($d = -.73$) and increasing quality of life ($d = .70$).

IMPLICATIONS FOR NURSING: A spiritual program may be feasible for reducing symptom severity in PTSD.

---

hypnosis or biofeedback should be considered for patients who have severe stress responses.

Psychological Domain

Assessment

Unlike assessment for other mental health problems, psychological assessment of the person under stress does not ordinarily include a mental status examination. Instead, psychological assessment focuses on the person's emotions and their severity, as well as his or her coping strategies. The assessment elicits the person's appraisal of risks and benefits, the personal meaning of the situation, and the person's commitment to a particular outcome. The nurse can then understand how vulnerable the person is to stress.

Using therapeutic communication techniques, a person's emotional state is assessed in a nurse–patient interview. By beginning the interview with a statement such as, "Let's talk about what you have been feeling," the nurse can elicit the feelings that the person has been experiencing. Identifying the person's emotions can be helpful in assessing the intensity of the stress being experienced. Negative emotions (anger, fright, anxiety, guilt, shame, sadness, envy, jealousy, and disgust) are usually associated with an inability to cope and severe stress.

After identifying the person's emotions, the nurse determines how the person reacts initially to them. For example, does the person who is angry respond by carrying out the innate urge to attack someone whom the person blames for the situation? Or does that person respond by thinking through the situation and overriding the initial innate urge to act? The person who tends to act impulsively has few real coping skills. For the person who can resist the innate urge to act and has developed coping skills, the focus of the assessment becomes determining their effectiveness.

In an assessment interview, it can be determined whether the person uses problem-focused or emotion-focused coping strategies effectively. Problem-focused coping is effective when the person can accurately assess the situation. In this case, the person sets goals, seeks information, masters new skills, and seeks help as needed. Emotion-focused coping is effective when the person has inaccurately assessed the situation and coping corrects the false interpretation.

Nursing Diagnoses for the Psychological Domain

The nurse should consider a nursing diagnosis of Ineffective Coping for patients experiencing stress who do not have the psychological resources to effectively manage the situation. Other useful nursing diagnoses include Disturbed Thought Processes, Disturbed Sensory Perception, Low Self-esteem, Fear, Hopelessness, and Powerlessness.

Interventions for the Psychological Domain

Numerous interventions help reduce stress and support coping efforts. All of the interventions are best carried out within the framework of a supportive nurse–patient relationship. Assisting patients to develop appropriate problem-solving strategies based on personal strengths and previous experiences is important in understanding and coping with stressful situations. Encouraging patients to examine times when coping has been successful and examine aspects of that situation can help in identifying strengths and strategies for the current problem. For example, a young mother was completely overwhelmed with feelings of inadequacy after the birth of her third child. Further assessment revealed that the patient's mother had helped during the 6 weeks after the other children had been born. The patient's mother was not available for the third birth. First, the nurse validated that having three children could be overwhelming for anyone. The nurse also explained the postpartum hormonal changes that were occurring, validating that the patient's feelings were typical of many mothers. Finally, together, the nurse and the patient identified resources in her environment that could support her during the postpartum period.

It is important to have the patient discuss the person–environment situation and develop alternative coping strategies. Some aspects of any situation cannot be changed, such as a family member's illness or a death of a loved one, but usually there are areas within the patient's control that can be changed. For example, a caregiver cannot reverse the family member's disability, but she can arrange for short-term respite.

Social Domain
Assessment

Social assessment data are invaluable in determining the person's resources for positive coping. The ability to make healthy lifestyle changes is strongly influenced by the person's health beliefs and family support system. Even the expression of stress is related to social factors, particularly cultural expectations and values.

Assessment should include use of the Recent Life Changes questionnaire (refer to Table 18.2) to determine the number and importance of life changes that the patient has experienced within the past year. If several recent life changes have occurred, the person–environment relationship has changed. The person is likely to be either at high risk for or already experiencing stress.

Social assessment also includes identification of the person's social network. Because employment is the mainstay of adulthood and the source of many personal contacts, assessment of any recent changes in employment status is important. If a person is unemployed, the nurse should determine the significance of the unemployment and its effects on the person's social network. For children and adolescents, nurses should note any recent changes in their attendance at school. The nurse should elicit the following data:

- Size and extent of the patient's social network, both relatives and nonrelatives, professional and nonprofessional, and how long known
- Functions that the network serves (e.g., intimacy, social integration, nurturance, reassurance of worth, guidance and advice, access to new contacts)
- Degree of reciprocity between the patient and other network members; that is, who provides support to the patient and who the patient supports
- Degree of interconnectedness; that is, how many of the network members know one another and are in contact

Nursing Diagnoses for the Social Domain

The nurse can generate several nursing diagnoses from the social assessment data that involve the person–environment interaction. The challenge of generating nursing diagnoses is to make sure that they are based on the person's appraisal of the situation. Some possible nursing diagnoses include Ineffective Role Performance, Impaired Parenting, Impaired Social Interaction, Social Isolation, and Disabled Family Coping.

Interventions for the Social Domain

Because the experience of stress and the ability to cope are a result of the appraisal of the person–environment relationship, interventions that affect the environment are important. People who are coping with stressful situations can often benefit from interventions that facilitate family unit functioning and promote the health and welfare of all family members. To intervene with the total family, the stressed person must agree for the family members to be involved. If the data gathered from the assessment of supportive and dissupportive factors indicate that the family members are not supportive, the nurse should assist the patient to consider expanding his or her social network. If the family is the major source of support, the nurse should design interventions that support the functioning of the family unit. Parent education can also be effective in supporting family unit functioning. If family therapy is needed, the nurse should refer the family to an advanced practice specialist.

Evaluation and Treatment Outcomes

The treatment outcomes established in the initial plan of care guide the evaluation. Individual outcomes relate to improved health, well-being, and social function. Depending on the level of intervention, there can also be family and network outcomes. Family outcomes may be related to improved communication or social support; for instance, caregiver stress is reduced when other members of the family help in the care of the ill member. Social network outcomes focus on modifying the social network to increase support for the individual.

SUMMARY OF KEY POINTS

- Stress affects everyone. Coping with stress can produce positive and negative outcomes. The person can learn and grow from the experience or maladaptation can occur.

- Stress is defined as an environmental pressure or force that put's strain on a person's system. Acute stress can lead to physiologic overload, which in turn can have a negative impact on a person's health, well-being, and social functioning. Chronic stress is clearly associated with negative health outcomes.

- Stress responses are determined by the person–environment relationship and the individual's cognitive appraisal of the risks and benefits of a situation. Stress responses are simultaneously emotional and physiologic, leading to an innate tendency to act.

- Many personal factors, such as personality patterns, beliefs, values, and commitment to an outcome, interact with environmental demands and constraints that produce a person–environment relationship.

- The concept of homeostasis is the body's tendency to resist physiological change and hold bodily functions relatively consistent, well-coordinated, and usually stable.

- When the brain interprets an event as a threat, physiological stability is challenged, and a "fight or flight" response occurs.

- Allostasis describes a dynamic regulatory process that maintains homeostasis through a process of adaptation. Physiological stability is achieved when the autonomic nervous system; the HPA; and the cardiovascular, metabolic, and immune systems respond to internal and external stimuli. As wear and tear on the brain and body occur, there is a corresponding increase in the number of abnormal biologic parameters called the allostatic load (AL). AL is an indication of chronic stress.

- Effective coping can be either problem focused or emotion focused. The outcome of successful coping is adaptation through enhanced health, psychological well-being, and social functioning.

- Within the social network, social support can help a person cope with stress.

- The overall goals in the nursing management of stress are to resolve the stressful person–environment situation, reduce the stress response, and develop positive coping skills.

CRITICAL THINKING CHALLENGES

1. Compare and contrast the concepts of homeostasis and allostasis.

2. Discuss the impact of acute stress versus chronic stress. Why is chronic stress of more concern than acute stress?

3. Explain why one person may experience the stress of losing a job differently from another.

4. A man is overweight, has hypertension and insomnia, and was recently widowed. The doctor has told him to lose weight and quit smoking. He seeks your advice. Would you recommend a problem-focused or an emotion-focused approach?

5. A woman at the local shelter announced to her group that she was returning to her husband because it was partly her fault that her husband beat her. Is this an example of problem-focused or emotion-focused coping? Justify your answer.

6. Using the Stress Coping and Adaptation Model (Figure 18.1), assess a patient and determine the cognitive appraisal of significant events.

 Noise (2007). David Owen (Tim Robbins) copes with the stressful noises of the city, specifically car alarms, by becoming aggressive and destructive. At first the noise is merely an irritant. Later, he interprets the noise as an assault on everyone. He becomes an activist, protecting others and gradually becomes very grandiose. As his grandiosity increases, he becomes more and more driven to damage vehicles with active care alarms.

VIEWING POINTS: What is the relationship between the physiological response to the noise and his eventual grandiose behavior? How would you help his reduce the stressful experience and cope positively? Observe your own feelings throughout the movie. Did you experience stress?

References

Aguilera, D. C. (1998). *Crisis intervention: Theory and methodology*, St. Louis: Mosby.

American Psychiatric Association. (2013). *Diagnostic and statistical manual of mental disorders* (5th ed). Arlington, VA: Author.

Azmitia, M., Syed, M., & Radmacher, K. (2008). On the intersection of personal and social identities: introduction and evidence from a longitudinal study of emerging adults. *New Directions for Child & Adolescent Development, 120*, 1–16.

Benjet, C., Borges, G., & Medina-Mora, M.E. (2010). Chronic childhood adversity and onset of psychopathology during three life stages: Childhood, adolescence and adulthood. *Journal of Psychiatric Research, 44*(11), 732–740.

Bryant-Lukosius, D. (2003). Review: Limited evidence exists on the effect of psychological coping styles on cancer survival or recurrence. *Evidence Based Nursing, 6*(3), 88.

Cannon W. B. (1932). *The wisdom of the body*. New York: Norton.

Carlson, E. D., & Chamberlain, R. M. (2005). Allostatic load and health disparities: A theoretical orientation. *Research in Nursing & Health, 28*, 306–315.

Clark, J. S., Bond, M. F., & Hecker, J. R. (2007). Environmental stress, psychological stress and allostatic load. *Psychology, Health & Medicine, 12*(1), 18–30.

de Castro, A. B., Voss, J. G., Ruppin, A., Dominguez, C. F., & Seixas, N. S (2010). Stressors among Latino day laborers. *American Association of Occupational Health Nurses, 58*(5), 185–196.

Friedman, M., & Rosenman, R. (1974). *Type A and your heart*. New York: Knopf.

Glover, D. A., Stuber, M., & Poland, R. E. (2006). Allostatic load in women with and without PTSD symptoms. *Psychiatry, 69*(3), 191–203.

Holmes, T., & Rahe, R. (1967). The Social Readjustment Patient Scale. *Journal of Psychosomatic Research, 11*(2), 213–218.

Juruena, M. F. (2013). Early-life stress and HPA axis trigger recurrent adulthood depression. *Epilepsy & Behavior*. http://dx.doi.org/10.1016/j.yebeh2013.10.020

Kendall, E., & Terry, D. (2009). Predicting emotional well-being following traumatic brain injury: a test of mediated and moderated models. *Social Science & Medicine, 69*(6), 947–954.

Kiecolt-Glaser, J. K., Loving, T. J., Stowell, J. R., Malarkey, W. B., Lemeshow, S., Dickinson, S. L., et al. (2005). Hostile marital interactions, proinflammatory cytokine production, and wound healing. *Archives of General Psychiatry, 62*(12), 1377–1384.

Kumari, M., Badrick, E., Sacker, A., Kirschbaum, C., Marmot, M., & Chandola, T. (2010). Identifying patterns in cortisol secretionin an older population. Finds from the Whitehall II study. *Psychoneuroendocrinology, 35*(7), 1091–1099.

Lalâ A., Bobîrnac, G., & Tipa, R. (2010). Stress levels, alexithymia, type A and type C personality patterns in undergraduate students. *Journal of Medicine & Life, 3*(2), 200–205.

Lazarus, R., & Folkman, S. (1984). *Stress, appraisal and coping.* New York: Springer.

Lazarus, R. S. (1999). *Stress and emotion: A new synthesis.* New York: Springer.

Lazarus, R. S. (2001). Relational meaning and discrete emotions. In K. R. Scherer, A. Schorr, & T. Johnstone (Eds.), *Appraisal processes in emotion: Theory, methods, research* (pp. 37–67). New York: Oxford University Press.

Li, Y., & Wu, S. (2010). Social networks and health among rural-urban migrants in China: A channel or a constraint? *Health Promotion International, 25*(3), 371–380.

Low, C. A., Thurston, R. C., & Matthews, K. A. (2010). Psychosocial factors in the development of heart disease in women: Current research and future directions. *Psychosomatic Medicine, 72*(9), 842–854.

Marchesi, C., Ossola, P., Scagnelli, F., Paglia, F., Aprile, S., Monici, A., et al. (2014). Type D personality in never-depressed patients and the development of major and minor depression after acute coronary syndrome. *Journal of Affective Disorders, 155,* 194–199.

McEwen, B. S. (2000). Allostasis and allostatic load: Implications for neuro-psychopharmacology. *Neuropsychopharmacology, 22,* 108–124.

McEwen, B. S. (2005). Stressed or stressed out: What is the difference? *Journal of Psychiatry Neuroscience, 30*(5), 315–318.

McEwen, B. S., & Bianaros, P. J. (2010). Central role of the brain in stress and adaptation: Links to socioeconomic status, health, and disease. *Annals of the New York Academy of Sciences, 118,* 190–222.

McVicar, A., Ravalier, J. J., & Greenwood, C. (2013). Biology of stress revisited: Intracellular mechanisms and the conceptualization of stress. *Stress & Health.* doi:10.1002/smi.2508

Mols, F., & Denollet, J. (2010). Type D personality in the general population: A systematic review of health status, mechanisms of disease, and work-related problems. *Health and Quality of Life Outcomes, 8,* 9.

Moran, C. C. (2001). Personal predictions of stress and stress reactions in firefighter recruits. *Disaster Prevention & Management, 10*(5), 356–365.

Peek, M. K., Cutchin, M. P., Salinas, J. J., Sheffield, K. M., Eschbach, K., Stowe, R. P., et al. (2010). Allostatic load among non-hispanic whites, non-hispanic blacks, and people of Mexican origin: Effects of ethnicity, nativity, and acculturation. *American Journal of Public Health, 100*(5), 940–946.

Rafanelli, C., Sirri, L., Grandi, S., & Fava, G. A. (2013). Is depression the wrong treatment target for improving outcome in coronary artery disease? *Psychotherapy and Psychosomatics, 82.* doi: 10.1159/000351586

Rahe, R. (1994). The more things change. *Psychosomatic Medicine, 56*(4), 306–307.

Rahe, R. H. (2000). Recent Life Changes Questionnaire (RLCQ).

Rahe, R. H., Taylor, C., Tolles, R. L., Newhall, L. M., Veach, T. L., & Bryson, S. (2002). A novel stress and coping workplace program reduces illness and healthcare utilization. *Psychosomatic Medicine, 64*(2), 278–286.

Seeman, T., Epel, E., Gruenewald, T., Karlamangla, A., & McEwen, B.S. (2010). Soci-economic differentials in peripheral biology: Cumulative allostatic load. *Annals of the New York Academy of Sciences, 1186,* 223–239.

Selye, H. (1956). *The stress of life.* New York: McGraw-Hill.

Selye, H. (1974). *Stress without distress.* Philadelphia: J. B. Lippincott.

Shen, B., Countryman, A. J., Spiro, A., & Niaura, R (2008). The prospective contribution of hostility characteristics to high fasting glucose levels. The moderating role of marital status. *Diabetes Care, 31*(7), 1293–1298.

Segerstrom, S. C. (2010). Resources, stress, and immunity: an ecological perspective on human psychoneuroimmunology [review]. *Annals of Behavioral Medicine, 40*(1), 114–125.

Seib, C., Whiteside, E., Lee, K., Humphreys, J., Tran, T. H., Chopin, L., et al. (2014). Stess, lifestyle, and quality of life in midlife and older Australian women: Results from the Stress and the Health of Women Study. *Women's Health Issues, 24*(1), e43–e52.

Sogaard, A. J., Dalgard, O. S., Holm, I., Roysamb, E., & Haheim, L. L. (2008). Associations between type A behavior pattern and psychological distress: 28 years of follow-up of the Oslo Study 1972/1973. *Social Psychiatry & Psychiatric Epidemiology, 43*(3), 216–223.

Sterling, P. (2012). Allostasis: A model of predictive regulation. *Physiology & Behavior,* 106, 5–15.

Stevenson, C. & Williams, L. (2014). Type D personality, quality of life and physical symptoms in the general population: A dimensional analysis. *Psychology & Health, 29*(3), 365–373.

Tamers, S. L., Okechukwu, C., Bohl, A. A., Gueguen, A., Goldberg, M., & Zins, M. (2014). The impact of stressul life events on excessive alcohol consumption in the French population: Findings from the GAZEL Cohort Study. *PLos One, 9*(1), e87654. www.plosone.org

Tishler, C. L., Bartholomae, S. & Rhodes, A. R. (2005). Personality profiles of normal healthy research volunteers: A potential concern for clinical drug trial investigators? *Medical Hypotheses, 65*(1), 1–7.

Whatley, A. D., Dilorio, C. K., & Yeager, K. (2010). Examining the relationships of depressive symptoms, stigma, social support and regimen-specific support on quality of life in adult patients with epilepsy. *Health Education Research, 25*(4), 575–584.

Zegwaard, M. I., Aartsen, M. J., Cuijpers, P, & Grypdonck, M. H. (2011, in press). Review: A conceptual model of perceived burden of informal caregivers for older persons with a severe functional psychiatric syndrome and concomitant problematic behavior. *Journal of Clinical Nursing.*

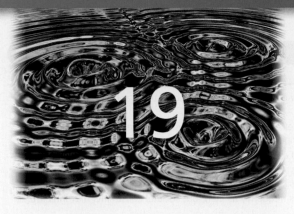

19

Management of Anger, Aggression, and Violence

Sandra P. Thomas

KEY CONCEPTS

- anger
- aggression
- gender, culture, and ethnic differences
- intervention fit
- violence

LEARNING OBJECTIVES

After studying this chapter, you will be able to:

1. Explore difference between healthy and maladaptive styles of anger.

2. Discuss principles of anger management as a psychoeducational intervention.

3. Discuss the factors that influence aggressive and violent behaviors.

4. Discuss theories used to explain anger, aggression, and violence.

5. Identify behaviors or actions that escalate and de-escalate violent behavior.

6. Recognize the risk for verbal and physical attacks on nurses.

7. Generate options for responding to the expression of anger, aggression, and violent behaviors in clinical nursing practice.

8. Apply the nursing process to the management of anger, aggression, and violence in patients

KEY TERMS

- anger management • catharsis • hostile aggression • instrumental aggression • inwardly directed anger
- maladaptive anger • outwardly directed anger

Maladaptive anger and potentially lethal violent behavior are increasingly evident in contemporary Western society. Temper tantrums of athletes, episodes of road rage, and school shootings often dominate the evening news. Clearly, mismanagement of angry emotion is a serious social problem.

Language pertaining to anger is imprecise and confusing. Some of the words used interchangeably with anger include *annoyance*, *frustration*, *temper*, *resentment*, *hostility*, *hatred*, and *rage*. To avoid perpetuating the confusion, three key concepts were selected for use in this chapter: *anger*, *aggression*, and *violence*. Anger, aggres-

sion, and violence should not be viewed as a continuum because one does not necessarily lead to another. That is a myth. In fact, cultural myths about anger abound (Table 19.1).

One goal of this chapter is to dispel confusion between anger as a normal, healthy response to violation of one's integrity and maladaptive anger that is detrimental to one's mental and physical health. Understanding this distinction is an important aspect of emotional intelligence.

A second goal of this chapter is to outline risk factors for aggression and violence and describe preventive interventions, particularly as they pertain to the

Table 19.1	CULTURAL MYTHS ABOUT ANGER	
Myth	**Truth**
Anger is a knee-jerk reaction to external events.	Humans can choose to slow down their reactions and to think and behave differently in response to events.
Anger can be uncontrollable, resulting in crimes of passion such as "involuntary manslaughter."	In societies that believe anger can be controlled, there are far fewer violent crimes than in the United States. Compare the statistics of Japan and the United States.
Anger behavior in adulthood is determined by temperament and childhood experiences.	Although temperament and early experiences are important, emotional development continues throughout life. Adults can acquire knowledge and skills to handle emotions more effectively.
Men are angrier than women.	Women experience anger as frequently as men, but societal constraints may inhibit their expression of it.
People have to behave aggressively to get what they want.	Making an assertive request is more likely to lead to the desired outcome.

nursing care environment. Assaults by patients toward the staff of hospitals and nursing homes are on the increase, and eight nurses were fatally injured while on duty during 2003–2009 (American Nurses Association, 2012). Aggression and violence occur across a wide spectrum of healthcare settings, requiring all nurses to develop expertise in prevention and management of aggression. Contrary to a popular misconception, patients who have psychiatric problems are not more violent than other patients, but astute clinicians need to know which patients *might* become aggressive given a combination of known risk factors with specific environmental conditions.

ANGER

Anger is an internal affective state, usually temporary rather than an enduring negative attitude. If expressed outwardly, anger behavior can be constructive or destructive. Whereas destructive anger alienates other people and invites retaliation, constructive anger can be a powerful force for asserting one's rights and achieving social justice.

> KEYCONCEPT   **Anger** is "a strong, uncomfortable emotional response to a provocation that is unwanted and incongruent with one's values, beliefs, or rights" (Thomas, 1998).

Anger is a signal that something is wrong in a situation; thus, the angry individual has the urge to take action (Lemay, Overall, & Clark, 2012). The situation is more distressing than a minor annoyance such as a slow grocery line. An interpersonal offense such as unjust or disrespectful treatment (a spouse lying, a coworker taking advantage) often provokes anger. The meaning of an angry episode depends on the relational context. For example, anger is more intense and intermingled with considerable hurt when loved ones violate the implicit relational contract ("If he loved me, how could he lie about that? How can I trust him again?") (Thomas, 2006).

Maladaptive anger (excessive outwardly directed anger or suppressed anger) is linked to psychiatric conditions, such as depression (Perugi, Fornaro, & Akiskal, 2011), as well as a plethora of medical conditions. For example, *excessive outwardly directed anger* is linked to coronary heart disease (Ketterer et al., 2011) and myocardial infarction (Mostofsky, Maclure, Tofler, Muller, & Mittleman, 2013). *Suppressed anger* is related to arthritis, breast and colorectal cancer, chronic pain, and hypertension (Burns, Quartana, & Bruehl, 2011; Thomas, 2009). Furthermore, suppressed anger was a predictor of early mortality for both men and women in a large 17-year study (Potpara & Lip, 2011).

In contrast to these maladaptive anger management styles, research shows that anger discussed with other people in a constructive way has a beneficial effect on blood pressure (Everson-Rose & Lewis, 2005; Thomas, 1997a), as well as statistically significant associations with better general health, a higher sense of self-efficacy, less depression, and a lower likelihood of obesity (Thomas, 1997b). Anger controlled through calming strategies is associated with faster wound healing and other health benefits (Gouin, Kiecolt-Glaser, Malarkey, & Glaser, 2008; Gross, Groer, & Thomas, in press). Thus, effective anger management is important in maintenance of holistic health.

Skillful anger control is essential to social and occupational success. People with poor anger control have more conflict at work, change jobs more frequently, take more unwise risks, and have more accidents than people with adaptive anger behavior (Bennett & Lowe, 2008).

The Experience of Anger

When you are angry, your heart pounds, your blood pressure rises, you breathe faster, your muscles tense, and you clench your jaw or fists as you experience an impulse to do something with this physical energy. Some individuals experience anger arousal as pleasurable, but others find its strong physical manifestations scary and unpleasant. People who were taught that anger is a sin may immediately try to ban it from awareness and deny its existence. However, suppression actually results in greater, more prolonged physiological arousal. A better option is finding a way to safely release the physical energy, either through vigorous physical activity (e.g., jogging) or through a calming activity (e.g., deep breathing). Later, at an opportune time, calmly discussing the incident with the provocateur permits clarification of misunderstandings and resolution of grievances. Box 19.1 invites the reader to explore variations in anger experience.

The physiology of anger involves the cerebral cortex, the sympathetic nervous system, the adrenal medulla (which secretes adrenaline and noradrenaline), the adrenal cortex (which secretes cortisol), the cardiovascular system, and even the immune system. From a biologic viewpoint, angry episodes may partially originate from developmental deficits, anoxia, malnutrition, toxins, tumors, neurodegenerative diseases, or trauma affecting the brain.

The Expression of Anger

While the physiological arousal of anger is similar in all people, ways of expressing anger differ. The most common modes, or styles, of anger expression are listed in Table 19.2.

In Western culture, control of anger was the dominant stance from Greco-Roman times to the 20th century. Anger was viewed as sinful, dangerous, and destructive—an irrational emotion to be contained, controlled, and denied. This pejorative view contributed to the development of a powerful taboo against feeling and expressing anger. People who have accepted this persistent taboo may have difficulty even knowing when they are angry. They may use euphemisms such as "a little upset."

In contrast to the denial or containment of angry emotion, some mental health care providers began to advocate the use of **catharsis** during the early 20th century, based on the animal research of ethologists and on Freud's conceptualization of "strangulated affect"; rather than holding in their anger, people were urged to "vent it," lest there be a dangerous "slush fund" of unexpressed anger building up in the body (Rubin, 1970). The legacy

Table 19.2	STYLES OF ANGER EXPRESSION	
Style	**Characteristic Behaviors**	**Gender Socialization Issues**
Anger suppression	Feeling anxious when anger is aroused Acting as though nothing happened Withdrawing from people when angry Conveying anger nonverbally by body language Sulking, pouting, or ruminating	In North America, girls are often discouraged from openly expressing anger, lest they hurt someone's feelings. Females are more likely than males to engage in passive-aggressive tactics; to ruminate about unresolved conflict; and to have somatic anger symptoms, such as headaches
Unhealthy outward anger expression	Flying off the handle Expressing anger in an attacking or blaming way Yelling, saying nasty things Calling the other person names or using profanity Using fists rather than words to express angry feelings	In North America, boys are encouraged to be aggressive and competitive, to express their anger in "manly" ways. Throughout life, males are more likely to express anger physically than females are.
Constructive anger discussion	Discussing the anger with a friend or family member even if the provocateur cannot be confronted at the time Approaching the person with whom one is angry and discussing the concern directly Using "I" language to describe feelings and request changes in another's behavior	Most research shows that females, more so than males, prefer to talk through anger episodes and restore relationship harmony. Both men and women may benefit from assertiveness training, problem-solving skills training, and conflict resolution workshops.

of the ill-advised "ventilationist movement" is still with us, visible in rude, uncivil behavior in the nation's classrooms, offices, roadways, and other public places, as well as in countless homes where loud arguments are a daily occurrence.

More ideally, the clear expression of honest anger may actually prevent aggression and help to resolve a situation (Thomas, 2009). Suppression of anger, prolonged rumination about the grievance, and malevolent fantasies of revenge do not resolve a problem and may result in negative consequences at a later time. Likewise, antagonistic anger toward an intimate partner or coworker only exacerbates the conflict (Lemay et al., 2012). In contrast, if anger is expressed assertively, beneficial outcomes are possible. In Averill's classic study (1983) of everyday anger, 76% of those who were on the receiving end of someone else's anger reported that they recognized their own faults as a result of the anger incident. Contrary to popular misconception, the relationship with the angry person was strengthened, not weakened.

Special Issues in the Nurse–Patient Relationship

Studies show that nurses often withdraw from angry patients and try to hide their own anger because "good nurses" do not get angry at patients (Farrell, Shafie, & Salmon, 2010). Coldness and distancing on the part of staff are acutely painful to patients (Carlsson, Dahlberg, Ekeburgh, & Dahlberg, 2006). What patients want are steady, dependable, confident caregivers who will remain connected with them when they are angry (Box 19.2).

Nurses' perceptions and beliefs about themselves as individuals and professionals influence their response to aggressive behaviors. For example, a nurse who considers any expression of anger inappropriate will approach an agitated patient differently from a nurse who considers agitated behavior to be meaningful. Understandably, nurses often shrink from patient anger when their own family backgrounds have been characterized by out-of-control anger or abuse. A nurse who has previously been assaulted by a patient is also more likely to have difficulty dealing with subsequent episodes of aggression.

Some patients have an uncanny ability to target a nurse's vulnerable characteristics. Although it is normal to become defensive when feeling vulnerable, maintaining personal control is a must. If not, the potential for punitive interventions is greater. Threatening an agitated patient (e.g., "You are going to get an injection if you don't calm down") will only worsen a volatile situation. Nurses must collaborate with other members of the treatment team when interacting with particularly challenging patients, obtaining consultation from supervisors if necessary.

BOX 19.2

Research for Best Practice: **What do Patients Want from Caregivers?**

Carlsson, G., Dahlberg, K., Ekebergh, M., & Dahlberg, H. (2006). *Patients longing for authentic personal care: A phenomenological study of violent encounters in psychiatric settings.* Issues in Mental Health Nursing, 27(3), 287–305.

THE QUESTION: How does the patient experience violent encounters?

METHODS: This qualitative study is approached from the reflective lifeworld approach. This methodology focuses on the patient experiences of their violent encounters. Seven men and two women, ages 20 to 38 years, agreed to interviews based on the reflective model. The interviews were transcribed verbatim, and the text was analyzed for meaning that was recorded and then transcribed. The goal of the analysis was to describe the essential structure of the phenomenon and its meaning.

FINDINGS: The researchers found that patients wanted steady, dependable, confident caregivers who remained connected with them when they were angry. When caregivers were cold and distant, patients felt a sense of despair, and their aggression increased:

- "My most lasting memory from these moments is the encounter with an expressionless, blank face with expressionless, cold eyes staring back at me" (p. 295).
- "I don't think they [the staff] really care whether I'm dead or alive . . . nobody is trying to help me to live, to stay alive" (p. 299).

In contrast, when caregivers displayed authentic sensitivity to their suffering, patients' aggression was diffused:

- "I could see in his face then that he liked me, he was not scared. . . . He was sort of calm and had loving eyes; it was very disarming" (p. 293).
- "You could tell that there is some warmth and authenticity. You can tell that she is serious, that she cares about you . . . it is authentic, not ingratiating just, so that I will behave" (p. 299).

IMPLICATIONS FOR NURSING: This study helps nurses understand the needs of patients who are violent. Being authentic and sensitive are valued nursing attributes. Demonstration of these attributes can help reduce patients' risk for aggressive behavior.

Assessment of Anger

Both **outwardly directed anger** (particularly the hostile, attacking forms) and **inwardly directed anger** (i.e., anger that is stifled despite strong arousal) produce adverse consequences, indicating a need for anger management intervention. Complicating matters, however, most people's anger styles cannot be neatly categorized as "anger-in" or "anger-out" because they behave differently in different environments (for example, yelling at secretaries in the office, stifling anger at spouse). Therefore, it is necessary to conduct a careful assessment of a patient's behavior pattern across various situations.

The manner of anger expression is not the only important aspect of assessment. The difficulty in regulating the **frequency** and **intensity** of anger must also be assessed along with the extent to which anger is creating problems in work or intimate relationships, and the presence or absence of coping techniques such as calming or diffusion through vigorous exercise. Given the current climate of evidence-based practice, it may be advantageous to administer a questionnaire that has been extensively used with thousands of people, permitting comparison of a particular client with established norms. The Spielberger State-Trait Anger Expression Inventory (STAXI) is one such tool (Spielberger, 1999). This instrument is particularly useful because it measures the general propensity to be angry (trait anger) as well as current feelings (state anger) and several styles of anger expression, including control through calming techniques.

Because anger and aggression can be symptomatic of many underlying psychiatric or medical disorders, from posttraumatic stress disorder (PTSD) and bipolar disorder to toxicities and head injuries, first any underlying disorder must be properly evaluated. At present, only one anger-related disorder, intermittent explosive disorder (IED), appears in the *Diagnostic and Statistical Manual of Mental Disorders (DSM-5)* (American Psychiatric Association [APA], 2013). This diagnosis is used when recurring aggressive outbursts cannot be attributed to any other condition. People with IED display aggressive behavior that is disproportionate to the precipitating event, usually a minor provocation by a family member or other close associate (APA, 2013). Once thought to be rare, new research shows that it is as common as many other psychiatric disorders (Coccaro, 2012). The disorder usually appears during the teen years and persists over the life course. A national study indicates that the average number of lifetime anger attacks per person is large (43 per person). Because the disorder involves inadequate production or functioning of serotonin, IED is commonly treated with selective serotonin reuptake inhibitors (SSRIs). However, behavior therapy should also be included. Only 28.8% of patients with IED ever receive treatment for their anger (Kessler, Coccaro, Fava, Jaeger, Jin, & Walters, 2006) although the IED population is just as responsive to treatment as are non-IED populations (McCloskey, Noblett, Deffenbacher, Gollan, & Coccaro, 2008).

Culture and Gender Considerations in Assessment

Anger is one of the six universal emotions with identifiable facial features and emotionally inflected speech. People across the globe experience the emotion of anger, along with the impulse to take action, but culture is perhaps the most important determinant of what angry individuals actually *do*. Thus, in Japan, a wife might indicate anger to her husband by creating a disorderly flower arrangement. Such a subtle nonverbal cue is unlikely to be understood (or even noticed) by a husband from another culture.

> **KEYCONCEPT** **Gender, culture, and ethnic differences** in the experience and expression of anger must be taken into consideration before planning interventions.

Cultural differences in anger behavior can emanate from the historical trajectories, religions, languages, and customs of a group of people (Thomas, 2006). The same event can provoke very different emotional responses in culturally different persons (e.g., a random act by a stranger could be perceived as insulting by one individual but dismissed with a laugh by someone from another culture).

Gender role socialization influences beliefs about the appropriateness of "owning" angry emotionality and revealing it to others.

Western cultures generally promote more aggressive behavior in males and more conciliatory behavior in females (see Table 19.2). However, these generalizations may not apply to marginalized individuals, such as ethnic minorities. For example, African American mothers often prepare their daughters to mobilize anger to cope with the harsh realities of racist treatment (Thomas & González-Prendes, 2009). Some clients from Eastern cultures disapprove of anger for both genders, particularly cultures emphasizing connectedness rather than individualism (e.g., Japanese). Therefore, clients in such cultures may ruminate for lengthy periods about anger episodes rather than verbalizing their feelings. A more extensive discussion of culture and gender factors can be found in Thomas (2006).

The essential element in a cultural assessment is exploration of what the client learned about anger and its display in his or her culture and family of origin (the primary bearer of that culture). Adult clients can be encouraged to transcend cultural imperatives and childhood admonitions when these no longer serve them well. For example, research has shown that using anger to cope with racism actually has a negative effect on African American well being (Pittman, 2011). Reflecting on negative outcomes of anger behaviors can motivate client adoption of new strategies. Referral to an anger management course or therapy may be useful.

Anger Interventions

Communication techniques that promote the expression of anger in nondestructive ways have been developed and validated through research (Davidson & Mostofsky, 2010;

Thomas, 2009). However, most people lack skill in handling anger constructively. Few people have healthy role models to observe while growing up. Therefore, education in anger management can be valuable, both for psychological growth and improved interpersonal relations.

Anger Management: A Psychoeducational Intervention

Anger management is an effective intervention that nurses can deliver to persons whose anger behavior is maladaptive in some way (i.e., interfering with success in work or relationships) but *not violent*. In recent years, there has been an increase in court-mandated "anger management" for persons whose behavior is violent as opposed to angry. When these individuals do not greatly benefit, a conclusion may be drawn that anger management is ineffective. However, psychoeducational anger management courses cannot be expected to modify *violent* behavior (interventions designed for aggressive and violent individuals are presented later in the chapter).

The desired outcomes of any anger management intervention are to teach people to (1) effectively modulate the physiological arousal of anger, (2) alter any irrational thoughts fueling the anger, and (3) modify maladaptive anger behaviors (e.g., blaming, attacking, or suppressing) that prevent problem solving in daily living. Group work is valuable to anger management clients because they need to practice new behaviors in an interpersonal context that offers feedback and support. The leader of an anger management group functions as a teacher and coach, not a therapist. Therefore, potential participants should be screened and referred to individual counseling or psychotherapy if their anger is deep seated and chronic. Exclusion criteria are paranoia, organic disorders, and severe personality disorders (Thomas, 2001). Candidates for psychoeducational anger management classes must have some insight that their behavior is problematic and some desire to enlarge their behavioral repertoire.

Clinicians achieve better outcomes when they follow empirically supported treatment manuals (Goldstein, Kemp, Leff, & Lochman, 2012; Goldstein et al., 2013). Anger management includes both didactic and experiential components. Educational handouts, videos, and workbooks are usually used. Ideally, participants commit to attendance for a series of weekly meetings, ranging from 4 to 10 weeks. Between the group meetings, participants are given homework assignments such as keeping an anger diary and applying the lessons of the class in their homes and work sites. Fresh anger incidents can be brought to the class for role-plays and group discussion. It may be useful to conduct for gender-specific or culturally specific groups (Thomas, 2001). Effectiveness of anger management has been demonstrated in studies of college students, angry

---

BOX 19.3

Research for Best Practice: **Anger Management for Family Members**

Son, J. Y., & Choi, Y. J. (2010). The effect of an anger management program for family members of patients with alcohol use disorders. Archives of Psychiatric Nursing, 24(1), 38–45.

THE QUESTION: Can a structured anger management program for family members of patients with alcohol use disorders promote effective anger expression and anger management?

METHODS: Sixty-three family members of patients with alcohol use disorders participated in anger management program of eight sessions with three groups for 2 months. Each session was held once a week for 2 hours by psychiatric–mental health nurse practitioners. Relaxation therapy was conducted at the beginning of each session. The goal of the anger management program was to have the participants express, ventilate, and cope with their anger in appropriate ways by using cognitive-behavioral techniques. The expression of anger was measured before and after the intervention by the Korean Anger Expression Inventory (based on the State-Trait Anger Expression Inventory).

FINDINGS: The total anger expression score of was significantly reduced at the end of the program, indicating that family members had improved their ability to effectively express anger.

IMPLICATIONS FOR NURSING: Anger management classes can be effective in helping family members of patients with substance use disorder learn to understand and modify their experience of anger through cognitive-behavior techniques.

---

drivers, angry veterans, various medical and psychiatric outpatients, and parents who have difficulty controlling anger toward their children (Kusmierska, 2012). Family members of patients with alcohol use disorders can also benefit from anger management (Box 19.3).

Studies show that individuals who are comfortable with religious/spiritual anger management strategies can successfully reduce maladaptive anger through prayer for the offender (Bremner, Koole, & Bushman, 2011) or forgiveness (Johnson, 2012; Mefford, Thomas, Callen, & Groer, in press).

Cognitive-Behavioral Therapy for Anger

Individuals who are not suitable candidates for a psychoeducational anger management intervention may benefit from cognitive-behavioral therapy delivered by an APN or psychologist. Deffenbacher (2011) recommends first establishing the therapeutic alliance because some angry individuals are not in a stage of readiness to change their behavior. When clients are more receptive, CBT involves avoidance of provoking stimuli, self-monitoring regarding cues of anger arousal, stimulus control, response disruption, and guided practice of more effective anger behaviors. Relaxation training is often introduced early in the treatment because it strengthens the therapeutic alliance and convinces clients that they can indeed learn to calm themselves when angry. When the body relaxes, there is less physical impetus to act impulsively in a way that one will later regret (Deffenbacher, 2011).

AGGRESSION AND VIOLENCE

Aggression and violence command the attention of the criminal justice system as well as the mental health care system. During periods when people are a danger to others, they may be separated from the larger society and confined in prisons or locked psychiatric units. Because nurses frequently practice in these settings, management of aggressive and violent behavior is an essential skill.

Factors That Influence Aggressive and Violent Behavior

The violent individual may feel trapped, frightened, or desperate, perhaps at the end of his or her rope. The nurse must remember that many violent individuals have experienced childhood abandonment, physical brutality, or sexual abuse. Confinement that replicates earlier experiences of degrading treatment may provoke aggressive response, but humane care may kindle hope of recovery and rehabilitation. The response of the nurse may be critical in determining whether aggression escalates or diminishes. Aggressive or violent behavior does not occur in a vacuum. Both the patient and the context must be considered. Therefore, a multidimensional framework (Figure 19.1) is essential for understanding and responding to these behaviors (Morrison & Love, 2003).

> **KEYCONCEPT** **Aggression** involves overt behavior intended to hurt, belittle, take revenge, or achieve domination and control. Aggression can be verbal (sarcasm, insults, threats) or physical (property damage, slapping, hitting). Mentally healthy people stop themselves from aggression by realizing the negative consequences to themselves or their relationships.

Impulsive aggression occurs in situations of anger and anxiety when the frontal cortex does not rein in the amygdala, resulting in behaviors comparable to "a wild horse." **Instrumental** aggression is premeditated and unrelated to immediate feelings of frustration or threat, as in acts committed "in cold blood" (Audenaert, 2013).

> **KEYCONCEPT** **Violence** is extreme aggression and involves the use of strong force or weapons to inflict bodily harm to another person and in some cases to kill. Violence connotes greater intensity and destruction than aggression. All violence is aggressive, but not all aggression is violent.

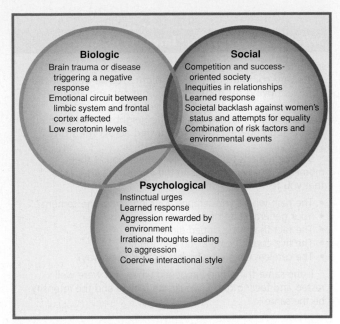

FIGURE 19.1 Biopsychosocial etiologies for patients with aggression.

Theories of Aggression and Violence

This section discusses some of the main theoretical explanations for aggression and violence. A single model or theory cannot fully explain aggression and violence; instead, choose the most useful theories for explaining a particular patient's experience and for planning interventions.

Biologic Theories

The brain structures most frequently associated with aggressive behavior are the limbic system and the cerebral cortex, particularly the frontal and temporal lobes. Patients with a history of damage to the cerebral cortex are more likely to exhibit increased impulsivity, decreased inhibition, and decreased judgment than are those who have not experienced such damage. The interaction of neurocognitive impairment and social history of abuse or family violence increases the risk for violent behavior (Siever, 2008).

An aggression-related gene (monoamine oxidase A), which affects norepinephrine, serotonin, and dopamine, may play a significant role in the violence enacted by abused children, especially boys (Siever, 2008). Low serotonin levels are also associated with irritability, increased pain sensitivity, impulsiveness, and aggression (Kuepper et al., 2010).

Sex hormones also play a role in some aggressive behavior. Violent male offenders have higher testosterone than control participants, and female offenders are

BOX 19.4
Self-Awareness Exercise: Intensity of Anger

Imagine this scene:
  You are coming home late at night. You've been at the library studying for midterm examinations and are tired. As you come up the front walk, you trip over a skateboard, probably left by one of the neighborhood children. Before you know it, you are sprawled across the front step.
  What emotions threaten to overwhelm you at that moment? What contributes to the intensity of the anger that you feel?

• The pain where you scraped your leg across the cement?
• Your general state of tiredness?
• The fact that you skipped dinner?
• The five cups of coffee you had today?
• The careless children who left a toy in your way?

  If the same thing had happened when you were well rested and feeling good, would the feeling and the intensity be the same?

more likely to commit crimes during the low progesterone phase of the menstrual cycle (Glenn & Raine, 2006). The odds of violent behavior also increase when separate risk factors, such as schizophrenia, substance abuse, and not taking prescribed medications, coexist in the same person. Before reading additional research evidence, try the anger exercise in Box 19.4. What does daily experience suggest about biologically based aspects of the experience and expression of anger?

NCLEXNOTE In caring for a potentially aggressive patient, the nurse should recognize that biochemical imbalance contributes to the person's inability to control aggression.

Psychological Theories

Several psychological explanations exist for aggressive and violent behaviors. This section discusses these theories and their treatment approaches.

Psychoanalytic Theories

Psychoanalytic theorists view emotions as instinctual drives. They view suppression of these drives as unhealthy and possible contributors to the development of psychosomatic or psychological disorders. Because the language of hydraulics is evident in Freud's use of terms such as cathexis (filling) and catharsis (release), some psychoanalysts recommended the use of cathartic approaches to release patients' pent-up anger. Following this theoretical formulation, nurses in the mid-20th century often used interventions that directed the patient to "let it out" by pounding a

pillow or ripping up telephone books (Thomas, 2009). However, studies did not support the theory that catharsis reduces aggression.

Contemporary psychoanalysts do not adhere to any single explanatory model of aggression, often focusing on patients' tendencies to reenact old childhood conflicts or their defensive attempts to deny vulnerability (Feindler & Byers, 2006). In working with angry patients, they focus on issues such as improved control over outbursts, heightened empathy for others, and repair of deficits in the personality structure. During analytic therapy, patients gradually achieve greater insight into unconscious processes (Feindler & Byers, 2006). Thus, they become aware of the reasons they developed maladaptive anger behaviors.

Behavioral Theories

As behavioral theories came into prominence, anger was viewed as a learned response to a stimulus rather than an instinctual drive. In the 1930s, the frustration-aggression hypothesis was advanced in which a person may experience anger and act violently in response to interference with or blocking of a goal. Laboratory experiments and the reality of everyday experience have proved the limitations of this theory (Thomas, 1990). Not all situations in which one's goal is blocked lead to anger or violence.

Social Learning Theory

In Bandura's social learning theory, he focuses on the role of learning and rewards in the expression of aggression and violence (Bandura, 2001). Children's observations of aggressive behaviors among family members and violence in their communities foster a context for learning that aggressive behavior is an acceptable way of getting what they want. According to this view, people develop aggressive and violent behaviors by participating in an environment that rewards aggression (Palazzolo, Roberto, & Babin, 2010).

General Aggression Model

The general aggression model (GAM) is a framework that accounts for the interaction of cognition, affect, and arousal during an aggressive episode (Anderson & Anderson, 2008) (Figure 19.2). In this model, an episode consists of *person and situation factors* in an ongoing *social interaction*. The episode is mediated through a person's thoughts, feelings, and intensity of arousal. Within this context, the individual appraises the episode and then makes a decision about a follow-up action. The outcome is either thoughtful or impulsive action. The *person factors* include characteristics such

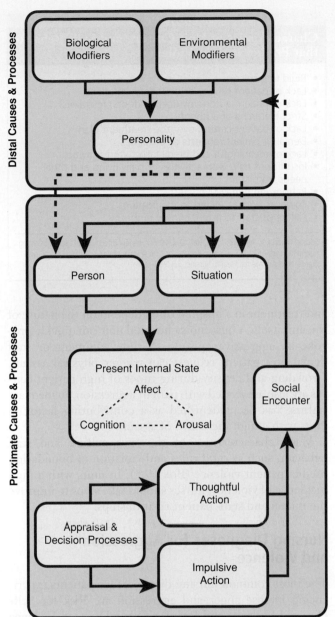

FIGURE 19.2 General aggression model overview. (Redrawn with permission from Anderson, C. A., & Anderson, K. B. [2008]. Men who target women: Specificity of target, generality of aggressive behavior. *Aggressive Behavior, 34*[6], 608.)

as gender, personality traits, beliefs and attitudes, values, goals, and behavior patterns. *Situational factors* include the actual provocation (insults, slights, verbal and physical aggression, interference with achieving goals) and cues that trigger memories of similar situations. *Cognition* includes hostile thoughts and scripts (previous behavior patterns and responses to similar episodes). Mood, emotion, and expressive motor responses (automatic reactions to specific emotions) represent the *affect component*. *Arousal* can be physiological, psychological, or both.

NURSING MANAGEMENT: Promoting Safety and Preventing Violence

Paramount aims of psychiatric nurses, particularly those staffing inpatient facilities, are promoting safety and preventing violence. The nurse works toward these goals by establishing therapeutic nurse–patient relationships and creating a therapeutic milieu. Intervening with a potentially violent patient begins with assessment of the history and the predictive factors outlined in the next section.

Assessment for Aggression and Violence

The patient's history is the most important predictor of potential for aggression and violence. Early life adverse circumstances, such as inadequate maternal nutrition, birth complications, traumatic brain injury, and lead exposure can contribute to risk for aggressive and criminal behaviors in adulthood (Liu, 2011). Important markers in the patient's history include previous episodes of rage and violent behavior, escalating irritability, intruding angry thoughts, and fear of losing control.

Characteristics Predictive of Aggression and Violence

The age, gender, and race of patients are *not* good predictors, but several research reports suggest that particular characteristics are predictive of violent behaviors. Involuntary hospitalization, suspiciousness, impulsivity, agitation, and unwillingness to follow unit rules are among the predictors identified in Johnson's (2004) systematic review of the literature about violence on inpatient psychiatric units. Those with diagnoses such as schizophrenia, bipolar disorder, brain injury, alcohol withdrawal, or attention deficit hyperactivity disorder are at increased risk for violent episodes (Zuzelo, Curran, & Zeserman, 2012).

Usually, there are some observable precursors to aggression and violence. In a study of aggressive episodes in an emergency department, the following behaviors indicated an impending aggressive episode: (1) *staring and eye contact* or glaring as a way of intimidation; (2) *tone and volume* of voice such as raised voices, sarcastic comments, and urgent or demeaning speech; (3) *anxiety* in patients, family or friends; (4) *mumbling* that shows increasing frustration; and (5) *pacing* that indicates increased agitation (Luck, Jackson, & Usher, 2007). Research by Bowers, James, Quirk, Wright, Williams, and Stewart (2013) points out that the "textbook picture" of gradual escalation of patient behavior does not always occur; aggression can have a sudden onset with no clear precipitant.

Impaired Communication

Impaired communication (including hearing loss and reduced visual acuity), disorientation, and depression have been found to be consistently associated with aggressive behavior among nursing home residents with dementia (Williams & Herman, 2011).

In patients with cognitive impairments, the nurse needs to know when the patient last voided and the pattern of bowel movements. The urge to void can be a powerful stimulus to agitated behavior. Regular toileting routines are not just interventions to prevent incontinence. Similarly, the anticipation of basic needs such as thirst and hunger is important, especially when working with adults and children who cannot readily express their needs. Other discomforts can arise from such conditions as ingrown toenails and adverse medication reactions.

Physical Condition

The patient's physical condition contributes to the likelihood of aggression. Patients with longstanding poor dietary habits (e.g., indigent patients, patients with alcoholism) often have deficiencies of thiamine and niacin. Increased irritability, disorientation, and paranoia may result. Assessing overall dietary intake is relevant, particularly of good tryptophan sources, such as wheat, flour, corn, milk, and eggs. Intake of caffeine, a potent stimulant, should be assessed and limited as necessary (Martin, Cook, Woodring, Burkhardt, Omar, & Kelly, 2008).

Social Factors

The nurse should evaluate social factors, such as crisis conditions in the patient's home, family, or community, that could lead to aggression or violent episodes. If assessment reveals stressful actions by family members, such as evicting the patient from the home, attention must be devoted to mobilizing resources for family and community support and alternative housing.

Are financial or legal troubles placing increased stress on the patient? Is the patient experiencing conflict with other patients on the unit or with certain staff? People reenact in new relationships the same behaviors that created problems in old ones. Thus, behavior in a mental health facility provides important clues to a patient's habitual responses to authority figures, opposite-sex peers, and same-sex peers. Assessment data provide direction for interventions such as reassigning roommates or caregivers.

Milieu and Environmental Factors

Angry or out-of-control behavior is highly influenced by contextual factors. Successful psychiatric stabilization

---

BOX 19.5

Characteristics of Unit Culture and Staff Behavior that Predict Patient Violence

- Rigid unit rules
- Lack of patient privacy or boundary violations
- Lack of patient autonomy (locked doors, restraints)
- Strict hierarchy of authority
- Lack of patient control over the treatment plan
- Denial of patient requests or privileges
- Lack of meaningful and predictable ward activities
- Insufficient help with activities of daily living and other needs from staff
- Patronizing behavior of staff
- Power struggles related to medications
- Failure of staff to listen, convey empathy

Source: Hamrin, V., Iennaco, J., & Olsen, D. (2009). A review of ecological factors affecting inpatient psychiatric unit violence: Implications for relational and unit cultural improvements. *Issues in Mental Health Nursing, 30,* 214–226.

---

and treatment in a hospital often depend on the nature of the unit itself. A busy, noisy hospital unit can quickly provoke an aggressive episode. A rude comment or staff denial of a patient request can trigger physical assault. Crowding and density during times of high patient census are also associated with patient aggression. Inadequate staffing has been identified as a contributing factor in units with a high incidence of assault.

Many characteristics of the unit culture and staff behavior, such as rigid rules and violation of boundaries, predict patient violence (Box 19.5). In units with a high incidence of violence, nurses should take steps to improve the milieu and staff–patient relationships.

Nursing Diagnoses for Aggression and Violence

The most common nursing diagnoses for patients experiencing intense anger and aggression are Risk for Self-Directed Violence and Risk for Other-Directed Violence (NANDA International, 2012). Outcomes focus on aggression control.

Interventions for Promoting Safety

Both patients and staff have a right to expect safety on a psychiatric unit. Nursing interventions focus on communication and development of the nurse–patient relationship, cognitive interventions, interventions for the milieu and environment, and violence prevention.

Communication and Development of the Therapeutic Nurse–Patient Relationship

Communicating with a patient who has the potential for aggression or violence follows the same principles discussed in Chapter 9. Aggressive behavior can be a patient's way to communicate a need for help (Finfgeld-Connett, 2009). Low self-esteem that has been further eroded during hospitalization or treatment may influence a patient to use force to meet his or her needs or to experience some sense of empowerment. The patient who behaves aggressively may receive rewards such as more frequent observation and more opportunities to discuss concerns with nurses. Clearly, this patient must be taught how to get his or her needs met in a more appropriate way.

Listening to the Patient's Illness Experience and Concerns

Development of the therapeutic nurse–patient relationship begins with listening. Some patient complaints are valid and deserve a respectful hearing. For example, disappointment with "playing little games with staff" or "attending classes" has been expressed by hospitalized psychiatric patients who longed for a deeper connection with nursing staff and more intensive insight-oriented therapies (Thomas, Shattell, & Martin, 2002). While patients and their family members are routinely requested to provide details about past medical treatments, medications, and hospitalizations, what is often overlooked is the subjective experience of the health problem (Thomas & Pollio, 2002). Many patients with persistent mental illness have had frightening medication reactions and unpleasant side effects of treatments (such as memory loss caused by electroconvulsive therapy). Understandably, they may harbor distrust of mental health clinicians and resent being hospitalized again. Inviting patients and families to talk about their experiences with the health care system may highlight both their concerns and resources. Simply listening to patients' concerns and "being with" them is often as significant as "doing for" them (Thomas & Pollio, 2002) (Box 19.6).

Validating

Patients who experience intense anger and rage can feel isolated and anxious. The nurse can acknowledge these intense feelings by reflecting "This must be scary for you." Empathic responding can reduce emotional arousal because the patient feels understood and supported (Jarry & Paivio, 2006). By drawing on past experience with other patients, the nurse can also reassure the patient that others have felt the same way.

Providing Choices

When possible, the nurse should provide the patient with choices, particularly patients who have little control over

their situation because of their condition. Offering concrete choices is better than offering open-ended options. For example, a patient who is experiencing a manic episode and is confined to her room may have few options in her daily schedule. However, she may be allowed to make choices about food, personal hygiene, and which pajamas to wear.

Cognitive Interventions to Address Aggression

Cognitive interventions are very useful in interacting with a potentially aggressive patient (see Chapter 12). These interventions are useful when the patient is in a nonaggressive state and willing to discuss the irrational thought process underlying aggressive episodes. These periods of interaction allow exploration of the patient's beliefs, and provision of reassurance, support, and education.

> **NCLEXNOTE**   The best time to teach the patient techniques for managing anger and aggression is when the patient is not experiencing the provoking event. Cognitive therapy approaches are useful and can be prioritized according to responses.

Providing Patient Education

Inpatient hospitalization offers opportunities for education of patients and families about a variety of topics. Nurses can seize "teachable moments" to convey important principles of anger management. For example, after an outburst of loud cursing by John, who mistakenly thought another patient (Jim) had stolen his cigarettes, the nurse helped him consider what he could have done differently in the situation. John was more amenable to learning about calming techniques and problem-solving strategies at this time because his behavior had resulted in adverse consequences (estrangement from Jim, disruption of the dayroom during a popular bingo game, and cancellation of his weekend pass). This incident could also be used for teaching in a subsequent group meeting of inpatients. Many units have daily meetings that permit processing of such conflicts. Jim could be invited to express his feelings about being falsely accused of stealing. Other patients may reveal how distressed they were when John was cursing loudly, providing John useful peer feedback about his outburst. Together, group members could generate ideas for more appropriate behavior.

Developing Prevention Strategies

Although patients are not always aware of it, escalation of feelings, thoughts, and behavior from

BOX 19.6 • THERAPEUTIC DIALOGUE • The Potentially Aggressive Patient

Paul is a 23-year-old patient in the high observation area of an inpatient unit. He is pacing back and forth. He is pounding one fist into his other hand. In the past 24 hours, Paul has been more cooperative and less agitated. The behavior the nurse observes now is more similar to the behavior that Paul displayed 2 days ago. Yesterday the psychiatrist told Paul that he would be granted more freedom in the unit if his behavior improved. The psychiatrist has just seen Paul and refused to change the restrictions on Paul's activities.

INEFFECTIVE APPROACH

Nurse: Paul, I can understand this is frustrating for you.

Paul: How can you understand? Have you ever been held like a prisoner?

Nurse: I do understand, Paul. Now you must calm down or more privileges will be removed.

Paul: [voice gets louder] But I was told that calm behavior would mean more privileges. Now you are telling me calm behavior only gets me what I have got! Can't you talk to the doctor for me?

Nurse: No, Paul, I can't talk to the doctor. [Paul appears more frustrated and agitated as the conversation continues.]

EFFECTIVE APPROACH

Nurse: Paul, you look upset (observation). What happened in your conversation with the psychiatrist? (seeking information)

Paul: Yesterday he said calmer behavior would mean more freedom in the unit. I have tried to be calmer and not to swear. You said you noticed the difference. But today he says "no" to more freedom.

Nurse: Some people might feel cheated if this happened to them. (validation). Is that how you feel?

Paul: Yeah, I feel real cheated. Nothing I do makes a difference. That's the way it is here, and that's the way it is when I am out of the hospital.

Nurse: Sounds like experiences like this leave you feeling pretty powerless. (validation)

Paul: I don't have any power, anywhere. Sometimes when I have no power I get mean. At least then people pay attention to me.

Nurse: In this situation with your doctor, what would help you feel that you had some power? (inviting patient partnership)

Paul: Well, if he would listen to me; if he would read my chart.

Nurse: I am a bit confused by the psychiatrist's decision. I won't make promises that your privileges will change, but would it be okay with you if I talk with him?

Paul: That would make me feel like someone is on my side.

CRITICAL THINKING CHALLENGE

- In the first scenario, how did the nurse escalate the situation?

- Compare the first scenario with the second. How are they different?

---

calmness to violence may follow a particular pattern. Disruption of the pattern can sometimes be a useful means for preventing escalation and helping the patient regain composure. Patients can be actively involved in development of an "early detection plan" based on identification of their own personal warning signs of aggression (Fluttert, Van Meijel, Webster, Nijman, Bartels, & Grypdonck, 2008). Although extant literature continues to focus on staff control of patient behavior, new research shows that aggressive patients would like to learn to handle their impulsive aggressive behavior themselves (deSchutter & Lodewijkx, 2013). Nurses can suggest strategies to interrupt patterns:

- Counting to 10
- Using a relaxation or breathing technique (see Chapter 13)
- Removing oneself from interactions or stimuli that may contribute to increased distress (voluntarily taking "time-out")
- Doing something different (e.g., reading, listening to quiet music, watching television)

Milieu and Environmental Interventions

The inpatient environment can be modified proactively to decrease the potential of aggressive and violent behaviors (Box 19.7).

BOX 19.7

Environmental Management: Violence Prevention

DEFINITION

Monitoring and manipulating the physical environment to decrease the potential of violent behavior directed toward self, others, or environment.

ACTIVITIES

- Remove potential weapons (e.g., sharps, ropelike objects) from the environment.
- Search the environment routinely to maintain it as hazard free.
- Search the patient and his or her belongings for weapons or potential weapons during inpatient admission procedures as appropriate.
- Monitor the safety of items that visitors bring to the environment.
- Instruct visitors and other caregivers about relevant patient safety issues.
- Limit patient use of potential weapons (e.g., sharps, ropelike objects).
- Monitor patient during use of potential weapons (e.g., razors).

- Place the patient with potential for self-harm with a roommate to decrease isolation and opportunity to act on self-harm thoughts, as appropriate.
- Assign a single room to the patient with potential for violence toward others.
- Place the patient in a bedroom located near a nursing station.
- Limit access to windows unless they are locked and shatter-proof, as appropriate.
- Lock utility and storage rooms.
- Provide paper dishes and plastic utensils at meals.
- Place the patient in the least restrictive environment that still allows for the necessary level of observation.
- Provide ongoing surveillance of all patient access areas to maintain patient safety and therapeutically intervene, as needed.
- Remove other individuals from the vicinity of a violent or potentially violent patient.
- Maintain a designated safe area (e.g., seclusion room) for patient to be placed when violent.
- Provide plastic, rather than metal, clothes hangers, as appropriate.

Adapted from Bulechek, G., Butcher, H.K., Dochterman, J. M., & Wagner, C. (2012). *Nursing interventions classification (NIC)* (6th ed). St. Louis: Mosby.

Reducing Stimulation

For people whose perceptions or thoughts are disordered from brain damage, degeneration, or other thought-processing difficulties, modification of the environment may be one of the main interventions. The patient with a brain injury, progressive dementia, or distorted vision may be experiencing intense and highly confusing stimulation even though the environment, from the nurse or family's perspective, seems calm and orderly.

Likewise, introducing more structure into a chaotic environment can help decrease the risk for aggressive behavior. It is possible to make stimuli meaningful or to simplify and interpret the environment in many practical ways, such as by identifying people or equipment that may be unfamiliar, providing cues as to what is expected (e.g., posting signs with directions, putting a toothbrush and toothpaste by the sink), and removing or silencing unnecessary stimuli (e.g., turning off paging systems).

Considering the environment from the patient's viewpoint is essential. For instance, if the surroundings are unfamiliar, the patient will need to process more information. Lack of a recognizable pattern or structure further taxes the patient's capacity to encode information. Appropriate interventions include clarifying the meaning and purpose of people and objects in the environment, enhancing the patient's sense of control and the predictability of the environment, and reducing other stimuli as much as possible (Bulechek, Butcher, Dochterman, & Wagner, 2012).

Creating a Culture of Nonviolence

Ultimately, nurses must strive to create cultures of nonviolence. One approach that shows promise is the Violence Prevention Community Meeting (VPCM) pioneered on an acute inpatient psychiatry unit at a veterans' hospital (Lanza, Rierdan, Forester, & Zeiss, 2009). Twice-weekly meetings, lasting 30 minutes, were attended by all patients and staff. Typical topics of discussion were boundary violations, ways of summoning assistance, and ways to air grievances and solve problems. A statistically significant reduction in patient violence resulted from implementation of the VPCM. Another approach illustrating the importance of administrative leadership is the daily interdisciplinary meeting held in the medical director's office at a New Hampshire hospital to review every incident of seclusion and restraint (SR) (Allen, de Nesnera, & Souther, 2009). Direct care staff provide firsthand reports about the incident followed by brainstorming about alternative strategies to be implemented in future incidents of aggressive and violent behavior. Approaches such as these are critical to the achievement of safer and more humane environments for psychiatric care.

Interventions for Managing Imminent Aggression and Violence

De-escalation

Authentic engagement with the patient is the core component in a therapeutic de-escalation by the nurse

(Finfgeld-Connett, 2009). Creative, patient-centered strategies, not techniques of physical restraint, are of paramount importance. Individualizing interventions is also emphasized by researchers Johnson and Delaney (2007); astute staff members realized that some patient behaviors (e.g., loudness, pacing) could be ignored and some "escalating" situations would actually subside without any staff intervention.

De-escalating potential aggression is always preferable to challenging or provoking a patient. De-escalating (commonly known as "talking the person down") is a skill that every nurse can develop. Trying to clarify what has upset the patient is important although not all patients are capable of articulating what provoked them, and some analyses will have to take place after a crisis has been diffused. The nurse can use therapeutic communication techniques to prevent a crisis or diffuse a critical situation (see Box 19.6).

The nurse who works with potentially aggressive patients should do so with respect and concern. The goal is to work with patients to find solutions, approaching these patients calmly, empathizing with the patient's perspective, and avoiding a power struggle. In dealing with aggression, as in other aspects of nursing practice, at times the best intervention is silence. It is easy to equate intervention with activity, the sense that "I must do something." But offering quiet calmness may be enough to help a patient regain control of his or her behavior.

KEYCONCEPT **Intervention fit** The nurse who intervenes from within the context of the therapeutic relationship must be cognizant of the fit of a particular intervention.

Interventions that are appropriate in early phases of escalation differ from those used when the patient's agitation is greater. The patient's affective, behavioral, and cognitive response to an intervention provides information about its effects and guides the nurse's next response (Figure 19.3). The following approaches are important in caring for patients who are aggressive or violent:

- Using nonthreatening body language
- Respecting the patient's personal space and boundaries
- Having immediate access to the door of the room in case you need to leave the room
- Choosing to leave the door open to an office while talking to a patient
- Knowing where colleagues are and making sure those colleagues know where you are
- Removing or not wearing clothing or accessories that could be used to harm you, such as scarves, necklaces, or dangling earrings

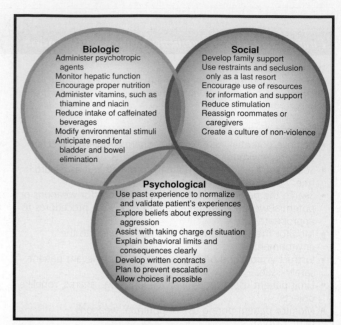

FIGURE 19.3 Biopsychosocial interventions for patients with aggression.

Administering and Monitoring PRN Medications

Patients with the potential for aggression and violence usually have a PRN (as-needed) medication order for agitation and aggression. Bowers et al. (2013), after analyzing multiple episodes of aggression, recommended that nurses use PRN medications more frequently although Smith et al. (2013) have cautioned against overexposing patients to psychotropic medications and/or giving medications for staff convenience. Administering a PRN medication is left to the discretion of the nurse, who makes a judgment about the patient after careful assessment.

Avoiding the Use of Seclusion and Restraint

Seclusion and restraint have been used by nurses when patients need to be separated from other patients on the unit. An integrative literature review by Laiho, Kattainen, Astedt-Kurki, Putkonen, Lindberg, and Kylma (2013) revealed that the decision to use SR is a dynamic process involving evaluation of the risk toward the patient, other patients, and the nurses themselves, as well as the need to maintain a therapeutic milieu.

Moylan (2009), an experienced clinician and researcher, reports that some of her patients verbalized positive feelings of safety after restraints were applied. She asserts that restraint can achieve a therapeutic outcome if no excessive force is used and the nurse conveys concern and respect for the patient throughout the period of confinement. Some patients surveyed by Canadian researchers found SR helpful when they felt out-of-control (Larue, Dumais, Boyer, Goulet, Bonin, & Baba, 2013). However, as noted in Chapter 10, SR are controversial interventions to be used judiciously and only when other interventions have failed to control the patient's behavior.

Recently, there has been recognition that SR interventions may be disproportionately applied to certain types of vulnerable patients, such as those who are deaf or hard of hearing. Hartman and Blalock (2011) found greater prevalence of SR interventions in hearing impaired patients than in a matched group of hearing individuals in a state mental hospital setting. SR interventions may cause considerable psychological damage by replicating childhood traumas. For example, seclusion may be extremely painful to a patient who has already experienced abandonment and rejection. Restraint may recreate trauma comparable to a rape ("They held me down, they pulled my drawers down") (Benson, Secker, Balfe, Lipsedge, Robinson, & Walk, 2003). Physical restraint may also produce injury or even death, due to catecholamine hyperstimulation, positional asphyxia, and/or preexisting medical conditions such as cardiac disease (Duxbury, Aiken, & Dale, 2013). Of 38 restraint-related deaths in the United Kingdom that were analyzed by Duxbury et al., 26 were attributable to asphyxia when the patient was held in a prone position. Supine position can also be problematic. Nurses involved in the physical restraint of patients feel conflicted about having to intervene in this manner, as shown in these excerpts from an interview study: "I felt instantly like a bully. I am awful, you know, look what I have done to this man;" "You kind of feel a bit dirty from the whole experience" (Bigwood & Crowe, 2008).

The controversy over SR interventions and their potential to be applied punitively provided impetus for issuance of federal guidelines for their use. American institutions that receive Medicare or Medicaid reimbursement must adhere to guidelines issued by the Center for Medicare and Medicaid Services. These guidelines specify that a registered nurse must verify the need for restraint or seclusion and then contact the physician or other licensed practitioner; within 1 hour, that practitioner must examine the patient (see Chapter 10). Individual states have also enacted laws to regulate the use of restraints, and professional organizations such as the International Society of Psychiatric-Mental Health Nurses (1999) and the American Psychiatric Nurses Association (2007) have released position statements on restraints as the last resort in an emergency.

Restraint-related injuries and deaths have prompted many facilities to ban their use entirely and train staff in alternative techniques. Examples of restraint-free units can be found in the literature. At one Pennsylvania hospital, the psychiatric unit has been restraint free for 2 years because the staff adopted person-centered, recovery-oriented care principles (Barton, Johnson, & Price, 2009). Although increased use of sedatives might be suspected, there has been a significant decrease in sedative–hypnotic drug administration as well. The old seclusion room was transformed into the Comfort Room and supplied with journaling materials and soothing music. Use of the room is voluntary, unlike staff-mandated "time-outs" or seclusion. Any patient may ask staff to use the room to decrease agitation and anxiety.

Comfort rooms are becoming more widespread, providing an appealing alternative to coercive interventions by unit staff. The majority (92.9%) of patients who used the comfort room at a rural tertiary mental hospital reported that its availability was helpful in reducing their distress (Sivak, 2012). Comfort rooms are more compatible with contemporary philosophies of person-centered, recovery-oriented care (Barton et al., 2009; Sivak, 2012).

Evaluation and Treatment Outcomes

Treatment outcomes can be considered at both individual and aggregate levels. The desired outcome at the individual level is for the patient to regain or maintain control over aggressive or potentially aggressive thoughts, feelings, and actions. The nurse may observe that the patient shows decreased psychomotor activity (e.g., less pacing), has a more relaxed posture, speaks more directly about feelings of anger and personal needs, requires less sedating medication, shows increased tolerance for frustration and the ability to consider alternatives, and makes effective use of other coping strategies.

Evidence of a reduction in risk factors in the treatment setting include decreased noise and confusion in the immediate environment; calmness on the part of nursing staff and others; and a climate of safety, clear expectations, and mutual acceptance and respect. In units, day hospitals, or group home settings, indicators of positive treatment outcomes include a reduction in the number and severity of assaults on staff and other patients, fewer incident reports, and increased staff competency in de-escalating potentially violent situations.

Examination of the interactions of the aggressor, victim, and environment has been proposed by Lanza and colleagues to get a complete picture of the incident (Lanza, Zeiss, & Rierdan, 2009). In the 360-degree interview, the incident becomes the center of a Venn diagram (Figure 19.4), and the victim, the assailant, supervisor, and coworkers are asked by a neutral party for information on the assault. All relevant participants may be asked to provide their perspective. This approach allows for a collaborative, community approach to preventing patient violence and avoids blaming one assailant for incidents that are provoked by a variety of contextual and interpersonal factors.

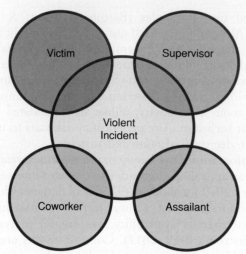

FIGURE 19.4 Application of 360-degree interviewing to a violent incident. (Redrawn with permission from Lanza, M. L., Zeiss, R. A., & Rierdan, J. [2009]. Multiple perspectives on assault: The 360-degree interview. *Journal of the American Psychiatric Nurses Association*, *14*[6], 413–420.)

Responding to Assault on Nurses

Because nurses have extended contact with patients during highly stressful circumstances, there is always the risk that they may be the recipients of patient aggression. Nurses and nurses' aides are the targets of patient violence more often than any other health care professionals (Janocha & Smith, 2010), and psychiatric nurses report higher rates of assault than nurses in other specialties (Hartley & Ridenour, 2011).

Assaults on nurses by patients can have both immediate and long-term consequences, as shown in Lanza's seminal research (1992) (Table 19.3). Reported assaults range from verbal abuse or threats and minor altercations to severe injuries, rape, and murder. Any assault can produce severe sequelae for the victim, including PTSD (Jacobowitz, 2013). After a violent incident, nurses struggle with their inclination to avoid the patient, and they watch for any signs of patient remorse; their response differs if the violent behavior was attributable to psychosis versus manipulative or volitional acting out (Zuzelo et al., 2012). Because of their role as caregivers, nurses may suppress the normal range of feelings after an assault, believing that it is wrong to experience strong feelings of anger and fear in this situation. This belief may relate to the conflict nurses experience in having to care for patients who have hurt them. The conflict between one's professional role as caregiver and one's own needs as an assault victim has been explored in a support group for nurses and nursing assistants who had been assaulted (Lanza, Demaio, & Benedict, 2005). The support group met twice per week for 6 weeks, allowing expression of anger, blame, and anxiety and concluding with develop-

Table 19.3	NURSES' RESPONSES TO ASSAULT	
Response Type	**Personal**	**Professional**
Affective	• Irritability • Depression • Anger • Anxiety • Apathy	• Erosion of feelings of competence, leading to increased anxiety and fear • Feelings of guilt or self-blame • Fear of potentially violent patients
Cognitive	• Suppressed or intrusive thoughts of assault	• Reduced confidence in judgment • Consideration of job change
Behavioral	• Social withdrawal	• Possible hesitation in responding to other violent situations • Possible overcontrolling • Possible hesitation to report future assaults • Possible withdrawal from colleagues • Questioning of capabilities by coworkers
Physiologic	• Disturbed sleep • Headaches • Stomach aches • Tension	• Increased absenteeism because of somatic complaints

ment of personal plans for working with potentially assaultive patients.

Unfortunately, patient aggression directed toward nurses is often minimized or tolerated by nurses as "part of the job" (Poster & Drew, 2006). Nurses seldom report attacks to the police or prosecute their attackers. Aggression by patients must be addressed more vigorously because it can threaten the other patients, other health care professionals, family members, and visitors, as well as the nursing staff. Reporting violent attacks increases public awareness and increases the likelihood that protective legislation will be enacted (Haun, 2013). Steps must be taken by institutions to reduce the incidence of patient assault. The environment should be modified with the addition of security alarms, video monitors, and de-escalation teams.

All nurses must be provided with training programs in the prevention and management of aggressive behavior. These programs, similar to courses on cardiopulmonary resuscitation (CPR), impart both knowledge and skills. Similar to CPR training, the courses need to be made available to nurses regularly, so that they have opportunities to reinforce and update what they have learned. Research shows that nurses who have participated in preventive training programs as students or as professionals become more confident in coping with patient aggression

(Jacobowitz, 2013). Jacobowitz recommends resilience-building sessions in which workers meet with a trained facilitator every 4 to 6 weeks. Some states have enacted legislation mandating workplace violence prevention programs, but the curricula vary, and the quality of training lacks systematic evaluation (Peek-Asa et al., 2009). Commercially marketed training programs have been criticized because they fail to consider the predatory aspect of some patients' violence and fail to cite nursing research.

RESEARCH AND POLICY INITIATIVES

Additional understanding of the phenomena of anger, aggression, and violence as they occur in the clinical setting is needed. Research studies that have illuminated this problem from a nursing perspective need to be continued and expanded. The links among biology, neurology, and psychology must be further elucidated. In addition, further explorations of the reciprocal influence of patient interactional style and treatment setting culture assist in the development and management of humane treatment settings. Finally, and perhaps most importantly, nurses must research the effectiveness of particular anger and aggression management interventions. Interventions aimed at specific populations, such as adolescent girls in residential placements, are being developed; however, outcomes have not yet been evaluated in randomized controlled trials (Goldstein et al., 2013).

Although much of this chapter focused on individuals who need to *down*regulate anger, the reader must remember that anger suppressors have a need to *up*regulate their anger and express it more assertively. Treatments should be tailored accordingly and patients' progress documented by administering questionnaires such as the STAXI both before and after the treatments. Feindler (2006) edited a useful practitioner's guide to comparative treatments of anger-related disorders. However, authors in this edited volume cautioned that research is sparse regarding the efficacy of some treatments, especially for culturally diverse clients whose heritage is quite different from the Euro-American heritage of most mental health clinicians in the United States. Thomas (2006) has pointed out the inadequacy of most training programs in preparing mental health professionals for work with culturally diverse clients. It is unknown what adaptations may be needed to deliver appropriate anger treatments to these individuals. Only by accruing sufficient empirical evidence can we obtain definitive guidance for clinical practice with angry and aggressive individuals.

There is a moral imperative for nurses to be involved in combating violence in the larger community. Lessening anger and violence in the workplace and the home demands involvement of all mental health professionals. Nurses can share their expertise with parents, children, teachers, and community agencies. Nurses are well positioned to teach health-promoting anger management classes in diverse practice settings, such as outpatient clinics, schools, and corporate sites. Classes for children and adolescents can be of great benefit because young people are forming the anger habits that will continue into adulthood (Puskar, Stark, Northcut, Williams, & Haley, 2011; Thomas, 2001).

Compelling scientific evidence is now available to show that violence portrayed in the media is harmful to children. As a result, television networks limit violent programming during hours when children are generally watching programs. However, this gain is offset by the growing availability of violent websites and videogames. Videogames actively involve players in violence and reward them for it. Nurses can add their voices to those of activists who object to the content of these games and to offensive media offerings. As concerned citizens, nurses can advocate for changes in public policy such as those recommended by the World Health Organization (2009) in its *Violence Prevention: The Evidence*.

Finally, nurses can support legislation to make assault on nurses a felony, similar to assault on lifeguards, bus drivers, jurors, umpires, and emergency medical technicians. Such legislation is in place in less than half of the United States. A vital first step is increased reporting of assaults because 80% are never reported (Haun, 2013). Nurses who provide indispensable services in the nation's psychiatric units, emergency rooms, and other settings deserve to be safe from violence in the enactment of their daily work.

SUMMARY OF KEY POINTS

- Anger is an emotional state, usually temporary, that can be expressed constructively or destructively. Destructive anger alienates other people and invites retaliation.

- Anger, aggression, and violence should not be viewed as a continuum. The anger of ordinary people seldom progresses to aggression or violence. Anger does not necessarily lead to aggression or violence.

- Anger management is a useful psychoeducational intervention that is effective with a wide variety of nonviolent individuals. However, anger management is not designed to modify violent behavior.

- Several theories explain anger, aggression, and violence and include neurobiologic and psychosocial theories. These theories serve as the basis of assessment and interventions.

■ The general aggression model accounts for the interaction of cognition, affect, and arousal during an aggressive episode.

■ There is no one factor that predicts aggression or violence. Factors that have been observed to be precursors are staring and eye contact, tone and volume of voice, anxiety, mumbling, and pacing.

■ Nursing interventions can be affective, cognitive, behavioral, or sociocultural. A therapeutic milieu supports a nonviolent culture.

■ If a violent incident occurs, using a 360-degree evaluation approach will help in understanding the interpersonal and contextual factors that led to the incident.

■ Seclusion or restraints should be used only as a last resort.

■ Patient aggression and violence are serious concerns for nurses in all areas of clinical practice. Training in and policies and procedures for the prevention and management of aggressive episodes should be available in all work settings.

CRITICAL THINKING CHALLENGES

1. Mary Jane, a 24-year-old single woman, has just been admitted to an inpatient psychiatry unit. She was transferred to the unit from the emergency department where she was treated for a drug overdose. She is sullen when she is introduced to her roommate and refuses to answer the questions the nurse has that are part of the admission procedure. The nurse tells Mary Jane that he will come back later to see how she is. A few minutes later, Mary Jane approaches the nursing station and asks in a demanding tone to talk with someone and complains that she has been completely ignored since she came into the unit. What frameworks can the nurse use to understand Mary Jane's behavior? At this point in time, what data does he have to develop a plan of care? What interventions might the nurse choose to use to help Mary Jane behave in a manner that is consistent with the norms of this inpatient unit?

2. Discuss the influence of gender and cultural norms on the expression of anger. When a nurse is caring for a patient from a culture that the nurse is not familiar with, what could the nurse ask to ensure that her or his expectations of the patient's behavior are consistent with the gender and cultural norms of the patient?

3. Under what circumstances should people who are aggressive or violent be held accountable for their behavior? Are there any exceptions?

4. When a nurse minimizes verbally abusive behavior by a patient, family member, or health care colleague, what implicit message does she or he send?

MOVIES *Mandela: Long Walk to Freedom:* 2013. South African icon Nelson Mandela displays the gamut of angry behaviors in this biographical epic: (1) righteous anger on behalf of his clients when he was a young lawyer; (2) fiery anger at the cruel persecution of blacks during apartheid; and (3) violence against the government after the failure of nonviolent protests to achieve freedom from oppression. Bomb throwing at government buildings results in 27 years of imprisonment, which could have created lasting bitterness against his oppressors. Yet after his release Mandela forgives those who had imprisoned him, becomes the first black president of his country, and receives the Nobel Peace Prize. This remarkable true story provides many lessons for all of us.

VIEWING POINTS: Although most of us will never be forced to endure such intolerable conditions, we all experience times of unfair or unkind treatment. How can we learn to use our anger productively or learn to let it go by forgiving those who wronged us?

References

Allen, D. E., deNesnera, A., & Souther, J. W. (2009). Executive-level reviews of seclusion and restraint promote interdisciplinary collaboration and innovation. *Journal of the American Psychiatric Nurses Association, 15*, 260–264.

American Nurses Association, & Nursing World. (2012). Workplace violence. Retrieved from www.nursingworld.org

American Psychiatric Association (APA). (2013). *Diagnostic and Statistical Manual of Mental Disorders DSM-5.* Arlington, VA: Author.

American Psychiatric Nurses Association. (2007). *2007 Position Statement on the Use of Seclusion and Restraint.* Arlington, VA: Author.

Anderson, C. A., & Anderson, K. B. (2008). Men who target women: specificity of target, generality of aggressive behavior. *Aggressive Behavior, 34*(6), 605–622.

Audenaert, K. (2013). Neurobiology of aggressive behavior: About wild horses and reins. *Proceedings of the 8th European congress on violence in clinical psychiatry* (pp. 44). Amsterdam: Kavanah.

Averill, J. R. (1983). Studies on anger and aggression: Implications for theories of emotion. *American Psychologist, 38*, 1145–1160.

Bandura, A. (2001). Social cognitive theory: An agentic perspective. *Annual Review of Psychology, 52*, 1–26.

Barton, S. A., Johnson, M. R., & Price, L. V. (2009). Achieving restraint-free on an inpatient behavioral health unit. *Journal of Psychosocial Nursing, 47*(1), 35–40.

Bennett, P., & Lowe, R. (2008). Emotions and their cognitive precursors: Responses to spontaneously identify stressful events among hospital nurses. *Journal of Health Psychology, 13*(4), 537–546.

Benson, A., Secker, I., Balfe, E., Lipsedge, M., Robinson, S., & Walker, J. (2003). Discourse of blame: Accounting for aggression and violence on an acute mental health inpatient unit. *Social Science and Medicine, 57*, 917–926.

Bigwood, S., & Crowe, M. (2008). "It's part of the job, but it spoils the job:" A phenomenological study of physical restraint. *International Journal of Mental Health Nursing, 17*, 215–222.

Bowers, L., James, K., Quirk, A., Wright, S., Williams, H., & Stewart, D. (2013). Identification of the "minimal triangle" and other common event-to-event transitions in conflict and containment incidents. *Issues in Mental Health Nursing, 34*, 514–523.

Bremner, R. H., Koole, S. L., & Bushman, B. J. (2011). "Pray for those who mistreat you": Effects of prayer on anger and aggression. *Personality and Social Psychology Bulletin, 37*, 830–837.

Bulechek, G., Butcher, H. K., Dochterman, J. M., & Wagner, C. (2012). *Nursing interventions classification (NIC)* (6th ed). St. Louis: Mosby.

Burns, J. W., Quartana, P., & Bruehl, S. (2011). Anger suppression and subsequent pain behaviors among chronic low back pain patients: Moderating effects of anger regulation style. *Annals of Behavioral Medicine, 42*, 42–54.

Carlsson, G., Dahlberg, K., Ekeburgh, M., & Dahlberg, H. (2006). Patients longing for authentic personal care: A phenomenological study of violent encounters in psychiatric settings. *Issues in Mental Health Nursing, 27*, 287–305.

Coccaro, E. F. (2012). Intermittent explosive disorder as a disorder of impulsive aggression for DSM-5. *American Journal of Psychiatry, 196*, 577–588.

Davidson, K., & Mostofsky, E. (2010). Anger expression and risk of coronary heart disease: Evidence from the Nova Scotia Health survey. *American Heart Journal, 159*(2), 199–206.

Deffenbacher, J. L. (2011). Cognitive-behavioral conceptualization and treatment of anger. *Cognitive and Behavioral Practice, 18*, 212–221.

deSchutter, M., & Lodewijkx, H. (2013). Psychiatric patients need a more active role in managing their own aggression. *Proceedings of the 8th European congress on violence in clinical psychiatry* (pp. 219–223). Amsterdam: Kavanah.

Duxbury, J., Aiken, F., & Dale, C. (2013). A review of theories of restraint-related deaths in the UK. *Proceedings of the 8th European congress on violence in clinical psychiatry* (pp. 46–50). Amsterdam: Kavanah.

Everson-Rose, S. A., & Lewis, T. T. (2005). Psychosocial factors and cardiovascular diseases. *Annual Review of Public Health, 26*, 469–500.

Farrell, G. A., Shafiei, T., & Salmon, P. (2010). Facing up to "challenging behavior": A model for training in staff-client interaction. *Journal of Advanced Nursing, 66*(7), 1644–1655.

Feindler, E. L. (2006). *Anger-related disorders: A practitioner's guide to comparative treatments*. New York: Springer.

Feindler, E. L., & Byers, A. (2006). Multiple perspectives on the conceptualization and treatment of anger-related disorders. In E. L. Feindler (Ed.), *Anger-related disorders: A practitioner's guide to comparative treatments* (pp. 303–320). New York: Springer.

Finfgeld-Connett, D. (2009). Model of therapeutic and non-therapeutic responses to patient aggression. *Issues in Mental Health Nursing, 30*(9), 530–537.

Fluttert, F., Van Meijel, B., Webster, C., Nijman, H., Bartels, A., & Grypdonck, M. (2008). Risk management by early recognition of warning signs in patients in forensic psychiatric care. *Archives of Psychiatric Nursing, 22*, 208–216.

Glenn, A. L., & Raine, A. (2008). The neurobiology of psychopathy. *Psychiatric Clinics of North America, 31*(3), 463–475.

Goldstein, N., Kemp, K., Leff, S., & Lochman, J. (2012). Guidelines for adapting manualized interventions for new target populations: A stepwise approach to using anger management as a model. *Clinical Psychology: Science, Practice, and Culture, 19*, 385–401.

Goldstein, N. E. S., Serico, J. M., Riggs Romaine, C. L., Zelechoski, A., Kalbeitzer, R., Kemp, K., et al. (2013). Development of the juvenile justice anger management treatment for girls. *Cognitive and Behavioral Practice, 20*, 171–188.

Gouin, J., Kiecolt-Glaser, J. K., Malarkey, W. B., & Glaser, R. (2008). The influence of anger expression on wound healing. *Brain, Behavior, and Immunity, 22*, 699–708.

Gross, R., Groer, M., & Thomas, S. P. (in press). Relationship of trait anger and anger expression to C-reactive protein in post-menopausal women. *Health Care for Women International*.

Hamrin, V., Iennaco, J., & Olsen, D. (2009). A review of ecological factors affecting inpatient psychiatric unit violence: Implications for relational and unit cultural improvements. *Issues in Mental Health Nursing, 30*, 214–226.

Harris, D., & Morrison, E. F. (1995). Managing violence without coercion. *Archives of Psychiatric Nursing, 9*(4), 203–210.

Hartley, D., & Ridenour, M. (2011). Workplace violence in the healthcare setting. National Institute for Occupational Safety and Health. Retrieved from www.medscape.com/view article/749441

Hartman, B., & Blalock, M. (2011). Comparison of seclusion and restraint prevalence between hearing patients and deaf or hard of hearing patients in a state hospital setting. *Issues in Mental Health Nursing, 32*, 42–45.

Haun, P. (2013). It's time to report workplace violence. *Tennessee Nurse, 76*(4), 12.

International Society of Psychiatric-Mental Health Nurses. (1999). *Position statement on the use of restraint and seclusion*. Philadelphia: Author.

Jacobowitz, W. (2013). PTSD in psychiatric nurses and other mental health providers: A review of the literature. *Issues in Mental Health Nursing, 34*, 787–795.

Jarry, J., & Paivio, S. (2006). Emotion-focused therapy for anger. In E. L. Feindler (Ed.), *Anger-related disorders: A practitioner's guide to comparative treatments* (pp. 203–229). New York: Springer.

Janocha, J. A., & Smith, R. T. (2010). *Workplace safety and health in the health care and social assistance industry, 2003–07*. Washington, DC: U.S. Bureau of Labor Statistics. Retrieved March 25, 2011, from http://www.bls.gov.opub/cwc.sh20100825ar01pl.htm

Johnson, A. (2012). Forgiveness: Moving from anger and shame to self-love. *Psychiatric Services, 63*, 311–312.

Johnson, M. E. (2004). Violence on inpatient psychiatric units: State of the science. *Journal of the American Psychiatric Nurses Association, 10*(3), 113–121.

Johnson, M. E., & Delaney, K. R. (2006). Keeping the unit safe: A grounded theory study. *Journal of the American Psychiatric Nurses Association, 12*(1), 13–21.

Johnson, M. E., & Delaney, K. R. (2007). Keeping the unit safe: The anatomy of escalation. *Journal of the American Psychiatric Nurses Association, 13*, 42–52.

Kessler, R., Coccaro, E., Fava, M., Jaeger, S., Jin, R., & Walters, E. (2006). The prevalence and correlates of DSM-IV intermittent explosive disorder in the National Comorbidity Survey replication. *Archives of General Psychiatry, 63*, 669–678.

Ketterer, M., Rose, B., Knysz, W., Farha, A., Deveshwar, S., Schairer, J., et al. (2011). Is social isolation/alienation confounded with, and non-independent of emotional distress in its association with early onset of coronary artery disease? *Psychology, Health, & Medicine, 16*(2), 238–247.

Kuepper, Y., Alexander, N., Osinsky, R., Kozyra, E., Schmitz, A., Netter, P., et al. (2010). Aggression—interactions of serotonin and testosterone in healthy men and women. *Behavior Brain Research, 206*(1), 93–100.

Kusmierska, G. (2012). Do anger management treatments help angry adults? A meta-analytic answer. *Dissertation Abstracts International; Section B: The Sciences and Engineering, 72*(12B), 7689.

Laiho, T., Kattainen, E., Astedt-Kurki, P., Putkonen, H., Lindberg, N., & Kylma, J. (2013). Clinical decision-making involved in secluding and restraining an adult psychiatric patient: An integrative literature review. *Journal of Psychiatric and Mental Health Nursing, 20*, 830–839.

Lanza, M. L. (1992). Nurses as patient assault victims: An update, synthesis, and recommendations. *Archives of Psychiatric Nursing, 6*(3), 163–171.

Lanza, M. L., Demaio, J., & Benedict, M. A. (2005). Patient assault support group: Achieving educational objectives. *Issues in Mental Health Nursing, 26*, 643–660.

Lanza, M. L., Rierdan, J., Forester, L., & Zeiss, R. A. (2009). Reducing violence against nurses: The Violence Prevention Community Meeting. *Issues in Mental Health Nursing*.

Lanza, M. L., Zeiss, R. A., & Rierdan, J. (2009). Multiple perspectives on assault: The 360-degree interview. *Journal of the American Psychiatric Nurses Association, 14*(6), 413–420.

Larue, C., Dumais, A., Boyer, R., Goulet, M-H., Bonin, J-P., & Baba, N. (2013). The experience of seclusion and restraint in psychiatric settings: Perspectives of patients. *Issues in Mental Health Nursing, 34*, 317–324.

Lemay, E. P., Overall, N. C., & Clark, M. S. (2012). Experiences and interpersonal consequences of hurt feelings and anger. *Journal of Personality and Social Psychology, 103*, 982–1006.

Liu, J. (2011). Early health risk factors for violence: Conceptualization, review of the evidence and implications. *Aggression & Violent Behaviors, 16*(1), 63–73.

Luck, L., Jackson, D., & Usher, K. (2007). STAMP: Components of observable behavior that indicate potential for patient violence in emergency departments. *Journal of Advanced Nursing, 59*, 11–19.

Martin, C. A., Cook, C., Woodring, J. H., Burkhardt, G., Omar, H. A., & Kelly, T. H. (2008). Caffeine use: Association with nicotine use, aggression, and other psychopathology in psychiatric and pediatric outpatient adolescents. *The Scientific World Journal, 8*, 512–516.

McCloskey, M. S., Noblett, K. L., Deffenbacher, J. L., Gollan, J. K., & Coccaro, E. F. (2008). Cognitive-behavioral therapy for intermittent explosive disorder: A pilot randomized trial. *Journal of Consulting and Clinical Psychology, 76*, 876–886.

Mefford, L., Thomas, S. P., Callen, B., & Groer, M. (in press). Religiousness-spirituality and anger management in community-dwelling older persons. *Issues in Mental Health Nursing*.

Mostofsky, E., Maclure, M., Tofler, G., Muller, J., & Mittleman, M. (2013). Relation of outbursts of anger and risk of acute myocardial infarction. *American Journal of Cardiology*. Retrieved from www.ajconline.org

Moylan, L. B. (2009). Physical restraint in acute care psychiatry: A humanistic and realistic nursing approach. *Journal of Psychosocial Nursing, 47*(3), 41–47.

NANDA International. (2012). *Nursing diagnoses: Definitions and classification 2012–2014.* Chichester, UK: Wiley Blackwell.

Palazzolo, K. E., Roberto, A. J., & Babin, E. A. (2010). The relationship between parents' verbal aggression and young adult children's intimate partner violence victimization and perpetration. *Health Communication, 25*(4), 357–364.

Peek-Asa, C., Casteel, C., Allareddy, V., Nocera, M., Goldmacher, S., Ohagan, E., et al. (2009). Workplace prevention programs in psychiatric units and facilities. *Archives of Psychiatric Nursing, 23*, 166–176.

Perugi, G., Fornaro, M., & Akiskal, H. S. (2011). Are atypical depression, borderline personality disorder and bipolar II disorder overlapping manifestations of a common cyclothymic diathesis? *World Psychiatry, 10*(1), 45–51.

Pittman, C. T. (2011). Getting mad but ending up sad: The mental health consequences for African Americans using anger to cope with racism. *Journal of Black Studies, 42*, 1106–1124.

Potpara, T. S., & Lip, G.Y. (2011). Lone atrial fibrillation: What is known and what is to come. *International Journal Clinical Practice, 65*(4), 446–457.

Poster, L., & Drew, B. (2006). Presidents' message. *American Psychiatric Nurses Association News, 18*(4), 2–3.

Puskar, K. R., Stark, K. H., Northcut, T., Williams, R., & Haley, T. (2011). Teaching kids to cope with anger: Peer education. *Journal of Child Health Care, 15*(1):5–13.

Rubin, T. I. (1970). *The angry book.* New York: Collier.

Siever, L. J. (2008). Neurobiology of aggression and violence. *American Journal of Psychiatry, 165*(4), 429–442.

Sivak, K. (2012). Implementation of comfort rooms to reduce seclusion, restraint use, and acting-out behaviors. *Journal of Psychiatric Nursing and Mental Health Services, 50*(2), 24–34.

Smith, G., Davis, R., Altenor, A., Tran, D. P., Wolfe, K. L., Deegan, J. A., et al. (2013). Psychiatric use of unscheduled medications in the Pennsylvania State Hospital System: Effects of discontinuing the use of PRN

orders. *Proceedings of the 8th European congress on violence in clinical psychiatry* (pp. 137). Amsterdam: Kavanah.

Spielberger, C. D. (1999). *Manual for the State Trait Anger Expression Inventory-2.* Odessa, FL: Psychological Assessment Resources.

Thomas, S. A., & González-Prendes, A. A. (2009). Powerlessness, anger, and stress in African American women: Implications for physical and emotional health. *Health Care for Women International, 30*(1–2), 93–113.

Thomas, S. P. (1990). Theoretical and empirical perspectives on anger. *Issues in Mental Health Nursing, 11*, 203–216.

Thomas, S. P. (1997a). Women's anger: Relationship of suppression to blood pressure. *Nursing Research, 46*, 324–330.

Thomas, S. P. (1997b). Angry? Let's talk about it! *Applied Nursing Research, 10*(2), 80–85.

Thomas, S. P. (1998). Assessing and intervening with anger disorders. *Nursing Clinics of North America, 33*(1), 121–133.

Thomas, S. P. (2001). Teaching healthy anger management. *Perspectives in Psychiatric Care, 37*(2), 41–48.

Thomas, S. P. (2005). Women's anger, aggression, and violence. *Health Care for Women International, 26*, 504–522.

Thomas, S. P. (2006). Cultural and gender considerations in the assessment and treatment of anger-related disorders. In E. L. Feindler (Ed.), *Anger-related disorders: A practitioner's guide to comparative treatments* (pp. 71–95). New York: Springer.

Thomas, S. P. (2009). *Transforming nurses' stress and anger* (3rd ed) New York: Springer.

Thomas, S. P., & Pollio, H. R. (2002). *Listening to patients.* New York: Springer.

Thomas, S. P., Shattell, M., & Martin, T. (2002). What's therapeutic about the therapeutic milieu? *Archives of Psychiatric Nursing, 16*(3), 99–107.

Williams, K. M., & Herman, R. E. (2011). Linking resident behavior to dementia care communication: Effects of emotional tone. *Behavior Therapy, 42*(1), 42–46.

World Health Organization. (2009). *Preventing violence: The evidence.* Geneva, Switzerland: Author.

Zuzelo, P., Curran, S., & Zeserman, M. (2012). Registered nurses' and behavior health associates' responses to violent inpatient interactions on behavioral health units. *Journal of the American Psychiatric Nurses Association, 18*(2), 112–126.

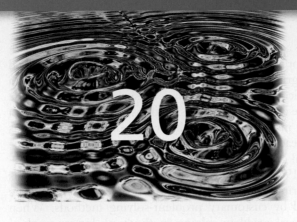

20

Crisis, Grief, and Disaster Management

Mary Ann Boyd

KEY CONCEPTS

- bereavement
- crisis
- grief
- disaster

LEARNING OBJECTIVES

After studying this chapter, you will be able to:

1. Describe the types of crises.

2. Differentiate between grief and bereavement.

3. Compare models of bereavement.

4. Discuss nursing management for persons experiencing crises, grief, and disaster.

5. Evaluate the effects of the crisis or disaster experience on lifestyle and survival.

6. Explain the psychological impact of disaster on victims of catastrophic events.

Successfully surviving crises and disaster may make a difference between being mentally healthy or mentally ill. This chapter explores the concepts of crisis, grief, and disaster management; broadens the scope and understanding of the responses of persons to crisis, loss, and disaster situations; and describes how the nursing process can be used to care for persons experiencing these events.

CRISIS

Adaptation and coping are a natural part of life (see Chapter 18). Crisis occurs when there is a perceived challenge or threat that overwhelms the capacity of the individual to cope effectively with the event. Life is disrupted, and unexpected emotional (e.g., depression) and biologic

(e.g., nausea, vomiting, diarrhea, headaches) responses occur. Functioning is severely impaired.

> **KEYCONCEPT** **Crisis** is a time-limited event that triggers adaptive or non-adaptive responses to maturational, situational, or traumatic experiences. A crisis results from stressful events for which coping mechanisms fail to provide adequate adaptive skills to address the perceived challenge or threat.

A crisis occurs when an individual is at a breaking point. A crisis is a turning point with either positive or negative outcomes. If positive, there is an opportunity for growth and change as new ways of coping are learned. If negative, suicide, homelessness, or depression can result. A crisis generally lasts no more than 4 to 6 weeks. At the end of that time, the person in crisis should have begun to come to grips with the event and begin to harness resources to cope with its long-term consequences. By definition, there is no such thing as a chronic crisis. People who live in constant turmoil are not in crisis but in chaos.

Many events evoke a crisis, such as natural disasters (e.g., floods, tornadoes, earthquakes) and human-made disasters (e.g., wars, bombings, airplane crashes) as well as traumatic experiences (e.g., rape, sexual abuse, assault). In addition, interpersonal events (divorce, marriage, birth of a child) create crises in the lives of any person.

Feelings of fear, desperation, and being out of control are common during a crisis, but the precipitating event and circumstances are unusual or rare, perceived as a threat, and specific to the individual. For example, a disagreement with a family member may escalate into a crisis for one person, but not another (Lyons, Hopley, Burton, & Horrocks, 2009). If the person is significantly distressed or social functioning is impaired, a diagnosis of acute stress disorder should be considered (American Psychiatric Association [APA], 2013). The person with an acute stress disorder has dissociative symptoms and persistently reexperiences the event (APA; see Chapter 26).

Historical Perspectives of Crisis

The basis of our understanding of a crisis began in the 1940s when Eric Lindemann (1944) studied bereavement reactions among the friends and relatives of the victims of the Cocoanut [sic] Grove nightclub fire in Boston in 1942. That fire, in which 493 people died, was the worst single building fire in the country's history at that time. Lindemann's goal was to develop prevention approaches at the community level that would maintain good health and prevent emotional disorganization. He described both grief and prolonged reactions as a result of loss of a significant person. He hypothesized that during the course of one's life, some situations, such as the birth of a child, marriage, and death, evoke adaptive mechanisms that lead either to mastery of a new situation (psychological growth) or impaired functioning.

In 1961, psychiatrist Gerald Caplan defined a crisis as occurring when a person faces a problem that cannot be solved by customary problem-solving methods. When the usual problem-solving methods no longer work, a person's life balance or equilibrium is upset. During the period of disequilibrium, there is a rise in inner tension and anxiety followed by emotional upset and an inability to function. This conceptualization of phases of a crisis is used today (Figure 20.1). According to Caplan, during a crisis, a person is open to learning new ways of coping to survive. The outcome of a crisis is governed by the kind of interaction that occurs between the person and available key social support systems.

Types of Crises

Research has focused on categorizing types of crisis events, understanding biopsychosocial responses to a crisis, and developing intervention models that support people through a crisis.

Developmental Crisis

While Lindemann and Caplan were creating their crisis model, Erik Erikson was formulating his ideas about crisis and development. He proposed that maturational

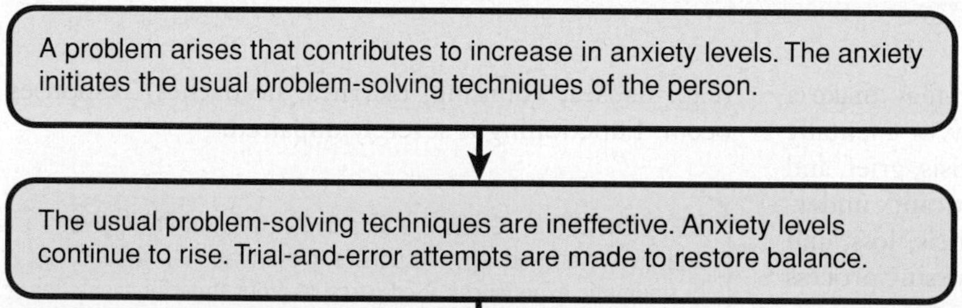

A problem arises that contributes to increase in anxiety levels. The anxiety initiates the usual problem-solving techniques of the person.

The usual problem-solving techniques are ineffective. Anxiety levels continue to rise. Trial-and-error attempts are made to restore balance.

The trial-and-error attempts fail. The anxiety escalates to severe or panic levels. The person adopts automatic relief behaviors.

When these measures do not reduce anxiety, anxiety can overwhelm the person and lead to serious personality disorganization, which signals the person is in crisis.

FIGURE 20.1 Phases of crisis.

crises are a normal part of growth and development and that successfully resolving a crisis at one stage allows the child to move to the next. According to this model, the child develops positive characteristics after experiencing a crisis. If he or she develops less desirable traits, the crisis is not resolved (see Chapter 7). The concept of **developmental crisis** continues to be used today to describe significant maturational events, such as leaving home for the first time, completing school, and accepting the responsibility of adulthood.

Situational Crisis

A **situational crisis** occurs whenever a specific stressful event threatens a person's biopsychosocial integrity and results in some degree of psychological disequilibrium. The event can be an internal one, such as a disease process, or any number of external threats. A move to another city, a job promotion, or graduation from high school can initiate a crisis even though they are positive events. Graduation from high school marks the end of an established routine of going to school, participating in school activities, and doing homework assignments. When starting a new job after graduation, the former student must learn an entirely different routine and acquire new knowledge and skills. If a person enters a new situation without adequate coping skills, a crisis may occur.

Traumatic Crisis

A **traumatic crisis** is initiated by unexpected, unusual events that can affect an individual or a multitude of people. In such situations, people face overwhelmingly hazardous events that entail injury, trauma, destruction, or sacrifice. Examples of events include national disasters (e.g., racial persecutions, riots, war), violent crimes (e.g., rape, murder, kidnappings, and assault and battery), and environmental disasters (e.g., earthquakes, floods, forest fires, hurricanes).

Grief and Bereavement

One of the most common crisis-provoking events is the death of a loved one. Although death is a certainty, much is unknown about the process of death. Fear of the unknown contributes to the mystique of death for the person who is dying, as well as the loved ones. The terms *grief* and *bereavement* are sometimes used interchangeably, but in this text, they are differentiated with grief being an intense biopsychosocial reaction and bereavement being the actual process of mourning and coping. Normally, the death of a loved one produces feelings of grief. Any subsequent loss can also reactivate these feelings.

> **KEYCONCEPT**   **Grief** is an intense, emotional reaction to the loss of a loved one. The reaction is a biopsychosocial response that often includes spontaneous expression of pain, sadness, and desolation. **Bereavement** is the process of mourning and coping with the loss of a loved one. It begins immediately after the loss, but it can last months or years. Individual differences and cultural practices influence grieving and bereavement.

Coping with Loss

Stage Theories

There has been wide acceptance that grief and bereavement follow stages (Bowlby & Parkes, 1970; Kubler-Ross, 1969). See Box 20.1. Although over time, the stage theory of grief and bereavement has been challenged and remains unsupported by empirical evidence today, it continues to be used by health care professionals.

Dual Process Model

The **dual process model** (DPM) offers another explanation of how grieving persons come to terms with their loss over time (Stroebe, Schut, & Boerner, 2010). According to DPM, the person adjusts to the loss by oscillating between **loss-oriented coping** (preoccupation with the deceased) and **restoration-oriented coping** (preoccupation with stressful events as a result of the death including financial issues, new identity as a widow[er]). **Oscillation** is the process of confronting (loss-oriented coping) and avoiding (restoration-oriented coping) the stresses associated with bereavement. At times, the bereaved person is confronted with the loss and memories, and at other times, the persons will be distracted and the thoughts and memories will be avoided. The bereaved experiences relief from the intense emotion associated with the loss by focusing on other things. For example, the bereaved person may be recalling a special moment in the relationship such as a wedding or imagining what the person would

---

BOX 20.1

Stages of Grief and Bereavement

1. *Shock:* denial and disbelief
2. *Acute mourning*
   a. Intense feeling states
   b. Social withdrawal
   c. Identification with the deceased
3. *Resolution:* acceptance of loss, awareness of having grieved, return to well-being, and ability to recall the deceased without subjective pain

Adapted from Zisook, S. (1987). Unresolved grief. In S. Zisook (Ed.), *Biopsychosocial aspects of bereavement* (p. 25). Washington, DC: American Psychiatric Press.

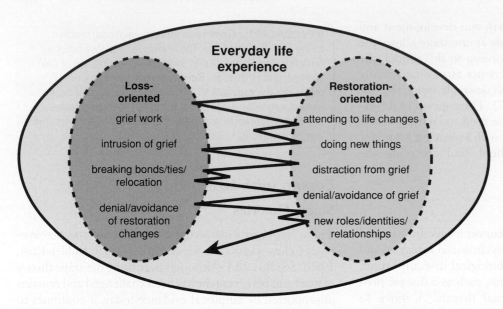

Everyday life experience

Loss-oriented
- grief work
- intrusion of grief
- breaking bonds/ties/relocation
- denial/avoidance of restoration changes

Restoration-oriented
- attending to life changes
- doing new things
- distraction from grief
- denial/avoidance of grief
- new roles/identities/relationships

FIGURE 20.2 Dual process model of coping with bereavement. (Redrawn from Stroebe, M., & Schut, H. [1999]. The dual process model of coping with bereavement: Rationale and description. *Death Studies*, 23, 213. Used with permission from Taylor & Francis Group.)

say about a current event but then switches to thinking about completing tasks that the deceased had previously undertaken (e.g., paying bills, cooking meals). In the loss-oriented coping mode, emotions relate to the relationship with the deceased person; in the restoration-oriented coping, the bereaved person's emotions relate to the stressful events associated with the responsibilities and changes as a result of the loss. Over time, after repeated confrontation with the loss, there is no longer a need to think about certain aspects of the loss (Caserta, Utz, Lund, Swenson, & de Vries, 2014). See Figure 20.2.

Types of Grief

Uncomplicated Grief

Most bereaved people experience normal or **uncomplicated grief** after the loss of a loved one. Uncomplicated grief is painful and disruptive. At the time of the loss, the grieving person may have a physical response such as tightening in the throat, choking, shortness of breath, a need to sigh, an empty feeling in the abdomen, and a lack of muscular power. A sense of unreality sets in, and there is increased emotional distance from others and an intense preoccupation with the image of the deceased person. Exaggerated feelings of guilt for minor negligence are common. Mourning rites and support from family and friends are helpful.

The most frequent initial reaction in grieving is yearning although disbelief and depression also occur during the first 2 years. Gradually, yearning, disbelief, and depression decline. Within the first 6 months after the loss, there may be signs of limited impairment during adaptation to new situations.

The bereavement process is often applied to other situations in which a loss occurs, not necessarily the death of a person, but has many of the same responses. The "empty nest syndrome" is an example of bereavement for children who have grown up and left home. This bereavement experience is less intense than that triggered by a loss through death, but the bereaved person has many of the same responses.

Most bereaved persons do not need clinical interventions and are able to find meaning and purpose in their lives. Their self-esteem and sense of competency remain intact. They gradually accept the sense of loss as a reality and are able to move on with their lives. There is little evidence that they need or benefit from counseling or therapy. Those who experience suicidal thoughts and gestures should be evaluated for depression and posttraumatic stress disorder (PTSD) (Bennett & Soulsby, 2012; Stroebe, Schut, & Stroebe, 2007; Zhang, El-Jawahri, & Prigerson, 2006).

Traumatic Grief

Traumatic grief is a term that is used for a more difficult and prolonged grief. In traumatic grieving, external factors influence the reactions and potential long-term outcomes. For example, memories of the traumatic death of the deceased may lead to more traumatic memories including the violent death scene (Mutabaruka, Séjourné, Bui, Birmes, & Chabro, 2012). The external circumstances of death associated with traumatic grief include (1) suddenness and lack of anticipation; (2) violence, mutilation and destruction; (3) degree of preventability or randomness of the death; (4) multiple deaths (bereavement overload); and (5) mourner's personal encounter with death involving a significant threat to personal survival or a massive and shocking confrontation with the deaths (or mutilation) of others (Bolton, Michalopoulos, Ahmed, Murray, & Bass, 2013; Reynolds, Stack, & Houle, 2011).

Bereavement of family members for those who committed suicide seems to differ from other sudden deaths. Common experiences during this bereavement process include stigmatization, shame and guilt, and a sense of rejection. The bereaved person may experience self-blame for contributing to the family member's death. Factors that influence bereavement after suicide include age of the deceased, quality of the relationship, the attitude of the bereaved to the loss, and cultural beliefs. These individuals benefit from psychological interventions (McKay & Tighe, 2013).

There is evidence that men experience grief differently than women, who are more likely to confront and express negative emotion (Pilling, Thege, Demetrovics, & Kopp, 2012; Stroebe, Stroebe, & Schut, 2006). Suicide bereavement may be different because of the survivor's questions regarding the family member's suicide and the impact of the suicide on the family (Barlow, Schiff, Chugh, Rawlinson, Hides, Leith, et al., 2010) (see Chapter 21). More research is needed in this area.

Complicated Grief

Complicated grief occurs in about 10% to 20% of bereaved persons (Fujisawa, Miyashita, Nakajima, Ito, Kato, & Kim, 2010). The person is frozen or stuck in a state of chronic mourning. The person feels bitter over the loss and wishes that his or her life could revert to the time they were together. In complicated grief there is an intense longing and yearning for the person who died that lasts for more than 6 months. Additionally, the person may have trouble accepting the death, an inability to trust others since the death, excessive bitterness related to the death, and feeling that life is meaningless without the deceased person (Claxton & Reynolds, 2012).

NURSING MANAGEMENT: Human Response to Crisis

The goal for people experiencing a crisis is to return to the pre-crisis level of functioning. The role of the nurse is to provide a framework of support systems that guide the patient through the crisis and facilitate the development and use of positive coping skills.

> **EMERGENCY CARE ALERT !** It is important to be acutely aware that a person in crisis may be at high risk for suicide or homicide. To determine the level of effectiveness of coping capabilities of the person, the nurse should complete a careful assessment for suicidal or homicidal risk. If a person is at high risk for either, the nurse should consider referral for admission to the hospital.

When assessing the coping ability of the client, the nurse should assess for unusual behaviors and determine the level of involvement of the person with the crisis. In addition, assess for evidence of self-mutilation activities that may indicate the use of self-preservation measures to avoid suicide. It is critical to assess the client's perception of the problem and the availability of support mechanisms (emotional and financial) for use by the person (Drenth, Herbst, & Strydom, 2010).

> **NCLEXNOTE**   During a crisis, the behaviors and verbalizations of a person may provide data that are indicative of a mental illness. Nursing care should be prioritized according to the severity of responses. After the crisis has been resolved, assess whether the abnormal thoughts or feelings disappear.

During an environmental crisis (e.g., flood, hurricane, forest fire) that affects the well-being of many people, nursing interventions will be a part of the community's efforts to respond to the event. This is covered in more detail in the section of the chapter on disasters. On the other hand, when a personal crisis occurs, the person in crisis may have only the nurse to respond to his or her needs. After the assessment, the nurse must decide whether to provide the care needed or to refer the person to a mental health specialist. Box 20.2 offers guidance in making this decision.

Biologic Domain

Assessment

Biologic assessment focuses on areas that usually undergo initial changes. Eliciting information about changes in

---

BOX 20.2

Decision Tree for Determining Referral

Situation: A 35-year-old woman is being seen in a clinic because of minor burns she received during a house fire. Her home was completely destroyed. She is tearful and withdrawn, and she complains of a great deal of pain from her minor burns. Biopsychosocial assessment is completed.

Assessment Result	Nursing Action
Patient has psychological distress but believes that her social support is adequate. She would like to talk to a nurse when she returns for her follow-up visit.	Provide counseling and support for the patient during her visit. Make an appointment for her return visit to the clinic for follow-up.
The patient is severely distressed. She has no social support. She does not know how she will survive.	Refer the patient to a mental health specialist. The patient will need crisis intervention strategies provided by a mental health specialist.

health practices provides important data that can be used to determine the severity of the disruption in functioning. Biologic functioning is important because a crisis can be physically exhausting. Disturbances in sleep and eating patterns and the reappearance of physical or psychiatric symptoms are common. Changes in body function may include tachycardia, tachypnea, profuse perspiration, nausea, vomiting, dilated pupils, and extreme shakiness. Some individuals may exhibit loss of control and have total disregard for their personal safety. These people are at high risk for injury, which may include infection, trauma, and head injuries (Betancourt et al., 2012). If sleep patterns are disturbed or nutrition is inadequate, the individual may not have the physical resources to deal with the crisis.

Nursing Diagnoses for the Biologic Domain

Biologic responses can be very severe during crises. All body systems can be affected. Possible Nursing Diagnoses may include Risk for Body Temperature Imbalance, Diarrhea, Impaired Urinary Elimination, and Stress Urinary Incontinence. In addition, the person may report a variety of somatic complaints. Implement appropriate nursing interventions to address the nursing diagnoses of assessed needs of the individual and make appropriate referrals.

Interventions for the Biologic Domain

Any negative physiological responses should be treated immediately. Be careful not to give unrealistic or false reassurances of positive outcomes over which you have no control. Other interventions focusing on the biologic domain will be those implemented for nursing diagnoses developed from assessment findings. Make referrals as appropriate (Davidhizar & Shearer, 2005). Pharmacological interventions may be needed to help maintain a high level of psychophysical functioning.

> **NCLEXNOTE** Individual responses to a crisis can be best understood by assessing the usual responses of the person to stressful events. The response to the crisis will also depend on the meaning of the event to the person. The use of therapeutic communication principles is a priority when caring for a person who has experienced a crisis or disaster.

Medication cannot resolve a crisis, but the judicious use of psychopharmacological agents can help reduce its emotional intensity. For example, Mrs. Brown has just learned that both of her parents have perished in an airplane crash. When she arrives at the emergency department to identify their bodies, she is shaking, sobbing, and unable to answer questions. The emergency physician

orders lorazepam (Ativan) (Box 20.3). The phases of treatment include initiation of treatment, assessment of stabilization from the treatment, and timeframe for maintenance of treatment.

1. **Initiation:** Because Mrs. Brown is overcome by grief and severe anxiety about seeing her parents' bodies, 2 mg of lorazepam is administered intramuscularly as ordered by the doctor. The nurse monitors the patient for onset of action and any side effects. If Mrs. Brown does not have some relief within 20 to 30 minutes, another injection can be given as ordered by the doctor.
2. **Stabilization:** During the next half hour, Mrs. Brown regains some of her composure. She is no longer shaking, and her crying is occasional. She is reluctant to identify her parents but can do so when accompanied by the nurse. After the paperwork is completed, Mrs. Brown is sent home with a prescription for lorazepam, 2 to 4 mg every 12 hours.
3. **Maintenance:** Mrs. Brown takes the medication during the next week as she plans and attends her parents' funeral and manages the affairs surrounding their deaths. The medication keeps her anxiety at a manageable level, enabling her to do the tasks required of her.
4. **Medication cessation:** Two weeks after the death of her parents, Mrs. Brown is no longer taking lorazepam. She is grieving normally and has periods of teariness and sadness about her loss, but she can cope. She visits with friends, reminisces with family members, and reads inspirational poems. All of these activities help her navigate the changes in her life brought about by her parents' sudden death.

This example demonstrates how a medication can be used to assist a person through a crisis. After that crisis has passed, the person can use his or her personal coping mechanisms to adapt.

Psychological Domain
Assessment

Psychological assessment focuses on the individual's emotions and coping strengths. In the beginning of the crisis, the person may report the feeling of numbness and shock. Responses to psychological distress should be differentiated from symptoms of psychiatric illnesses that may be present. Later, as the reality of the crisis sinks in, the person will be able to recognize and describe the felt emotions. The nurse should expect these emotions to be intense and be sure to provide some support during their expression. At the beginning of a crisis, assess the individual for behaviors that indicate a depressed state, the presence of confusion, uncontrolled weeping or screaming, disorientation, or aggression. The person may be suffering from a loss of feelings of well-being and safety. In addition, panic responses, anxiety, and fear may be

BOX 20.3

Drug Profile: Lorazepam (Ativan)

DRUG CLASS: Benzodiazepine; antianxiety/sedative hypnotic agent

RECEPTOR AFFINITY: Acts mainly at the subcortical levels of the central nervous system (CNS), leaving the cortex relatively unaffected. Main sites of action may be the limbic system and reticular formation. It potentiates the effects of α-aminobutyric acid, an inhibitory neurotransmitter. The exact mechanism of action is unknown.

INDICATIONS: Management of anxiety disorders or for short-term relief of symptoms of anxiety or anxiety associated with depression (oral forms). Also used as preanesthetic medication in adults to produce sedation, relieve anxiety, and decrease recall of events related to surgery (parenteral form). Unlabeled parenteral uses for management of acute alcohol withdrawal.

ROUTE AND DOSAGE: Available in 0.5-, 1-, and 2-mg tablets; 2 mg/mL concentrated oral solution and 2 mg/mL and 4 mg/mL solutions for injection.

Adults: Usually 2–6 mg/d orally, with a range of 1–10 mg/d in divided doses, with the largest dose given at night. 0.05 mg/kg intramuscularly (IM) up to a maximum of 4 mg administered at least 2 h before surgery. Initially 2 mg total or 0.044 mg/kg intravenously (IV) (whichever is smaller). Doses as high as 0.05 mg/kg up to a total of 4 mg may be given 15–20 min before the procedure to those benefiting by a greater lack of recall.

Geriatric patients: Dosage not to exceed adult IV dose. Orally, 1–2 mg/d in divided doses initially, adjusted as needed and tolerated.

Children: Drug should not be used in children younger than 12 years.

HALF-LIFE (PEAK EFFECT): 10–20 h (1–6 h [oral]; 60–90 min IM; 10–15 min IV).

SELECTED ADVERSE REACTIONS: Transient mild drowsiness, sedation, depression, lethargy, apathy, fatigue, light-headedness, disorientation, anger, hostility, restlessness, confusion, crying, headache, mild paradoxical excitatory reactions during first 2 weeks of treatment, constipation, dry mouth, diarrhea, nausea, bradycardia, hypotension, cardiovascular collapse, urinary retention, and drug dependence with withdrawal symptoms.

WARNINGS: Contraindicated in psychoses; acute narrow angle glaucoma; shock; acute alcoholic intoxication with depression of vital signs; and during pregnancy, labor and delivery, and while breastfeeding. Use cautiously in patients with impaired liver or kidney function and those who are debilitated. When given with theophylline, there is a decreased effect of lorazepam. When using the drug IV, it must be diluted immediately before use and administered by direct injection slowly or infused at a maximum rate of 2 mg/min. When giving narcotic analgesics, reduce its dose by at least half in patients who have received lorazepam.

SPECIFIC PATIENT AND FAMILY EDUCATION
- Take the drug exactly as prescribed; do not stop taking the drug abruptly.
- Avoid alcohol and other CNS depressants.
- Avoid driving and other activities that require alertness.
- Notify the prescriber before taking any other prescription or over-the-counter drug.
- Change your position slowly and sit at the edge of the bed for a few minutes before arising.
- Report to the prescriber any severe dizziness, weakness, drowsiness that persists, rash or skin lesions, palpitations, edema of the extremities, visual changes, or difficulty urinating.

---

present (Fischer, Postmes, Koeppl, Conway, & Fredriksson, 2011). The ability to cope by problem solving may be disrupted. By assessing the person's ability to solve problems, the nurse can evaluate whether he or she can cognitively cope with the crisis situation and determine the kind and amount of support needed.

Nursing Diagnoses for the Psychological Domain

Many nursing diagnoses generated from assessment of the psychological domain may be appropriate for the person experiencing the crisis. The nursing diagnoses may include Grieving, Post-Trauma Syndrome, Confusion, Ineffective Coping, Risk for Violence (self-directed or directed toward others), Impaired Communication, Interrupted Family Processes, Anxiety, Powerlessness, and many other diagnoses. The nurse should make sure that the diagnoses are based on the person's appraisal of the situation. In addition, any diagnosis should be determined from the assessment data that have been clustered and prioritized to address identified needs.

Interventions for the Psychological Domain

Safety interventions to protect the person in crisis from harm should include preventing the person from committing suicide or homicide, arranging for food and shelter (if needed), and mobilizing social support. After the person's safety needs have been met, the psychosocial aspects of the crisis can be addressed and the individual can be prepared for recovery. Guidelines for crisis intervention and examples are presented in Table 20.1. Individuals should be encouraged to report any depression, anxiety, or interpersonal difficulties during the recovery period.

Counseling reinforces healthy coping behaviors and interaction patterns. Counseling, which focuses on identifying emotions and positive coping strategies for the corresponding nursing diagnosis, helps the person to integrate the effects of the crisis into a real life experience. Responses to crisis differ with individuals. Some may present with behaviors that indicate transient disruptions in their ability to cope. Others may be totally devastated.

Table 20.1 GUIDELINES FOR CRISIS INTERVENTION		
Approach	**Rationale**	**Example**
Support the expression (or non-expression) of feelings according to cultural or ethnic practices.	Emotional support helps the person face reality. The emotional expression by the victim may be culturally driven.	Accompany the husband to view the body of his deceased wife.
Help the person think clearly and focus on one implication at a time.	Focusing on all the implications at once can be too overwhelming.	A woman left her husband because of abuse. At first, focus only on her living arrangements and safety. At another time, discuss the other implications of the separation.
Avoid giving false reassurances, such as "It will be all right."	Giving false reassurances blocks communication. It may not be all right.	Patient: "My doctor told me that I have a terminal illness." Nurse: "What does that mean to you?"
Clarify fantasies with facts.	Accurate information is needed to problem solve.	A young mother believes that her comatose child will regain consciousness although the medical evidence contradicts it. Gently clarify the meaning of the medical evidence.
Link the person and family with community resources, as needed.	Strengthening the person's social network so social support can be obtained reduces the effect of the crisis.	Provide information about a meeting of a support group such as that of the American Cancer Society.

Adapted from Lazarus, R. (1991). *Emotion and adaptation* (p. 122). New York: Oxford University Press.

At times, telephone counseling may provide the person with enough help that face-to-face counseling is not necessary. If counseling strategies do not work, other stress reduction and coping enhancement interventions can be used (see Chapter 18). The nurse should refer anyone who cannot cope with a crisis to a mental health specialist for an evaluation.

Social Domain

Assessment

Assessment of the impact of the crisis on an individual's social functioning is essential because a crisis usually severely disrupts social proficiencies. The nurse should assess the severity of the crisis to determine the capability of the individual or the community to respond in a supportive way.

Nursing Diagnoses for the Social Domain

Nursing diagnoses associated with the social domain include Impaired Adjustment, Impaired Social Interaction, and Impaired Interrupted Family Processes. Other diagnoses may be Ineffective Role Performance and Relocation Stress Syndrome. Any nursing diagnosis generated will depend on the assessment findings related to the needs of the patient.

Interventions for the Social Domain

The nursing interventions for the social domain can focus on the individual, the family, and the community.

A crisis often disrupts a person's social network, leading to changes in available social support. Development of a new social support network may help the person cope more effectively with the crisis. Supporting the development of new support contacts within the context of available social networks can be done by contacting available local and state agencies for assistance as well as specific private support groups and religious groups.

Telephone Hotlines

Public and private funding and the efforts of trained volunteers permit most communities to provide crisis services to the public. For example, telephone hotlines for problems ranging from child abuse to suicide are a part of health delivery systems of most communities. Crisis services permit immediate access to the mental health system for people who are experiencing an emergency (such as threatened suicide) or for those who need help with stress or a crisis.

Residential Crisis Services

Many communities provide, as part of the health care network, residential crisis services for people who need short-term housing. The specific residential crisis services available within a community reflect the problems that the community members judge as particularly important. For example, some communities provide shelter for teenage runaways; others offer shelter for abused spouses. Still others provide shelter for people who would otherwise require acute psychiatric hospitalization. These settings provide residents with a place to stay in a supportive, homelike atmosphere. The people who use these services are linked to other community services such as financial aid.

Evaluation and Treatment Outcomes

Outcomes developed in cooperation with the person experiencing the crisis guide the evaluation. Once assessment data are clustered and prioritized the nursing diagnosis and the outcomes are determined. Once interventions are developed and implemented in cooperation with the individual in crisis, the person should come through the crisis with improved health, well-being, and social function. If complications occur, the nurse should make appropriate alterations in the entire nursing process or make appropriate referrals.

DISASTER AND TERRORISM

A disaster is a sudden ecological or human-made phenomenon that is of sufficient magnitude to require external help to address the psychosocial needs as well as the physical needs of the victims. Acts of terrorism present situations that mimic disasters and can be categorized as a type of disaster.

> **KEYCONCEPT**   A **disaster** is a sudden overwhelming catastrophic event that causes great damage and destruction that may involve mass casualties and human suffering requiring assistance from all available resources.

Although crises and disasters are usually viewed as negative experiences, the outcomes can be positive. Some survivors of disasters draw on resources that they never realized they had and grow from those experiences (Osofsky & Osofsky, 2013). However, the survivors of disasters may have severe psychological problems. Fear, anger, and distress elevate severe anxiety to the panic level, which can result in a severe mental illnesses. Unresolved crisis or disastrous events can lead to disorganized thinking and responses that are inappropriate and traumatic for the person experiencing the situation (Wisnivesky et al., 2011). In addition, the victims may experience the development of acute stress disorder (that has a strong emphasis on dissociative symptoms) and PTSD.

Historical Perspectives of Disasters in the United States

Throughout history, disasters have been portrayed from a fatalistic perspective that humans have little control over catastrophic events. Some cultures contend that natural disasters are acts of God. Other cultures express their belief that natural disaster events can be attributed to gods dwelling within such places as volcanoes, with eruptions being an expression of the gods' anger (van Griensven et al., 2006). Although often caused by nature, disasters can have human origins. Wars and civil disturbances that destroy homelands and displace people are included among the causes of disasters. Other causes include a building collapse, blizzard, drought, earthquake, epidemic, explosion, famine, fire, flood, hazardous material or transportation incident (such as a chemical spill), hurricane, nuclear incident, terrorist attack, and tornado. Often, the unpredictability of such disasters causes fear, confusion, and stress that can have lasting effects on the health of affected communities and their sense of well-being (Wisnivesky et al., 2011).

In recent history, we have experienced several attacks of violence and terrorism that are unprecedented in North America. The destruction of the World Trade Center in New York and the attack on the Pentagon in Washington, DC, on September 11, 2001, the dispersal of anthrax spores in the United States mail, the Sandy Hook school tragedy, and the Boston bombing shattered North Americans' sense of safety and security.

Since September 11, 2001, the emergency response planning of federal, state, and local agencies has focused on possible terrorist attacks with chemical, biologic, radiologic, nuclear, or high-yield explosive weapons. Before September 11, 2001, government agencies and public health leaders had not incorporated mental health into their overall response plans to bioterrorism. But in the aftermath of the mass destruction of human life and property in 2001, government and health care leaders are recognizing the need for monumental mental health efforts to be implemented during episodes of terrorism and disaster. The psychological and behavioral consequences of a terrorist attack are now included in most disaster plans.

The earthquake and tsunami in Japan in 2011 and the Hurricane Katrina disaster in the United States in 2005 highlight the importance of government preparedness for natural disasters as well as terrorism. In the United States, the lack of government response and breakdown in communication during Katrina resulted in thousands of hurricane victims being displaced and injured. The Japan disaster became a cascade of disasters, resulting in the death of thousands of residents and contamination from the damaged nuclear site. Consequences of these disasters will still be occurring months and years after the initial events.

Phases of Disaster

Natural and human-made disaster can be conceptualized in three phases:

1. *Prewarning of the disaster*. This phase entails preparing the community for possible evacuation of the

environment, mobilization of resources, and review of community disaster plans. In some disasters, such as in the 2011 earthquake in Japan, there is very little warning.

2. *The disaster event occurs.* In this phase, the rescuers provide resources, assistance, and support as needed to preserve the biopsychosocial functioning and survival of the victims. In large disasters, the rescuers and health care professionals also experience the traumatic event as both residents and health care providers. These individuals are more likely to experience greater physical and psychological trauma than those who experience the event solely as a civilian or as a professional (Leitch, Vanslyke, & Allen, 2009). The victims experience the initial trauma and threats that occur immediately after the disaster such confusion (communication breakdown), lack of safety (no available law enforcement), and lack of health care services.

3. *Recuperative effort.* In the third phase, the focus is on implementing strategies for healing sick and injured people, preventing complications of health problems, repairing damages, and reconstructing the community. The disruption effects can be traumatic to the community residents. The debris, lack of trust of the government, fragmentation of families, financial problems, lack of adequate housing, inadequate temporary housing, and fear of another disaster contribute to the long-term negative effects of disasters.

Long-term mental health consequences are evident in most disasters. For example, in a follow-up study of alcohol use among survivors of 10 disasters, the majority of post-disaster alcohol use disorders represented the continuation or recurrence of preexisting problems. Those with an alcohol abuse disorder were four times more likely to cope by drinking alcohol than those who did not have a substance abuse problem, indicating that this group could benefit from mental health interventions (North, Ringwalt, Downs, Derzon, & Galvin, 2011).

Even though serious mental health problems are known to exist or be exacerbated after a disaster, research has shown few people access mental health services (Noorthoorn, Havenaar, de Haan, van Rood, & van Stiphout, 2010). In a follow-up study of Hurricane Katrina survivors, one-third had evidence of a mood or anxiety disorder, but fewer than 35% of those had used mental health services (Springgate et al., 2011; Wang et al., 2007). Undertreatment of these disorders was evident.

NURSING MANAGEMENT: Human Response to Disaster or Terrorism

Psychiatric nurses encounter three different types of disaster victims. The first category is the victims who may or may not survive. If they survive, the victims often experience severe physical injuries. The more serious the physical injury, the more likely the victim will experience a mental health problem such as PTSD, depression, anxiety, or other mental health problems (Noorthoorn et al., 2010). Victims and families need ongoing health care to prevent complications related to both their physical and mental health (Springgate, et al., 2011).

The second category of victims includes the professional rescuers. These are persons who are less likely to experience physical injury but who often experience psychological stress. The professional rescuers, such as police officers, firefighters, nurses, and so on, have more effective coping skills than do volunteer rescuers who are not prepared for the emotional impact of a disaster. However, many professional responders report experiencing PTSD for many months after the traumatic event in which they were involved (Haugen, Evces, & Weiss, 2012).

The third category includes everyone else involved in the disaster. Psychological effects may be experienced worldwide by millions of people as they experience terrorism or disaster vicariously or as direct victims of the terrorism/disaster event. After an act of terrorism, most people will experience some psychological stress, including an altered sense of safety, hypervigilance, sadness, anger, fear, decreased concentration, and difficulty sleeping. Others may alter their behavior by traveling less, staying at home, avoiding public events, keeping children out of school, or increasing smoking and alcohol use. In a nationwide interview of 560 adults after September 11, 2001, 90% reported at least one stress symptom and 44% had several symptoms of stress (Schuster et al., 2001). In New York State, almost half a million people reported symptoms that would meet the criteria for acute PTSD (see Chapter 26). In Manhattan, the estimated prevalence of acute PTSD was 11.2%, increasing to 20% in people living close to the World Trade Center (Galea et al., 2002; Schlenger et al., 2002). However, in analysis of suicide rates after September 11, 2001 and the Oklahoma City bombing, there appears to be no support for an increase or decrease in suicides following these events (Pridemore, Trahan, & Chamlin, 2009).

The role of the behavioral health care worker in disasters, specifically a nuclear detonation in a U.S. city is the support of lifesaving activities and the prevention of additional casualties from fallout. There are six broad categories of interventions including promoting appropriate protective actions, discouraging dangerous behaviors, managing patient/survivor flow to facilitate the best use of scarce resources, supporting first responders, assisting with triage, and delivering palliative care when appropriate (Dodgen Norwood, Becker, Perez, & Hansen, 2011).

Victims experiencing head injuries or psychic trauma after a disaster may have to be hospitalized. During a disaster, a victim with a mental illness may experience regression to his or her pretreatment condition. If community mental health facilities are available, they should be directed to seek assistance from mental health care professionals. The victims should receive follow-up care for the disaster response after they are discharged.

Biologic Domain

Assessment

The nurse should assess physical reactions that may involve many changes in body functions, such as tachycardia, tachypnea, profuse perspiration, nausea, vomiting, dilated pupils, and extreme shakiness. Virtually any organ may be involved. Some victims may exhibit panic reactions and loss of control and have a total disregard for their personal safety. The victims may be suicidal or homicidal and are at high risk for injuries that may include infection, trauma, and head injuries. During the rescue, medical care is a priority. Any medical or psychiatric disorders should be assessed and information communicated to the rest of the health care team.

Unexplained physical symptoms such as headache, fatigue, pain, chest pain, and gastrointestinal disturbances have been reported in the aftermath of a disaster in both traumatized and non-traumatized populations. Possible risk factors for the development of unexplained physical symptoms include female gender, high physical damage, and PTSD (Anwar, Mpofu, Matthews, & Brock, 2013; Bonanno et al., 2012).

Nursing Diagnoses for the Biologic Domain

Because the responses to disaster are so varied, almost any nursing diagnosis can be generated from the assessment data. Ineffective Thermoregulation, Ineffective Breathing Patterns, Insomnia and Risk for Self-harm are examples of possible nursing diagnoses.

Interventions for the Biologic Domain

Any physiological problems or injuries should be treated quickly. During the emergency response, individuals will be triaged to the appropriate level of care. Victims who are primarily distressed and may have somatic symptoms will be treated after those suffering from exposure with critical injuries. The primary public health concern is clean drinking water, food, shelter, and medical care. Natural disasters do not usually cause an increase in infectious disease outbreaks, but contaminated water and food and lack of shelter and medical care may worsen illnesses that already exist (Migl & Powell, 2010). All

patients need to be reassured of the caring and commitment of the nurse to their safety, comfort, and well-being throughout the triage process. Ideally, a mental health specialist is an integral member of the triage team. Many of the same interventions used for persons experiencing stress or crisis will be used for these victims. See also Chapter 29 for discussion of somatization.

Psychological Domain

Assessment

Therapeutic communication is key to understanding the extent of the psychological responses to a disaster and to establishing a bridge of trust that communicates respect, commitment, and acceptance. Developing rapport with the victim or victims communicates reassurance and support. The victims should be assessed for behaviors that indicate a depressed state, presence of confusion, uncontrolled weeping or screaming, disorientation, or aggressive behavior. Ideally, the nurse should assess the coping strategies the victim uses to normally manage stressful situations.

During a disaster, fear and hopelessness can immobilize victims. The victims may suffer from loss of feelings of well-being and various psychological problems, including panic responses, anxiety, and fear. Dissociation and fear are predictive of later developing PTSD and depressive symptoms. Victims witnessing others suffer are especially high risk for future mental health problems and should be assessed for the details of the disaster (Rosendal, Salcioğlu, Andersen, & Mortensen, 2011).

The survivors of the disaster may experience traumatic bereavement because of their feelings of guilt that they survived the disaster (Bolton et al., 2013; Viswanath et al., 2012). Responses to psychological distress need to be differentiated from any psychiatric illness that the person may be experiencing. A response to a disaster may leave the person feeling overwhelmed, incapacitated, and disoriented.

Nursing Diagnoses for the Psychological Domain

Initially, fear and hopelessness can be expected. Depending on the long-term impact of the disaster and the type of disaster (e.g., terrorist attack or tsunami), there could be any number of nursing diagnosis such as Grieving, Impaired Resilience, Low Self-Esteem, or Risk for Suicide.

Interventions for the Psychological Domain

The **ABCs of psychological first aid** include focusing on A (arousal), B (behavior), and C (cognition). When arousal is present, the intervention goal is to decrease excitement by providing safety, comfort, and consolation. When abnormal or irrational behavior is present, survivors should be assisted to function more effectively in the disaster, and when cognitive disorientation occurs, reality testing and clear information should be provided. In the initial phases, the nurse should assist the victim in focusing on the reality of problems that are immediate, with specific goals that are consistent with available resources as well as the culture and lifestyle of the victim.

After the initial interventions, the nurse should support the development of resilience, coping, and recovery while providing technical assistance, training, and consultation. During the treatment process, it may become necessary to administer an antianxiety medication or sedative, especially in the early phases of recovery (Centers for Disease Control and Prevention [CDC], 2005). The goals of care include helping the victims prioritize and match available resources with their needs, preventing further complications, monitoring the environment, disseminating information, and implementing disease control strategies (CDC, 2012).

Debriefing (the reconstruction of the traumatic events by the victim) may be helpful for some. Long a common practice, debriefing was believed to be necessary in order for the person to develop a healthy perspective of the event and ultimately prevent PTSD. However, research does not support debriefing as a useful treatment for the prevention of PTSD after traumatic incidents. Additionally, different cultural groups respond differently to traumatic events, and many non-Western ethnic groups present symptoms somatically rather than psychologically. Therefore, compulsory debriefing is not recommended (Hawker, Durkin, & Hawker, 2011).

If the victim has symptoms of PTSD, referral to a mental health clinic for additional evaluation and treatment is important (see Chapter 26). The nurse should prepare the victim for recovery by teaching about the effects of stress and helping the victim identify personal strengths and coping skills. Positive coping skills should be supported. The victims should be encouraged to report any depression, anxiety, or interpersonal difficulty during the recovery period. After most disasters, support groups are established that help victims and their families deal with the psychological effects of the disaster.

Women exhibit higher levels of distress than men after a disaster, especially pregnant women and older women (Tong, Zotti, & Hsia, 2011; Viswanath et al., 2012). Assess the ages of the female victims, their capability to participate in problem-solving activities related to the devastation left by the disaster, and their level of self-confidence or self-esteem that would allow each to participate as a team member or a team leader in addressing the needs of others. This includes encouraging the victims to do necessary chores and participate in decision making and to take advantage of the opportunity to serve as leaders or team members, as dictated by their abilities.

Outreach is especially important because research shows that disaster victims do not access mental health systems. Peer-delivered mental health services are especially effective in identifying and connecting with victims, especially those with pre-disaster psychiatric problems (North & Pfefferbaum, 2013).

Educating the public and emphasizing the natural recovery process is important. Information gaps and rumors add to the anxiety and stress of the situation. Giving information and direction helps the public and victims to use the coping skills they already possess. Initially, the event may leave individuals and families in a stage of ambiguity with frantic, disorganized behavior. In addition, individuals and family members are concerned about their own physical and psychological responses to the disastrous event. Children are especially vulnerable to disasters and respond according to their ages and family experiences. Traumatized children and adolescents are high risk victims of a wide range of behavioral, psychological, and neurologic problems after experiencing various traumatic events (Osofsky & Osofsky, 2013; Pfefferbaum & North, 2013).

When the nurse explains anticipated reactions and behaviors, this helps the victims gain control and improve coping. For example, after a major disaster, they may have excessive worry, preoccupation with the event, and changes in eating and sleeping patterns. With time, counseling, and group work, these symptoms will lessen. Active coping strategies can be presented in multiple media forums, such as television and radio. After the initial shock, victims react by trying to do something to resolve the situation. When victims begin working to remedy the disaster situation, their physical responses become less exaggerated, and they are more able to work with less tension and fear.

Social Domain

Assessment

The nurse should assess the kind and severity of a natural or human-made disaster or terrorist act to determine the capability of individuals and communities to respond in a supportive way. The nurse should maintain a calm demeanor, obtain and distribute information about the disaster and the victims, and reunite victims and their families. In addition, there is a need to monitor the news media's impact on the mental health of the victims of the crisis. Sometimes the persistence of the news media diminishes the ability of the survivors to achieve closure to the crisis (McGinty, Webster, Jarlenski, & Barry, 2014). Constant rehashing of the disaster in the newspapers and on television can increase and prolong the severity or initiate feelings of anxiety and depression.

Cultural values and beliefs help define the significance and meaning of a disaster. In some instances, a disaster can slow development, but usually the customs, beliefs, and value systems remain the same. It is important that first responders and health care teams are sensitive to the cultural and religious beliefs of the community. In many instances, victims' spiritual beliefs and religious faith help them cope with the disaster (Varghese, 2010).

In a disaster, the victims may experience economic distress because of job loss and loss of other resources. This may ultimately lead to psychological distress. In addition, acts of aggression and other mental health problems may emerge (Ozbay, Heyde, Reissman, & Sharma, 2013; Wisnivesky et al., 2011). Again, shelter, money, and food may not be available. The absence of basic human needs such as food, a place to live, or immediate transportation quickly becomes a priority that may precipitate acts of violence.

Nursing Diagnoses for the Social Domain

Nursing diagnoses associated with the social domain include Impaired Adjustment, Impaired Social Interaction, and Interrupted Family Processes. Ineffective Role Performance and Relocation Stress Syndrome are also diagnoses that could be generated during a disaster. Other nursing diagnoses can be generated from the assessment findings according to the needs of the victims.

Interventions for the Social Domain

The focus of nursing interventions for the social domain include the individual, family, and community. The individual should learn about the community resources that can be made available. Family support systems may need to be reestablished. The health care community should actively reach out to the media and keep the press engaged. Direct attention to stories that inform and help the public respond should be encouraged. Some federal agencies assist victims of disasters. This assistance is available for individual, families, and communities. One of these agencies is the Federal Emergency Management Agency (FEMA). When a disaster occurs, FEMA sends a team of specialists who review the devastation of disaster. They provide counseling and mental health services and arrange for many of the victims to access other services needed for survival, including training programs. In addition, the Substance Abuse and Mental Health Services Administration (SAMHSA) of the Department of Health and Human Services is available to assist both victims of and responders to the disaster. When a disaster disrupts the victim's social network, other resources must be made available for social support. The social support system provides an environment in which the victims experience respect and caring from the caregivers, the opportunity

to ventilate and examine personal feelings regarding the tragedy, and the opportunity to begin the healing and recovery process. Supporting the development of more contacts within the social network can be done by organizing support groups within the area of the disaster that address grief and loss, trauma, psychoeducational needs, and substance abuse. In addition, the nurse may refer the victims to nearby support groups or religious groups that are appropriate to meet their needs.

Evaluation and Treatment Outcomes

To determine the effectiveness of nursing interventions, the nurse should evaluate the outcomes based on the success of resolution of the disaster. The outcomes will depend on the specific disaster and its meaning (appraisal) to the survivors. For example, are the survivors in a safe place? Are the victims able to cope with the disaster? Were the appropriate supports given, so the victims could draw upon their own strengths?

SUMMARY OF KEY POINTS

- A crisis is a time-limited event that occurs when coping mechanisms fail to provide adaptive skills to address a perceived challenge or threat.

- Grief is an intense emotional response to loss, and bereavement is the process of mourning. There are variations in grief responses that are influenced by the characteristics of the individual and the situation of loss.

- Stage theories of grief although popular, lack evidence. The dual process model explains bereavement as an oscillation between loss-oriented coping and restoration-oriented coping. Over time, there is less of a need to think about the loss.

- Most persons grieve normally and do not need counseling. Complicated grief occurs in about 10% to 20% of bereaved persons. Interventions are required for this group.

- Biopsychosocial assessment reveals changes in domains. Interventions are designed to support people through crises by helping them identify the resources they need and how to get them.

- Disaster is a sudden, overwhelming catastrophic event that causes great damage and may cause mass casualties and human suffering that require assistance from all available resources.

- Depending on the disaster, interventions are provided to individuals, families, and communities.

CRITICAL THINKING CHALLENGES

1. Compare nursing interventions used for crises with those used for disasters. What are the similarities? What are the differences?

2. After the death of his mother, a 24-year-old single man with schizophrenia moves into an apartment. He continues to take his medication but feels sad about his mother's death. He is not adjusting well to living alone and tells his nurse that he no longer wants to go to work. In tears, he admits that he is lonely and can no longer cope with the apartment. The nurse generates the following nursing diagnosis: Ineffective Coping related to inadequate support system. Develop a plan of care for this young man.

3. Compare the evidence for the stage theories of grieving with the dual process model. What are the pros and cons of each?

4. Discuss the role of medication when used in crises.

5. Compare normal grief with complicated grief. How would you recognize the difference? When would it be appropriate to refer a bereaved person to a mental health specialist?

6. There is a terrorist threat in your community. A patient appears in the emergency department convinced that he is going to die. How would you proceed with assessing this patient?

Grace is Gone (2007): Stanley Phillips (John Cusack) is a manager of a home-supply store and parent of two girls, 12-year-old Heidi (Shelan O'Keefe) and 8-year-old Dawn (Gracie Bednarczyk). His wife is a soldier in Iraq, but the viewers know her by her message left on the family answering machine. When an army captain and chaplain deliver the news that Grace had died bravely in combat, Stanley becomes numb. He impulsively takes his girls to wherever they desire—a theme park in Florida. Most of the movie follows the three on the trip and the father's attempt to delay and deny his wife's death.

VIEWING POINTS: Describe Stanley's reaction when he receives the news of his wife's death. What clues are present that Heidi gradually understands that something terrible has happened?

References

American Psychiatric Association. (2013). *Diagnostic and statistical manual of mental disorders* (5th ed.). Arlington, VA: Author.

Anwar, J., Mpofu, E., Matthews, L. R., Brock, K. D. (2013). Risk factors of posttraumatic stress disorder after an earthquake disaster. *Journal of Nervous & Mental Disorders, 201*(12), 1045–1052.

Barlow, C. A., Schiff, J. W., Chugh, U., Rawlinson, D., Hides, E., & Leith, J. (2010). An evaluation of a suicide bereavement peer support program. *Death Studies, 34*(10), 915–930.

Bennett, K. M., & Soulsby, L. K. (2012). Wellbeing in bereavement and widowhood illness. *Crisis and Loss, 20*(14), 321–337.

Betancourt, T. S., Newnham, E. A., Layne, C. M., Kim, S., Steinberg, A. M., Ellis, H., et al. (2012). Trauma history and psychopathology in war-affected refugee children referred for trauma-related mental health services in the United States. *Journal of Traumatic Stress, 25*(6), 682–690.

Bolton, P., Michalopoulos, L., Ahmed, A. M., Murray, L. K., & Bass, J. (2013). The mental health and psychosocial problems of survivors of torture and genocide in Kurdistan, Northern Iraq: A brief qualitative study. *Torture, 23*(1), 1–14.

Bonanno, G. A., Mancini, A. D., Horton, J. L., Powell, T. M., Leardmann, C. A., Boyko, E. J., et al. (2012). Trajectories of trauma symptoms and resilience in deployed US military service members: Prospective cohort study. *The British Journal of Psychiatry, 200*(4), 317–323.

Bowlby, J., & Parkes, C. M. (1970). Separation and loss within the family. In E. J. Anthony (Ed.), *The child in his family.* New York: Wiley.

Caffo, E., Forresi, B., & Lievers, L. S. (2005). Impact, psychological sequelae and management of trauma affecting children and adolescents. *Current Opinion in Psychiatry, 18*(4), 422–428.

Caserta, M., Utz, R., Lund, D., Swenson, K. L., & de Vries, B. (2014). Coping processes among bereaved spouses. *Death Studies, 38*(3), 145–155.

Caplan, G. (1961). *An approach to community mental health.* New York: Grune & Stratton.

Centers for Disease Control and Prevention. (2012). Disaster mental health for states: Key principles, issues, and questions. *Emergency Preparedness and Response.* Retrieved from http://emergency.cdc.gov/mentalhealth/states.asp.

Claxton, R. & Reynolds, C. F. 3rd. (2012). Complicated grief #254. *Journal of Palliative Medicine, 15*(7), 829–830.

Dodgen, D., Norwood, A. D., Becker, S. M., Perez, J. T., & Hansen, C. K. (2011). Social, psychological, and behavioral responses to a nuclear detonation in a U.S. city: Implications for health care planning and delivery. *Disaster Medicine & Public Health Preparedness, 5*(suppl 1), S54–S64.

Drenth, C. M., Herbst, A .F., & Strydom, H. (2010). A complicated grief intervention model. *Health SA Gesondheid, 15*(1), 1–8. doi:10.4102/hsaf. v15i1.415

Fischer, P., Postmes, T., Koeppl, J., Conway, L., & Fredriksson, T. (2011). The meaning of collective terrorist threat: Understanding the subjective causes of terrorism reduces its negative psychological impact. *Journal of Interpersonal Violence, 26*(7), 1432–1445.

Fujisawa, D., Miyashita, M., Nakajima, S., Ito, M., Kato, M. & Kim, Y. (2010). Prevalence and determinants of complicated grief in general population. *Journal of Affective Disorders, 127*(1–3), 352–358.

Galea, S., Ahern, J., Resnick, H., Kilpatrick, D., Bucuvalas, M., Gold, J., & Vlahov, D. (2002). Psychological sequelae of the September 11 terrorist attacks in New York City. *New England Journal of Medicine, 346*(13), 982–987.

Haugen, P. T., Evces, M., & Weiss, D. S. (2012). Treating posttraumatic stress disorder in first responders: A systematic review. *Clinical Psychology Review, 32*(5), 370–380.

Hawker, D. M., Durkin, J., & Hawker, D. S. (2011). To debrief or not to debrief our heroes: That is the question. *Clinical Psychology and Psychotherapy, 18*(6), 453–463.

Kubler-Ross, E. (1969). *On death and dying.* New York: Macmillan Publishing Company.

Lazarus, R. (1991). *Emotion and adaptation* (p. 122). New York: Oxford University Press.

Leitch, M. L., Vanslyke, J., & Alleln, M. (2009). Somatic experiencing treatment with social service workers following hurricanes Katrina and Rita. *Social Work, 54*(1), 9–18.

Lindemann, E. (1944). Symptomatology and management of acute grief. *American Journal of Psychiatry, 101*, 141–148.

Lyons, C., Hopley, P., Burton, C. R., & Horrocks, J. (2009). Mental health crisis and respite services: Service user and carer aspirations. *Journal of Psychiatric and Mental Health Nursing, 16*, 424–433.

McGinty, E. E., Webster, D. W., Jarlenski, M., & Barry, C. (2014). News media framing of serious mental illness and gun violence in the United States, 1997–2012. *American Journal of Public Health, 104*(3), 406–413.

McKay, K., & Tighe, J. (2013). Talking through the dead: The impact and interplay of lived grief after suicide. *Omega, 68*(2), 111–121.

Migl, K. S., & Pwell, R. M. (2010). Physical and environmental considerations for first responders. *Critical Care Nursing Clinics of North America, 22*(4), 445–454.

Mutabaruka, J., Séjourné, N., Bui, E., Birmes, P., & Chabro, H. (2012). Traumatic grief and traumatic stress in survivors 12 years after the genocide in Rwanda. *Stress and Health. 28*(4), 289–296.

Noorthoorn, E. O., Havenaar, J. M., de Haan, H.A., van Rood, Y. R., & van Stiphout, W. H. J. (2010). Mental health service use and outcomes after the Enschede Fireworks disaster: A naturalistic follow-up study. *Psychiatric Services, 61*(11), 1138–1143.

North, C. S., & Pfefferbaum, B. (2013). Mental health response to community disasters: A systematic review. *JAMA, 310*(5), 507–518.

North, C. S., Ringwalt, C. L., Downs, D., Derzon, J., & Galvin, D. (2011). Postsidadter course of alcohol use disorders in systematically studied survivors of 10 disasters. *Archives of General Psychiatry, 68*(2), 173–180.

Osofsky, H. J., & Osofsky, J. D. (2013). Hurricane Katrina and the gulf oil spill: Lessons learned. *Psychiatric Clinics of North America, 36*(3), 371–382.

Ozbay, F., Auf der H. T., Reissman, D., Sharma, V. (2013). The enduring mental health impact of the September 11th terrorist attacks: Challenges and lessons learned. *Psychiatric Clinics of North America, 36*(3), 417–429.

Pfefferbaum, B. & North, C. S. (2013). Assessing children's disaster reactions and mental health needs: Screening and clinical evaluation. *Canadian Journal of Psychiatry, 58*(3), 135–142.

Pilling, J., Thege, B. K., Demetrovics, Z., & Kopp, M. S. (2012). Alcolhol use in the first three years of bereavement: A national representative survey. *Substance Abuse Treatment, Prevention, and Policy*, 7, 1–5. http://www.substanceabusepolicy.com/content/7/1/3

Pridemore, W. A., Trahan, A., & Chamlin, M. B. (2009). No evidence of suicide increase following terrorist attacks in the United States: An interrupted time-series analysis of September 11 and Oklahoma City. *Suicide & Life-threatening Behavior, 39*(6), 659–670.

Reynolds C. F., Stack J., & Houle J. Healing. (2011). Emotions After Loss (HEAL): Diagnosis and treatment of complicated grief. UPMC Synergies. Available at: http://healstudy.org/wp-content/uploads/2010/10/S270-Synergies_GR_Spring_2011.pdf. Accessed May 21, 2014.

Rosendal, S., Salcioğlu, E., Andersen, H. S., & Mortensen, E. L. (2011). Exposure characteristics and peri-trauma emotional reactions during the 2004 tsunami in Southeast Asia: What predicts posttraumatic stress and depressive symptoms? *Comprehensive Psychiatry*, in press.

Schlenger, W. E., Caddell, J. M., Ebert, L., Jordan, B. K., Rourke, K. M., Wilson, D., et al. (2002). Psychological reactions to terrorist attacks: Findings from the national study of Americans' reactions to September 11. *Journal of the American Medical Association, 288*(5), 581–588.

Schuster, M. A., Stein, B. D., Jaycox, L., Collins, R. L., Marshall, G. N., Elliott, M. N., et al. (2001). A national survey of stress reactions after September 11, 2001, terrorist attacks. *New England Journal of Medicine, 345*(20), 1507–1512.

Springgate, B. F., Wennerstrom, A., Meyers, D., Allen, C. E., Vannoy, S. D., Bentham, W., Wells, K. B. (2011). Building community resilience through mental health infrastructure and training in post-Katrina New Orleans. *Ethnicity & Disease, 21*(3 Suppl 1), S1–20–29.

Stroebe, M., & Schut, H. (1999). The dual process model of coping with bereavement: Rationale and description. *Death Studies, 23*, 197–224.

Stroebe, M., Schut, H., & Boerner, K. (2010). Continuing bonds in adaptation to bereavement: Toward theoretical integration. *Clinical Psychology Review, 30*, 259–268.

Stroebe, M., Schut, D., & Stroebe, W. (2007). Health outcomes of bereavement: A review. *Lancet, 270*(9603), 1960–1973.

Stroebe, M., Stroebe, W., & Schut, D. (2006). Bereavement research: methodological issues and ethical concerns, *Palliative Medicine, 17*(3), 235–240.

Tong, V. T., Zotti, M. E., & Hsia, J. (2011). Impact of the Red River catastrophic flood on women giving birth in North Dakota, 1994–2000. *Maternal & Child Health Journal, 15*(3), 281–288.

van Den Berg, B., Grievink, L., Yzermans, J. & Lebret, E. (2005). Medically unexplained physical symptoms in the aftermath of disasters. *Epidemiologic Reviews, 27*, 92–106.

Varghese, S. B. (2010). Cultural, ethical, and spiritual implications of natural disasters from the survivors' perspective. *Critical Care Nursing Clinics of North America, 22*(4), 515–522.

Viswanath, B., Maroky, A. S., Math, S. B., John, J. R., Benegal, V., Hamza, A., et al. (2012). Psychological impact of the tsunami on elderly survivors. *American Journal of Geriatric Psychiatry, 20*(5), 402–407.

Wang, P. S., Gruber, J. J., Powers, R. E., Schoenbaum, M., Speier, A. H., Wells, K. B., & Kessler, R. C. (2007). Mental health service use among Hurricane Katrina survivors in the eight months after the disaster. *Psychiatric Services, 58*(11), 1403–1411.

Wisnivesky, J. P., Teitelbaum, S. L., Todd, A. C., Boffetta, P., Crane, M., Crowley, L., et al. (2011). Persistence of multiple illnesses in World Trade Center rescue and recovery workers: A cohort study. *Lancet, 387*(9794), 888–897.

Zhang, B., El-Jawahri, A., & Prigerson, H. G. (2006). Update on bereavement research: Evidence-based guidelines for the diagnosis and treatment of complicated bereavement. *Journal of Palliative Medicine, 9*(5), 1188–1203.

Zisook, S. (1987). Unresolved grief. In S. Zisook (Ed.), *Biopsychosocial aspects of bereavement* (pp. 21–34). Washington, DC: American Psychiatric Press.

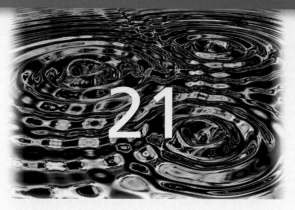

21

Suicide Prevention
Screening, Assessment, and Intervention

Emily J. Hauenstein

KEY CONCEPTS

- hopelessness
- lethality
- suicide

LEARNING OBJECTIVES

After studying this chapter, you will be able to:

1. Identify suicide as a major mental health problem in the United States.

2. Define *suicide, suicidality, suicide attempt, parasuicide,* and *suicidal ideation.*

3. Describe population groups that have high rates of suicide.

4. Describe risk factors associated with suicide completion.

5. Identify key factors associated with specific suicide acts.

6. Describe evidence-based interventions used to reduce imminent and ongoing suicide risk.

7. Explain the importance of documentation and reporting when caring for patients who may be at risk of suicide.

KEY TERMS

- case finding • commitment to treatment statement • parasuicide • suicidal ideation • suicidality
- suicide attempt • suicide contagion

Suicide is one of the major health problems in the United States, accounting for 38,000 deaths each year. For every suicide death, an additional 25 suicide attempts are made. More than half of people complete suicide in their first attempt, and more than 30% will have a repeat attempt. The public health problem of suicidal behavior is so important that several goals stated in *Healthy People 2010* and retained in *Healthy People 2020* directly target the reduction of deaths by suicide (U.S. Department of Health and Human Services [U.S. DHHS], 2010).

More than 90% of suicides in the United States are associated with mental illness or alcohol and substance abuse (Insel, 2010). The subsequent visibility of the mental disorder discredits the person, leaving him or her open to stigmatization. Suicide is so rejected in contemporary society that people with strong suicidal thoughts do not seek treatment for fear of being stigmatized by others. Reports and portrayals of suicide in the popular media and television further stigmatize those who consider or attempt suicide. Society's unwillingness to talk openly about suicide also contributes to the common misperceptions resulting in many myths regarding suicide (Murphy, Fatoye, & Wibberley, 2013). Box 21.1 presents several myths and facts about suicide.

Suicides are preventable deaths when immediate friends and family and health care providers identify symptoms and use effective interventions. All practicing nurses will come into contact with patients who are thinking about suicide and often can prevent suicides by identifying and intervening with those at risk. Through individual and public education, nurses also can do much to demystify suicide and reduce stigma for those at risk. To reduce the devastating public impact of suicide on those at risk and their families, nurses must be knowledgeable about suicide and be able to implement effective preventive interventions. This chapter contains tools that

BOX 21.1

Myths and Facts about Suicide

Myth: People who talk about suicide do not complete suicide.

Fact: Many people who die by suicide have given definite warnings of their intentions. Always take any comment about suicide seriously.

Myth: Suicide happens without warning.

Fact: Most suicidal people give many clues and warning signs regarding their suicidal intention.

Myth: Suicidal people are fully intent on dying.

Fact: Most suicidal people are undecided about living or dying. A part of them wants to live; however, death seems like the only way out of their pain or situation. They may allow themselves to "gamble" with death, leaving it up to others to save them.

Myth: Suicides occur more frequently during holidays.

Fact: The suicide rate is lowest in December. The rate peaks in the spring and fall.

Myth: Improvement after a suicide crisis means that the risk is over.

Fact: Most suicides occur within 3 months of "improvement" when the individual has the energy and motivation to actually follow through with his or her suicidal thoughts.

Source: Suicide.org. (2011). *Suicide myths. Suicide prevention, awareness and support.* Retrieved July 9, 2012, from http://www.suicide.org/suicide-myths.html.

can be used to reduce the broad effects of suicide and provide appropriate care for suicidal patients.

SUICIDE AND SUICIDE ATTEMPT

KEYCONCEPT   Suicide is the voluntary act of killing oneself. It is a fatal, self-inflicted destructive act with explicit or inferred intent to die. It is sometimes called suicide completion.

This behavioral definition of suicide is limited and does not consider the complexity of the underlying depressive illness, personal motivations, and situational and family factors that provoke the suicide act. Except for the very young, suicide occurs in all age groups, social classes, and cultures (CDC, 2014a).

The term **suicidality** refers to all suicide-related behaviors and thoughts of completing or attempting suicide and suicide ideation. **Suicidal ideation** is thinking about and planning one's own death. Population studies show that suicidal ideation ranges between 3% and 10% but varies by characteristics of the participants and the way suicidal ideation is measured. Although suicide ideation often does not progress, about 4% to 18% will eventually attempt suicide, with each subsequent attempt associated with greater lethality (Nakagawa Grunebaum, Ocuendo, Burke, Kashima, & Mann, 2009).

A **suicide attempt** is a nonfatal, self-inflicted destructive act with explicit or implicit intent to die. Only recently have data on suicide attempts been compiled. In 2010,

650,000 people visited a hospital for injuries due to self-harm behavior (American Foundation for Suicide Prevention [AFSP], 2014). Adolescents make more attempts than do adults, but they generally are less successful. Suicide ideation, recent psychiatric hospitalization, and a previous attempt are significant predictors of a completed suicide (Selby, Yen, & Spirito, 2013; De Leo, Draper, Snowdon, & Kolves, 2013).

Parasuicide is a voluntary, apparent attempt at suicide, commonly called a suicidal gesture, in which the aim is not death (e.g., taking a sublethal drug). Parasuicidal behavior varies by intent. Some people truly wish to die, but others simply wish to feel nothing for a while. Still others want to send a message about their emotional state. Parasuicide behavior is never normal and should always be taken seriously. Parasuicide occurs frequently in younger age groups but declines after the age of 44 years.

KEYCONCEPT   Lethality refers to the probability that a person will successfully complete suicide. Lethality is determined by the seriousness of the person's intent and the likelihood that the planned method of death will succeed. A plan to use an accessible firearm to commit suicide has greater lethality than a suicide plan that involves superficial cuts of the wrist.

Suicide is ranked as the 10th leading cause of death and accounts for 12.1 deaths per 100,000 population (Centers for Disease Control and Prevention [CDC], 2014a). A suicide occurs every 13.7 minutes in the United States: a rate of 80 completed successful suicides per day. The suicide rate in the United States has been stable for several years despite a significant increase in the rate of suicide attempts. Mountain regions have the highest rate of suicide (Figure 21.1). Its overall prevalence may be underestimated because suicide can be disguised as vehicular accidents or homicide, especially in young people (CDC, 2014a).

Suicide Across the Life Span

Children, Adolescents, and Young Adults

Among adolescents 15 to 24 years of age, there are approximately 100 to 200 attempts for every completed suicide (CDC, 2014b). Approximately, 15% of high school students have seriously considered suicide and 7% have attempted to take their own life (CDC, 2014a). Among American Indian and Alaskan natives ages 15 to 34 years, suicide is the second leading cause of death (CDC, 2014b).

Mental disorders can lead to school failure, alcohol or other drug abuse, family discord, violence, and suicide. Approximately 20% of U.S. children and adolescents are affected by mental disorders in their lifetime. In 2011,

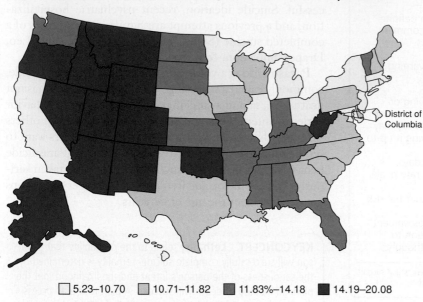

Suicide Rate
2000–2006, United States
Age-adjusted Death Rates per 100,000 Population

▷ District of Columbia

☐ 5.23–10.70 ▨ 10.71–11.82 ▨ 11.83%–14.18 ■ 14.19–20.08

Note: Reports for All Ages include those of unknown age.   *Data courtesy of CDC*

FIGURE 21.1 Number of deaths attributable to suicide in the United States per 100,000 population, 2007. (From Kaiser Family Foundation, statehealthfacts.org. Retrieved from http://www.nimh.nih.gov/statistics/4NAT_MAP.shtml: Centers for Disease Control and Prevention, National Center for Health Statistics, Division of Vital Statistics. (2010, May)

1.8% of youths (grades 9 to 12) reported that they had seriously considered attempting suicide during the preceding 12 months; 12% made a plan, and 7.8% attempted (CDC, 2014a). Suicide attempts vary according to racial and ethnic groups. In 2011 white non-Hispanic adolescents had the lowest rate of suicide attempts in the past 12 months, 1.9% compared to 3.2% Hispanic, 4.5% for Asian and 6.6% for American Indian or Alaska Native. A lower proportion of adolescent males reported suicide attempts in the past 12 months, 1.9% compared to females, 2.9% (U.S. DHHS).

Adults and Older Adults

In adults, death rates from suicide range from 12.3 to 17.2 deaths per 100,000 with the highest rates occurring in the 45- to 54-year age group (CDC, 2014b). Suicide rates peak during middle age, and a second peak occurs in those age 75 years and older. Physical illness and financial difficulties are important precipitants to suicide in older adults (Van Orden & Conwell, 2011).

Suicide death is a leading cause of death among armed service members deployed to Iraq and Afghanistan. Recent studies comparing suicide risk of veterans with the general population show excess risk for firearm suicide deaths. With the repeated deployment of military personnel that occurred, suicide behavior among soldiers remains a significant concern. There are several factors thought to contribute to the suicide rate. Combat exposure is one of the leading factors for both men and women military members. For women, military sexual trauma also contributes to the suicide ideation and attempts (Boyd, Bradshaw, & Robinson, 2013; Mitchell, Gallaway, Millikan, & Bell, 2012).

Epidemiology and Risk Factors

Mental illness is an important factor contributing to suicide in adults. Most young adults who commit suicide also have a depressive disorder, and many have personality disorders. Adolescents who have panic attacks are particularly at risk for suicide. Auditory hallucinations increase the risk for suicide because of the possibility of individuals impulsively responding to "voices" directing them to kill themselves. Substance abuse increases the likelihood that suicidal ideation will result in both parasuicidal and suicidal behaviors. Box 21.2 identifies risk factors for suicide (Goldston et al., 2009; U.S. DHHS, 2010).

Medical illnesses increase the likelihood of chronic depression, which in turn contributes to the increased suicide rate of those older than the age of 65 years (De Leo et al., 2013; Liu, Kraines, Puzia, Massing-Schaffer, & M. Kleiman, 2013; Kim et al., 2011). Additionally, symptoms of comorbid illnesses often are similar to those of depressive disorder, making recognition of depressive disorder by primary care providers difficult. Patients are often reticent to disclose their suicidal thoughts, further

---

BOX 21.2

Factors Enhancing Suicide Risk

VULNERABILITY
Primary family member who has completed suicide
Psychiatric disorder
Previous attempt by the patient
Loss (e.g., death of significant other, divorce, job loss)
Unrelenting physical illness

RISK
White or Native American man
Older man
Adolescent non-Hispanic white or Native American male
Gay, lesbian, or bisexual orientation
Access to firearms
Middle-aged woman

INTENT
Suicide plan and means of executing it
Inability to commit to treatment

DISINHIBITION
Impulsivity
Isolation
Psychotic thoughts
Drug or alcohol use

---

complicating detection. Consequently, health professionals fail to identify many patients who are experiencing suicidal ideation. In one study, 12.4% of persons visiting their primary care physicians for routine medical care had suicidal ideation, yet only 2.1% disclosed that information to their physicians (Bryan, Corso, Rudd, & Cordero, 2008).

Psychological Risk Factors

Internal distress, low self-esteem, and interpersonal distress have long been associated with suicide. Childhood physical and sexual abuse are linked to suicide, suicide ideation, and parasuicide. Cognitive risk factors include problem-solving deficits, impulsivity, rumination, and hopelessness. Impulsivity, anger, and reduced inhibition increase the risk of suicide. Recent purchase of a handgun increases the risk of self-harm (Hawkins & Cougle, 2013; Pompili et al., 2013; Zhang & Li, 2013).

Social Risk Factors

Social isolation is a primary risk factor for suicide. Social distress leads to despair and can be caused by family discord, parental neglect, abuse, parental suicide, and divorce. Social distress can prevent the patient from accessing the support necessary to prevent suicidal acts. Other social factors associated with suicide risk include economic deprivation, unemployment, and poverty, especially among youth. More poorly educated men also have an enhanced risk for suicide (Walsh, Clayton, Liu, & Hodges, 2009; Ando et al., 2013; CDC, 2014).

Gender

Males have a higher suicide completion rate than females. For men, suicide is the eighth leading cause of death, with a rate of 19.9 per 100,000 in 2010, more than four times the rate in women (AFSP, 2014). Men complete 79% of all suicides; 57.5% of these deaths are by firearms. Men are more likely to use means that have a higher rate of success, such as firearms and hanging (U.S. DHHS, 2014). Rural men have a much higher risk of suicide than urban men, and that gap is widening, perhaps attributable to the higher rates of gun ownership in rural areas (McCarthy, Blow, Ignacio, Ilgen, Austin, Valenstein, et al., 2012). Most suicide deaths occur in men with psychiatric disorders, primarily depression, in many cases complicated by substance abuse (Schmutte et al., 2009). Substance abuse, aggression, hopelessness, emotion-focused coping, social isolation, and having little purpose in life have been associated with suicidal behavior in men. Unmarried, unsociable men between the ages of 42 and 77 years with minimal social networks and no close relatives have a significantly increased risk for committing suicide (Walsh et al., 2009). White and American Indian/Alaska native men had the highest rates of any racial/ethnic population in this *older* age group. Suicide attempts are often lethal in this age group because men in this age group and in all racial and ethnic groups except those of Asian descent use firearms to commit suicide (U.S. DHHS, 2014).

Women across age and racial and ethnic groups are less likely to die from suicide than are men but are more likely to attempt suicide. Women make three attempts to every attempt by men. Adolescent girls and women ages 10 to 44 years have the highest rate of suicide attempts. Women are less likely to complete a suicide, partly because they are more likely to choose less lethal methods. For women, whereas current or previous exposure to violence, sexual assault, or both increases a woman's risk for suicidal behavior, having a small child reduces risk (Stack & Wasserman, 2009).

Sexuality

The lesbian, gay, bisexual, and transgender (LGBT) population is at increased risk for suicide (Mustanski & Liu, 2013; Ploderi et al., 2013). Other risk factors include early disclosure of their sexual orientation and early onset of sexual activity (Paul et al., 2002). A cross-national study meta-analysis showed that lifetime suicide ideation was more common among gay men (40%–55%) compared with heterosexual men (18%–30%) as were lifetime suicide attempts (8%–25% for gay men versus 1%–13% in heterosexual men) (Lewis, 2009). Depressive symptoms and suicidality rates in early adolescence are higher among sexual minority youth than among heterosexual youth and these disparities persist into young adulthood. These disparities are largest for females and bisexually-identified youth (Marshal et al., 2013). In lesbian, gay, and bisexual older adults, there are high levels of poor general health disability and depression (Fredriksen-Goldsen et al., 2013).

Race and Ethnicity

There is considerable variation in the profile of suicide rates across racial groups, including the age when rates are at their peak and the duration of high rates across several age groups (Figure 21.2). The suicide rate per 100,000 (both men and women) is 14.1 for whites, 5.1 for African Americans, and 5.9 for Hispanics living in the United States (Wadsworth & Kubrin, 2007).

White adolescents and men have high rates from the age of 15 years onward, but the peak suicide rate is among those older than 75 years. Access to firearms is associated with the risk of completed suicides, particularly for white males. In 2009, 51.8% of deaths from suicide were firearm related and most suicides occur in the victim's home. Firearm ownership in more prevalent in the United States than in any other country—approximately 35% to 39% of households have firearms (Anglemyer, Horvath, & Rutherford, 2014).

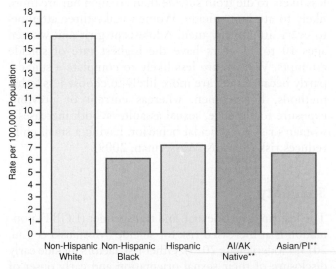

FIGURE 21.2 Suicide rates among persons ages 10 years and older, by race or ethnicity, United States, 2002–2005. During 2005 to 2009, the highest suicide rates were among American Indian or Alaskan natives, and non-Hispanic whites. All rates are age-adjusted to the standard 2000 population. Rates are based on less than 20 deaths are not shown as they are statistically unreliable. AI, American India; AK, Alaskan; PI, Pacific Islander. (From Centers for Disease Control and Prevention. (2014) *Injury prevention & control: Violence prevention*. National Statistics at a Glance. Retrieved from http://www.cdc.gov/violenceprevention/suicide/statistics/rates01.html.)

Although the overall suicide rate for African Americans is low, young African American men take their lives at a rate considerably above that of other age groups. Family cohesion and social support in African American families contribute to the lower rates in this group. Higher rates of suicide in younger men is associated with being in foster care, early aggressive behavior, depression, and dissatisfaction with life (Liu et al., 2013; Wang, Lightsey, Tran, & Bonapart, 2013).

Even though the suicide rate for Hispanics (Latinos) is less than half of the overall U.S. rate, suicide is the 12th leading cause of death for Hispanics of all ages and third leading cause of death for Hispanic males ages 15 to 34. Among Hispanic ethnic subgroups in the United States, Puerto Rican adults have the highest rates of suicide attempts. Hispanics born in the United States have higher rates of suicidal ideation and attempts than Hispanic immigrants (Suicide Prevention Resource Center [SPRC], 2013a).

Suicide is the eighth leading cause of death for American Indians/Alaska Natives of all ages and the second leading cause of death among youth ages 10 to 24. Men and women ages 35 to 64 had a greater percentage increase in suicide rates between 1999 and 2012 than any other racial/ethnic group. Lifetime rates of having attempted suicide reported by adolescents ranged from 21.8% in girls to 11.8% in boys. Adolescent suicide attempts are significantly higher among youth (both sexes) raised on reservations (17.6%) compared to youth raised in urban areas (14.3%). Whereas exposure to suicide and access to alcohol and drugs contribute to suicide rates for Native Americans, family support and cultural and tribal orientation are protective (SPRC, 2013b).

The scant literature on suicide among Asian populations shows that suicide ideation, plans, and attempts are more common than popularly believed and vary within Asian ethnic groups. For example Native Hawaiians living in Hawaii who were between the ages of 15 and 44 had a significantly higher suicide death rate than other racial/ethnic groups, but those over 45 had a much lower rate than Whites, the same rate as Japanese, and a higher rate than Filipinos. Asians who immigrated to the United States as children have higher rates of suicidal ideation and suicide attempts than U.S. born Asians. Cultural identification with the Asian culture (sense of belonging and affiliation with spiritual, material, intellectual, and emotional features) is associated with a 69% reduction in the risk of suicide attempt (SPRC, 2013c).

The reasons for racial and ethnic variations are unclear. The rates of depressive disorder, a major risk factor for suicide, vary across racial group. Cultural stress, perceived discrimination, and vulnerability are thought to contribute to the risk of suicide (Gomez, Miranda, & Polanco, 2011).

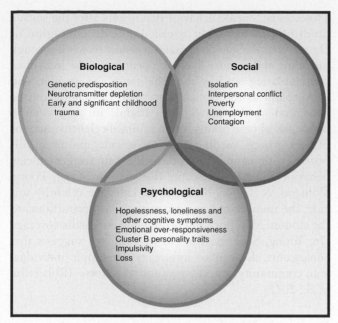

Biological

Genetic predisposition
Neurotransmitter depletion
Early and significant childhood
trauma

Social

Isolation
Interpersonal conflict
Poverty
Unemployment
Contagion

Psychological

Hopelessness, loneliness and
other cognitive symptoms
Emotional over-responsiveness
Cluster B personality traits
Impulsivity
Loss

FIGURE 21.3 Biopsychosocial causes of suicide.

Etiology

The convergence of biologic, psychological, and social factors can be directly linked to suicidal behavior (Figure 21.3). In genetically and physiologically vulnerable individuals, thoughts, feelings, and personality factors can interfere with personal problem solving, promote impulsivity, and support suicidal behavior. Poverty, unemployment, and social conflict also contribute to suicidal behavior in those at risk for suicide.

Biologic Theories

Depression and severe childhood trauma are linked to suicide. Those who complete suicide often have extremely low levels of the neurotransmitter serotonin. Impairments in the serotonergic system contribute to suicidal behavior. Additionally, people who make near-lethal suicide attempts have much lower levels of the neurotransmitter dopamine and noradrenaline (Fernandez-Navarro et al., 2012).

Physiological Effects of Child Abuse

Child abuse has been described as a specific vulnerability for psychopathology and suicide. Enhanced vulnerability to depressive disorder and suicide associated with child abuse apparently is attributable to altered serotonin and dopamine metabolism and subsequent hypothalamic–pituitary–adrenal dysregulation that occurs coincident with the intractable stress of the abuse experience (Guillaume et al., 2013). Twin studies further establish the independent contribution of childhood sexual abuse to

biologic alterations that lead to suicidal behavior in adolescence and adults in genetically vulnerability individuals (Roy, Sarchiopone, & Carli, 2009).

Genetic Factors

Suicide runs in families. First-degree relatives of individuals who have completed suicide have a two to eight times higher risk for suicide than do individuals in the general population. Suicide of a first-degree relative is highly predictive of a serious attempt in another first-degree relative. Children of depressed and suicidal parents have higher rates of suicidal behavior themselves. The genetic link to suicide is evident in twin studies. Suicidal behavior has a 50% concordance for completed suicide (Tidemalm et al., 2011).

Psychological Theories

Cognitive Theories

Most evidence on the psychological contributions to suicidal behavior point to cognitive, affective, behavioral, and personality factors that intensify the experience of hopelessness and disconnection from others. Aaron Beck first identified the cognitive triad of hopelessness, helplessness, and worthlessness as integral to the experience of depression (Beck, Rush, Shaw, & Emery, 1979). Since then, a significant evidence base has been established linking hopelessness, loneliness, and other cognitive symptoms to suicide (van Dulmen & Goossens, 2013). Depressed persons who are hopeless are more likely to consider suicide than those who are depressed but hopeful about the future. Furthermore, it appears that lack of positive thoughts about the future is more likely to predict suicidal behavior than negative thoughts even though both contribute to hopelessness (Zhang & Li, 2013). The importance of specific cognitive symptoms to suicide risk varies by age and the suicide attempt history of the individual.

> **KEYCONCEPT** **Hopelessness** is the pervasive belief that undesirable events are likely to occur coupled with the belief that one's situation is unlikely to improve (Ellis & Rutherford, 2008).

Emotional factors and personality traits also play a role in suicidal behavior by enhancing perceptions of helplessness and hopelessness, contributing to poor self-esteem, and interfering with coping efforts. Shame, guilt, despair, and emotion-focused coping have been linked to suicidal behavior (Guerreiro, Cruz, Frasquilho, Santos, Figueira, & Sampaio, 2013; Upthegrove, Ross, Brunet, McCollum, & Jones, 2014). Loss and grief are also important considerations. Emotional distress often is potentiated by personality traits such as in borderline personality disorder (see Chapter 27) that contribute to poor self esteem, impulsivity, and suicidal behavior. Poor self-esteem in turn has been linked to suicide ideation, attempts, and deaths (Capron, Norr, Macatee, & Schmidt, 2013).

Interpersonal–Psychological Theory of Suicidal Behavior

The interpersonal–psychological theory of suicidal behavior (Joiner & Van Orden, 2008; Joiner, et al., 2009) provides a basis for discriminating between those who are thinking about suicide versus those who are likely to engage in suicidal acts. The theory postulates that those most at risk are those who have engaged in previous acts of self-harm, believe they are alienated from social relationships, and perceive themselves to be a burden to those they love. Together these beliefs lead to the misperception that others would be better off without them and the idea that sacrificing themselves is the appropriate action to take. Additionally, recent evidence suggests that over arousal for someone who has developed the capacity for suicide can be particularly significant in identifying potential suicide victims (Ribeiro, Silva, & Joiner, 2014).

Social Theories

Before the turn of the 20th century, Emile Durkheim (1897) linked suicide to the social conditions in which people live. Both a lack of social connectedness and social conditions contribute to suicidal behavior. People who are socially connected are less likely to engage in suicidal behavior. When an individual has others he or she can depend on, suicide can be prevented, even among those at significant risk. Even among people with social bonds, however, lack of community and social resources can interact with physiological and psychological risk to increase the likelihood of suicide.

Social Distress

A lack of social connection contributes to suicide ideation, attempts, and deaths across the age span. Among adults, those who are single, never married, separated, widowed, and homeless without religious affiliation report loneliness or otherwise are socially isolated are also more likely to engage in suicidal behavior (Mezuk, Rock, Lohman, & Choi, 2014; Séquin, Beauchamp, Robert, Dimambro, & Turecki, 2014). Being socially connected, however, does not in itself reduce risk. Interpersonal conflict and being a victim of bullying can contribute to suicidal behavior, especially in adolescents and young adults (Messias, Kindrick, & Castro, 2014).

Suicide Contagion

Social exposure to suicide is associated with an increased personal risk for suicidal behavior, particularly among adolescents. Suicide behavior that occurs after the suicide death of a known other is called **suicide contagion** or cluster suicide. Suicide contagion seems to work through modeling and is more likely to occur when the individual contemplating suicide is of the same age, gender, and background as the person who died. Contagion can be prompted by the suicide of a friend, an acquaintance, online social networking, or an idolized celebrity. Actions of peer groups, media reports of suicide, and even billboards with content about suicide can trigger suicide behavior among adolescents (Robertson, Skegg, Poore, Williams, & Taylor, 2012). In the case of a celebrity suicide, the number of "copycat suicides" is proportional to the amount, duration, and prominence of media coverage (Ju, Young, Seok, & Yip, 2014). Evidence suggests that adolescents also can be influenced by simple individual and community suicide prevention efforts (Robertson et al., 2012).

Economic Disadvantage

Poverty and economic disadvantage are associated with depression, suicide ideation, and suicide mortality. Individuals who are not employed, not married, and with low education and low income have a higher risk of suicide. Suicide risk is greater for low income females in socially deprived areas and males living alone in materially deprived areas (Burrows, Auger, Gamache, & Hamel, 2013). Adolescents from impoverished neighborhoods have more suicidal ideation and attempts, and suicides increase as the percentage of boarded-up buildings in a neighborhood increases, particularly if the individuals have a mental disorder (Page et al., 2014).

In impoverished communities, lack of good schools and employment opportunities lead to unemployment and loss of meaningful social roles. Low-income men are at risk for suicide when they lose their jobs, especially when their wives obtain jobs to support their families (Ying & Chang, 2009). Additionally, access to health care is limited in these communities, and there is an increased exposure to others exhibiting suicidal behavior that enhances suicide risk (Bernburg, Thorlindsson, & Sigfusdottir, 2009).

Family Response to Suicide

Suicide has devastating effects on everyone it touches, especially family and close friends. One suicide is estimated to leave at least six survivors who are significantly impacted by the loss (Andriessen & Krysinska, 2012). In the aftermath of a family member's suicide, survivors experience more grief, anxiety and depression, guilt, shame, self-blame, and dysfunction than families whose loss was because of other reasons and the personal and familial disruption often lasts for years. Although recovery from a loved one's suicide is an ongoing task, survivors who are emotionally healthy before the suicide act and who have social support are able to manage the psychological trauma associated with suicide. Still, the intensity and duration of the postsuicide grief process for many survivors has led to the development of family intervention programs. Although the evidence base for these interventions is still small, strategies that support a positive sense of self, enhance problem-solving, promote the formation of a suicide story, encourage social reintegration, reduce stigma, use journaling, or permit the survivor to debrief may be effective in reducing subjective distress and to resolve grief (Andriessen & Krysinska, 2012; Buus, Caspersen, Hansen, Stenager, & Fleischer, 2013). These strategies may be most effective delivered in survivor peer help groups.

TREATMENT AND NURSING CARE FOR SUICIDE PREVENTION

Interdisciplinary Treatment and Recovery

The challenges of preventing suicides and promoting healthy coping belong to all disciplines. An interdisciplinary treatment or recovery approach along with peer support is needed for managing the threats of suicide.

Priority Care Issues

EMERGENCY CARE ALERT ! A true psychiatric emergency exists when an individual presents with one or more symptoms associated with imminent risk for suicidal behavior. Immediate and focused action is needed to prevent the patient's death.

The first priority is to provide for the patient's safety while initiating the *least* restrictive care possible. In contrast, an example of the *most* restrictive care is an outpatient who is admitted to a locked unit with one staff member who is assigned to observe the person at all times. Hospitalization should be reserved for those whose safety cannot be ensured in an outpatient environment.

NURSING MANAGEMENT: Preventing Suicide and Promoting Mental Health

Suicidal ideation, planning, and acts are not easily predicted and therefore are difficult to study. As a result, few evidence-based treatments exist that are known to prevent suicide and manage suicidal behavior. There is growing consensus that the suicidal act is part of a continuum of behaviors that extend long before and after a specific suicide behavioral incident. The beginning evidence points to four steps in preventing suicide and promoting long-term mental health: identification of those

thinking about suicide (case finding), assessment to determine an imminent suicidal threat, intervening to change suicidal behavior associated with a specific suicidal threat, and institution of effective interventions to prevent future episodes of suicidal behavior (Catanese, John, Di Battista, & Clarke, 2009).

Assessment

Case Finding

Case finding refers to identifying people who are at risk for suicide so proper treatment can be initiated. People who are contemplating suicide often do not share their ideation. This lack of disclosure often means that family, friends, and health professionals are unable to intervene until the suicidal ideation and planning have progressed. Yet early identification of suicidal ideation may reduce suicide deaths. Nurses can play important roles in suicide prevention by recognizing the warning signs. See Box 21.3 for the warning signs developed by the American Association of Suicidology (2014); the mnemonic IS PATH WARM can serve as a useful memory aide for these signs.

Case finding requires careful and concerned questioning and listening that make the patient feel valued and cared about (Box 21.4). Most standardized health questionnaires have questions about suicide thoughts. Many nurses are concerned that asking patients about their suicidal thoughts will provoke a suicide attempt. This belief simply is not true. The patient expressing suicidal ideation often has had these thoughts for some time and may feel more socially connected when another recognizes the seriousness of the situation. Under no circumstances should a patient be promised secrecy about suicidal

---

BOX 21.3

Warning Signs for Suicide

I—Ideation: Talking or writing about death, dying, or suicide
Threatening or talking of wanting to hurt or kill self
Looking for ways to kill self: seeking access to firearms, available pills, or other means
S—Substance abuse: Increased substance (alcohol or drug) use
P—Purposelessness: No perceived reason for living; no sense of purpose in life
A—Anxiety: Anxiety, agitation, unable to sleep or sleeping all the time
T—Trapped: Feeling trapped (like there is no way out)
H—Hopelessness
W—Withdrawal: Withdrawal from friends, family, and society
A—Anger: Rage, uncontrolled anger, seeking revenge
R—Recklessness: Acting reckless or engaging in risky activities, seemingly without thinking
M—Mood change: Dramatic mood changes

Adapted from American Association of Suicidology. (2014). *Know the warning signs.* Retrieved from http://www.suicidology.org/web/guest/stats-and-tools/warning-signs.

BOX 21.4 • THERAPEUTIC DIALOGUE: • Suicide

When Caroline sought medical care for a cold from her nurse practitioner, the nurse observed more than a cough and runny nose. Caroline appeared downcast and unusually sad. As the nurse and patient talked, the subject of family life came up, whereupon Caroline began to cry softly. As words tumbled out, she said she had been unhappy at home for a long time. When she was very young, she recalled being happy, but things changed when her brother was born, 4 years after her. Her father began to abuse her sexually, starting when Caroline was 5 years old and continuing until he moved out of the house when she was 12 years old. Caroline suspects her mother knew of the abuse, although she did nothing about it.

Two years ago, Caroline's father committed suicide. Caroline feels relieved about his death but frustrated that she never got a chance to tell him how angry she was with him. Caroline's relationship with her mother has not improved. Caroline says her mother favors her brother and is always telling her she won't amount to anything. Caroline begins to cry harder.

INEFFECTIVE APPROACH

Nurse: Clearly, many things are troubling you. Don't you think that things seem worse now because you have a cold?

Caroline: Well, that could be. What are you going to do to make me feel better?

Nurse: Give you some medicine to help you sleep and clear your nose. I think you should see a psychiatrist, too.

Caroline: I don't need a psychiatrist. I came here for my cold.

Nurse: I know you did, but you seem to be depressed.

Caroline: What are you, some kind of social worker? I am just tired.

Nurse: I am a nurse, and you seem down to me. Are you thinking about suicide?

Caroline: I don't think you know what you're talking about. I want to go now. Could you give me my medicine?

EFFECTIVE APPROACH

Nurse: It seems as though many things have been piling up on you. Does it seem that way to you, too?

Caroline: It sure does. I've just been trying to get through one day at a time, but now with this cold and no sleep, I feel like I can't go on.

Nurse: When you say you can't go on, what does that mean to you?

Caroline: Lately, I have been thinking about running away to some place where I can't be found and maybe starting over. But then I think, where would I go? Where would I stay? Who would take care of me?

Nurse: When you think that your plan for escape won't work, what happens?

Caroline: (Starting to cry again.) Then I think that maybe it would be better if I just did what my father did. I really don't think anyone would miss me.

Nurse: So you think you might take your life, like your Dad did?

Caroline: Yeah, and what really scares me is lately I have been thinking about that a lot. I keep saying to myself, "You're just tired," but I am so exhausted now that I can't chase the thoughts away.

Nurse: So, do you think about suicide every day?

Caroline: It seems like I never stop thinking about it.

Nurse: Is there anything you can do to make the thoughts go away?

Caroline: Nothing. (Silence.)

Nurse: What would you do?

Caroline: I think I would get as many pills as I could find, drink a lot of alcohol, and maybe smoke some pot and just go to sleep.

Nurse: Do you have enough pills at home to kill yourself?

Caroline (wan smile): I was hoping that the sleeping medicine you would give me might do the job.

Nurse: It sounds like you need some help getting through this time in your life. Would you like some?

Caroline: I honestly don't know—I just want to sleep for a long time.

CRITICAL THINKING CHALLENGE

- In the first interaction, the nurse made two key blunders. What were they? What effect did they have on the patient? How did they interfere with the patient's care?

- What did Caroline do that might have contributed to the nurse's behavior in the first interaction?

- In the second interaction, the nurse did several things that ensured reporting of Caroline's suicidal ideation. What were they? What differences in attitude might differentiate the nurse in the first interaction from the nurse in the second?

thoughts, plans, or acts. Instead, tell patients that disclosure of suicidal intent will be shared with other interdisciplinary team members so the safety of the patient can be ensured.

Assessing Risk

After suicide ideation has been established, the next step is to determine the risk for a suicide attempt. Suicide risk assessment is difficult and whenever possible should proceed only with the assistance of other members of the interdisciplinary treatment team. Assessing for risk includes determining the seriousness of the suicidal ideation, degree of hopelessness, disorders, previous attempt, suicide planning and implementation, and availability and lethality of suicide method. Risk assessment also includes the patient's resources, including coping skills and social supports, that can be used to counter suicidal impulses. Box 21.5 lists some questions that might be asked in assessing the risk for suicide.

The greatest predictor of a future suicide attempt is a previous attempt, partly because the individual already has broken the "taboo" around suicidal behavior. Repeated episodes of self-harm with or without suicidal intent also increase immediate risk because they increase an individual's capacity to complete suicide (Ribeiro et al., 2014). Other important signs of high risk are the presence of suicide planning behaviors (detailed plan, availability of means, opportunity, and capability) and engaging in final acts such as giving away prized possessions and saying goodbye to loved ones. Although the presence of a specific psychiatric disorder such as depression is an important consideration in risk assessment, anxiety, agitation,

---

BOX 21.5

Assessment of Suicidal Episode

INTENT TO DIE

1. Have you been thinking about hurting or killing yourself?
2. How seriously do you want to die?
3. Have you attempted suicide before?
4. Are there people or things in your life who might keep you from killing yourself?

SEVERITY OF IDEATION

1. How often do you have these thoughts?
2. How long do they last?
3. How much do the thoughts distress you?
4. Can you dismiss them or do they tend to return?
5. Are they increasing in intensity and frequency?

DEGREE OF PLANNING

1. Have you made any plans to kill yourself? If yes, what are they?
2. Do you have access to the materials (e.g., gun, poison, pills) that you plan to use to kill yourself?
3. How likely is it that you could actually carry out the plan?
4. Have you done anything to put the plan into action?
5. Could you stop yourself from killing yourself?

---

alcohol use, and impulsivity may be better indicators of immediate risk. On the other hand, support from important others, religious prohibitions, responsibility for young children, and employment may provide protection from suicidal impulses.

Ideally, an interdisciplinary team conducts suicide risk assessment in an emergency department or outpatient facility with multiple supports. Nurses practicing in more isolated situations should keep a list of contacts in settings that routinely conduct suicide risk assessments so the contacts may be consulted if a seriously suicidal individual appears in the nurse's setting.

> **NCLEXNOTE** Suicide assessment is always considered a priority. Practice by asking patients about suicidal thoughts and plans. Develop a plan with a suicidal patient that focuses on resisting the suicidal impulse. Apply the assessment process that delineates the (1) intent to die, (2) severity of ideation, (3) availability of means, and (4) degree of planning.

Nursing Diagnoses and Outcome Identification

Several nursing diagnoses may be applied when dealing with a suicidal patient, including Risk for Suicide, Interrupted Family Processes, Anxiety, Ineffective Health Maintenance, Risk for Self-Directed Violence, Impaired Social Interaction, Ineffective Coping, Chronic Low Self-Esteem, Insomnia, Social Isolation, and Spiritual Distress.

Interventions for Imminent, Intermediate, and Long-Term Suicide Prevention

Interventions for Those at Imminent Risk

There are three urgent priorities for care of a person who is at imminent risk for suicide: reconnecting the patient to other people and instilling hope, restoring emotional stability and reducing suicidal behavior, and ensuring safety. Reconnecting the patient interpersonally includes listening intently and without judgment to the patient's thoughts and feelings and validating his or her experience and suffering. This intervention directly challenges the patient's belief that no one cares. Using cognitive interventions can help the client to regain hope (see Chapter 12). These actions help reestablish links between the patient's presuicidal past and helps the patient begin establishing goals for the future (Gudmundsdottir & Thome, 2014).

Ensuring Patient Safety

Helping patients develop strategies for making safer choices when distressed is an important goal. Nurses caring for patients who are emerging from the initial hours and days of a suicide attempt can support the patient and focus on managing suicidal urges and developing protective strategies. As the nurse connects with the patient, together they can create a list of personal and professional resources that can be used when the individual is in crisis. With the nurse's help, the patient can visualize "emotional spaces that are safe places to go" when distressed.

Until recently, the no-suicide contract was a staple of psychiatric nursing practice and widely used across disciplines as a means of preventing suicide among those at risk. No-suicide contracts are verbal and written "contracts" between the individual at imminent risk for suicide and a health care provider that contain an agreement that the patient will not commit suicide during a specific time period. Careful evaluation of this practice has not established its efficacy in preventing suicidal behavior and suicide deaths. As a consequence, the nurse should avoid engaging in a no-suicide contract with a patient (Puskar & Urda, 2011).

Inpatient Safety Considerations

When hospitalization is considered the best option to ensure the safety of the patient, the nurse has responsibility for providing a safe, therapeutic environment in which human connection, instilling hope, and changing suicidal behavior can occur. There are no evidence-based guidelines for preventing suicides in hospitals. Inpatient suicides do occur. Between January 1995 and June 30, 2008, 641 of 5,208 sentinel events (12.3%) were inpatient suicides (Janofsky, 2009), a rate that continues to present challenges for the inpatient nursing staff. The vast majority of inpatient suicides take place in psychiatric facilities, and the method used in 75% of these events is hanging (Tishler & Reiss, 2009).

Removal of dangerous items and environmental hazards, continuous or intermittent observation of at-risk patients by hospital personnel trained in observation methods, and limitation of outpatient passes are the mainstays of hospital interventions. Observation procedures vary from facility to facility. For patients who require constant supervision, a staff member will be assigned only to the high-risk patient. For less risky patients, observation may entail close or intermittent observations.

Observation is not, in itself, therapeutic. An observation becomes therapeutic when interaction occurs with the patient. Psychiatric intensive care of this kind and restriction of freedom can be very upsetting to the patient who is withdrawn and isolated. Nurses can help patients reestablish personal control by including them in decisions about their care and restricting their behavior only as necessary. Nurses can also reduce the patient's stress while ensuring the patient's safety by intruding as little as possible on the person's exercise of free will. Observational periods can be used to help patients express a broad range of feelings and strengthen their belief in their own abilities to keep themselves safe. During observation, the

BOX 21.6
Using Reflection

THERAPEUTIC OBSERVATION

INCIDENT • An inpatient is angry about being under continual observation and keeps trying to get away from the nurse. He starts yelling at the nurse, staff, and other patients and threatens to kill himself the first chance he gets.

REFLECTION • Upon reflection, the nurse realized that she had been preoccupied with issues that were occurring in her personal life. Although she kept the patient under constant supervision, she hadn't really spoken with him much. In focusing on her own problems, the nurse recognized that she had inadvertently made the patient feel even more isolated and disconnected. The nurse also realized that she had missed an opportunity to help the patient feel more hopeful and to engage him in planning for his own safety.

nurse can help the patient describe feelings and identify ways to manage safety needs (Box 21.6).

Interventions for Intermediate and Long-Term Risk

Patients who are suicidal may need ongoing preventive interventions. The risk varies with the genetic, psychiatric, and psychological profile of the patient and the extent of his or her social support. Discouragement and hopelessness often persist long past the suicidal episode. Episodes of hopelessness should be anticipated and planned for in the patient's care. Patients should be taught to expect setbacks and times when they are unable to see much of a future for themselves. They should be encouraged to think of times in their lives when they were not so hopeless and consider how they may feel similarly in the future. Helping patients review the goals they already have achieved and at the same time set goals that can be achieved in the immediate future can help them manage periods of discouragement and hopelessness.

Interventions for the Biologic Domain

Patients who have survived a suicide attempt often need physical care of their self-inflicted injury. Overdose, gunshot wounds, and skin wounds are common. For both groups, there will be biologic interventions for the underlying psychiatric disorder (see Unit 6).

Medication Management

Medication management focuses on treating the underlying psychiatric disorder. In schizophrenia and schizoaffective disorder, evidence suggests that antipsychotic use is related to decreased mortality compared with those not taking an antipsychotic, but only clozapine has been shown to have a protective effect (De Hert, Corell, & Cohen, 2010). For depression, a nonlethal antidepressant, such as a selective serotonin reuptake inhibitor, usually will be prescribed.

Electroconvulsive Therapy

Electroconvulsive therapy (ECT) has been used in both inpatient and outpatient settings to alleviate severe depression, especially in medically compromised groups such older adults, who may not tolerate conventional pharmacotherapy for depression (see Chapter 11). Rapid reduction in depression often leads to a decreased suicide drive (Fink, 2014). More research is needed to determine the role ECT may play in managing suicidal behavior. At this time, ECT is among several strategies used to decrease suicidal behavior over the long term.

Interventions for the Psychological Domain

The goals of treatment in the psychological domain include reducing the capacity for suicidal behavior, increasing tolerance for distress, expanding coping abilities, and developing effective crisis management strategies. During the early part of a hospitalization, the most important way to reduce stress is to help the patient feel more secure and hopeful. As patients become more comfortable in their environment, the nurse can provide education about emotions, help patients explore and link presuicidal beliefs to a positive and hopeful future, support the application of new skills in managing negative thoughts, and help develop effective problem-solving skills.

Challenging the Suicidal Mindset

Teaching patients to distract themselves when thinking about suicide or engaging in negative self-evaluation can help to diminish suicidal ideation, dysfunctional thinking, and emotional reactivity. Simple distracting techniques such as reminding oneself to think of other things or engaging in other activities such as talking on the telephone, reading, or watching a movie are excellent temporary means of distracting the patient from negative cognitive states. See Boxes 21.7 and 21.8 for additional information for educating patients and their families about suicide prevention.

Validating the patient and teaching the patient to self-validate are powerful means of reducing suicidal thinking. Patients can learn that everyone experiences emotional distress and can begin to recognize it a routine event. To manage emotional distress and increase tolerance for it, patients can be taught simple anxiety management strategies such as relaxation and visualization. The

BOX 21.7

Psychoeducation Checklist: **Suicide Prevention**

When teaching the patient and family about suicide and its prevention, be sure to address the following topics:
- Importance of emotional connections to family and friends
- Importance of instilling hope
- Discouraging suicidal ideation, rumination, self-harming behaviors
- Self-validation
- Emotional distress management
- Finding alternatives to suicidal behavior
- Establishing and using a crisis management plan
- Reestablishing the social network of the patient.
- Information about treatment of underlying psychiatric disorders

patient can be encouraged to write about his or her emotional experiences.

Patients engage in suicidal behavior because they view it as their only option. When negative thoughts and emotions coexist, they reinforce each other and contribute to

BOX 21.8

Educational Resources for Suicidal Patients and Families

Biebel, D. B., & Foster, S. L. (2005). *Finding your way after the suicide of someone you love.* Grand Rapids, MI: Zondervan Publishing Company.
Bryson, K. (2006). *Those they left behind: Interviews, stories, essays, and poems by survivors of suicide.* Raleigh, NC: Lulu.com.
Colt, G. (2006). *November of the soul: The enigma of suicide.* New York: Scribner.
Conroy, D. (2006). *Out of the nightmare: Recovery from depression and suicidal pain.* Lincoln, NE: Authors Choice Press.
Crook, M. (2004). *Out of the darkness: Teens talk about suicide.* Vancouver, British Columbia: Arsenal Pulp Press.
Fox, J., & Roldan, M. (2008). *Voices of strength: Sons and daughters of suicide speak out.* Far Hills, NJ: New Horizon Press.
Hays, H. (2005). *Surviving suicide: Help to heal your heart.* Dallas: Brown Books Publishing Group.
Joiner, T. (2005). *Why people die by suicide.* Cambridge: Harvard University Press.
Linn-Gust, M. (2010). *Rocky roads: The journeys of families through suicide grief.* Albuquerque, NM: Chellehead Works.
Lukas, C., & Seiden, H. (2007). *Silent grief: Living in the wake of suicide.* Philadelphia: Jessica Kingsley Publishers.
Myers, M., & Fine, C. (2006). *Touched by suicide: Hope and healing after loss.* New York: Gotham Publishing.
Nelson, R., Galas, J., & Cobain, B. (2006). *The power to prevent suicide: A guide for teens helping teens.* St. Paul, MN: Free Spirit Publishing.
Requarth, M. (2008). *After a parent's suicide: Helping children heal.* Sebastopol, CA: Healing Hearts Press.
Robinson, D. (2008). *Suicide is not a dirty word.* Glasgow, Scotland: SHN publishers.
Rogers, D. (2007). *My child's final act: Suicide.* Frederick, MD: PublishAmerica.

hopelessness, which in turn increases the likelihood of a serious suicidal attempt (Catanese et al., 2009). Individuals who are suicidal often believe they are a burden to their family, who would be better off without them. Nurses can challenge negative beliefs, especially the patient's idea that he or she is a burden to others (see Chapter 12). Ask the patient to describe the events that led to specific suicidal behavior so the patient can be engaged in developing alternative solutions. For each event, work with the patient to identify specific strategies that could be used to manage his or her distress, sense of disconnection, extreme focus on suicidal ideas, and other experiences that led the person to believe he or she had no option other than to die.

Developing New Coping Strategies

Preventing suicidal behavior requires that patients develop crisis management strategies, generate solutions to difficult life circumstances other than suicide, engage in effective interpersonal interactions, and maintain hope. The nurse can help the patient develop a written plan that can be used as a blueprint for action when the patient feels like he or she is losing control. The plan should include strategies that the patient can use to self-soothe; friends and family members that could be called, including multiple phone numbers where they can be reached; self-help groups and services such as suicide hotlines; and professional resources, including emergency departments and outpatient emergency psychiatric services.

Commitment to Treatment

Patients are usually ambivalent about wanting to die. The **commitment to treatment statement** (CTS) directly addresses ambivalence about treatment by asking the patient to engage in treatment by making a commitment to try new approaches. Different from the no-suicide contract, the CTS does not restrict the patient's rights regarding the option of suicide. Instead, the patient agrees to engage in treatment and access emergency service if needed. Underlying the CTS is the expectation that the patient will communicate openly and honestly about all aspects of treatment, including suicide. This commitment is written and signed by the patient. The efficacy of this approach has yet to be established by systematic research. Whether using the CTS or other means, be observant for lapses in the patient's participation in treatment and discuss them with the patient and other members of the interdisciplinary team.

Interventions for the Social Domain

Poor social skills may interfere with the patient's ability to engage others. The nurse should assess the patient's social capability early in treatment and make necessary provisions for social skills training. The interpersonal relationship with the nurse is an ideal place to begin shaping social behaviors that will help the patient to establish a social network that will sustain him or her during periods of discouragement or crisis. Participation in support networks such as recovery groups, clubhouses, drop-in centers, self-help groups, or other therapeutic social engagement will help the patient become connected to others.

Patients need to anticipate that even some of the people closest to them will feel uncomfortable with their suicidal behavior. Helping the patient to anticipate the stigmatizing behavior of others and how to manage it will go far in reintegrating the patient into a supportive social community. The nurse can also explore the patient's participation in specific social activities such as attending church or community activities.

Evaluation and Treatment Outcomes

The most desirable treatment outcome is the patient's recovery with no future suicide attempts. Short-term outcomes include maintaining the patient's safety, averting suicide, and mobilizing the patient's resources. Whether the patient is hospitalized or cared for in the community, his or her emotional distress must be reduced. Long-term outcomes must focus on maintaining the patient in psychiatric treatment, enabling the patient and family to identify and manage suicidal crises effectively, and widening the patient's support network.

Continuum of Care

Whether the suicide prevention plan is instituted in the hospital or in an outpatient setting, the patient cannot be released to home until a workable plan of care is in place. The care plan includes scheduling an appointment for outpatient treatment, providing for continuing somatic treatments until the first outpatient treatment visit, ensuring post-release contact between the patient and significant other, providing for access to emergency psychiatric care, and arranging the patient's environment so it provides both structure and safety.

At the first follow-up visit, the patient and health care provider can establish a plan of care that specifies the intensity of outpatient care. Very unstable patients may need frequent supervision (e.g., telephone or face-to-face meetings or both) in the early days after hospitalization to maintain the patient's safety in the community. These contacts often can be short; their purpose is to convey the ongoing concern and caring of professionals involved in the patient's care. In arranging outpatient care, be certain to refer the patient to a provider who can provide the intensity of care the patient may need.

The patient's outpatient environment should be made as safe as possible before discharge. The nurse must share the care plan with family members so they can remove any objects in the patient's environment that could be used to engage in self-harm. The nurse should explain this measure to the patient to reinforce his or her sense of self-control. It is important to be reasonable in deciding what to remove from the environment. Patients who are truly determined to kill themselves after discharge will succeed in doing so, using whatever means are available.

Documentation and Reporting

The nurse must thoroughly document encounters with suicidal patients. This action is for the patient's ongoing treatment and the nurse's protection. Lawsuits for malpractice in psychiatric settings often involve completed suicides. The medical record must reflect that the nurse took every reasonable action to provide for the patient's safety.

The record should describe the patient's history, assessment, and interventions agreed upon by the patient and nurse. The nurse should document the presence or absence of suicidal thoughts, intent, plan, and available means to illustrate the patient's current and ongoing suicide risk. If the patient denies any suicidal ideation, it is important that the denial is documented. Documentation must include any use of drugs, alcohol, or prescription medications by the patient during the 6 hours before the assessment. It should include the use of antidepressants that are especially lethal (e.g., tricyclics), as well as any medication that might impair the patient's judgment (e.g., a sleep medication). Notes should reflect the level of the patient's judgment and ability to be a partner in treatment.

The documentation should reflect if any medications were prescribed, the dosages, and the number of pills dispensed. Notes should reflect the plan for ongoing treatment, including the time of the next appointment with the provider, instructions given to the patient about obtaining emergency care if needed, and the names of family members and friends who will act as supports if the patient needs them.

NURSES' REFLECTION

Caring for suicidal patients is highly stressful and can lead to secondary trauma for the nurse. Nurses who care for suicidal patients must regularly share their experiences and feelings with one another. Talking about how the situations or actions of patients make them feel will help alleviate symptoms of stress. Some nurses find outpatient therapy helpful because it enhances their understanding of what situations are most likely to trigger secondary trauma. By demonstrating how to manage effectively the stressors in their own lives, nurses can be powerful role models for their patients.

SUMMARY OF KEY POINTS

- Suicide is a common and major public health problem.

- Suicide completion is more common in white men, especially older men.

- Parasuicide is more common among women than men.

- People who attempt suicide and fail are likely to try again without treatment.

- Suicidal behavior has genetic and biologic origins.

- A suicide assessment focuses on the intention to die, hopelessness, available means, previous attempts and self-harm behavior, and degree of planning.

- Patients who are in crisis, depressed, or use substances are at risk for suicide.

- The major objectives of brief hospital care are to maintain the patient's safety, reestablish the patient's biologic equilibrium, help the patient reconnect to others, instill hope, strengthen the patient's cognitive coping skills, and develop an outpatient support system.

- The nurse who cares for suicidal patients is vulnerable to secondary trauma and must take steps to maintain personal mental health.

CRITICAL THINKING CHALLENGES

1. A religious African American woman who lives with her three children, husband, and mother comes to her primary care provider. She is tearful and very depressed. What factors should be investigated to determine her risk for suicide and need for hospitalization?

2. A poor woman with no insurance is hospitalized after her third suicide attempt. Antidepressant medication is prescribed. What kinds of treatment will be most effective in preventing future suicidal behavior?

3. A young man enters his workplace inebriated and carrying a gun. He does not threaten anyone but says that he must end it all. Assuming that he can be disarmed, what civil rights must be considered in taking further action in managing his suicidal risk?

4. You are a nurse in a large outpatient primary care setting responsible for an impoverished population. You want to implement a case-finding program for suicide prevention. Discuss how you would proceed and some potential problems you might face.

 Daughter of a Suicide: 1996 (Documentary). This personal documentary is the story of a woman whose mother committed suicide when the daughter was 18 years old. The daughter recounts the emotional struggle and depression left as the lifelong legacy of suicide and explores her efforts to heal. Combining digital video, 16-mm, and super-8 film, *Daughter of a Suicide* uses interviews with family and friends to tell the story of both mother and daughter.

VIEWING POINTS: How does this movie show that the effects of suicide do not end with a person's death?

The Virgin Suicides: 1999. After the suicide death of their 13-year-old daughter Cecilia, the Lisbon family becomes recluses. The remaining daughters try to resume their life by defying the withdrawal of their parents. Unsuccessful, the movie climaxes with the suicide deaths of the three remaining teenage girls.

VIEWING POINTS: What conditions in the girls family led the girls to take their lives?

Paradise Now: 2005. This movie traces the motivations of two suicide bombers in Palestine. It explores how the two young men came to the decision to kill themselves and others and their ambivalence about their impending deaths. Ultimately, one decides to live, and the movie ends with an ambiguous fate of the other. This movie provides insight into the background and troubled thoughts that precede a suicidal act.

VIEWING POINTS: Can suicide be a political act? What other factors in these young men's lives might have contributed to their decision to volunteer as suicide bombers?

References

American Association of Suicidology. (2014). *Understanding and helping the suicidal individual. Fact sheet.* Retrieved May 28, 2014, from http://www.suicidology.com.

American Foundation for Suicide Prevention. (2014). Facts and figures. *Understanding and preventing suicide through research, education, and advocacy.* Retrieved from http://www.afsp.org/understanding-suicide/facts-and-figures. Retrieved on May 24, 2014.

American Foundation for Suicide Prevention. (2014). Facts and figures. *Understanding and preventing suicide through research, education, and advocacy.* Retrieved from http://www.afsp.org/understanding-suicide/facts-and-figures. Retrieved on May 24, 2014.

Ando, S., Kasai, K., Matamura, M., Hasegawa, Y., Hirakawa, H., Asukai, N. (2013). Psychosocial factors associated with suicidal ideation in clinical patients with depression. *Journal of Affective Disorders, 151*(2), 561–565.

Andriessen, K., & Krysinska, K. (2012). Essential questions on suicide bereavement and postvention. *International Journal of Environmental Research and Public Health, 9*(1), 24–32.

Anglemyer, A., Horvath, T., & Rutherford, G. (2014). The accessibility of firearms and risk for suicide and homicide victimization among household members. *Annals of Internal Medicine, 160*(2), 101–110.

Beck, A. T., Rush, A. J., Shaw, B. F., & Emery, G. F. (1979). *Cognitive therapy of depression.* New York: The Guildford Press.

Bernburg, J. G., Thorlindsson, T., & Sigfusdottir, I. D. (2009). The spreading of suicidal behavior: The contextual effect of community household poverty on adolescent suicidal behavior or/and the mediating. *Social Science & Medicine, 68*(2), 380–389.

Boyd, M. A., Bradshaw, W., & Robinson, M. (2013). Mental health issues of women deployed to Iraq and Afghanistan. *Archives of Psychiatric Nursing, 27*(1), 10–22.

Bryan, C. J., Corso, K. A., Rudd, M., & Cordero, L. (2008). Improving detection of suicidal patients in primary care through routine screening. *Primary Care & Community Psychiatry, 13*(4), 143–147.

Burrows, S., Auger, N., Gamache, P., Hamel, D. (2013). Leading causes of unintentional injury and suicide mortality in Canadian adults across the urban-rural continuum. *Public Health Reports, 128*(6), 443–453.

Buus, N., Caspersen, J., Hansen, R., Stenager, E., & Fleischer, E. (2013). Experiences of parents whose sons or daughters have (had) attempted suicide. *Journal of Advanced Nursing, 70*(4), 823–832.

Capron, D. W., Norr, A. M., Macatee, R. J., & Schmidt, N. B. (2013). Distress tolerance and anxiety sensitivity cognitive concerns: Testing the incremental contributions of affect dysregulation constructs on suicidal ideation and suicide attempt. *Behavior Therapy, 44*(3), 349–358.

Catanese, A. A., John, M. S., Di Battista, J., & Clarke, D.M. (2009). Acute cognitive therapy in reducing suicide risk following a presentation to an emergency department. *Behaviour Change, 26*(1), 16–26.

Centers for Disease Control and Prevention, National Center for Injury Prevention and Control. (2014a). *Suicide facts at a glance* 2012. Retrieved May 25, 2014, from http://www.cdc.gov/violenceprevention/pdf/Suicide_DataSheet-a.pdf.

Center for Disease Control. (2014b). Surveillance for violent deaths - National Violent Death Reporting System, 16 states, 2010. *Morbidity and Mortality Weekly Report, 63*(1), 1–33.

De Hert, M., Correll, C. U., & Cohen, D. (2010). Do antipsychotic medications reduce or increase mortality in schizophrenia? A critical appraisal of the FIN-11 study. *Schizophrenia Research, 117*(1), 68–74.

De Leo, D., Draper, B. M., Snowdon, J., & Kolves, K. (2013). Suicides in older adults: A case-control psychological autopsy study in Australia. *Journal of Psychiatric Research, 47*(7), 980–988.

Durkheim, E. (1951 [1897]). *Suicide.* New York: Free Press.

Ellis, T. E., & Rutherford, B. (2008). Cognition and suicide: Two decades of progress. *International Journal of Cognitive Therapy, 1*(1), 47–68.

Fernández-Navarro, P., Vaquero-Lorenzo, C., Blasco-Fontecilla, H., Díaz-Hernández, M., Gratacòs, M., Estivill, X., et al. (2012). Genetic epistasis in female suicide attempters. *Progress in Neuro-Psychopharmacology & Biological Psychiatry, 38*(2), 294–301.

Fink, M. (2014). What was learned: Studies by the consortium for research in ECT (CORE) 1997-2011. *Acta Psychiatrica Scandinavia, 129*(6), 416–426.

Fredriksen-Goldsen, K. I., Emlet, C. A., Kim, H. J., Muraco, A., Erosheva, E. A., Goldsen, J., et al. (2013). The physical and mental health of lesbian, gay male, and bisexual (LGB) older adults: The role of key health indicators and risk and protective factors. *The Gerontologist, 53*(4), 664–675.

Goldston, D. B., Daniel, S. S., Erkanli, A., Reboussin, B. A., Mayfield, A., Frazier, P. H., & Treadway, S. L. (2009). Psychiatric diagnoses as contemporaneous risk factors for suicide attempts among adolescents and young adults: Developmental changes. *Journal of Consulting & Clinical Psychology, 77*(2), 281–290.

Gomez, J., Miranda, R., & Polanco, L. (2011). Acculturative stress, perceived discrimination, and vulnerability to suicide attempts among emerging adults. *Journal of Youth & Adolescence, 40*(11), 1465–1476.

Gudmundsdottir, R. M., & Thome, M. (2014). Evaluation of the effects of individual and group cognitive behavioural therapy and of psychiatric rehabilitation on hopelessness of depressed adults: A comparative analysis. *Journal of Psychiatric & Mental Health Nursing,* doi:10.1111/jpm.12157

Guerreiro, D. F., Cruz, D., Frasquilho, D., Santos, J. C., Figueira, M. L., & Sampaio, D. (2013). Association between deliberate self-harm and coping in adolescents: A critical review of the last 10 years' literature. *Archives of Suicide Research, 17*(2), 91–105.

Guillaume, S., Perroud, N., Jollant, F., Jaussent, I., Olie, E., Malafosse, A., et al. (2013). HPA axis genes may modulate the effect of childhood adversities on decision-making in suicide attempters. *Journal of Psychiatric Research, 47*(2), 259–265.

Hawkins, K. A., & Cougle, J. R. (2013). A test of the unique and interactive roles of anger experience and expression in suicidality: Findings from a population-based study. *Journal of Nervous & Mental Disease, 201*(11), 959–963.

Insel, T. (2010). The under-recognized public health crisis of suicide. *Director's posts about suicide prevention.* Retrieved September 10, 2010, from http://www.nimh.nih.gov/about/directo/index-suicide-prevention.shtml.

Janofsky, J. S. (2009). Reducing inpatient suicide risk: Using human factors analysis to improve observation practices. *Journal of the American Academy of Psychiatry and the Law, 37*(1), 15–24.

Joe, S., & Niedermeier, D. M. (2008). Social work research on African-Americans and suicidal behavior: A systematic 25 year review. *Health and Social Work, 33*(4), 249–257.

Joiner, T. E., & Van Orden, K. A. (2008). The interpersonal-psychological theory of suicidal behavior indicates specific and crucial psychotherapeutic targets. *International Journal of Cognitive Therapy, 1*(1), 80–89.

Joiner, T. E., Van Orden, K. A., Witte, T. K., Selby, E. garroutte A., Ribeiro, J. D., Lewis, R., & Rudd, M. D. (2009). Main predictions of the interpersonal-psychological theory of suicidal behavior: Empirical tests in two samples of young adults. *Journal of Abnormal Psychology, 118*(3), 634–646.

Ju, J. N., Young, L. W., Seok, N. M., & Yip, P. S. (2014). The impact of indiscriminate media coverage of a celebrity suicide on a society with a high suicide rate: Epidemiological findings on copycat suicides from South Korea. *Journal of Affective Disorders, 156*, 56–61. doi:10.1016/j.ad.2013.11.015

Kim, Y. R., Choi, K. H., Oh, Y., Lee, H. K., Kweon, Y. S., Lee, C.T., et al. (2011). Elderly suicide attempters by self-poisoning in Korea. *International Psychogeriatrics, 23*(6), 979–985.

Lewis, N. M. (2009). Mental health in sexual minorities: Recent indicators, trends, and their relationship to place in North American and Europe. *Health & Place, 15*(4), 1029–1045.

Liu, R. T., Kraines, M. A., Puzia, M. E., Massing-Schaffer, M., & Kleiman, E. M. (2013). Sociodemographic predictors of suicide means in a population-based surveillance system: Findings from the national violent Death Reporting system. *Journal of Affective Disorders, 151*(2), 449–454.

Marshal, M. P., Dermody, S. S., Cheong, J., Burton, C. M., Friedman, M. S., Aranda, F., et al. (2013). Trajectories of depressive symptoms and suicidality among heterosexual and sexual minority youth. *Journal of Youth and Adolescence, 42*(8), 1243–1256.

McCarthy, J. F., Blow, F. X., Ignacio, R. V., Ilgen, M. A., Austin, K. L., & Valenstein, M. (2012). Suicide among patients in the Veterans Affairs health system: Rural-urban differences in rates, risks, and methods. *American Journal of Public Health, 102*(suppl 1), 11–17.

Messias, E., Kindrick, K., & Castro, J. (2014). School bullying, cyberbullying, or both: Correlates of teen suicidality in the 2011 CDC youth risk behavior survey. *Comprehensive Psychiatry, doi:10.1016/comppsych.2014.02.005*

Mezuk, B., Rock, A., Lohman, M. C., & Choi, M. (2014). Suicide risk in long-term care facilities: A systematic review. *International Journal of Geriatric Psychiatry. doi:10.1002/gps.4142*

Mitchell, M. M., Gallaway, M. S., Millikan, A. M., & Bell, M. (2012). Interaction of combat exposure and unit cohesion in predicting suicide-related ideation among post-deployment soldiers. *Suicide & Life threatening Behavior, 42*(5), 486–494.

Mustanski, B., & Liu, R. T. (2013). A longitudinal study of predictors of suicide attempts among lesbian, gay, bisexual, and transgender youth. *Archives of Sexual Behavior, 42*(3), 437–448.

Murphy, N. A., Fatoye, F., & Wibberley, C. (2013). The changing face of newspaper representations of the mentally ill. *Journal of Mental Health, 22*(3), 271–282.

Page, A., Lewis, G., Kidger, J., Heron, J., Chittleborough, C., Evans, J., Gunnell, D. (2014). Parental socio-economic position during childhood as a determinant of self-harm in adolescence. *Social Psychiatry & Psychiatric Epidemiology, 49*(2), 193–203.

Paul, J. P., Catania, J., Pollack, L., Moskowitz, J., Conchola, J., Mills, T., et al. (2002). Suicide attempts among gay and bisexual men: Lifetime prevalence and antecedents. *American Journal of Public Health, 92*(8), 1338–1345.

Ploderi, M., Wagenmakers, E. J., Tremblay, P., Ramsay, R., Kralovec, K., Fartacek, C., et al. (2013). Suicide risk and sexual orientation: A critical review. *Archives of Sexual Behavior, 42*(5), 715–727.

Pompili, M., Innamorati, M., Gonda, X., Serafini, G., Sarno, S., Erbuto, D., et al. (2013). Affective temperaments and hopelessness as predictors of health and social functioning in mood disorder patients: A prospective follow-up study. *Journal of Affective Disorders, 150*(2), 216–222.

Puskar, K., & Urda, B. (2011). Examining the efficacy of no-suicide contracts in inpatient psychiatric settings: Implications for psychiatric nursing. *Issues in Mental Health Nursing, 32*(12), 785–788.

Ribeiro, J. D., Silva, C., & Joiner, T. E. (2014). Overarousal interacts with a sense of fearlessness about death to predict suicide risk in a sample of clinical outpatients. *Psychiatry Research, 218*, 106–112. *doi:10.1016/j.psychres.2014.03.036*

Robertson, L., Skegg, K., Poore, M., Williams, S., & Taylor, B. (2012). An adolescent suicide cluster and the possible role of electronic communication technology. *Crisis, 33*(4), 239–245.

Schmutte, T., O'Connell, M., Weiland, M., Lawless, S., & Davidson, L. (2009). Stemming the tide of suicide in older white men: A call to action. *American Journal of Men's Health, 3*(3), 189–200.

Séquin, M., Beauchamp, G., Robert, M., Dimambro, M., & Turecki, G. (2014). Developmental model of suicide trajectories. *British Journal of Psychiatry.* PMID: 24809398.

Selby, E. A., Yen, S., & Spirito, A. (2013). Time varying prediction of thoughts of death and suicidal ideation in adolescents: Weekly rating over 6-month follow-up. *Journal of Clinical Child & Adolescent Psychology, 42*(4), 481–495.

Stack, S., & Wasserman, I. (2009). Gender and suicide risk: The role of wound site. *Suicide and Life-Threatening Behavior, 39*(1), 13–20.

Suicide Prevention Resource Center (SPRC). (2013a). *Suicide among racial/ethnic populations in the U.S.: Hispanics.* Waltham, MA: Education Development Center, Inc.

Suicide Prevention Resource Center (SPRC). (2013b). *Suicide among racial/ethnic populations in the U.S.: American Indians/Alaska Natives.* Waltham, MA: Education Development Center, Inc.

Suicide Prevention Resource Center (SPRC). (2013c). *Suicide among racial/ethnic populations in the U.S.: Asians,* Pacific Islanders, and Native Hawaiians. Waltham, MA: Education Development Center, Inc.

Tidemalm, D., Runeson, B., Waern, M., Frisell, T., Carlstrom, E., Lichtenstein, P., et al. (2011). Familial clustering of suicide risk: A total population study of 11.4 million individuals. *Psychological Medicine, 41*(12), 2527–2534.

Tishler, C. L., & Reiss, N. S. (2009). Inpatient suicide: preventing a common sentinel event. *General Hospital Psychiatry, 31*(2), 103–109.

Upthegrove, R., Ross, K., Brunet, K., McCollum, R., & Jones, J. (2014). Depression in first episode psychosis: The role of subordination and shame. *Psychiatry Research, 217*(3), 177–184.

Ukrowicz, K. C., Ekblad, A. G. Cheavens, J. S., Rosenthal, M. Z., & Lynch, T. R. (2008). Coping and thought suppression as predictors of suicidal ideation in depressed older adults with personality disorders. *Aging and Mental Health, 12*(1), 149–157.

United States Department of Health and Human Services. (2010). *Healthy people 2020.* Retrieved from http://www.healthypeople.gov. Retrieved on May 25, 2014.

Valentiner, D. P., Gutierrez, P. M., & Blacker, D. (2002). Anxiety measures and their relationship to adolescent suicidal ideation and behavior. *Journal of Anxiety Disorders, 16*(1):11–32.

van Dulmen, M. H., & Goossens, L. (2013). *Loneliness trajectories, Journal of Adolescence, 36*(6), 1247–1249.

van Hooijdonk, C., Droomers, M., Deerenberg, I. M., Mackenbach, J. P., & Kunst, A. E. (2008). The diversity in associations between community social capital and health per health outcome, population group and location studied. *International Journal of Epidemiology, 27*(6), 1384–1392.

Van Orden, K. A., & Conwell, Y. (2011). Suicides in late life. *Current Psychiatry Reports.*

Wadsworth, T., & Kubrin, C. E. (2007). Hispanic suicide in U.S. metropolitan areas: Examining the effects of immigration, assimilation, affluence, and disadvantage. *American Journal of Sociology, 112*(6), 1848–1885.

Walsh, S., Clayton, R., Liu, L., & Hodges, S. (2009). Divergence in contributing factors for suicide among men and women in Kentucky: Recommendations to raise public awareness. *Public Health Reports, 124*(6), 861–867.

Wang, M. C., Lightsey, O. R., Tran, K. K., Bonaparte, T. S. (2013). Examining suicide protective factors among black college students. *Death Studies, 37*(3), 228–247.

Webb, R. T., Marshall, C. E., & Abel, K. M. (2011). Teenage motherhood and risk of premature death: Long-term follow-up in the ONS longitudinal study. *Psychological Medicine, 41*(9), 1867–1877.

Ying, Y. H., & Chang, K. Y. (2009). A study of suicide and socioeconomic factors. *Suicide and Life-Threatening Behavior, 39*(2), 214–226.

Zhang, J., & Li, Z. (2013). The association between depression and suicide when hopelessness is controlled for. *Comprehensive Psychiatry, 54*(7), 790–796.

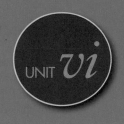
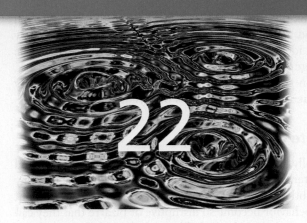

22

Schizophrenia
Management of Thought Disorders

Andrea C. Bostrom and Mary Ann Boyd

KEY CONCEPTS

- disorganized symptoms
- negative symptoms
- neurocognitive impairment
- positive symptoms

LEARNING OBJECTIVES

After studying this chapter, you will be able to:

1. Identify key symptoms of schizophrenia.

2. Analyze the prevailing theories relevant to schizophrenia.

3. Analyze the human response to schizophrenia with emphasis on hallucinations, delusions, and social isolation.

4. Formulate nursing diagnoses based on an assessment of people with schizophrenia.

5. Develop recovery-oriented nursing interventions for patients with psychotic disorders.

6. Analyze the implementation and evaluation of psychotherapeutic drugs used to treat people with schizophrenia and their impact on nursing care planning and intervening.

7. Analyze special concerns within the nurse–patient relationship common to caring for those with schizophrenia.

8. Identify expected outcomes and their evaluation for patients with schizophrenia.

KEY TERMS

- affective lability - aggression - agitation - agranulocytosis - akathisia - alogia - ambivalence - anhedonia
- apathy - autistic thinking - avolition - catatonic excitement - circumstantiality - clang association - concrete thinking - confused speech and thinking - delusions - diminished emotional expression - echolalia - echopraxia
- extrapyramidal side effects - flight of ideas - hallucinations - hypervigilance - hypofrontality - illusions
- loose associations - metonymic speech - neologisms - neuroleptic malignant syndrome - oculogyric crisis
- paranoia - polyuria - pressured speech - prodromal - psychosis - referential thinking - regressed behavior
- retrocollis - stereotypy - stilted language - tangentiality - tardive dyskinesia - torticollis - verbigeration
- waxy flexibility - word salad

One of the most fascinating groups of disorders is the schizophrenia spectrum disorders that have confounded scientists and philosophers for centuries. Schizophrenia spectrum disorders are some of the most severe mental illnesses and are present in all cultures, races, and socioeconomic groups. Their symptoms have been attributed to possession by demons, considered punishment by gods for evils done, or accepted as evidence of the inhumanity of its sufferers. These explanations have resulted in enduring stigma for people diagnosed with the disorder. Today the stigma persists although it has less to do with demonic possession than with society's unwillingness to shoulder the tremendous costs associated with housing, treating, and rehabilitating persons with schizophrenia. Schizophrenia is the highlighted disorder in this chapter, followed by a discussion of other psychotic disorders, including schizoaffective and delusional disorders in Chapter 23.

OVERVIEW OF SCHIZOPHRENIA

In the late 1800s, Emil Kraepelin first described the course of the disorder he called *dementia praecox* because of its early onset and notable changes in an individual's cognitive functioning. In the early 1900s, Eugen Bleuler renamed the disorder *schizophrenia*, meaning *split minds*, and began to determine that there was not just one type of schizophrenia but rather a group of schizophrenias. More recently, Kurt Schneider differentiated behaviors associated with schizophrenia as "first rank" symptoms (psychotic delusions, hallucinations) and "second rank" symptoms (all other experiences and behaviors associated with the disorder). These pioneering physicians had a great influence on the current diagnostic conceptualizations of schizophrenia that emphasize the heterogeneity of the disorder in terms of symptoms, course of illness, and positive and negative symptoms.

Clinical Course

The natural progression of schizophrenia is usually described as a chronic illness that deteriorates with time and with an eventual plateau in the symptoms. Only for older adults with schizophrenia has it been suggested that improvement might occur. In reality, no one really knows what the course of schizophrenia would be if patients were able to adhere to a treatment regimen throughout their lives. Only recently have medications been relatively effective, with manageable side effects. The clinical picture of schizophrenia is complex, individuals differ from one another, and the experience for a single individual may be different from episode to episode.

Prodromal Period

A recent discussion in the literature suggests that a prodromal period for psychosis (hallucinations, delusions) and possible schizophrenia might be identifiable (Barajas et al., 2013; Tarbox et al., 2013). The benefit of discovering the presence of symptoms early, before they have solidified into a major disorder, is that treatments might be initiated early. The risks of proposing this period as a specific diagnosis category are that people might be stigmatized and that, if misdiagnosed (because several psychiatric disorders besides schizophrenia begin with psychotic symptoms), patients may be subjected to medications that were unnecessary or harmful. A prodromal period for individuals with schizophrenia has usually been identified in retrospect and is evidenced by some change in overall function (difficulties in school or work, within relationships, or daily activities) accompanied by transient or weak symptoms of psychosis.

Acute Illness

Initially, the illness behaviors may be both confusing and frightening to the patient and the family. The changes may be subtle; however, at some point, the changes in thought and behavior become so disruptive or bizarre that they can no longer be overlooked. These might include episodes of staying up all night for several nights, incoherent conversations, or aggressive acts against oneself or others. For example, one patient's parents reported their son walking around the apartment for several days holding his arms and hands as if they were a machine gun, pointing them at his parents and siblings, and saying "rat-a-tat-tat, you're dead." Another father described his son's first delusional–hallucination episode as so convincing that it was frightening. His son began visiting cemeteries and making "mind contact" with the deceased. He saw his deceased grandmother walking around in the home and was certain that there were pipe bombs in objects in his home.

As symptoms progress, patients are less and less able to care for their basic needs, such as eating, sleeping, and bathing. Substance use is common. Functioning at school or work deteriorates. Dependence on family and friends increases, and those individuals recognize the patients' need for treatment. In the acute phase, these individuals with schizophrenia are at high risk for suicide. Patients are hospitalized usually to protect themselves or others.

The initial treatment focuses on alleviation of symptoms through initiation of medications, decreasing the risk of suicide through safety measures, normalizing sleep, and reducing substance use. Functional deficits persist during this period, and the patient and family must begin to learn to cope with these deficits. Emotional blunting diminishes the ability and desire to engage in hobbies, vocational activities, and relationships. Limited participation in social activities spirals into numerous skill deficits, such as difficulty engaging others interpersonally. Cognitive deficits lead to problems recognizing patterns in situations and transferring learning and behaviors from one circumstance to another similar one.

Stabilization

After the initial diagnosis of schizophrenia and initiation of treatment, stabilization of symptoms becomes the focus. Symptoms become less acute but may be present. Treatment is intense during this period as medication regimens are established and patients and their families begin to adjust to the idea of a family member having a long-term severe mental illness. Ideally, the use of substances is eliminated. Socialization with others begins to increase, and rehabilitation begins.

Recovery

After the patient's condition is stabilized, the patient focuses on regaining the previous level of functioning and quality of life. Medication treatment of individuals with schizophrenia has generally contributed to an improvement in the lifestyles of people with this disorder; however, no medication has cured it. Faithful medication management tends to make the impairments in functioning less severe when they occur and provides a smoother road to recovery. As with any chronic illness, stresses of life and major crises can contribute to exacerbations of symptoms.

Family support and involvement are extremely important at this time. After the initial diagnosis has been made, patients and families must be educated to anticipate and expect relapse and know how to cope with it. This is one of the important themes throughout the nursing process for people with schizophrenia.

Relapses

Relapses can occur at any time during treatment and recovery. They are very detrimental to the successful management of this disorder. Relapse is not inevitable; however, it occurs with sufficient regularity to be a major concern in the treatment of schizophrenia. With each relapse, there is a longer period of time to recover. Combining medications and psychosocial treatment greatly diminishes the severity and frequency of recurrent relapses (Guo et al., 2010).

One of the major reasons for relapse is failure to follow the medication regimen. Even with newer medications, adherence continues to be a problem (Kaplan, Casoy, & Zummo, 2013). Discontinuing medications almost certainly leads to a relapse and may actually be a stressor that causes a severe and rapid relapse (Acosta, Hernández, Pereira, Herrera, & Rodríguez, 2012). Lower relapse rates are found, for the most part, among groups who follow a treatment regimen.

Many other factors trigger relapse. Impairment in cognition and coping leaves patients vulnerable to stressors. Limited accessibility of community resources, such as public transportation, housing, entry-level and low-stress employment, and social services leaves individuals without access to social support. Income supports that can buffer the day-to-day stressors of living may be inadequate. The degree of stigmatization that the community holds for mental illness attacks the self-concept of patients. The level of responsiveness from family members, friends, and supportive others (such as peers and professionals) when patients need help also has an impact.

Diagnostic Criteria

Schizophrenia is a mixture of core symptoms that are present for a significant portion of a 1-month period but with continuous signs of disturbance persisting for at least 6 months. Core symptoms include positive symptoms (hallucinations and delusions), negative symptoms (diminished emotional expression and avolition), and other possible co-occurring symptoms (disorganization, abnormal psychomotor behavior, impaired cognition, depression, and mania). Positive symptoms can be thought of as symptoms that exist but should not and negative symptoms as ones that should be there but are not (American Psychiatric Association [APA], 2013). See Key Diagnostic Characteristics 22.1.

> **KEYCONCEPT** **Positive symptoms** reflect an excess or distortion of normal functions, including delusions and hallucinations. **Negative symptoms** reflect a lessening or loss of normal functions, such as restriction or flattening in the range and intensity of emotion (**diminished emotional expression**), reduced fluency and productivity of thought and speech (alogia), withdrawal and inability to initiate and persist in goal-directed activity (**avolition**), and inability to experience pleasure (**anhedonia**).

As the study of schizophrenia and its symptoms, causes, and responses to treatment has progressed, the importance of assessing core symptoms (i.e., positive and negative symptoms) associated with the disorder is gaining prominence. Assessing the existence and degree of core symptoms over a period of time (e.g., the past month) serves as the basis for determining diagnosis, treatment methods, and evaluation of response to treatment.

Positive Symptoms of Schizophrenia

Delusions are erroneous fixed, false beliefs that cannot be changed by reasonable argument. They usually involve a misinterpretation of experience. For example, the patient believes someone is reading his or her thoughts or plotting against him or her. Various types of delusions include the following:

- *Grandiose:* the belief that one has exceptional powers, wealth, skill, influence, or destiny
- *Nihilistic:* the belief that one is dead or a calamity is impending
- *Persecutory:* the belief that one is being watched, ridiculed, harmed, or plotted against
- *Somatic:* beliefs about abnormalities in bodily functions or structures

KEY DIAGNOSTIC CHARACTERISTICS 22.1 • SCHIZOPHRENIA

DIAGNOSTIC CRITERIA

A. Two (or more) of the following, each present for a significant portion of time during a 1-month period (or less if successfully treated). At least one of these must be (1), (2), or (3):
1. Delusions.
2. Hallucinations.
3. Disorganized speech (e.g., frequent derailment or incoherence).
4. Grossly disorganized or catatonic behavior.
5. Negative symptoms (i.e., diminished emotional expression or avolition).

B. For a significant portion of the time since the onset of the disturbance, level of functioning in one or more major areas, such as work, interpersonal relations, or self-care, is markedly below the level achieved prior to the onset (or when the onset is in childhood or adolescence, there is failure to achieve expected level of interpersonal, academic, or occupational functioning).

C. Continuous signs of the disturbance persist for at least 6 months. This 6-month period must include at least 1 month of symptoms (or less if successfully treated) that meet Criterion A (i.e., active-phase symptoms) and may include periods of prodromal or residual symptoms. During these prodromal or residual periods, the signs of the disturbance may be manifested by only negative symptoms or by two or more symptoms listed in Criterion A present in an attenuated form (e.g., odd beliefs, unusual perceptual experiences).

D. Schizoaffective disorder and depressive or bipolar disorder with psychotic features have been ruled out because either 1) no major depressive or manic episodes have occurred concurrently with the active-phase symptoms, or 2) if mood episodes have occurred during active-phase symptoms, they have been present for a minority of the total duration of the active and residual periods of the illness.

E. The disturbance is not attributable to the physiological effects of a substance (e.g., a drug of abuse, a medication) or another medical condition.

F. If there is a history of autism spectrum disorder or a communication disorder of childhood onset, the additional diagnosis of schizophrenia is made only if prominent delusions or hallucinations, in addition to the other required symptoms of schizophrenia, are also present for at least 1 month (or less if successfully treated).

TARGET SYMPTOMS AND ASSOCIATED FINDINGS

- Inappropriate affect
- Loss of interest or pleasure
- Dysphoric mood (anger, anxiety, or depression)
- Disturbed sleep patterns
- Lack of interest in eating or refusal of food
- Difficulty concentrating
- Some cognitive dysfunction, such as confusion, disorientation, or memory impairment
- Lack of insight
- Depersonalization, derealization, and somatic concerns
- Motor abnormalities

Associated Physical Examination Findings

- Physically awkward
- Poor coordination or mirroring
- Motor abnormalities
- Cigarette-related pathologies, such as emphysema and other pulmonary and cardiac problems

Associated Laboratory Findings

- Enlarged ventricular system and prominent sulci in the brain cortex
- Decreased temporal and hippocampal size
- Increased size of basal ganglia
- Decreased cerebral size
- Slowed reaction times
- Abnormalities in eye tracking

Reprinted with permission from the *Diagnostic and Statistical Manual of Mental Disorders*, Fifth Edition (Copyright ©2013). American Psychiatric Association. All Rights Reserved.

Hallucinations are perceptual experiences that occur without actual external sensory stimuli. They can involve any of the five senses, but they are usually *visual* or *auditory*. Auditory hallucinations are more common than visual ones. For example, the patient hears voices carrying on a discussion about his or her own thoughts or behaviors.

Negative Symptoms of Schizophrenia

Negative symptoms are not as dramatic as positive symptoms, but they can interfere greatly with the patient's ability to function day to day. Because expressing emotion is difficult for them, people with schizophrenia laugh, cry, and get angry less often. Their affect is flat, and they may show little or no emotion when personal loss occurs. They also experience ambivalence, which is the concurrent experience of equally strong opposing feelings so that it is impossible to make a decision. The avolition may be so profound that simple activities of daily living, such as dressing or combing hair, may not get done. Anhedonia prevents the person with schizo-

phrenia from enjoying activities. People with schizophrenia may have limited speech and difficulty saying anything new or carrying on a conversation. These negative symptoms cause the person with schizophrenia to withdraw and experience feelings of severe isolation.

Neurocognitive Impairment

Neurocognitive impairment exists in people with schizophrenia and may be independent of positive and negative symptoms. Neurocognition includes memory (short and long term); vigilance or sustained attention; verbal fluency or the ability to generate new words; and executive functioning, which includes volition, planning, purposive action, and self-monitoring behavior. Working memory is a concept that includes short-term memory and the ability to store and process information.

KEYCONCEPT **Neurocognitive impairment** in memory, vigilance, and executive functioning is related to poor functional outcome in schizophrenia (Fanning, Bell, & Fiszdon, 2012).

This impairment is independent of the positive symptoms. That is, cognitive dysfunction can exist even if the positive symptoms are in remission. Not all areas of cognitive functioning are impaired. Long-term memory and intellectual functioning are not necessarily affected. However, low intellectual functioning is common and may be related to a lack of educational opportunities. Neurocognitive dysfunction often is manifested in disorganized symptoms.

> **KEYCONCEPT** **Disorganized symptoms** of schizophrenia are things that make it difficult for the person to understand and respond to the ordinary sights and sounds of daily living. These include confused speech and thinking and disorganized behavior.

Disorganized Thinking

The following are examples of **confused speech and thinking** patterns:

- **Echolalia**—repetition of another's words that is parrot-like and inappropriate
- **Circumstantiality**—extremely detailed and lengthy discourse about a topic
- **Loose associations**—absence of the normal connectedness of thoughts, ideas, and topics; sudden shifts without apparent relationship to preceding topics
- **Tangentiality**—the topic of conversation is changed to an entirely different topic that is a logical progression but causes a permanent detour from the original focus

- **Flight of ideas**—the topic of conversation changes repeatedly and rapidly, generally after just one sentence or phrase
- **Word salad**—string of words that are not connected in any way
- **Neologisms**—words that are made up that have no common meaning and are not recognized
- **Paranoia**—suspiciousness and guardedness that are unrealistic and often accompanied by grandiosity
- **Referential thinking**—belief that neutral stimuli have special meaning to the individual, such as the television commentator speaking directly to the individual
- **Autistic thinking**—restricts thinking to the literal and immediate so that the individual has private rules of logic and reasoning that make no sense to anyone else
- **Concrete thinking**—lack of abstraction in thinking; inability to understand punch lines, metaphors, and analogies
- **Verbigeration**—purposeless repetition of words or phrases
- **Metonymic speech**—use of words interchangeably with similar meanings
- **Clang association**—repetition of words or phrases that are similar in sound but in no other way, for example, right, light, sight, might
- **Stilted language**—overly and inappropriately artificial formal language
- **Pressured speech**—speaking as if the words are being forced out

Disorganized perceptions often create oversensitivity to colors, shapes, and background activities. **Illusions** occur when the person misperceives or exaggerates stimuli that actually exist in the external environment. This is in contrast to hallucinations, which are perceptions in the absence of environmental stimuli. Ancillary symptoms that may accompany schizophrenia include anxiety, depression, and hostility.

Disorganized Behavior

Disorganized behavior (which may manifest as very slow, rhythmic, or ritualistic movement) coupled with disorganized speech make it difficult for the person to partake in daily activities. Examples of disorganized behavior include the following:

- **Aggression**—behaviors or attitudes that reflect rage, hostility, and the potential for physical or verbal destructiveness (usually comes about if the person believes someone is going to do him or her harm)
- **Agitation**—inability to sit still or attend to others, accompanied by heightened emotions and tension
- **Catatonic excitement**—a hyperactivity characterized by purposeless activity and abnormal movements such as grimacing and posturing

- **Echopraxia**—involuntary imitation of another person's movements and gestures
- **Regressed behavior**—behaving in a manner of a less mature life stage; childlike and immature behavior
- **Stereotypy**—repetitive, purposeless movements that are idiosyncratic to the individual and to some degree outside of the individual's control
- **Hypervigilance**—sustained attention to external stimuli as if expecting something important or frightening to happen
- **Waxy flexibility**—posture held in odd or unusual fixed position for extended periods of time

Schizophrenia Across the Life Span

Children

The diagnosis of schizophrenia is rare in children before adolescence. When it does occur in children ages 5 or 6 years, the symptoms are essentially the same as in adults. In this age group, hallucinations tend to be visual and delusions less developed. Because disorganized speech and behavior may be explained better by other disorders that are more common in childhood, those disorders should be considered before applying the diagnosis of schizophrenia to a child.

However, new studies suggest that the likelihood of children later experiencing schizophrenia can be predicted. Developmental abnormalities in childhood, including delays in attainment of speech and motor development, problems in social adjustment, and poorer academic and cognitive performance, have been found to be present in individuals who experience schizophrenia in adulthood. Specific factors that appear to predict schizophrenia in adulthood include problems in motor and neurologic development, deficits in attention and verbal short-term memory, poor social competence, positive formal thought disorder–like symptoms, and severe instability of early rearing environment (Meier et al., 2014).

Older Adults

People with schizophrenia do get older and others develop schizophrenia in late life. For older patients who have had schizophrenia since young adulthood, this may be a time in which they experience some improvement in symptoms or decrease in relapse fluctuations. There is some evidence that suggests that older adults with schizophrenia may be more likely to develop cognitive impairment than those without mental disorders (Loewenstein, Czaja, Bowie, & Harvey, 2012). However, their lifestyle probably is dependent on the effectiveness of earlier treatment, the support systems that are in place (including relationships with family members and professionals), and the interaction between environmental stressors and the patient's functional impairments. The cost of caring for older patients with schizophrenia remains high because many are no longer cared for in institutions, and community-based treatment has developed more slowly for this age group than for younger adults.

Epidemiology

Schizophrenia occurs in all cultures and countries, is prevalent in about 0.7% of the worldwide population, and is listed within the top 20 illnesses for life lost from premature death and years lived in less than full health (Department of Health Statistics & Information Systems, 2013). Its economic costs are enormous. Direct costs include treatment expenses, and indirect costs include lost wages, premature death, and incarceration. In addition, employment among people with schizophrenia is one of the lowest of any group with disabilities. The costs of schizophrenia in terms of individual and family suffering probably are inestimable.

People with schizophrenia tend to cluster in the lowest social classes in industrialized countries and urban communities. The symptoms of the illness are so pervasive that it is difficult for these individuals to maintain any type of gainful employment. Homelessness is a problem for people with severe mental illness (e.g., schizophrenia or bipolar illness). People with schizophrenia are more likely to remain homeless with few opportunities for employment (Auquier et al., 2013). (See also Chapter 38.)

Risk Factors

Genetic factors related to cognitive and brain function and brain structure are known risks for schizophrenia. Early neurologic problems, stressful life events, and nonhereditary genetic factors also contribute to the likelihood of developing the disorder. Environmental factors include migrant status, having an older father, *Toxoplasmosis gondii* antibodies, prenatal famine, lifetime cannabis use, obstetrical complications, urban rearing, and winter or spring birth (Brown, 2011).

Age of Onset

Schizophrenia is usually diagnosed in late adolescence and early adulthood. Men tend to be diagnosed between the ages of 18 and 25 years and women between the ages of 25 and 35 years. The earlier the diagnosis and the longer the psychosis is untreated, the more severe the disorder (Fraguas et al., 2014).

Gender Differences

Men tend to be diagnosed earlier and have a poorer prognosis than women. This may be a sex-linked outcome, but it may also reflect the poorer prognosis for any individual who develops the disorder at an early age (Goldstein, Cherkerzian, Tsuang, & Petryshen, 2013).

Ethnic and Cultural Differences

Increasingly, efforts are being made to consider culture and ethnic origin when diagnosing and treating individuals with schizophrenia. Racial groups may have varying diagnosis rates of schizophrenia. However, it is not clear if these findings represent correct diagnosis or misdiagnosis of the disorder based on a cultural bias of the clinician. For instance, schizophrenia has been consistently overdiagnosed among African Americans. African American and Hispanic individuals with bipolar disorder are more likely to have misdiagnoses of schizophrenia than are white individuals. Serious mental disorders may be unrecognized in Asian Americans because of stereotypical beliefs that they are "problem free" (Cohen & Marino, 2013).

Familial Differences

First-degree biologic relatives (children, siblings, parents) of an individual with schizophrenia have a 10 times estimated greater risk for schizophrenia than the general population. Other relatives may have an increased risk for related disorders such as schizoaffective disorder and schizotypal personality disorder (Boshes, Manschreck, & Konigsberg, 2012).

Comorbidity

Several somatic and psychological disorders coexist with schizophrenia. This results in significant morbidity and mortality for people with schizophrenia, with individuals who have this diagnosis dying up to 20 years earlier than the general population. Physical health conditions and illnesses to which people with schizophrenia are particularly susceptible include tuberculosis, HIV, hepatitis B and C, osteoporosis, poor dentition, impaired lung function, altered (reduced) pain sensitivity, sexual dysfunction, obstetric complications, cardiovascular problems, hyperpigmentation, obesity, diabetes, metabolic syndrome with hyperlipidemia, polydipsia, thyroid dysfunction, and hyperprolactinemia (Carliner, Collins, Cabassa, McNallen, Joestl, & Lewis-Fernández, 2014; Laursen, Nordentoft, & Mortensen, 2014). Several health system factors contribute to this, including barriers to obtaining primary care, the insufficient preparation of mental health practitioners in managing physical illness, the tendency for mental health providers to fail to ask about physical health, and the absence of standards of care that include screening and monitoring medical issues.

Substance Abuse and Depression

Among the behavioral comorbidities, substance abuse is common. Depression may also be observed in patients with schizophrenia. This is an important symptom for several reasons. First, depression may be evidence that the diagnosis of a mood disorder is more appropriate. Second, depression is not unusual in chronic stages of schizophrenia and deserves attention. Third, the suicide rate (4.9%) among individuals with schizophrenia is higher than that of the general population. Risk factors for suicide are untreated psychosis, history of suicide attempt, age younger than 28 years, severity of depression, and substance abuse (Austad, Joa, Johannessen, & Larsen, 2013; Challis, Nielssen, Harris, & Large, 2013).

Diabetes Mellitus

There is a renewed interest in the relationship of diabetes mellitus and schizophrenia. Years ago, an association was established between glucose regulation and psychiatric disorders, suggesting that people with schizophrenia may be more prone to type II diabetes than is the general public (Franzen, 1970; Schimmelbusch, Mueller, & Sheps, 1971). Evidence that supports this view includes a higher rate of type II diabetes in first-degree relatives of people with schizophrenia and higher rates of impaired glucose tolerance and insulin resistance among people with schizophrenia. However, obesity, which is associated with type II diabetes, is a growing problem in the United States in general and is complicated in schizophrenia treatment by the tendency of individuals to gain weight after their disease is managed with medications. Weight gain in some individuals may be attributed to a return to a healthier living situation in which regular meals are available and symptoms that interfere with obtaining food regularly (e.g., delusions) are decreased. For others, weight gain may be a medication side effect.

Disordered Water Balance

Patients with schizophrenia who have an abnormality in the hippocampus may experience disordered water balance in which individuals drink compulsively as a result of neuroendocrine dysfunction (Goldman et al., 2011). The prevalence rate of disordered water balance reportedly ranges around 5% to 20% (Hawken, Crookall, Reddick, Millson, Milev, & Delva, 2009). Often a benign condition, disordered water balance may go undetected for months to years; however, ingesting large amounts of water over a prolonged period may lead to complications, such as renal dysfunction, urinary incontinence, cardiac failure, malnutrition, or permanent brain damage (Valente & Fisher, 2010).

Disordered water balance can progress to water intoxication for a few, but notable number of, individuals. This is a life-threatening complication of unknown cause when a patient ingests an unusually large volume of water, the kidneys' capacity to excrete water is overwhelmed, serum sodium levels rapidly fall below the normal range of 135 to 145 mEq/L to a level of 120 mEq/L or less, and the rapid decrease in sodium produces neurologic signs such as muscle twitching and irritability, putting the patient at risk for seizures or coma or possibly death. Box 22.1 presents the physiologic signs and symptoms of disordered water balance and its progression.

Behaviorally, these patients seem to be "driven to drink" (polydipsia) and may consume between 4 and 10 liters of fluid a day. They carry soda cans and water bottles with them, hoard cups or other water containers, and drink frequently from fountains and showers and sometimes from toilets. They make frequent trips to the bathroom because of the excessive need to urinate (**polyuria**). Generally, the amount of urine excreted reflects the amount of fluid ingested. The patient's urine becomes very dilute with a very low specific gravity (1.008 or lower). Because of increased urgency and incontinence, especially at nighttime, the patient's clothing and room may smell like urine. Some patients may become highly agitated when efforts are made to limit access to water and other fluids. Other emotional or behavioral responses, such as increased psychotic symptoms, irritability, and lability, are caused by changes in sodium levels and the rapidity with which they occur.

BOX 22.1

Physiologic Signs and Symptoms of Disordered Water Balance

MILD DISORDERED WATER BALANCE
- Increased diurnal weight gain
- Specific urine gravity (1.011–1.025)
- Normal serum sodium (135–145 mEq/L)

MODERATE DISORDERED WATER BALANCE
- Increased diurnal weight gain
- Specific urine gravity (1.010–1.003)
- Possible facial puffiness
- Periodic nocturia

SEVERE DISORDERED WATER BALANCE
- Possible evidence of stomach or bladder dilation
- Specific urine gravity (1.003–1.000)
- Frequent signs of nausea, vomiting
- Possible history of major motor seizure
- Possible change in blood pressure or pulse
- Polyuria
- Polydipsia
- Urinary incontinence during the night

From Snider, K., & Boyd, M. A. (1991). When they drink too much: Nursing interventions for patients with disordered water balance. *Journal of Psychosocial Nursing and Mental Health Services, 29*(7), 13.

BOX 22.2

Deficits That Cause Vulnerability in Schizophrenia

COGNITIVE DEFICITS
- Deficits in processing complex information
- Deficits in maintaining a steady focus of attention
- Inability to distinguish between relevant and irrelevant stimuli
- Difficulty forming consistent abstractions
- Impaired memory

PSYCHOPHYSIOLOGIC DEFICITS
- Deficits in sensory inhibition
- Poor control of autonomic responsiveness

SOCIAL SKILLS DEFICITS
- Impairments in processing interpersonal stimuli, such as eye contact or assertiveness
- Deficits in conversational capacity
- Deficits in initiating activities
- Deficits in experiencing pleasure

COPING SKILLS DEFICITS
- Overassessment of threat
- Underassessment of personal resources
- Overuse of denial

Adapted from McGlashan, T. H. (1994). Psychosocial treatments of schizophrenia: The potential relationships. In N. C. Andreasen (Ed.), *Schizophrenia: From mind to molecule* (pp. 189–215). Washington, DC: American Psychiatric Press.

Etiology

Schizophrenia is believed to be caused by the interaction of a biologic predisposition or vulnerability and environmental stressors (see the diathesis–stress model discussed in Chapter 18). Environmental risk factors include pregnancy or obstetric complications and social adversity such as migration, unemployment, urban living, childhood abuse, and social isolation or absence of close friends (Box 22.2 and Fig. 22.1) (Goff, 2013).

Biologic Theories

Neuroanatomic Findings

The lateral and third ventricles are somewhat larger, and total brain volume is somewhat smaller in persons with schizophrenia compared with those without schizophrenia. The thalamus and the medial temporal lobe structures, including the hippocampus, superior temporal, and prefrontal cortices, tend to be smaller also (Birnbaum & Weinberger, 2013; Johnson et al., 2013).

Familial Patterns

The likelihood of first-degree relatives (including siblings and children) developing schizophrenia has long been recognized as 10 times more likely than are individuals in the general population. While this likelihood clearly suggests

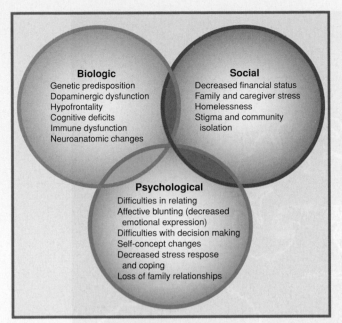

Biologic
Genetic predisposition
Dopaminergic dysfunction
Hypofrontality
Cognitive deficits
Immune dysfunction
Neuroanatomic changes

Social
Decreased financial status
Family and caregiver stress
Homelessness
Stigma and community
  isolation

Psychological
Difficulties in relating
Affective blunting (decreased
  emotional expression)
Difficulties with decision making
Self-concept changes
Decreased stress respose
  and coping
Loss of family relationships

FIGURE 22.1 Biopsychosocial etiologies for patients with schizophrenia.

a strong genetic factor, the concordance for schizophrenia among monozygotic (identical) twins is 50%, suggesting that there are also environmental factors (Bonsch, Wunschel, Lenz, Janssen, Weisbrod, & Sauer, 2012).

Genetic Associations

Genetic associations have been identified in a number of regions of the brain, and some have already been tied to altered dopamine transmission. However, these associations are more likely related to the susceptibility of developing the schizophrenia disorder rather than the cause (Birnbaum et al., 2013).

Neurodevelopment

The neurodevelopmental hypothesis explains the etiology of schizophrenia as pathologic processes caused by genetic and environmental factors that begin before the brain reaches its adult state. Evidence suggests that in utero during the first or second trimester, genes involved with cell migration, cell proliferation, axonal outgrowth, and myelination may be affected by neurologic insults such as viral infections. That is, early neurodevelopmental insults may lead to dysfunction of specific networks that become obvious at adolescence during the normal loss of some plasticity and synapse (Goff, 2013).

Neurotransmitters, Pathways, and Receptors

Positron emission tomography (PET) scan findings suggest that in schizophrenia, there is a general reduction in

brain metabolism, with a relative hypermetabolism in the left side of the brain and in the left temporal lobe. Abnormalities exist in specific areas of the brain in frontal, temporal, and cingulate regions (Smieskova et al., 2013). These findings support further exploration of differential brain hemisphere function in people with schizophrenia (Fig. 22.2). Other PET studies show **hypofrontality,** or a reduced cerebral blood flow and glucose metabolism in the prefrontal cortex of people with schizophrenia and hyperactivity in the limbic area (Figs. 22.3 and 22.4) (Buchsbaum, 1990; Buchsbaum, et al., 2007).

Dopamine Dysregulation

Positive symptoms of schizophrenia, specifically, hallucinations and delusions, are thought to be related to dopamine *hyperactivity* in the mesolimbic tract at the D_2 receptor site in the striatal area where memory and emotion are regulated. Dopamine dysfunction is thought to be involved not only in schizophrenia, but also in psychosis in other disorders. If there is no psychosis, it is unlikely that there is an overactivity of dopamine in the striatal region.

On the other hand, chronic low levels of dopamine in the prefrontal cortex are thought to underlie cognitive dysfunction in schizophrenia. Cognitive and negative symptoms of schizophrenia, once thought to be related to dopamine dysfunction on a single pathway, are now thought to be associated with transmitter or neural connectivity systems. In many cases, these dysfunctions precede the onset of psychosis (Lau, Wang, Hsu, & Liu, 2013).

Role of Other Receptors

Other receptors are also involved in dopamine neurotransmission, especially serotonergic receptors. It is becoming clear that schizophrenia does not result from dysregulation of a single neurotransmitter or biogenic amine (e.g., norepinephrine, dopamine, or serotonin). Investigators are also hypothesizing a role for glutamate and gamma-aminobutyric acid (GABA) because of the complex interconnections of neuronal transmission and the complexity and heterogeneity of schizophrenia symptoms. The N-methyl-D-aspartate (NMDA) class of glutamate receptors is being studied because of the actions of phencyclidine (PCP) at these sites and the similarity of the psychotic behaviors that are produced when someone takes PCP (see Figs. 22.2–22.4) (Goff, 2013).

Psychosocial Theories

There are no accepted psychosocial theories that explain the cause of schizophrenia. However, social stressors cannot be ignored because they can contribute to the changes in brain function that result in schizophrenia and add to the day-to-day challenges of living with a mental illness.

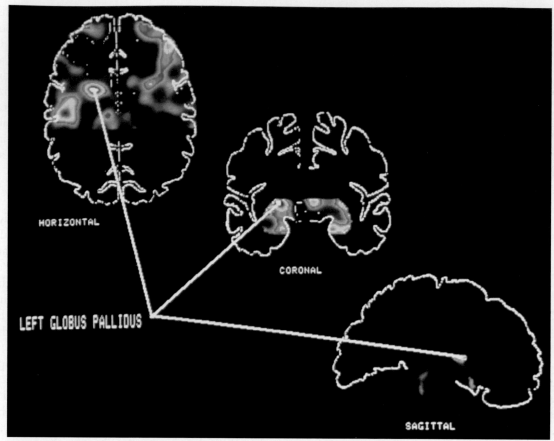

FIGURE 22.2 Area of abnormal functioning in a person with schizophrenia. These three views show the excessive neuronal activity in the left globus pallidus (portion of the basal ganglia next to the putamen). (Courtesy of John W. Haller, PhD, Departments of Psychiatry and Radiology, Washington University, St. Louis.)

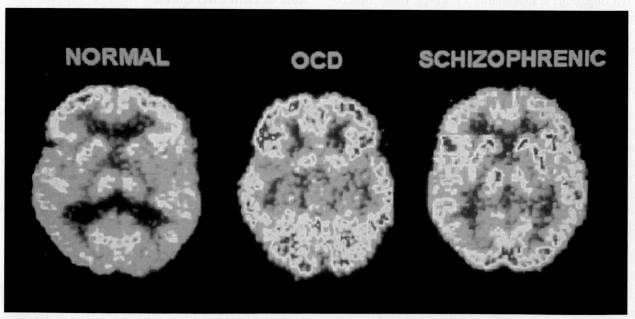

FIGURE 22.3 Metabolic activity in a control subject (**left**), a subject with obsessive–compulsive disorder (**center**), and a subject with schizophrenia (**right**). (Courtesy of Monte S. Buchsbaum, MD, The Mount Sinai Medical Center and School of Medicine, New York.)

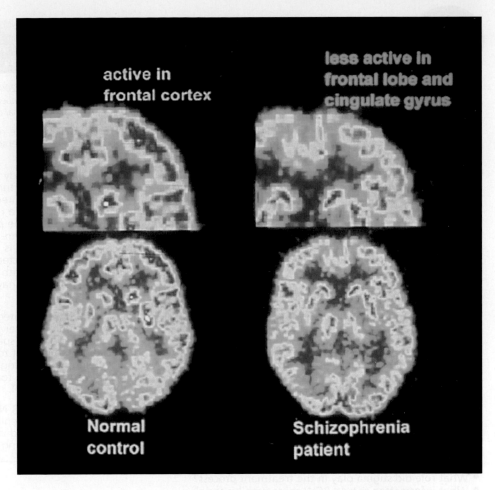

FIGURE 22.4 Positron emission tomography scan with 18F-deoxyglucose shows metabolic activity in a horizontal section of the brain in a control subject (**left**) and in an unmedicated patient with schizophrenia (**right**). *Red* and *yellow* indicate areas of high metabolic activity in the cortex; *green* and *blue* indicate lower activity in the white matter areas of the brain. The frontal lobe is magnified to show reduced frontal activity in the prefrontal cortex of the patient with schizophrenia. (Courtesy of Monte S. Buchsbaum, MD, The Mount Sinai Medical Center and School of Medicine, New York.)

They can also create barriers to obtaining necessary treatment and recovery.

One of the major social stressors is the social stigma that surrounds mental illnesses (see Chapter 2). The clinical vignette in Box 22.3 describes the impact of living with a stigmatizing illness. Another is the absence of good, affordable, and supportive housing in many communities. With 2010's enactment of insurance parity for mental illness, it is hoped that quality and continuity of care will be enhanced. Finally, the mental health service delivery system is fragmented, and the quality and types of services vary from community to community (National Alliance on Mental Illness, 2013).

Family Response to Disorder

Initially, families usually experience disbelief, shock, and fear along with concern for the family member. Families may attribute the episode to taking illicit drugs or to extraordinary stress or fatigue and hope that this is an isolated or transient event. They may be fearful of the behaviors and respond to patient anger and hostility with fear, confusion, and anxiety. They may deny the severity

and chronicity of the illness and only partially engage in treatment. As families begin to acknowledge the disorder and the long-term care nature of recovery, they may feel overwhelmed, angry, and depressed. See Box 22.4 for discussion of recovery-oriented interventions.

TREATMENT AND NURSING CARE FOR PATIENTS WITH SCHIZOPHRENIA

Interdisciplinary Treatment and Recovery

The most effective treatment approach for individuals with schizophrenia involves a variety of disciplines, including nursing (both generalist and advanced practice psychiatric nurses), psychiatry, psychology, social work, occupational and recreational therapy, and pastoral counseling. Pharmacologic management is the responsibility of the physicians and nurses; various psychosocial interventions can be implemented by all of the members of the mental health team. Individuals with general education in psychology, sociology, and social work often serve as case managers, nursing aids or technicians, and other support personnel in hospitals and community treatment

Clinical Vignette

BOX 22.3
GRADUATE STUDENT IN PERIL

BGW, born in 1973, spent most of his teenage years using drugs and alcohol, behavior that started when he was 11 years old. He and his small group of friends spent their teenage years outside of school running around on bicycles. He failed 8th grade, repeated it, and made it to 10th grade. He was removed permanently from school at the age of 16 years. His dress included a dirty denim jacket or Army fatigues, torn tee shirts with rock band logos, and tight-fitting jeans. At age 16, he was hospitalized for a psychotic episode initiated by LSD; it was the scariest moment of his life. His mind had been getting fuzzier every day; he had dabbled with black magic and Satanism. Later, he admitted that for years he had been trapped in a fantasy land, only partially explained by his drug use.

Years of treatment followed, and even with abstinence from drugs, his mental status fluctuated. After antipsychotic agents were prescribed, he began to feel like himself. He was motivated to complete his GED and entered college. He kept his mental illness a secret. While in graduate school, his thoughts, feelings, and behaviors began to change. His thinking became delusional, his moods unpredictable, and his behaviors illogical. Finally, he was hospitalized again, and his condition was stabilized with medication. Currently, he is reapplying to graduate school and this time vowing to keep people close to him aware of his mental status.

What Do You Think?
- What role did stigma play in the treatment process?
- What information should BGW share with his social network about his mental illness and treatment?

Adapted from First person account: Graduate student in peril. (2002). *Schizophrenia Bulletin, 28*(4), 745–755.

BOX 22.4
Research for Best Practice: **Recovery for People With Schizophrenia and Their Families**

Noiseux, S., & Ricard, N. (2008). Recovery as perceived by people with schizophrenia, family members, and health professionals: A grounded theory. *International Journal of Nursing Studies, 45*(8), 1148–1162.

THE QUESTION: Are recovery concepts consistent with the experiences of persons with schizophrenia and their families?

METHODS: This study used a grounded theory approach. Semi-structured interviews of 41 participants were conducted in three different settings: a hospital, a self-help group, and a community setting. Selection criteria included that the person with schizophrenia is in stable health, sees him- or herself as being in the process of recovery, and is able to speak about it. Family members were expected to display a strong bond with their relative living with schizophrenia, and the health professionals had to have at least 3 years mental health nursing experience.

FINDINGS: Seven categories emerged from the interviews, including perceiving schizophrenia as a "descent into hell," igniting a spark of hope, developing insight, activating the instinct to fight back, discovering keys to well-being, maintaining a constant equilibrium between internal and external forces, and finally, seeing light at the end of the tunnel.

IMPLICATIONS FOR NURSING: A person and family living with schizophrenia need mental health promotion and recovery-oriented interventions to support inner resources in developing an individual's potential.

---

agencies. These varied professionals and paraprofessionals are necessary because of the complex nature of the symptoms and chronic course of schizophrenia. See Interdisciplinary Treatment/Recovery Plan 22.1.

Priority Care Issues

Several special concerns exist when working with people with schizophrenia. A suicide assessment always should be done with a person who is experiencing a psychotic episode. In an inpatient unit, patient safety concerns extend to potential aggressive actions toward staff and other patients during episodes of psychosis. During times of acute illness, a priority of care is treatment with antipsychotic medications and, in some instances, hospitalization.

Patients need help in accepting and understanding their illness and developing a support system that encourages their recovery. Recovery-oriented strategies can address any hopelessness associated with suicide attempts and encourage an independent lifestyle.

Nursing Management: Human Response to Schizophrenia

Nursing management of the patient with schizophrenia lasts many years. Different phases of the illness require various nursing interventions. During exacerbation of symptoms, many patients are hospitalized for stabilization. During periods of relative stability, the nurse supports the patient in implementing a therapeutic regimen, developing recovery-oriented strategies, and coping with stress (Nursing Care Plan 22.1, pp. 347–349).

Biologic Domain
Biologic Assessment

Current and Past Health Status and Physical Examination

It is important to conduct a thorough history and physical examination to rule out medical illness or substance and to screen for comorbid medical illnesses, such as diabetes mellitus, hypertension, and cardiac disease, or a family history of such disorders. People with schizophrenia have a higher mortality rate from physical illness and

INTERDISCIPLINARY TREATMENT/RECOVERY PLAN 22.1

Patient With Schizophrenia

Admission Date	Date of This Plan	Type of Plan: Check Appropriate Box					
		☐ Initial	☐ Master	☐ 30	☐ 60	☐ 90	☐ Other

Treatment Team Present
A. Barton, MD; J. Jones, RNC; C. Anderson, CNS; B. Thomas, PhD; T. Toon, Mental Health Technician (MHT); J. Barker, MHT; J.T., with mother and father

DIAGNOSIS: SCHIZOPHRENIA

ASSETS (MEDICAL, PSYCHOLOGICAL, SOCIAL, EDUCATIONAL, VOCATIONAL, RECREATIONAL)

1. First episode of psychosis. No evidence of drug use.
2. Premorbid functional level appears to be normal.
3. Maintained good grades in high school.
4. Has supportive family members.

Prob. No	Date	Problem/Need	Code	Change Code	Change Date
1	3/5/14	Is hallucinating and had delusional thoughts. Unable to communicate with parents or staff.		T	
2	3/5/14	Is aggressive and is striking out at staff and unfamiliar people.		T	
3	3/5/14	Dropped out of college because of thoughts and behaviors.		X	
4	3/4/14	Family members are very upset about their son's psychiatric symptoms.		T	

CODE   T = Problem must be addressed in treatment.
N = Problem noted and will be monitored.
X = Problem noted, but deferred/inactive/no action necessary.
O = Problem to be addressed in aftercare/continuing care.
I = Problem incorporated into another problem.
R = Resolved.

INDIVIDUAL TREATMENT PLAN PROBLEM SHEET

#1 Problem/Need	Date Identified	Problem Resolved Discontinuation Date
Is hallucinating and has delusional thoughts. Unable to communicate with parents or staff.	3/5/14	

Objective(s)/Short-Term Goals	Target Date	Achievement Date
1. Reduce report and observations of hallucinations and delusions.	3/15/14	
Treatment Interventions	**Frequency**	**Person Responsible**
1. Antipsychotic therapy for hallucinations and delusions. Administer and monitor for adherence, effect, and side effects.	As prescribed	MD/RN
2. Monitor frequency of hallucinations and delusions.	Close observation for 24–48 hours; then according to RN judgment	RN/MHT
3. Attend symptom management group as symptoms subside.	Daily	

Continued

INTERDISCIPLINARY TREATMENT/RECOVERY PLAN 22.1 *(Continued)*

#2 Problem/Need	Date Identified	Problem Resolved/ Discontinuation Date
Is aggressive and is hitting out at staff and unfamiliar people.	3/5/14	

Objective(s)/Short-Term Goals	Target Date	Achievement Date
1. De-escalate aggressive behavior.	3/15/14	

Treatment interventions	Frequency	Person Responsible
1. Keep patient in a quiet, nonstimulating environment. Assign private room.	Ongoing	RN
2. Administer antianxiety medication as needed.	PRN	MD/RN
3. Use de-escalation techniques when approaching patient.	Ongoing	Everyone
4. Assign to anger management group if needed when psychotic symptoms decrease.	In 1 week	CNS

#3 Problem/Need	Date Identified	Problem Resolved/ Discontinuation Date
Family members are very upset about their son's psychiatric symptoms.	3/5/14	

Objective(s)/Short-Term Goals	Target Date	Achievement Date
Increase family's comfort levels with mental illness.	3/15/14	

Treatment Interventions	Frequency	Person Responsible
1. Meet with family each time they visit. Provide counseling and education to family.	Ongoing	CNS/RN/MD/PhD
2. Encourage to attend family support group.	Weekly	PhD
3. Provide community resources for the treatment of mental illness.	When visiting	CNS

Responsible QMHP	**Client or Guardian**	**Staff Physician**
Signature Date	Signature Date	Signature Date

often have smoking-related illnesses, such as emphysema, and other pulmonary and cardiac problems.

Physical Functioning

Self-care often deteriorates, and sleep may be nonexistent during acute phases. Information regarding physical functioning may best be collected from family members.

> **NCLEXNOTE** When assessing a patient with schizophrenia, the nurse should prioritize the severity of the current responses to the disorder. If hallucinations are impairing function, then managing hallucinations is a priority, and medications are needed immediately. If hallucinations are not a problem, coping with the negative symptoms becomes a priority.

Nutritional Assessment

A nutritional history should be completed to determine baseline eating habits and preferences. Medications can alter normal nutrition, and the patient may need to limit calories or fat consumption.

Pharmacologic Assessment

Baseline information about initial psychological and physical functioning should be obtained before initiation of medication (or as early as possible). Before medication begins, standardized assessment of abnormal motor movements should be conducted using one of several assessment tools designed for that purpose, such as the Abnormal Involuntary Movement Scale (AIMS) (see Appendix B),

NURSING CARE PLAN 22.1

The Patient With Schizophrenia

JT is a 19-year-old African American man who was brought to the hospital after his return from college where he had locked himself in his room for 3 days. He was talking to nonexistent people in a strange language. His room was covered with small pieces of taped paper with single words on them. His parents immediately made arrangements for him to be hospitalized.

Setting: Psychiatric Intensive Care Unit

Baseline Assessment: JT is a 6'1", 145-lb young man whose appearance is disheveled. He has not slept for 4 days and appears frightened. He is hypervigilant, pacing, and mumbling to himself. He is vague about past drug use, but his parents do not believe that he has used drugs. He appears to be hallucinating, conversing as if someone is in the room. He is confused and unable to write, speak, or think coherently. He is disoriented to time and place. Lab values are within normal limits except hemoglobin, 10.2, and hematocrit, 32. He has not eaten for several days.

Associated Psychiatric Diagnoses	Medications
Schizophrenia	Risperidone (Risperdal), 2 mg bid Lorazepam (Ativan), 2 mg PO or IM for agitation PRN

Nursing Diagnosis 1: Disturbed Thought Processes

Defining Characteristics

- Delusional thinking (people are thinking his thoughts; CIA agents are searching for him because of the plan he has developed)
- Suspiciousness
- Hallucinations (responding to voices that are not heard by others)
- Cognitive impairment: attention, memory, and executive function impairments

Related Factors

- Uncompensated alterations in brain activity

Outcomes

Initial

- Decreased delusional thinking through accurate interpretation of environment
- Conversations include fewer references to thought broadcasting and concerns about the CIA
- Expresses less suspiciousness about staff and other patients
- Decreased evidence of talking to people that others can't see (fewer vocalizations and observations of responding to sounds that others can't hear)
- Able to participate in activities of increasing length and complexity (e.g., sitting through group and group activities, able to make projects that require increased concentration and contain more steps)

Long Term

- Able to identify, monitor, and recognize antecedents to delusional thinking and hallucinations
- Able to use coping mechanisms that will help to minimize or control symptoms of delusions and hallucinations, particularly reaching out to peer, professional, and family support systems
- Able to participate in conversations with others that stay on topic and contain little delusional content
- Able to demonstrate stable cognitive functioning through self-care activities, participation in recreational and vocational activities, and support connections to important others

Continued

NURSING CARE PLAN 22.1 *(Continued)*

Interventions

Interventions	Rationale	Ongoing Assessment
• Initiate a nurse–patient relationship by using an accepting, nonjudgmental approach. • Be patient.	• A therapeutic relationship will provide patient support as JT begins to deal with a devastating disorder. • Be patient because his brain is not processing information normally.	• Determine the extent to which JT is willing to trust and engage in a relationship. • Determine the length of time JT can attend to conversation or activity with others.
• Administer risperidone as prescribed. Observe for affect, side effects, and adverse effects. Begin teaching about the medication and its importance after symptoms subside.	• Risperidone is a D_2 and 5-HT_{2A} antagonist and is indicated for the treatment of schizophrenia.	• Make sure JT swallows pills. Monitor for relief of positive symptoms using a standardized measure such as the SAPS. Assess side effects, especially extrapyramidal. Monitor blood pressure for orthostatic hypotension and body temperature increase (NMS).
• During hallucinations and delusional thinking, assess significance (what feelings is JT experiencing; what actions do the voices or his thoughts suggest he accomplish?). Reassure JT that you will keep him safe and that you are aware that his experiences are very real to him even though you may not be having the same experiences. (Do not try to convince JT that his hallucinations are not real or his delusions are not true.) Redirect JT to here-and-now activities and experiences. • Assess ability for self-care activities.	• It is important to understand the experience and context of the hallucinations and delusions to be able to provide appropriate interventions and redirect the patient to more reality-based activities. By avoiding arguments about the content of the patient's delusional beliefs or the experiences of patient's hallucinations, the nurse will enhance communication. Arguing about delusional thoughts or hallucinatory experiences just places the patient in a position to defend his beliefs. • Disturbed thinking may interfere with JT's ability to carry out ADLs.	• Assess the meaning of the hallucinations or delusions of the patient. Determine whether he is a danger to himself or others. Determine whether patient can be directed to a more reality-based activity. • Continue to assess: Determine whether JT can manage his own self-care.

Evaluation

Outcomes	Revised Outcomes	Interventions
• Hallucinations and delusions began to decrease within 3 days. • Is oriented to time, place, and person. Attention and memory improving.	• Participate in unit activities according to ITP. • Agree to continue to take antipsychotic medication as prescribed.	• Encourage attendance at treatment activities. • Teach JT about medications. • Teach JT about schizophrenia.

Nursing Diagnosis 2: Risk for Violence

Defining Characteristics	Related Factors
• Assaultive toward others, self, and environment • Presence of pathophysiologic risk factors: delusional thinking and auditory hallucinations	• Frightened, secondary to auditory hallucinations and delusional thinking • Poor impulse control • Dysfunctional communication patterns

Outcomes

Initial	Long-term
• Avoid hurting self or assaulting other patients or staff. • Decrease agitation and aggression.	• Control behavior with assistance from staff and parents.

Continued

NURSING CARE PLAN 22.1 (*Continued*)

Interventions

Interventions	Rationale	Ongoing Assessment
• Acknowledge patient's fear resulting from the experience of hallucinations and delusional thoughts.	• Hallucinations and delusions change an individual's experience of environmental stimuli.	• Assess the patient's ability to hear you and respond appropriately to your comments and requests; assess the patient's ability to concentrate on what is being said and happening around him.
• Be genuine and empathic.	• The patient will benefit from your ability to understand his experience and express that understanding while presenting reality.	• Assess for evidence that the client is less frightened with less potential for striking out.
• Offer the patient choices of maintaining safety, including helping the patient to be less overwhelmed by the environment: minimize the noise and people around the patient.	• By having choices, he will begin to develop a sense of control over his behavior.	• Observe the patient's nonverbal communication for evidence of increased agitation.
• Use medications to help the patient relax and maintain more calm: administer lorazepam, 2 mg, for agitation. The PO route is preferable to injection, so offer the patient this choice long before he has lost control.	• Exact mechanisms of action are not understood, but medication is believed to potentiate the inhibitory neurotransmitter GABA, relieving anxiety and producing sedation.	• Observe for a decrease in agitated behavior. • Offering this to the patient early, as fear and agitation are beginning to become evident, prevents the potential for the patient to lose control.

Evaluation

Outcomes	Revised Outcomes	Interventions
• JT gradually decreased agitated behavior. • Lorazepam was given regularly for first 2 days.	• Demonstrate control of behavior by resisting auditory command hallucinations and delusional thoughts that cause suspicion and fear of others.	• Teach JT about the effects of hallucinations and delusions. • Problem solve ways of controlling response to hallucinations when they occur. • Problem solve ways to refrain from discussing delusional beliefs with people who are unfamiliar with the patient. • Emphasize the importance of taking prescribed antipsychotic medication.

ADL, activity of daily living; bid, twice a day; GABA, gamma-aminobutyric acid; IM, intramuscular; ITP, interdisciplinary treatment plan; NMS, neuroleptic malignant syndrome; PO, oral; SAPS, Scale for the Assessment of Positive Symptoms.

the Dyskinesia Identification System (DISCUS) (Sprague & Kalachnik, 1991) (Box 22.5, p. 350), or the Simpson–Angus Rating Scale (Simpson & Angus, 1970), which is designed for Parkinson's symptoms.

Nursing Diagnoses for Biologic Domain

Typical nursing diagnoses focusing on the biologic domain for the person during all phases of schizophrenia include Self-Care Deficit and Disturbed Sleep Pattern. During a relapse, Ineffective Therapeutic Regimen Management, Imbalanced Nutrition, Excess Fluid

Volume, and Sexual Dysfunction are possible diagnoses. Constipation may occur if the patient takes anticholinergic medications.

Interventions for Biologic Domain

Nursing interventions during the initial acute phase of schizophrenia include prompt, safe, and informed administration of antipsychotic medications (Table 22.1). During any stage, attention to self-care needs and the patient's ability to maintain hygiene and adequate nutrition are important.

BOX 22.5

The Dyskinesia Identification System: Condensed User Scale (DISCUS)

| NAME | | I.D. | |

| (facility)

Dyskinesia Identification System: Condensed User Scale (DISCUS)

CURRENT PSYCHOTROPICS/ANTI-CHOLINERGIC AND TOTAL MG/DAY

_____ _____mg
_____ _____mg
_____ _____mg
_____ _____mg

See Instructions on Other Side | EXAM TYPE (check one)
☐ 1. Baseline
☐ 2. Annual
☐ 3. Semi-annual
☐ 4. D/C—1 mo
☐ 5. D/C—2 mo
☐ 6. D/C—3 mo
☐ 7. Admission
☐ 8. Other

COOPERATION (check one)
☐ 1. None
☐ 2. Partial
☐ 3. Full | SCORING
0—**Not present** (movements not observed or some movements observed but not considered abnormal)
1—**Minimal** (abnormal movements are difficult to detect or movements are easy to detect but occur only once or twice in a short nonrepetitive manner)
2—**Mild** (abnormal movements occur infrequently and are easy to detect)
3—**Moderate** (abnormal movements occur frequently and are easy to detect)
4—**Severe** (abnormal movements occur almost continuously **and** are easy to detect)
NA—**Not assessed** (an assessment for an item is not able to be made) | |

ASSESSMENT
DISCUS Item and Score (circle one score for each item)

FACE
1. Tics.................................... 0 1 2 3 4 NA
2. Grimaces........................... 0 1 2 3 4 NA

EYES
3. Blinking............................ 0 1 2 3 4 NA

ORAL
4. Chewing/Lip Smacking......... 0 1 2 3 4 NA
5. Puckering/Sucking/Thrusting Lower Lip............... 0 1 2 3 4 NA

LINGUAL
6. Tongue Thrusting/Tongue in Cheek.................. 0 1 2 3 4 NA
7. Tonic Tongue....................... 0 1 2 3 4 NA
8. Tongue Tremor..................... 0 1 2 3 4 NA
9. Athetoid/Myokymic/Lateral Tongue.................... 0 1 2 3 4 NA

HEAD/NECK/TRUNK
10. Retrocollis/Torticollis............. 0 1 2 3 4 NA
11. Shoulder/Hip Torsion........... 0 1 2 3 4 NA

UPPER LIMB
12. Athetoid/Myokymic Finger–Wrist–Arm................. 0 1 2 3 4 NA
13. Pill Rolling .... 0 1 2 3 4 NA

LOWER LIMB
14. Ankle Flexion/Foot Tapping....................... 0 1 2 3 4 NA
15. Toe Movement................... 0 1 2 3 4 NA

EVALUATION (see Appendix C)

1. Greater than 90 d neuroleptic exposure? : YES NO
2. Scoring/intensity level met? : YES NO
3. Other diagnostic conditions? : YES NO
(if yes, specify)
_____
_____

4. Last exam date: _____
Last total score: _____
Last conclusion: _____

Preparer signature and title for items 1–4 (if different from physician):

5. Conclusion (circle one):
A. No TD (if scoring prerequisite met, list other diagnostic condition or explain in comments)
B. Probable TD
C. Masked TD
D. Withdrawal TD
E. Persistent TD
F. Remitted TD
G. Other (specify in comments)

6. Comments:
_____
_____
_____
_____
_____
_____

COMMENTS/OTHER
_____
_____
_____
_____
_____

| TOTAL SCORE
(items 1–15 only) | |
| EXAM DATE | |

| RATER SIGNATURE AND TITLE | NET EXAM DATE | CLINICIAN SIGNATURE | DATE |

From Sprague, R. L., & Kalachnik, J. E. (1991). Reliability, validity, and a total score cutoff for the Dyskinesia Identification System, Condensed User Scale (DISCUS) with mentally ill and mentally retarded populations. *Psychopharmacology Bulletin, 27*(1), 51–58.

Table 22.1 SELECTED ANTIPSYCHOTIC DRUGS

Generic Name	Trade Name	Dosage Range for Adults (mg/d)
Second-Generation Antipsychotics		
Aripiprazole	Abilify	10–15
Clozapine	Clozaril	200–600
Iloperidone	Fanapt	12–24
Risperidone	Risperdal	4–16
Olanzapine	Zyprexa	10–20
Paliperidone	Invega	3–12
Quetiapine	Seroquel	300–400
Ziprasidone	Geodon	40–160
Lurasidone	Latuda	40–80
Selected First-Generation Antipsychotic Drugs Used to Treat Psychosis in the United States		
Chlorpromazine	NA[a]	30–800
Fluphenazine	NA	0.5–20
Haloperidol	Haldol	1–15
Loxapine	Loxitane	20–250
Perphenazine	NA	4–32
Pimozide[c]	NA	1–10
Prochlorperazine[b]	—	15–25
Thiothixene	Navane	5–25
Trifluoperazine	Stelazine	5–25

[a]Not Applicable. No longer available by trade name.

[b]Approved in the United States for Tourette's syndrome.

[c]Adapted from Stahl, S. (2013). *Essential psychopharmacology: Neuroscientific basis and practical application* (4th ed.). Cambridge, UK: Cambridge University Press.

NCLEXNOTE Monitoring actions and side effects of medications are priority nursing interventions. Second-generation antipsychotics are used with increasing frequency and should be easily recognized. The older first-generation medications are used occasionally.

Promotion of Self-Care Activities

For many people with schizophrenia, the plan of care will include specific interventions to enhance self-care, nutrition, and overall health knowledge. Negative symptoms commonly leave patients unable to initiate these seemingly simple activities. Developing a daily schedule of routine activities (such as showering and shaving) can help the patient structure the day. Most patients actually know how to perform self-care activities (e.g., hygiene, grooming) but lack motivation (avolition) to carry them out consistently. Interventions include developing a schedule with the patient for various hygiene activities and emphasizing the importance of maintaining appropriate self-care activities. Given the problems related to attention and memory in people with schizophrenia, education about these areas requires careful planning.

Activity, Exercise, and Nutritional Interventions

Encouraging activity and exercise is necessary, not only to maintain a healthy lifestyle but also to counteract the side effects of psychiatric medications that cause weight gain. Because the diagnosis is usually made in late adolescence or early adulthood, it is possible to establish solid exercise patterns early.

During episodes of acute psychosis, patients are unable to focus on eating. Often when patients begin antipsychotic medication, normal satiety and hunger responses change, and overeating or weight gain can become a problem. Promoting healthy nutrition is a key intervention. Maintaining healthy nutrition and monitoring calorie intake also become important because of the effect many medications have on eating habits. Patients report that their appetites increase and cravings for food develop when some medications are initiated.

Weight gain is one of the reasons some patients stop taking medication. Increased weight places patients at greater risk for several health problems, such as type II diabetes mellitus and early death. Monitoring for diabetes and managing weight are important activities for all care providers. Patients should be screened for risk factors of diabetes, such as family history, obesity as indicated by a body mass index (BMI) exceeding or equal to 27, and age older than 45 years. Patients' weight should be measured at regular intervals and the BMI calculated. Blood pressure readings should be taken regularly. Laboratory findings for triglycerides, high-density lipoprotein cholesterol, and glucose level should be monitored and reviewed regularly. All providers should be alert to the development of hyperglycemia, particularly in patients known to have diabetes who begin taking second-generation antipsychotic agents. A program to address weight gain should be initiated at the earliest sign of weight gain (probably between 5 and 10 pounds over desired body weight). Reduced caloric intake may be accomplished by increasing the patient's access to affordable, healthful, and easy-to-prepare foods. Behavioral management of weight gain includes keeping a food diary, diet teaching, and support groups (Koch & Scott, 2012).

Thermoregulation Interventions

Patients with schizophrenia may have disturbed body temperature regulation. In winter, they may seem to be oblivious to cold weather. In the heat of summer, they may dress for winter. Observing patients' responses to temperatures helps in identifying problems in this area. In patients who are taking psychiatric medications, body temperature needs to be monitored, and the patient needs to be protected from extremes in temperature.

Promotion of Normal Fluid Balance and Prevention of Water Intoxication

Nursing interventions for disordered water balance include teaching and assisting the patient to develop self-monitoring skills. Fluid intake and weight gain should be monitored to control fluid intake and reduce the likelihood of developing water intoxication. Patients with mild disordered water balance are easily treated in outpatient settings and benefit from educational programs that teach them to monitor their own urine specific gravity and daily weight gains. Patients with moderate disordered water balance may respond well to education but have a more difficult time controlling their own fluid intake, which requires more careful monitoring of intake and weight throughout the day. Patients with severe disordered water balance require considerable assistance, probably on an inpatient unit, to restrict their continual water-seeking behavior. These patients may create disruption on the unit, so they are best managed by one-on-one observation to redirect their behavior.

Pharmacologic Interventions: Antipsychotics

Antipsychotic drugs have the general effect of blocking dopamine transmission in the brain by blocking D_2 receptors to some degree (see Chapter 11). Some also block other dopamine receptors and receptors of other neurotransmitters to varying degrees. For the most part, the antidopamine effects are not specific to the mesolimbic and mesocortical tracts associated with schizophrenia but instead travel to all the dopamine receptor sites throughout the brain. This results in desirable antipsychotic effects but also creates some unpleasant and undesirable side effects. The actions of these drugs on other neurotransmitter systems account for additional side effects.

The second-generation antipsychotic drugs risperidone (Risperdal) (Box 22.6), olanzapine (Zyprexa), quetiapine (Seroquel), paliperidone (Invega), ziprasidone (Geodon), aripiprazole (Abilify), iloperidone (Fanapt), asenapine (Saphris), and Lurasidone (Latuda) are available in a variety of formulations. They are effective in treating negative and positive symptoms. These newer drugs also affect several other neurotransmitter systems, including serotonin. This is believed to contribute to their antipsychotic effectiveness (see Chapter 11).

Monitoring and Administering Medications

Antipsychotic medications are the treatment of choice for patients with psychosis. The use of first-generation

---

BOX 22.6

Drug Profile: Risperidone (Risperdal)

DRUG CLASS: Atypical antipsychotic

RECEPTOR AFFINITY: Antagonist with high affinity for D_2 and 5-HT_2, also histamine (H_1) and α_1-, α_2-adrenergic receptors, weak affinity for D_1 and other serotonin receptor subtypes; no affinity for acetylcholine or β-adrenergic receptors

INDICATIONS: Treatment of schizophrenia; short-term treatment of acute manic or mixed episodes associated with bipolar I disorder; and irritability associated with autistic disorder in children and adolescents, including symptoms of aggression toward others, deliberate self-injuriousness, temper tantrums, and quickly changing moods

ROUTES AND DOSAGE: 0.25-, 0.5-, 1-, 2-, 3-, and 4-mg tablets and liquid concentrate (1 mg/mL); 0.5-, 1-, 2-, 3-, and 4-mg orally disintegrating tablets

Adult: Schizophrenia: Initial dose: typically 1 mg bid. Maximal effect at 6 mg/d. Safety not established above 16 mg/d. Use lowest possible dose to alleviate symptoms

Bipolar mania: 2 to 3 mg/d

Children: 0.25 mg/d for patients <20 kg and 0.5 mg/d for patients >20 kg

HALF-LIFE (PEAK EFFECT): Mean, 20 h (1 h; peak active metabolite = 3–17 h)

SELECT ADVERSE REACTIONS: Insomnia, agitation, anxiety, extrapyramidal symptoms, headache, rhinitis, somnolence, dizziness, headache, constipation, nausea, dyspepsia, vomiting, abdominal pain, hypersalivation, tachycardia, orthostatic hypotension, fever, chest pain, coughing, photosensitivity, weight gain

BOXED WARNING: Increased mortality in elderly patients with dementia-related psychosis

WARNING: Rare development of neuroleptic malignant syndrome. Observe frequently for early signs of tardive dyskinesia. Use caution with individuals who have cardiovascular disease; risperidone can cause electrocardiographic changes. Avoid use during pregnancy or while breastfeeding. Hepatic or renal impairments increase plasma concentration

SPECIFIC PATIENT/FAMILY EDUCATION
- Notify your prescriber if tremor, motor restlessness, abnormal movements, chest pain, or other unusual symptoms develop.
- Avoid alcohol and other CNS depressant drugs.
- Notify your prescriber if pregnancy is possible or planning to become pregnant. Do not breastfeed while taking this medication.
- Notify your prescriber before taking any other prescription or OTC medication.
- May impair judgment, thinking, or motor skills; avoid driving or other hazardous tasks.
- During titration, the individual may experience orthostatic hypotension and should change positions slowly.
- Do not abruptly discontinue.

bid, twice a day; CNS, central nervous system; OTC, over the counter.

antipsychotics (e.g., haloperidol, chlorpromazine) decreased dramatically with the introduction of the second generation of antipsychotics. However, it is important that medication choice be individualized based on each patient's experience and preference as well as the side effect profiles of selected drugs rather than limit drug selection to one type or class of antipsychotic medication. This is particularly true during the acute phase of the illness for people with schizophrenia who are known to be treatment responsive.

Generally, it takes about 1 to 2 weeks for antipsychotic drugs to effect a change in symptoms. During the stabilization period, the selected drug should be given an adequate trial, generally 6 to 12 weeks before considering a change in the drug prescription. If treatment effects are not seen, another antipsychotic agent may be tried. Clozapine (Clozaril) is used when no other second-generation antipsychotic is effective; see Box 22.7 for more information about clozapine.

Adherence to a prescribed medication regimen is the best approach to preventing relapse. Unfortunately, patient treatment adherence with second-generation antipsychotic agents is not improved from that with conventional antipsychotic agents (Guo et al., 2011). The use of long-acting injectables is expected to improve compliance outcomes (Altamura et al., 2012). Box 22.8 provides information about interventions to promote medication adherence for patients with schizophrenia.

Patients with schizophrenia generally face a lifetime of taking antipsychotic medications. Rarely is discontinuation of medications prescribed; however, many patients stop taking medications on their own. Some situations that require the cessation of medication use are neuroleptic malignant syndrome (see later discussion) or agranulocytosis (dangerously low level of circulating neutrophils). Discontinuation is an option when tardive dyskinesia develops. Discontinuation of medications, other than in circumstances of a medical emergency, should be achieved

---

BOX 22.7

Drug Profile: Clozapine (Clozaril)

DRUG CLASS: Atypical antipsychotic

RECEPTOR AFFINITY: D_1 and D_2 blockade, antagonist for 5-HT_2, histamine (H_1), α-adrenergic, and acetylcholine. These additional antagonist effects may contribute to some of its therapeutic effects. Produces fewer extrapyramidal effects than standard antipsychotics with lower risk for tardive dyskinesia

INDICATIONS: Severely ill individuals who have schizophrenia and have not responded to standard antipsychotic treatment; reduction in risk of recurrent suicidal behavior in schizophrenia or schizoaffective disorders

ROUTES AND DOSAGE: Available only in tablet form, 25- and 100-mg doses

Adult Dosage: Initial dose 25 mg PO bid or qid, may gradually increase in 25–50 mg/d increments, if tolerated, to a dose of 300–450 mg/d by the end of the second week. Additional increases should occur no more than once or twice weekly. Do not exceed 900 mg/d. For maintenance, reduce dosage to lowest effective level

Children: Safety and efficacy with children younger than age 16 years have not been established

HALF-LIFE (PEAK EFFECT): 12 h (1–6 h)

SELECT ADVERSE REACTIONS: Drowsiness, dizziness, headache, hypersalivation, tachycardia, hypo- or hypertension, constipation, dry mouth, heartburn, nausea or vomiting, blurred vision, diaphoresis, fever, weight gain, hematologic changes, seizures, tremor, akathisia

BOXED WARNING: Agranulocytosis, defined as a granulocyte count of <500 mm³, occurs at about a cumulative 1-year incidence of 1.3%, most often within 4–10 weeks of exposure, but may occur at any time; WBC count before initiation, and weekly WBC counts while taking the drug and for 4 weeks after discontinuation

Seizures, myocarditis, and other adverse cardiovascular and respiratory effects (orthostatic hypotension)

WARNING: Increased mortality in elderly patients with dementia-related psychosis; rare development of NMS; *hyperglycemia and diab*etes, tardive dyskinesia, cases of sudden, unexplained death have been reported; avoid use during pregnancy and while breastfeeding

PRECAUTIONS: Fever, pulmonary embolism, hepatitis, anticholinergic toxicity, and interference with cognitive and motor functions

SPECIFIC PATIENT/FAMILY EDUCATION
- Need informed consent regarding risk for agranulocytosis. Weekly or biweekly blood draws are required. Notify your prescriber immediately if lethargy, weakness, sore throat, malaise, or other flu-like symptoms develop.
- You should not take Clozaril if you are taking other medicines that cause the same serious bone marrow side effects.
- Inform the patient of risk of seizures, hyperglycemia and diabetes, and orthostatic hypotension. It may potentiate the hypotensive effects of antihypertensive drugs and anticholinergic effects of atropine-type drugs.
- Administration of epinephrine should be avoided in the treatment of drug-induced hypotension.
- Notify your prescriber if pregnancy is possible or planning to become pregnant. Do not breastfeed while taking this medication.
- Notify your prescriber before taking any other prescription or OTC medication. Avoid alcohol or other CNS depressant drugs.
- May cause drowsiness and seizures; avoid driving or other hazardous tasks.
- During titration, the individual may experience orthostatic hypotension and should change positions slowly.
- Do not abruptly discontinue.

---

bid, twice a day; CNS, central nervous system; NMS, neuroleptic malignant syndrome; OTC, over the counter; qid, four times a day; WBC, white blood cell.

BOX 22.8

Research for Best Practice: **Medication Adherence in People With Schizophrenia**

Gray, R., White, J., Schulz, M., & Abderhalden, C. (2010). Enhancing medication adherence in people with schizophrenia: An international programme of research. International Journal of Mental Health Nursing, 19(1), 36–44.

THE QUESTION: Do adherence therapy interventions improve adherence?

METHODS: Adherence therapy facilitates shared decision making between patients and clinicians. This paper reviewed the results of four adherence therapy trials that had mixed results. The authors then developed an adherence intervention based on six adherence-modifying factors: efficacy of medication, side effect management, clinician characteristics, medication side effects, experiences of medication and illness, and beliefs and attitudes about medications.

FINDINGS: Two studies showed improvement in symptoms and quality of life through implementing adherence therapy session over 8 weeks starting in the inpatient unit before discharge to the community. In adherence therapy, there are five key exercises that broadly follow a sequence: structured medication problem solving (practical problems, such as side effects), looking back (review past experiences of illness and treatment), exploring ambivalence, discussing beliefs and concerns, and looking forward (life goals).

IMPLICATIONS FOR NURSING: The authors confirm that people with schizophrenia need to be more involved in the decision making and in control of their own medications. Future studies are needed to evaluate the effectiveness of interventions that enhance the feeling of being in control over medication.

---

by gradually lowering the dose over time. This diminishes the likelihood of withdrawal symptoms, which include withdrawal dyskinesias and withdrawal psychosis.

Monitoring Extrapyramidal Side Effects

Parkinsonism that is caused by antipsychotic drugs is identical in appearance to Parkinson disease and tends to occur in older patients. The symptoms are believed to be caused by the blockade of D_2 receptors in the basal ganglia, which throws off the normal balance between acetylcholine and dopamine in this area of the brain and effectively increases acetylcholine transmission.

The symptoms are managed by reestablishing the balance between acetylcholine and dopamine by either reducing the dosage of the antipsychotic (thereby increasing dopamine activity) or adding an anticholinergic drug (decreasing acetylcholine activity), such as benztropine mesylate or trihexyphenidyl.

Abrupt discontinuation of anticholinergic drugs can cause a cholinergic rebound and result in withdrawal symptoms, such as vomiting, excessive sweating, and altered dreams and nightmares. Thus, the anticholinergic drug dosage should be reduced gradually (tapered)

over several days. If a patient experiences akathisia (physical restlessness), an anticholinergic medication may not be particularly helpful. Table 22.2 lists anticholinergic side effects of antiparkinson drugs and several antipsychotic medications and interventions to manage them.

Dystonic reactions are also believed to result from the imbalance of dopamine and acetylcholine, with the latter dominant. Young men seem to be more vulnerable to this particular extrapyramidal side effect. This side effect, which develops rapidly and dramatically, can be very frightening for patients as their muscles tense and their body contorts. The experience often starts with **oculogyric crisis,** in which the muscles that control eye movements tense and pull the eyeball so that the patient is looking toward the ceiling. This may be followed rapidly by **torticollis,** in which the neck muscles pull the head to the side, or **retrocollis,** in which the head is pulled back, or orolaryngeal–pharyngeal hypertonus, in which the patient has extreme difficulty swallowing. The patient may also experience contorted extremities. These symptoms occur early in antipsychotic drug treatment, when the patient may still be experiencing psychotic symptoms. This compounds the patient's fear and anxiety and requires a quick response. The immediate treatment is to administer benztropine mesylate, 1 to 2 mg, or diphenhydramine, 25 to 50 mg, intramuscularly or intravenously. This is followed by daily administration of anticholinergic drugs and, possibly, by a decrease in antipsychotic medication. See Box 22.9 for more information about benztropine.

Table 22.2	NURSING INTERVENTIONS FOR ANTICHOLINERGIC SIDE EFFECTS
Effect	**Intervention**
Dry mouth	Provide sips of water, hard candies, and chewing gum (preferably sugar free)
Blurred vision	Avoid dangerous tasks; teach patient that this side effect will diminish in a few weeks
Decreased lacrimation	Use artificial tears if necessary
Mydriasis	May aggravate glaucoma; teach patient to report eye pain
Photophobia	Wear sunglasses
Constipation	High-fiber diet; increased fluid intake; laxatives as prescribed
Urinary hesitancy	Privacy; run water in sink; warm water over perineum
Urinary retention	Regular voiding (at least every 2–3 h) and whenever urge is present; catheterize for residual; record intake and output; evaluate for benign prostatic hypertrophy
Tachycardia	Evaluate for pre-existing cardiovascular disease; sudden death has occurred with thioridazine (Mellaril)

BOX 22.9

Drug Profile: **Benztropine Mesylate**

DRUG CLASS: Antiparkinson agent

RECEPTOR AFFINITY: Blocks cholinergic (acetylcholine) activity, which is believed to restore the balance of acetylcholine and dopamine in the basal ganglia.

INDICATIONS: Used in psychiatry to reduce extrapyramidal symptoms (acute medication-related movement disorders), including pseudoparkinsonism, dystonia, and akathisia (not tardive syndromes) caused by neuroleptic drugs such as haloperidol. Most effective with acute dystonia.

ROUTES AND DOSAGE: Available in tablet form, 0.5-, 1-, and 2-mg doses, also injectable 1 mg/mL (Cogentin).

Adult dosage: For acute dystonia, 1–2 mg IM or IV usually provides rapid relief. No significant difference in onset of action after IM or IV injection. Treatment of emergent symptoms may be relieved in 1 or 2 days, with 1–2 mg PO 2–3 times/d. Maximum daily dose is 6 mg/d. After 1–2 weeks, withdraw drug to see if continued treatment is needed. Medication-related movement disorders that develop slowly may not respond to this treatment.

Geriatric: Older adults and very thin patients cannot tolerate large doses.

Children: Do not use in children younger than 3 years of age. Use with caution in older children.

HALF-LIFE: 12–24 h; very little pharmacokinetic information is available.

SELECT ADVERSE REACTIONS: Dry mouth, blurred vision, tachycardia, nausea, constipation, flushing or elevated temperature, decreased sweating, muscular weakness or cramping, urinary retention, urinary hesitancy, dizziness, headache, disorientation, confusion, memory loss, hallucinations, psychoses, and agitation in toxic reactions, which are more pronounced in elderly adults and occur at smaller doses.

WARNING: Avoid use during pregnancy and while breastfeeding. Give with caution in hot weather because of possible heatstroke. Contraindicated with angle-closure glaucoma, pyloric or duodenal obstruction, stenosing peptic ulcers, prostatic hypertrophy or bladder neck obstructions, myasthenia gravis, megacolon, and megaesophagus. May aggravate the symptoms of tardive dyskinesia and other chronic forms of medication-related movement disorder. Concomitant use of other anticholinergic drugs may increase side effects and risk for toxicity. Coadministration of haloperidol or phenothiazines may reduce serum levels of these drugs.

SPECIFIC PATIENT/FAMILY EDUCATION
- Take with meals to reduce dry mouth and gastric irritation.
- Dry mouth may be alleviated by sucking sugarless candies, adequate fluid intake, or good oral hygiene; increase fiber and fluids in diet to avoid constipation; stool softeners may be required. Notify your prescriber if urinary hesitancy or constipation persists.
- Notify your prescriber if rapid or pounding heartbeat, confusion, eye pain, rash, or other adverse symptoms develop.
- May cause drowsiness, dizziness, or blurred vision; use caution driving or performing other hazardous tasks requiring alertness. Avoid alcohol and other CNS depressants.
- Do not abruptly stop this medication because a flu-like syndrome may develop.
- Use caution in hot weather. Ensure adequate hydration. May increase susceptibility to heat stroke.

CNS, central nervous system; IM, intramuscular; IV, intravenous; PO, oral.

Akathisia appears to be caused by the same biologic mechanism as other **extrapyramidal side effects.** Patients are restless and report they feel driven to keep moving. They are very uncomfortable. Frequently, this response is misinterpreted as anxiety or increased psychotic symptoms, and the patient may be inappropriately given increased dosages of antipsychotic drug, which only perpetuates the side effect. If possible, the dose of antipsychotic drug should be reduced. A β-adrenergic blocker such as propranolol (Inderal), 20 to 120 mg, may be required. Failure to manage this side effect is a leading cause of patients ceasing to take antipsychotic medications (see Chapter 11).

Tardive dyskinesia, tardive dystonia, and tardive akathisia are less likely but still possible to appear in individuals taking second-generation, rather than first-generation, antipsychotics. Table 22.3 describes these and associated motor abnormalities. **Tardive dyskinesia** is late-appearing abnormal involuntary movements (dyskinesia). It can be viewed as the opposite of parkinsonism both in observable movements and in etiology. Whereas muscle rigidity and absence of movement characterize parkinsonism, constant movement characterizes tardive dyskinesia. Typical movements involve the mouth, tongue, and jaw and include lip smacking, sucking, puckering, tongue protrusion, the bonbon sign (where the tongue rolls around in the mouth and protrudes into the cheek as if the patient were sucking on a piece of hard candy), athetoid (worm-like) movements in the tongue, and chewing. Other facial movements, such as grimacing and eye blinking, also may be present.

Movements in the trunk and limbs are frequently observable. These include rocking from the hips, athetoid movements of the fingers and toes, jerking movements of the fingers and toes, guitar strumming movements of the fingers, and foot tapping. The long-term health problems for people with tardive dyskinesia are choking associated with loss of control of muscles used for swallowing and compromised respiratory function leading to infections and possibly respiratory alkalosis.

Because the movements resemble the dyskinetic movements of some patients who have idiopathic Parkinson's disease and who have received long-term treatment with L-DOPA (a direct-acting dopamine agonist that crosses

Table 22.3	EXTRAPYRAMIDAL SIDE EFFECTS OF ANTIPSYCHOTIC DRUGS	
Side Effect	Period of Onset	Symptoms
Acute Motor Abnormalities		
Parkinsonism or pseudoparkinsonism	5–30 d	Resting tremor, rigidity, bradykinesia or akinesia, masklike face, shuffling gait, decreased arm swing
Acute dystonia	1–5 d	Intermittent or fixed abnormal postures of the eyes, face, tongue, neck, trunk, and extremities
Akathisia	1–30 d	Obvious motor restlessness evidenced by pacing, rocking, shifting from foot to foot; subjective sense of not being able to sit or be still; these symptoms may occur together or separately
Late-Appearing Motor Abnormalities		
Tardive dyskinesia	Months to years	Abnormal dyskinetic movements of the face, mouth, and jaw; choreoathetoid movements of the legs, arms, and trunk
Tardive dystonia	Months to years	Persistent sustained abnormal postures in the face, eyes, tongue, neck, trunk, and limbs
Tardive akathisia	Months to years	Persisting, unabating sense of subjective and objective restlessness

Adapted from Casey, D. E. (1994). Schizophrenia: Psychopharmacology. In J. W. Jefferson & J. H. Greist (Eds.), *The Psychiatric Clinics of North America Annual of Drug Therapy* (Vol. 1, pp. 81–100). Philadelphia, PA: W. B. Saunders.

the blood–brain barrier), the suggested hypothesis for tardive dyskinesia includes the supersensitivity of the dopamine receptors in the basal ganglia.

There is no consistently effective treatment; however, antipsychotic drugs mask the movements of tardive dyskinesia and have periodically been suggested as a treatment. This is counterintuitive because these are the drugs that cause the disorder. Second-generation antipsychotic drugs, such as clozapine, may be less likely to cause the disorder. The best management remains prevention through using the lowest possible dose of antipsychotic drug over time that minimizes the symptoms of schizophrenia (see Table 22.3).

Monitoring Other Side Effects

Orthostatic hypotension is another side effect of antipsychotic drugs. Primarily an antiadrenergic effect, decreased blood pressure may be general or orthostatic. Patients may be protected from falls by teaching them to rise slowly and by monitoring blood pressure before giving the medication. The nurse should monitor and document lying, sitting, and standing blood pressures when any antipsychotic drug therapy begins.

Hyperprolactinemia can occur. When dopamine is blocked in the tuberoinfundibular tract, it can no longer repress prolactin, the neurohormone that regulates lactation and mammary function. The prolactin level increases and, in some individuals, side effects appear. Gynecomastia (enlarged breasts) can occur in people of both sexes and is understandably distressing to individuals who may be experiencing delusional or hallucinatory body image disturbances. Galactorrhea (lactation) also may occur. Menstrual irregularities and sexual dysfunction are also possible. If these symptoms appear, the medication

should be reduced or changed to another antipsychotic agent. Hyperprolactinemia is associated with the use of haloperidol and risperidone.

Sedation is another possible side effect of antipsychotic medication. Patients should be monitored for the sedating effects of antipsychotic agents. In elderly patients, sedation can be associated with falls.

Weight gain is related to antipsychotic agents, especially olanzapine and clozapine. Patients may gain as much as 20 or 30 pounds within 1 year. Increased appetite and weight gain are distressing to patients. Diet teaching and monitoring may have some effect. Another solution is to increase the accessibility of healthful, easy-to-prepare food.

New-onset diabetes should be assessed in patients taking antipsychotic drugs. There is an association between new-onset diabetes mellitus and the administration of second-generation antipsychotic agents, especially after weight gain. Patients should be monitored for clinical symptoms of diabetes. Fasting blood glucose tests are commonly ordered for these individuals.

Cardiac arrhythmias may also occur. Prolongation of the QTc interval is associated with torsades de pointes (polymorphic ventricular tachycardia) or ventricular fibrillation. The potential for drug-induced prolonged QT interval is associated with many drugs. Ziprasidone (Geodon) is more likely than other second-generation antipsychotics to prolong the QT interval and change the heart rhythm. For these patients, baseline electrocardiograms may be ordered. Nurses should observe these patients for cardiac arrhythmias.

Agranulocytosis is a reduction in the number of circulating granulocytes and decreased production of granulocytes in the bone marrow that limits one's ability to fight infection. Agranulocytosis can develop with the use of all antipsychotic drugs, but it is most likely to develop with clozapine use. Although laboratory values below 500 cells/mm³ are indicative of agranulocytosis, often granulocyte counts drop to below 200 cells/mm³ with this syndrome.

Patients taking clozapine should have regular blood tests. White blood cell and granulocyte counts should be measured before treatment is initiated and at least weekly or twice weekly after treatment begins. Initial white blood cell counts should be above 3,500 cells/mm³ before treatment initiation; in patients with counts of 3,500 and 5,000 cells/mm³, cell counts should be monitored three times a week if clozapine is prescribed. Any time the white blood cell count drops below 3,500 cells/mm³ or granulocytes drop below 1,500 cells/mm³, use of clozapine should be stopped, and the patient should be monitored for infection.

However, a faithfully implemented program of blood monitoring should not replace careful observation of the patient. It is not unusual for blood cell counts to drop precipitously in a period of 2 to 3 days. This may not be discovered when the patient is on a strict weekly blood monitoring schedule. Any reported symptoms that are suggestive of a bacterial infection (fever, pharyngitis, and weakness) should be cause for concern, and immediate evaluation of blood count status should be undertaken. Because patients are frequently discharged before the critical period of risk for agranulocytosis, patient education about these symptoms is also essential so that they will report these symptoms and obtain blood monitoring. In general, granulocytes return to normal within 2 to 4 weeks after discontinuation of use of the medication.

Preventing Drug–Drug Interactions

Several potential drug–drug interactions are possible when administering antipsychotic medications. One of the cytochrome P450 enzymes responsible for the metabolism of olanzapine and clozapine is 1A2. If either olanzapine or clozapine is given with another medication that inhibits this enzyme, such as fluvoxamine (Luvox), the antipsychotic blood level could increase and possibly become toxic. On the other hand, cigarette smoking can also induce 1A2 and lower concentration of drugs metabolized by this enzyme, such as olanzapine and clozapine. Smokers may require a higher dose of these medications than do nonsmokers (Stahl, 2013).

Several second-generation antipsychotic agents, including clozapine, quetiapine, and ziprasidone, are metabolized by the 3A4 enzyme. Weak inhibitors of this enzyme include the antidepressants fluvoxamine, nefazodone, and norfluoxetine (an active metabolite of fluoxetine). Potent inhibitors of 3A4 enzyme include ketoconazole (antifungal), protease inhibitors, and eryth-

romycin. If these drugs are given with clozapine, quetiapine, aripiprazole, or ziprasidone, the antipsychotic level will rise. In addition, the mood stabilizer carbamazepine (Tegretol) is a 3A4 inducer. When this drug is given with clozapine, quetiapine, or ziprasidone, the antipsychotic dose should be increased to compensate for the 3A4 induction. If the use of carbamazepine is discontinued, dosage of the antipsychotic agent needs to be adjusted (Stahl, 2013).

Risperidone, clozapine, aripiprazole, and olanzapine are substrates for the enzyme 2D6. Theoretically, antidepressants (fluoxetine and paroxetine) that inhibit this enzyme could increase levels of these antipsychotics. However, this is not usually clinically significant (Stahl, 2013).

Pharmacologic Interventions: Anticholinergics

Anticholinergics are administered for parkinsonism and dystonia secondary to antipsychotic medication (see Chapter 11). There is also potential for abuse of anticholinergic drugs. Some patients may find the anticholinergic effects of these drugs on mood, memory, and perception pleasurable. Although at toxic dosages, patients may experience disorientation and hallucinations, lesser doses may cause patients to experience greater sociability and euphoria.

Teaching Points

Nonadherence to the medication regimen is an important factor in relapse; the family must be made aware of the importance of the patient consistently taking medications. Medication education should cover the association between medications and the amelioration of symptoms, side effects and their management, and interpersonal skills that help the patient and family report medication effects.

Management of Complications

Neuroleptic Malignant Syndrome
Neuroleptic malignant syndrome (NMS) is a life-threatening condition that can develop in reaction to antipsychotic medications. Patients develop severe muscle rigidity with elevated temperature and a rapidly accelerating cascade of symptoms (occurring during the next 48 to 72 hours), which can include two or more of the following: hypertension, tachycardia, tachypnea, prominent diaphoresis, incontinence, mutism, leukocytosis, changes in level of consciousness ranging from confusion to coma, and laboratory evidence of muscle injury (e.g., elevated creatinine phosphokinase). The incidence of NMS has decreased recently from 3% to 0.02% probably because of an increased awareness of the symptoms and

earlier interventions such as stopping the offending medication (Margetic & Margetic, 2010). As many as one third of these patients may die as a result of the syndrome. NMS is probably underreported and may account for unexplained emergency department deaths of patients taking these drugs because their symptoms do not seem serious. The presenting symptom is a temperature greater than 99.5°F (usually between 101°F and 103°F) with no apparent cause.

The most important aspects of nursing care for patients with NMS relate to recognizing symptoms early, holding any antipsychotic (any dopamine-blocking agent) medications, and initiating supportive nursing care (Fig. 22.5). In any patient with fever, fluctuating vital signs, abrupt changes in levels of consciousness, or any of the symptoms presented in Box 22.10, NMS should be suspected. The nurse should be especially alert for early signs and symptoms of NMS in high-risk patients, such as those who are agitated, physically exhausted, or dehydrated or who have an existing medical or neurologic illness. Patients receiving parenteral or higher doses of neuroleptic drugs or lithium concurrently must also be carefully assessed. The nurse should carefully monitor fluid intake and fluid and electrolyte status.

> **NCLEXNOTE** Recognition of side effects, including movement disorders, tardive dyskinesia, and weight gain, should lead to interventions. NMS is a medical emergency.

Medical treatment includes administering dopamine agonist drugs, such as bromocriptine (modest success), and muscle relaxants, such as dantrolene or benzodiazepine. Antiparkinsonism drugs are not particularly useful. Some patients experience improvement with electroconvulsive therapy (ECT).

The nurse must frequently monitor vital signs of the patient with symptoms of NMS. In addition, it is important to check the results of the patient's laboratory tests for increased creatine phosphokinase, an elevated white blood cell count, elevated liver enzymes, or myoglobinuria. The nurse must be prepared to initiate supportive measures or anticipate emergency transfer of the patient to a medical–surgical or an intensive care unit.

Treating high temperature (which frequently exceeds 103°F) is an important priority for these patients. High body temperature may be reduced with a cooling blanket and acetaminophen. Because many of these patients experience diaphoresis, temperature elevation, or dysphagia, it

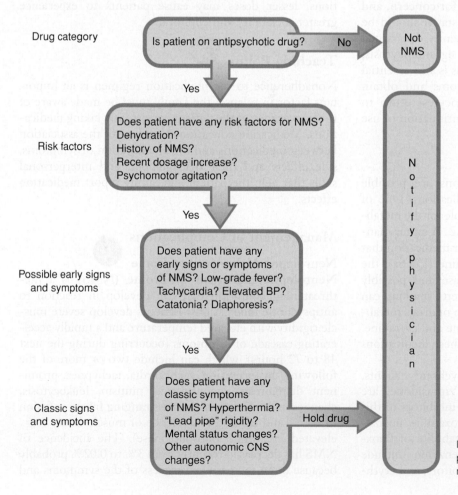

FIGURE 22.5 Action tree for "holding" an antipsychotic drug because of suspected neuroleptic malignant syndrome.

BOX 22.10

Recognizing Neuroleptic Malignant Syndrome

ONSET: 2 weeks after initiation of antipsychotic treatment or change in dose

RISK FACTORS: Male gender, pre-existing medical or neurologic disorders, depot administration, and high ambient temperature

IMMINENT INDICATORS
- Hyperthermia
- Muscle rigidity
- Change in mental status
- Tachycardia
- Hypertension or hypotension
- Tachypnea or hypoxia
- Diaphoresis or sialorrhea
- Tremor
- Incontinence
- Creatinine phosphokinase elevation or myoglobinuria
- Leukocytosis
- Metabolic acidosis

Sources: Agar, L. (2010). Recognizing neuroleptic malignant syndrome in the emergency department: A case study. *Perspectives in Psychiatric Care, 46*(2), 143–151.
Gillman, P. K. (2010). Neuroleptic malignant syndrome: Mechanisms, interactions, and causality. *Movement Disorders, 25*(12), 1780–1790.
Trollor, J. N., Chen, X., & Sachdev, P. S. (2009). Neuroleptic malignant syndrome associated with atypical antipsychotic drugs. *CNS Drugs, 23*(6), 477–492.

is important to monitor fluid hydration. Another important aspect of care for patients with NMS is safety. Joints and extremities that are rigid or spastic must be protected from injury. The treatment of these patients depends on the facility and availability of medical support services. In general, patients in psychiatric inpatient units that are separated from general hospitals are transferred to medical–surgical settings for treatment.

Anticholinergic Crisis

An anticholinergic crisis is a potentially life-threatening medical emergency caused by an overdose of or sensitivity to drugs with anticholinergic properties. This syndrome (also called anticholinergic delirium) may result from an accidental or intentional overdose of antimuscarinic drugs, including atropine, scopolamine, or belladonna alkaloids, which are present in numerous prescription drugs and over-the-counter medicines. The syndrome may also occur in psychiatric patients who are receiving therapeutic doses of anticholinergic drugs, especially when such agents are combined with other psychotropic drugs that produce anticholinergic side effects. Numerous drugs commonly prescribed in psychiatric settings, including tricyclic antidepressants and some antipsychotics, produce anticholinergic side effects. As a result of either drug overdose or sensitivity, these anticholinergic substances may produce an acute delirium or a psychotic reaction resembling schizophrenia.

More severe anticholinergic effects may occur in older patients, even at therapeutic levels (Stahl, 2013).

The signs and symptoms of anticholinergic crisis are dramatic and physically uncomfortable (Box 22.11). This disorder is characterized by elevated temperature; parched mouth; burning thirst; hot, dry skin; decreased salivation; decreased bronchial and nasal secretions; widely dilated eyes (bright light is painful); decreased ability to accommodate visually; increased heart rate; constipation; difficulty urinating; and hypertension or hypotension. The face, neck, and upper arms may become flushed because of a reflex blood vessel dilation. In addition to peripheral symptoms, patients with anticholinergic psychosis may experience neuropsychiatric symptoms of anxiety, agitation, delirium, hyperactivity, confusion, hallucinations (especially visual), speech difficulties, psychotic symptoms, or seizures. The acute psychotic reaction that is produced resembles schizophrenia. The classic description of anticholinergic crisis is summarized in the following mnemonic: "Hot as a hare, blind as a bat, mad as a hatter, dry as a bone."

In general, episodes of anticholinergic crisis are self-limiting, usually subsiding in 3 days. However, if untreated, the associated fever and delirium may progress to coma or cardiac and respiratory depression. Although rare, death is generally caused by hyperpyrexia and brain stem depression. After use of the offending drug is discontinued, improvement usually occurs within 24 to 36 hours.

A specific and effective antidote, physostigmine, an inhibitor of anticholinesterase, is frequently used for treating and diagnosing anticholinergic crisis. Administration of this drug rapidly reduces both the behavioral and physiologic symptoms. However, the usual adult dose of physostigmine is 1 to 2 mg intravenously given slowly during a period of 5 minutes because rapid injection of physostigmine may cause seizures, profound bradycardia, or heart block. Physostigmine is relatively short acting, so it may need to be given several times during the course of treatment. This drug provides relief from symptoms for a period of 2 to 3 hours. In addition to receiving physostigmine, patients

BOX 22.11

Signs and Symptoms of Anticholinergic Crisis

- **Neuropsychiatric signs:** confusion; recent memory loss; agitation; dysarthria; incoherent speech; pressured speech; delusions; ataxia; periods of hyperactivity alternating with somnolence, paranoia, anxiety, or coma
- **Hallucinations:** accompanied by "picking," plucking, or grasping motions; delusions; or disorientation
- **Physical signs:** nonreactive dilated pupils; blurred vision; hot, dry, flushed skin; facial flushing; dry mucous membranes; difficulty swallowing; fever; tachycardia; hypertension; decreased bowel sounds; urinary retention; nausea; vomiting; seizures; or coma

who intentionally overdose on large amounts of anticholinergic drugs are treated by gastric lavage, administration of charcoal, and catharsis. The dose may be repeated after 20 or 30 minutes.

It is important for the nurse to be alert for signs and symptoms of anticholinergic crisis, especially in elderly and pediatric patients, who are much more sensitive to the anticholinergic effects of drugs, and in patients who are receiving multiple medications with anticholinergic effects. If signs and symptoms of the syndrome occur, the nurse should discontinue use of the offending drug and notify the physician immediately.

Electroconvulsive Therapy

ECT is suggested as a possible alternative when the patient's schizophrenia is not being successfully treated by medication alone. For the most part, this is not indicated unless the patient is catatonic or has depression that is not treatable by other means. In general, ECT is not used often for the treatment of schizophrenia, but it may be useful for those persons who are medication resistant, assaultive, and psychotic (Kristensen, Brandt-Christensen, Ockelmann, & Jorgensen, 2012).

Psychological Domain

Although schizophrenia is a brain disorder, the psychological manifestations are the most difficult to assess and treat. Many of these psychological manifestations improve with the use of medications, but they are not necessarily eliminated.

Psychological Assessment

Several assessment scales have been developed to help evaluate positive and negative symptom clusters in schizophrenia. Box 22.12 lists standardized instruments used in assessing symptoms of patients with schizophrenia. These include the Scale for the Assessment of Positive Symptoms (SAPS) (Box 22.13), Scale for the Assessment of Negative Symptoms (SANS) (Box 22.14, p. 362), and Positive and Negative Syndrome Scale (PANSS) (Kay, Fiszbein, & Opler, 1987), which assesses both symptom clusters in the same instrument. Tools that list symptoms, such as the Brief Psychiatric Rating Scale (see Appendix A), SANS, or SAPS can also be used to help patients self-monitor their symptoms.

Usually, information about prediagnosis experiences requires retrospective reporting by the patient or the family. This reporting is reliable for the frankly psychotic symptoms of delusions and hallucinations; however, negative symptoms are more difficult to date. In fact, negative symptoms vary from a slight deviation from normal to a clear impairment. Negative symptoms probably occur earlier than positive symptoms but are less easily recognized (Box 22.15, p. 363).

BOX 22.12

Rating Scales for Use With Schizophrenia

SCALE FOR THE ASSESSMENT OF NEGATIVE SYMPTOMS (SANS)
Andreasen, N. C. (1984). Scale for the assessment of negative symptoms. SANS. Iowa: Dept of Psychiatry, College of Medicine, the University of Iowa. Copyright 1984. *See Box 22–14.*

SCALE FOR THE ASSESSMENT OF POSITIVE SYMPTOMS (SAPS)
Andreasen, N. C. (1981). Scale for the assessment of positive symptoms. SANS. Iowa: Dept of Psychiatry, College of Medicine, the University of Iowa. *See Box 22.13.*

POSITIVE AND NEGATIVE SYNDROME SCALE (PANSS)
Kay, S. R., Fiszbein, A., & Opler, L. A. (1987). The Positive and Negative Syndrome Scale (PANSS) for Schizophrenia. *Schizophrenia Bulletin, 13,* 261–276. Available from first author.

ABNORMAL INVOLUNTARY MOVEMENT SCALE (AIMS)
Guy, W. (1976). *ECDEU: Assessment manual for psychopharmacology* (DHEW Publication No. 76–338). Washington, DC: Department of Health, Education, and Welfare, Psychopharmacology Branch. *See Appendix B.*

BRIEF PSYCHIATRIC RATING SCALE (BPRS)
Overall, J. E., & Gorham, D. R. (1988). The Brief Psychiatric Rating Scale (BPRS): Recent developments in ascertainment and scaling. *Psychopharmacology Bulletin, 24,* 97–99. *See Appendix A.*

DYSKINESIA IDENTIFICATION SYSTEM: CONDENSED USER SCALE (DISCUS)
Sprague, R. L., & Kalachnik, J. E. (1991). Reliability, validity, and a total score cutoff for the Dyskinesia Identification Scale System: Condensed User Scale (DISCUS) with mentally ill and mentally retarded populations. *Psychopharmacology Bulletin, 27*(1), 51–58. See Box 22.5.

SIMPSON–ANGUS RATING SCALE
Simpson, G. M., & Angus, J. W. S. L. (1970). A rating scale for extrapyramidal side effects. *Acta Psychiatrica Scandinavica, 212*(suppl), 11–19. Copyright 1970. Munksgaard International Publishers, Ltd.

Responses to Mental Health Problems

Schizophrenia robs people of mental health and imposes social stigma. People with schizophrenia struggle to maintain control of their symptoms, which affect every aspect of their lives. The person with schizophrenia displays a variety of interrelated symptoms and experiences deficits in several areas. More than half of patients report the following prodromal symptoms (in order of frequency): tension and nervousness, lack of interest in eating, difficulty concentrating, disturbed sleep, decreased enjoyment and loss of interest, restlessness, forgetfulness, depression, social withdrawal from friends, feeling laughed at, more religious thinking, feeling bad for no reason, feeling too excited, and hearing voices or seeing things.

Because schizophrenia is a disorder of thoughts, perceptions, and behavior, it is sometimes not recognized as an illness by the person experiencing the symptoms. Many people with thought disorders do not believe that

BOX 22.13

Scale for the Assessment of Positive Symptoms (SAPS)

0 = None   1 = Questionable   2 = Mild   3 = Moderate
            4 = Marked   5 = Severe

HALLUCINATIONS

1 *Auditory Hallucinations*   0 1 2 3 4 5
   The patient reports voices, noises, or other sources that no
   one else hears.
2 *Voices Commenting*   0 1 2 3 4 5
   The patient reports a voice that makes a running commen-
   tary on his behavior or thoughts.
3 *Voices Conversing*   0 1 2 3 4 5
   The patient reports hearing two or more voices conversing.
4 *Somatic or Tactile Hallucinations*   0 1 2 3 4 5
   The patient reports experiencing peculiar physical sensations in the body.
5 *Olfactory Hallucinations*   0 1 2 3 4 5
   The patient reports experiencing unusual smells that no
   one else notices.
6 *Visual Hallucinations*   0 1 2 3 4 5
   The patient sees shapes or people that are not actually
   present.
7 *Global Rating of Hallucinations*   0 1 2 3 4 5
   This rating should be based on the duration and severity of
   the hallucinations and their effect on the patient's life.

DELUSIONS

8 *Persecutory Delusions*   0 1 2 3 4 5
   The patient believes he is being conspired against or perse-
   cuted in some way.
9 *Delusions of Jealousy*   0 1 2 3 4 5
   The patient believes his spouse is having an affair with
   someone.
10 *Delusions of Guilt or Sin*   0 1 2 3 4 5
   The patient believes that he has committed some terrible
   sin or done something unforgivable.
11 *Grandiose Delusions*   0 1 2 3 4 5
   The patient believes he has special powers or abilities.
12 *Religious Delusions*   0 1 2 3 4 5
   The patient is preoccupied with false beliefs of a religious
   nature.
13 *Somatic Delusions*   0 1 2 3 4 5
   The patient believes that somehow his body is diseased,
   abnormal, or changed.
14 *Delusions of Reference*   0 1 2 3 4 5
   The patient believes that insignificant remarks or events
   refer to him or have some special meaning.
15 *Delusions of Being Controlled*   0 1 2 3 4 5
   The patient feels that his feelings or actions are controlled
   by some outside force.
16 *Delusions of Mind Reading*   0 1 2 3 4 5
   The patient feels that people can read his mind or know
   his thoughts.
17 *Thought Broadcasting*   0 1 2 3 4 5
   The patient believes that his thoughts are broadcast so
   that he or others can hear them.
18 *Thought Insertion*   0 1 2 3 4 5
   The patient believes that thoughts that are not his own
   have been inserted into his mind.

19 *Thought Withdrawal*   0 1 2 3 4 5
   The patient believes that thoughts have been taken away
   from his mind.
20 *Global Rating of Delusions*   0 1 2 3 4 5
   This rating should be based on the duration and persistence
   of the delusions and their effects on the patient's life.

BIZARRE BEHAVIOR

21 *Clothing and Appearance*   0 1 2 3 4 5
   The patient dresses in an unusual manner or does other
   strange things to alter his appearance.
22 *Social and Sexual Behavior*   0 1 2 3 4 5
   The patient may do things considered inappropriate according to usual social norms (e.g., masturbating in public).
23 *Aggressive and Agitated Behavior*   0 1 2 3 4 5
   The patient may behave in an aggressive, agitated manner,
   often unpredictably.
24 *Repetitive or Stereotyped Behavior*   0 1 2 3 4 5
   The patient develops a set of repetitive actions or rituals
   that he must perform over and over.
25 *Global Rating of Bizarre Behavior*   0 1 2 3 4 5
   This rating should reflect the type of behavior and the
   extent to which it deviates from social norms.

POSITIVE FORMAL THOUGHT DISORDER

26 *Derailment*   0 1 2 3 4 5
   A pattern of speech in which ideas slip off track onto
   ideas obliquely related or unrelated.
27 *Tangentiality*   0 1 2 3 4 5
   Replying to a question in an oblique or irrelevant manner.
28 *Incoherence*   0 1 2 3 4 5
   A pattern of speech that is essentially incomprehensible at
   times.
29 *Illogicality*   0 1 2 3 4 5
   A pattern of speech in which conclusions are reached that
   do not follow logically.
30 *Circumstantiality*   0 1 2 3 4 5
   A pattern of speech that is very indirect and delayed in
   reaching its goal idea.
31 *Pressure of Speech*   0 1 2 3 4 5
   The patient's speech is rapid and difficult to interrupt; the
   amount of speech produced is greater than that considered normal.
32 *Distractible Speech*   0 1 2 3 4 5
   The patient is distracted by nearby stimuli that interrupt his
   flow of speech.
33 *Clanging*   0 1 2 3 4 5
   A pattern of speech in which sounds rather than meaningful relationships govern word choice.
34 *Global Rating of Positive Formal
   Thought Disorder*   0 1 2 3 4 5
   This rating should reflect the frequency of abnormality and
   degree to which it affects the patient's ability to communicate.

INAPPROPRIATE AFFECT

35 *Inappropriate Affect*   0 1 2 3 4 5
   The patient's affect is inappropriate or incongruous, not
   simply flat or blunted.

From Nancy C. Andreasen, MD, PhD, Department of Psychiatry, College of Medicine. The University of Iowa, Iowa City, IA 52242. Copyright 1984 Nancy C. Andreasen. Reprinted with permission.

BOX 22.14

Scale for the Assessment of Negative Symptoms (SANS)

0 = None   1 = Questionable   2 = Mild   3 = Moderate
           4 = Marked   5 = Severe

AFFECTIVE FLATTENING OR BLUNTING

1 *Unchanging Facial Expression*   0 1 2 3 4 5
The patient's face appears wooden, changes less than expected as emotional content of discourse changes.

2 *Decreased Spontaneous Movements*   0 1 2 3 4 5
The patient shows few or no spontaneous movements, does not shift position, move extremities, etc.

3 *Paucity of Expressive Gestures*   0 1 2 3 4 5
The patient does not use hand gestures, body position, etc., as an aid to expressing ideas.

4 *Poor Eye Contact*   0 1 2 3 4 5
The patient avoids eye contact or "stares through" interviewer even when speaking.

5 *Affective Nonresponsivity*   0 1 2 3 4 5
The patient fails to smile or laugh when prompted.

6 *Lack of Vocal Inflections*   0 1 2 3 4 5
The patient fails to show normal vocal emphasis patterns, is often monotonic.

7 *Global Rating of Affective Flattening*   0 1 2 3 4 5
This rating should focus on overall severity of symptoms, especially unresponsiveness, eye contact, facial expression, and vocal inflections.

ALOGIA

8 *Poverty of Speech*   0 1 2 3 4 5
The patient's replies to questions are restricted in amount; tend to be brief, concrete, and unelaborated.

9 *Poverty of Content of Speech*   0 1 2 3 4 5
The patient's replies are adequate in amount but tend to be vague, overconcrete, or overgeneralized, and convey little information.

10 *Blocking*   0 1 2 3 4 5
The patient indicates, either spontaneously or with prompting, that his train of thought was interrupted.

11 *Increased Latency of Response*   0 1 2 3 4 5
The patient takes a long time to reply to questions; prompting indicates that the patient is aware of the question.

12 *Global Rating of Alogia*   0 1 2 3 4 5
The core features of alogia are poverty of speech and poverty of content.

AVOLITION—APATHY

13 *Grooming and Hygiene*   0 1 2 3 4 5
The patient's clothes may be sloppy or soiled, and patient may have greasy hair, body odor, etc.

14 *Impersistence at Work or School*   0 1 2 3 4 5
The patient has difficulty seeking or maintaining employment, completing school work, keeping house, etc. If an inpatient, cannot persist at ward activities, such as OT, playing cards, etc.

15 *Physical Anergia*   0 1 2 3 4 5
The patient tends to be physically inert. May sit for hours and does not initiate spontaneous activity.

16 *Global Rating of Avolition—Apathy*   0 1 2 3 4 5
Strong weight may be given to one or two prominent symptoms if particularly striking.

ANHEDONIA—ASOCIALITY

17 *Recreational Interests and Activities*   0 1 2 3 4 5
The patient may have few or no interests. Both the quality and quantity of interests should be taken into account.

18 *Sexual Activity*   0 1 2 3 4 5
The patient may show a decrease in sexual interest and activity, or enjoyment when active.

19 *Ability to Feel Intimacy and Closeness*   0 1 2 3 4 5
The patient may display an inability to form close or intimate relationships, especially with the opposite sex and family.

20 *Relationships With Friends and Peers*   0 1 2 3 4 5
The patient may have few or no friends and may prefer to spend all of time isolated.

21 *Global Rating of Anhedonia–Asociality*   0 1 2 3 4 5
This rating should reflect overall severity, taking into account the patient's age, family status, etc.

ATTENTION

22 *Social Inattentiveness*   0 1 2 3 4 5
The patient appears uninvolved or unengaged. May seem "spacey."

23 *Inattentiveness During Mental Status Testing*   0 1 2 3 4 5
Tests of "serial 7's" (at least five subtractions) and spelling "world" backward: Score: 2 = 1 error; 3 = 2 errors; 4 = 3 errors.

24 *Global Rating of Attention*   0 1 2 3 4 5
This rating should assess the patient's overall concentration, clinically and on tests.

From Nancy C. Andreasen, MD, PhD, Department of Psychiatry, College of Medicine, The University of Iowa, Iowa City, IA 52242. Copyright 1984 Nancy C. Andreasen. Reprinted with permission.

---

they have a mental illness. Their denial of mental illness and the need for treatment poses problems for the family and clinicians. Ideally, in lucid moments, patients recognize that their thoughts are really delusions, that their perceptions are hallucinations, and that their behavior is disorganized. In reality, many patients do not believe that they have a mental illness but agree to treatment to please family and clinicians.

Mental Status and Appearance

The patient may look eccentric or disheveled or have poor hygiene and bizarre dress. The patient's posture may suggest lethargy or stupor.

Mood and Affect

Patients with schizophrenia often display altered mood states. In some cases, they may show heightened emotional activity; others may display severely limited emotional responses. Affect, the outward expression of mood, is categorized on a continuum: flat (emotional expression entirely absent), blunted (expression of emotions present but greatly diminished), and full range. Inappropriate affect is marked by incongruence between the emotional expression and the thoughts expressed. Other common emotional symptoms include the following:

- **Affective lability**—abrupt, dramatic, unprovoked changes in type of emotions expressed

are those not sanctioned or held by a cultural or religious subgroup.

BOX 22.15

Understanding a Son's Symptoms of Schizophrenia

Dr. Willick (1994) described his reactions and observations of his son diagnosed with schizophrenia:

"... Struggling as he does with many of what we now call the 'negative symptoms,' he has lost that gleam in his eye, that joyous good humor, that zest for life which he once showed. Today, it is hard for him to feel things strongly, or to enjoy his music, sports, or being with his family. . . . There has also been a significant cognitive impairment. Things that he was easily able to grasp when he was 14 years old are now much harder for him. He has lost considerable capacity for abstract thinking. His language is very concrete and has lost the richness and subtlety of expression it once had. He has a hard time following a moderately complicated plot of an article he reads or a movie he sees, and he can describe it only in a superficial and concrete way (pp. 8–9).

"I know that I should be most proud of Gary, and I can often feel that. The problem is that it is not easy to see that he is displaying great courage in coping with what has happened to him. The symptoms of the illness make him appear lacking in motivation, initiative, and will, and even he accuses himself of not trying hard enough. It is hard for an observer to see how difficult it must be for him to get up every day, hoping to feel different, only to awake with the same feeling of anhedonia. In some ways, those admirable qualities that he possessed before he became ill are no doubt serving him well as he tries to fight an illness that none of us, let alone Gary himself, can really comprehend" (pp. 11–12).

From Willick, M. S. (1994). Schizophrenia: A parent's perspective—mourning without end. In N.C. Andreasen (Ed.), *Schizophrenia: From mind to molecule* (pp. 5–19). Washington, DC: American Psychiatric Press.

- **Ambivalence**—the presence and expression of two opposing feelings, leading to inaction
- **Apathy**—reactions to stimuli are decreased; diminished interest and desire

Speech

Speech patterns may reflect obsessions, delusions, pressured thinking, loose associations, or flight of ideas and neologisms. Speech is an indicator of thought content and other mental processes and is usually altered. An assessment of speech should note any difficulty articulating words (dysarthria) and difficulty swallowing (dysphagia) as indicators of medication side effects. In many instances, what an individual says is as important as how it is said. Both content and speech patterns should be noted.

Thought Processes and Delusions

Delusions can be distinguished from strongly held ideas by the person continuing to hold the belief in spite of contradictory evidence (APA, 2013). Culture must be considered when evaluating delusions. Delusional beliefs

It can often be difficult to distinguish between bizarre and nonbizarre delusions. Nonbizarre delusions generally have themes of jealousy and persecution and are derived from ordinary life experiences. Examples include a woman believes that her husband, from whom she has recently separated, is trying to poison her or a man believes that members of the Mafia are trying to kill him because, when he was in high school, he reported to the principal that several of his classmates were selling drugs at school (APA, 2013).

Bizarre delusions are those that are impossible, illogical, and not derived from ordinary life experiences. Bizarre delusions often include delusions of control (that some outside force controls thoughts and actions), thought broadcasting (that others can read or hear one's thoughts), thought insertion (that someone has placed thoughts into one's mind), and thought withdrawal (that someone is removing thoughts from one's mind) (APA, 2013). For example, a patient who has been with a hypnotist for 2 months reports that the hypnotist continued to read his mind and was "picking his brain away piece by piece." Another patient was convinced that a computer chip was placed in her vagina during a gynecologic examination and that this somehow directly influenced her physical movements and her thoughts.

Assessing and judging the content of the delusion and exploring other aspects of the delusional experience are helpful in understanding the significance of these false beliefs. The underlying feeling that accompanies the delusion should be identified. Other aspects to consider include the conviction with which the delusion is held; the extent other aspects of the individual's life are incorporated or affected by the delusion; the degree of internal consistency, organization, and logic evidenced in the delusion; and evaluating the amount of pressure (in terms of preoccupation and concern) individuals feel in their lives as a result of the delusion (Box 22.16).

Hallucinations

Hallucinations are the most common example of disturbed sensory perception observed in patients with schizophrenia. Hallucinations can be experienced in all sensory modalities; however, auditory hallucinations are the most common in schizophrenia. Some specific hallucinations may be sufficient to diagnose schizophrenia, such as hearing voices conversing with each other or carrying on a discussion with someone who is not there. Because most individuals will not spontaneously share their hallucinatory experiences with an interviewer, the nurse may need to rely on indirect evidence in the patient's behavior, such

BOX 22.16 • THERAPEUTIC DIALOGUE • The Patient With Delusions

John joined the nurse in a game of pool. The following conversation occurred as they played.

INEFFECTIVE APPROACH

John: The CIA put a transmitter in my molar, here (points to his right cheek).

Nurse: No one would put a transmitter in your tooth; come on, the CIA isn't looking for you.

John: Yeah, they want to monitor me while I'm here. I know that they have the real Jenna Bush here in the hospital. They are trying to get George Bush to intervene with the Michigan Militia. Mark from Michigan told me that.

Nurse: Jenna Bush can't possibly be here; I saw her on television this morning.

John: Maybe—she does have darker hair and has different colored contacts to disguise her eyes, but they're just trying to keep people from knowing what they're doing.

Nurse: John, Jenna Bush isn't in the hospital; if she were, I would know it because I work here.

John: (With anger) You don't know anything! You are probably from the CIA also. I have nothing else to say to you.

EFFECTIVE APPROACH

John: The CIA put a transmitter in my molar, here (points to his right cheek).

Nurse: Oh. Which balls are mine?

John: You get the striped ones. Yeah, they want to monitor me while I'm here. I know that they have the real Jenna Bush here in the hospital. They are trying to get George Bush to intervene with the Michigan Militia. Mark from Michigan told me that.

Nurse: I suppose it could be Jenna Bush, but do you suppose that it could just be someone who looks like her?

John: Maybe—she does have darker hair and has different colored contacts to disguise her eyes. But they're just trying to keep people from knowing what they're doing.

Nurse: You sound a little overwhelmed with all the information you have.

John: No, no. I can handle it. The CIA can't do anything to me. I'll never talk.

Nurse: I thought they could hear you when you talk to me.

John: Huh? Oh, that transmitter is so that they can send me misinformation. They send a tower of babble to my brain. They are trying to confuse me so that I stay away from Jenna Bush. They all think they can keep me from my mission.

Nurse: Who're they?

John: Everyone in the government. The CIA, FBI, ATF, IRS—all those alphabets.

Nurse: So everyone in the government is trying to get to you?

John: Well, maybe not everybody. Just the ones that care about money and the militia. I don't think they care about me much in Commerce or Health and Human Services. Although they'd care too if they knew.

Nurse: I would think that's pretty frightening to have all these people out looking for you. You must be scared a lot.

John: It's scary, but I can handle it. I've handled it all my life.

Nurse: You've been in scary situations all your life?

John: Yeah. I don't know. Maybe not scary, just hard. I never seemed to be able to do as well as my parents wanted—or as I wanted.

CRITICAL THINKING CHALLENGE

• How did the nurse's argumentative responses cause the patient to react in the first scenario?

• What effective communication techniques did the nurse use in the second scenario?

---

as (1) pauses during conversations in which the individual seems preoccupied or appears to be listening to someone other than the interviewer, (2) looking toward the perceived source of a voice, or (3) responding to the voices in some manner. Although patients may not spontaneously share their hallucinations, many validate observations of the examiner or admit to a history of hallucinations when asked (Box 22.17).

Disorganized Communication

The other aspect of thought content and processes that may be altered in schizophrenia is the organization of expressed thoughts. Impaired verbal fluency (ability to produce spontaneous speech) is commonly present. Abrupt shifts in the focus of conversation are a typical symptom of disorganized thinking. The most

BOX 22.17 • THERAPEUTIC DIALOGUE • The Patient With Hallucinations

The following conversation took place in a dayroom with several staff in the room. The patient was potentially very violent. Although it is a good example of dealing with someone who is hallucinating, it is not a situation that should be taken lightly. Always make certain that you have a means to leave a situation (i.e., that you are not in the corner of a room), that the patient does not have a potential weapon, and that you have sufficient staff close by so that you are safe.

Jason approached the nurse and asked to play pool. The nurse debated about playing but chose to play because Jason appeared distracted, and the game might give him something to focus on.

INEFFECTIVE APPROACH

Nurse: Shall I break?

Jason: (Had been looking off to his right but turns and looks directly at the nurse.) Yeah, go ahead. (Looks at the table briefly and then turns to look out the door and down the hallway.)

Nurse: (Breaking the pool balls without putting any in a pocket.) It's your turn. You can hit any that you'd like.

Jason: (Turning back to the table.) Huh? (Shaking his head as he stared at the table.) What?

Nurse: You know, Jason, you really should pay attention.

Jason: (Hits a ball in and moves to the other side of the table. Stops in line with the next shot but doesn't bend down to take aim. Stands very still and then shakes his head slightly and quickly. Leans down to take aim and then stands up again.)

Nurse: Jason. (Looks at nurse.) Jason! Are you going to play or not? I don't have all day.

Jason: Oh yeah. (Leans down, takes aim, and misses.)

Nurse: (Moves to where the next shot is. Position is near where Jason is standing. Nurse watches him carefully, moving closer to him.) Please move over, Jason.

Jason: No. (Doesn't move. In peripheral vision, nurse sees Jason's lips move, and he again looks to his right and shakes his head in a staccato motion, as if trying to shake something out of his head.)

EFFECTIVE APPROACH

Nurse: Shall I break?

Jason: (Had been looking off to his right but turns and looks directly at the nurse.) Yeah, go ahead. (Looks at the table briefly and then turns to look out the door and down the hallway.)

Nurse: (Breaking the pool balls without putting any in a pocket.) Your turn; you can hit any that you'd like.

Jason: (Turning back to the table.) Huh? (Shakes his head as he stares at the table.) What?

Nurse: You can hit any ball you like. I didn't get any.

Jason: (Hits a ball in and moves to the other side of the table. Stops in line with the next shot but doesn't bend down to take aim. Stands very still and then shakes his head slightly and quickly. Leans down to take aim and then stands up again.)

Nurse: Jason. (He looks at the nurse.) Are you aiming at the 10th ball?

Jason: Oh yeah. (Leans down, takes aim, and misses.)

Nurse: (Moving to where her next shot is. The position is very close to where Jason is standing. The nurse watches him carefully while moving closer to him.) Here, let me take this shot.

Jason: Oh. (Moves back. In peripheral vision, nurse sees Jason's lips move, and again he looks to his right and shakes his head in a staccato motion as if trying to shake something out of his head.)

Nurse: I missed again. (Moves away from table and turns to Jason, who moves up to the table. He leans down and then stands up again. His lips move again as he turns his head to the right and then looks over his back toward the doorway.) Jason. Jason. (He looks at the nurse.) You have the striped ones.

Jason: (Nods and leans down to take a shot, which he makes. He then misses the next shot. He stands up and moves back from the table, again looking back toward the doorway. He shakes his head.) No!

Nurse: (Watches him closely and moves to the opposite side of the table, making the next shot. Lining up the next shot, Jason leans the pool cue against the table, looks past the nurse, and turns and walks away toward the door. He looks down the hallway, takes a few steps, stops for a minute or so, turns back into the room, and again looks past the nurse. He sits down and shakes his head again. He holds his head in his hands with his hands covering his ears. The nurse picks up his pool cue and places both against the wall out of the way. The nurse sits next to another staff member at a vantage point from which Jason can still be watched.)

CRITICAL THINKING CHALLENGE

• How did the nurse's impatience translate into Jason's behavior in the first scenario?

• What effective communicating techniques did the nurse use in the second scenario?

severe shifts in focus may occur after only one or two words (word salad), after one or two phrases or sentences (flight of ideas or loose associations), or somewhat less severely as a shift that occurs when a new topic is repeatedly suggested and pursued from the current topic (tangentiality).

Cognitive Impairments

Although cognitive impairments in schizophrenia vary widely from patient to patient, several primary problems have been identified:

- Attention may be increased and sustained on external stimuli over a period of time (hypervigilance).
- The ability to distinguish and focus on relevant stimuli may be diminished.
- Familiar cues may go unrecognized or be improperly encoded.
- Information processing may be diminished, leading to inappropriate or illogical conclusions from available observations and information (Baker et al., 2014; Lepage, Bodmar, & Bowie, 2014).

Cognitive impairments are not easy to recognize. By relying only on clinical assessment, the nurse can miss the extent of the impairment. Using a standardized instrument can provide a screening measurement of cognitive function (see Chapter 10). If impairment exists, neuropsychological testing by a qualified psychologist may be necessary.

Memory and Orientation

Impairments in orientation, memory, and abstract thinking may be observed. Orientation to time, place, and person may remain relatively intact unless the patient is particularly preoccupied with delusions and hallucinations. Although all aspects of memory may be affected in schizophrenia, registration or the recall within seconds of newly learned information may be particularly diminished. This affects the individual's short- and long-term memory. The ability to engage in abstract thinking may be impaired.

Insight and Judgment

Individuals display insight when they display evidence of knowing their own thoughts, the reality of external objects, and their relationship to these. Judgment is the ability to decide or act about a situation. Insight and judgment are closely related to each other and depend on cognitive functions that are frequently impaired in people with schizophrenia.

Behavioral Responses

During periods of psychosis, unusual or bizarre behavior often occurs. These behaviors can usually be understood within the context of the patient's disturbed thinking. The nurse needs to understand the significance of the behavior to the individual. One patient moved the family furniture into the yard because he thought that evil spirits were hiding in the furniture. His bizarre behavior was an attempt to protect his family. Another patient painted a sequence of numbers on his bedroom walls. He said that the numbers were the language of the angels. His delusional thoughts were at the basis of his behavior.

Because of the negative symptoms, specifically, avolition, patients may not seem interested or organized to complete normal daily activities. They may stay in bed most of the day or refuse to take a shower. Many times, they agree to get up in the morning and go to work, but they never get around to it. Several specific behaviors are associated with schizophrenia, including stereotypy (idiosyncratic repetitive, purposeless movements), echopraxia (involuntary imitation of others' movements), and waxy flexibility (posture held in odd or unusual fixed positions for extended periods). In some cases, certain behaviors need to be evaluated carefully to distinguish them from movements that are associated with medication side effects, such as grimacing, stereotypical behavior, or agitation.

Self-Concept

In schizophrenia, self-concept is usually poor. Patients often are aware that they are hearing voices others do not hear. They recognize that they are different from others and are often scared of "going crazy." Many are aware of the loss of expectations for their future achievements. The pervasive stigma associated with having a mental illness contributes to the poor self-concept. Body image can be disturbed, especially during periods of hallucinations or delusions. One patient believed that her body was infected with germs, and she could feel them eating away her insides.

Stress and Coping Patterns

Stressful events are often linked to psychiatric symptoms (see Chapter 18 for a discussion of the diathesis–stress model). It is important to determine stresses from the patient's perspective because a stressful event for one may not be stressful for another (see Chapter 18). It is also important to determine typical coping patterns, especially negative coping strategies, such as the use of substances or aggressive behavior.

Risk Assessment

Because of high suicide and attempted suicide rates among patients with schizophrenia, the nurse needs to assess the patient's risk for self-injury: Does the patient speak of suicide, have delusional thinking that could lead to dangerous behavior, or have command hallucinations telling him or her to harm self or others? Does the patient have homicidal ideations? Does the patient lack social support and the skills to be meaningfully engaged with other people or a vocation? Substance-related disorders are also common among patients with schizophrenia, and nurses should assess for substance abuse.

Nursing Diagnoses for Psychological Domain

Many nursing diagnoses can be generated from data collected assessing the psychological domain. Disturbed thought processes can be used for delusions, confusion, and disorganized thinking (Fig. 22.6). Disturbed Sensory Perception is appropriate for hallucinations or illusions. Other examples of diagnoses include Chronic Low Self-esteem, Personal Identity Disturbance, Risk for Violence, Ineffective Coping, and Knowledge Deficit.

Interventions for Psychological Domain

All of the psychological interventions, such as counseling, conflict resolution, behavior therapy, and cognitive interventions, are appropriate for patients with schizophrenia. The following discussion focuses on applying these interventions.

Developing the Nurse–Patient Relationship

The development of the nurse–patient relationship with patients with schizophrenia centers on developing trust, accepting the person as a worthy human being, and infusing the relationship with hope. People with schizophrenia are often reluctant to engage in any relationship because of previous rejection and, in some instances, an underlying suspiciousness that is a part of the illness. If they are having hallucinations, their images of other people may be distorted and frightening. They are struggling to trust their own thoughts and perceptions, and engaging in an interaction with another human being may prove too overwhelming.

The nurse should approach the patient in a calm and caring manner. Engaging the patient in a relationship may take time. Short, time-limited interactions are best for a patient who is experiencing psychosis. Being consistent in

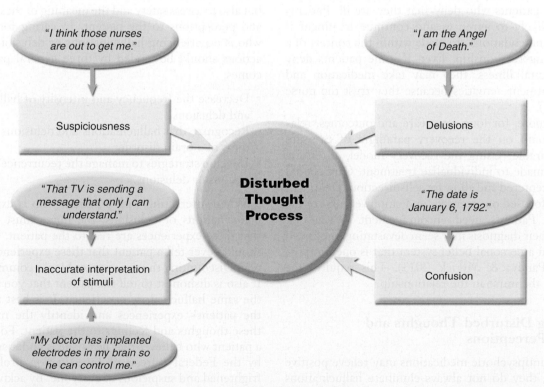

FIGURE 22.6 Nursing diagnosis concept map: Disturbed Thought Process.

BOX 22.18

A Brother's Perspective

A sibling describes his brother with schizophrenia and the importance of both medications and relationships.

In 1998, at the age of 40 years, Robert was admitted to a psychiatric hospital. His brother was told at the time that he would never be able to live independently, and even if discharged, would only be repeatedly hospitalized. Robert had a long history of treatment and in 1998 had received all types of antipsychotic medications, but he had not received any of the "new atypical variety." He was prescribed one of these drugs, and within months, the staff who had predicted the most discouraging of outcomes told Robert's brother that he was in the midst of a miraculous recovery—his thinking was clear and free of delusions and they were preparing Robert's discharge.

A few weeks into the discharge planning, Robert called his brother distressed because his social worker, whom Robert had known for years from a prior hospitalization, was leaving. The social worker had been abruptly transferred to another hospital. Robert deteriorated rapidly into tantrums, hallucinations, and dangerous behaviors. His discharge was put on hold. Robert's brother's rhetorical question was, "What was the difference between Robert on the same medication on Monday, when he was alright, and Tuesday, when he no longer was?" His answer for Robert was the loss of an important relationship.

Robert is now living in a community-based home where the dedicated staff members have shown that they can keep rehospitalization rates below 3%.

Robert's brother has interviewed many former psychiatric patients for a book. He found that every one of his interviewees, while attributing their recovery to medications or finding God or a particular program, also identified an important relationship with one human being who believed in their ability to recover. Most of the time, this person was a professional such as a social worker, a nurse, or a doctor. Sometimes it was a clergy or family member. A believing relationship....

Robert's brother concluded, "Let's provide a range of medications, and let's study their effectiveness, but let's remember that the pill is the ultimate downsizing. Let's find resources to give people afflicted with mental illness what all of us need: fellow human beings upon whom we can depend to help us through our dark times and, once through, to emerge into gloriously imperfect lives."

For nurses, it is important to remember that it is not what we do to people, but rather, what we do with people: give hope, listen to their dreams, help them find ways to get as close as they can.

Adapted from Neugeboren, J. (2006). Meds alone couldn't bring Robert back. *Newsweek*. Retrieved June 17, 2014, from www.power/article/recovery/meds.html

---

interactions and following through on promises will help establish trust within the relationship.

Establishing a therapeutic relationship is crucial, especially with patients who deny that they are ill. Patients are more likely to agree to and continue treatment if these recommendations are made within the context of a safe, trusting relationship. Even if some patients deny having mental illness, they may take medication and attend treatment activities because they trust the nurse (Box 22.18).

Furthermore, for long-term care and outcomes, relationships built on the recovery paradigm of care are highly desirable. Using the recovery model, all efforts should be made to individualize treatment. Care should be person centered and allow for self-direction. Treatment should be focused on strengths and empowerment of the individual. Patients need encouragement to see that although their diagnosis may seem devastating, they need to maintain a personal belief system that is open to possibilities (Pandya & Myrick, 2013). This requires the same from the nurse in the relationship.

Managing Disturbed Thoughts and Sensory Perceptions

Although antipsychotic medications may relieve positive symptoms, they do not always eliminate hallucinations and delusions. The nurse must continue helping the patient develop creative strategies for dealing with these sensory and thought disturbances. Information about the content of the hallucinations and delusions is needed, not only to determine whether the medications are effective but also to assess safety and the meaning of these thoughts and perceptions to the patient. In caring for a patient who is experiencing hallucinations or delusions, nursing actions should be guided by three general patient outcomes:

- Decrease the frequency and intensity of hallucinations and delusions.
- Recognize that hallucinations and delusions are symptoms of a brain disorder.
- Develop strategies to manage the recurrence of hallucinations or delusions.

When interacting with a patient who is experiencing hallucinations or delusions, the nurse must remember that these experiences are real to the patient. The nurse should never tell a patient that these experiences are not real. Discounting the experiences blocks communication. It also is dishonest to tell the patient that you are having the same hallucinatory experience. It is best to validate the patient's experiences and identify the meaning of these thoughts and feelings to the patient. For example, a patient who believes that he or she is under surveillance by the Federal Bureau of Investigation probably feels frightened and suspicious of everyone. By acknowledging how frightening it must be to always feel like you are being watched, the nurse focuses on the feelings that are

Using Reflection

DELUSIONAL THINKING

INCIDENT • A patient was convinced that he married a famous movie star.

REFLECTION • At first the nurse discounted the delusion as being trivial and insignificant. Upon further analysis, the nurse realized that by being married to a famous person, the patient would also believe that he was an important, special person. The nurse developed a new perspective of the patient, who was probably suffering from low self-esteem.

generated by the delusion, not the delusion itself. The nurse can then offer to help the patient feel safe within this environment. The patient, in turn, begins to feel that someone understands him or her (Box 22.19).

Teaching About Symptoms

Teaching patients that hallucinations and delusions are part of the disorder becomes easier after the medication begins working. When patients believe and acknowledge that they have a mental illness and that some of their thoughts are delusions and some of their perceptions are hallucinations, they can develop strategies to manage their symptoms.

Patients benefit greatly by learning recovery strategies of self-regulation, symptom monitoring, and relapse prevention. By monitoring events, time, place, and stimuli surrounding the appearance of symptoms, the patient can begin to predict high-risk times for symptom recurrence. Cognitive behavioral therapy is often used in helping patients monitor and identify their emerging symptoms to prevent relapse (Mueser, Deavers, Penn, & Cassisi, 2013).

Another important nursing intervention is to help the patient identify to whom and where to talk about delusional or hallucinatory material. Because self-disclosure of these symptoms immediately labels someone as having a mental illness, patients should be encouraged to evaluate the environment for negative consequences of disclosing these symptoms. For example, it may be fine to talk about it at home but not at the grocery store.

Enhancing Cognitive Functioning

After identifying deficits in cognitive functioning, the nurse and patient can develop interventions that target specific deficits. The most effective interventions usually involve the whole treatment team. If the ability to focus or attend is an issue, patients can be encouraged to select activities that improve attention, such as computer games.

For memory problems, patients can be encouraged to make lists and to write down important information.

Executive functioning problems are the most challenging for these patients. Patients who cannot manage daily problems may have planning and problem-solving impairments. For these patients, developing interventions that closely simulate real-world problems may help. Through coaching, the nurse can teach and support the development of problem-solving skills. For example, during hospitalizations, patients are given medications and reminded to take them on time. They are often instructed in a classroom setting but rarely have an opportunity to practice self-medication and figure out what to do if their prescription expires, the medications are lost, or they forget their medications. Yet, when discharged, patients are expected to take medication at the prescribed dose at the prescribed time. Interventions designed to have patients actively engage in problem-solving behavior with real problems are needed (Box 22.20).

Other approaches to helping patients solve problems and learn new strategies for dealing with problems include solution-focused therapy, which focuses on the strengths and positive attributes that exist within each person, and cognitive behavioral therapy (Mueser et al., 2013), which focuses directly on collaboratively determined symptoms and strategies to address them. These therapies involve years of training to master, but certain techniques can be used. For example, the nurse can ask patients to identify the most important problem from

BOX 22.20
Research for Best Practice: Telenursing Interventions

Beebe, L. H., Smith, K., Crye, D., Addonizio, C., Strunk, D. J., Martin, W., & Poche, J. (2008). Telenursing interventions increases psychiatric medication adherence in schizophrenia outpatients. Journal of the American Psychiatric Nurses Association, 14(3), 217–224.

THE QUESTION: Will outpatients who participate in telephone intervention problem solving for outpatients with schizophrenia (TIPS) have significantly higher objective adherence than those who receive care as usual?

METHODS: This experimental study evaluated the effectiveness of TIPS in improving medication adherence in 25 outpatients with schizophrenia randomly assigned to an experimental group (13) and a control group (12) during a 3-month period. Medication adherence was measured by pill count and record review. TIPS is a weekly telephone nursing intervention that fosters problem solving, offers coping alternatives, provides reminders to use alternatives, and assesses the effectiveness of coping efforts.

FINDINGS: The group participating in TIPS had improved adherence to psychiatric medications.

IMPLICATIONS FOR NURSING: Telenursing appears to be an effective intervention that improves adherence to medication and other treatment requirements. More research is needed.

their perspective. This focuses the patient on an important issue for him or her.

Using Behavioral Interventions

Behavioral interventions can be very effective in helping patients improve motivation and organize routine, daily activities, such as maintaining a regular schedule and completing activities. Reinforcement of positive behaviors (getting up on time, completing hygiene, going to treatment activities) can easily be included in a treatment plan. In the hospital, patients gain unit privileges by following an agreed-on treatment plan. A social learning intervention called a token economy, which is built on positive reinforcement principles, has a large supportive base of evidence for its success (McDonnell et al., 2013). Unfortunately, behavioral interventions have fallen out of favor because of practitioner attitudes and some problematic past implementations. Their use should be reconsidered.

Teaching How to Cope With Stress

Developing skills to cope with personal, social, and environmental stresses is important to everyone but particularly to those with a severe mental illness. Stresses can easily trigger symptoms that patients are trying to avoid. Establishing regular counseling sessions to support the development of positive coping skills is helpful for both hospitalized patients and those living in the community.

Providing Patient Education

Cognitive deficits (difficulty in processing complex information, maintaining steady focus of attention, distinguishing between relevant and irrelevant stimuli, and forming abstractions), may challenge the nurse planning educational activities. Evidence indicates that people with schizophrenia may learn best in an errorless learning environment (Leshner, Tom, & Kern, 2013). That is, they are directly given correct information and then encouraged to write it down. Errorless learning is an educational intervention based on the principle of operant conditioning that learning is stronger and more likely to last if it occurs in the absence of errors. Asking questions that encourage guessing is not as effective in helping them retain information. Trial-and-error learning is avoided.

Teaching and explaining should occur in an environment with minimal distractions. Terminology should be clear and unambiguous. Visual aids can supplement verbal information, but these materials should have simple information stated in simple language. The nurse takes care not to overcrowd the visual material or incorporate images that draw attention away from important content. Teaching should occur in small segments with fre-

quent reinforcement. Most important of all, teaching should occur when the patient is ready. Regular assessments of cognitive abilities with standardized instruments can help determine this readiness. These suggestions can be adapted for teaching during any phase of the illness.

Skill-training interventions should be designed to compensate for cognitive deficits. To help patients learn to process complex activities, such as catching a bus, preparing a meal, or shopping for food or clothing, nurses should break the activity into small parts or steps and list them for the patient's reference, for example:

- Leave your apartment with your keys in hand.
- Make sure you have correct bus fare in your pocket.
- Close the door.
- Walk to the corner.
- Turn right and walk three blocks to the bus stop.

Providing Family Education

Because having a family member with schizophrenia is a life-changing event for the family and friends who provide care and support, educating patients and their families is crucial. It is a primary concern for the psychiatric–mental health nurse. Family support is crucial to help patients maintain treatment. Education should include information about the disease course, treatment regimens, support systems, and life management skills (Box 22.21). The most important factor to stress during patient and family education is the consistent taking of medication.

Social Domain

Social Assessment

Several difficulties with social functioning occur in schizophrenia. As the disorder progresses, individuals can

---

BOX 22.21

Psychoeducation Checklist: **Schizophrenia**

When caring for the patient with schizophrenia, be sure to include the caregiver as appropriate and address the following topic areas in the teaching plan:

- Psychopharmacologic agents, including drug action, dosage, frequency, and possible adverse effects; stress the importance of adherence to the prescribed regimen
- Management of hallucinations
- Recovery strategies
- Coping strategies such as self-talk, getting busy
- Management of the environment
- Use of contracts that detail expected behaviors, with goals and consequences
- Community resources

become increasingly socially isolated. On a one-to-one basis, this occurs as the individual seems unable to connect with people in his or her environment. Several aspects of the symptoms already discussed can contribute to this. For example, emotional blunting and anhedonia (the inability to form emotional attachment and experience pleasure) result in an experience of not being engaged in activities and relationships.

Cognitive deficits that contribute to difficult social functioning include problems with face and affect recognition, deficiencies in recall of past interactions, problems with decision making and judgment in conflictual interactions, and poverty of speech and language. Poor functioning and the inability to complete activities of daily living are manifested in poor hygiene, malnutrition, and social isolation.

Functional Status

Functional status of patients with schizophrenia should be assessed initially and at regular periods. Level of independence, ability to work, ability to maintain an independent living environment, and self-care should be evaluated.

Social Systems

In schizophrenia, support systems become very important in maintaining the patient in the community. The individual may become socially isolated if the treatment and management occur in long-term care facilities and group homes away from family and friends. One challenge in treating patients with schizophrenia is to identify and maintain the patient's links with family and significant others. Assessment of the formal support (e.g., family, providers) and informal support (e.g., neighbors, friends) should be conducted.

Quality of Life

People with schizophrenia often have a poor quality of life, especially older people, who may have spent many years in long-term hospitals. The nurse should assess the patient's quality of life and how it could be improved. Simple changes, such as arranging for a different roommate or improving access to social activities by meeting transportation needs, can greatly improve a patient's quality of life.

Family Assessment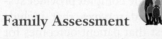

The assessment of the family could take many forms, and the family assessment guide presented in Chapter 14 can be used. In some instances, the patient is young and living with his or her parents. Often, the nurse's

first contact with the patient and family is in the initial phases of the disorder. The family is dealing with the shock and disbelief of having a child with a mental illness that has lifelong consequences. In these cases, the assessment process may be extended over several sessions to provide the family with support and education about the disorder.

Because women with schizophrenia generally have better treatment outcomes than do men, many marry and have children. These women experience the same life stresses as other women and may find themselves single parents, raising children in poverty-stricken conditions. Managing a psychiatric illness and trying to be an effective parent in a socially stigmatizing society are almost impossible because of the lack of financial resources and social support. This family will need an extensive assessment of financial need and social support. The family life cycle model presented in Chapter 14 can also be used as a framework for the assessment.

Nursing Diagnoses for Social Domain

The nursing diagnoses generated from the assessment of the social domain are typically Impaired Social Interaction, Ineffective Role Performance, Disabled Family Coping, or Interrupted Family Processes. Outcomes depend on the specific diagnostic area.

Interventions for Social Domain

Promoting Patient Safety

Although violence is not a consistent behavior of people with schizophrenia, it is always a concern during the initial phase when hallucinations or delusions may put patients at risk for harming themselves or others. Nonviolent patients who are experiencing hallucinations and delusions can also be at risk for victimization by more aggressive patients. The patient who is hallucinating needs to be protected. This protection may include increased staff monitoring and, if necessary, a safer environment in a secluded area.

Identifying patient risk factors for violence, such as a history of violence, can alert the nursing staff of a potential for engagement in aggressive behavior, but careful assessment and management of the immediate environment and treating the psychiatric symptoms are more important in avoiding aggression (Chu, Thomas, Ogloff, & Daffern, 2013). The nurse's best approach to avoiding violence or aggression is to demonstrate respect for the patient and the patient's personal space, assess and monitor for signs of fear and agitation, and use preventive interventions before the patient loses control. Patients should be encouraged to discuss their anger and be involved in their treatment decisions. Medications should be administered as ordered. Because most antipsychotic and antidepressant medications take 1 to 2 weeks to begin moderating behavior, the nurse must be vigilant during the acute illness.

If the patient loses control and is a danger to self or others, restraints and seclusion may be used as a last resort. Health Care Financing Administration (HCFA) guidelines and hospital policy must be followed (see Chapter 4), and staff should be trained in the proper use of seclusion and restraints. In addition, staff need to have planned sessions after all incidents of violence or physical management to analyze the event. These sessions allow staff to learn how better to manage these situations and evaluate patients' cues. With sensitive leadership, these sessions can help staff to learn more about the interaction of patient and staff characteristics that can contribute to these incidents.

Convening Support Groups

People with mental illness benefit from support groups that focus on daily problems and the stress of dealing with a mental illness. These groups are useful throughout the continuum of care and help reduce the risk of suicide. In the hospital setting, the focus of the group can be simply sharing the experience of living with a mental illness. In the community, a regular support group can provide interaction with people with similar problems and issues. Friendships often develop from these groups. Using peer counseling and support groups is also supported within the recovery model of care (Pratt, Macgregor, Reid, & Given, 2012).

Implementing Milieu Therapy

Individuals with schizophrenia can be hospitalized or live in group homes for a long period of time. The challenge is helping people who are unable to live with family members to live harmoniously with strangers who have similar interpersonal difficulties. Arranging the treatment environment to maximize therapy is crucial to the rehabilitation of the patient.

Developing Recovery-Oriented Rehabilitation Strategies

Rehabilitation strategies are used to support the individual's recovery and integration into the community (see Chapter 5). Community-based psychosocial rehabilitation programs usually offer long-term intensive case management services to adults with schizophrenia. Programs provide a continuum of services to meet the changing needs of people with psychiatric disabilities. Patients set rehabilitation goals, and services are then provided to help "clients" (most programs do not use the term "patients") reach their goals. Services range from daily home visits to providing transportation, occupational training, and group support. Assertive community treatment (ACT) is one example of these types of services and has a solid base of evidence to support its use (Mueser et al., 2013).

Social skills training, provided either individually or in groups, is also useful when working with patients who have schizophrenia (Mueser et al., 2013). This training teaches patients specific behaviors needed for social interactions. The skills are taught by lecture, demonstration, role-playing, and homework assignments. Nurses may be team members and be involved in case management or provision of services. Furthermore, efforts to offer supportive employment experiences (Mueser et al., 2013) that incorporate patient preferences, rapid job search and employment, and ongoing job supports have shown effectiveness. Although long-term self-sufficiency has not necessarily been achieved, supportive employment has been the most effective vocational rehabilitation method.

Implementing Family Interventions

When schizophrenia first becomes apparent, the patient and family must negotiate the mental health system for the first time (in most cases), a challenge that almost equals that of confronting the family member's illness. In most states, the mental health system is huge and is usually ignored unless an adult foster care home moves into a neighborhood or a family member becomes seriously mentally ill. The system includes private inpatient and outpatient clinics supported by insurance and public community mental health clinics and hospitals supported by public funds. Because mental health coverage in most insurance packages is insufficient for someone with schizophrenia, most families eventually deal with the public mental health system. If the patient is aggressive, many private facilities encourage hospitalization in a public sector facility even for the first admission.

Family members should be encouraged to participate in support groups that help them deal with the realities of living with a loved one with a mental illness (see Chapter 14). Family members should receive information about local community and state resources and organizations such as mental health associations and those that can help families negotiate the complex provider systems. Evidence for family-based services that include support and education suggest that patient outcomes for medication management, symptom control, stress, and functional status are improved (Mueser et al., 2103).

Evaluation and Treatment Outcomes

Outcome research related to schizophrenia has redefined previous ways of thinking about the course of the disorder. Schizophrenia was once considered to have a progressively long-term and downward course, but it is now known that people with schizophrenia can be successfully treated and managed. In one older but significant study, the researchers interviewed patients 20 to 25 years after diagnosis and found that 50% to 66% experienced significant improvement or recovery (Harding, Zubin, & Strauss, 1987). This study is important because it occurred before the development of second-generation antipsychotic agents. Today, we can be hopeful that even more people can experience improvement or recover from schizophrenia.

Continuum of Care

Continuity of care has been identified as a major goal of recovery for patients with schizophrenia because they are at risk for becoming "lost" to services if left alone after discharge. Discharge planning encourages follow-up care in the community. In fact, many state mental health systems require an outpatient appointment before discharge. Treatment of people with schizophrenia occurs across a variety of settings. Not only inpatient hospitalization but also partial hospitalization, day treatment, and crisis stabilization can be used effectively.

Inpatient-Focused Care

Much of the previous discussion concerns care in the inpatient setting. Today, inpatient hospitalizations are brief and focus on patient stabilization. Many times, patients are involuntarily admitted for a short period (see Chapter 4). During the stabilization period, the status is changed to voluntary admission whereby the patient agrees to treatment.

Emergency Care

Emergency care ideally takes place in a hospital emergency department, but often the crisis occurs in the home. Patients are usually relapsing and do not recognize their bizarre or aggressive behaviors as symptoms. A specially trained crisis team is sent to assess the emergency and recommend further treatment. In the emergency department, patients are brought not only because of relapse but also because of medication side effects or water intoxication. Nurses should refer to the previous discussion for nursing management.

Community Care

Most of the care of patients with schizophrenia is provided in the community through publicly supported

---

BOX 22.22

Research for Best Practice: **The Process of Self-Recovery**

Shea, J. M. (2010). Coming back normal: The process of self-recovery in those with schizophrenia. *Journal of the American Psychiatric Nurses Association, 16*(1), 43–51.

THE QUESTION: How is the process of self-identity (important for recovery) reconstructed in people with schizophrenia?

METHODS: A grounded theory study was conducted with 10 participants representing three categories of community adjustment and four significant others. Nineteen semi-structured interviews were completed.

FINDINGS: The final results supported the use of the term recovery rather than reconstruction of self because the process involved more than simply putting the pieces together. The self-recovery process included six stages: entering the territory, struggling for control, active self-care, finding a social fit, checking out the self, and coming back to normal.

IMPLICATIONS FOR NURSING: This process has a direct impact on the daily struggles of those with schizophrenia. Using this model, the nurse can understand where the person with schizophrenia is in the recovery journey.

---

recovery-oriented mental health delivery systems. The recovery journey can be long and require a variety of services such as ACT; outpatient therapy; case management; and psychosocial rehabilitation, including clubhouse programs (Box 22.22). While the patient is in the community, his or her health care should be integrated with physical health care. Nurses should be especially vigilant that patients with mental illnesses receive proper primary and medical health care.

NCLEXNOTE Priorities in the patient with acute symptoms of schizophrenia include managing psychosis and keeping the patient safe and free from harming him- or herself or others. In the community, the priorities are preventing relapse, maintaining psychosocial functioning, engaging in psychoeducation, improving quality of life, and instilling hope.

Mental Health Promotion

In some cases, it is not the disorder itself that threatens the mental health of the person with schizophrenia but the stresses of trying to receive care and services. Health care systems are complex and are often at the mercy of a system rule that is outdated. Development of assertiveness and conflict resolution skills can help the person in negotiating access to systems that will provide services. Developing a positive support system for stressful periods helps promote a positive outcome (Fig. 22.7).

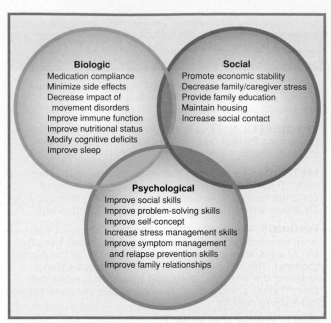

Biologic
Medication compliance
Minimize side effects
Decrease impact of
 movement disorders
Improve immune function
Improve nutritional status
Modify cognitive deficits
Improve sleep

Social
Promote economic stability
Decrease family/caregiver stress
Provide family education
Maintain housing
Increase social contact

Psychological
Improve social skills
Improve problem-solving skills
Improve self-concept
Increase stress management skills
Improve symptom management
 and relapse prevention skills
Improve family relationships

FIGURE 22.7 Biopsychosocial outcomes for patients with schizophrenia.

SUMMARY OF KEY POINTS

- The person with schizophrenia displays a complex of myriad symptoms typically categorized as positive symptoms (those that exist but should not), such as delusions or hallucinations and disorganized thinking and behavior, and negative symptoms (characteristics that should be there but are lacking), such as alogia, avolition, anhedonia, and diminished emotional expression.

- In the past, the diagnosis and treatment of schizophrenia focused on the more observable and dramatic positive symptoms (i.e., delusions and hallucinations), but recently scientists have shifted their focus to the disorganizing symptoms of cognition. The recovery model now focuses on the individual patient and the instillation of hope.

- The clinical presentation of schizophrenia occurs in three phases: phase 1 entails initial diagnosis and first treatment, phase 2 includes periods of relative calm between episodes of overt signs and symptoms but during which the patient needs sustained treatment, and phase 3 includes periods of exacerbation or relapse that require hospitalization or more frequent contacts with mental health professionals and increased use of resources. A prodromal risk period may be identifiable.

- Biologic theories of what causes schizophrenia include genetic, neurodevelopment, and neurotransmission imbalances. The last is supported by the advanced technology of PET scan findings and the understanding of the mechanisms of antipsychotic medications.

- Biologic assessment of the patient with schizophrenia must include a thorough history and physical examination to rule out any medical illness or substance abuse problem that might be the cause of the patient's symptoms, assessment of risk for self-injury or injury to others, and creation of baseline health information before medications are administered. Several standardized assessment tools are available to help assess characteristic abnormal motor movements.

- Several nursing interventions address the biologic domain, including promotion of self-care activities, activity, exercise, nutritional, thermoregulation, and fluid balance interventions. In general, the antipsychotic drugs used to treat patients with schizophrenia block dopamine transmission in the brain but also cause some troublesome and sometimes serious side effects, primarily anticholinergic side effects and extrapyramidal side effects (motor abnormalities). Newer second-generation antipsychotic agents block serotonin as well as dopamine. The nurse should be familiar with these drugs, their possible side effects, and the interventions required to manage or control side effects.

- The extrapyramidal side effects of antipsychotic drugs can appear early in drug treatment and include acute parkinsonism or pseudoparkinsonism, acute dystonia, and akathisia, or they can appear late in treatment after months or years. The primary example of late-appearing extrapyramidal side effects is tardive dyskinesia, which is a severe syndrome of abnormal motor movements of the mouth, tongue, jaw, trunk, fingers, and toes.

- Psychological assessment must include equal attention to manifestations of both positive and negative symptoms and a concentrated focus on the cognitive impairments that make it so difficult for these patients to manage their disorder. Several standardized assessment tools assess for positive and negative symptoms. Development of the nurse–patient relationship is key in helping patients manage the disturbed thoughts and sensory perceptions. Interventions should be designed to enhance cognitive functioning. Patient and family education are critical interventions for the person with schizophrenia.

- Because schizophrenia is a lifetime disorder and patients require the continued support and care of mental health professionals and family or friends, one of the primary nursing interventions is ensuring that patients and families are properly educated regarding the course of the disorder, importance of drug maintenance, and need for consistent care and support. Research is demonstrating that interaction between patients and their families is key to the success of long-term treatments and outcomes.

CRITICAL THINKING CHALLENGES

1. Delusions are often based on beliefs not held by others. Occasionally delusions are based on cultural beliefs that are outside of those held by the majority of society. Describe steps that professional psychiatric caregivers should use to make sure their responses consider the cultural basis of a patient's delusions.

2. Delusions and hallucinations are based to varying degrees on patients' experiences and emotional responses to them. What experiences and emotions might form the basis of delusions that are grandiose or persecutory? What might form the basis of auditory hallucinations that tell patients of their importance or their need to harm themselves?

3. What steps might the nurse take to develop trust in a patient who has hallucinations and delusions and is frightened of other people?

4. Given that a patient with mental illness requires extra efforts at confidentiality and that patients with schizophrenia are often suspicious of their family members, explain ways you can help families and patients take advantage of the social support that may be available only from each other.

5. What steps can be taken in the community to enhance the living circumstances of people with schizophrenia?

6. Discuss how therapeutic communication might have to change when working with a person with schizophrenia who is displaying primarily negative symptoms. How will you deal with the person's diminished response to you (both verbally and emotionally) when you are teaching or giving instructions for activities? How will you help the person compensate for some of his or her cognitive deficits?

7. A person who has schizophrenia is admitted during a relapse with an advance directive requesting specific medications to be used and family to be contacted. The physician leading the treatment team refuses to follow this advance directive. How might you respond?

A Beautiful Mind: 2001. This Academy Award–winning movie starring Russell Crowe is based on the biography by Sylvia Nasar of the mathematician and Nobel Laureate John Nash. It presents the life and experiences of this man as he experienced schizophrenia. It shows how his life and work were altered and the effects on his relationships with family and colleagues. The movie depicts how this man came to terms with his illness.

VIEWING POINTS: How does the treatment John Nash received in the 1950s differ from treatment today? How would you classify his symptoms according to the *DSM-IV-TR*? What is typical or problematic about Mr. Nash's relationship with the medications prescribed for him?

The Soloist: 2009. Based on a true story, this movie portrays the experience of Steve Lopez (played by Robert Downey, Jr.) when he befriends Nathaniel Anthony Ayers, "the soloist" (played by Jamie Foxx), who has severe, persistent, and untreated schizophrenia—and more importantly, exceptional musical talent. Once a student at the prestigious Juilliard School of Music, Ayers lives on the streets of Los Angeles playing his two-string violin. See also the book by the same title.

VIEWING POINTS: What are the risks and rewards of taking on such a personal relationship? How best can nurses advocate for individuals with severe mental illness (and their family and friends) when community resources are inadequate?

MOVIE viewing GUIDES related to this chapter are available at: http://thePoint.lww.com/Boyd5eUpdate.

A related Psychiatric-Mental Health Nursing video on the topic of Schizophrenia is available at: http://thePoint.lww.com/Boyd5eUpdate.

References

Acosta, F. J., Hernández, J. L., Pereira, J., Herrera, J., & Rodríguez, C. J. (2012) Medication adherence in schizophrenia. *World Journal of Psychiatry*, 2(5), 74–82. doi:10.5498/wjp.v2.i5.74

Altamura, A. C., Aguglia, E., Bassi, M., Bogetto, F., Cappellari, L., De Giorgi, S., et al. (2012). Rethinking the role of long-acting atypical antipsychotics in the community setting (Review). *International Clinical Psychopharmacology*, 27(6), 336–349.

American Psychiatric Association. (2013). *Diagnostic and statistical manual of mental disorders* (5th ed). Arlington, VA: Author.

Auquier, P., Tinland, A., Fortanier, C., Loundou, A., Baumstarck, K., Lanson, C., et al. (2013). Toward meeting the needs of homeless people with schizophrenia: The validity of quality of life measurement. *PLOS One*, 8(10), 1–9.

Austad, F., Joa, I., Johannessen, J. O., & Larsen, T. K. (2013). Gender differences in suicidal behavior in patients with first-episode psychosis. *Early Intervention Psychiatry*, doi:10.1111/eip.12113

Baker, J. T., Holmes, A. J., Masters, G. A., Yeo, B. T., Krienen, F., Buckner, R. L., et al. (2014). Disruption of cortical association networks in schizophrenia and psychotic bipolar disorder. *JAMA Psychiatry*, 71(2), 109–118.

Barajas, A., Usall, J., Baños, I., Dolz, M., Villalta-Gil, V., Vilaplana, M., et al. (2013). Three-factor model of premorbid adjustment in a sample with chronic schizophrenia and first-episode psychosis. *Schizophrenia Research*, 151(1–3), 252–258.

Birnbaum, R., & Weinberger, D. R. (2013). Functional neuroimaging and schizophrenia: A view towards effective connectivity modeling and polygenic risk. *Dialogues in Clinical Neuroscience*, 15(3), 279–289.

Bonsch, D., Wunschel, M., Lenz, B., Janssen, G., Weisbrod, M., & Sauer, H. (2012). Methylation matters? Decreased methylation status of genomic DNA in the blood of schizophrenic twins. *Psychiatry Research*, 19(3), 533–537.

Boshes, R. A., Manschreck, T. C., & Konigsberg, W. (2012). Genetics of the schizophrenias: A model accounting for their persistence and myriad phenotypes. *Harvard Review of Psychiatry*, 20(3), 119–129.

Brown, A. S. (2011). The environment and susceptibility to schizophrenia. *Progress in Neurobiology*, 93(1), 23–58. doi:10.1016/j.pneurobio.2010.09.003

Buchsbaum, M. (1990). The frontal lobes, basal ganglia, and temporal lobes as a site for schizophrenia. *Schizophrenia Bulletin*, 16, 377–387.

Buchsbaum, M. S., Buchsbaum, B. R., Hazlett, E. A., Haznedar, M. M., Newmark, R., Tang, C. Y., et al. (2007). Relative glucose metabolic rate higher in white matter in patients with schizophrenia. *American Journal of Psychiatry*, 164(7), 1072–1081.

Carliner, H., Collins, P. Y., Cabassa, L. J., McNallen, A., Joestl, S. S., & Lewis-Fernández, R. (2014). Prevalence of cardiovascular risk factors among racial and ethnic minorities with schizophrenia spectrum and bipolar disorders: A critical literature review. *Comprehensive Psychiatry, 55,* 233–247. doi:10.1016/j.comppsych.2013.09.009.

Challis, S., Nielssen, O., Harris, A., & Large, M. (2013). Systematic meta-analysis of the risk factors for deliberate self-harm before and after treatment for first-episode psychosis. *Acta Psychiatrica Scandinavica, 127*(6), 442–454.

Chu, C. M., Thomas, S. D., Ogloff, J., & Daffern, M. (2013). The short-to medium-term predictive accuracy of static and dynamic risk assessment measures in a secure forensic hospital. *Assessment, 20*(2), 230–241.

Cohen, C. I., & Marino, L. (2013). Racial and ethnic differences in the prevalence of psychotic symptoms in the general population. *Psychiatric Services, 64*(11), 1103–1109.

Department of Health Statistics and Information Systems. (2013). *WHO methods and data sources for global burden of disease estimates 2000–2011.* Geneva: World Health Organization.

Fanning, J. R., Bell, M. D., & Fiszdon, J. M. (2012). Is it possible to have impaired neurocognition but good social cognition in schizophrenia? *Schizophrenia Research, 135*(1–3), 68–71.

Fraguas, D., Del Rey-Mejias, A., Morenos, C., Castro-Fornieles, J., Graell, M., Otero, S., et al. (2014). Duration of untreated psychosis predicts functional and clinical outcome of children and adolescents with first-episode psychosis: A 20 year longitudinal study. *Schizophrenia Research, 152,* 130–138. doi:10/1016/j.schres.2013.11.018

Franzen, G. (1970). Plasma free fatty acids before and after an intravenous insulin injection in acute schizophrenic men. *British Journal of Psychiatry, 116*(531), 173–177.

Goff, D. C. (2013). Future perspectives on the treatment of cognitive deficits and negative symptoms in schizophrenia. *World Psychiatry, 12,* 99–107.

Goldman, M. B., Wang, L., Wachi, C., Daudi, S. Csernansky, J., Marlow-O'Connor, M., et al. (2011). Structural pathology underlying neuroendocrine dysfunction in schizophrenia. *Behavioural Brain Research, 218*(1), 106–113.

Goldstein, J. M, Cherkerzian, S., Tsuang, M. T., & Petryshen, T. L. (2013). Sex differences in the genetic risk for schizophrenia: History of the evidence for sex-specific and sex-dependent effects. *American Journal of Medical Genetics, Part B, Neuropsychiatric Genetics, 162B,* 698–710. doi:10.1002/ajmg.b.32159

Gray, R., White, J., Schulz, M., & Abderhalden, C. (2010). Enhancing medication adherence in people with schizophrenia: An international programme of research. *International Journal of Mental Health Nursing, 19*(1), 36–44.

Guo, X., Fang, M., Zhai, J., Wang, B., Wang, C., Hu, B., et al. (2011). Effectiveness of maintenance treatments with atypical and typical antipsychotics in stable schizophrenia with early stage: 1-year naturalistic study. *Psychopharmacology, 216*(4), 475–484.

Guo, X., Zhai, J., Fang, M., Wang, B., Wang, C., Hu, B., et al. (2010). Effect of antipsychotic medication alone vs. combined with psychosocial intervention on outcomes of early-stage schizophrenia: A randomized, 1-year study. *Archives of General Psychiatry, 67*(9), 895–904.

Harding, C., Zubin, J., & Strauss, J. (1987). Chronicity in schizophrenia: Fact, partial fact or artifact? *Hospital and Community Psychiatry, 38*(5), 477–486.

Hawken, E. R., Crookall, J. M., Reddick, D., Millson, R. C., Milev, R., & Delva, M. (2009). Morality over a 20-year period in patients with primary polydipsia associated with schizophrenia: A retrospective study. *Schizophrenia Research, 107*(2–3), 128–133.

Johnson, S. L. M., Wang, L., Alpert, K. I., Greenstein, D., Clasen, L., Lalonde, F., et al. (2013). Hippocampal shape abnormalities of patients with childhood-onset schizophrenia and their unaffected siblings. *Journal of the American Academy of Child & Adolescent Psychiatry, 52*(5), 527–536.e2.

Kaplan, G., Casoy, J., & Zummo, J. (2013). Impact of long-acting injectable antipsychotics on medication adherence and clinical, functional, and economic outcomes of schizophrenia. *Patient Preference and Adherence, 7,* 1171–1180. doi:10.2147/PPA.S53795

Kay, S. R., Fiszbein, A., & Opler, L. A. (1987). The Positive and Negative Syndrome Scale (PANSS) for schizophrenia. *Schizophrenia Bulletin, 13,* 261–276.

Kristensen, D., Brandt-Christensen, M., Ockelmann, H. M., & Jorgensen, M. S. (2012). The use of electroconvulsive therapy in a cohort of forensic psychiatric patients with schizophrenia. *Criminal Behavior and Mental Health, 22*(2), 148–156.

Koch, D. A., & Scott, A. J. (2012). Weight gain and lipid-glucose profiles among patients taking antipsychotic medications: Comparisons for prescriptions administered using algorithms versus usual care. *Journal of Psychiatric & Mental Health Nursing, 19*(5), 389–394.

Lau, C. I., Wang, H. C., Hsu, J. L., & Liu, M. E. (2013). Does the dopamine hypothesis explain schizophrenia? *Reviews in the Neurosciences, 24*(4), 389–400.

Laursen, T. M., Nordentoft, M., & Mortensen, P. B. (2014). Excess early mortality in schizophrenia. *Annual Review of Clinical Psychology, 10,* 425–448. doi:10.1146/annurev-clinpsy-032813-153657

Lepage, M., Bodmar, M., & Bowie, C. R. (2014). Neurocognition: Clinical and functional oucomes in schizophrenia. *Canadian Journal of Psychiatry, 59*(1), 5–12.

Leshner, A. F, Tom, S. R., & Kern, R. S. (2013). Errorless learning and social problem solving ability in schizophrenia: An examination of the compensatory effects of training. *Psychiatry Research, 206*(1), 1–7.

Loewenstein, D. A., Czaja, S. J., Bowie, C. R., & Harvey, P. D. (2012). Age-associated differences in cognitive performance in older patients with schizophrenia: A comparison with health older adults. *American Journal of Geriatric Psychiatry, 20*(1), 29–40.

MacKinnon, K., Newman-Taylor, K., & Stopa, L. (2011). Persecutory delusions and the self: An investigation of implicit and explicit self-esteem. *Journal of Behavior Therapy and Experimental Psychiatry, 42*(1), 54–64.

Margetic′, B. & Margetic′, B. A. (2010). Neuroleptic malignant syndrome and its controversies. *Pharmacopepidemiology and Drug Safety, 19*(5), 429–435.

McDonnell, M. G., Strbnik, D., Angerl, F., McPherson, S., Lowe, J. J., Sugar, A., Short, R. A., et al. (2013). Randomized controlled trial of contingency management of stimulant use in community mental health patients with serious mental illness. *American Journal of Psychiatry, 170*(1), 94–101.

Meier, M. H., Caspi, A., Reichenberg, A., Keefe, R. S. E., Fisher, H. L., Harrington, H. L., et al. (2014). Neuropsychological decline in schizophrenia from the premorbid to the postonset period: Evidence from a population-representative longitudinal study. *American Journal of Psychiatry, 171,* 91–101. doi:10.1176/appi.ajp.2013.12111438

Mueser, K. T., Deavers, F., Penn, D. L., & Cassisi, J. E. (2013). Psychosocial treatment for schizophrenia (Review). *Annual Review of clinical Psychology, 9,* 465–497.

National Alliance on Mental Illness (NAMI). (2013). *Trends, themes and best practices in state mental health legislation.* Arlington, VA: NAMI.

Neugeboren, J. (2006). Meds alone couldn't bring Robert back. *Newsweek.* Retrieved June 17, 2014, from www.power/article/recovery/meds.html

Noiseux, S., & Ricard, N. (2008). Recovery as perceived by people with schizophrenia, family members and health professionals: A grounded theory. *International Journal of Nursing Studies, 45*(8), 1148–1162.

Pandya, A., & Myrick, K. (2013). Wellness and recovery programs: A model of self-advocacy for people living with mental illness (Review). *Journal of Psychiatric Practice, 19*(3), 242–246.

Pratt, R., Macgregor, A., Reid, S., & Given, L. (2012). Wellness Recovery Action Planning (WRAP) in self-help and mutual support groups. *Psychiatric Rehabilitation Journal, 15*(5), 403–405.

Schimmelbusch, W. H., Mueller, P. S., & Sheps, J. (1971). The positive correlation between insulin resistance and duration of hospitalization in untreated schizophrenia. *British Journal of Psychiatry, 118*(545), 429–436.

Shea, J. M. (2010). Coming back normal: The process of self-recovery in those with schizophrenia. *Journal of the American Psychiatric Nurses Association, 16*(1), 43–51.

Simpson, G. M., & Angus, J. W. (1970). A rating scale for extrapyramidal side effects. *Acta Psychiatrica Scandinavica. Supplementum, 212,* 11–19.

Smieskova, R., Marmy, J., Schmidt, A., Bendfeldt, K., Riecher-Rossler, A., Walter, M., et al. (2013). Do subjects a clinical high risk for psychosis differ from those with a genetic high risk?—A systematic review of structural and functional brain abnormalities. *Current Medicinal Chemistry, 20*(3), 467–481.

Snider, K., & Boyd, M. (1991). When they drink too much: Nursing interventions for patients with disordered water balance. *Journal of Psychosocial Nursing, 29*(7), 13.

Sprague, R. L., & Kalachnik, J. E. (1991). Reliability, validity, and a total score cutoff for the Dyskinesia Identification Scale System: Condensed User Scale (DISCUS) with mentally ill and mentally retarded populations. *Psychopharmacology Bulletin, 27,* 51–58.

Stahl, S. (2013). *Stahl's essential psychopharmacology: Neuroscientific basis and practical application* (4th ed). Cambridge, UK: Cambridge University Press.

Tarbox, S. I., Addington, J., Cadenhead, K. S., Cannon, T. D., Cornblatt, B. A., Perkins, D. O., et al. (2013). Premorbid functional development and conversion to psychosis in clinical high-risk youths. *Development and Psychopathology, 25*(4 Pt 1), 1171–1186.

Valente, S., & Fisher, D. (2010). Recognizing and managing psychogenic polydipsia in mental health. *The Journal for Nurse Practitioners, 6*(7), 546–552

Willick, M. S. (1994). Schizophrenia: A patient's perspective – journey without end. In N. C. Andressen (Ed.), *Schizophrenia: From mind to molecule* (pp. 5–19). Washington, DC: American Psychiatric Press.

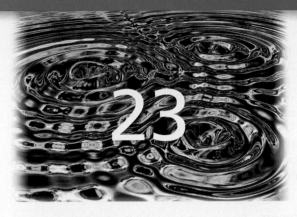

23

Schizoaffective, Delusional, and Other Psychotic Disorders
Management of Thoughts and Moods

Nan Roberts and Roberta Stock

KEY CONCEPTS

- Psychosis
- Delusions

LEARNING OBJECTIVES

After studying this chapter, you will be able to:

1. Define schizoaffective disorder and distinguish the major differences among schizophrenia, schizoaffective, and mood disorders.

2. Discuss the important epidemiological findings related to schizoaffective disorder.

3. Explain the primary etiologic factors regarding schizoaffective disorder.

4. Explain the primary elements involved in assessment, nursing diagnoses, nursing interventions, and evaluation of patients with schizoaffective disorder.

5. Define delusional disorder and its subtypes.

6. Explain the important epidemiologic findings regarding delusional disorder.

7. Discuss the primary etiologic factors of delusional disorder.

8. Explain the nursing care of patients with delusional disorder.

9. Identify other disorders defined by the presence of psychosis, including schizophreniform, and brief psychotic, as well as psychotic disorders attributable to a substance.

KEY TERMS

- delusional disorder • erotomanic • persecutory delusions • schizoaffective disorder (SAD)
- thymoleptic

Psychiatric–mental health nurses care for patients who have psychiatric disorders involving underlying psychoses other than schizophrenia and mood disorders. This chapter introduces these other psychotic disorders and describes the associated nursing care. Central to understanding the problems of these patients is the concept of **psychosis**, a term used to describe a state in which an individual experiences positive symptoms, also known as psychotic symptoms (hallucinations; delusions; or disorganized thoughts, speech, or behavior) (see Chapter 22).

> **KEYCONCEPT** **Psychosis**, a state in which a person experiences symptoms including hallucinations; delusions; or disorganized thoughts, speech, or behavior, is the key distinguishing factor in psychotic disorders.

Other psychotic disorders defined by the presence of psychosis include schizoaffective, delusional, schizophreniform, and brief psychotic disorders. Psychotic disorders may also be induced by drugs or alcohol.

Recognizing and understanding psychotic disorders is crucial to providing meaningful care. For example, schizoaffective disorder is one of the more complex psychotic disorders to identify but is also one of the more common diagnoses that the generalist psychiatric nurse is likely to encounter. Nurses practicing in nonpsychiatric settings, on the other hand, have a key role to play in identifying delusional disorders because persons with delusional disorder are more likely to be treated in a medical-surgical setting and are rarely seen by psychiatrists, so the disorder often remains undiagnosed.

SCHIZOAFFECTIVE DISORDER

Schizoaffective disorder (SAD) is a complex and persistent psychiatric illness. This disorder was recognized in 1933 by Kasanin, who described varying degrees of symptoms of both schizophrenia and mood disorders beginning in youth. All of his patients were well adjusted before the sudden onset of symptoms that erupted after the occurrence of a specific environmental stressor. Since Kasanin's time, debate and controversy about the status of this disorder have been extensive, resulting in many different definitions and classifications (Malhi, 2013). More than 50 years after SAD was first described, the diagnosis was finally officially confirmed by the psychiatric community and included in the American Psychiatric Association (APA, 1980) *Diagnostic and Statistical Manual of Mental Disorders*, 3rd Edition, Revision (*DSM-III-R*). Box 23.1 reflects the history of this debate. Even since, however, it has been argued that this disorder should be named either schizophrenia with mood symptoms or mood disorder with schizophrenic symptoms (Malhi, 2013).

Clinical Course

SAD is characterized by periods of intense symptom exacerbation alternating with quiescent periods, during

---

BOX 23.1

History of the Diagnosis: Schizoaffective

- 1933: Kasanin first coined the phrase *schizoaffective psychosis.*
- 1980: The *DSM-III* did not include diagnostic criteria for schizoaffective disorder.
- 1987: Schizoaffective disorder was first recognized as a separate diagnosis in the *DSM-III-R;* the definition included length of time in relationship to symptoms.
- 1994: Schizoaffective disorder was maintained as a separate disorder in the *DSM-IV.*
- 2000: Schizoaffective disorder was maintained as a separate disorder in the *DSM-IV-TR.*
- 2013: Schizoaffective disorder continues to be diagnosed as a separate disorder in *DSM-5.*

---

which psychosocial functioning is adequate. This disorder is at times marked by psychosis; at other times, by mood disturbance. When psychosis and mood disturbance occur at the same time, a diagnosis of schizoaffective disorder is made (APA, 2013). Patients with SAD are more likely to exhibit persistent psychosis than are patients with a mood disorder. They feel that they are on a "chronic roller coaster ride" of symptoms that are often difficult to manage.

> **NCLEXNOTE** Patients with schizoaffective disorder have many similar responses to their disorder as people with schizophrenia, with one exception. These patients have many more "mood" responses and are very susceptible to suicide.

The long-term outcome of SAD is generally better than that of schizophrenia but worse than that of mood disorder (Möller, Jäger, Riedel, Obermeier, Strauss, & Bottlender, 2010). These patients resemble the mood disorder group in work function and the schizophrenia group in social function. In one study, patients with SAD were less likely to recover and more likely to have persistent psychosis, with or without mood symptoms than those with bipolar disorder. Persons with SAD usually have higher functioning than those with schizophrenia with severe negative symptoms and early onset of illness (Bora, Yucel, & Pantelis, 2009).

Diagnostic Criteria

Mental health providers find SAD difficult to conceptualize, diagnose, and treat because of the variable clinical course. Patients are often misdiagnosed as having schizophrenia. The difficulty in conceptualizing SAD is reflected in the controversy regarding the diagnostic criteria discussed earlier.

To be diagnosed with SAD, a patient must have an uninterrupted period of illness when there is a major depressive, manic, or mixed episode along with two of the following symptoms of schizophrenia: delusions, hallucinations, disorganized speech, disorganized or catatonic behavior, or negative symptoms (e.g., diminished emotional expression, alogia, or avolition). In addition, the positive symptoms (delusions or hallucinations) must be present without the mood symptoms at some time during this period (for at least 2 weeks). Two related subtypes of SAD have been identified: bipolar and depressive. In the bipolar type, the patient exhibits manic symptoms alone or a mix of manic and depressive symptoms. Patients with the depressive type display only symptoms of a major depressive episode (APA, 2013).

Epidemiology and Risk Factors

The lifetime prevalence of SAD is estimated to be less than 0.3% (APA, 2013). This disorder occurs less commonly than does schizophrenia. The incidence of SAD is relatively constant across populations in varied geographic, climatic, industrial, and social environments. Environmental contributions are minimal.

Patients with SAD are at risk for suicide. The risk for suicide in patients with psychosis is increased by the presence of depression. Risk factors for suicide increase with the use of alcohol or substances, cigarette smoking, previous suicide attempts and hospitalizations (Bolton & Robinson, 2010).

Lack of regular social contact may be a factor that confers a long-term risk for suicidal behavior, which may be reduced by treatments designed to enhance social networks and contact and help patients to protect themselves against environmental stressors (Reutfors et al., 2010).

Age of Onset

SAD can affect all age groups. In children, the disorder is rare and is often indistinguishable from schizophrenia. In older adults, this disorder becomes complicated because of frequent comorbid medical conditions. The typical age of onset for this disorder is early adulthood, and the most common type presented is bipolar. Other studies have reported a relatively late onset of SAD of mainly the depressive type (APA, 2013).

Gender

SAD is more likely to occur in females than in males, which may be accounted for by a greater incidence of the depressive type in females (APA, 2013).

Ethnicity and Culture

Most patients are white. Although some reports have indicated a connection between SAD and social class, others support no specific association with race, geographic area, or class. There is evidence that African Americans are more likely to receive a diagnosis of schizophrenia but not necessarily SAD disorder (Anglin & Malaspina, 2008).

Family

Relatives of patients diagnosed with SAD appear to be at increased risk for this disorder, schizophrenia, or bipolar disorder. Some initial genome evidence indicates that if there is a familial association, it is more likely related to the mother than the father (Wiener et al., 2013). There is also some evidence of an increased risk of development of SAD if a first-degree relative has mental illness of some form.

Comorbidity

SAD may be associated with substance abuse including alcohol, cigarettes, and other recreational drugs. Similar to other severe mental disorders, these individuals also die approximately 25 years earlier than the general population (Hartz et al., 2014).

Etiology

Biologic Theories

Although the etiologies of schizophrenia and mood disorder have been investigated extensively, the etiology of SAD remains unresolved. Research to locate a biologic marker has been limited. Variables may be structural as well as neurochemical.

Neuropathologic

Magnetic resonance imaging (MRI) and computed tomography scans have been used in the study of SAD for more than 25 years (Takahashi et al., 2009). Midline brain abnormalities, especially in women, have been found. In SAD, changes in brain structure appear to be similar to those seen in other psychotic disorders, such as schizophrenia (Takahashi et al., 2009). Whether midline structural abnormality is directly causal, indirectly contributory, or an intriguing phenomenon in SAD is unclear.

Genetic

The etiology is believed to be primarily genetic. Results from family, twin, and adoption studies vary but suggest that SAD may consist of phenotypic variations or expressions of a genetic interform between schizophrenia and affective psychoses (Wiener et al., 2013).

Biochemical

The studies of neurotransmitter dysfunction in schizoaffective disorder are found within the schizophrenia research. There is strong evidence that excessive dopaminergic activity and glutaminergic dysfunction are involved in the clinical symptoms of schizoaffective disorder (Abi-Dargham & Meyer, 2014). More studies are needed to further explain the biochemical involvement.

Psychological and Social Theories

Psychological, psychodynamic, environmental, and interpersonal factors may have a precipitating role when they coincide with a biomedical diathesis that creates vulnerability to this disorder (see Chapter 7 for an explanation of the diathesis-stress theory). No current psychodynamic behavioral, cognitive, or developmental theories of causation explain SAD. Family dynamics do not appear to affect the development of this disorder except for the strong genetic predisposition, which is virtually unexplained.

Interdisciplinary Treatment

Patients with SAD benefit from comprehensive treatment. Because this disorder is persistent, these individuals are constantly trying to manage complex symptoms. Ideally, most of the treatment occurs within the patient's natural environment, and hospitalizations are limited to times of symptom exacerbation, when symptoms are so severe or persistent that extended care in a protected environment is necessary.

Pharmacologic intervention is needed to stabilize the symptoms and presents specific challenges. Long-term atypical antipsychotic agents, now the mainstay of pharmacologic treatment, are as effective as the traditional combination of a standard antipsychotic agent and an antidepressant drug. Mood stabilizers, such as lithium or valproic acid (see Chapter 11), may be used. A combination of antipsychotic and antidepressant agents is often used.

After the patient's condition has stabilized (i.e., the patient exhibits a decrease in positive and negative symptoms), the treatment that led to remission of symptoms should be continued. Titrating antipsychotic agents to the lowest dose that provides suitable protection may enable optimal psychosocial functioning while slowing the recurrence of new episodes. Patients diagnosed with SAD are unlikely to be medication free. Electroconvulsive therapy is considered when symptoms are refractory to other interventions or when the patient's life is at risk and a rapid response is required. Ongoing maintenance may be necessary to avoid relapse (Huuhka et al., 2012).

The treatment plan is revised regularly, and symptoms are monitored to guide medication management. Psychiatric nursing interventions are guided by the nursing diagnoses. After the patient is released from the hospital, home visits may be needed. Psychotherapy helps manage interpersonal relationships and mood changes. Social services are needed to obtain disability benefits or services. Use of advanced practice clinicians helps to provide continuity of care.

Priority Care Issues

Patients with SAD are highly susceptible to suicide (Pompili et al., 2011). Living with a persistent psychotic disorder that has a mood component makes suicide a risk.

NURSING MANAGEMENT: Human Response to Schizoaffective Disorder

Nursing care for patients with SAD is focused on minimizing psychiatric symptoms through promoting medication maintenance and on helping patients maintain optimal levels of functioning. Interventions center on developing social and coping skills through supportive, nurturing, and nonconfrontational approaches. The nurse must be constantly attuned to the mood state of the patient and help the patient learn to solve problems, resolve conflict, and cope with social situations that trigger anxiety.

Biologic Domain
Assessment

Assessment of patients with SAD is similar to assessment of those with schizophrenia and mood disorders. A careful history from the patient and family is crucial and should contain a description of the full range and duration of symptoms the patient has experienced and those observed by the family. A patient who has had symptoms for a relatively long period of time has increased difficulty overcoming effects of the psychosis, which can cause function to deteriorate.

A thorough systems assessment is important to discover any physiologic problems the patient is experiencing, such as sleep pattern disturbances, difficulties with self-care, or poor nutritional habits.

Nursing Diagnoses for the Biologic Domain

Common nursing diagnoses for the biologic domain are Disturbed Thought Process, Disturbed Sensory Perception, and Insomnia, but almost any nursing diagnosis can be generated because of the variety of problems that patients with SAD face. The persistent nature of this disorder lends itself to numerous and varied problems that must all be addressed (see Nursing Care Plan 23.1).

Interventions for the Biologic Domain
Pharmacologic Interventions

An in-depth medication history is important in evaluating response to past medications and predicting response to the present regimen. The nurse should investigate adherence to past treatment to determine the probability of compliance. The nurse should develop a plan to increase compliance based on previous problems with adherence. For example, the nurse can use medication boxes and calendars and obtain help from others in managing the medication. Recognizing medication side

(text continues on page 384)

NURSING CARE PLAN 23.1

The Patient With Schizoaffective Disorder

Ms. B is a 28-year-old divorced woman with a 4-year-old daughter. They reside with Ms. B's parents. Ms. B is a hairdresser and tries to work, but she becomes stressed in the workplace, which results in her being fired. She has never applied for disability. Her parents are stressed because of the exacerbations of her illness and caring for her child.

Ms. B has had numerous hospitalizations for aggressive behavior, noncompliance with medications, and receiving medications from various physicians, which result in inappropriate psychiatric management. She is medication seeking and is often prescribed benzodiazepines and diet pills by her primary care physician.

The patient has an ingrained delusional system that makes it hard to introduce reality orientation and feedback. She believes that her ex-husband has sexually abused their child. She has gone to numerous attorneys to try and prosecute the ex-husband to no avail because of the lack of evidence to prove any abuse.

For the past 2 years, Ms. B has believed that a bank guard is in love with her. She is adamant about him protecting her and her child. She states that he watches over them. They have no contact other than speaking to each other when she enters the bank. She has been seeing a man the past 9 months but states that she really does not care much for him, and it is hard for her to move forward in the relationship because she loves the bank guard.

Medications have included antidepressants, antipsychotics (typical and atypical), mood stabilizers, benzodiazepines, sleep medications, and anticonvulsants. She often complains of being depressed, yet she does not take antidepressant medications as prescribed.

Setting: Intensive Care Psychiatric Unit in a General Hospital

Baseline Assessment: Ms. B is admitted to the hospital through the emergency department. She was hearing voices and was delusional. She has not been taking medications for several months. She is oriented in all spheres and well nourished but unkempt. She is verbalizing delusions about a man at the bank. She cannot sleep well and reportedly goes outdoors at night and yells at a bank guard. Reality feedback increases her agitation. She denies any problems.

Associated Psychiatric Diagnosis	Medications
Schizoaffective disorder	None

Nursing Diagnosis 1: Ineffective Individual Coping

Defining Characteristics	Related Factors
Inability to meet role expectations	Chronicity of the condition
Anxiety	Inadequate psychological resources secondary to delusions
Delusions	Inadequate coping skills
Inability to problem solve	Inadequate psychological resources to adapt to residential setting

Outcomes

Initial	Discharge
1. Identify coping pattern	5. Manage own behavior
2. Identify stressors	6. Medication compliance
3. Identify personal strengths	7. Reduction of delusions
4. Accept support through the nursing relationship	

Continued

NURSING CARE PLAN 23.1 *(Continued)*

Interventions

Interventions	Rationale	Ongoing Assessment
Initiate a nurse–patient relationship to develop trust.	Through the use of the nurse–patient relationship, the patient will be able to maintain compliance with the treatment plan.	Determine whether the patient is able to relate to the nurse.
Facilitate the identification of stressors in the patient's environment.	To be able to cope with stressors, they need to be identified by the patient.	Assess whether the patient is able to identify and verbalize stressors.
Develop coping strategies to manage environmental stressors.	The patient needs to develop realistic strategies to handle environmental stressors.	Determine whether patient-identified strategies are realistic.
Help the patient to identify personal strengths.	By identifying personal strengths, the patient will increase confidence in using coping strategies.	Assess the patient's ability to incorporate coping strategies into her daily routine.
Assist the patient to understand the disorder and its management.	By understanding the disorder, the patient can develop ways to manage her disorder.	Assess the patient's level of understanding of the disease.
Facilitate emotional support for the family.	A supported family is better equipped to support the patient.	Assess the family's ability to seek emotional support from the staff.
Teach coping skills.	By developing positive coping skills, anxiety and agitation will decrease.	Assess the patient's ability to learn the skills to manage stressors.
After discharge, refer to community support group (i.e., coping skills group).	The client often experiences regression on discharge from the inpatient setting and needs increased support to continue to develop positive coping skills.	Determine the client's attendance and participation in the group.
Refer for psychiatric follow-up care.	Provide medication monitoring with adjustments needed on a regular basis to ensure continued progress.	Determine the client's response to medications related to effectiveness and side effects.
Refer to outpatient Transitional Treatment Program.	Transitional services provide a bridge between inpatient and community settings and allow the client to develop coping skills and a safe environment.	Determine the client's ability to identify stressors in home and community and negative coping skills.

Evaluation

Outcomes	Revised Outcomes	Interventions
Within the nursing relationship, Ms. B was able to understand how coping skills can reduce stressors.	Support the patient's ability to recognize stressor and apply coping skills.	Discuss stressors and means of applying coping skills.
Increased insight into what behavior is appropriate has helped the patient to decrease verbalization of delusions.	Provide ongoing support to maintain the present level of functioning.	Discuss behavior and provide reality feedback.
The client attends and participates in groups, giving examples of use of positive coping skills.	Reinforce positive coping skills and assist the client to overcome obstacles that prevent development.	Provide ongoing education and support.
The client attends psychiatric follow-up appointments and has increase in antipsychotic medications because of symptom exacerbation.	Continue assessment of reaction to medications.	Provide education and support to the client.
The client attends the Transitional Treatment Program.	Offer the client to continue program at decreasing time intervals.	Provide support for positive behavior changes.

Continued

NURSING CARE PLAN 23.1 *(Continued)*

Nursing Diagnosis 2: Disturbed Thought Processes

Defining Characteristics	Related Factors
Delusions Impulsivity Medication noncompliance	Ingrained delusions Decreased ability to process secondary to delusions

Outcomes

Initial	Discharge
1. Maintain reality orientation. 2. Communicate clearly with others. 3. Expresses delusional material less frequently.	4. Identify situations that contribute to delusions. 5. Identify how delusions affect life situations. 6. Use coping strategies to deal with delusions. 7. Recognize changes in behavior.

Interventions

Interventions	Rationale	Ongoing Assessment
Promote medication compliance.	Compliance will reduce delusions.	Assess for side effects: heat intolerance, neuroleptic malignant syndrome, renal failure, constipation, dry mouth, increased appetite, salivation, nausea, vomiting, tardive dyskinesia, seizures, somnolence, agitation, insomnia, dizziness.
Teach actions, effects, and side effects of medications.	The more knowledgeable patients are about medication, the more likely they will comply.	Assess the client's ability to understand information.
Support reality testing through helping the patient to differentiate thoughts and feelings in relationship to situations.	When comparing thoughts with the situations, patients can develop skills to refute delusions.	Assess for medication compliance.
Monitor verbalization of delusional material.	Determine whether medication is reducing delusional thoughts.	Assess verbalization of delusional material.
Identify stressors that promote delusions.	If the patient is able to identify stressors that promote delusions, she can manage the stressors to effectively decrease delusions.	Assess the patient's ability to recognize stressors when they occur.
Assist the patient in developing skills to deal with delusions (recognizing delusional themes can help the patient in distinguishing between reality- and nonreality-based patterns).	Even though medication can reduce the occurrence of delusions, they may continue in some people with decreased intensity. Cognitive behavioral skills are important in dealing with these altered thoughts.	Monitor the patient's ability to handle delusions.
Refer to community support services that focus on reality testing (i.e., Transitional Treatment Program).	The client's delusions often continue but verbalization decreases.	Assess for indicators of continued delusions.

Evaluation

Outcomes	Revised Outcomes	Interventions
Delusions will be less ingrained.	Continue to practice skills in reality orientation and communication.	Support verbalization of reality-based thoughts.
The patient verbalized action, effect, dosage, and side effects of medications.	Take prescribed medication regularly.	Give positive feedback for understanding of medication.
The client attends programs but continues to voices some delusions.	Encourage the client to consider doubt about the reality of delusions.	Continue focus on reality testing and support client gains.
Medication compliance		Initiate pill counts.

Continued

NURSING CARE PLAN 23.1 *(Continued)*

Summary: Ms. B was discharged from the hospital. Verbalization of delusions had not decreased. She was less anxious. She is presently taking 30 mg of Abilify at bedtime, 75 mg of Effexor XR in the morning, 0.5 mg of Xanax in the morning, and 50 mg of Seroquel at bedtime. Mother is helping by filling a weekly medication box. At times, Ms B is questioning her delusions.

Nursing Diagnosis 3: Ineffective Family Coping

Defining Characteristics	Related Factors
Unable to meet physical, emotional, and spiritual needs of family members. Withdrawal from client at time of need. Poor communication of family boundaries, rules, and expectations.	Inadequate understanding of individual's illness. Progression of individual symptoms that exhaust positive coping skills of family members.

Outcomes

Initial	Discharge
1. Family members will identify their own reactions to the individual and illness. 2. Family members will identify the needs of family members.	3. Family members will identify behavioral expectations of the individual upon her return home. 4. The family and client will meet with a counselor before discharge to identify a working plan to assist the client in functioning in the home environment.

Interventions

Interventions	Rationale	Ongoing Assessment
Assist family members to develop problem-solving skills. Assist family members with their behavioral response to the client's behavior. Educate the family about the client's illness and treatment of her illness.	Client behavior can create conflict within the family and a need for conflict resolution skills. Each family member's behavior has an effect on other family members' behavior. Knowledge about illness will assist family members in coping with client behaviors.	Determine the ability of family members to develop problem-solving skills. Assess family members' ability to identify their own reactions. Assess family members' ability to understand the illness, treatment, and goals.

Evaluation

Outcomes	Revised Outcomes	Interventions
Family members are willing to work on problems solving skills but verbalize feeling overwhelmed. Family members are willing to identify their own behavior. Family members verbalize realization of client's behavior as an illness and not "making things up."	Support family members and offer continued educational and support services. Support the ability of family members to identify any negative reactions to the client's behavior. Support the family and provide for continued knowledge and skills.	Refer family members to family support group (e.g., National Alliance on Mental Illness). Assist family members to identify methods to increase their own positive coping skills. Give written information and websites related to the client's illness and refer her to the local mental health association.

effects quickly and intervening promptly to alleviate them will promote patient compliance. Understanding the need for medications is essential to the patient.

Mood and psychotic symptoms are of equal importance and are evaluated throughout treatment. Atypical antipsychotic agents are generally prescribed because of their efficacy for psychosis and for their **thymoleptic** (mood stabilizing) properties (Kantrowitz & Citrome, 2011). Clozapine, reported effective for SAD by several authorities, can reduce hospitalizations and risk for suicide (Pompili et al., 2011). Dosages are the same as those used for treating schizophrenia.

In many cases, symptoms of depression disappear when psychotic symptoms decrease. If depressive symptoms persist, use of an antidepressant agent may be helpful. Successful use of anticonvulsant agents for people with this disorder has been documented in several clinical trials (Kantrowitz & Citrome, 2011). Mood stabilizers, which decrease the frequency and intensity of episodes, can be an alternative adjunctive medication for mood states associated with the bipolar type.

Administering and Monitoring Medications

The greatest challenge in pharmacologic interventions is monitoring target symptoms and identifying changes in symptom pattern. Patients can switch from being relatively calm to being very emotional. Careful observation and documentation to determine whether the patient is overreacting to an environmental event or experiences a change in mood symptoms will help determine when a medication change is required.

Adherence to medication regimens is critical to a successful outcome. Patients need an opportunity to discuss barriers to compliance.

Managing Side Effects

Monitoring medication side effects in patients with SAD is similar to that in patients with schizophrenia. Extrapyramidal side effects, weight gain, and sedation are assessed and documented.

Monitoring for Drug Interactions

Avoid using lithium with antipsychotic medications. A few patients taking haloperidol and lithium have experienced an encephalopathic syndrome followed by irreversible brain damage. Lithium may interact similarly with other antipsychotic agents. It may also prolong the effects of neuromuscular blocking agents. Use of nonsteroidal antiinflammatory drugs may increase plasma lithium levels. Diuretics and angiotensin-converting enzyme inhibitors should be prescribed cautiously with lithium, which is excreted through the kidneys (see Chapter 11 for more information).

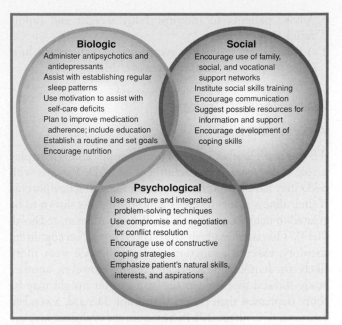

FIGURE 23.1 Biopsychosocial interventions for patients with schizoaffective disorder.

Patient Education

Interventions are based on the needs identified by the biopsychosocial assessment (Figure 23.1). Establishing a regular sleep pattern by setting a routine can help to promote or reestablish normal patterns of rest. Educating the patient about the food groups in MyPlate and about what constitutes good nutrition can improve nutritional status. Help the patient to identify self-care deficits, especially those caused by lack of motivation. For deficits created by severe mood symptoms, establishing a routine and setting goals are useful.

Additional teaching points specifically related to patient medication use include:

- Instruct patients on the prescribed medication regimen.
- Determine whether the patient has sufficient resources to purchase and obtain medications.
- Have the patient write down the prescribed medication and time of administration.
- Explain the target symptom for each medication (e.g., psychosis and mood for atypical antipsychotic agents, mood for antidepressant and mood stabilizer drugs).
- Caution patients about orthostatic hypotension and instruct them to get up slowly from lying and sitting positions. Also advise them to maintain adequate fluid intake.
- Advise patients to contact their case managers or health care providers if they experience dramatic changes in body temperature (neuroleptic malignant syndrome [NMS]), inability to control motor movement (dystonia), or dizziness.
- Advise patients to avoid over-the-counter medications unless a prescriber is consulted.

- Advise patients to monitor body weight and report rapid weight gains.
- Advise patients to report symptoms of diabetes mellitus (e.g., frequent urination, excessive thirst).

Psychological Domain
Assessment

The patient's level of insight into his or her illness may play a role in the course and treatment of SAD. Patients with SAD may have better insight than those with schizophrenia if their illness is less severe. Clinical insight is shown to be related to neurocognition (Nair, Palmer, Aleman, & David, 2014). That is, individuals who scored higher on cognition, memory, executive function, and intelligence were more likely to demonstrate clinical insight. However, another study showed that individuals with greater insight may be more depressed than others (Misdrahi, Denard, Swendsn, Jaussent, & Courtet, 2014). Stressors are evaluated because they may trigger symptoms. Uncovering or exploratory techniques are generally avoided. Mental status and reality contact may be compromised. Assessment of anxiety level or reactions to stressful situations is important because the combination of these symptoms with psychosis increases the patient's risk for suicide (Box 23.2).

Nursing Diagnoses for the Psychological Domain

In SAD, individuals vacillate between mood dysregulation and disturbed thinking. Typical nursing diagnoses for

BOX 23.2
Using Reflection

OVERREACTING TO STRESSES

INCIDENT • A patient living in the community told a community health nurse that she refused to let her children go to school because of a terrorist threat in another state.

REFLECTION • At first, the nurse thought that the patient had overslept and had made an excuse for not sending her children to school. Upon further analysis, the nurse realized that the patient was overreacting to a stressful situation. Overreaction is one of the characteristics of schizoaffective disorder. The patient was experiencing extreme stress and needed to develop coping strategies for her overreaction to these types of events.

this domain include Hopelessness, Powerlessness, Ineffective Coping, Low Self-esteem, and Impaired Social Interaction (Figure 23.2).

Interventions for the Psychological Domain

Using appropriate interpersonal modalities is important to help the patient, family, and social and vocational support networks cope with the onslaught of acute episodes and recuperative periods. Therapeutic relationships are critical in helping these individuals move toward recovery (Roche, Madigan, Lyne, Feeney, & O'Donoghue, 2014). Patients with SAD have fewer awareness deficits than those with schizophrenia. Structured, integrated, and problem-solving psychotherapeutic interventions are

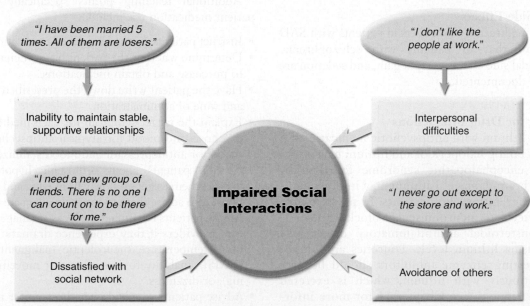

FIGURE 23.2 Nursing diagnosis concept map: Impaired Social Interactions.

used to develop or increase the patient's insight. Psychoeducational interventions can help to decrease symptoms, enhance recognition of early regression, and hone psychosocial skills (Box 23.3).

Social Domain

Assessment

Social dysfunction is common with SAD. Premorbid adjustment, such as marital status and adolescent social adjustment, may influence patients' levels of functioning at the time of diagnosis and their prognoses. Assess for social skill deficits and problems with interpersonal conflicts, particularly in males. Assessment of an adult patient's childhood may give a clue to his or her current level of social functioning. Assess the patient's use of fantasy and fighting as a means of coping. Patients who report the most severe peer rejection present with the angriest dispositions and display antisocial behaviors.

Nursing Diagnoses for the Social Domain

Because of mood and thought disturbances, these individuals have significant problems in the social domain. Typical nursing diagnoses include Compromised Family Coping, Impaired Home Maintenance, and Social Isolation.

Interventions for the Social Domain

Social skills training is useful for remediating social deficits and may result in positive social adjustment. Positive results include improved interpersonal competence and decreased symptom severity. Identifying feelings and developing realistic goals, along with supportive therapy, can integrate insight into the

disease process. Education focusing on conflict resolution skills, promoting compromise, negotiation, and expression of negative feelings help the patient achieve positive social adjustment. Social skills can be improved through role-playing and assertiveness training. Supportive, nurturing, and nonconfrontational interventions help to minimize anxiety and improve understanding (Box 23.4).

Helping to develop coping skills is essential. Teach communication skills to decrease conflicts and environmental negativity. Memory is linked with development of social skills; psychotic symptoms interfere with retention of skills, resulting in slowed learning requiring long-term and intense social training.

Families are at risk for ineffective coping. Family members face many of the same issues faced by families of patients with schizophrenia and are often puzzled by the patient's emotional overreaction to normal daily stresses. Frequent arguments may lead to verbal and physical abuse.

Evaluation and Treatment Outcomes

Teaching skills to patients with SAD often takes longer. Psychoeducation results in increased knowledge of the illness and treatment, increased medication compliance, fewer relapses and hospitalizations, briefer inpatient stays, increased social function, decreased family tension, and lighter family burdens (Vieta, 2010). Maintain realistic outcomes and praise small successes to promote positive outcomes (Figure 23.3).

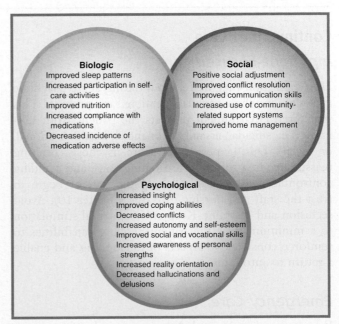

FIGURE 23.3 Biopsychosocial outcomes for patients with schizoaffective disorder.

BOX 23.4 • THERAPEUTIC DIALOGUE • Ms. B's "Delusions"

INEFFECTIVE COMMUNICATION

Nurse: Hello, Ms. B. What has been happening?

Patient: The guy from the bank keeps me up all night.

Nurse: That's not possible.

Patient: He's there all the time to look after me.

Nurse: No, he's not. You just think that.

Patient: No, he really is. He is helping me.

Nurse: He does not even know who you are.

EFFECTIVE COMMUNICATION

Nurse: Hello, Ms. B. How have you been?

Patient: That guy from the bank is really bothering me.

Nurse: What is he doing?

Patient: He keeps me up all night. I go out in the street to yell at him.

Nurse: Have you actually seen him at night?

Patient: No, but I know he is there.

Nurse: How can he be there when you cannot see him?

Patient: He can't.

Nurse: Does it seem that the thoughts about him come from your mind?

Patient: This might be.

Nurse: Your illness often causes thoughts that are not reality based.

Patient: It seems real but yet so unreal. Those are sort of stupid thoughts.

CRITICAL THINKING CHALLENGE

- How could the nurse's approach in the first scenario have prevented development of a therapeutic relationship?
- How can the second scenario benefit the patient in developing insight into her delusions?
- Discuss the differences between the two approaches.

Continuum of Care

Inpatient-Focused Care

Hospitalization may be required during acute psychotic episodes or when suicidal ideations are present. This structured environment protects the patient from self-harm (i.e., suicidal, assaultive, financial, legal, vocational, or social). During periods of acute psychosis, offering reassurance in a soft, nonthreatening voice and avoiding confrontational stances will help the patient begin to trust the staff and nursing care (see Chapter 10). Avoid seclusion and restraint. Keep environmental stimulation to a minimum. Use the patient's coping capabilities to reinforce constructive aspects of functioning and enable a return to autonomy.

Emergency Care

Emergency care is needed during periods of symptom exacerbation. Psychosis, mood disturbance, and medication-related adverse effects account for most emergency situations. During an exacerbation of psychosis, patients may become agitated or aggressive. Assaultive behavior is managed by using therapeutic techniques (see Chapter 19) and pharmacologic management. If medications are used, benzodiazepines such as lorazepam or atypical antipsychotics such as Geodon are usually given. Possible medication-related adverse effects include NMS as a reaction to dopamine antagonists or serotonin intoxication, especially if the patient is taking an atypical antipsychotic agent and a selective serotonin reuptake inhibitor (see Chapter 22).

Family Intervention

Helping families support the patient in the home or a community placement is an integral part of nursing care. With patient permission, key family members can be included in home visits to learn about symptoms, medications, and side effects. By collaborating with family members, the patient's willingness to follow treatment, monitor symptoms, and continue with rehabilitation and recovery can be strengthened.

Community Treatment

After release from the hospital, graduated levels of care (i.e., partial hospitalization, day treatment, and group home) can help the patient return to a more manageable environment. Programs that foster building and practicing social and vocational skills are appropriate. These incorporate the patient's natural skills, interests, and aspirations.

Because this illness is episodic, the person with SAD requires close and continued follow-up in the outpatient setting by psychiatrists, nurses, and therapists. These patients require ongoing medication management, supportive and cognitive therapy, and symptom management. If symptoms intensify, hospitalization may be required until they are brought under control.

DELUSIONAL DISORDER

Delusional disorder is a psychotic disorder characterized by stable, and well-systematized delusions that occur in the absence of other psychiatric disorders. **Delusions** are false, fixed beliefs unchanged by conflicting evidence. Delusions can be a possible situation that could occur in real life (spouse having an affair) and are plausible in the context of the person's ethnic and cultural background or they can be bizarre and clearly impossible (alien from outer space) (APA, 2013).

> **KEYCONCEPT   Delusions** are fixed, false beliefs that cannot be changed by conflicting evidence. They can be situations that could occur in real life and are plausible in the context of the person's ethnic and cultural background or clearly impossible.

Examples of real-life situations include being followed, poisoned, infected, loved at a distance, or deceived by a spouse or lover. A diagnosis of delusional disorder is based on the presence of one or more delusions for at least 1 month (APA, 2013). Delusions are the primary symptom of this disorder. Apart from the direct impact of the delusion, psychosocial functioning is not markedly impaired.

Clinical Course

The course of delusional disorder is variable. The onset can be acute, or the disorder can occur gradually and become chronic. Patients usually live with delusions for

BOX 23.5

Using Reflection

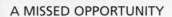

A MISSED OPPORTUNITY

INCIDENT • A patient in primary care insists that he is being stalked by his former boss, who wants the patient's newly developed computer program. He refuses to see any mental health professionals. The nurse focuses on the patient's physical problems and ignores his delusional thoughts.

REFLECTION • Later, the nurse reflected on the meaning and significance of the patient's beliefs. Could the patient be a victim of stalking? Does the patient have a delusional disorder and need treatment? Does he need further evaluation? Would he hurt anyone? Unfortunately, the nurse will not know the meaning or significance of the statement without further assessment.

years, rarely receiving psychiatric treatment unless their delusion relates to their health (somatic delusion), or they act on the basis of their delusion and violate legal or social rules (Box 23.5). Full remissions can be followed by relapses.

Apart from the direct impact of the delusion, psychosocial functioning is not markedly impaired. Behavior is remarkably normal except when the patient focuses on the delusion. At that time, thinking, attitudes, and mood may change abruptly. Personality does not usually change, but the patient is gradually, progressively involved with the delusional concern (APA, 2013).

Diagnostic Criteria

Delusional disorder includes several subtypes: erotomanic, grandiose, jealous, persecutory, somatic, mixed, and unspecified. The subtype represents the prominent theme of the delusion. A patient who has met criteria A for schizophrenia does not receive a diagnosis of delusional disorder (see Chapter 22 for criteria A). Although hallucinations may be present, they are not prominent (APA, 2013).

If mood episodes occur with this disorder, the duration of the mood episode is relatively brief compared with the duration of the delusional period. Delusions are not caused by the direct physiologic effects of substances (i.e., cocaine, amphetamines, marijuana) or a general medical condition (i.e., Alzheimer's disease, systemic lupus erythematosus). Delusional disorder is a diagnosis of exclusion requiring careful evaluation. Distinguishing this disorder from schizophrenia and mood disorders with psychotic features is difficult (APA, 2013).

The prevalence of delusional disorder is about 0.2% in the general population. Research data are limited because numbers of recorded case studies and participants are small, and the studies lack systematic description, assessment, and diagnosis. Delusional disorder may be associated with dysfunction in the frontal-subcortical systems and with temporal dysfunction, particularly on the left side (Marneros et al., 2012).

Erotomanic Delusions

The **erotomanic** subtype is characterized by the delusional belief that the patient is loved intensely by the "loved object," who is usually married, of a higher socioeconomic status, or otherwise unattainable. The patient believes that the loved object's position in life would be in jeopardy if his or her true feelings were known. In addition, the patient is convinced that he or she is in amorous communication with the loved object. The loved object is often a public figure (e.g., movie star, politician) but may also be a common stranger. The patient believes that the loved object was the first to make advances and fall in love. The patient may entertain some delusional beliefs about a sexual relationship with the loved object, yet the beliefs are unfounded. The delusion, which often idealizes romantic love and spiritual union rather than sexual attraction, becomes the central focus of the patient's existence.

The patient may have minimal or no contact with the loved object and often keeps the delusion secret, but efforts to contact the loved object through letters, telephone calls, gifts, visits, surveillance, and stalking are also common. The patient may in many cases transfer his or her delusion to another loved object. There is some evidence that celebrity worship is associated with cognitive deficits (McCutcheon, Ashe, Houran, & Maltby, 2003).

Patients with erotomanic delusional disorder are often lower level employees; lead withdrawn, lonely lives; are single with poor interpersonal relationships; and have limited sexual contacts or are sexually repressed. Clinical patients are mostly women, who do not usually act out their delusions. Forensic patients are mostly men, who tend to be more aggressive and can become violent in pursuit of the loved object although the loved object may not be the object of the aggression. Men in particular come into contact with the law in their pursuit of the loved object or in a misguided effort to rescue the loved object from some imagined danger. Orders of protection are generally ineffective, and criminal charges of stalking or harassment that lead to incarceration are ineffective as a long-term solution to the problem (Rosenfeld, 2003). The result is repeated arrests and psychiatric examinations followed by ineffective treatment. Patients are rarely motivated to seek psychiatric treatment. This disorder is difficult to control, contain, or treat. Separation from the loved object is the only satisfactory means of intervention (APA, 2013).

Grandiose Delusions

Patients presenting with grandiose delusions are convinced they have a great, unrecognized talent or have made an important discovery. A less common presentation is the delusion of a special relationship with a prominent person (i.e., an adviser to the president) or of actually being a prominent person (i.e., the president). In the latter case, the person with the delusion may regard the actual prominent person as an impostor. Other grandiose delusions may be religious in nature, such as a delusional belief that he or she has a special message from a deity (APA, 2013).

Jealous Delusions

The central theme of the jealous subtype is the unfaithfulness or infidelity of a spouse or lover. The belief arises without cause and is based on incorrect inferences justified by "evidence" (i.e., rumpled clothing, spots on sheets) the patient has collected. The patient usually confronts the spouse or lover with a host of such evidence. An associated feature is paranoia. The patient may attempt to intervene in the imagined infidelity by secretly following the spouse or lover or by investigating the imagined lover (Marneros et al., 2012).

Delusions of jealousy are difficult to treat and may diminish only with separation, divorce, or the death of the spouse or lover. Except in older adults, such patients generally are male. Jealousy is a powerful, potentially dangerous emotion. Aggression or even violent behavior may result. Litigious behavior is common, and symptoms with forensic aspects are often seen. Care is essential in determining how to deal with the patient.

Somatic Delusions

Somatic delusions, a mix of psychotic and somatic symptoms, have been described for more than 100 years. The central theme of somatic delusions involves bodily functions or sensations. These patients believe they have physical ailments. Delusions of this nature are fixed, inarguable, and intense, with the patient totally convinced of the physical nature of the somatic complaint. Medication can cause tactile hallucinations that result directly from the physiologic effects of the medication; when the medication or drug is removed, the symptoms disappear. Somatic delusions are manifested in the following beliefs (APA, 2013):

- A foul odor is coming from the skin, mouth (delusions of halitosis), rectum, or vagina
- Insects have infested the skin (delusional parasitosis)
- Internal parasites have infested the digestive system

- A certain body part is misshapen or ugly (contrary to visible evidence)
- Parts of the body are not functioning (e.g., large intestine, bowels)

The delusion of infestation by insects cannot occur without sensory perceptions, which constitute tactile hallucinations. The patient vividly describes crawling, itching, burning, swarming, and jumping on the skin surface or below the skin. The patient maintains the conviction that he or she is infested with parasites in the absence of objective evidence to the contrary.

Patients with somatic delusions use excessive health care resources. They seek repeated medical consultations with dermatologists, entomologists, infectious disease specialists, and general practitioners. They seek treatment from primary care physicians and refuse psychiatric referral. Even if they seek psychiatric help, these patients typically do not comply with long-term psychiatric intervention. Patients often go through elaborate rituals to cleanse themselves or their surroundings of the perceived pests, collecting hair, scabs, and skin flakes as evidence of an infection. Anger and hostility are common among this group, and behavioral characteristics include shame, depression, and avoidance.

The somatic subtype is rare but may be underdiagnosed. Both genders are affected equally, but when onset occurs in late middle age, female patients tend to predominate. Studies of somatic delusions have been marred by methodologic uncertainties, and factors limiting investigation include rarity of the disease, lack of contact with psychiatrists, and noncompliance with the medication regimen.

Persecutory Delusions

The central theme of **persecutory delusions** is the patient's belief that he or she is being conspired against, cheated, spied on, followed, poisoned, drugged, maliciously maligned, harassed, or obstructed in pursuit of long-term goals. This is the most common subtype (APA, 2013).

The focus of persecutory delusions is often on some injustice that must be remedied by legal action (querulous paranoia). Patients often seek satisfaction by repeatedly appealing to courts and other government agencies (MacKinnon, Newman-Taylor, & Stopa, 2011). These patients are often angry and resentful and may even behave violently toward the people they are persecuting them. The course may be chronic although the patient's preoccupation with the delusional belief often waxes and wanes. The clarity, logic, and systematic elaboration of this delusional theme leave a remarkable stamp on this condition (APA, 2013).

Mixed and Unspecified Delusions

In the mixed subtype, no one delusional theme predominates, and the patient presents with two or more types of delusions. In the unspecified subtype, the delusional beliefs cannot be clearly determined, or the predominant delusion is not described as a specific type. Patients are usually females who experience feelings of depersonalization and derealization and have negative-associated paranoid features (APA, 2013).

Epidemiology and Risk Factors

Delusional disorder is relatively uncommon in clinical settings. The best estimate of its prevalence in the population is about 0.2% (APA, 2013).

Few risk factors are associated with delusional disorder. Patients can live with their delusions without psychiatric intervention because their behavior is normal although if delusions are somatic, patients risk unnecessary medical interventions. Acting on delusions carries a risk for intervention by law enforcement agencies or the legal system. Suicide attempts are neither more nor less common than in the general population (Kovacs, Voros, & Fekete, 2005).

Age of Onset

Delusional disorder can begin in adolescence and occurs in middle to later adulthood. Onset occurs at a later age than among patients with schizophrenia (APA, 2013).

Gender

Gender does not appear to affect the overall frequency of most delusional disorders (APA, 2013). Patients with erotomanic delusions are generally women; in forensic settings, most people with this disorder are men. Men also tend to experience more jealous delusions, except in the older adult population, in which women outnumber men.

Ethnicity and Culture

A person's ethnic, cultural, and religious background must be considered in evaluating the presence of delusional disorder. The content of delusions varies among cultures and subcultures (APA, 2013).

Family

An increased familial risk and familial genetic factors are unknown.

Comorbidity

Mood disorders are frequently found in patients with delusional disorders. Typically, mild symptoms of depression such as irritable or dysphoric mood are present. Delusional disorder may also be associated with obsessive-compulsive disorder and paranoid, schizoid, or avoidant personality disorder (APA, 2013; González-Rodríguez, Molina-Andreu, Navarro, Gastó, Penadés, & Catalán, 2014).

Etiology

The cause of delusional disorder is unknown. The only major feature of this condition is the formation and persistence of the delusions. Few have investigated possible neurophysiologic and neuropsychological causes of delusional disorder, and theories of causation are contradictory. No psychological or social theories of causation are addressed in the literature.

Biologic Theories

Neuropathologic

In patients with delusional disorder, MRI shows a degree of temporal lobe asymmetry. However, these differences are subtle, so delusional disorder may involve a neurodegenerative component (Ota, Mizukami, Katano, Sato, Takeda, & Asada, 2003). The tactile hallucinations of somatic delusions may arise from sensory alterations in the nervous system or from sensory input that has been misinterpreted because of subtle cortical changes associated with aging.

Biochemical

Delusional disorder is probably biologically distinct from other psychotic disorders. Delusions may involve faulty processing of essentially intact perceptions whereby perceptions become linked with an interpretation that has deep emotional significance but no verifiable basis). Alternately, a complex, malfunctioning dopaminergic system may lead to delusions (Marneros, et al., 2012). This explanation could lead to the argument that a particular delusion depends on the "circuit" that is malfunctioning. Denial of reality has been linked to right posterior cortical dysfunction. Some authors have proposed a combination of biologic and early life experiences as etiological components (Bentall, Corcoran, Howard, Blackwood, & Kinderman, 2001). It has also been theorized that delusions may arise from dysfunction in the entorhinal cortex, which is located in the inner parts of the temporal lobes and serves as a relay between the prefrontal cortex and the hippocampus (Arehart-Treichel, 2004).

Interdisciplinary Treatment

Few, if any, interdisciplinary treatments are associated with delusional disorder. Pharmacologic intervention is often based on symptoms. For example, patients with somatic delusions are treated for the specific complaints with which they present. Use of benzodiazepines may be common with this disorder because complaints are vague.

Priority Care Issues

By the time a patient with a diagnosis of delusional disorder is seen in a psychiatric setting, he or she has generally had the delusion for a long time. It is deeply ingrained and many times unshakable even with psychopharmacologic intervention. These patients rarely comply with medication regimens.

Male patients who have the erotomanic subtype are likely to require special care because they are more likely than other patients to act on their delusions (for example, by continued attempts to contact the loved object or stalking). This group is generally seen in forensic settings.

NURSING MANAGEMENT: Human Response to Delusional Disorder

Biologic Domain

Assessment

Body systems are assessed to evaluate any physical problems. In people with somatic delusional disorder, assessment may be tedious because of the number and variety of presenting symptoms. Complaints are explored to develop a complete symptom history and to determine whether symptoms have a physical basis or are delusional. Past history of each complaint should be determined because this information may affect the outcome. The more recent the onset, the more favorable the prognosis.

> **NCLEXNOTE** By definition, delusions are fixed, false beliefs that cannot be changed by reasonable arguments. The nurse should assess the patient's delusion to evaluate its significance to the patient and the patient's safety and the safety of others. The nurse should not dwell on the delusion or try to change it.

Most patients who receive diagnoses of delusional disorder do not experience functional difficulties or impairments. Self-care patterns may be disrupted in patients with the somatic subtype by the elaborate processes used to treat perceived illness (e.g., bathing rituals, creams). Sleep may be disrupted because of the central and overpowering nature of the delusions.

A complete medication history, past and present, is also important to determine the patient's past response and what agents the individual perceives as effective. Examining the patient's records for tests and procedures may help to substantiate the individual's complaints and symptoms.

Nursing Diagnoses for the Biologic Domain

The nursing diagnoses for the biologic domain depend on the type of delusions that are manifested and the response to these symptoms. For example, for a woman with the somatic delusion that insects are crawling on her, Disturbed Sensory Perception (Tactile) would be appropriate. For others who are fearful of poisoning, Imbalanced Nutrition, Less Than Body Requirements, may be a useful diagnosis. Refusal of medication may support a nursing diagnosis of Ineffective Therapeutic Regimen Management.

Interventions for the Biologic Domain

Interventions are based on the problems identified during assessment (Figure 23.4). The nurse helps the patient establish routines that can resolve problems and promote healthy functioning. A mechanism for managing the patient's medication regimen is developed.

Somatic Interventions

Treating somatic disorder is difficult because of the patient's insistence that the problem is not psychiatrically related. Many patients with delusional disorder are seen

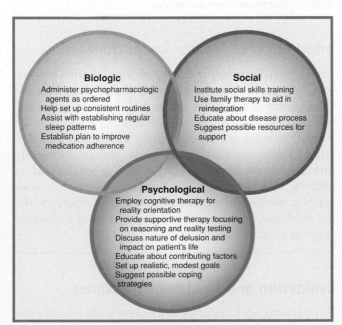

FIGURE 23.4 Biopsychosocial interventions for patients with delusional disorder.

Biologic
Administer psychopharmacologic agents as ordered
Help set up consistent routines
Assist with establishing regular sleep patterns
Establish plan to improve medication adherence

Social
Institute social skills training
Use family therapy to aid in reintegration
Educate about disease process
Suggest possible resources for support

Psychological
Employ cognitive therapy for reality orientation
Provide supportive therapy focusing on reasoning and reality testing
Discuss nature of delusion and impact on patient's life
Educate about contributing factors
Set up realistic, modest goals
Suggest possible coping strategies

only by nonpsychiatric specialists, who use expensive and ineffective treatments. Patients with this disorder may adhere poorly to psychiatric pharmacotherapy, which is most likely related to the lack of insight about their illness (Nose, Barbui, & Tansella, 2003). Realistic and modest goals are most sensible. Establishing a therapeutic relationship is fundamental but far from simple.

Pharmacologic Interventions

Sparse literature is available about using psychiatric medications in delusional disorder. Antipsychotic agents are useful in improving acute symptoms by decreasing agitation and the intensity of the delusion.

Administering and Monitoring Medications
Compliance in this population is problematic. Patients do not adhere to medication regimens and require monitoring of target symptoms. Look for an opportunity to discuss medications and barriers to compliance.

Managing Side Effects
Management of side effects is similar to that in other disorders that have a delusional component. The nurse assesses for neuroleptic malignant syndrome, extrapyramidal side effects, weight gain, and sedation.

Monitoring for Drug Interactions
Interactions are similar to those seen with medications for other disorders. A detailed list of prior and current medications must be elicited from these patients, especially those with somatic delusions because they may be receiving medications from many different practitioners.

Teaching Points
Instruct patients to take medication as prescribed. Determine whether the patient has sufficient resources to purchase and obtain medications and explain target symptoms for each medication. Caution patients not to take over-the-counter medications without consulting their providers.

Psychological Domain

Assessment

Patients with delusional disorder show few if any psychological deficits, and those that do occur are generally related directly to the delusion. In these patients, average or marginally low intelligence is characteristic. Use of the Minnesota Multiphasic Personality Inventory, a clinical scale that identifies paranoid symptom deviation, may be useful in substantiating the diagnosis.

Mental status is not generally affected. Thinking, orientation, affect, attention, memory, perception, and personality are generally intact. Presenting reality-based evidence in an attempt to change the person's delusion can be helpful in determining whether the belief can be altered with sufficient evidence. If mental status is altered, this fact is generally brought to the health professional's attention by a third party. In these cases, the person has usually acted in some manner to draw attention to him- or herself. Talk with the person to grasp the nature of the delusional thinking: theme, impact on the person's life, complexity, systematization, and related features.

Nursing Diagnoses for the Psychological Domain

Numerous nursing diagnoses could be generated based on assessment of the psychological domain. Ineffective Denial, Impaired Verbal Communication, Deficient Knowledge, and Risk for Loneliness are some examples. The nursing diagnoses of Readiness for Enhanced Self-concept, Chronic Low Self-esteem, Anxiety, Fear, and Powerlessness may also be generated.

Interventions for the Psychological Domain

Patients with delusional disorder are treated most effectively in outpatient settings with supportive therapy that allays the person's anxiety. Initiating discussion of the troubling experiences and consequences of the delusion and suggesting a means for coping may be successful. Assisting the person toward a more satisfying general adjustment is desirable (Box 23.6).

Insight-oriented therapy is not useful because there is no benefit in trying to prove the delusion is not true. Cognitive therapy with supportive therapy that focuses on reasoning or reality testing to decrease delusional thinking, or modifying the delusion itself, may be helpful. Educational interventions can aid the patient in understanding how factors such as sensory impairment, social and physical isolation, and stress contribute to the intensity of this disorder.

Social Domain
Assessment

A common characteristic of individuals with delusional disorder is normal behavior and appearance. Ethnic and cultural systems have different beliefs that are accepted within their individual context but not outside their group. Problems can occur in social, occupational, or interpersonal areas. Social function is generally impaired, and social isolation is common among this group. Most are employed, but they generally hold low-level jobs. Many are married.

In general, the person's social and marital functioning is more likely to be impaired than his or her intellectual or occupational functioning.

Assessing the person's capacity to act in response to the delusion is important. What is the person's level of impulsiveness (i.e., related to behaviors of suicide, homicide, aggression, or violence)? Establishing as complete a picture of the person as possible, including the person's subjective private experiences and concrete psychopathologic symptoms, helps to reduce uncertainty in the assessment process.

Nursing Diagnoses for the Social Domain

Several nursing diagnoses can be generated from the assessment data for the social domain. Ineffective Coping, Interrupted Family Processes, and Ineffective Role Performance are examples.

Interventions for the Social Domain

People with diagnoses of delusional disorder often become socially isolated. The secretiveness of their delusions and the importance the delusions have in their life are central to this phenomenon. Social skills training tailored to the patient's specific deficits can help to improve social adaptation. Family therapy can help the person reintegrate into the family; family education and patient education enhance understanding. Families face many of the same issues as families of patients with other disorders involving delusions, but the stress of dealing with this disorder is not as great.

Evaluation and Treatment Outcomes

For patients with delusional disorders, the greater the lack of insight and the poorer the compliance with medication regimens, the more difficult it is to teach

---

BOX 23.6

Psychoeducation Checklist: **Delusional Disorder**

When caring for the patient with delusional disorder, be sure to include the caregiver, as appropriate, and address the following topic areas in the teaching plan:

- Psychopharmacologic agents (antipsychotic or antidepressants), if used, including drug action, dosage, frequency, and possible adverse effects
- Identification of troubling experiences
- Consequences of delusions
- Realistic goal setting
- Positive coping strategies
- Safety measures
- Social training skills
- Family participation in therapy

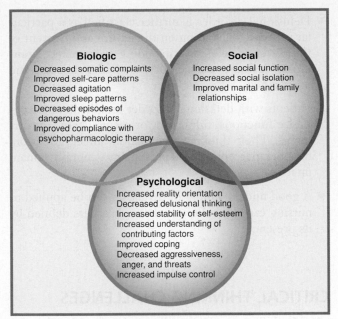

FIGURE 23.5 Biopsychosocial outcomes for patients with delusional disorder.

the individual. Resistance is typical, and the person is not amenable to interventions. The patient rarely, if ever, develops full insight, and the symptoms related to the original diagnosis are not likely to disappear completely. In evaluating progress, the nurse must remember that outcomes are often not met completely. The nurse should maintain realistic outcomes and praise small successes to promote positive outcomes (Figure 23.5).

Continuum of Care

Inpatient-Focused Care

Hospitalization rarely occurs and is usually initiated by the legal or social violations. The hospital environment protects the patient from further legal intervention. Insight-oriented interventions help the patient to understand his or her situation. Avoid confrontational situations; use the patient's coping abilities to reinforce constructive aspects of functioning to enable a return to autonomy.

Emergency Care

Emergency care is seldom required unless the patient has had an incident with the law or legal system.

Family Intervention

Family therapy may be helpful. By helping the family to develop mechanisms to cope with the patient's delusions, nurses help the family to be more supportive and understanding of the patient.

Community Treatment

Patients with diagnoses of delusional disorder are treated most effectively in an outpatient setting. Insight-oriented therapy to develop an understanding of the patient's delusion may be helpful. Medications are not often used with delusional disorder, but antipsychotic agents or benzodiazepines are helpful during exacerbations. Other treatments include supportive therapy, development of coping skills, cognitive therapy, and social skills training. Family therapy may be helpful.

OTHER PSYCHOTIC DISORDERS

Other disorders have psychoses as their defining features. The nursing care of patients with these disorders is not discussed specifically, but the generalist psychiatric nurse has the ability to apply care used with other disorders to the disorders presented here.

Schizophreniform Disorder

The essential features of schizophreniform disorder are identical to those of criteria A for schizophrenia, with the exception of the duration of the illness, which can be less than 6 months. Symptoms must be present for at least 1 month to be classified as a schizophreniform disorder. About one-third of the individuals recover with the other two-thirds developing schizophrenia (APA, 2013).

Altered social or occupational functioning may occur but is not necessary. Most patients experience interruption in one or more areas of daily functioning (APA, 2013).

Brief Psychotic Disorder

In brief psychotic disorder, the length of the episode is at least 1 day but less than 1 month. The onset is sudden and includes at least one of the positive symptoms of criteria A for schizophrenia found in Chapter 22. Differentiating this illness from bipolar SAD is important. The person generally experiences emotional turmoil or overwhelming confusion and rapid, intense shifts of affect (APA, 2013). Although episodes are brief, impairment can be severe, and supervision may be required to protect the person. Suicide is a risk, especially in younger patients. This disorder accounts for 9% of the cases of first onset (APA, 2013).

Psychotic Disorders Attributable to a Substance

Patients with a psychotic disorder attributable to a substance present with prominent hallucinations or delusions that are the direct physiologic effects of a substance (e.g., drug abuse, toxin exposure) (APA, 2013). During intoxication, symptoms continue as long as the use of the substance continues. Withdrawal symptoms can occur for as long as 4 weeks. Differential diagnosis is recommended.

SUMMARY OF KEY POINTS

- Schizoaffective disorder (SAD) has symptoms typical of both schizophrenia and mood disorders but is a separate disorder. Although these patients experience mood problems most of the time, the diagnosis of SAD depends on the presence of positive symptoms (i.e., delusions or hallucinations) and mood symptoms at some time during the uninterrupted period of illness.

- Although controversy and discussion continue about whether SAD is truly a separate disorder, the *DSM-5* currently identifies it as separate.

- Patients with SAD will likely never be medication free.

- Patients with SAD have fewer awareness deficits and appear to have more insight than do patients with true schizophrenia, a fact that can be used in teaching patients to control symptoms, recognize early regression, and develop psychosocial skills.

- Nursing care for patients with SAD is focused on minimizing psychiatric symptoms through promoting medication maintenance and on helping patients maintain optimal levels of functioning. Interventions center on developing social and coping skills through supportive, nurturing, and nonconfrontational approaches. The nurse must be constantly attuned to the mood state of the patient and help the patient learn to solve problems, resolve conflict, and cope with social situations that trigger anxiety.

- Delusional disorder is characterized by fixed, false delusions that could either occur in real life and are plausible in the context of the patient's ethnic and cultural background or are completely implausible. These delusions may or may not interfere with an individual's ability to function socially. Patients typically deny any psychiatric basis for their problem and refuse to seek psychiatric care. Patients whose delusions relate to somatic complaints are often seen in medical-surgical units of hospitals. Diagnosis otherwise is often made only when patients act on the basis of their delusions and violate the law or social rules.

- Delusional disorder is further classified as a particular subtype, depending on the nature and content of the patient's delusions, including erotomanic, grandiose, jealous, persecutory, somatic, mixed, and unspecified.

- Patients with delusional disorder usually do not experience functional difficulties or mental status impairments. Their thinking, orientation, affect, attention, memory, perception, and personality generally remain intact.

- A good understanding of psychoses can be applied to nursing care for other psychotic disorders defined by its presence.

CRITICAL THINKING CHALLENGES

1. Mr. J first received a diagnosis of schizophrenia, but after experiencing extreme mood disturbances, he finally received a diagnosis of SAD. During a recent outpatient visit, he confides to a nurse that he just has stress and does not think that he really has any psychiatric problems. Identify assessment areas that should be pursued before the patient leaves his appointment. How would you confront the denial?

2. Ms. S believed that she had bipolar disorder. At a recent clinic visit, she was told that she most probably had schizoaffective disorder. The patient asked the nurse how a bipolar disorder could turn into schizoaffective disorder. Identify three appropriate responses to her question.

3. A patient with schizoaffective disorder is prescribed an antipsychotic agent (Risperdal) and a mood stabilizer (Depakote). The patient asks you why both medications are needed. Develop the best response for this question. Be thorough.

4. At an interdisciplinary treatment team meeting, the nurse recommends that a woman with schizoaffective disorder attend an anger management group. The rest of the team believes that only a mood stabilizer is needed. Develop the rationale for attending the anger management group in addition to medication supplementation.

5. A patient was prescribed olanzapine (Zyprexa) and an antidepressant (Lexapro) for the treatment of schizoaffective disorder. Since her last monthly visit, she gained 15 pounds. She is considering discontinuing her medication regimen because of the weight gain. Develop a plan to address her weight gain and her intention to discontinue her medication regimen.

6. Patient A has received a diagnosis of schizoaffective disorder, and patient B has received a diagnosis of delusional disorder. How would the symptoms differ? Would there be any similarities? If so, what would they be?

7. Identify and explain each of the subtypes of delusional disorder.

8. An older adult in a nursing home has a delusion that her husband is having an affair with her sister. Discuss nonpharmacologic nursing interventions that should be implemented with this patient. How would you explain her delusion to her husband? Choose one of the subtypes of delusion and develop a plan for clinical management, focusing on psychiatric nursing care, for a patient experiencing this condition.

9. A patient convincingly informs you that she is having an affair with a famous actor. They both attended the same college about the same time. How would you determine if this patient's belief is a delusion or reality? Is it important that the nurse understand whether the relationship is real? Explain the rationale for your answer.

10. A patient informs a student nurse that he is a member of the Secret Service and that he is undercover. He asks the nurse to keep the secret. The student considers several possible responses, including redirecting the patient to a different topic and confronting him with the reality of his hospitalization. Discuss the best response to this patient's comment.

Misery: 1990. This movie stars James Caan as Paul Sheldon and Kathy Bates as Annie Wilkes. Sheldon is the writer of a popular mystery series who finishes his last novel in a secluded cabin in Colorado. After being rescued in a blizzard by Annie Wilkes, he becomes her prisoner when she prevents him from leaving his cabin. Annie is in love with him but is demanding and possessive. She identifies with the heroine in his latest novel and is outraged with the conclusion of the novel.

SIGNIFICANCE: Annie demonstrates the thinking patterns associated with delusional disorder.

VIEWING POINTS: Identify the disturbed thinking that Annie demonstrates. Part of Annie's behavior seems normal, and other behaviors are illogical. How are they linked?

References

Abi-Dargham, A., & Meyer, J. M. (2014). Schizophrenia: The role of dopamine and glutamate. *The Journal of Clinical Psychiatry.* doi:10.4088/JCP.13078co7c

American Psychiatric Association. (1980). *Diagnostic and statistical manual of mental disorders* (3rd ed.). Washington, DC: Author.

American Psychiatric Association. (2013). *Diagnostic and statistical manual of mental disorders* (5th ed.). Arlington, VA: Author.

Anglin, D. M., & Malaspina, D. (2008). Ethnicity effects on clinical diagnoses compared to best-estimate research diagnoses in patients with psychosis: A retrospective medical chart review. *Journal of Clinical Psychiatry, 69*(6), 941–945.

Arehart-Treichel, J. (2004). Delusions linked to brain region, but why? *Psychiatric News, 39*(19), 21.

Bentall, R. P., Corcoran, R., Howard, R., Blackwood, N., & Kinderman, P. (2001). Persecutory delusions: A review and theoretical integration. *Clinical Psychology Review, 21*(8), 1143–1192.

Bolton, J. M., & Robinson, J. (2010). Population-attributable fractions of Axis I and Axis II mental disorders for suicide attempts: Findings from a representative sample of the adult, noninstitutionalized US population. *American journal of public health, 100*(12) 2473–2480.

Bora, E., Yucel, M., & Pantelis, C. (2009). Cognitive functioning in schizophrenia, schizoaffective disorder and affective psychoses: Meta-analytic study. *British Journal of Psychiatry, 195*(6), 475–482.

González-Rodríguez, A., Molina-Andreu, O., Navarro, V., Gastó, C., Penadés, R., & Catalán, R. (2014). Delusional disorder: No gender differences in age at onset, suicidal ideation, or suicidal behavior. *Revista Brasileira de Psiquiatria.* doi:10.1590/1516-4446-2013-1205

Hartz, S. M., Pato, C. N., Medeiros, H., Cavazos-Rehg, P., Sobell, J. L., Knowles, J. A., et al. (2014). Comorbidity of severe psychotic disorders with measures of substance use. *JAMA Psychiatry, 71*(3), 248–254.

Huuhka, K., Viikki, M., Tammentie, T., Tuohimaa, K., Björkqvist, M., Alanen, H., et al. (2012). One-year follow-up after discontinuing maintenance electroconvulsive therapy. *Journal of ECT, 28*(4), 225–228.

Kantrowitz, J., & Citrome, L. (2011). Schizoaffective disorder. A review of current research themes and pharmacological management. *CNS Drugs, 25*(4), 317–331.

Kasanin, J. (1933). The acute schizo-affective psychoses. *American Journal of Psychiatry, 13,* 97–126.

Kovacs, A., Voros, V., & Fekete, S. (2005). Suicide attempt and melancholic depression in a male with erotomania: Case report. *Archives of Suicide Research, 9*(4), 369–372.

MacKinnon, K., Newman-Taylor, K., & Stopa, L. (2011). Persecutory delusions and the self: An investigation of implicit and explicit self-esteem. *Journal of Behavior Therapy and Experimental Psychiatry, 42*(1), 54–64.

Malhi, F. S. (2013). Making up schizoaffective disorder: Cosmet changes to a sad creation. *Australian & New Zealand Journal of Psychiatry, 47*(10), 891–894.

Marneros, A., Pillmann, F., & Wustmann, T. (2012). Delusional disorders — Are they simply paranoid schizophrenia? *Schizophrenia Bulletin, 38*(3), 561–568.

McCutcheon, L. E., Ashe, D. D., Houran, J., & Maltby, J. (2003). A cognitive profile of individuals who tend to worship celebrities. *The Journal of Psychology, 137*(4), 309–322.

Misdrahi, D., Denard, S., Swendsen, J., Jaussent, I., & Courtet, P. (2014). *Psychiatry Research,* http://dx.doi.org/10.1016/j.psychres.2014.01.039

Möller, H. J., Jäger, M., Riedel, M., Obermeier, M., Strauss, A., & Bottlender, R. (2010). The Munich 15-year follow-up study (MUFUSSAD) on first-hospitalized patients with schizophrenic or affective disorders: Comparison of psychopathological and psychosocial course and outcome and prediction of chronicity. *European Archives of Psychiatry & Clinical Neuroscience, 260*(5), 367–384.

Nair, A., Palmer, E. C., Aleman, A., & David, A. S. (2014). Relationship between cognition, clinical and cognitive insight in psychotic disorders: A review and meta-analysis. *Schizophrenia Research, 152*(1), 191–200.

Nose, M., Barbui, C., & Tansella, M. (2003). How often do patients with psychosis fail to adhere to treatment programmes? A systematic review. *Psychological Medicine, 33*(7), 1149–1160.

Ota, M., Mizukami, K., Katano, T., Sato, S., Takeda, T., & Asada, T. (2003). A case of delusional disorder, somatic type with remarkable improvement of clinical symptoms and single photon emission computed tomography findings following modified electroconvulsive therapy. *Progress in Neuro-psychopharmacology & Biological Psychiatry, 27*(5), 881–884.

Pompili, M. 1., Serafini, G., Innamorati, M., Lester, D., Shrivastava, A., Girardi, P., et al. (2011). Suicide risk in first episode psychosis: A selective review of the current literature. *Schizophrenia Research, 129*(1), 1–11.

Reutfors, J., Bahmanyar, S., Jönsson, E. G., Ekbom, A., Nordström, P., Brandt, L., et al. (2010). Diagnostic profile and suicide risk in schizophrenia spectrum disorder. *Schizophrenia Research, 123*(2–3), 251–256.

Roche, E., Madigan, K., Lyne, J. P., Feeney, L., & O'Donoghue, B. (2014). The therapeutic relationship after psychiatric admission. *The Journal of Nervous and Mental Disease, 202*(3), 186–192.

Rosenfeld, B. (2003). Recidivism in stalking and obsessional harassment. *Law & Human Behavior, 27*(3), 251–265.

Takahashi, T., Wood, S. J., Soulsby, B., Kawasaki, Y., McGorry, P. D., Suzuki, M., et al. (2009). An MRI study of the superior temporal subregions in first-episode patients. *Schizophrenia Research, 113*(2), 158–166.

Vieta, E. (2010). Developing an individualized treatment plan for patients with schizoaffective disorders: From pharmacotherapy to psychoeducation. *Journal of Clinical Psychiatry, 71*(suppl 2), 14–19.

Wiener, H., Klei, L., Calkins, M., Wood, J., Nimgaonkar, V., Gur, R., et al. (2013). Principal components of heritability from neurocognitive domains differ between families with schizophrenia and control subjects. *Schizophrenia Bulletin, 39*(2), 464–471.

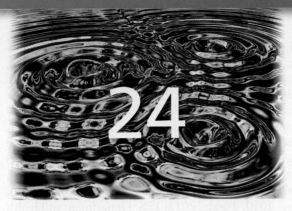

24

Depression
Management of Depressive Moods and Suicidal Behavior

Barbara Jones Warren

KEY CONCEPTS

- depression
- mood
- mood disorders
- suicidal behavior

LEARNING OBJECTIVES

After studying this chapter, you will be able to:

1. Describe the prevalence and incidence of depressive disorders and suicide within American society.

2. Delineate the clinical symptoms and course of depressive disorders and suicidal behavior.

3. Analyze the biopsychosocial theories of depressive disorders and suicidal behavior.

4. Assess the human responses to depressive disorders.

5. Formulate nursing diagnoses with recovery-oriented strategies, interventions, and evaluative approaches that address the cultural needs of persons diagnosed with depressive disorders and for those who exhibit suicidal behavior.

KEY TERMS

- affect • anhedonia • depressive disorder • depression not otherwise specified • persistent dysthymic disorder
- major depressive episodes • mood episode

Most people have bad days or times of feeling sad and overwhelmed. When depressed feelings interfere with daily activities and relationships, this mood can impair judgment and contribute to negative views of the world. In some instances, depression is a symptom of a depressive disorder. This chapter discusses the concept of depressive moods and disorders and the related serious issue of suicidal behavior.

OVERVIEW OF MOOD AND DEPRESSION

> **KEYCONCEPT** **Mood** is a pervasive and sustained emotion that influences one's perception of the world and how one functions.

Normal variations in mood occur in response to life events. Normal mood variations, such as sadness, euphoria, and anxiety, are time limited and are not usually associated with significant functional impairment. Normal range of mood or **affect**, the expression of mood, varies considerably both within and among different cultures (Pedersen, Draguus, Lonner, & Trimble, 2008; Purnell, 2012; Rosenquist, Fowler, & Christakis, 2011; Warren, 2012, 2011a; Warren & Broome, 2011). Several terms are used to describe affect or outward emotional expression, including the following:

- *Blunted:* significantly reduced intensity of emotional expression
- *Flat:* absent or nearly absent affective expression
- *Inappropriate:* discordant affective expression accompanying the content of speech or ideation

- *Labile:* varied, rapid, and abrupt shifts in affective expression
- *Restricted or constricted:* mildly reduced in the range and intensity of emotional expression

When a mood interferes with daily life, a mood disorder may exist that will benefit from treatment. Mood disorders are diagnosed if there is a **mood episode**, a severe mood change that lasts at least 2 weeks that causes clinically significant distress or impairment. According to the current DSM-5 (American Psychiatric Association [APA], 2013) depression and other categories of depression are now discussed as a stand-alone diagnostic category labeled depressive disorders. Earlier versions of the DSM discussed depression in the same diagnostic category as bipolar disorders (APA, 2013). There are a number of subdiagnostic categories within major depressive disorders. These consist of disruptive mood dysregulation, persistent depressive (dysthymia), premenstrual dysphoric, substance/medication-induced, other specified depressive and unspecified depressive disorders (APA, 2013). This chapter focuses on depressive disorders; Chapter 25 presents bipolar disorders.

Depression is the primary mood of depressive disorders. Depression can be overwhelming. Unless appropriately treated, depression persists over time, has a significant negative effect on quality of life, and increases the risk of suicide.

> **KEYCONCEPT** **Depression** is a common mental state characterized by sadness, loss of interest or pleasure, feelings of guilt or low self-worth, disturbed sleep or appetite, low energy, and poor concentration (APA, 2013; McEnany, 2011; World Health Organization [WHO], 2014).

DEPRESSIVE DISORDERS

The primary symptoms of **depressive disorders** include sad, empty, or irritable mood with somatic and cognitive changes. There are several types of depressive disorders which are differentiated by duration, timing, and causes (APA, 2013). Major depressive disorder is highlighted in this chapter. The clinical symptoms and course of depressive phenomena are complex, dynamic biopsychosocial processes involving life span and cultural aspects. Persons with depressive disorders experience a lower quality of life and are at greater risk for development of physical health problems than those who are not depressed. Depressive disorders are so widespread that they are mostly diagnosed and treated in the primary care setting. Every nurse will have an opportunity to impact this pandemic health concern (WHO, 2014).

Depressive disorders are characterized by severe and debilitating depressive episodes. Depressive disorders are associated with high levels of impairment in occupational, social, and physical functioning and cause as much disability and distress to patients as chronic medical disorders. Frequently, they are undetected and untreated. Because suicide is a significant risk, these disorders are associated with premature death. The incidence of misdiagnosis is often greater for persons who are treated by someone from culturally and ethnically different populations because their explanation of their symptomatology may be expressed using different terminology than used persons who are not from these populations (Munoz, Primm, Ananth, & Ruiz, 2007; Tsai, Lin, Chang, Chang, & Chou, 2010; Tusaie, 2013; U.S. Department of Health and Human Services [U.S. DHHS], 2001).

Clinical Course

Major depressive disorder is commonly a progressive, recurrent illness. With time, episodes tend to occur more frequently, become more severe, and are of a longer duration. The onset of depression may occur at any age. However, the initial onset may occur in puberty; the highest onset occurs within persons within their 20s (APA, 2013). Reoccurrences of depression are related to age of onset, increased intensity and severity of symptoms and presence of psychosis, anxiety, and/or personality features. The risk for relapse is higher in persons who experienced initial symptoms at a younger age and incur other mental disorders (Warren, in press).

Diagnostic Criteria

The primary diagnostic criterion for major depressive disorder is one or more **major depressive episodes**, which is either a depressed mood or a loss of interest or pleasure in nearly all activities for at least 2 weeks. Four of seven additional symptoms must be present: disruption in sleep, appetite (or weight), concentration, or energy; psychomotor agitation or retardation; excessive guilt or feelings of worthlessness; and suicidal ideation (Key Diagnostic Characteristics 24.1). Individuals often describe themselves as depressed, sad, hopeless, discouraged, or "down in the dumps." If individuals complain of feeling "blah," having no feelings, constantly tired, or feeling anxious, a depressed mood can sometimes be inferred from their facial expression and demeanor (APA, 2013). The current DSM-5 lists **persistent depressive disorder (dysthymic disorder)** as a long duration mood disorder that has a lower intensity of depressive symptomatology (APA, 2013).

Depressive Disorders Across the Life Span
Children and Adolescents

Children with depressive disorders have similar symptoms to those seen in adults with a few exceptions. They are more likely to have anxiety symptoms, such as fear of separation, and somatic symptoms, such as stomach aches

296.2X MAJOR DEPRESSIVE DISORDER, SINGLE EPISODE
296.3X MAJOR DEPRESSIVE DISORDER, RECURRENT

Diagnostic Criteria

A. Five (or more) of the following symptoms have been present during the same 2-week period and represent a change from previous functioning; at least one of the symptoms is either (1) depressed mood or (2) loss of interest or pleasure.
  • **Note:** Do not include symptoms that are clearly attributable to another medical condition.
  1. Depressed mood most of the day, nearly every day, as indicated by either subjective report (e.g., feels sad, empty, hopeless) or observation made by others (e.g., appears tearful). (**Note:** In children and adolescents, can be irritable mood.)
  2. Markedly diminished interest or pleasure in all, or almost all, activities most of the day, nearly every day (as indicated by either subjective account or observation).
  3. Significant weight loss when not dieting or weight gain (e.g., a change of more than 5% of body weight in a month), or decrease or increase in appetite nearly every day. (**Note:** In children, consider failure to make expected weight gain.)
  4. Insomnia or hypersomnia nearly every day.
  5. Psychomotor agitation or retardation nearly every day (observable by others, not merely subjective feelings of restlessness or being slowed down).
  6. Fatigue or loss of energy nearly every day.
  7. Feelings of worthlessness or excessive or inappropriate guilt (which may be delusional) nearly every day (not merely self-reproach or guilt about being sick).
  8. Diminished ability to think or concentrate, or indecisiveness, nearly every day (either by subjective account or as observed by others).
  9. Recurrent thoughts of death (not just fear of dying), recurrent suicidal ideation without a specific plan, or a suicide attempt or a specific plan for committing suicide.
B. The symptoms cause clinically significant distress or impairment in social, occupational, or other important areas of functioning.
C. The episode is not attributable to the physiological effects of a substance or to another medical condition.

Note: Criteria A–C represent a major depressive episode.
Note: Responses to a significant loss (e.g., bereavement, financial ruin, losses from a natural disaster, a serious medical illness or disability) may include the feelings of intense sadness, rumination about the loss, insomnia, poor appetite, and weight loss noted in Criterion A, which may resemble a depressive episode. Although such symptoms may be understandable or considered appropriate to the loss, the presence of a major depressive episode in addition to the normal response to a significant loss should also be carefully considered. This decision inevitably requires the exercise of clinical judgment based on the individual's history and the cultural norms for the expression of distress in the context of loss.
D. The occurrence of the major depressive episode is not better explained by schizoaffective disorder, schizophrenia, schizophreniform disorder, delusional disorder, or other specified and unspecified schizophrenia spectrum and other psychotic disorders.
E. There has never been a manic episode or a hypomanic episode.
  • **Note:** This exclusion does not apply if all of the manic-like or hypomanic-like episodes are substance-induced or are attributable to the physiological effects of another medical condition.

Associated Findings
• Tearfulness, irritability, brooding, obsessive rumination, anxiety, phobias, excessive worry over physical health, and complaints of pain
• Possible panic attacks
• Difficulty with intimate relationships
• Difficulties with sexual functioning
• Marital problems
• Occupational problems
• Substance abuse, such as alcohol
• High mortality rate; death by suicide
• Increased pain and physical illness
• Decreased physical, social, and role functioning
• May be preceded by dysthymic disorder

and headaches. They may have less interaction with their peers and avoid play and recreational activities that they previously enjoyed. Mood may be irritable, rather than sad, especially in adolescents. The risk of suicide, which peaks during the midadolescent years, is very real in children and adolescents. Mortality from suicide, which increases steadily through the teens, is the third leading cause of death for that age group. Findings from research indicate that deaths caused by illegal drug use and automobile crashes may be the outcome of adolescent depression and suicidal ideation (Dulcan & Lake, 2012; Liehr & Diaz, 2010; Warren, in press). Disruptive mood dysregulation disorder is a new depressive disorder diagnostic category in the DSM-5.

Older Adults

Most older patients with symptoms of depression do not meet the full criteria for major depression. However, it is estimated that 8% to 20% of older adults in the community and as many as 37% in primary care settings experience depressive symptoms. Treatment is successful in 60% to 80%, but response to treatment is slower than in younger adults. Depression in older adults often is associated with chronic illnesses, such as heart disease, stroke, and cancer; symptoms may have a more somatic focus. Depressive symptomatology in this group may be confused with symptoms of dementia or cerebrovascular accidents. Hence, differential diagnosis may be required to ascertain the root and cause of symptoms. Suicide is a very serious risk for older adults, especially men. People older than 65 years have the highest suicide rates of any age group. There is a greater likelihood of death during or after a suicide attempt in older adults. In those 85 years and older, the suicide rate is the highest, at 21 suicides per 100,000 persons (Blazer & Steffens, 2009).

Epidemiology and Risk Factors

The prevalence of major depressive disorder within the United States population is approximately 7% within a 12-month time period. Individuals between the ages of 18 and 29 years have a three times higher prevalence rate than those persons aged 60 and older (APA, 2013). The prevalence rates for females and males differ with females experiencing "a 1.5- to 3-fold higher rate than males beginning in early adolescence" (APA, 2013, p. 165). The recurrence of major depressive disorder is contingent upon the severity and persistence of symptoms, younger age of initial occurrence, and presence of comorbid psychiatric illness (APA, 2013; Josey & Neidert, 2013; Tarraza, 2013). An estimated 17 million Americans experience a depressive disorder on an annual basis.

Data from the WHO indicate that depression is the leading cause of years lost because of disability. More than 50% of persons who recover from an initial episode of depression experience another episode within 5 to 10 years (WHO, 2014).

Risk factors for the development of depression include the following:

- Prior episode of depression
- Family history of depressive disorder
- Lack of social support
- Lack of coping abilities
- Presence of life and environmental stressors
- Current substance use or abuse
- Medical and/or mental illness comorbidity

Age of Onset and Gender

The mean age of onset for major depressive disorder is about 40 years; 50% of all patients have an onset between the ages of 20 and 50 years. During a 20-year period, the mean number of episodes is five or six. Symptoms usually develop during a period of days to months. About 50% of patients have significant depressive symptoms before the first identified episode. An untreated episode typically lasts 6 to 13 months, regardless of the age of onset.

It appears that the chances of experiencing major depressive disorder are increasing in progressively younger age groups. Major depressive disorder is twice as common in adolescent and adult women as in adolescent and adult men. Prepubertal boys and girls are equally affected (National Institutes of Mental Health [NIMH], 2009).

Ethnicity and Culture

Prevalence rates of depressive disorders are unrelated to race. Culture can influence the experience and communication of symptoms of depression. Persons from culturally and ethnically diverse populations may formulate and describe their depressive symptomatology differently than the clinical language used for diagnosis. For example, expressions such as "heartbrokenness" (Native American and Middle Eastern), "brain fog" (persons from the West Indies), "zar," and "running amok" may be used in place of such terms as "depressed," "sad," "hopeless," and "discouraged" (Beeber, Lewis, Cooper, Maxwell, & Sandelowski, 2010; Herrera, Lawson, Sramek, 1999; Warren, 2013a, 2013b, 2013c; Warren & Lutz, 2007).

In some cultures, somatic symptoms, rather than sadness or guilt, may predominate. Individuals from various Asian cultural groups may have complaints of weakness, tiredness, or imbalance. "Problems of the heart" (in Middle Eastern cultures) or of being "heartbroken" (among Hopi Indians) may be the way that persons from these cultural groups express their depressive experiences. Culturally distinctive experiences need to be assessed to ascertain any presence of depressive disorder from a "normal" cultural emotional response (Munoz et al., 2007; Pedersen et al., 2008).

Comorbidity

Major depressive disorders often co-occur with other psychiatric disorders including substance-related ones. Depression often is associated with a variety of medical conditions, particularly endocrine disorders, cardiovascular disease, neurologic disorders, autoimmune conditions, viral or other infectious diseases, certain cancers, and nutritional deficiencies, or as a direct physiologic effect of a substance (e.g., a drug of abuse, a medication, other somatic treatment for depression, or toxin exposure) (Gonzales, Vega, Williams, Tarraf, West, & Neighbors, 2010). Grief and bereavement represent a very different combination of symptoms than major depression. The former conditions are associated with emptiness and loss while major depression is associated with ongoing emptiness, loss, and anhedonia (APA, 2013).

Etiology
Biologic Theories
Genetic

Family, twin, and adoption studies demonstrate that genetic influences undoubtedly play a substantial role in the etiology of mood disorders. Major depressive disorder is more common among first-degree biologic relatives of people with this disorder than among the general population. Currently, a major research effort is focusing on developing a more accurate paradigm regarding the contribution of genetic factors to the development of mood disorders (Shi et al., 2011).

Neurobiologic Hypotheses

Neurobiologic theories of the etiology of depression emerged in the 1950s. These theories posit that major depression is caused by a deficiency or dysregulation in central nervous system (CNS) concentrations of the neurotransmitters norepinephrine, dopamine, and serotonin or in their receptor functions. These hypotheses arose in part from observations that some pharmacologic agents elevated mood, and subsequent studies identified their mechanisms of action. All antidepressants currently available have their therapeutic effects on these neurotransmitters or receptors. Current research focuses on the synthesis, storage, release, and uptake of these neurotransmitters, as well as on postsynaptic events (e.g., second-messenger systems) (Stahl, 2013a, 2013b; Yudofsky & Hales, 2010).

Neuroendocrine and Neuropeptide Hypotheses

Major depressive disorder is associated with multiple endocrine alterations, specifically of the hypothalamic–pituitary–adrenal axis, the hypothalamic–pituitary–thyroid axis, the hypothalamic–growth hormone axis, and the hypothalamic–pituitary–gonadal axis. In addition, mounting evidence indicates that components of neuroendocrine axes (e.g., neuromodulatory peptides such as corticotropin-releasing factor) may themselves contribute to depressive symptoms. Evidence also suggests that the secretion of these hypothalamic and growth hormones is controlled by many of the neurotransmitters implicated in the pathophysiology of depression (Stahl, 2013a; Yudofsky & Hales, 2010).

Psychoneuroimmunology

Psychoneuroimmunology is a recent area of research into a diverse group of proteins known as *chemical messengers* between immune cells. These messengers, called cytokines, signal the brain and serve as mediators between immune and nerve cells. The brain is capable of influencing immune processes, and conversely, immunologic response can result in changes in brain activity (Shi et al., 2011; Yudofsky & Hales, 2010). The specific role of these mechanisms in psychiatric disease pathogenesis remains unknown.

Psychological Theories

Psychodynamic Factors

Most psychodynamic theorists acknowledge some debt to Freud's original conceptualization of the psychodynamics of depression, which ascribes the etiology to an early lack of love, care, warmth, and protection and resultant anger, guilt, helplessness, and fear regarding the loss of love. The ensuing conflict between wanting to be loved and fear of rejection engenders pathologic self-

punitiveness (also conceptualized as aggression turned inward), self-rejection, low self-esteem, and depressive symptoms (see Chapter 7).

Behavioral Factors

The behaviorists hold that depression occurs primarily as the result of a severe reduction in rewarding activities or an increase in unpleasant events in one's life. The resultant depression then leads to further restriction of activity, thereby decreasing the likelihood of experiencing pleasurable activities, which, in turn, intensifies the mood disturbance.

Cognitive Factors

The cognitive approach maintains that irrational beliefs and negative distortions of thought about the self, the environment, and the future engender and perpetuate depressive effects (see Chapter 7).

Developmental Factors

Developmental theorists posit that depression may be the result of loss of a parent through death or separation or lack of emotionally adequate parenting. These factors may delay or prohibit the realization of appropriate developmental milestones.

Social Theories

Family Factors

Family theorists ascribe maladaptive patterns in family interactions and as contributing to the onset of depression particularly in the onset and occurrence of depression in younger individuals (Warren, in press). See Chapter 14.

Social Factors

Depression has long been understood as a multifactorial disorder that occurs when environmental factors (e.g., death of family member) interact with the biologic and psychological makeup of the individual. Major depression may follow adverse or traumatic life events, especially those that involve the loss of an important human relationship or role in life. Social isolation, deprivation, and financial deprivation are risk factors (APA, 2013). Recent evidence suggests that depression in one person is associated with similar symptoms in friends, coworkers, siblings, spouses, and neighbors. Female friends seem to be especially influential in the spread of depression from one friend to another (Rosenquist et al., 2011).

Family Response to Disorder

Depression in one member affects the whole family. Spouses, children, parents, siblings, and friends experience frustration, guilt, and anger when a family member is immobilized and cannot function. It is often hard for others to understand the depth of the mood and how disabling it can be. Financial hardship can occur when the family member cannot go to work and spends days in bed. The lack of understanding and difficulty of living with a depressed person can lead to abuse. Women between the ages of 18 and 45 years constitute the majority of those experiencing depression. This incidence may affect women's ability to not only have productive lives and take care of themselves but to also take care of their children or other family members they may have responsibility for. Moreover, research indicates that the incidence of depression may be higher in children whose mothers experience depression (Lutz & Warren, 2007; U.S. DHHS, 2001; Warren & Lutz, 2007).

Interdisciplinary Treatment

Although depressive disorders are the most commonly occurring mental disorders, they are usually treated within the primary care setting, not the psychiatric setting. Individuals with depression enter mental health settings when their symptoms become so severe that hospitalization is needed, usually for suicide attempts, or if they self-refer because of incapacitation. Interdisciplinary treatment of these disorders, which is often lifelong, needs to include a wide array of health professionals in all areas. The specific goals of treatment are:

- Reduce or control symptoms and, if possible, eliminate signs and symptoms of the depressive syndrome.
- Improve occupational and psychosocial function as much as possible.
- Reduce the likelihood of relapse and recurrence through recovery-oriented strategies.

Priority Care Issues

The overriding concern for people with mood disorders is safety because these individuals may experience self-destructive thoughts and suicidal ideations. Hence, the assessment of possible suicide risk should be routinely conducted in any person who is incurring depressive symptomatology (see Chapter 21).

NURSING MANAGEMENT: Human Response to Depressive Disorder

An awareness of the risk factors for depression, a comprehensive and culturally competent biopsychosocial assessment, history of illness, and past treatment are key to formulating a treatment or recovery plan and to evaluating outcomes (Nursing Care Plan 24.1). Interviewing a family member or close friend about the patient's day-to-day functioning and specific symptoms may be helpful in determining the course of the illness, current symptoms, and level of functioning.

Biologic Domain
Assessment

Because some symptoms of depression are similar to those of some medical problems or side effects of medication therapies, biologic assessment must include a physical systems review and thorough history of medical problems, with special attention to CNS function, endocrine function, anemia, chronic pain, autoimmune illness, diabetes, or menopause. Additional medical history includes surgeries; medical hospitalizations; head injuries; episodes of loss of consciousness; and pregnancies, childbirths, miscarriages, and abortions. A complete list of prescribed and over-the-counter medications should be compiled, including the reason a medication was prescribed or its use discontinued. A physical examination is recommended with baseline vital signs and baseline laboratory tests, including a comprehensive blood chemistry panel, complete blood counts, liver function tests, thyroid function tests, urinalysis, and electrocardiograms (Chapter 10). Biologic assessment also includes evaluating the patient for the characteristic neurovegetative symptoms listed below.

> **NCLEXNOTE** In determining severity of depressive symptoms, nursing assessment should explore physical changes in appetite and sleep patterns and decreased energy. And considering the possibility of suicide should always be a priority with patients who are depressed. Assessment and documentation of suicide risk should always be included in patient care.

- *Appetite and weight changes:* In major depression, changes from baseline include a decrease or increase in appetite with or without significant weight loss or gain (i.e., a change of more than 5% of body weight in 1 month). Weight loss occurs when the person not dieting. Older adults with moderate to severe depression need to be assessed for dehydration as well as weight changes.
- *Sleep disturbance:* The most common sleep disturbance associated with major depression is insomnia which is categorized according to three categories: initial insomnia (difficulty falling asleep), middle insomnia (waking up during the night and having difficulty returning to sleep), and terminal insomnia (waking too early and being unable to return to sleep). Less frequently, the sleep disturbance is hypersomnia (prolonged sleep episodes at night or increased daytime sleep). The individual with either insomnia or hypersomnia complains of not feeling rested upon awakening.
- *Decreased energy, tiredness, and fatigue:* Fatigue associated with depression is a subjective experience of feeling tired regardless of how much sleep or physical activity a person has had. Even the smallest tasks require substantial effort.

> **NCLEXNOTE** Remember the three major assessment categories listed above. A question may state several patient symptoms and expect the student to recognize that the patient being described is depressed.

NURSING CARE PLAN 24.1

The Patient With Depressive Disorder

BC is a 55-year-old man who lost his wife to cancer 18 months ago. Since his wife's death, he continued to live in their family home with his dog. His dog died 2 weeks ago, and he has been despondent since then. His children found him sitting on the side of his bed with a loaded gun. He had already written a note that he did not want to be a burden and that his children would be better off without him. His family brought him to the emergency department for evaluation.

Setting: Intensive Care Psychiatric Unit in a General Hospital

Baseline Assessment: BC looks older than his stated age of 55 years. He is dressed in wrinkled clothes, has a slight body odor, and needs a shave. He says that his life was over when his wife died and he was just hanging around to take care of the dog. He has two grown children living in the area and several friends from his local church. He denies any health problems. According to his children, he received treatment for depression 10 years ago after the traumatic death of a son who was deployed in Iraq. He reports that he is not hungry and has lost 10 pounds in the past month. He also reports he has been unable to sleep through the night since his wife died. He denies using substances.

Associated Psychiatric Diagnosis	Medications
Diagnostic features: Sadness, suicidal ideation, loss of weight, sleep disruption Other conditions for focus of clinical attention: Recent loss of wife, 10 years ago had depression episode after death of son who was deployed to Iraq Principal diagnosis: Major depressive disorder, recurrent, moderate to severe symptoms	Escitalopram (Lexapro) 20 mg/day

Nursing Diagnosis 1: Risk for Suicide

Defining Characteristics	Related Factors
Attempts to inflict life-threatening injury to self Feelings of hopelessness Expresses desire to die Lethal means available	Single male Recently lost wife Believes he is a burden to family

Outcomes

Initial	Discharge
1. Remain free from self-harm. 2. Identify factors that led to suicidal intent and methods for managing suicidal impulses if they return. 3. Accept treatment of depression by trying the SSRI antidepressants.	1. Agrees to continue with outpatient therapy. 2. Agrees to take antidepressant. 3. Agrees that family can remove gun(s) from home.

Interventions

Interventions	Rationale	Ongoing Assessment
Initiate a nurse–patient relationship by demonstrating an acceptance of BC as a worthwhile human being through the use of nonjudgmental statements and behavior.	A sense of worthlessness often underlies suicide ideation. The positive therapeutic relationship can support hopefulness.	Assess the stages of the relationship and determine whether a therapeutic relationship is actually being formed. Identify indicators of trust.
Initiate suicide precautions per hospital policy.	Safety of the individual is a priority with people who have suicide ideation (see Chapter 21).	Determine intent to harm self—plan and means.
Discuss with the family members removal of lethal weapons from home.	Suicidal behavior is often impulsive. Removing means of suicide may prevent persons from acting on impulsive thoughts.	Follow-up with the patient and family member about removing lethal weapons.

Continued

NURSING CARE PLAN 24.1 *(Continued)*

Evaluation

Outcomes	Revised Outcomes	Interventions
Has not harmed self.	Identify strategies to resist suicide attempts in the future.	Discuss antecedents that led to the suicide attempt. Discuss initiation of an antidepressant.

Nursing Diagnosis 2: Hopelessness

Defining Characteristics	Related Factors
Decreased affect Decreased appetite Insomnia Lack of initiative States he has no reason to live	Loss of wife Loss of dog Loss of son

Outcomes

Initial	Discharge
Accept support through the nurse–patient relationship. Identify hopelessness as a pervasive feeling.	Express feelings of being hopeful for the future.

Interventions

Interventions	Rationale	Ongoing Assessment
Establish a trusting therapeutic relationship. Enhance BC's sense of hope by being attentive, validating your interpretation of what is being said or experienced, and helping him verbalize what she is expressing nonverbally. Assist to reframe and redefine negative statements ("not a burden but missing your wife"). Participate in a recovery group focusing on hope.	Therapeutic relationships are effective in instilling hope. By showing respect for the patient as a human being who is worth listening to, the nurse can support and help build the patient's sense of self. Reframing an event positively rather than negatively can help the patient view the situation in an alternative way. Group support can be very effective in discussing hope and identifying strategies to establish hopefulness.	Observe verbal and nonverbal cues that increase communications. Determine whether the patient confirms interpretation of situation and if he can verbalize what he is expressing nonverbally. Assess whether BC is feeling more hopeful. Determine if the patient is attending group sessions and participating in discussions.

Evaluation

Outcomes	Revised Outcomes	Interventions
Able to discuss future events in a positive manner. Attending recovery group regularly.	Discuss specific plans for future events. None.	Continue with cognitive approaches when discussing future events.

GAF, Global Assessment of Functioning; SSRI, selective serotonin reuptake inhibitor.

In addition to a physical assessment, including weight and appetite, sleep habits, and fatigue factors, an assessment of current medications should be completed. The frequency and dosage of prescribed medications, over-the-counter medications, and use of herbal or culturally related medication treatments should be explored. In depression, the nurse must always assess the lethality of the medication the patient is taking. For example, if a patient has sleeping medications at home, the individual should be further queried about the number of pills in the bottle. Patients also need to be assessed for their use of alcohol, marijuana, and other mood-altering medications, as well as herbal substances because of the potential for drug–drug interactions. For example, patients taking antidepressants that affect serotonin regulation could also be taking St. John's wort (*Hypericum perforatum*) to fight depression. The combined drug and herb could interact to cause serotonin syndrome (altered mental status, autonomic dysfunction, and neuromuscular abnormalities). SAMe (S-adenosylmethionine) is another herbal preparation that patients may be taking. Patients need to be advised regarding possible adverse side effects of SAMe with any prescribed antidepressant because the exact action of this herb is unknown.

Nursing Diagnoses for the Biologic Domain

Several nursing diagnoses could be formulated based on assessment data, including Insomnia, Imbalanced Nutrition, Fatigue, Self-Care Deficit, and Nausea. Other diagnoses that should be considered are Disturbed Thought Processes and Sexual Dysfunction.

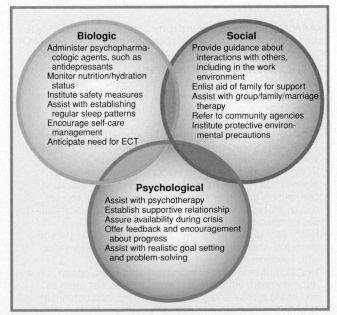

FIGURE 24.1 Biopsychosocial interventions for patients with major depressive disorder. ECT, electroconvulsive therapy.

BOX 24.1

Research for Best Practice: **Home-based Deep Breathing for Depression in Patients With Coronary Heart Disease**

Chung, L. J., Tsai, P. S., Liu, B. Y., Kuei-Ru, C., Wei-Hsiang, L., Yuh-Kae, S., & Mei-Yeh, W. (2010). Home-based deep breathing for depression in patients with coronary heart disease: a randomized controlled trial. International Journal of Nursing Studies, 47(11), 1346–1353.

THE QUESTION: How effective is a home-based deep-breathing training program compared with weekly telephone support in patients with coronary heart disease (CHD)?

METHODS: In a controlled trial, 62 patients with CHD with Beck Depression Inventory-II (BDI-II) scores above 10 were randomized to receive either home-based deep breathing training (n = 28) or weekly telephone support (n = 34). The deep breathing exercise consisted of diaphragmatic breathing with four to six slow and deep breaths per minute, three times per day. Participants and raters were blinded to the study hypothesis. Depressive symptoms were assessed with the BDI-II and the Patient Health Questionnaire-9 (PHQ-9) at baseline and 2 weeks after the test.

FINDINGS: The group using the deep breathing exercise has significantly lower depression scores than the control group.

IMPLICATIONS FOR NURSING: Nurses should consider teaching patients who are depressed deep breathing exercises to their improve mood and reduce their depressive symptoms.

Interventions for the Biologic Domain

Biologic interventions center around education, pharmacologic interventions, and other somatic interventions (Fig. 24.1).

Teaching Physical Care

Because weeks or months of disturbed sleep patterns and nutritional imbalance only make depression worse, counseling and education should aim to establish normal sleep patterns and healthy nutrition. Encouraging patients to practice positive sleep hygiene and eat well-balanced meals regularly helps the patient move toward remission or recovery.

Deep-breathing exercises three times a day have been shown to reduce self-report depressive symptoms within 4 weeks in patients with coronary heart disease (Box 24.1). Activity and exercise are also important for improving depressed mood state. Most people find that regular exercise is hard to maintain. People who are depressed may find it impossible. When teaching about exercise, it is important to start with the current level of patient activity and increase it slowly. For example, if the patient is spending most of the time in bed, encouraging the patient to get dressed every day and walk for 5 or

10 minutes may be all that patient can tolerate. Gradually, patients should be encouraged to have a regular exercise program and to slowly increase their food intake.

Pharmacologic Interventions

An antidepressant is selected based primarily on an individual patient's target symptoms; genetic factors; responses related to cultural, racial, and ethnic influences; and an individual agent's side effect profile (Posmontier, 2013; Warren, 2011a). Other factors that may influence choice include prior medication response, drug interactions and contraindications, concurrent medical and psychiatric disorders, patient age, and cost of medication. Failure to consider these influences may increase the risk of aversive and injurious side effects (Dollard, 2013).

> **NCLEXNOTE** Patients may be reluctant to take prescribed antidepressant medications or may self-treat depression based on their cultural beliefs and values (Institute of Medicine [IOM], 2003; Munoz et al., 2007; Warren, 2013a, 2013b, 2013c). A culturally competent nursing care and teaching plan needs to address the importance for adherence to a medication regimen and emphasize any potential drug–drug interactions.

Medication therapy should be reviewed on a regular basis to ascertain whether changes or discontinuation of medications might be needed (Leahy & Kohler, 2013; Limandri, 2013). The treatment and clinical management of patients with psychiatric disorders are divided into the acute phase; continuation phase; maintenance phase; and, when indicated, discontinuation of medication use.

- *Acute phase.* The primary goal of therapy for the acute phase is symptom reduction or remission. The objective is to choose the right match of medication and dosage for the patient. Careful monitoring and follow-up are essential during this phase to assess patient response to medications, adjust the dosage if necessary, identify and address side effects, and provide patient support and education.
- *Continuation phase.* The goal of this treatment phase is to decrease the risk for relapse (a return of the current episode of depression). If a patient experiences a response to an adequate trial of medication, use of the medication generally is continued at the same dosage for at least 4 to 9 months after the patient returns to a clinically well state (Stahl, 2013a, 2013b).

BOX 24.2

Drug Profile: Escitalopram Oxalate (Lexapro)

DRUG CLASS: Antidepressant

RECEPTOR AFFINITY: A highly selective serotonin reuptake inhibitor with low affinity for 5HT 1–7 or α- and β-adrenergic, dopamine D1–5, histamine H1–3, muscarinic M1–5, and benzodiazepine receptors or for Na^+, K^+, Cl^-, and Ca^{++} ion channels that have been associated with various anticholinergic, sedative, and cardiovascular side effects

INDICATIONS: Treatment of major depressive disorder, generalized anxiety disorder

ROUTES AND DOSAGES: Available as 5-, 10-, and 20-mg oral tablets

Adults: Initially 10 mg once a day. May increase to 20 mg after a minimum of 1 week. Trials have not shown greater benefit at the 20-mg dose

Geriatric: The 10-mg dose is recommended. Adjust dosage related to the drug's longer half-life and the slower liver metabolism of older adult patients

Renal impairment: No dosage adjustment is necessary for mild to moderate renal impairment

Children: Safety and efficacy have not been established in this population

HALF LIFE (PEAK EFFECT): 27–32 h (4–7 h)

SELECTED ADVERSE REACTIONS: Most common adverse events include insomnia, ejaculation disorder, diarrhea, nausea, fatigue, increased sweating, dry mouth, somnolence, dizziness, and constipation. Most serious adverse events include ejaculation disorder in men; fetal abnormalities and decreased fetal weight in pregnant patients; and serotonin syndrome if coadministered with MAOIs, St. John's wort, or SSRIs, including citalopram (Celexa), of which escitalopram (Lexapro) is the active isomer

BOXED WARNING: Suicidality in children, adolescents, and young adults

WARNING: There is potential for interaction with MAOIs. Lexapro should not be used in combination with an MAOI or within 14 days of discontinuing an MAOI

SPECIFIC PATIENT AND FAMILY EDUCATION
- Do not take in combination with citalopram (Celexa) or other SSRIs or MAOIs. A 2-week washout period between escitalopram and SSRIs or MAOIs is recommended to avoid serotonin syndrome.
- Families and caregivers should be advised of the need for close observation and communication with the prescriber.
- Notify your prescriber if pregnancy is possible or being planned. Do not breast-feed while taking this medication.
- Use caution driving or operating machinery until you are certain that escitalopram does not alter your physical abilities or mental alertness.
- Notify your prescriber of any OTC medications, herbal supplements, and home remedies being used in combination with escitalopram.
- Ingestion of alcohol in combination with escitalopram is not recommended, although escitalopram does not seem to potentiate mental and motor impairments associated with alcohol.

MAOI, monoamine oxidase inhibitor; OTC, over the counter; SSRI, selective serotonin reuptake inhibitor.
Source: RX List available at http://www.rxlist.com/cgi/generic/lexapro.htm.

- *Maintenance phase.* For patients who are at high risk for recurrence (see Risk Factors), the optimal duration of maintenance treatment is unknown but is measured in years, and full-dose therapy is required for effective prophylaxis (Schatzberg & Nemeroff, 2009).
- *Discontinuation of medication use.* The decision to discontinue active treatment should be based on the same factors considered in the decision to initiate maintenance treatment. These factors include the frequency and severity of past episodes, the persistence of dysthymic symptoms after recovery, the presence of comorbid disorders, and patient preference. Many patients continue taking medications for their lifetime.

Administering Medications

Antidepressant medications have proved effective in all forms of major depression. To date, controlled trials have shown no single antidepressant drug to have greater efficacy in the treatment of major depressive disorder. Antidepressant medications can be grouped as follows:

- Selective serotonin reuptake inhibitors (SSRIs), which currently include escitalopram oxalate (Lexapro), fluoxetine (Prozac), sertraline (Zoloft), fluvoxamine (Luvox), paroxetine (Paxil), and citalopram (Celexa) (Box 24.2), and serotonin norepinephrine reuptake inhibitors (SNRIs), which include venlafaxine (Effexor), nefazodone (Serzone), duloxetine (Cymbalta), and desvenlafaxine (Pristiq)
- Cyclic antidepressants, which include the tricyclic antidepressants (TCAs), and maprotiline (a tetracyclic)
- Monoamine oxidase inhibitors (MAOIs), which include phenelzine (Nardil), tranylcypromine (Parnate), isocarboxazid (Marplan), and selegiline (Emsam)
- Other antidepressants, which include bupropion (Wellbutrin), a norepinephrine dopamine reuptake inhibitor; mirtazapine (Remeron), an α_2-antagonist; and trazodone (Desyrel), a serotonin-2 antagonist/reuptake inhibitor

See Chapter 11 for a list of antidepressant medications, usual dosage range, half-life, and therapeutic blood levels. For more information, see Box 24.3.

The first-generation drugs, the TCAs and MAOIs, are being used less often than the second-generation drugs, the SSRIs and atypical antidepressants. Second-generation drugs selectively target the neurotransmitters and receptors thought to be associated with depression and to minimize side effects. The side effect profiles of the two generations of drugs are significantly different as well (Table 24.1). The efficacy of the MAOIs is well established. Evidence suggests their distinct advantage in treating a specific subtype of depression, so-called atypical depression (characterized by increased appetite, reverse diurnal mood variation, and hypersomnia), depression

with panic symptoms, and social phobia (Schatzberg & Nemeroff, 2009). Given their dietary restrictions, MAOIs usually are reserved for patients whose depression fails to respond to other antidepressants or patients who cannot tolerate typical antidepressants.

Monitoring Medications

Observations, vital signs, patients' subjective reports, and rating scales are the nursing tools for monitoring medication effects. The nurse is responsible for ensuring that patients are receiving a therapeutic dosage, assessing

---

BOX 24.3

Drug Profile: Mirtazapine (Remeron)

DRUG CLASS: Antidepressant

RECEPTOR AFFINITY: Believed to enhance central noradrenergic and serotonergic activity antagonizing central presynaptic α_2-adrenergic receptors. Mechanism of action is unknown

INDICATIONS: Treatment of depression

ROUTES AND DOSAGE: Available as 15- and 30-mg tablets

Adults: Initially, 15 mg/d as a single dose preferably in the evening before sleeping. Maximum dosage is 45 mg/d

Geriatric: Use with caution; reduced dosage may be needed

Children: Safety and efficacy is not established

HALF-LIFE (PEAK EFFECT): 20–40 h (2 h)

SELECTED ADVERSE REACTIONS: Somnolence, increased appetite, dizziness, weight gain, elevated cholesterol or triglyceride and transaminase levels, malaise, abdominal pain, hypertension, vasodilation, vomiting, anorexia, thirst, myasthenia, arthralgia, hypoesthesia, apathy, depression, vertigo, twitching, agitation, anxiety, amnesia, increased cough, sinusitis, pruritus, rash, urinary tract infection, mania (rare), agranulocytosis (rare)

BOXED WARNING: Suicidality in children, adolescents, and young adults

WARNING: Contraindicated in patients with known hypersensitivity. Use with caution in older adults, patients who are breast-feeding, and patients with impaired hepatic function. Avoid concomitant use with alcohol or diazepam, which can cause additive impairment of cognitive and motor skills

SPECIFIC PATIENT AND FAMILY EDUCATION
- Take the dose once a day in the evening before sleep.
- Families and caregivers should be advised of the need for dose observation and communication with the prescriber.
- Avoid driving and performing other tasks requiring alertness.
- Notify your prescriber before taking any OTC or other prescription drugs.
- Avoid alcohol and other CNS depressants.
- Notify your prescriber if pregnancy is possible or planned.
- Monitor temperature and report any fever, lethargy, weakness, sore throat, malaise, or other "flu-like" symptoms.
- Maintain medical follow-up, including any appointments for blood counts and liver studies.

CNS, central nervous system; OTC, over the counter.

Table 24.1 SIDE EFFECTS OF ANTIDEPRESSANT MEDICATIONS

Generic (Trade) Drug Name	Side Effects				
	Anticholinergic	Sedation	Orthostatic Hypotension	Gastrointestinal Distress	Weight Gain
Tricyclics: Tertiary Amines					
Amitriptyline	+4	+4	2	0	+4
Clomipramine (Anafranil)	+3	+3	+2	+1	+4
Imipramine (Tofranil)	+2	+2	+3	+1	+3
Tricyclics: Secondary Amines					
Amoxapine	+3	+2	+1	0	+1
Desipramine (Norpramin)	+1	+1	+1	0	+1
Nortriptyline (Pamelor)	+2	+2	+1	0	+1
Selective Serotonin Reuptake Inhibitors					
Fluoxetine (Prozac)	0/+1	0/+1	0/+1	+3	0
Sertraline (Zoloft)	0	0/+1	0	+3	0
Paroxetine (Paxil)	0	0/+1	0	+3	0
Fluvoxamine (Luvox)	0/+1	0/+1	0/+1	+3	0
Citalopram (Celexa)	0/+1	0/+1	0/+1	+3	0
Escitalopram (Lexapro)	0/+1	0/+1	0/+1	+3	0
Atypical: Antidepressants					
Venlafaxine (Effexor)	0	0	0	+3	0
Trazodone (Oleptro)	0	+1	+3	+1	+1
Nefazodone	0/+1	+1	+2	+2	0/+1
Bupropion (Wellbutrin)	+2	+2	+1	0	0/+1
Mirtazapine (Remeron)	+3	+4	+3	+3	+2
Desvenlafaxine (Pristiq)	+0	+0	+0	+3	+0

0, absent or rare; 0/+1, lowest likelihood; +4, highest likelihood.

BOX 24.4

Guidelines for Administering and Monitoring Antidepressant Medications

Nurses should do the following in administering and monitoring antidepressant medications:

- Observe the patient for checking or saving medications for a later suicide attempt.
- Monitor vital signs (such as orthostatic vital signs and temperature): obtain baseline data before the initiation of medications.
- Monitor periodically liver and thyroid function tests, blood chemistry, and complete blood count as appropriate and compare with baseline values.
- Monitor the patient symptoms for therapeutic response and report inadequate response to prescriber.
- Monitor the patient for side effects and report to the prescriber serious side effects or those that are chronic and problematic for the patient. (Table 24.2 indicates pharmacologic and nonpharmacologic interventions for common side effects.)
- Monitor drug levels as appropriate. (Therapeutic drug levels for antidepressants are listed in Chapter 11.)
- Monitor dietary intake as appropriate, especially with regard to MAOI antidepressants.
- Inquire about patient use of other medications, alcohol, "street" drugs, OTC medications, and herbal supplements that might alter the desired effects of prescribed antidepressants.

MAOI, monoamine oxidase inhibitor; OTC, over the counter.

medication adherence, and evaluating side effects. Patients should be carefully observed when taking antidepressant medications (Box 24.4). In the depths of depression, saving medication for a later suicide attempt is quite common. During antidepressant treatment, the nurse should monitor and document vital signs, plasma drug levels as appropriate, liver and thyroid function tests, complete blood counts, and blood chemistry to make sure that patients are receiving a therapeutic dosage and are adherent to the prescribed regimen. Results of these tests also help evaluate for toxicity (see Chapter 11 for therapeutic blood levels).

Baseline orthostatic vital signs should be obtained before initiation of any medication, and in the case of medications known to have an impact on vital signs, such as TCAs, MAOIs, or venlafaxine, they should be monitored on a regular basis. If these medications are administered to children or older adults, the dosage should be lowered to accommodate the physiologic state of the individual.

Individualizing dosages is essential for achieving optimal efficacy. When the newer antidepressants are used, this is usually done by fine-tuning medication dosage based on patient feedback. The TCAs, including imipramine (Tofranil), desipramine (Norpramin), amitriptyline

Table 24.2	INTERVENTIONS TO RELIEVE SIDE EFFECTS OF ANTIDEPRESSANTS	
Side Effect	**Pharmacologic Intervention**	**Nonpharmacologic Intervention**
Dry mouth, caries, inflammation of the mouth	Bethanechol 10–30 mg tid Pilocarpine drops	Sugarless gum Sugarless lozenges 6–8 cups of water per day Toothpaste for dry mouth
Nausea, vomiting	Change medication	Take medication with food Soda crackers, toast, tea
Weight gain	Change medication	Nutritionally balanced diet Daily exercise
Urinary hesitation Constipation	Bethanechol 10–30 mg tid Stool softener	6–8 cups of water per day Bulk laxative Daily exercise 6–8 cups of water per day Diet rich in fresh fruits, vegetables, and grains
Diarrhea	OTC antidiarrheal	Maintain fluid intake
Orthostatic hypotension		Increase hydration Sit or stand up slowly
Drowsiness	Shift dosing time Lower medication dose Change medication	One caffeinated beverage at strategic time Do not drive when drowsy No alcohol or other recreational drugs Plan for rest time
Fatigue	Lower medication dose Change medication	Daily exercise
Blurred vision	Bethanechol 10–30 mg tid Pilocarpine eyedrops	Temporary use of magnifying lenses until body adjusts to medication
Flushing, sweating	Terazosin 1 mg qd Lower medication dose Change medication	Frequent bathing Lightweight clothing
Tremor	β-blockers Lower medication dose	Reassure the patient that tremor may decrease as the patient adjusts to medication. Notify the caregiver if tremor interferes with daily functioning.

OTC, over the counter; qd, every day; tid, three times a day.

(Elavil), and nortriptyline (Pamelor), have standardized valid plasma levels that can be useful in determining therapeutic dosages, although therapeutic plasma levels may vary from individual to individual. Blood samples should be drawn as close as possible to 12 hours away from the last dose. The newer antidepressants do not have established standardized ranges, and optimal dosing is based on efficacy and tolerability.

Managing Side Effects
Ideally, side effects are minimal and can be alleviated by nonpharmacologic interventions. For example, if patient is having difficulty going to sleep, caffeinated products should avoid (Table 24.2). For those taking, MAOIs, close attention to diet restrictions should be given. See Chapter 11 for tyramine-restricted diets.

First-Generation Antidepressants: TCAs and MAOIs.
The most common side effects associated with TCAs are the antihistaminic side effects (sedation and weight gain) and anticholinergic side effects (potentiation of

CNS drugs, blurred vision, dry mouth, constipation, urinary retention, sinus tachycardia, and decreased memory).

> **EMERGENCY CARE ALERT !** If possible, TCAs should not be prescribed for patients at risk for suicide. Lethal doses of TCAs are only three to five times the therapeutic dose, and more than 1 g of a TCA is often toxic and may be fatal. Death may result from cardiac arrhythmia, hypotension, or uncontrollable seizures.

Serum TCA levels should be evaluated when overdose is suspected. In acute overdose, almost all symptoms develop within 12 hours. Anticholinergic effects are prominent and include dry mucous membranes, warm and dry skin, blurred vision, decreased bowel motility, and urinary retention. CNS suppression (ranging from drowsiness to coma) or an agitated delirium may occur. Basic overdose treatment includes induction of emesis, gastric lavage, and cardiorespiratory supportive care.

The most common side effects of MAOIs are headache, drowsiness, dry mouth and throat, constipation, blurred vision, and orthostatic hypotension. Additional selected adverse effects of MAOIs include insomnia, nausea, agitation, dizziness, asthenia, weight loss, and postural hypotension. Although priapism was not reported during clinical trials, the MAOIs are structurally similar to trazodone, which has been associated with priapism (prolonged painful erection).

> **EMERGENCY CARE ALERT !** If coadministered with food or other substances containing tyramine (e.g., aged cheese, beer, red wine), MAOIs can trigger a hypertensive crisis that may be life-threatening. Symptoms include a sudden, severe pounding or explosive headache in the back of the head or temples, racing pulse, flushing, stiff neck, chest pain, nausea and vomiting, and profuse sweating.

MAOIs are more lethal in overdose than are the newer antidepressants and thus should be prescribed with caution if the patient's suicide potential is elevated (see Chapter 11). An MAOI generally is given in divided doses to minimize side effects.

Second-Generation Antidepressants: SSRIs and Other Antidepressants. Serotonin syndrome is a potentially serious side effect caused by drug-induced excess of intrasynaptic serotonin (5-hydroxytryptamine [5-HT]; see Chapter 11) (Box 24.5). First reported in the 1950s, it

---

BOX 24.5

Serotonin Syndrome

CAUSE: Excessive intrasynaptic serotonin

HOW IT HAPPENS: Combining medications that increase CNS serotonin levels, such as SSRIs + MAOIs; SSRIs + St. John's wort; or SSRIs + diet pills; dextromethorphan or alcohol, especially red wine; or SSRI + street drugs, such as LSD, MMDA, or Ecstasy

SYMPTOMS: Mental status changes, agitation, ataxia, myoclonus, hyperreflexia, fever, shivering, diaphoresis, diarrhea

TREATMENT
- Assess all medication, supplements, foods, and recreational drugs ingested to determine the offending substances.
- Discontinue any substances that may be causative factors. If symptoms are mild, treat supportively on an outpatient basis with propranolol and lorazepam and follow-up with the prescriber.
- If symptoms are moderate to severe, hospitalization may be needed with monitoring of vital signs and treatment with intravenous fluids, antipyretics, and cooling blankets.

FURTHER USE: Assess on a case-by-case basis and minimize risk factors for further medication therapy.

CNS, central nervous system; LSD, lysergic acid diethylamide; MAOI, monoamine oxidase inhibitor; MMDA, 3-methoxy-4,5-methylenedioxyamphetamine; SSRI, selective serotonin reuptake inhibitor.

---

was relatively rare until the introduction of the SSRIs. Serotonin syndrome is most often reported in patients taking two or more medications that increase CNS serotonin levels by different mechanisms (Stahl, 2013a). The most common drug combinations associated with serotonin syndrome involve the MAOIs, the SSRIs, and the TCAs.

Although serotonin syndrome can cause death, it is mild in most patients, who usually recover with supportive care alone. Unlike neuroleptic malignant syndrome, which develops within 3 to 9 days after the introduction of neuroleptic medications (see Chapter 22), serotonin syndrome tends to develop within hours or days after initiating or increasing the dose of serotonergic medication or adding a drug with serotomimetic properties. The symptoms include altered mental status, autonomic dysfunction, and neuromuscular abnormalities. At least three of the following must be present for a diagnosis: mental status changes, agitation, myoclonus, hyperreflexia, fever, shivering, diaphoresis, ataxia, and diarrhea. In patients who also have peripheral vascular disease or atherosclerosis, severe vasospasm and hypertension may occur in the presence of elevated serotonin levels. In addition, in a patient who is a slow metabolizer of SSRIs, higher-than-normal levels of these antidepressants may circulate in the blood. Medications that are not usually considered serotonergic, such as dextromethorphan (Pertussin) and meperidine (Demerol), have been associated with the syndrome (Alpern & Henretig, 2010).

> **EMERGENCY CARE ALERT !** The most important emergency interventions are stopping use of the offending drug, notifying the prescriber, and providing necessary supportive care (e.g., intravenous fluids, antipyretics, cooling blanket). Severe symptoms have been successfully treated with antiserotonergic agents, such as cyproheptadine (Levin et al., 2008).

Although the SSRIs and newer atypical antidepressants produce fewer and generally milder side effects, there are some side effects to note. Among the most common are:

- Insomnia and activation
- Headaches
- Gastrointestinal symptoms
- Weight gain

Sexual side effects, primarily diminished interest and performance, are also reported with some SSRIs, particularly sertraline. The most potentially harmful, but preventable, side effect or interaction of SSRIs is serotonin syndrome (see Box 24.5). The atypical antidepressant nefazodone (once a more popular medication) has been shown to raise hepatic enzyme levels in some patients, potentially leading to hepatic failure. Trazodone administration has been associated with erectile dysfunction and priapism. Bupropion can cause seizures, particularly in patients at risk for seizures. Bupropion has also been associated with the development of psychosis because it is dopaminergic, and its use should be avoided in patients with schizophrenia. Venlafaxine can cause blood pressure to increase, although this side effect appears to be dose related and can be controlled by lowering the dose (APA, 2013).

Monitoring for Drug Interactions

Potential drug interactions associated with agents that are metabolized by the cytochrome P450 systems should be considered when children or older adults are treated (see Chapter 11). Five of the most important enzyme systems are 1A2, 2D6, 2C9, 2C19, and 3A4. The 1A2 system is inhibited by the SSRI fluvoxamine. Thus, other drugs that use the 1A2 system will no longer be metabolized as efficiently. For example, if fluvoxamine is given with theophylline, the theophylline dosage must be lowered or blood levels of theophylline will rise and cause possible side effects or toxic reactions, such as seizures. Fluvoxamine also affects the metabolism of atypical antipsychotics. On the other hand, smoking and caffeine can induce 1A2 system activity. This means that smokers may need to be given a higher dose of

medications that are metabolized by this system (Stahl, 2013a, 2013b).

Fluoxetine (Prozac) and paroxetine (Paxil) are potent inhibitors of 2D6. One of the most significant drug interactions is caused by SSRI inhibition of 2D6 that in turn causes an increase in plasma levels of TCAs. If there is concomitant administration of an SSRI and a TCA, the plasma drug level of TCA should be monitored and probably reduced. In the 3A4 system, some SSRIs (fluoxetine, fluvoxamine, and nefazodone) raise the levels of alprazolam (Xanax) or triazolam (Halcion) through enzyme inhibition, requiring reduction of dosage of the benzodiazepine. For more information, see Table 24.3.

Teaching Points

If depression goes untreated or is inadequately treated, episodes can become more frequent, more severe, and longer in duration and can lead to suicide. Patient education involves explaining this pattern and the importance of continuing medication use after the acute phase of treatment to decrease the risk for future episodes. Patient concerns regarding long-term antidepressant therapy need to be assessed and addressed. All teaching points need to be developed and delivered using a culturally competent approach to enhance patient adherence (U.S. DHHS, 2001; Warren, 2008).

Table 24.3	DRUG–DRUG INTERACTIONS: ANTIDEPRESSANTS	
Antidepressant	**Other Drug**	**Effect of Interaction or Treatment**
Fluvoxamine	Theophylline	Increased theophylline level: seizures. Tx: Reduce theophylline levels when administering with fluvoxamine.
Fluoxetine Paroxetine	TCAs Benzodiazepines Phenothiazines	Increased in plasma levels of TCA. Tx: Reduce TCA levels when giving with fluoxetine or paroxetine.
Fluoxetine Fluvoxamine Nefazodone	Alprazolam Benzodiazepines	Increased plasma levels of alprazolam. Tx: Reduce dose of alprazolam when administered with benzodiazepines.
Nefazodone	Digoxin Phenothiazines Antihistamines	Increased levels of digoxin, antihistamines, and benzodiazepines. Tx: Reduce dose of nefazodone when giving with these medications.
Fluvoxamine	Caffeine Nicotine	Lowered levels of fluvoxamine. Tx: Increase dose of fluvoxamine in smokers or patients whose coffee, tea, or caffeinated drink intake is high.
SSRIs	Warfarin	Increased prothrombin time, bleeding. Tx: Monitor closely; decrease dose of warfarin if giving with SSRIs.
SSRIs	Lithium TCAs Barbiturates	Increased CNS effects of SSRIs. Tx: Adjust dosage of SSRI.
SSRIs	Phenytoin	Increased serum levels of phenytoin. Tx: Adjust dosage of phenytoin.

CNS, central nervous system; SSRI, selective serotonin reuptake inhibitor; TCA, tricyclic antidepressant; Tx, treatment.

Source: Stahl, S. M. (2013a). *Stahl's essential psychopharmacology: Neuroscientific basis and practical applications* (4th ed.). New York: Cambridge Press.

Even after the first episode of major depression, medication should be continued for at least 6 months to 1 year after the patient achieves complete remission of symptoms. If the patient experiences a recurrence after tapering the first course of treatment, the regimen should be reinstituted for at least another year, and if the illness reoccurs, medication should be continued indefinitely (Schatzberg & Nemeroff, 2009).

Patients should also be advised not to take herbal substances such as St. John's wort or SAMe if they are also taking prescribed antidepressants. St. John's wort also should not be taken if the patient is taking nasal decongestants, hay fever and asthma medications containing monoamines, amino acid supplements containing phenylalanine, or tyrosine. The combination may cause hypertension. The exact mechanism of SAMe is unknown, but some serious safety concerns (e.g., development of coronary atherosclerosis, altered thought process, mania) have been reported in persons using the herb substance.

Other Somatic Therapies

Electroconvulsive Therapy

Although its therapeutic mechanism of action is unknown, electroconvulsive therapy (ECT) is an effective treatment for patients with severe depression. It is generally reserved for patients whose disorder is refractory or intolerant to initial drug treatments and who are so severely ill that rapid treatment is required (e.g., patients with malnutrition, catatonia, or suicidality).

ECT is contraindicated for patients with increased intracranial pressure. Other high-risk patients include those with recent myocardial infarction, recent cerebrovascular accident, retinal detachment, or pheochromocytoma (a tumor on the adrenal cortex or other tumors) and those at risk for complications of anesthesia. Older age has been associated with a favorable response to ECT, but the effectiveness and safety in this group have not been shown. Because depression can increase the mortality risk for older adults, in particular, and some older adults do not respond well to medication, effective treatment is especially important for this age group (Van der Wurff, Stek, Hoogendijk, & Beekman, 2003).

The role of the nurse in the care of the patient undergoing ECT is to provide educational and emotional support for the patient and family, assess baseline or pretreatment levels of function, prepare the patient for the ECT process, monitor and evaluate the patient's response to ECT, provide assessment data with the ECT team, and modify treatment as needed (see Chapter 11 for more information). The actual procedure, possible therapeutic mechanisms of action, potential adverse effects, contraindications, and nursing interventions are described in detail in Chapter 11.

Light Therapy (Phototherapy)

Light therapy is described in Chapter 8. Given current research, light therapy is an option for well-documented mild to moderate seasonal, nonpsychotic, winter depressive episodes in patients with recurrent major depressive disorders, including children and adolescents. Evidence also indicates that light therapy can modestly improve symptoms in nonseasonal depression, especially when administered during the first week of treatment in the morning for those experiencing sleep deprivation (Lewy, Lefler, Emens, & Bauer, 2006).

Repetitive Transcranial Magnetic Stimulation

In 2008, the U.S. Food and Drug Administration approved repetitive transcranial magnetic stimulation (rTMS) for the treatment of patients with mild treatment-resistant depression. In rTMS, a magnetic coil placed on the scalp at the site of the left motor cortex releases small electrical pulses that stimulate the site of the left dorsolateral prefrontal cortex in the superficial cortex. This rapidly changing magnetic field stimulates the brain sufficiently to depolarize neurons and exert effects across synapses. These pulses (similar in type and strength as a magnetic resonance imaging machine) easily pass through the hair, skin, and skull, requiring much less electricity than ECT. The patient is awake, reclining in an rTMS chair during the procedure, and can resume normal activities immediately after the procedure. Because anesthesia is not required, there are no risks associated with sedation. Treatment of depression typically consists of 20 to 30 sessions, lasting 37 minutes each over 4 to 6 weeks. Depending on the level of practice and training, the nurse's role the use of the rTMS varies from education, preparation, and postprocedure care to performing the procedure (Bernard, Westmand, Dutton, & Lanocha, 2009).

Psychological Domain

Assessment

The mental status examination is an effective clinical tool to evaluate the psychological aspects of major depression because the focus is on disturbances of mood and affect, thought processes and content, cognition, memory, and attention. The comprehensive mental status examination is described in detail in Chapter 10.

Mood and Affect

The person with depression has a sustained period of feeling depressed, sad, or hopeless and may experience

anhedonia (loss of interest or pleasure). The patient may report "not caring anymore" or not feeling any enjoyment in activities that were previously considered pleasurable. In some individuals, this may include a decrease in or loss of libido (sexual interest or desire) and sexual function. In others, irritability and anger are signs of depression, especially in those who deny being depressed.

Numerous assessment scales are available for assessing depression. Easily administered self-report questionnaires can be valuable detection tools. These questionnaires cannot be the sole basis for making a diagnosis of major depressive episode, but they are sensitive to depressive symptoms. The following are five commonly used self-report scales:

- General Health Questionnaire (GHQ)
- Center for Epidemiological Studies Depression Scale (CES-D)
- Beck Depression Inventory (BDI)
- Zung Self-Rating Depression Scale (SDS)
- PRIME-MD

Clinician-completed rating scales may be more sensitive to improvement in the course of treatment, can assess symptoms in relationship to the depressive diagnostic criteria, and may have a slightly greater specificity than do self-report questionnaires in detecting depression. These include the following:

- Hamilton Rating Scale for Depression (HAM-D)
- Montgomery-Asberg Depression Rating Scale (MADRS)
- National Institute of Mental Health Diagnostic Interview Schedule (DIS)

Thought Content

Depressed individuals often have an unrealistic negative evaluation of their worth or have guilty preoccupations or ruminations about minor past failings. Such individuals often misinterpret neutral or trivial day-to-day events as evidence of personal defects, and they have an exaggerated sense of responsibility for untoward events. As a result, they feel hopeless, helpless, worthless, and powerless. The possibility of disorganized thought processes (e.g., tangential or circumstantial thinking) and perceptual disturbances (e.g., hallucinations, delusions) should also be included in the assessment.

Suicidal Behavior

Patients with major depression are at increased risk for suicide. The development of suicide behavior is a complex phenomenon, and symptoms are often hidden or veiled by somatic symptoms.

> **KEYCONCEPT** **Suicidal behavior** is the occurrence of persistent thought patterns and actions that indicate a person is thinking about, planning, or enacting suicide.

Suicidal ideation includes thoughts that range from a belief that others would be better off if the person were dead or thoughts of death (passive suicidal ideation) to actual specific plans for committing suicide (active suicidal ideation). See Chapter 21. The frequency, intensity, and lethality of these thoughts can vary and can help to determine the seriousness of intent. The more specific the plan and the more accessible the means, the more serious is the intent. The risk for suicide needs to be initially assessed in patients who incur depressive disorders as well as reassessed throughout the course of treatment.

Suicidal ideation is not a normal reaction to stress. Persons who express any suicidal ideation need immediate mental health assessment regarding the depth of their thoughts and intentions. More than 90% of persons who complete suicide have one or more of the following risk factors: lack of availability and inadequacy of social supports; family violence, including physical or sexual abuse; past history of suicidal ideation or behavior; presence of psychosis or substance use or abuse; and decreased ability to control suicidal impulses (NIMH, 2009).

There are ethnic and cultural differences regarding suicide behavior. Men often use firearms, and women often use of pills or other poisonous substances to commit suicide. Children often use suffocation. Data on suicide completion rates are reported highest in persons from American Indian, Alaskan Natives, and non Hispanic white descent. These rates are lowest for persons from Hispanic, non-Hispanic black, and Asian and Pacific Islander descent. Ongoing research regarding suicide in veterans indicates that they have a risk twice that of persons in the general population. Psychological stress and previously diagnosed psychiatric disorders are chief risk factors for veterans. Counseling and supportive services need to be provided to family and friends of persons who attempt or commit suicide because family and friends may experience feelings of grief, guilt, anger, and confusion (Cerel, Jordan, & Duberstien, 2008).

Cognition and Memory

Many individuals with depression report an impaired ability to think, concentrate, or make decisions. They may appear easily distracted or complain of memory difficulties. In older adults with major depression, memory difficulties may be the chief complaint and may be mistaken for early signs of dementia (pseudodementia) (APA, 2013; Blazer & Steffens, 2009). When the depression is fully treated, the memory problem often improves or fully resolves.

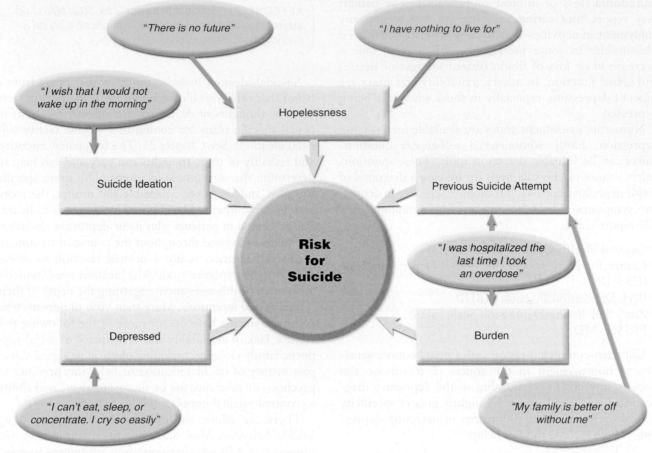

FIGURE 24.2 Nursing diagnosis concept map: Risk for Suicide.

Nursing Diagnoses for the Psychological Domain

Nursing diagnoses focusing on the psychological domain for the patient with a depressive disorder are numerous. If patient data lead to the diagnosis of Risk for Suicide, the patient should be further assessed for plan, intent, and accessibility of means (Fig. 24.2). Other nursing diagnoses include Hopelessness, Low Self-Esteem, Ineffective Individual Coping, Decisional Conflict, Spiritual Distress, and Dysfunctional Grieving.

Interventions for the Psychological Domain

For patients with severe or recurrent major depressive disorder, the combination of psychotherapy (including interpersonal, cognitive behavioral, behavior, brief dynamic, or dialectical behavioral therapies) and pharmacotherapy has been found to be superior to treatment with a single modality. Recent studies suggest that short-term cognitive and interpersonal therapies may be as effective as pharmacotherapy in milder depressions. In many instances, cognitive behavioral therapy is an effective strategy for preventing relapse in patients who have

had only a partial response to pharmacotherapy alone (APA, 2013). Clinical practice guidelines suggest that the combination of medication and psychotherapy is particularly useful in more complex situations (e.g., depression in the context of concurrent, chronic general-medical or other psychiatric disorders, or in patients who fail to experience complete response to either treatment alone). Psychotherapy in combination with medication is also used to address collateral issues, such as medication adherence or secondary psychosocial problems (Apostolo & Kolcaba, 2009).

> **NCLEXNOTE** A cognitive therapy approach is recommended for helping persons restructure the negative thinking processes related to a person's concept of self, others, and the future. This approach should be included in most nursing care plans for patients with depression.

Therapeutic Relationship

One of the most effective therapeutic tools for caring for any person with a psychiatric disorder is the therapeutic relationship. For a person who is depressed, there are a number of effective approaches:

BOX 24.6 • THERAPEUTIC DIALOGUE • Approaching the Depressed Patient

George Sadder is a 70-year-old retired businessman who has been admitted to a day treatment program because of complaints of stomach pains, insomnia, and hopelessness. He has withdrawn from social activities he previously enjoyed, such as golfing and going out to eat with his wife and friends. This morning he sits in a chair by himself rather than joining a group activity.

INEFFECTIVE APPROACH

Nurse: Hi, Mr. Sadder. My name is Sally. How are you feeling today?

Mr. S: Lousy, just lousy! I didn't sleep well last night, and my stomach is killing me!

Nurse: Oh, that is too bad! Have you had any breakfast?

Mr. S: No! Didn't I say that my stomach is killing me?

Nurse: Maybe eating breakfast would help your stomach pain.

Mr. S: You don't know anything about my pain! (Gets up and walks away.)

EFFECTIVE APPROACH

Nurse: Hi. My name is Sally.

Mr. S: Hello, Sally. My name is George Sadder.

Nurse: I'd like to sit down with you, if that is OK.

Mr. S: If you want, but I am not much of a talker.

Nurse: That's OK. We can talk or not, whatever you wish.

Mr. S: (Patient winces)

Nurse: You just winced. Are you in pain?

Mr. S: Yes, my stomach has been killing me lately.

Nurse: What do you usually do to ease the pain?

Mr. S: I usually take an antacid with my meals but forgot this morning.

Nurse: I'll see if I can get some for you now.

Mr. S: Thanks. When my stomach settles down, maybe we can talk.

Nurse: That would be fine. I'll check back with you in a few minutes.

CRITICAL THINKING CHALLENGE

• What ineffective techniques did the nurse use in the first scenario, and how did they impair communication?

• What effective techniques did the nurse use in the second scenario, and how did they facilitate communication?

• Establishment and maintenance of a supportive relationship based on the incorporation of culturally competent interventions and strategies
• Availability in times of crisis
• Vigilance regarding dangerousness to self and others
• Education about the illness and treatment goals
• Encouragement and feedback concerning progress
• Guidance regarding the patient's interactions with the personal and work environment
• Realistic goal setting and monitoring

Interacting with depressed individuals is challenging because they tend to be withdrawn and have difficulty expressing feelings and engaging in interpersonal interactions. The therapeutic relationship can be strengthened through the use of cognitive interventions as well as the nurse's ability to win the patient's trust through the use of culturally competent strategies in the context of empathy (Box 24.6).

Cheerleading, or being overly cheerful to a person who is depressed, blocks communication and can be quite irritating. Nurses should avoid approaching patients with depression with an overly cheerful attitude. Instead, a calm, supportive empathic approach helps keep communication open.

> NCLEXNOTE Establishing the patient–nurse relationship with a person who is depressed requires an empathic, quiet approach that is grounded in the nurse's understanding of the cultural needs of the patient.

Cognitive Interventions

Cognitive interventions such as thought stopping and positive self-talk can dispel irrational beliefs and distorted attitudes and in turn reduce depressive symptoms during the acute phase of major depression (see Chapter 12). Nurses should consider using cognitive approaches when caring for persons who are depressed. The use of cognitive interventions in the acute phase of treatment combined with medication is now considered first-line treatment for mildly to moderately depressed outpatients.

Behavioral Interventions

Behavioral interventions are effective in the acute treatment of patients with mild to moderately severe depression, especially when combined with pharmacotherapy. Therapeutic techniques include activity scheduling, social skills training, and problem solving. Behavior therapy techniques are described in Chapter 7.

Interpersonal Therapy

Interpersonal therapy seeks to recognize, explore, and resolve the interpersonal losses, role confusion and transitions, social isolation, and deficits in social skills that may precipitate depressive states. It maintains that losses must be mourned and related affects appreciated, role confusion and transitions must be recognized and resolved, and social skills deficits must be overcome to acquire social supports. Some evidence in controlled studies suggests that interpersonal therapy is more effective in reducing depressive symptoms with certain populations, such as depressed patients with human immunodeficiency virus infection, and less successful with patients who have personality disorders (see Chapter 28).

Family and Marital Therapy

Patients who perceive high family stress are at risk for greater future severity of illness, higher use of health services, and higher health care expense. Marital and family problems are common among patients with mood disorders; comprehensive treatment requires that these problems be assessed and addressed. They may be a consequence of the major depression but may also predispose persons to develop depressive symptoms or inhibit recovery and resilience processes. Research suggests that marital and family therapy may reduce depressive symptoms and the risk for relapse in patients with marital and family problems. The depressed spouse's depression has marked impact on the marital adjustment of the nondepressed spouse. It is recommended that treatment approaches be designed to help couples be supportive of each other, to adapt, and to cope with the depressive symptoms within the framework of their ongoing marital relations. Many family nursing interventions (discussed in detail in

Chapter 14) may be used by the psychiatric nurse in providing targeted family-centered care. These include:

- Monitoring patient and family for indicators of stress
- Teaching stress management techniques
- Counseling family members on coping skills for their own use
- Providing necessary knowledge of options and support services
- Facilitating family routines and rituals
- Assisting the family to resolve feelings of guilt
- Assisting the family with conflict resolution
- Identifying family strengths and resources with family members
- Facilitating communication among family members

Group Interventions

Individuals who are depressed can receive emotional support in groups and learn how others deal with similar problems and issues. As group members serve as role models for new group members, they also benefit as their self-esteem increases, which strengthens their ability to address their issues (see Chapter 13). Group interventions are often used to help an individual cope with depression associated with bereavement or chronic medical illness. Group interventions are also commonly used to educate patients and families about their disorder and medications.

Teaching Patients and Families

Patients with depression and their significant others often incorrectly believe that their illness is their own fault and that they should be able to "pull themselves up by their boot straps and snap out of it." Persons from some cultural groups believe that the symptoms of depression may be a result of someone placing a hex on the affected person because the person has done something evil (Warren, 2008). It is vital to be culturally competent to be effective in teaching patients and their families about the treatment modalities for depression.

Patients need to know the full range of suitable treatment options before consenting to participate in treatment. Information empowers patients to ask questions, weigh risks and benefits, and make the best treatment choices. The nurse can provide opportunities for patients to question, discuss, and explore their feelings about past, current, and planned use of medications and other treatments. Developing strategies to enhance adherence and to raise awareness of early signs of relapse can be important aids to increasing treatment efficacy and promoting recovery (Box 24.7).

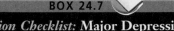

BOX 24.7

Psychoeducation Checklist: **Major Depressive Disorder**

When caring for the patient with a major depressive disorder, be sure to include the following topic areas in the teaching plan:

- Psychopharmacologic agents, including drug action, dosing frequency, and possible adverse effects
- Risk factors for recurrence; signs of recurrence
- Adherence to therapy and treatment program
- Recovery strategies
- Nutrition
- Sleep measures
- Self-care management
- Goal setting and problem solving
- Social interaction skills
- Follow-up appointments
- Community support services

Social Domain

Assessment

Social assessment focuses on the individual's developmental history, family psychiatric history, patterns of relationships, quality of support system, education, work history, and impact of physical or sexual abuse on interpersonal function (see Chapter 14). Including a family member or close friend in the assessment process can be helpful. Changes in patterns of relating (especially social withdrawal) and changes in level of occupational functioning are commonly reported and may represent a significant deterioration from baseline behavior. Increased use of "sick days" may occur. The family's level of support and understanding of the disorder also need to be assessed. For people who are depressed, special attention should be given to the individual's spiritual dimension and religious background (Box 24.8).

BOX 24.8
Using Reflection

ASSESSMENT OF SPIRITUAL DISTRESS

INCIDENT • A patient expresses extreme guilt over a childhood incident involving a teenage pregnancy that resulted in her child being anonymously adopted. The child is now an adult and is trying to contact her. She tells the nurse that she has committed an unforgivable sin.

REFLECTION • The nurse listened for several minutes and reflected on the meaning of the patient's statements and observed how distraught the patient appeared. The nurse then asked the patient if she would want to see the hospital chaplain for further clarification. The patient was greatly relieved and requested help from a chaplain.

Nursing Diagnoses for the Social Domain

Nursing diagnoses common for the social domain include Ineffective Family Coping, Ineffective Role Performance, Interrupted Family Processes, and Caregiver Role Strain (if the patient is also a caregiver).

Interventions for the Social Domain

Individuals experiencing depression have often withdrawn from daily activities, such as engaging in family activities, attending work, and participating in community activities. During hospitalization, patients often withdraw to their rooms and refuse to participate in unit activity. Nurses help the patient balance the need for privacy with the need to return to normal social functioning. Even though depressed patients should not be approached in an overly enthusiastic manner, they should be encouraged to set realistic goals to reconnect with their families and communities. Explain to patients that attending social activities, even though they do not feel like it, will promote the recovery process and help them achieve their goals.

Milieu Therapy

While hospitalized, milieu therapy (see Chapter 10) helps depressed patients maintain socialization skills and continue to interact with others. When depressed, people are often unaware of the environment and withdraw into themselves. On a psychiatric unit, depressed patients should be encouraged to attend and participate in unit activities. These individuals have decreased energy levels and thus may be moving more slowly than others, however, their efforts should be praised.

Safety

In many cases, patients are admitted to the psychiatric hospital because of a suicide attempt. Suicidality should continually be evaluated, and the patient should be protected from self-harm (see Chapter 21). During the depths of depression, patients may not have the energy to complete a suicide. As patients begin to feel better and have increased energy, they may be at a greater risk for suicide. If a previously depressed patient appears to become energized overnight, he or she may have made a decision to commit suicide and thus may be relieved that the decision is finally made. The nurse may misinterpret the mood improvement as a positive move toward recovery; however, this patient may be very intent on suicide. These individuals should be carefully monitored to maintain their safety.

Interventions for Family Members

The family needs education and support during and after the treatment of family members. Because major depressive disorder is a recurring disorder, the family needs information about specific antecedents to a family member's depression and what steps to take. For example, one patient may routinely become depressed during the fall of each year, with one of the first symptoms being excessive sleepiness. For another patient, a major loss, such as a child going to college or the death of a pet, may precipitate a depressive episode. Families of older adults need to be aware of the possibility of depression and related symptoms, which often occurs after the deaths of friends and relatives. Families of children who are depressed often misinterpret depression as behavior problems.

Nurses are exceptionally well positioned to engage patients and their families in the active process of improving daily functioning, increasing knowledge and skill acquisition, and increasing independent living. Consumer-oriented support groups can help to enhance the self-esteem and the support network of participating patients and their families. Advice, encouragement, and the sense of group camaraderie may make an impor-

tant contribution to recovery (APA, 2013). Organizations providing support and information include the Depression and Bipolar Support Network (DBSA), National Alliance on Mental Illness (NAMI), and the Mental Health Association and Recovery, Inc. (a self-help group).

Evaluation and Treatment Outcomes

The major goals of treatment are to help the patient to be as independent as possible and to achieve stability, remission, and recovery from major depression. It is often a lifelong struggle for the individual. Ongoing evaluation of the patient's symptoms, functioning, and quality of life should be carefully documented in the patient's record in order to monitor outcomes of treatment.

Continuum of Care

Mild to moderate depression is often first recognized in primary care settings. Primary care nurses should be able to recognize depression in these patients and make appropriate interventions or referrals. Those with more severe depressive symptoms may be directly admitted to inpatient and outpatient mental health settings or emergency departments. The continuum of care beyond these settings may include partial hospitalization or day treatment programs; individual, family, or group psychotherapy; and home visits. Although most patients with major depression are treated in outpatient settings, brief hospitalization may be required if the patient is suicidal or psychotic (Dollard, 2013; Mitchell, Kane, Kameg, Spino, & Hong, 2013).

Nurses working on inpatient units provide a wide range of direct services, including administering and monitoring medications and target symptoms; conducting psychoeducational groups; and more generally, structuring and maintaining a therapeutic environment. Nurses providing home care have an excellent opportunity to detect undiagnosed depressive disorders and make appropriate referrals.

Nursing practice requires a coordinated, ongoing interaction among patients, families, and providers to deliver comprehensive services. This includes using the complementary skills of both psychiatric and medical care colleagues for forming overall goals, plans, and decisions and for providing continuity of care as needed. Collaborative care between the primary care provider and mental health specialist is also key to achieving remission of symptoms and physical well-being, restoring baseline occupational and psychosocial functioning, and reducing the likelihood of relapse or recurrence.

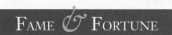

FAME & FORTUNE

Wilbur Wright (1867–1912)

Genius inventor

PUBLIC PERSONA

Of the Wright brothers, Wilbur and Orville, Wilbur Wright is viewed as the real genius and the one who developed intellectual control over the problem of flight. Although his brother, Orville, had inventive skills and was an ideal counterpart, Wilbur was the one who envisioned things that others could not see. Together, the brothers had the skill to build what they imagined. They once built a wagon that reduced the wheel friction so it could haul 10 times as much as before. In his early teens, Wilbur invented a machine to fold newspapers, and Orville built a small printing press for a newspaper he started.

PERSONAL REALITIES

Wilbur Wright had depression that started after a childhood injury he sustained when he was hit in the face with a bat during a game. Complications followed from the medication he received, which affected his heart. He then developed an intestinal disorder, which caused him to abandon his college plans and remain secluded for 4 years. He thought he could never realize his goal of becoming a clergyman. During his poor health and seclusion, he cared for his mother, who was ill with tuberculosis, which eventually caused her death. After his mother died, Wilbur emerged from his depression, and he and his brother went into the printing business together. Later, they focused on airplanes and flying.

Source: Crouch, T. D. (1990). *The bishop's boys: A life of Wilbur and Orville Wright*. New York: W.W. Norton & Company.

SUMMARY OF KEY POINTS

- Moods influence perception of life events and functioning. Depressive disorders are characterized by persistent or recurring disturbances in mood that cause significant psychological distress and functional impairment (typified by feelings of sadness, hopelessness, loss of interest, and fatigue).

- Depressive disorders include both major depressive disorder (depression) and persistent depressive disorder (dysthymic disorder).

- Risk factors include a family history of depressive disorders, prior depressive episodes; lack of social support; stressful life events; substance use; and medical problems, particularly chronic or terminal illnesses.

- The recommended depression treatment guidelines include antidepressant medication, alone or with psychotherapeutic management or psychotherapy, and electroconvulsive therapy for severe depression.

- Nurses must be knowledgeable regarding culturally competent strategies related to the use of antidepressant medications, pharmacologic therapeutic effects and associated side effects, toxicity, dosage ranges, and contraindications. Nurses must also be familiar with electroconvulsive therapy protocols and associated interventions. Patient education and the provision of emotional support during the course of treatment are also nursing responsibilities.

- Many symptoms of depression, such as weight and appetite changes, sleep disturbance, decreased energy, and fatigue, are similar to those of medical illnesses. Assessment includes a thorough medical history and physical examination to detect or rule out medical or psychiatric comorbidity.

- Biopsychosocial assessment includes assessing mood; speech patterns; thought processes and thought content; suicidal or homicidal thoughts; cognition and memory; and social factors, such as patterns of relationships, quality of support systems, and changes in occupational functioning. Several self-report scales are helpful in evaluating depressive symptoms.

- Establishing and maintaining a therapeutic, culturally competent nurse–patient relationship is key to successful outcomes. Nursing interventions that foster the therapeutic relationship include being available in times of crisis, providing understanding and education to patients and their families regarding goals of treatment, providing encouragement and feedback concerning the patient's progress, providing guidance in the patient's interpersonal interactions with others and work environment, and helping to set and monitor realistic goals.

- Psychosocial interventions for depressive disorders include self-care management, cognitive therapy, behavior therapy, interpersonal therapy, patient and family education regarding the nature of the disorder and treatment goals, marital and family therapy, and group therapy that includes medication maintenance support groups and other consumer-oriented support groups.

CRITICAL THINKING CHALLENGES

1. Describe how you would do a suicide assessment on a patient who comes into a primary care office and is distraught and expressing concerns about her ability to cope with her current situation.

2. Describe how you would approach the patient described in the previous Thinking Challenge if you determined that she was suicidal.

3. Discuss difficulties in the differential diagnosis of depressive disorder from other medical and psychiatric disorders. List the information you would use to rule out the other diagnosis when dealing with a patient who appears to be depressed.

4. Describe how you would approach a patient who is expressing concern that the diagnosis of depressive disorder will negatively affect her social and work relationships.

5. Your depressed patient does not seem inclined to talk about his depression. Describe the measures you would take to initiate a therapeutic relationship with him.

6. Think about all of the above situations and relate them to persons from culturally and ethnically diverse populations (e.g., African, Latino, or Asian descent; Jewish or Jehovah Witness religions; across the life-span individuals from children to older adult populations).

About Schmidt: 2002. This movie is about a 67-year-old man, Warren Schmidt, played by Jack Nicholson, who retires from his job as an insurance company executive. He experiences work withdrawal and a lack of direction for his retirement. His wife, Helen, irritates him, and he has no idea what to do to fill his days. While watching television one day, he is moved to sponsor a child in Africa with whom he begins a long, one-sided correspondence. When his wife dies unexpectedly, he is initially numb, then sad, and finally angry when he discovers that she had an affair with his best friend many years ago.

He is estranged from his only daughter, Jeanie, whose wedding to Randall, a man he thinks is beneath her, is imminent. The movie follows Warren as he searches for connection and meaning in his life.

SIGNIFICANCE: Warren Schmidt demonstrates a common phenomenon among the older adults when they retire. He also shows the impact of grief superimposed on initial dysthymia or depression.

VIEWING POINTS: Look for the changes in Schmidt's manifestations of depression in different situations. Note how he experiences the various stages of grieving. What do you think about Schmidt's search for significance and meaning in his life?

Dead Poet's Society: 1989. This film portrays John Keating, played by Robin Williams, as a charismatic English teacher in a conservative New England prep school for boys in 1959. John brings his love of poetry to the students and encourages them to follow their dreams and talents and make the most of every day. His efforts put him at odds with the administration of the school, particularly the headmaster, played by Norman Lloyd, as well as Tom Perry, the father of one of his students, played by Kurtwood Smith. Tom's son, Neil, played by Robert Sean Leonard, chooses to act in a school play despite the objection of his father to any extracurricular activities. When Neil cannot reconcile his love of theater and his father's expectations that he pursue a career in medicine, he kills himself. John Keating blames himself for the death, as does the school administration. He is fired by the administration but has a moment of pride when his students demonstrate their ability to think and act for themselves.

SIGNIFICANCE: This film accurately portrays the sensitivity of adolescents and their longing for worthwhile role models. It also shows adolescent growth and development in a realistic manner. It demonstrates the combination of factors that accompany a decision to commit suicide. We can see how Neil feels caught between his desires and the demands of his father. In the cultural context of the late 1950s, few children or adolescents dared to challenge or defy their parents, especially such a domineering man as Tom Perry.

VIEWING POINTS: Look for the differences in Neil's behavior with his peers and his father or other adults besides Mr. Keating. What, if any, clues do you get that Neil might attempt suicide? What actions by any of the main characters might have prevented his suicide?

MOVIE viewing GUIDES related to this chapter are available at http://thePoint.lww.com/Boyd5eUpdate.

A related Psychiatric-Mental Health Nursing video on the topic of Depression is available at: http://thePoint.lww.com/Boyd5eUpdate.

References

Alpern, E. R., & Henretig, F. M. (2010). Fever. In G. R. Fleisher & S. Ludwig (Eds.). *Textbook of pediatric emergency* (pp. 273–274). Philadelphia: Wolters Kluwer.

American Psychiatric Association (APA). (2013). *Diagnostic and statistical manual of mental disorders DSM-5* (5th ed.). Arlington, VA: Author.

Apostolo, J. L., & Kolcaba, K. (2009). The effects of guided imagery on comfort, depression, anxiety, and stress of psychiatric inpatients with depressive disorders. *Archives of Psychiatric Nursing, 23*(6), 403–411.

Beeber, L. S., Lewis, V. S., Cooper, C., Maxwell, L., & Sandelowski, M. (2010). Meeting the "now" need: PMH-APRN- Interpreter teams provide in-home mental health intervention for depressed Latina mothers with limited English proficiency. *Journal of the American Psychiatric Nurses Association, 15*(4), 249–259.

Bernard, S., Westmand, G., Dutton, P. R., & Lanocha, K. (2009). A psychiatric nurse's perspective: Helping patients undergo repetitive transcranial magnetic stimulation (rTMS) for depression. *Journal of the American Psychiatric Nurses Association, 15*(5), 325–337.

Blazer, D. G., & Steffens, D. C. (2009). *The American Psychiatric Publishing textbook of geriatric psychiatry* (4th ed.). Washington, DC: American Psychiatric Publishing.

Cerel, J., Jordan, J. R., & Duberstien, P. R. (2008). The impact of suicide on the family. *Crisis, 29*, 38–44.

Dollard, M. K. (2013). Psychopharmacology in psychiatric emergency. In L. G. Leahy & C. G. Kohler (Eds.), *Manual of clinical psychopharmacology for nurses* (Chapter 1, pp. 301–329). Washington, DC: American Psychiatric Publishing.

Dulcan, M. K., & Lake, M. (2012). *Concise guide to child and adolescent psychiatry* (4th ed.). Washington, DC: American Psychiatric Publishing.

Gonzalez, H. M., Vega, W. A., Williams, D. R., Tarraf, W., West, B. T., & Neighbors, H. (2010). Depression care in the United States. *Archives of General Psychiatry, 67*(1), 37–46.

Herrera, J. M., Lawson, W. B., & Sramek, J. J. (Eds.). (1999). *Cross cultural psychiatry*. New York: John Wiley & Sons.

Institute of Medicine. (2003). *Unequal treatment: Confronting racial and ethnic disparities in health care*. Washington, DC: National Academies Press.

Josey, L. M., & Neidert, E. M. (2013). Depressive disorders. In L. G. Leahy & C. G. Kohler (Eds.), *Manual of clinical psychopharmacology for nurses* (Chapter 3, pp. 59–84). Washington, DC: American Psychiatric Publishing.

Limandri, B. J. (2013). Management of metabolic side effects of psychotropic medications. In L. G. Leahy & C. G. Kohler (Eds.), *Manual of clinical psychopharmacology for nurses* (Chapter 12, pp. 331–352). Washington, DC: American Psychiatric Publishing.

Leahy, L. G., & Kohler, C. G. (2013). Introduction to clinical psychopharmacology for nurses. In L. G. Leahy & C. G. Kohler (Eds.), *Manual of clinical psychopharmacology for nurses* (Chapter 1, pp. 1–27). Washington, DC: American Psychiatric Publishing.

Lewy, A. J., Lefler, B. J., Emens, J. S., & Bauer, V. K. (2006). The circadian basis of winter depression. Retrieved from http://www.pnas.org/cgi/doi/10.1073/pnas.0602425103

Levin, T. T., Cortes-Ladino, A., Weiss, M., & Palomba, M. L. (2008). Life threatening toxicity due to a citalopram-fluconazole drug intraction, case reports and discussion. *General Hospital Psychiatry, 30*(4), 372–377.

Liehr, P., & Diaz, N. (2010). A pilot study examining the effect of mindfulness on depression and anxiety for minority children. *Archives of Psychiatric Nursing, 24*(1), 69–71.

Lutz, W. J., & Warren, B. J. (2007). The state of nursing science: Cultural and lifespan issues depression part II: Focus on children and adolescents. *Issues in Mental Health Nursing, 28*(7), 749–764.

McEnany, G. P. (2011). Sleep in psychiatric mental health settings. In N. S. Redeker & G. P. McEnany (Eds.), *Sleep disorders and sleep promotion in nursing practice,* (Chapter 19, pp. 309–320). Washington, DC: American Psychiatric Publishing.

Mitchell, A. M., Kane, I., Kameg, K. M., Spino, E. R., & Hong, B. (2013). Integrated management of self-directed injury. In K. R. Tusaie & J. J. Fitzpatrick (Eds.), *Advanced practice psychiatric nursing: Integrating psychotherapy, psychopharmacology, and complementary and alternative approaches* (Chapter 15, pp. 362–387). New York: Springer Publishing Company.

Munoz, R., Primm, A., Ananth, J., & Ruiz, P. (2007). *Life in color: Culture in American psychiatry*. Chicago, IL: Hilton Publishing.

National Institutes of Mental Health. (2009). *Suicide in the U.S: Statistics and prevention*. Retrieved from http://www.nimh.nih.gov/health/publications/suicide-in-the-us-statistics-and-prevention/index.shtml

Pedersen, C. A., Draguus, J. G., Lonner, W. J., & Trimble, J. E. (2008). *Counseling across cultures* (6th ed.). Thousand Oaks, CA: Sage Publishing.

Posmontier, B. (2013). Complementary and alternative pharmacotherapies. In L. G. Leahy & C. G. Kohler (Eds.), *Manual of clinical psychopharmacology for nurses* (Chapter 13, pp. 353–377). Washington, DC: American Psychiatric Publishing.

Purnell, L. D. (2012). *Transcultural health care* (4th ed.). Philadelphia: F. A. Davis.

Rosenquist, J. N., Fowler, J. H., & Christakis, N. A. (2011). Social network determinants of depression. *Molecular Psychiatry, 16*(3), 273–281.

Schatzberg, A. F., & Nemeroff, C. B. (2009). *Textbook of psychopharmacology* (4th ed.) Washington, DC: American Psychiatric Publishing.

Shi, J., Potash, S. J., Knowles, J. A., Weissman, M. M., Coryyell, W., Lawson, W. B., et al. (2011). Genome-wide association study of recurrent early-onset major depressive disorder. *Molecular Psychiatry, 16*(2), 193–201.

Stahl, S. M. (2013a). *Stahl's essential psychopharmacology: Neuroscientific basis and practical applications* (4th ed.). New York: Cambridge Press.

Stahl, S. M. (2013b). *Stahl's essential psychopharmacology: The prescriber's guide* (4th ed.). New York: Cambridge Press.

Tarraza, M. (2013). Medical problems and psychiatric syndromes. In K. R. Tusaie & J. J. Fitzpatrick (Eds.), *Advanced practice psychiatric nursing: Integrating psychotherapy, psychopharmacology, and complementary and alternative approaches* (Chapter 18, pp. 468–485). New York: Springer Publishing Company.

Tsai, W. P., Lin, L. Y., Chang, W. L., Chang, H. C., & Chou, M. C. (2010). The effects of suicide awareness program in enhancing community volunteers' of suicide warning signs. *Archives of Psychiatric Nursing, 24*(1), 63–68.

Tusaie, K. R. (2013). Integrative management of disordered mood. In K. R. Tusaie & J. J. Fitzpatrick (Eds.), *Advanced practice psychiatric nursing: Integrating psychotherapy, psychopharmacology, and complementary and alternative approaches* (Chapter 8, pp. 122–157). New York: Springer Publishing Company.

United States Department of Health and Human Services (USDHHS). (1999). *Mental health: A report of the Surgeon General.* Rockville, MD: United States Department of Health and Human Services, Substance Abuse and Mental Health Services Administration, Center for Mental Health Services, National Institutes of Health, National Institute of Mental Health.

Van der Wurff, F. B., Stek, M., Hoogendijk W., & Beekman A. (2003). Electroconvulsive therapy for the depressed elderly. *Cochrane Database of Systematic Reviews,* (2), CD003593.

Warren, B. J. (in press). Substance abuse. In B. Melnyk & P. Jensen (Eds.), *The Guide to Child and Adolescent Mental Health Screening, Early Intervention and Health Promotion* (2nd ed.). Cherry Hill, NJ: National Association of Pediatric Nurse Practitioners (NAPNAP).

Warren, B. J. (2008). Cultural and ethnic considerations. In D. Antai-Otong (Ed.), *Psychiatric nursing: Biological and behavioral concepts* (2nd ed., pp. 174–193). Clifton Park, NJ: Thomson Delmar Learning.

Warren, B. J. (2011a). Guest Editor. CNE Series: Two sides of the coin: The bully and the bullied. *Journal of Psychosocial Nursing and Mental Health Services, 49*(10), 22–29.

Warren, B. J. (2011b). Cultural competence in psychiatric nursing. In N. L. Keltner, C. E. Bostrom, & T. McGuinness (Eds.), *Psychiatric nursing* (6th ed., Chapter 14, pp. 164–172). St. Louis, MO: Mosby.

Warren, B. J., & Broome, B. (2011). CNE Series: The culture of adolescents with urologic dysfunction: Mental health, wellness, and illness awareness. *Urologic Nursing, 31*(2), 95–104.

Warren, B. J. (2012). Depression: Management of depressive disorders and suicidal behavior. In M. A. Boyd (Ed.), *Psychiatric nursing: Contemporary practice* (5th ed., Chapter 24, pp. 401–425). Philadelphia: Wolters Kluwer, Lippincott Williams & Wilkins.

Warren, B. J. (2013a). How culture is assessed in the *DSM-5. Journal of Psychosocial Nursing, 51*(4), 40–45.

Warren, B. J. (2013b). Culturally sensitive psychopharmacology. In L. G. Leahy & C. G. Kohler (Eds.), *Clinical manual of psychopharmacology for nurses* (Chapter 14, pp. 379–402). Washington, DC: American Psychiatric Publishing, Inc.

Warren, B. J. (2013c) Ethnopharmacology. In B. Cockerman (Ed.), *Blackwell encyclopaedia health and society medical anthropology.* Somerset, NJ: Wiley.

Warren, B. J., & Lutz, W. J. (2007). The state of nursing science: Cultural and lifespan issues depression Part II: Focus on adults. *Issues in Mental Health Nursing, 28*(7), 707–748.

World Health Organization (WHO). (2014). Evidence-based recommendations for management of depression in non-specialized health settings. Retrieved from http://www.who.int/mental_health/mhgap/evidence/depression/en/index.html

Yudofsky, S. C., & Hales, R. E. (2010). *Essentials of neuropsychiatry and behavioral neurosciences* (6th ed.). Washington, DC: American Psychiatric Publishing.

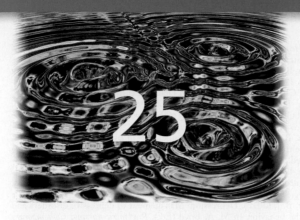

25 Bipolar Disorders
Management of Mood Lability

Mary Ann Boyd

KEY CONCEPTS

- bipolar disorders
- mania
- mood lability

LEARNING OBJECTIVES

After studying this chapter, you will be able to:

1. Describe the prevalence and incidence of bipolar disorders.
2. Delineate the clinical symptoms of bipolar disorders with emphasis on mood lability.
3. Analyze the biopsychosocial theories explaining bipolar disorder and mood lability.
4. Identify evidence-based interventions for patients diagnosed with bipolar disorders and for those who exhibit mood lability.
5. Develop recovery-oriented strategies that address the needs of persons diagnosed with bipolar disorders and for those who exhibit mood lability.

KEY TERMS

- bipolar I • bipolar II • elation • elevated mood • euphoria • expansive mood • hypomania
- hypomanic episode • grandiosity • irritable mood • manic episode • mixed episode • rapid cycling

Everyone has ups and downs. Mood changes are a part of everyday life, and expression of feeling is integral to communication. But when moods are so pervasive that they cloud reasoning and judgment, they become problematic and interfere with interpersonal relationships. In some instances, extreme moods such as mania are symptoms of mental disorders. This chapter discusses bipolar disorders that are characterized by severe mood changes with bipolar I highlighted.

MANIA DEFINED

Mania is one of the primary symptoms of bipolar disorders. It is recognized by an elevated, expansive, or irritable mood.

KEYCONCEPT **Mania** is primarily characterized by an abnormally and persistently elevated, expansive, or irritable mood.

Mania is easily recognized by the cognitive changes that occur. Elevated self-esteem is expressed as **grandiosity** (exaggerating personal importance) and may range from unusual self-confidence to grandiose delusions. Speech is pressured; the person is more talkative than usual and at times is difficult to interrupt. There is often a flight of ideas (illogical connections between thoughts) or racing thoughts. Distractibility increases.

In mania, the need for sleep is decreased, and energy is increased. The individual often remains awake for long periods or wakes up several times at night full of energy. Initially, there is an increase in goal-directed activity that is

BOX 25.1
THE PATIENT WITH MANIA

Mr. Bell was a day trader on the stock market. Initially, he was quite successful and, as a result, upgraded his lifestyle with a more expensive car; a larger, more luxurious house; and a boat. When the stock market declined dramatically, Mr. Bell continued to trade, saying that if he could just find the "right" stock he could earn back all of the money he had lost. He spent his days and nights in front of his computer screen, taking little or no time to eat or sleep. He defaulted on his mortgage and car and boat payments and was talking nonstop to his wife. She brought him to the hospital for evaluation.

What Do You Think?
- What behavioral symptoms of mania does Mr. Bell exhibit?
- What cognitive symptoms of mania does Mr. Bell exhibit?

purposeful (e.g., cleaning the house), but it deteriorates into hyperactivity, agitation, and disorganized behavior. Social activities, occupational functioning, and interpersonal relationships are eventually impaired. There can be excessive involvement in pleasurable activities with little regard for painful consequences (e.g., excessive spending, risky sexual behavior, drug or alcohol use) (Box 25.1). Persons with mania are often hospitalized to prevent self-harm.

A **manic episode** is defined as a distinct period (of at least 1 week or less if hospitalized) of abnormally and persistently elevated, expansive, or irritable mood with abnormally increased goal-directed behavior or energy (American Psychiatric Association [APA], 2013). An **elevated mood** can be expressed as **euphoria** (exaggerated feelings of well-being) or **elation** (feeling "high," "ecstatic," "on top of the world," or "up in the clouds"). An **expansive mood** is characterized by lack of restraint in expressing feelings; an overvalued sense of self importance; and a constant and indiscriminate enthusiasm for interpersonal, sexual, or occupational interactions.

For some, an **irritable mood** instead of an elevated mood is pervasive during mania. These individuals are easily annoyed and provoked to anger, particularly when their wishes are challenged or thwarted. Maintaining social relationships during these episodes is difficult.

Even though mania is primarily associated with bipolar disorders, other psychiatric disorders, such as schizophrenia, schizoaffective disorder, anxiety disorders, some personality disorders (borderline personality disorder and histrionic personality disorder), substance abuse involving stimulants, and adolescent conduct disorders, can have symptoms that mimic a manic episode. Mania can also be caused by medical disorders or their treatments, certain metabolic abnormalities, neurologic disorders, central nervous system CNS tumors, and medications.

BIPOLAR DISORDERS

The bipolar disorder group of disorders includes bipolar I (periods of major depressive, manic, or mixed episodes), bipolar II (periods of major depression and hypomania), and cyclothymic disorder (periods of hypomanic episodes and depressive episodes that do not meet the full criteria for a major depressive episode).

> **KEYCONCEPT** **Bipolar disorders** are characterized by periods of mania or hypomania that alternate with depression. These disorders can be further designated as bipolar I, bipolar II, and cyclothymic disorder depending on the severity of the manic and depressive symptoms.

Mood lability is the term used for the rapid shifts in moods that often occur in bipolar disorder. One month a person is happy, and the next he or she is in the depth of depression. These mood shifts leave everyone confused and interfere with social interaction.

> **KEYCONCEPT** **Mood lability** is alterations in moods with little or no change in external events.

Rapid cycling is an extreme form of mood lability and can occur in both bipolar I and bipolar II disorders. In its most severe form, rapid cycling includes continuous cycling between subthreshold mania and depression or hypomania and depression. The essential feature of rapid cycling is the occurrence of four or more mood episodes that meet criteria for manic, mixed, hypomanic, or depressive episode during the previous 12 months (APA, 2013).

Clinical Course

Bipolar disorder is a chronic, cyclic disorder. Those with an earlier onset have more frequent episodes than persons who develop the illness later in life. An early onset and a family history of illness are associated with multiple episodes or continuous symptoms. Symptoms of the illness can be unpredictable and variable. Bipolar disorder can lead to severe functional impairment such as alienation from family, friends, and coworkers; indebtedness; job loss; divorce; and other problems of living (Lee et al., 2010).

Diagnostic Criteria

To be diagnosed with **bipolar I**, at least one manic episode or mixed episode and a depressive episode have to occur. See Key Diagnostic Characteristics 25.1. The term **mixed episode** is used when mania and depression occur at the same time, which leads to extreme anxiety,

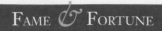

FAME & FORTUNE

Vincent Van Gogh (1853–1890)
Post-Impressionist Artist

PUBLIC PERSONA

Vincent Van Gogh, born in Holland, was the son of a pastor and grew up to be one of the most important artists in Western culture. His works are found in museums worldwide.

PERSONAL REALITIES

As a child, Van Gogh lacked self-confidence and was described as highly emotional. As an adult, he was unsuccessful in relationships and was unable to maintain friendships. His moods vacillated between high-energy periods, when he would produce his multiple works, and exhaustion and then depression. Because of his mood lability, many believe that he had bipolar disorder. He also had episodes of psychosis, delusions, and seizures. During one of his episodes, he cut off a lobe of his ear. Ultimately, he committed suicide at a very young age.

agitation, and irritability. These individuals are clearly miserable and are at high risk for suicide.

Bipolar II is not as easily recognized as bipolar I because the symptoms are less dramatic. **Hypomania**, a mild form of mania, is characteristic of bipolar II. A **hypomanic episode** is less intense, and there is little impairment in social or occupational functioning. Normal judgment is mostly intact.

In a cyclothymic disorder, hypomanic symptoms occur alternating with numerous periods of depressive symptoms. However, these symptoms are less severe than the bipolar disorders. To be diagnosed with this disorder, the symptoms have to be present for at least 2 years of numerous periods.

Bipolar Disorders Across the Life Span

Children and Adolescents

Bipolar disorder in children has been recognized only recently. Although it is not well studied, depression usually appears first. Somewhat different than in adults, the hallmark of childhood bipolar disorder is intense rage. Children may display seemingly unprovoked rage episodes for as long as 2 to 3 hours. The symptoms of bipolar disorder reflect the developmental level of the child. Children younger than 9 years exhibit more irritability and emotional lability; older children exhibit more classic symptoms, such as euphoria and grandiosity. The first contact with the mental health system often occurs when the behavior becomes disruptive, possibly 5 to 10 years after its onset. These children often have other psychiatric disorders, such as attention deficit hyperactivity disorder or conduct disorder (Chen et al., 2013; Wozniak, Faraone, Mick, Monuteaux, Coville, & Biederman, 2010) (see Chapter 35).

Older Adults

Older adults with bipolar disorder have more neurologic abnormalities and cognitive disturbances (confusion and disorientation) than do younger patients. The incidence of mania decreases with age, but the onset of bipolar disorder can also occur in older adults. Symptoms are similar to the earlier onset bipolar disorder (Chu et al., 2010).

Epidemiology and Risk Factors

Risk factors for bipolar disorders include a family history of mood disorders; prior mood episodes; lack of social support; stressful life events; substance use; and medical problems, particularly chronic or terminal illnesses.

Age of Onset

Bipolar disorder has a lifetime prevalence of 1.1% for bipolar I and 1.4% for bipolar II (Kessler, Petukhova, Sampson, Zaslavsky, & Wittchen, 2012). Most patients with bipolar disorder experience significant symptoms before age 25 years. The estimated mean age of onset is between 21 and 30 years. Nearly 20% of those with bipolar disorder have symptoms before the age of 19 years. Estimates of the prevalence of bipolar disorder in older adults decline with age (Byers, Yaffe, Covinsky, Friedman, & Bruce, 2010).

Gender

Although no significant gender differences have been found in the incidence of bipolar I and II diagnoses, gender differences have been reported in phenomenology, course, and treatment response. In addition, some data show that female patients with bipolar disorder are at greater risk for depression and rapid cycling than are male patients, but male patients are at greater risk for manic episodes.

Ethnicity and Culture

No significant differences have been found based on race or ethnicity (Perron, Fries, Kilbourne, Vaughn, & Bauer, 2010).

Comorbidity

The two most common comorbid conditions are anxiety disorders (panic disorder and social phobia are the most prevalent) and substance use (most commonly alcohol and marijuana). Individuals with a comorbid anxiety disorder are more likely to experience a more severe course. A history of substance use further complicates the course of illness and results in less chance for remission and poorer treatment compliance (Kessler et al., 2012; Kenneson, Fundeburk, & Maisto, 2013).

KEY DIAGNOSTIC CHARACTERISTICS 25.1 • BIPOLAR I DISORDER 296.XX

296.4X—BIPOLAR I, CURRENT OR MOST RECENT EPISODE MANIC
296.4X—BIPOLAR I, CURRENT OR MOST RECENT EPISODE HYPOMANIC
296.4X—BIPOLAR I, CURRENT OR MOST RECENT EPISODE DEPRESSED

Diagnostic Criteria

For a diagnosis of bipolar I disorder, it is necessary to meet the following criteria for a manic episode. The manic episode may have been preceded by and may be followed by hypomanic or major depressive episodes (See Major Depressive Disorder Diagnostic Criteria). Major depressive episodes are common in bipolar I disorder but are not required for the diagnosis of bipolar I disorder.

Manic Episode

A. A distinct period of abnormally and persistently elevated, expansive, or irritable mood and abnormally and persistently increased goal-directed activity or energy, lasting at least 1 week and present most of the day, nearly every day (or any duration if hospitalization is necessary).

B. During the period of mood disturbance and increased energy or activity, three (or more) of the following symptoms (four if the mood is only irritable) are present to a significant degree and represent a noticeable change from usual behavior:
1. Inflated self-esteem or grandiosity.
2. Decreased need for sleep (e.g., feels rested after only 3 hours of sleep).
3. More talkative than usual or pressure to keep talking.
4. Flight of ideas or subjective experience that thoughts are racing.
5. Distractibility (i.e., attention too easily drawn to unimportant or irrelevant external stimuli), as reported or observed.
6. Increase in goal-directed activity (either socially, at work or school, or sexually) or psychomotor agitation (i.e., purposeless non–goal-directed activity).
7. Excessive involvement in activities that have a high potential for painful consequences (e.g., engaging in unrestrained buying sprees, sexual indiscretions, or foolish business investments).

C. The mood disturbance is sufficiently severe to cause marked impairment in social or occupational functioning or to necessitate hospitalization to prevent harm to self or others, or there are psychotic features.

D. The episode is not attributable to the physiological effects of a substance (e.g., a drug of abuse, a medication, other treatment) or to another medical condition.
- **Note:** A full manic episode that emerges during antidepressant treatment (e.g., medication, electroconvulsive therapy) but persists at a fully syndromal level beyond the physiological effect of that treatment is sufficient evidence for a manic episode and, therefore, a bipolar I diagnosis.

Note: Criteria A–D constitute a manic episode. At least one lifetime manic episode is required for the diagnosis of bipolar I disorder.

Hypomanic Episode

A. A distinct period of abnormally and persistently elevated, expansive, or irritable mood and abnormally and persistently increased activity or energy, lasting at least 4 consecutive days and present most of the day, nearly every day.

B. During the period of mood disturbance and increased energy and activity, three (or more) of the following symptoms (four if the mood is only irritable) have persisted, represent a noticeable change from usual behavior, and have been present to a significant degree:
1. Inflated self-esteem or grandiosity.
2. Decreased need for sleep (e.g., feels rested after only 3 hours of sleep).
3. More talkative than usual or pressure to keep talking.
4. Flight of ideas or subjective experience that thoughts are racing.
5. Distractibility (i.e., attention too easily drawn to unimportant or irrelevant external stimuli), as reported or observed.
6. Increase in goal-directed activity (either socially, at work or school, or sexually) or psychomotor agitation.
7. Excessive involvement in activities that have a high potential for painful consequences (e.g., engaging in unrestrained buying sprees, sexual indiscretions, or foolish business investments).

C. The episode is associated with an unequivocal change in functioning that is uncharacteristic of the individual when not symptomatic.

D. The disturbance in mood and the change in functioning are observable by others.

E. The episode is not severe enough to cause marked impairment in social or occupational functioning or to necessitate hospitalization. If there are psychotic features, the episode is, by definition, manic.

F. The episode is not attributable to the physiological effects of a substance (e.g., a drug of abuse, a medication, other treatment).
- **Note:** A full hypomanic episode that emerges during antidepressant treatment (e.g., medication, electroconvulsive therapy) but persists at a fully syndromal level beyond the physiological effect of that treatment is sufficient evidence for a hypomanic episode diagnosis. However, caution is indicated so that one or two symptoms (particularly increased irritability, edginess, or agitation following antidepressant use) are not taken as sufficient for diagnosis of a hypomanic episode, nor necessarily indicative of a bipolar diathesis.

Note: Criteria A–F constitute a hypomanic episode. Hypomanic episodes are common in bipolar I disorder but are not required for the diagnosis of bipolar I disorder.

Bipolar I Disorder

A. Criteria have been met for at least one manic episode (Criteria A–D under "Manic Episode" above).

B. The occurrence of the manic and major depressive episode(s) is not better explained by schizoaffective disorder, schizophrenia, schizophreniform disorder, delusional disorder, or other specified or unspecified schizophrenia spectrum and other psychotic disorder.

Etiology

The etiology of mood disorders is unknown, but the current thinking is that bipolar disorder results when there is an interaction between the genetic predisposition and psychosocial stress such as abuse or trauma (Hashimoto, 2010; Liu, 2010).

Biologic Theories

Chronobiologic Theories

Sleep disturbance is common in individuals with bipolar disorder, especially mania. Sleep patterns appear to be regulated by an internal biologic clock center in the hypothalamus. Artificially induced sleep deprivation is known to precipitate mania in some patients with bipolar disorder. It is possible that circadian dysregulation underlies the sleep–wake disturbances of bipolar disorder. Seasonal changes in light exposure also trigger affective episodes in some patients, typically depression in winter and hypomania in the summer in the northern hemisphere (Salvatore, Indic, Murray, & Baldessarini, 2012).

Genetic Factors

Results from family, adoption, and twin studies indicate that bipolar disorder is highly heritable. Studies of monozygotic twins show risks from 40% to 90% of acquiring the illness if their identical twin has the disorder range (Craddock & Sklar, 2009). No one gene or sequence of genes is responsible for the pathology of bipolar disorder. Evidence suggests that there is an overlap in the genetic etiology of schizophrenia and bipolar disorders (Lee et al., 2013).

Chronic Stress and Kindling

The role of an allostatic load or wear and tear on the body (see Chapter 18) is thought to contribute to cognitive impairment, comorbidity, and eventual mortality of those with bipolar disorder (Vieta et al., 2013). In this model, bipolar disorder is viewed as a disorder where the allostatic load increases as the number of mood episodes increases leading to an increase in physical and mental health problems. An interaction between stress and brain development is viewed as dynamic and individuals have different kinds of stress adaptation depending on their neurobiologic responses (Brietzke, Mansur, Soczynska, Powell, & McIntyre, 2012).

A closely related concept is the kindling theory that posits that as genetically predisposed individuals experience repetitive, subthreshold stressors at vulnerable times, mood symptoms of increasing intensity and duration occur. Eventually, a full-blown depressive or manic episode erupts. Each episode leaves a trace and increases the person's vulnerability or sensitizes the person to have another episode

with less stimulation. In later episodes, there may be little or no stress before the depression or mania. The disorder takes on a life of its own, and over time, the time between episodes decreases (Bender & Alloy, 2011).

Psychological and Social Theories

Psychosocial theories are useful in planning recovery-oriented interventions that focus on reducing environmental stress and trauma in genetically vulnerable individuals. It is now generally accepted that psychosocial and environmental events contribute to the severity of the disorder and the frequency of the mood episodes (Bender & Alloy, 2011). Two promising theories are currently receiving research support.

The behavioral approach system dysregulation theory proposed that individuals with bipolar disorder are overly sensitive and overreact to relevant cues when approaching a reward. That is, the intensity of the goal-motivated behavior can lead to manic symptoms such as euphoria, decreased need for sleep, and excessive self-confidence. On the other hand, the system can be deactivated and lead to depressive symptoms such as decreased energy, hopelessness, and sadness (Bender & Alloy, 2011).

The social rhythm disruption theory is consistent with the research on the impact of the circadian rhythm dysregulation previously discussed. In our environment, there are patterned social events such as meal times, exercise times, and regular companionship. Individuals with bipolar disorder have less regular social rhythms than those without bipolar disorder. This theory suggests that when patterned social events are disrupted, mood episodes are more likely to appear (Bender & Alloy, 2011).

Family Response to Disorder

Bipolar disorder can devastate families, who often feel that they are on an emotional merry-go-round, particularly if they have difficulty understanding the mood shifts. A major problem for family members is dealing with the consequences of impulsive behavior during manic episodes, such as excessive debt, assault charges, and sexual infidelities.

Interdisciplinary Treatment and Recovery

An important recovery goal is to minimize and prevent either manic or depressive episodes, which tend to accelerate over time. The fewer the episodes, the more likely the person can live a normal, productive life. Patients with bipolar disorder have a complex set of issues and have the best chance of recovery by working with an interdisciplinary team (see Interdisciplinary Treatment/Recovery Plan 25.1). Nurses, physicians, social workers, psychologists, and activity therapists all have valuable expertise. For children with bipolar disorder, school teachers and counselors are included in the team. For older adult patients, the

INTERDISCIPLINARY TREATMENT/RECOVERY PLAN 25.1

Patient With Bipolar Disorder Community Mental Health Center Treatment Program for JR, a 43-Year-Old Female

Admission Date	Date of This Plan	Type of Plan: Check Appropriate Box
		☐ Initial ☐ Master ☐ 30 ☐ 60 ☐ 90 ☐ Other

Treatment Team Present:
J. R., M. Jones, MD; S. Smith, RNC; T. Thompson, PhD (psychologist); G. Bond, LCSW (social worker); V. Stevens, BA (rehabilitation counselor)

DIAGNOSIS

Bipolar I

ASSETS (MEDICAL, PSYCHOLOGICAL, SOCIAL, EDUCATIONAL, VOCATIONAL, RECREATIONAL)

1. Controls illness through medication and monthly visits for brief counseling and stress management.
2. Lives independently in apartment.
3. Works at a library and has good relationships with boss and coworkers.
4. Easily makes friends.

MASTER PROBLEM LIST

Prob No.	Date	Problem	Code	Change Code	Change Date
1	1/12/15	Ineffective coping: Does not want to go to work because of intense grief for mother's death.		R	2/12/12
2	1/12/15	Mood disturbance. Patient is very depressed, not eating or sleeping.		R	4/14/12
3	6/12/15	Mood changes with the seasons. Needs monitoring of mood.		T	
4	6/12/15	Interpersonal issues interfering with ability to work at library		T	

CODE T = Problem must be addressed in treatment.
   N = Problem noted and will be monitored.
   X = Problem noted but deferred/inactive/no action necessary.
   O = Problem to be addressed in aftercare/continuing care.
   I = Problem incorporated into another problem.
   R = Resolved.

INDIVIDUAL TREATMENT PLAN PROBLEM SHEET

#1 Problem/Need	Date Identified	Problem Resolved/Discontinuation Date
Cyclic mood changes, usually according to the season. Medication needs to be re-evaluated and adjusted according to mood changes. Stress is often the precipitant to mood changes. Needs updating on information about bipolar disorder.	1/12/15	Ongoing

Continued

INTERDISCIPLINARY TREATMENT/RECOVERY PLAN 25.1 *(Continued)*

Patient With Bipolar Disorder Community Mental Health Center Treatment Program for JR, a 43-Year-Old Female

Objective(s)/Short-Term Goals	Target Date	Achievement Date
1. Monitor mood changes. 2. Adjust medications as needed.	Every 3 months	

Treatment Interventions	Frequency	Person Responsible
1. Evaluate mood changes.	Every 3 months or as needed.	RN
2. Adjust medications.	Every 3 months or as needed.	MD
3. Medication education.	Weekly class.	RN
4. Stress management techniques.	Weekly class for 6 weeks.	Psychologist

Responsible QMHP	**Patient or Guardian**	**Staff Physician**
Signature Date	Signature Date	Signature Date

primary care physician becomes part of the team. Helping the patient and family to learn about the disorder and manage it throughout a lifetime is critical for recovery.

Priority Care Issues

During a manic episode, patient safety is a priority. Risk of suicide is always present for those having a depressive or manic episode. During a depressive episode, the patient may believe that life is not worth living. During a manic episode, the patient may believe that he or she has supernatural powers, such as the ability to fly. As patients recover from a manic episode, they may be so devastated by the consequences of impulsive behavior and poor judgment during the episode that suicide seems like the only option.

During a manic episode, poor judgment and impulsivity lead to risk-taking behaviors that can have dire consequences for the patient and family. For example, when one patient gambled all of his family's money away, he blamed his partner for letting him have access to the money. A physical confrontation with the partner resulted.

NURSING MANAGEMENT: Human Response to Bipolar Disorder

The nursing care of patients with a bipolar disorder is one of the most interesting yet greatest challenges in psychiatric nursing. In general, the behavior of patients with bipolar disorder is normal between mood episodes. The nurse's first contact with the patient is usually during a manic or depressive episode. Recovery-oriented nursing care begins with the initial assessment through engaging the patient in a partnership and empowering the person to make decisions in setting overall goals of care (Box 25.2). During acute episodes, the patient's judgment may be impaired,

but as the manic or depressive symptoms subside, the person will be able to participate in care decisions.

Biologic Domain

Assessment

Symptoms of mania (or depression), especially changes in activity, eating, and sleep patterns, are evaluated for severity. The patient may not sleep, resulting in irritability and physical exhaustion. Diet and body weight usually change during a manic or depressive episode. Laboratory studies, such as thyroid function and electrolytes, should be completed to detect evidence of malnutrition and fluid imbalance. Abnormal thyroid functioning can be responsible for

---

BOX 25.2

Research for Best Practice: **Promoting Choice for People with Bipolar Disorder**

Jones, M., & Jones, A. (2008). Promotion of choice in the care of people with bipolar disorder: A mental health nursing perspective. *Journal of Psychiatric & Mental Health Nursing, 15(2), 87–92.*

THE QUESTION: What key issues arise with persons diagnosed with bipolar disorder?

METHODS: This case study was a detailed account of interviews with a person who was hospitalized for 4 weeks for bipolar mania.

FINDINGS: The nurse and the patient negotiated throughout the 4 weeks to reach the best medication regimen. The nurse found that partnering with the patient and promoting a shared decision-making approach was important in reducing the symptoms and focusing on recovery. A multidisciplinary approach is recommended.

IMPLICATIONS FOR NURSING: Promoting patient choice in treatment selection results in successful reduction of symptoms and helps the patient learn to manage the illness.

the mood and behavioral disturbances. In mania, patients often become hypersexual and engage in risky sexual practices. Changes in sexual practices should be included in the assessment. For depression, the assessment should follow the process explained in Chapter 24.

Many times, manic or depressive episodes occur after patients stop taking their medication. Exploring the reasons for discontinuing the medication will help in planning adherence strategies in the future. Some stop taking their medications because of side effects; others do not believe they have a mental disorder. The use of alcohol and other substances should be carefully assessed. Usually, a drug screen is ordered. In some instances, patients have been taking an antidepressant as prescribed for depression without realizing that a bipolar disorder existed.

Nursing Diagnoses for the Biologic Domain

Among nursing diagnoses in this domain are Insomnia; Sleep Deprivation; Imbalanced Nutrition; Hypothermia, Deficient Fluid Volume; and Non-adherence if patients have stopped taking their medication (Figure 25.1). If patients are in the depressive phase of illness, the previously discussed diagnoses for depression should be considered.

Interventions for the Biologic Domain

Teaching Physical Care

In a state of mania, the patient's physical needs are rest, adequate hydration and nutrition, and reestablishment of physical well-being. Self-care has usually deteriorated. For a patient who is unable to sit long enough to eat, snacks and high-energy foods should be provided that can be eaten while moving. Alcohol should be avoided. Sleep hygiene is a priority but may not be realistic until medications take effect. Limiting stimuli can be helpful in decreasing agitation and promoting sleep.

> **NCLEXNOTE** Protection of patients with mania is always a priority. Ongoing assessment should focus on irritability, fatigue, and the potential for harming self or others.

After the patient's mood stabilizes, the nurse should focus on monitoring changes in physical functioning in sleep or eating behavior and teaching patients to identify antecedents to mood episodes such as a family argument or a financial problem. Strategies for dealing with future events can then be identified. The patient can

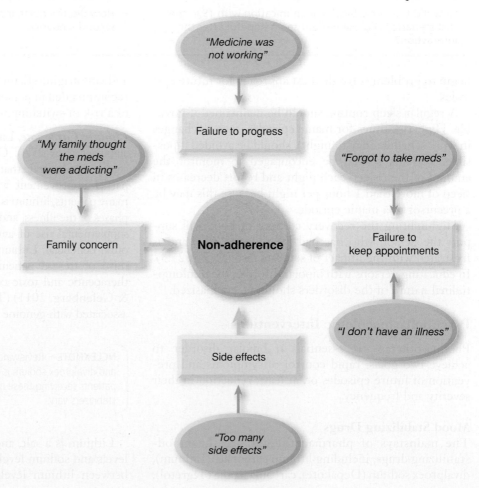

FIGURE 25.1 Nursing diagnosis concept map: non-adherence.

BOX 25.3 • THERAPEUTIC DIALOGUE • Instilling Hope

TS is a 26-year-old veteran who was recently diagnosed with bipolar disorder. He was admitted to the hospital for erratic behavior at home and work. His wife and children will stay with him only if his behavior and angry outbursts improve. He has threatened to kill himself if his family leaves him.

INEFFECTIVE APPROACH

Nurse: Mr. S, you must commit to staying on your medicine or you will lose your family.

TS: No one understands what it is like to get so angry. I don't see how a little pill and seeing a shrink will help.

Nurse: Well, it is your chance to keep your family.

TS: You don't understand.

EFFECTIVE APPROACH

Nurse: Mr. S, I hope that you are feeling better.

TS: No one understands what it is like to get so angry. I don't see how a little pill and seeing a shrink will help.

Nurse: It is interesting that medication is an effective treatment for bipolar disorder, but it is important to take it. There is evidence that medication has helped others to control moods. Following up with your provider will give you an opportunity to discuss the effects of the medication and how you are managing your illness.

TS: What do you mean, manage my illness?

Nurse: People with bipolar disorder learn to manage their illness through recognizing how stress impacts their moods, staying on their medications, and learning about the disorder. Then it is possible to lead a normal, independent productive life.

TS: Really? Let me think about this.

CRITICAL THINKING CHALLENGE

- How did the nurse block communication with TS in the first scenario? Did the patient seem hopeful after the interaction?

- How did the nurse instill hope in TS in the second scenario?

begin to problem solve the best approach for future episodes.

A regular sleep routine should be maintained if possible. High-risk times for manic episodes, such as changes in work schedule (day to night), should be avoided if possible. Patients should be encouraged to monitor the amount of their sleep each night and report decreases in sleep of more than 1 hour per night because this may be a precursor to a manic episode.

Highlighting the recovery concept of hope will support the person who has had multiple episodes and is frustrated with the impact of several episodes (Box 25.3). In educating persons with bipolar disorder, the nonlongitudinal nature of the disorders should be emphasized.

Psychopharmacologic Interventions

Pharmacotherapy is essential in bipolar disorder to achieve two goals: rapid control of symptoms and prevention of future episodes or, at least, reduction in their severity and frequency.

Mood Stabilizing Drugs

The mainstays of pharmacotherapy are the mood-stabilizing drugs, including lithium carbonate (Lithium), divalproex sodium (Depakote), carbamazepine (Tegretol),

and lamotrigine (Lamictal). Antidepressant therapy is not recommended in persons with bipolar depression because of a risk of switching to mania.

Lithium Carbonate. Lithium is the most widely used mood stabilizer (Box 25.4). Combined response rates from five studies demonstrate that 70% of patients experienced at least partial improvement with lithium therapy. However, for many patients, lithium is not a fully adequate treatment for all phases of the illness, and particularly during the acute phase, supplemental use of antipsychotics and benzodiazepines is often beneficial. Lithium is poorly tolerated in at least one third of treated patients and has a narrow gap between therapeutic and toxic concentrations (Freeman, Wiegand, & Gelenberg, 2011) (Table 25.1). Response to lithium is associated with genome variations (Chen et al., 2014).

> **NCLEXNOTE** Reviewing blood levels of lithium carbonate and divalproex sodium is an ongoing nursing assessment for patients receiving these medications. Side effects of mood stabilizers vary.

Lithium is a salt, and the interaction between lithium levels and sodium levels in the body and the relationship between lithium levels and fluid volume in the body

BOX 25.4

Drug Profile: Lithium (Eskalith)

DRUG CLASS: Mood stabilizer

RECEPTOR AFFINITY: Alters sodium transport in nerve and muscle cells, increases norepinephrine uptake and serotonin receptor sensitivity, slightly increases intraneuronal stores of catecholamines, delays some second messenger systems. Mechanism of action is unknown.

INDICATIONS: Treatment and prevention of manic episodes in bipolar affective disorder

ROUTES AND DOSAGE: 150-, 300-, and 600-mg capsules. Lithobid, 300-mg slow-release tablets; Eskalith CR, 450-mg controlled-release tablets; lithium citrate, 300-mg/5 mL liquid form

Adult: In acute mania, optimal response is usually 600 mg tid or 900 mg bid. Obtain serum levels twice weekly in acute phase. Maintenance: Use lowest possible dose to alleviate symptoms and maintain serum level of 0.6–1.2 mEq/L. In uncomplicated maintenance, obtain serum levels every 2–3 months. Do not rely on serum levels alone. Monitor patient side effects.

Geriatric: Increased risk for toxic effects; use lower doses; monitor frequently

Children: Safety and efficacy in children younger than 12 years of age has not been established.

HALF-LIFE (PEAK EFFECT): Mean, 24 h (peak serum levels in 1–4 h). Steady state reached in 5–7 d.

SELECTED ADVERSE REACTIONS: Weight gain

WARNING: Avoid use during pregnancy or while breastfeeding. Hepatic or renal impairments increase plasma concentration.

SPECIFIC PATIENT/FAMILY EDUCATION
- Avoid alcohol and other CNS depressant drugs.
- Notify your prescriber if pregnancy is possible or planned. Do not breastfeed while taking this medication.
- Notify your prescriber before taking any other prescriptions, OTC medications, or herbal supplements.
- May impair judgment, thinking, or motor skills; avoid driving or other hazardous tasks.
- Do not abruptly discontinue use.

bid, twice a day; CNS, central nervous system; OTC, over the counter; tid, three times a day.

EMERGENCY CARE ALERT ! If symptoms of moderate or severe toxicity (e.g., cardiac arrhythmias, blackouts, tremors, seizures) are noted, withhold additional doses of lithium, immediately obtain a blood sample to analyze the lithium level, and push fluids if the patient can take fluids. Contact the physician for further direction about relieving the symptoms.

Mild side effects tend to subside or can be managed by nursing measures (Table 25.3).

Divalproex Sodium. Divalproex sodium (Depakote), an anticonvulsant, has a broader spectrum of efficacy and has about equal benefit for patients with pure mania as for those with other forms of bipolar disorder (i.e., mixed mania, rapid cycling, comorbid substance abuse, and secondary mania) (Box 25.5). Divalproex is usually initiated at 250 mg twice a day or lower. In the inpatient setting, it can be initiated in an oral loading dose using 20 to

Table 25.1	LITHIUM BLOOD LEVELS AND ASSOCIATED SIDE EFFECTS
Plasma Level	**Side Effects or Symptoms of Toxicity**
<1.5 mEq/L Mild side effects	Metallic taste in mouth
	Fine hand tremor (resting)
	Nausea
	Polyuria
	Polydipsia
	Diarrhea or loose stools
	Muscular weakness or fatigue
	Weight gain
	Edema
	Memory impairments
1.5–2.5 mEq/L Moderate toxicity	Severe diarrhea
	Dry mouth
	Nausea and vomiting
	Mild to moderate ataxia
	Incoordination
	Dizziness, sluggishness, giddiness, vertigo
	Slurred speech
	Tinnitus
	Blurred vision
	Increasing tremor
	Muscle irritability or twitching
	Asymmetric deep tendon reflexes
	Increased muscle tone
>2.5 mEq/L Severe toxicity	Cardiac arrhythmias
	Blackouts
	Nystagmus
	Coarse tremor
	Fasciculations
	Visual or tactile hallucinations
	Oliguria, renal failure
	Peripheral vascular collapse
	Confusion
	Seizures
	Coma and death

remain crucial issues in its safe, effective use. The higher the sodium levels, the lower the lithium level will be and vice versa. Thus, changes in dietary sodium intake can affect lithium blood levels that, in turn, may affect therapeutic results or increase the incidence of side effects. The same applies to fluid volume. If body fluid decreases significantly because of a hot climate, strenuous exercise, vomiting, diarrhea, or drastic reduction in fluid intake, then lithium levels can rise sharply, causing an increase in side effects, progressing to lethal lithium toxicity. The key is to start the dose low and increase it slowly to maximize the therapeutic response and avoid overshooting the therapeutic window. See Table 25.2 for lithium interactions with other drugs. See Chapter 11 for further discussion of lithium's possible mechanisms of action, pharmacokinetics, side effects, and toxicity.

Table 25.2	LITHIUM INTERACTIONS WITH MEDICATIONS AND OTHER SUBSTANCES
Substance	**Effect of Interaction**
ACE inhibitors, such as: • Captopril • Lisinopril • Quinapril	Increase serum lithium; may cause toxicity and impaired kidney function
Acetazolamide	Increases renal excretion of lithium; decreases lithium levels
Alcohol	May increase serum lithium level
Caffeine	Increases lithium excretion; increases lithium tremor
Carbamazepine	Increases neurotoxicity despite normal serum levels and dosage
Fluoxetine	Increases serum lithium levels
Haloperidol	Increases neurotoxicity despite normal serum levels and dosage
Loop diuretics, such as furosemide	Increase lithium serum levels but may be safer than thiazide diuretics; potassium-sparing diuretics (amiloride, spirolactone) are safest
Methyldopa	Increases neurotoxicity without increasing serum lithium levels
NSAIDs, such as: • Diclofenac • Ibuprofen • Indomethacin • Piroxicam	Decrease renal clearance of lithium Increase serum lithium levels by 30%–60% in 3–10 days Aspirin and sulindac do not appear to have the same effect
Osmotic diuretics, such as: • Urea • Mannitol • Isosorbide	Increases renal excretion of lithium and decreases lithium levels
Sodium chloride	High sodium intake decreases lithium levels; low sodium diets may increase lithium levels and lead to toxicity
Thiazide diuretics, such as: • Chlorothiazide • Hydrochlorothiazide	Promote sodium and potassium excretion; increase lithium serum levels; may produce cardiotoxicity and neurotoxicity
TCAs	Increases tremor; potentiates pharmacologic effects of tricyclic antidepressants

ACE, angiotensin-converting enzyme; NSAID, nonsteroidal antiinflammatory drug; TCA, tricyclic antidepressant.

years of use. Some cases were described as hemorrhagic, with a rapid progression from onset to death. If pancreatitis is diagnosed, valproate use should be discontinued.

Carbamazepine. Carbamazepine, an anticonvulsant, also has mood-stabilizing effects. Data from various studies suggest that it may be effective in patients who experience no response to lithium. Carbamazepine is metabolized by CYP3A4 and induces CYP1A2 and 3A4. The most common side effects of carbamazepine are dizziness, drowsiness, nausea, and vomiting, which may be avoided with slow incremental dosing. Carbamazepine has a boxed

Table 25.3	INTERVENTIONS FOR LITHIUM SIDE EFFECTS
Side Effect	**Intervention**
Edema of feet or hands	Monitor intake and output; check for possible decreased urinary output. Monitor sodium intake. Patient should elevate legs when sitting or lying. Monitor weight.
Fine hand tremor	Provide support and reassurance if it does not interfere with daily activities. Tremor worsens with anxiety and intentional movements; minimize stressors. Notify prescriber if it interferes with patient's work and compliance will be an issue. More frequent smaller doses of lithium may also help.
Mild diarrhea	Take lithium with meals. Provide for fluid replacement. Notify prescriber if becomes severe; may need a change in medication preparation or may be early sign of toxicity.
Muscle weakness, fatigue, or memory and concentration difficulties	Provide support and reassurance; this side effect will usually pass after a few weeks of treatment. Short-term memory aids such as lists or reminder calls may be helpful. Notify prescriber if becomes severe or interferes with the patient's desire to continue treatment.
Metallic taste	Suggest sugarless candies or throat lozenges. Encourage frequent oral hygiene.
Nausea or abdominal discomfort	Consider dividing the medication into smaller doses or give it at more frequent intervals. Give medication with meals.
Polydipsia	Reassure patient that this is a normal mechanism to cope with polyuria.
Polyuria	Monitor intake and output. Provide reassurance and explain the nature of this side effect. Also explain that this causes no physical damage to the kidneys.
Toxicity	Withhold medication. Notify prescriber. Use symptomatic treatments.

30 mg/kg body weight. Baseline liver function tests and a complete blood count with platelets should be obtained before starting therapy, and patients with known liver disease should not be given divalproex sodium. There is a boxed warning for hepatotoxicity. Optimal blood levels appear to be in the range of 50 to 150 ng/mL. Levels may be obtained weekly until the patient is stable and then every 6 months. Divalproex sodium is associated with increased risk for birth defects. Cases of life-threatening pancreatitis have been reported in adults and children receiving valproate, either initially or after several

BOX 25.5

Drug Profile: **Divalproex Sodium (Depakote)**

DRUG CLASS: Antimania agent

RECEPTOR AFFINITY: Thought to increase level of inhibitory neurotransmitter, GABA, to brain neurons. Mechanism of action is unknown.

INDICATIONS: Mania, epilepsy, migraine.

ROUTES AND DOSAGE: Available in 125-mg delayed-release capsules, and 125-, 250-, and 500-mg enteric-coated tablets.

Adult Dosage: Dosage depends on symptoms and clinical picture presented; initially, the dosage is low and gradually increased depending on the clinical presentation

HALF-LIFE (PEAK EFFECT): 6–16 h (1–4 h)

SELECTED ADVERSE REACTIONS: Sedation, tremor (may be dose related), nausea, vomiting, indigestion, abdominal cramps, anorexia with weight loss, slight elevations in liver enzymes, hepatic failure, thrombocytopenia, transient increases in hair loss

BOXED WARNING: Hepatotoxicity, teratogenicity, pancreatitis

WARNING: Use cautiously during pregnancy and lactation. Contraindicated in patients with hepatic disease or significant hepatic dysfunction. Administer cautiously with salicylates; may increase serum levels and result in toxicity.

SPECIFIC PATIENT AND FAMILY EDUCATION
- Take with food if gastrointestinal upset occurs.
- Swallow tablets or capsules whole to prevent local irritation of mouth and throat.
- Notify your prescriber before taking any other prescription or OTC medications or herbal supplements.
- Avoid alcohol and sleep-inducing or OTC products.
- Avoid driving or performing activities that require alertness.
- Do not abruptly discontinue use.
- Keep appointments for follow-up, including blood tests to monitor response.

GABA, gamma-aminobutyric acid; OTC, over the counter.

warning for aplastic anemia and agranulocytosis, but frequent clinically unimportant decreases in white blood cell counts occur. Estimates of the rate of severe blood dyscrasias vary from one in 10,000 patients treated to a more recent estimate of one in 125,000 (Schatzberg, Cole, & DeBattista, 2010). Mild, nonprogressive elevations of liver function test results are relatively common. Carbamazepine is associated with increased risk for birth defects.

In patients older than 12 years, carbamazepine is begun at 200 mg once or twice a day. The dosage is increased by no more than 200 mg every 2 to 4 days, to 800 to 1,000 mg a day or until therapeutic levels or effects are achieved. It is important to monitor for blood dyscrasias and liver damage. Liver function tests and complete blood counts with differential are minimal

pretreatment laboratory tests and should be repeated about 1 month after initiating treatment and at 3 months, 6 months, and yearly. Other yearly tests should include electrolytes, blood urea nitrogen, thyroid function tests, urinalysis, and eye examinations. Carbamazepine levels are measured monthly until the patient is on a stable dosage. Studies suggest that blood levels in the range of 8 to 12 ng/mL correspond to therapeutic efficacy. See Table 25.4 for carbamazepine's interactions with other drugs. See Chapter 11 for further discussion of carbamazepine's possible mechanisms of action, pharmacokinetics, side effects, and toxicity.

EMERGENCY CARE ALERT !   Both valproate and carbamazepine may be lethal if high doses are ingested. Toxic symptoms appear in 1 to 3 hours and include neuromuscular disturbances, dizziness, stupor, agitation, disorientation, nystagmus, urinary retention, nausea and vomiting, tachycardia, hypotension or hypertension, cardiovascular shock, coma, and respiratory depression.

Lamotrigine. For a depressive episode, mood stabilizers such as lamotrigine (Lamictal) that requires a dose titration are frequently prescribed (Box 25.6). Lamotrigine (Lamictal) is approved by the U.S. Food and Drug Administration for the maintenance treatment of bipolar disorder. It may be particularly effective for rapid cycling and in the depressed phase of bipolar illness. If

Table 25.4	SELECTED MEDICATION INTERACTIONS WITH CARBAMAZEPINE	
Interaction	**Drug Interacting With Carbamazepine**
Increased carbamazepine levels	Erythromycin Cimetidine Propoxyphene Isoniazid Calcium channel blockers (verapamil) Fluoxetine Danazol Diltiazem Nicotinamide
Decreased carbamazepine levels	Phenobarbital Primidone Phenytoin
Drugs whose levels are decreased by carbamazepine	Oral contraceptives Warfarin, oral anticoagulants Doxycycline Theophylline Haloperidol Divalproex sodium Tricyclic antidepressants Acetaminophen: increased metabolism but also increased risk for hepatotoxicity

---

BOX 25.6
Drug Profile: Lamotrigine (Lamictal)

DRUG CLASS: Antiepileptic

RECEPTOR AFFINITY: Lamotrigine had a weak inhibitory effect on the serotonin 5-HT$_3$ receptor. It does not exhibit high-affinity binding: adenosine A$_1$ and A$_2$; adrenergic α_1, α_2, and β; dopamine D$_1$ and D$_2$; GABA A and B; histamine H$_1$; kappa opioid; muscarinic acetylcholine; and serotonin 5-HT$_2$.

INDICATIONS: Epilepsy, bipolar disorder (acute mood with standard therapy)

ROUTES AND DOSAGE: Available in tablets: 25 mg, 100 mg, 150 mg, and 200 mg scored. (3.1, 16)

CHEWABLE DISPERSIBLE TABLETS: 2 mg, 5 mg, and 25 mg. (3.2, 16)

HALF-LIFE (PEAK EFFECT): 32 hours, but can be increased if taking valproate.

SELECTED ADVERSE REACTIONS: Dizziness, somnolence, and other symptoms and signs of CNS depression.

BOXED WARNING: Serious rashes requiring hospitalization and discontinuation of treatment; the incidence of these rashes, which have included Stevens-Johnson syndrome, is 0.08% (0.8 per 1,000) in adult patients receiving

WARNINGS: Hypersensitivity reaction, multiorgan failure, blood dyscrasias, and suicidal behavior and ideation have occurred.

SPECIFIC PATIENT AND FAMILY EDUCATION
- Do not drive a car or to operate other complex machinery until you have gained sufficient experience taking lamotrigine.
- Lamotrigine may cause a serious skin rash that may cause you to be hospitalized or to stop lamotrigine; it may rarely cause death.

CNS, central nervous system; GABA, gamma-aminobutyric acid

---

lamotrigine is given with valproic acid (Depakote), the dose should be reduced. Depakote decreases the clearance of lamotrigine. Lamotrigine does have a "boxed warning" for skin rash. Nurses should be especially vigilant for the appearance of any skin rash. If a rash does appear, it is most likely benign. However, it is not possible to predict whether the rash is benign or serious (Stevens-Johnson syndrome).

Antipsychotics

Antipsychotics are prescribed for either adjunct or monotherapy. These agents provide some of the broadest efficacy and are more likely used as the only medication to treat bipolar disorder than the mood stabilizers (Stahl, 2013).

Administering and Monitoring Medications

During acute mania, patients may not believe that they have a psychiatric disorder and refuse to take medication.

Because their energy is still high, they can be very creative in avoiding medication. Through patience and the development of a trusting relationships, patients will be more likely begin to participate in a shared decision-making process. It is important for patients to have a sense of empowerment and participation in treatment even during the most acute episodes. After patients begin to take medications, symptom improvement should be evident. If a patient is very agitated, a benzodiazepine may be given for a short period.

Managing Side Effects

Patients with bipolar disorder order are usually treated with several medications. Additionally, patients may be taking other "nonpsychiatric" medications. In some instances, one agent is used to augment the effects of another, such as supplemental thyroid hormone to boost antidepressant response in depression. Possible side effects for each medication should be listed and cross-referenced. When a side effect appears, the nurse should document the side effect and notify the prescriber, so that further evaluation can be made. In some instances, medications should be changed.

Monitoring for Drug Interactions

It is a well-established practice to combine mood stabilizers with antidepressants or antipsychotics. The previously discussed drug interactions should be considered when caring for a person with bipolar disorder. A big challenge is monitoring alcohol, drugs, over-the-counter medications, and herbal supplements. A complete list of all medications should be maintained and evaluated for any potential interaction.

Promoting Adherence

Adherence to a complex medication regimen over months to years is difficult. Yet, one of the primary reasons that acute symptoms reappear is because of discontinuation of medications. It is important to recognize that taking medication as prescribed over time is difficult. Nurses can help patients and families incorporate taking medications into their lifestyles by developing realistic plans. The use of pill boxes, reminders, and other cues will increase the likelihood of adherence.

Teaching Points

For patients who are taking lithium, it is important to explain that a change in salt intake can affect the therapeutic blood level. If there is a reduction in salt intake, the body will naturally retain lithium to maintain homeostasis. This increase in lithium retention can lead to toxicity. After the patient has been stabilized on a lithium dose, salt intake should remain constant. This is fairly easy to do except during the summer, when excessive perspiration can occur. Patients should increase salt intake during periods of perspiration, increased exercise, and dehydration. Most mood stabilizers and antidepressants can cause weight gain. Patients should be alerted to this potential side effect and should be instructed to monitor any changes in eating, appetite, or weight. Weight reduction techniques may need to be instituted. Patients also should be clearly instructed to check with the nurse or physician before taking any over-the-counter medications, herbal supplements, or any other complementary and alternative treatment approaches.

Other Somatic Therapies

Electroconvulsive therapy (ECT) may be a treatment alternative for patients with severe mania who exhibit unremitting, frenzied physical activity. Other indications for ECT are acute mania that is unresponsive to antimanic agents or high suicide risk. ECT is safe and effective in patients receiving antipsychotic drugs. Use of valproate or carbamazepine will elevate the seizure threshold, requiring some adjustments in treatment.

Psychological Domain
Assessment

The assessment of the psychological domain should follow the process explained in Chapter 10. Individuals with bipolar disorder can usually participate fully in this part of the assessment.

Mood

By definition, bipolar disorder is a disturbance of mood. If the patient is depressed, using an assessment tool for depression may help determine the severity of depression. If mania predominates, evaluating the quality of the mood (elated, grandiose, irritated, or agitated) becomes important. Usually, mania is determined by clinical observation.

Cognition

In a depressive episode, the individual may not be able to concentrate enough to complete cognitive tasks, such as those called for in a mental status assessment. During the acute phase of a manic or depressive episode, mental status may be abnormal, and in a manic phase, judgment is impaired by extremely rapid, disjointed, and distorted thinking. Moreover, feelings such as grandiosity can interfere with normal executive functioning.

Thought Disturbances

Psychosis commonly occurs in patients with bipolar disorder, especially during acute episodes of mania. Auditory hallucinations and delusional thinking are part of the clinical picture. In children and adolescents, psychosis is not so easily disclosed.

Stress and Coping

Stress and coping are critical assessment areas for a person with bipolar disorder. A stressful event often triggers a manic or depressive episode. In some instances, there are no particular stresses that preceded the episode, but it is important to discuss the possibility. Determining the patient's usual coping skills for stresses lays the groundwork for developing interventional strategies. Negative coping skills, such as substance use or aggression, should be identified because these skills need to be replaced with positive coping skills.

Risk Assessment

Patients with bipolar disorder are at high risk for injury to themselves and others, with 10% to 15% of patients completing suicide. Child abuse, spouse abuse, or other violent behaviors may occur during severe manic or depressive episodes; thus, patients should be assessed for suicidal or homicidal risk. Additionally, they are high risk for comorbid mental disorders such as substance abuse and anxiety disorders. Significant risks for cardiovascular and metabolic disease are found in this group. Smoking is also a major health hazard (Parks, Radke, & Mazade, 2008).

Nursing Diagnoses for the Psychological Domain

Nursing diagnoses associated with the psychological domain of bipolar disorder include Disturbed Sensory Perception, Disturbed Thought Processes, Defensive Coping, Risk for Suicide, Risk for Violence, Ineffective Coping, and Nonadherence (Noncompliance) (see Figure 25.1).

Interventions for the Psychological Domain

Pharmacotherapy is necessary for treatment of people with bipolar disorder, but it is only one aspect of recovery. Psychosocial strategies are critical in successful treatment and prevention of relapse. Psychoeducation, individual cognitive behavioral therapy, individual interpersonal therapy, and adjunctive therapies (such as those for substance use) are all recommended psychotherapeutic approaches (Crowe et al., 2010; Hoberg et al., 2013) (Box 25.7).

BOX 25.7

Research for Best Practice: **Psychosocial Interventions for People With Bipolar Disorder**

Crowe, M., Whitehead, L., Wilson, L., Carlyle, D., O'Brien, A., Inder, M., & Joyce, P. (2010). Disorder-specific psychosocial interventions for bipolar disorder—A systematic review of the evidence for mental health nursing practice. International Journal of Nursing Studies, 47, 896–908.

THE QUESTION: Are psychosocial interventions for bipolar disorder efficacious for medication adherence?

METHODS: An extensive review of literature using Medline, CINAHL and PsycINFO databases resulted in the selection of 35 relevant research studies.

FINDINGS: Psychopharmacologic-only interventions are not effective for the management of bipolar disorder because of high-rates of non-adherence. Group psycho-education, interpersonal social rhythm therapy, family interventions, and cognitive behavioral therapy are all effective when use as an adjunct to psychotherapy. The common factors of these interventions were that they were all structured and adhered to manualized protocols for up to 2 years.

IMPLICATIONS FOR NURSING: Psychiatric mental health nurses are in excellent position to integrate psychosocial interventions into their clinical practice settings. These interventions require about 2 years to teach the patients the skills that are needed to manage bipolar disorder.

Several risk factors associated with bipolar disorders make patients more vulnerable to relapses and resistant to recovery. Among these are high rates of nonadherence to medication therapy, obesity, marital conflict, separation, divorce, unemployment, and underemployment. Even those who take their medication regularly are likely to experience recurrences and have difficulty keeping jobs and maintaining significant relationships.

Important goals of psychosocial interventions are identifying risk factors and developing strategies to address them. It is also important to help the patient understand the disorder and manage the mood lability and dysfunctional thoughts that are often precursors to a manic or depressive episode. The nurse partners with the patient in developing strategies to remember to take medications, identify therapeutic and side effects, and know when and how to contact a clinician. Particularly important are enhancing social and occupational functioning, improving quality of life, increasing the patient and family's acceptance of the disorder, and reducing the suicide risk (Crowe et al., 2010).

Psychotherapy

Long-term psychotherapy may help prevent both mania and depression by reducing the stresses that trigger episodes and increasing the patient's acceptance of the need

for medication. Patients should be encouraged to keep their appointments with the therapist, be honest and open, do the assigned homework, and give the therapist feedback on whether the treatment is effective.

Teaching Patients and Family

Psychoeducation is designed to provide information on bipolar disorder and successful treatment and recovery. The nurse can provide information about the illness and obstacles to recovery. Helping the patient recognize warning signs and symptoms of relapse and to cope with residual symptoms and functional impairment are important interventions. Watching for early warning signs and triggers can mean early treatment. Family members should be included in developing an emergency plan for recognizing and intervening if relapse symptoms occur (Box 25.8).

In the interest of improved medication adherence, listening carefully to the patient's concerns about the medication, dosing schedules and dose changes, and side effects is helpful. Resistance to accepting the illness and to taking medication, the symbolic meaning of medication taking, and worries about the future can be discussed openly. Health teaching and weight management should be components of any psychoeducation program. In addition to individual variations in body weight, many of the medications (divalproex sodium, lithium, antidepressants, and atypical antipsychotics)

BOX 25.8

Relapse Prevention and Emergency Plan

COMMON INDICATORS FOR RELAPSE

Mania
Reading several books or newspapers at once
Cannot concentrate on one topic
Talking faster than usual
Feeling irritable
Hungry all the time
Friends remark on changes in mood
More energy than usual

Depression
Quit cooking, cleaning, daily chores
Avoid people
Crave foods (i.e., chocolate)
Headaches
Do not care about other people
Sleeping more or restless sleep
People are irritating to be around

EMERGENCY PLAN
Keep a list of emergency contacts (provider, close family members).
Keep a current list of all medications, including their dosages.
Information about other health problems
Symptoms that indicate others need to take responsibility for care
Treatment preferences (who, where, medications, advanced directive location)

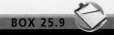

BOX 25.9

Psychoeducation Checklist: **Bipolar I Disorder**

When caring for the patient with a bipolar I disorder, be sure to include the following topic areas in the teaching plan:

- Psychopharmacologic agents, including drug action, dosage, frequency, and possible adverse effects
- Medication regimen adherence
- Recovery plan
- Relapse prevention plan
- Strategies to decrease agitation and restlessness
- Safety measures
- Self-care management
- Follow-up laboratory testing
- Support services

are associated with weight gain. Monitoring weight and developing individual weight management plans can reduce the risk of relapse and increase the possibility of medication adherence. Box 25.9 provides a checklist for psychoeducation.

Social Domain

Assessment

One of the tragedies of bipolar disorder is its effect on social and occupational functioning. Cultural views of mental illness influence the patient's acceptance of the disorder. During illness episodes, patients often behave in ways that jeopardize their social relationships. Losing a job and going through a divorce are common events. When performing an assessment of social function, the nurse should identify changes resulting from a manic or depressive episode.

Nursing Diagnoses for the Social Domain

Nursing diagnoses for adults can include Ineffective Role Performance, Interrupted Family Processes, Impaired Social Interaction, Impaired Parenting, and Compromised Family Coping. The diagnoses for children and adolescents can include Delayed Growth and Development and Caregiver Role Strain in family coping with a member with a bipolar disorder.

Interventions for the Social Domain

Interventions focusing on the social domain are integral to nursing care for all ages. During mania, patients usually violate others' boundaries. For example, roommate selection for patients requiring hospital admittance needs to be carefully considered. If possible, a private room is ideal because patients with bipolar disorder tend to irritate others, who quickly tire of the intrusiveness. These patients

may miss the cues indicating anger and aggression from others. The nurse should protect the manic patient from self-harm, as well as harm from other patients.

Support Groups

Support groups are helpful for people with this disorder. Participating in groups allows the person to meet others with the same disorder and learn management and preventive strategies. Support groups also are helpful in dealing with the stigma associated with mental illnesses.

Interventions for Family Members

Marital and family interventions are often needed at different periods in the life of a person with bipolar disorder. For the family with a child with this disorder, additional parenting skills are needed to manage the behaviors. The goals of family interventions are to help the family understand and cope with the disorder. Interventions may range from occasional counseling sessions to intensive family therapy.

Family psychoeducation strategies have been shown to be particularly useful in decreasing the risk of relapse and hospitalization. The sooner the education is begun, the more effective this approach is (Popovic et al., 2013; Reinares, Sánchez-Moreno, & Fountoulakis, 2014).

Evaluation and Treatment Outcomes

Desired treatment outcomes are stabilization of mood and enhanced quality of life. Primary tools for evaluating outcomes are nursing observation and patient self-report (see Nursing Care Plan 25.1).

Continuum of Care

Inpatient-Focused Care

Inpatient admission is the treatment setting of choice for patients who are severely psychotic or who are an immediate threat to themselves or others. In acute mania, nursing interventions focus on patient safety because patients are prone to injury because of hyperactivity and are often are unaware of injuries they sustain. Distraction may also be effective when a patient is talking or acting inappropriately. Removal to a quieter environment may be necessary if other interventions have not been successful, but the patient should be carefully monitored. During acute mania, patients are often impulsive, disinhibited, and interpersonally inappropriate, so the nurse should avoid direct confrontations or challenges.

(text continues on page 444)

NURSING CARE PLAN 25.1

The Patient With Bipolar I Disorder

JR, a 43-year-old, single woman, lives in a metropolitan city and works for a large travel agency booking corporate business trips. She has a history of alcohol abuse that began when she was in high school. Initially, she relied on alcohol for stress reduction but gradually began abusing it. Her mother, grandfather, and sister all committed suicide within the past several years. JR's father has remarried and moved out of the area. JR has one brother whom she sees occasionally.

Three years ago, JR left her husband after 15 years of an unhappy marriage and moved into a small condominium in a less affluent neighborhood. She began having symptoms of bipolar mixed disorder at that time, when she sold all her clothes, bleached her hair blonde, and began cruising the bars. She would consume excessive amounts of alcohol and often end up spending the night with a stranger. At first her behavior was attributed to her recent divorce. When she began missing work and charging excessively on her credit cards, her friends

and two children became concerned and convinced her to seek help for her behavior.

JR received a diagnosis of manic episode, and treatment with lithium carbonate was initiated. Her mood stabilized briefly, but she had two more manic episodes within the next 18 months. Shortly after her last manic episode, she became severely depressed and attempted suicide. Antidepressants were tried, but she discontinued taking them after a significant weight gain. Once her depression lifted, her mood was stable for several months.

About 2 months ago, JR began missing work again because of depression. She refused to take any antidepressants and just wanted to "wait it out." She often boasted that her one success in life was helping people travel and have a good time. Last week she was told that her position was being eliminated because of a company issue. Now she believes that she is a failure as a wife, as an employee, and as a woman. She became despondent and finally took an overdose to "end it all."

Setting: Intensive Care Psychiatric Unit In A General Hospital

Baseline Assessment: JR is a 43-year-old single woman transferred from ICU after a 3-day hospitalization following a suicide attempt with an overdose of multiple prescriptions and alcohol. She had her first manic episode 3 years before, and subsequently has had symptoms of a mixed bipolar mood disorder most of the time. Medication with lithium carbonate has not protected her from mood swings, and prior trials of antidepressants have been unsuccessful. She is currently depressed, with pressured speech, agitation, irritability, sensory overload, inability to sleep, and anorexia.

Associated Psychiatric Diagnosis	Medications
Bipolar I disorder, most recent episode depressed severe, without psychotic features	Lithium carbonate 300 mg tid × 2 years L-thyroxine 0.1 mg q AM × 1 d Clonazepam 0.5 mg bid for sleep and agitation Lamotrigine added on transfer to be titrated up to 100 mg per day

Nursing Diagnosis 1: Risk Suicide

Defining Characteristics	Related Factors
Attempts to inflict life-threatening injury to self Expresses desire to die Poor impulse control Lack of support system	Feelings of helplessness and hopelessness secondary to bipolar disorder Depression Loss secondary to finances/job, divorce

Outcomes

Initial	Discharge
1. Remain free from self-harm. 2. Identify factors that led to suicidal intent and methods for managing suicidal impulses if they return. 3. Accept treatment of depression by trying the SSRI antidepressants.	4. Discuss the management of bipolar disorder. 5. Identify the antecedents to depression.

Continued

NURSING CARE PLAN 25.1 (Continued)

Interventions

Interventions	Rationale	Ongoing Assessment
Initiate a nurse–patient relationship by demonstrating an acceptance of JR as a worthwhile human being through the use of nonjudgmental statements and behavior. Initiate suicide precautions per hospital policy.	A sense of worthlessness often underlies suicide ideation. The positive therapeutic relationship can maintain the patient's dignity. Safety of the individual is a priority with people who have suicide ideation (see Chapter 21).	Assess the stages of the relationship and determine whether a therapeutic relationship is actually being formed. Identify indicators of trust. Determine intent to harm self—plan and means.

Evaluation

Outcomes	Revised Outcomes	Interventions
Has not harmed self, denies suicidal thought/intent after realizing that she is still alive. JR agreed to try to treat her depression by initiating treatment with lamotrigine.	Absence of suicidal intent will continue.	Discontinue suicide precautions; maintain ongoing assessment for suicidality.

Nursing Diagnosis 2: Chronic Low Self-Esteem

Defining Characteristics	Related Factors
Long-standing self-negating verbalizations Expressions of shame and guilt Evaluates self as unable to deal with events Frequent lack of success in work and relationships Poor body presentation (eye contact, posture, movements) Nonassertive/passive	Failure to stabilize mood Unmet dependency needs Feelings of abandonment secondary to separation from significant other Feelings of failure secondary to loss of job, relationship problems Unrealistic expectations of self

Outcomes

Initial	Discharge
1. Identify positive aspects of self. 2. Modify excessive and unrealistic expectations of self.	3. Verbalize acceptance of personal limitations. 4. Report freedom from most symptoms of depression. 5. Begin to take verbal and behavioral risks.

Interventions

Interventions	Rationale	Ongoing Assessment
Enhance JR's sense of self by being attentive, validating your interpretation of what is being said or experienced, and helping her verbalize what she is expressing nonverbally. Assist to reframe and redefine negative statements ("not a failure, but a setback"). Problem solve with patient about how to approach finding another job.	By showing respect for the patient as a human being who is worth listening to, the nurse can support and help build the patient's sense of self. Reframing an event positively rather than negatively can help the patient view the situation in an alternative way. Work is very important to adults. Losing a job can decrease self-esteem. Focusing on the possibility of a future job will provide hope for the patient.	Determine whether patient confirms interpretation of situation and if she can verbalize what she is expressing nonverbally. Assess whether the patient can actually view the world in a different way. Assess the patient's ability to problem solve. Determine whether she is realistic in her expectations.

Continued

NURSING CARE PLAN 25.1 *(Continued)*

Interventions

Interventions	Rationale	Ongoing Assessment
Encourage positive physical habits (healthy food and eating patterns, exercise, proper sleep).	A healthy lifestyle promotes well-being, increasing self-esteem.	Determine JR's willingness to consider making lifestyle changes.
Teach patient to validate consensually with others.	Low self-esteem is generated by negative interpretations of the world. Through consensual validation, the patient can determine whether others view situations in the same way.	Assess JR's ability to participate in this process.
Teach esteem-building exercises (self-affirmations, imagery, use of humor, meditation/prayer, relaxation).	There are many different approaches that can be practiced to increase self-esteem.	Assess JR's energy level and ability to focus on learning new skills.
Assist in establishing appropriate personal boundaries.	In an attempt to meet their own needs, people with low self-esteem often violate other people's boundaries and allow others to take advantage of them. Helping patients establish their own boundaries will improve the likelihood of needs being met in an appropriate manner.	Assess JR's ability to understand the concept of boundary violation and its significance.
Provide an opportunity within the therapeutic relationship to express thoughts and feelings. Use open-ended statements and questions. Encourage expression of both positive and negative statements. Use movement, art, and music as means of expression.	The individual with low self-esteem may have difficulty expressing thoughts and feelings. Providing them with several different outlets for expression helps to develop skills for expressing thoughts and feelings.	Monitor thoughts and feelings that are expressed in order to help the patient examine them.
Explore opportunities for positive socialization.	Individuals with low self-esteem may be in social situations that reinforce negative valuation of self. Helping patient identify new positive situations will give other options.	Assess whether the new situations are potentially positive or are a re-creation of other negative situations.
JR began to identify positive aspects of self as she began to modify excessive and unrealistic expectations of self.	Strengthen ability to affirm positive aspects and examine expectations related to work and relationships.	Refer to mental health clinic for cognitive-behavioral psychotherapy with a feminist perspective.
She verbalized that she would probably never work for the company again and that it would never be the same. She verbalized that she would need more assertiveness skills in her relationships.	Identify important aspects of job, so that she can begin looking for a job that had those characteristics.	Attend a women's group that focuses on assertiveness skills.
As JR's mood improved, she was able to sleep through the night, and she began eating again—began feeling better about herself.	Maintain a stable mood to promote positive self-concept.	Monitor mood and identify antecedents to depression.

Nursing Diagnosis 3: Ineffective Individual Coping

Defining Characteristics	Related Factors
Verbalization in inability to cope or ask for help Reported difficulty with life stressors Inability to problem solve Alteration in social participation Destructive behavior toward self Frequent illnesses Substance abuse	Altered mood (depression) caused by changes secondary to body chemistry (bipolar disorder) Altered mood caused by changes secondary to intake of mood-altering substance (alcohol) Unsatisfactory support system Sensory overload secondary to excessive activity Inadequate psychological resources to adapt to changes in job status

Continued

Outcomes

Initial	Discharge
1. Accept support through the nurse–patient relationship. 2. Identify areas of ineffective coping. 3. Examine the current efforts at coping. 4. Identify areas of strength. 5. Learn new coping skills.	6. Practice new coping skills. 7. Focus on strengths.

Interventions

Interventions	Rationale	Ongoing Assessment
Identify current stresses in JR's life, including her suicide attempt and the bipolar disorder.	When areas of concern are verbalized by the patient, she will be able to focus on one issue at a time. If she identifies the mental disorder as a stressor, she will more likely be able to develop strategies to deal with it.	Determine whether JR is able to identify problem areas realistically. Continue to assess for suicidality.
Identify JR's strengths in dealing with past stressors.	By focusing on past successes, she can identify strengths and build on them in the future.	Assess if JR can identify any previous successes in her life.
Assess current level of depression using Beck's Depression Inventory or a similar one and intervene according to assessed level.	Severely depressed or suicidal individuals need assistance with decision making, grooming and hygiene, and nutrition.	Continue to assess for mood and suicidality.
Assist JR in discussing, selecting, and practicing positive coping skills (jogging, yoga, thought stopping).	New coping skills take a conscious effort to learn and will at first seem strange and unnatural. Practicing these skills will help the patient incorporate them into her coping strategy repertoire.	Assess whether JR follows through on learning new skills.
Educate regarding the use of alcohol and its relationship to depression.	Alcohol is an ineffective coping strategy because it actually exacerbates the depression.	Assess for the patient's willingness to address her drinking problem.
Assist patient in coping with bipolar disorder, beginning with education about it.	A mood disorder is a major stressor in a patient's life. To manage the stress, the patient needs a knowledge base.	Determine JR's knowledge about bipolar disorder.
Administer lithium as ordered (give with food or milk). Reinforce the action, dosage, and side effects. Review laboratory results to determine whether lithium is within therapeutic limits. Assess for toxicity. Recommend a normal diet with normal salt intake; maintenance of adequate fluid intake.	Lithium carbonate is effective in the treatment of bipolar disorder but must be managed. Patient should have a thorough knowledge of the medication and side effects.	Assess for target action, side effects, and toxicity.
Administer lamotrigine as ordered, to be titrated up to 100 mg per day. Observe for presence of hypersensitivity to the drug. Teach about action, dosage, and side effects.	Lamotrigine can be effective in bipolar disorder.	Assess for target action, side effects, and toxicity. Assess skin daily for changes or presence of rash.
Administer thyroid supplement as ordered. Review laboratory results of thyroid functioning. Discuss the symptoms of hypothyroidism and how they are similar to depression. Emphasize the importance of taking lithium and L-thyroxine. Explain about the long-term effects of lithium on thyroid functioning.	Hypothyroidism can be a side effect of lithium carbonate and also mimics symptoms of depression.	Determine whether patient understands the relationship between thyroid dysfunction and lithium carbonate.

Continued

NURSING CARE PLAN 25.1 *(Continued)*

Evaluation

Outcomes	Revised Outcomes	Interventions
Clonazepam 0.5 mg bid for sleep and agitation.		
JR easily engaged in a therapeutic relationship. She examined the areas in her life where she coped ineffectively.	Establish a therapeutic relationship with a therapist at the mental health clinic.	Refer to mental health clinic.
She identified her strengths and how she coped with stressors and especially her illness in the past. She is willing to try antidepressants again, in hopes of not having the weight gain.	Continue to view illness as a potential stressor that can disrupt life.	Seek advice immediately if there are any problems with medications.
She learned new problem-solving skills and reported that she learned a lot about her medication. She is committed to complying with her medication regimen. She identified new coping skills that she could realistically do. She will focus on strengths.	Continue to practice new coping skills as stressful situations arise.	Discuss with therapist the outcomes of using new coping skills. Attend Alcoholics Anonymous if alcohol is used as a stress reliever.

The length of stay in an inpatient unit will be relatively short, 3 to 5 days. The plan of care will focus on medication management (Figure 25.2), including control of side effects, initiation or revision of a recovery plan, psychoeducation, and promotion of self-care. Nurses should be familiar with drug–drug interactions and with interventions to help control side effects.

Intensive Outpatient Programs

Intensive outpatient programs for several weeks of acute-phase care during a manic or depressive episode are used when hospitalization is not necessary or to prevent or shorten hospitalization. These programs are usually called partial hospitalization. Close medication monitoring and milieu therapies that foster restoration of a patient's previous adaptive abilities are the major nursing responsibilities in these settings.

Setting up frequent office visits and crisis telephone calls are additional nursing interventions that can help to shorten or prevent hospitalization during the acute phase of a manic episode. Family sessions or psychoeducation that includes the patient are alternatives. Severely and persistently ill patients may need ongoing intensive treatment, but the frequency of visits can be decreased for patients whose conditions stabilize and who enter the continuation or the maintenance phase of treatment.

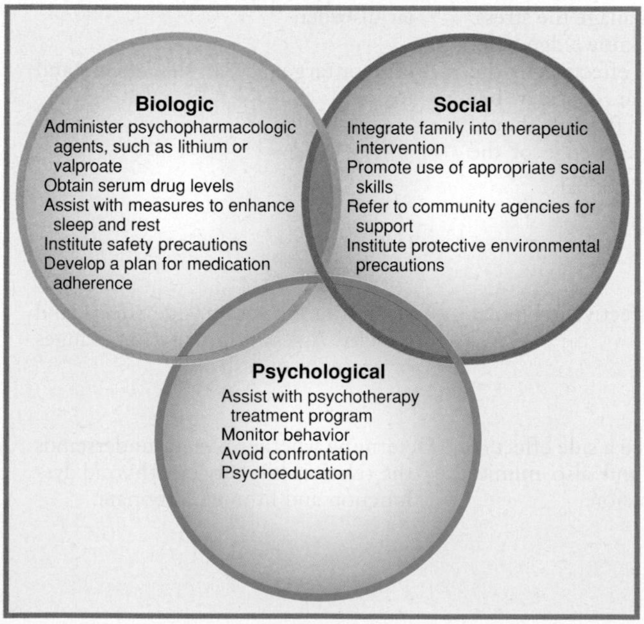

Spectrum of Care

In today's health care climate, with efforts to reduce hospitalization, most patients with bipolar disorder are treated in a community setting. Hospitalizations are usually brief, and recovery is emphasized. Medication regimens that promote adherence, psychoeducation about management of the illness, and supportive psychotherapy help move these individuals function in the coin their recovery. Patients need extended and continued follow-up to monitor medication trials and side effects, reinforce self-care management, and provide continued psychosocial support.

Mental Health Promotion

Mental health promotion activities should be the focus during remissions. During this period, patients have an opportunity to learn new coping skills that promote

FIGURE 25.2 Biopsychosocial interventions for patients with bipolar I disorder.

positive mental health. Stress management and relaxation techniques can be practiced for use when needed. A plan for managing emerging symptoms can also be developed during this period.

SUMMARY OF KEY POINTS

- Bipolar disorders are characterized by one or more manic episodes or mixed mania (co-occurrence of manic and depressive states) that cause marked impairment in social activities, occupational functioning, and interpersonal relationships and may require hospitalization to prevent self-harm.

- Manic episodes are periods in which the individual experiences abnormally and persistently elevated, expansive, or irritable mood characterized by inflated self-esteem, decreased need to sleep, excessive energy or hyperactivity, racing thoughts, easy distractibility, and an inability to stay focused. Other symptoms can include hypersexuality and impulsivity.

- Bipolar disorders are underreported and are often misdiagnosed. Bipolar I disorder is more dramatic than bipolar II and is easier to diagnosis.

- Genetics play a role in the etiology of bipolar disorders. Risk factors include a family history of mood disorders; prior mood episodes; lack of social support; stressful life events; substance use; and medical problems, particularly chronic or terminal illnesses.

- Biopsychosocial assessment includes assessing mood; speech patterns; thought processes and thought content; suicidal or homicidal thoughts; cognition and memory; and social factors, such as patterns of relationships, quality of support systems, and changes in occupational functioning. Several self-report scales are helpful in evaluating depressive symptoms.

- Many symptoms of bipolar depression, such as weight and appetite changes, sleep disturbance, decreased energy, and fatigue, are similar to those of medical illnesses. Assessment includes a thorough medical history and physical examination to detect or rule out medical or psychiatric comorbidity.

- Establishing and maintaining a therapeutic nurse–patient relationship is key to successful outcomes. Shared decision making with the patient leads to positive outcomes. Recovery-oriented nursing interventions that foster the therapeutic relationship include being available in times of crisis, providing understanding and education to patients and their families regarding goals of treatment and recovery, providing encouragement and feedback concerning the patient's progress, providing guidance in the patient's interpersonal interactions with others and work environment, and helping to set and monitor realistic goals.

- Pharmacotherapy includes mood stabilizers used alone or in combination with antipsychotics or benzodiazepines if psychosis, agitation, or insomnia. Electroconvulsive therapy is a valuable alternative for patients with severe mania that does not respond to other treatment.

- Recent major advances in bipolar disorder treatment research validate the efficacy of integrated psychosocial and pharmacologic treatment involving family or couples therapies, psychoeducational programs, and individual cognitive behavioral or interpersonal therapies.

- Psychosocial interventions for bipolar disorders include self-care management, cognitive therapy, behavior therapy, interpersonal therapy, patient and family education regarding the nature of the disorder and treatment goals, marital and family therapy, and group therapy that includes medication maintenance support groups and other consumer-oriented support groups.

CRITICAL THINKING CHALLENGES

1. A patient tells you that he no longer needs medication because he has special powers that protect him from evil forces. He no longer needs sleep and can see things that others do not see. What approaches would you use to help the patient decide to take his medication?

2. Describe how you would approach a patient who is expressing concern that the diagnosis of bipolar disorder will negatively affect her social and work relationships.

3. Your patient with mania is experiencing physical hyperactivity that is interfering with his sleep and nutrition. Describe the actions you would take to meet the patient's needs for nutrition and rest.

4. Prepare a hypothetical discussion with a patient with potential bipolar disorder concerning the advantages and disadvantages of lithium versus divalproex sodium for treatment of bipolar disorder.

5. Think about all of the above situations and relate them to persons from culturally and ethnically diverse populations (e.g., African, Latino, or Asian descent; Jewish or Jehovah Witness religions; across the life-span individuals from children to older adult populations).

Michael Clayton: 2007. Arthur Edens (Tom Wilkinson), a successful corporate lawyer, is experiencing the stress of a high-profile legal case and stops taking his medication. Consequently, he has a manic episode with delusions about one of the jurors, who he eventually contacts. The story traces the attempts by his colleague and friend Michael Clayton (George Clooney) to repair the damage Arthur's behavior has caused to the lawsuit and to get his friend treated before his mania further damages his life.

Sɪɢɴɪꜰɪᴄᴀɴᴄᴇ: Viewers can gain insight into the devastating impact of mental illness on the successful career of a well-respected attorney. This film depicts the poor judgment, impulsivity, and consequences of a full-blown mania episode.

Vɪᴇᴡɪɴɢ Pᴏɪɴᴛs: Identify the mania symptoms that Arthur displays. What feelings are evoked when you see the strange behavior that he exhibits? If Arthur were your patient, how would you approach him, and what medication would you expect him to be prescribed?

Mᴏᴠɪᴇ viewing GUIDES related to this chapter are available at http://thePoint.lww.com/Boyd5eUpdate.

A related Psychiatric-Mental Health Nursing video on the topic of Bipolar Disorders is available at: http://thePoint.lww.com/Boyd5eUpdate.

References

American Psychiatric Association. (2013). *Diagnostic and statistical manual of mental disorders* (5th ed.). Arlington, VA: Author.

Bender, R. E., & Alloy, L. B. (2011). Life stress and kindling in bipolar disorder: Review of the evidence and integration with emerging biopsychosocial theories. *Clinical Psychology Review, 31*(3), 383–398.

Brietzke, E., Mansur, R. B., Soczynska, J., Powell, A. M., & McIntyre, R. S. (2012). A theoretical framework informing research about the role of stress in the pathophysiology of bipolar disorder. *Progress in Neuro-Psychopharmacology & Biological Psychiatry, 39*(1), 1–8.

Byers, A. L., Yaffe, K., Covinsky, K. E., Friedman, M. B., & Bruce, J. L. (2010). The occurrence of mood and anxiety disorders among older adults. *Archives of General Psychiatry, 67*(5), 489–496.

Chen, C. H., Lee, C. S., Lee, M. T., Ouyang, W. C., Chen, C. C., Chong, M. Y., et al. (2014). Variant GADL1 and response to lithium therapy in bipolar I disorder. *The New England Journal of Medicine, 370*(2), 119–128.

Chen, M. H., Su, T. P., Chen, Y. S., Hsu, J. W., Huang, K. L., Chang, W. H., et al. (2013). Higher risk of developing mood disorders among adolescents with comorbidity of attention deficit hyperactivity disorder and disruptive behavior disorder: A nationwide study. *Journal of Psychiatric Research, 47*(8), 1019–1023.

Chu, D., Gildengers, A. G., Houck, P. R., Anderson, S. J., Mulsant, B. H., Reynolds, C. F., et al. (2010), Does age at onset have clinical significance in older adults with bipolar disorder? *International Journal of Geriatric Psychiatry, 25*(12), 1266–1271.

Craddock, N. & Sklar, P. (2009). Genetics of bipolar disorder: Successful start to a long journey. *Trends in Genetics, 25*(2), 99–105.

Crowe, M., Whitehead, L., Wilson, L., Carlyle, D., O'Brien, A., Inder, M., et al. (2010). Disorder-specific psychosocial interventions for bipolar disorder—A systematic review of the evidence for mental health nursing practice. *International Journal of Nursing Studies, 47*(7), 896–908.

Freeman, M. P., Wiegand, C. B., & Gelenberg, A. J. (2011). Lithium. In A. F. Schatzberg & C. B. Nemeroff (Eds.), *The American Psychiatric Publishing textbook of psychopharmacology* (4th ed). Washington, DC: American Psychiatric Publishing.

Hashimoto, K. (2010). Brain-derived neurotrophic factor as a biomarker for mood disorders: An historical overview and future directions. *Psychiatry and Clinical Neurosciences, 64*(4), 341–357.

Hoberg, A. A., Vickers, K. S., Ericksen, J., Bauer, G., Kung, S., Stone, R., et al. (2013). Feasibility evaluation of and interpersonal and social rhythm therapy group delivery model. *Archives of Psychiatric Nursing, 27*(6), 271–277.

Kenneson, A., Funderburk, F. S., & Maisto, S. A. (2013). Risk factors for secondary substance use disorders in people with childhood and adolescent-onset bipolar disorder. Opportunities for prevention. *Comprehensive Psychiatry, 54*(5), 439–446.

Kessler, R. C., Petukhova, M., Sampson, N. A., Zaslavsky, A. M., & Wittchen, H. (2012). Twelve-month and lifetime prevalence and lifetime morbid risk of anxiety and mood disorders in the United States. *International Journal of Methods in Psychiatric Research, 21*(3), 169–184.

Lee, S. H., Ripke, S., Neale, B. M., Faraone, S. V., Purcell, S. M., Cross-Disorder Group of the Psychiatric Genomics Consortium, et al. (2013). Genetic relationship between five psychiatric disorders estimated from genome-wide SNPs. *Nature Genetics, 45*(9), 984–994.

Lee, S., Tsang, A., Kessler, R. C., Jin, R., Sampson, N., Andrade, L., et al. (2010). Rapid-cycling bipolar disorders: Cross-national community study. *British Journal of Psychiatry, 196*, 217–225.

Liu, R. T. (2010). Early life stressors and genetic influences on the development of bipolar disorder: The roles of childhood abuse and brain-derived neurotrophic factor. *Child Abuse & Neglect, 34*(7), 516–522.

Parks, J., Radke, A. Q., & Mazade, N. A. (2008). *Measurement of health status for people with serious mental illnesses (technical support)*. Alexandria, VA: National Association of State Mental Health Program Directors, Medical Directors Council.

Perron, B. D., Fries, L. E., Kilbourne, A. M., Vaughn, M. G., & Bauer, M. (2010). Racial/ethnic group differences in bipolar symptomatology in a community sample of persons with bipolar I disorder. *The Journal of Nervous and Mental Disease, 198*(1), 16–21.

Popovic, D., Reinares, M., Scott, J., Nivoli, A., Murru, A., Pacchiarotti, I., et al. (2013). Polarity index of psychological interventions in maintenance treatment of bipolar disorder. *Psychotherapy and Psychosomatics, 82*(5), 292–298.

Reinares, M., Sánchez-Moreno, J., & Fountoulakis, K. N. (2014). Psychosocial interventions in bipolar disorder: What, for whom, and when. *Journal of Affective Disorders, 156*, 46–55.

Salvatore, P., Indic, P., Murray, G., & Baldessarini, R. J. (2012). Biological rhythms and mood disorders. *Dialogues in Clinical Neuroscience, 14*(4), 369–379.

Schatzberg, A. F., Cole, J. O., & DeBattista, C. (2010). *Manual of clinical psychopharmacology* (7th ed). Washington, DC: American Psychiatric Publishing.

Stahl, S. M. (2013). *Stahl's essential psychopharmacology* (4th ed). New York: Cambridge University Press.

Vieta, E., Popovic, D., Rosa, A. R., Solé, B., Grande, I., Frey, B. N., et al. (2013). The clinical implications of cognitive impairment and allostatic load in bipolar disorder. *European Psychiatry, 28*(1), 21–29.

Wozniak, J., Faraone, S. V., Mick, E., Monuteaux, C., Coville, A., & Biederman, J. (2010). A controlled family study of children with DSM: Bipolar-I disorder and psychiatric co-morbidity. *Psychological Medicine, 40*(7), 1079–1088.

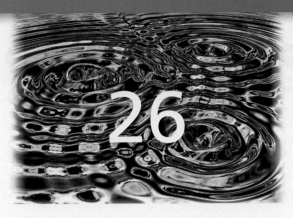

26

Anxiety, Obsessive-Compulsive, Trauma, and Stressor-Related Disorders

Management of Anxiety, Panic, and Trauma-Related Stress

Judith M. Erickson and Mary Ann Boyd

KEY CONCEPTS

- anxiety
- compulsions
- obsessions
- panic
- traumatic event

LEARNING OBJECTIVES

After studying this chapter, you will be able to:

1. Differentiate normal anxiety responses from those suggestive of an anxiety disorder.

2. Identify biopsychosocial indicators for four levels of anxiety and nursing interventions appropriate for each level.

3. Describe the prevalence and incidence of anxiety, obsessive-compulsive, and trauma–stress-related disorders.

4. Delineate clinical symptoms and course of anxiety, obsessive-compulsive, and trauma–stress-related disorders.

5. Analyze biopsychosocial theories of anxiety, obsessive-compulsive, and trauma–stress-related disorders.

6. Apply nursing process with recovery-oriented interventions for persons with anxiety, obsessive-compulsive, and trauma–stress-related disorders.

KEY TERMS

- acute stress disorder • agoraphobia • depersonalization • derealization • distraction • dissociation • exposure therapy • flooding • hyperarousal • implosive therapy • intrusion • kindling • panic attacks • panic control treatment • panicogenic • phobias • positive self-talk • posttraumatic stress disorder • systematic desensitization

There are several mental disorders related to anxiety, stress, and trauma. At one time, these disorders were all categorized as "Anxiety Disorders." Now, obsessive-compulsive disorder (OCD) and trauma–stressor-related disorder are categorized separately (APA, 2013) (see Table 26.1). This chapter will discuss four categories of related disorders including anxiety, obsessive-compulsive, trauma and stressor, and dissociative disorders. Panic disorder, OCD, and posttraumatic stress disorder (PTSD)

receive particular attention in this chapter because of the frequency with which people experience these disorders.

NORMAL VERSUS ABNORMAL ANXIETY RESPONSE

Anxiety is an unavoidable, human condition that takes many forms and serves different purposes. Anxiety can be positive and motivate one to act, or it can produce

Anxiety Disorders	Obsessive-Compulsive Disorders	Trauma- and Stressor-Related Disorders	Dissociative Disorders
Table 26.1 DSM-5 ANXIETY, OBSESSIVE-COMPULSIVE, AND TRAUMA/STRESSOR-RELATED DISORDERS			
Separation anxiety disorder	Obsessive-compulsive disorder	Reactive attachment disorder	Dissociative identity disorder
Selective mutism	Body dysmorphic disorder	Disinhibited social engagement disorder	Dissociative amnesia
Specific phobias	Hoarding disorder	Posttraumatic stress disorder	Depersonalization/derealization disorder
Social anxiety disorder (social phobia)	Trichotillomania (hair-pulling) disorder	Acute stress disorder	Other dissociative disorders
Panic disorder	Excoriation (skin-picking) disorder	Adjustment disorders	
Agoraphobia	Substance/medication induced obsessive-compulsive disorder	Other trauma- and stressor-related disorders	
Generalized anxiety disorder			
Substance/medication-induced anxiety disorder			
Other specified anxiety disorder			

paralyzing fear, causing inaction. Normal anxiety is described as being of realistic intensity and duration for the situation and is followed by relief behaviors intended to reduce or prevent more anxiety (Peplau, 1989). Normal anxiety response is appropriate to the situation, can be dealt with without repression, and can be used to help the individual identify what underlying problem has caused the anxiety.

> **KEYCONCEPT Anxiety** is an uncomfortable feeling of apprehension or dread that occurs in response to internal or external stimuli and can result in physical, emotional, cognitive, and behavioral symptoms.

During a perceived threat, rising anxiety levels cause physical and emotional changes in all individuals. A normal emotional response to anxiety consists of three parts: physiologic arousal, cognitive processes, and coping strategies. Physiologic arousal, or the fight-or-flight response, is the signal that an individual is facing a threat. Cognitive processes decipher the situation and decide whether the perceived threat should be approached or avoided. Coping strategies are used to resolve the threat. Box 26.1 summarizes many physical, affective, cognitive, and behavioral symptoms associated with anxiety. The factors that determine whether anxiety is a symptom of a mental disorder are the intensity of anxiety relative to the situation, the trigger for the anxiety, and the particular symptom clusters that manifest the anxiety. Table 26.2 describes the four degrees of anxiety and associated perceptual changes and patterns of behavior. Anxiety is a component of all of the disorders discussed in this chapter.

OVERVIEW OF ANXIETY DISORDERS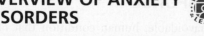

The primary symptoms of anxiety disorders are fear and anxiety. Even though symptoms of anxiety disorders can

be found in healthy individuals, an anxiety disorder is diagnosed when the fear or anxiety is excessive or out of proportion to the situation. An individual's ability to work or interpersonal relationships are impaired. Anxiety disorders occur more frequently in women than men (2:1). Anxiety disorders are differentiated by the situation or objects that provoke the fear, anxiety, or avoidance behavior and the cognitive thoughts (APA, 2013).

Anxiety disorders are the most common of the psychiatric illnesses treated by health care providers. Approximately 40 million American adults (older than 18 years old) or about 18.1% of this age group within a given year have an anxiety disorder. Direct and indirect costs of treating anxiety disorders are in the tens of billions of dollars. Women experience anxiety disorders more often than do men. Anxiety disorders may also be associated with other mental or physical comorbidities such as heart disease, respiratory disease, and mood disorders (Stein et al., 2014; Tully & Baune, 2014). There is a particularly strong relationship between the coexistence of depression and anxiety disorders. A single patient may concurrently have more than one anxiety disorder or other psychiatric disorders as well.

Anxiety disorders tend to be chronic and persistent illnesses, with full recovery more likely among those who do not have other mental or physical disorders (Ayazi, Lien, Eide, Swartz, & Hauff, 2014). Three quarters of those with an anxiety disorder have their first episode by age 21.5 years.

Anxiety Disorders Across the Life Span

Prompt identification, diagnosis, and treatment of individuals with anxiety disorders may be difficult for special populations such as children and older adult patients. Often, the symptoms suggestive of anxiety disorders may go unnoticed by caregivers or are misdiagnosed because they mimic cardiac or pulmonary pathology rather than a psychological disturbance.

BOX 26.1

Symptoms of Anxiety

PHYSICAL SYMPTOMS
Cardiovascular
Sympathetic
Palpitations
Heart racing
Increased blood pressure

Parasympathetic
Actual fainting
Decreased blood pressure
Decreased pulse rate

Respiratory
Rapid breathing
Difficulty getting air
Shortness of breath
Pressure of chest
Shallow breathing
Lump in throat
Choking sensations
Gasping
Spasm of bronchi

Neuromuscular
Increased reflexes
Startle reaction
Eyelid twitching
Insomnia
Tremors
Rigidity
Spasm
Fidgeting

Pacing
Strained face
Unsteadiness
Generalized weakness
Wobbly legs
Clumsy motions

Skin
Flushed face
Pale face
Localized sweating (palm region)
Generalized sweating
Hot and cold spells
Itching

Gastrointestinal
Loss of appetite
Revulsion toward food
Abdominal discomfort
Diarrhea
Abdominal pain
Nausea
Heartburn
Vomiting

Eyes
Dilated pupils

Urinary Tract
Parasympathetic
Pressure to urinate
Increased frequency of urination

AFFECTIVE SYMPTOMS
Edgy
Impatient
Uneasy
Nervous
Tense
Wound-up
Anxious
Fearful
Apprehensive
Scared
Frightened
Alarmed
Terrified
Jittery
Jumpy

COGNITIVE SYMPTOMS
Sensory-Perceptual
Mind is hazy, cloudy, foggy, dazed
Objects seem blurred or distant
Environment seems different or unreal
Feelings of unreality
Self-consciousness
Hypervigilance

Thinking Difficulties
Cannot recall important things
Confused

Unable to control thinking
Difficulty concentrating
Difficulty focusing attention
Distractibility
Blocking
Difficulty reasoning
Loss of objectivity and perspective
Tunnel vision

Conceptual
Cognitive distortion
Fear of losing control
Fear of not being able to cope
Fear of physical injury or death
Fear of mental disorder
Fear of negative evaluations
Frightening visual images
Repetitive fearful ideation

BEHAVIORAL SYMPTOMS
Inhibited
Tonic immobility
Flight
Avoidance
Speech dysfluency
Impaired coordination
Restlessness
Postural collapse
Hyperventilation

Adapted from Beck, A. T., & Emery, C. (1985). *Anxiety disorders and phobias: A cognitive perspective* (pp. 23–27). New York: Basic Books.

Table 26.2   DEGREES OF ANXIETY

Degree of Anxiety	Effects on Perceptual Field and on Ability to Focus Attention	Observable Behavior
Mild	Perceptual field widens slightly. Able to observe more than before and to see relationships (make connection among data). Learning is possible.	Is aware, alerted, sees, hears, and grasps more than before. Usually able to recognize and name anxiety easily.
Moderate	Perceptual field narrows slightly. Selective inattention: does not notice what goes on peripheral to the immediate focus but can do so if attention is directed there by another observer.	Sees, hears, and grasps less than previously. Can attend to more if directed to do so. Able to sustain attention on a particular focus; selectively inattentive to contents outside the focal area. Usually able to state, "I am anxious now."
Severe	Perceptual field is greatly reduced. Tendency toward dissociation: to not notice what is going on outside the current reduced focus of attention; largely unable to do so when another observer suggests it.	Sees, hears, and grasps far less than previously. Attention is focused on a small area of a given event. Inferences drawn may be distorted because of inadequacy of observed data. May be unaware of and unable to name anxiety. Relief behaviors generally used.
Panic (terror, horror, dread, uncanniness, awe)	Perceptual field is reduced to a detail, which is usually "blown up," i.e., elaborated by distortion (exaggeration), or the focus is on scattered details; the speed of the scattering tends to increase. Massive dissociation, especially of contents of self-system. Felt as enormous threat to survival. Learning is impossible.	Says, "I'm in a million pieces," "I'm gone," or "What is happening to me?" Perplexity, self-absorption. Feelings of unreality. Flights of ideas or confusion. Fear. Repeats a detail. Many relief behaviors used automatically (without thought). The enormous energy produced by panic must be used and may be mobilized as rage. May pace, run, or fight violently. With dissociation of contents of self-system, there may be a very rapid reorganization of the self, usually going along pathologic lines (e.g., a "psychotic break" is usually preceded by panic).

Adapted from Peplau, H. (1989). Theoretical constructs: Anxiety, self, and hallucinations. In A. O'Tool & S. Welt (Eds.), *Interpersonal theory in nursing practice: Selected works of Hildegarde. E. Peplau*. New York: Springer.

Children and Adolescents

Children and adolescents do experience anxiety disorders. Anxiety disorders include some of the most common conditions of children and adolescents (CDC, 2013; Kessler et al., 2012a). If left untreated, symptoms persist and gradually worsen and sometimes lead to suicidal ideation and suicide attempts, early parenthood, drug and alcohol dependence, and educational underachievement later in life (Kessler et al., 2012b).

Separation anxiety disorder, excessive fear or anxiety concerning separation from home or attachment figures, usually occurs in childhood. These children experience extreme distress when separated from home or attachment figures, worry about them when separated from them, and worry about untoward events (i.e., getting lost) and what will happen to them. This disorder is discussed in Chapter 35.

A rare disorder typically seen in childhood is *selective mutism* where children do not initiate speech or respond when spoken to by others (APA, 2013). Children with this disorder are often very anxious when asked to speak in school or read aloud. They can suffer academic impairment because of their inability to communicate with others.

Older Adults

Generally speaking, the prevalence of anxiety disorders declines with age. However, in the older adult population, rates of anxiety disorders are as high as mood disorders, which commonly co-occur. This combination of depressive and anxiety symptoms has been shown to decrease social functioning, increase somatic (physical) symptoms, and increase depressive symptoms (King-Kallimanis, Gum, & Kohn, 2009). In one study nearly half of primary care patients with chronic pain had at least one anxiety disorder. Detecting and treating anxiety is an important component of pain management (Kroenke et al., 2013). Because the older adult population is at risk for suicide, special assessment of anxiety symptoms is essential.

PANIC DISORDER

Panic is an extreme, overwhelming form of anxiety often experienced when an individual is placed in a real or perceived life-threatening situation. Panic is normal during periods of threat but is abnormal when it is continuously experienced in situations that pose no real physical or psychological threat. Some people experience heightened anxiety because they fear experiencing another panic attack. This type of panic interferes with the individual's ability to function in everyday life and is characteristic of panic disorder.

KEYCONCEPT **Panic** is a normal but extreme overwhelming form of anxiety often experienced when an individual is placed in a real or perceived life-threatening situation.

Clinical Course

The onset of panic disorder is typically between 20 to 24 years of age. The disorder can surface in childhood or after the fourth decade of life but does not usually manifest after the third decade of life. Panic disorder is treatable, but studies have shown that even after years of treatment, many people remain symptomatic. In some cases, symptoms may even worsen (American Psychiatric Association [APA], 2013).

Panic Attacks

Panic attacks are sudden, discrete periods of intense fear or discomfort that reaches its peak within a few minutes and is accompanied by significant physical and cognitive symptoms (APA, 2013). They usually peak in about 10 minutes but can last as long as 30 minutes before returning to normal functioning. The physical symptoms include palpitations, chest discomfort, rapid pulse, nausea, dizziness, sweating, paresthesias, trembling or shaking, and a feeling of suffocation or shortness of breath. Cognitive symptoms include disorganized thinking, irrational fears, **depersonalization** (being detached from oneself), and a decreased ability to communicate. Usually, there are feelings of impending doom or death, fear of going crazy or losing control, and desperation.

The physical symptoms can mimic those of a heart attack. Individuals often seek emergency medical care because they feel as if they are dying, but most have negative cardiac workup results. People experiencing panic attacks may also believe that the attacks stem from an underlying major medical illness (APA, 2013). Even with sound medical testing and assurance of no underlying disease, they often remain unconvinced.

NCLEXNOTE Physical symptoms of panic attack are similar to cardiac emergencies. These symptoms are physically taxing and psychologically frightening to patients. Recognition of the seriousness of panic attacks should be communicated to the patient.

Individuals with panic disorder experience recurrent, unexpected panic attacks followed by persistent concern about experiencing subsequent panic attacks. They fear implications of the attacks, and they have behavioral changes related to the attacks (APA, 2013). Panic attacks are either *expected* with an obvious cue or trigger or *unexpected* with no obvious cue. The first panic attack is usually associated with an identifiable cue (e.g., anxiety-provoking medical conditions, such as asthma, or in

Clinical Vignette

BOX 26.2
PANIC DISORDER

M, a 22-year-old man, has experienced several life changes, including a recent engagement, loss of his father to cancer and heart disease, graduation from college, and entrance to the workforce as a computer engineer in a large inner-city company. Because of his active lifestyle, his sleep habits have been poor. He frequently uses sleeping aids at night and now drinks a full pot of coffee to start each day. He continues to smoke to "relieve the stress." While sitting in heavy traffic on the way to work, he suddenly experienced chest tightness, sweating, shortness of breath, feelings of being "trapped," and foreboding that he was going to die. Fearing a heart attack, he went to an emergency department, where his discomfort subsided within a half hour. After several hours of testing, the doctor informed him that his heart was healthy. During the next few weeks, he experienced several episodes of feeling trapped and slight chest discomfort on his drive to work. He fears future "attacks" while sitting in traffic and while in his crowded office cubicle.

What Do You Think?

- What risk factors does M have that might contribute to the development of panic attacks?
- What lifestyle changes do you think would help M reduce stress?

FAME & FORTUNE

Charles Darwin (1809–1882)
Theory of Evolution

PUBLIC PERSONA

Charles Darwin, credited as the first scientist to gain wide acceptance of the theory of natural selection, might never have published his seminal work, *Origin of the Species*, had it not been for his psychiatric illness. Born in England, Charles Darwin, the grandson of a famous poet, inventor, and physician, was expected to accomplish great things. However, his childhood years were troublesome. When he was sent to Cambridge to study medicine, card playing and drinking became his main activities. After meeting a botanist, however, his life changed, and he embarked on a 5-year expedition to the Pacific coast of South America.

PERSONAL REALITIES

Darwin described his sensation of fear, accompanied by troubled beating of the heart, sweat, and trembling of muscles. Thought to have panic disorder, he constantly worried about what he thought he knew until he finally published his ideas on paper. In 1859, *The Origin of Species by Means of Natural Selection* was published. In 1882, he died and was buried in Westminster Abbey.

Source: Darwin, C. (1887). *The life and letters of Charles Darwin.* New York: Appleton & Co.

---

initial trials of illicit substance use) but subsequent attacks are often unexpected without any obvious cue (Box 26.2). Panic attacks not only occur in panic disorder, but also occur in other mental disorders such as depression, bipolar, eating disorders, and some medical conditions such as cardiac or respiratory disorders (APA, 2013).

Diagnostic Criteria

Panic disorder is a chronic condition that has several exacerbations and remissions during the course of the disease. It is characterized by the appearance of disabling attacks of panic that often lead to other symptoms, such as phobias.

Physical or psychological symptoms include palpitations, sweating, shaking, shortness of breath or smothering, sensations of choking, chest pain, nausea or abdominal distress, dizziness, derealization or depersonalization, fear of going crazy, fear of dying, paresthesias, and chills or hot flashes (APA, 2013) (see Key Diagnostic Characteristics 26.1).

Epidemiology and Risk Factors

In the National Epidemiologic Survey on Alcohol and Related Conditions 2001–2002, which had 43,093 participants, 5.1% of those reporting had experienced panic disorder in their lifetimes, and 2.1% experienced panic disorder in the year preceding the survey. Increased risk is associated with being female; middle aged; of low socioeconomic status; and widowed, separated, or divorced

(Grant et al., 2006). In another study combining three major epidemiological databases, the authors found significantly higher rates of panic disorder among whites than among African Americans, Asians, and Latinos (Asnaani, Gutner, Hinton, & Hofmann, 2009). The estimates of isolated panic attacks are 22.7% of the population.

Family history, substance and stimulant use or abuse, smoking tobacco, and severe stressors are risk factors for panic disorder. People who have several anxiety symptoms and those who experience separation anxiety during childhood often develop panic disorder later in life. Early life traumas, a history of physical or sexual abuse, socioeconomic or personal disadvantages, and behavioral inhibition by adults have been associated with an increased risk for anxiety disorders in children (Benjamin, Beidas, Comer, Puliafico, & Kendall, 2011; Jovanovic et al., 2011).

Comorbidity

Patients may experience more than one anxiety disorder, depression, eating disorder, substance use or abuse, or schizophrenia (Torres et al., 2014). Although people with panic disorder are thought to have more somatic complaints than the general population, panic disorder correlates with certain medical conditions, including vertigo, cardiac disease, gastrointestinal disorders, asthma, and cigarette smoking. In one study, the 12-month prevalence of panic

---

KEY DIAGNOSTIC CHARACTERISTICS 26.1 • PANIC DISORDER

Diagnostic Criteria

A. Recurrent unexpected panic attacks. A panic attack is an abrupt surge of intense fear or intense discomfort that reaches a peak within minutes, and during which time four (or more) of the following symptoms occur:
Note: The abrupt surge can occur from a calm state or an anxious state.

1. Palpitations, pounding heart, or accelerated heart rate.
2. Sweating.
3. Trembling or shaking.
4. Sensations of shortness of breath or smothering.
5. Feelings of choking.
6. Chest pain or discomfort.
7. Nausea or abdominal distress.
8. Feeling dizzy, unsteady, light-headed, or faint.
9. Chills or heat sensations.
10. Paresthesias (numbness or tingling sensations).
11. Derealization (feelings of unreality) or depersonalization (being detached from oneself).
12. Fear of losing control or "going crazy."
13. Fear of dying.

   • **Note:** Culture-specific symptoms (e.g., tinnitus, neck soreness, headache, uncontrollable screaming or crying) may be seen. Such symptoms should not count as one of the four required symptoms.

B. At least one of the attacks has been followed by 1 month (or more) of one or both of the following:
   1. Persistent concern or worry about additional panic attacks or their consequences (e.g., losing control, having a heart attack, "going crazy").
   2. A significant maladaptive change in behavior related to the attacks (e.g., behaviors designed to avoid having panic attacks, such as avoidance of exercise or unfamiliar situations).

C. The disturbance is not attributable to the physiological effects of a substance (e.g., a drug of abuse, a medication) or another medical condition (e.g., hyperthyroidism, cardiopulmonary disorders).

D. The disturbance is not better explained by another mental disorder (e.g., the panic attacks do not occur only in response to feared social situations, as in social anxiety disorder; in response to circumscribed phobic objects or situations, as in specific phobia; in response to obsessions, as in obsessive-compulsive disorder; in response to reminders of traumatic events, as in posttraumatic stress disorder; or in response to separation from attachment figures, as in separation anxiety disorder).

Target Symptoms

• Discrete period of intense fear or discomfort with four (or more) of the following symptoms that develop abruptly and reach a peak within 10 minutes:
   • Palpitations, pounding heart, or accelerated heart rate
   • Sweating
   • Trembling or shaking
   • Sensations of shortness of breath or smothering
   • Feelings of choking
   • Chest pain or discomfort
   • Nausea or vomiting
   • Feeling dizzy, unsteady, lightheaded, or faint
   • Derealization (feeling of unreality) or depersonalization (being detached from oneself)
   • Fear of losing control or going crazy
   • Fear of dying
   • Paresthesias (numbness or tingling sensations)
   • Chills or hot flushes
• Great apprehension about the outcome of routine activities and experiences
• Loss or disruption of important interpersonal relationships
• Demoralization
• Possible major depressive episode

Associated Findings

• Nocturnal panic attack (waking from sleep in a state of panic)
• Constant or intermittent feelings of anxiety related to health and mental health
• Pervasive concerns about abilities to complete daily tasks or withstand daily stressors
• Excessive use of drugs or other means to control panic attacks

Associated Physical Examination Findings
• Transient tachycardia
• Moderate elevation of systolic blood pressure

Associated Laboratory Findings
• Compensated respiratory alkalosis (decreased carbon dioxide, decreased bicarbonate levels, almost normal pH)

Other Targets for Treatment
• Loss or disruption of important interpersonal or occupational activities
• Demoralization
• Possible major depressive episode

Reprinted with permission from the *Diagnostic and Statistical Manual of Mental Disorders,* Fifth Edition (Copyright ©2013). American Psychiatric Association. All Rights Reserved.

---

disorder among patients with cardiac disease was found to be significantly higher than among those without cardiac disease (6.0% compared with 3.4%). Furthermore, these patients used emergency departments at a significantly higher rate (Korczak, Goldstein, & Levitt, 2007).

Etiology

Biologic Theories

Genetic Factors

There appears to be a substantial familial predisposition to panic disorder with an estimated heritability of 48%.

Research findings are establishing associations between the neurotransmitter pathways involved in regulation of the monoamine mechanism (Konishi et al., 2014). More research is needed to analyze genetic factors in the etiology of panic disorders.

Neuroanatomic Theories

Certain neurologic abnormalities have also been identified in patients with panic disorder. The most common abnormalities are found in the "fear network" of the brain, that is, the amygdala, hippocampus, thalamus, midbrain, pons, medulla, and cerebellum. Research shows a reduction in volume in some areas and increases in different brain area (Del Casale et al., 2013).

Biochemical Theories

Identification of neurotransmitter involvement in panic disorder has evolved from the neurochemical studies with **panicogenic** substances known to produce panic attacks, such as yohimbine, fenfluramine, norepinephrine, epinephrine, sodium lactate, and carbon dioxide. These substances are often used in studies to stimulate a panic attack (Zwanzger, Domschke, & Bradwejn, 2012).

Serotonin and Norepinephrine

Serotonin and norepinephrine are both implicated in panic disorders. Norepinephrine effects acts on those systems most affected by a panic attack—the cardiovascular, respiratory, and gastrointestinal systems. Serotonergic neurons are distributed in central autonomic and emotional motor control systems regulating anxiety states and anxiety-related physiologic and behavioral responses (Ravindran & Stein, 2010).

Gamma-Aminobutyric Acid

Gamma-aminobutyric acid (GABA) is the most abundant inhibitory neurotransmitter in the brain. GABA receptor stimulation causes several effects, including neurocognitive effects, reduction of anxiety, and sedation. GABA stimulation also results in increased seizure threshold. Abnormalities in the benzodiazepine–GABA–chloride ion channel complex have been implicated in panic disorder (Stein, Steckler, Lightfoot, Hay, & Goddard, 2010).

Hypothalamic–Pituitary–Adrenal Axis

Recent research implicates a role of the hypothalamic–pituitary–adrenal axis (HPA) axis in panic disorders. A current explanation is that as stress hormones are activated, anxiety increases, which can lead to a panic attack (Pace & Heim, 2011). See Chapter 18.

Psychological and Social Theories

Psychoanalytic and Psychodynamic Theories

Psychodynamic theories explain that anxiety develops after separation and loss. A great number of patients link their initial panic attack with recent personal losses. However, at this point the empirical evidence is inadequate for a psychodynamic explanation. It remains unclear why some patients develop panic disorder while others with similar experiences develop other disorders (Pilecki, Arentoft, & McKay, 2011).

Cognitive Behavioral Theories

Learning theory underlies most cognitive behavioral explanations of panic disorder. Classic conditioning theory suggests that one learns a fear response by linking an adverse or fear-provoking event, such as a car accident, with a previously neutral event, such as crossing a bridge. One becomes conditioned to associate fear with crossing a bridge. Applying this theory to people with panic disorder has limitations. Phobic avoidance is not always developed secondary to an adverse event.

Further development of this theory led to an understanding of **interoceptive conditioning**, which pairs a somatic discomfort, such as dizziness or palpitations, with an impending panic attack. For example, during a car accident, the individual may experience rapid heartbeat, dizziness, shortness of breath, and panic. Subsequent experiences of dizziness or palpitations, unrelated to an anxiety-provoking situation, incite anxiety and panic. Furthermore, people with panic disorder may misinterpret mild physical sensations (sweating, dizziness) as being catastrophic, causing panic as a result of learned fear (catastrophic interpretation). Some researchers hypothesize that individuals with a low sense of control over their environment or with a particular sensitivity to anxiety are vulnerable to misinterpreting normal stress. Controlled exposure to anxiety-provoking situations and cognitive countering techniques has proven successful in reducing the symptoms of panic.

Family Response to Disorder

Families with panic disorder have difficulty with overall communication. Parents with panic disorder may inadvertently cause excessive fears, phobias, or excessive worry in their children. Individuals need a tremendous amount of support and encouragement from significant others.

Pharmacologic treatment for panic disorder also affects the family in other ways. Medications used to treat panic disorder readily cross the placenta and are excreted in breast milk, potentially barring women who are pregnant or breastfeeding from receiving treatment. Pregnancy may actually protect against certain anxiety disorders, but postpartum onset of such disorders is common. Decisions about taking medications during pregnancy and breastfeeding may lead to guilt, anxiety, and an exacerbation of symptoms.

Interdisciplinary Treatment and Recovery

Nurses are pivotal in stabilizing the inpatient by providing a safe and therapeutic environment. The nurse also administers medication, monitors its effects, and develops an individual care plan to meet the patient's needs. Advanced practice nurses, licensed clinical social workers, or licensed counselors provide individual psychotherapy sessions as appropriate. Often, a clinical psychologist administers psychological testing and interprets the test results to assist with appropriate diagnosis and to tailor treatment.

Priority Care Issues

People with panic disorder are often depressed and consequently are at high risk for suicide. Adolescents with panic disorder may be at higher risk for suicidal thoughts or attempt suicide more often than other adolescents (Katz, Yaseen, Mojtabai, Cohen, & Galynker, 2011). As many as 15% of patients with panic disorder commit suicide; women with both panic disorder and depression or panic disorder and substance abuse are especially at risk (APA, 2013; Katz et al., 2011).

NURSING MANAGEMENT: Human Response to Panic Disorder

Physiologic symptoms tend to be the impetus for patients to seek medical assistance because the symptoms overlap with other medical and psychiatric illnesses. Often, patients are seen in emergency departments as they seek treatment for their physical symptoms. Biologic, psychological, and social assessments unveil potential underlying pathology and guide the nurse to an accurate nursing diagnosis.

Biologic Domain

Assessment

Skillful assessment is required to rule out life-threatening causes, including cardiac or neurologic involvement. After it has been determined that the patient does not have other medical problems, the nurse should assess for the characteristic symptoms of a panic attack. If the panic attack occurs in the presence of the nurse, direct assessment of the symptoms should be made and documented. Questions to ask the patient might include the following:

- What did you experience preceding and during the panic episode, including physical symptoms, feelings, and thoughts?
- When did you begin to feel that way? How long did it last?
- What is it that caused you to feel and think that way?
- Have you experienced these symptoms in the past? If so, under what circumstances?
- Has anyone in your family ever had similar experiences?
- What do you do when you have these experiences that help you to feel safe?
- Have the feelings and sensations ever gone away on their own?

Substance Use

Assessment for panicogenic substance use, such as sources of caffeine, pseudoephedrine, amphetamines, cocaine, or other stimulants, may rule out contributory issues either related or unrelated to panic disorder. Tobacco use can also contribute to the risk for panic symptoms. Many individuals with panic disorder use alcohol or central nervous system (CNS) depressants in an effort to self-medicate anxiety symptoms, and withdrawal from CNS depressants may produce symptoms of panic.

Sleep Patterns

Sleep is often disturbed in patients with panic disorder. In fact, panic attacks can occur during sleep, and the patient may fear sleep for this reason. Nurses should closely assess the impact of sleep disturbance because fatigue may increase anxiety and susceptibility to panic attacks.

Physical Activity

Active participation in a routine exercise program requires assessment. If the patient does not exercise routinely, define the barriers. If exercise is avoided because of chronic muscle tension, poor muscle tone, muscle cramps, general fatigue, exhaustion, or shortness of breath, the symptoms may indicate poor physical health.

Pregnancy

Because panic disorder manifests during the childbearing years, pregnant patients should be assessed carefully for an underlying panic disorder. Although pregnancy may actually protect the mother from developing panic symptoms, postpartum onset of panic disorder requires particular attention. During a time that tremendous effort is spent on family, postpartum onset of panic disorder negatively affects lifestyle and decreases self-esteem in affected women, leading to feelings of overwhelming personal disappointment.

Nursing Diagnoses for the Biologic Domain

Appropriate nursing diagnoses for the individual with panic disorder include Anxiety, Risk for Self-Harm, Social Isolation, Powerlessness, and Ineffective Family Coping. Other diagnoses may apply after the nurse has completed a thorough psychiatric nursing assessment and developed an individual services plan (care plan).

Interventions for the Biologic Domain

The course of panic disorder culminates in phobic avoidance as the affected person attempts to avoid situations that increase panic. Because identifying and avoiding anxiety-provoking situations are important during therapy, drastically changing lifestyle to avoid situations does not aid recovery. Interventions that focus on the physical aspects of anxiety and panic are particularly helpful in reducing the number and severity of the attacks, giving patients a rapid sense of accomplishment and control.

Teaching Breathing Control

Hyperventilation is common. Often, people are unaware that they take rapid, shallow breaths when they become anxious.

Teaching patients breathing control can be helpful. Focus on the breathing and help them to identify the rate, pattern, and depth. If the breathing is rapid and shallow, reassure the patient that exercise and breathing practice can help change this breathing pattern. Then assist the patient in practicing abdominal breathing by performing the following exercises:

- Instruct the patient to breathe deeply by inhaling slowly through the nose. Have him or her place a hand on the abdomen just beneath the rib cage.
- Instruct the patient to observe that when one is breathing deeply, the hand on the abdomen will actually rise.
- After the patient understands this process, ask him or her to inhale slowly through the nose while counting to five, pause, and then exhale slowly through pursed lips.
- While the patient exhales, direct attention to feeling the muscles relax, focusing on "letting go."
- Have the patient repeat the deep abdominal breathing for 10 breaths, pausing between each inhalation and exhalation. Count slowly. If the patient complains of lightheadedness, reassure him or her that this is a normal feeling while deep breathing. Instruct the patient to stop for 30 seconds, breathe normally, and then start again.
- The patient should stop between each cycle of 10 breaths and monitor normal breathing for 30 seconds.
- This series of 10 slow abdominal breaths followed by 30 seconds of normal breathing should be repeated for 3 to 5 minutes.
- Help the patient to establish a time for daily practice of abdominal breathing.

Abdominal breathing may also be used to interrupt an episode of panic as it begins. After patients have learned to identify their own early signs of panic, they can learn the four-square method of breathing, which helps divert or decrease the severity of the attack. Patients should be instructed as follows:

- Advise the patient to practice during calm periods and to begin by inhaling slowly through the nose, count to four, and then hold the breath for a count of four.
- Direct the patient to exhale slowly through pursed lips to a count of four and then rest for a count of four (no breath).
- Finally, the patient may take two normal breaths and repeat the sequence.

After patients practice the skill, the nurse should assist them in identifying the physical cues that will alert them to use this calming technique.

Teaching Nutritional Planning

Maintaining regular and balanced eating habits reduces the likelihood of hypoglycemic episodes, lightheadedness, and fatigue. To help teach the patient about healthful eating and ways to minimize physical factors contributing to anxiety:

- Advise the patient to reduce or eliminate substances in the diet that promote anxiety and panic, such as food coloring, monosodium glutamate, and caffeine (withdrawal from which may stimulate panic). Patients need to plan to reduce caffeine consumption and then eliminate it from their diet. Many over-the-counter (OTC) remedies are now used to boost energy or increase mental performance, and some of these contain caffeine. A thorough assessment should be made of all OTC products to assess the potential of anxiety-provoking ingredients.
- Instruct the patient to check each substance consumed and note whether symptoms of anxiety occur and whether the symptoms are relieved by not consuming the product.

Teaching Relaxation Techniques

Teaching the patient relaxation techniques is another way to help individuals with panic and anxiety disorders. Some are unaware of the tension in their bodies and first need to learn to monitor their own tension. Isometric exercises and progressive muscle relaxation are helpful methods to learn to differentiate muscle tension from muscle relaxation. This method of relaxation is also helpful when patients have difficulty clearing the mind, focusing, or visualizing a scene, which are often required in other forms of relaxation, such as meditation. Box 26.3 provides one method of progressive muscle relaxation.

Promoting Increased Physical Activity

Physical exercise can effectively decrease the occurrence of panic attacks by reducing muscle tension, increasing metabolism, and relieving stress. Exercise programs reduce many of the precipitants of anxiety by improving circulation, digestion, endorphin stimulation, and tissue oxygenation. In addition, exercise lowers cholesterol levels, blood pressure, and weight. After assessing for contraindications to physical exercise, assist the patient in establishing a routine exercise program. Engaging in 10- to 20-minute sessions on treadmills or stationary bicycles two to three times weekly is ideal during the winter months. Casual walking or bike riding during warmer weather promotes health. Help the patient to identify community resources that promote exercise.

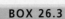

BOX 26.3

Teaching Progressive Muscle Relaxation

Choose a quiet, comfortable location where you will not be disturbed for 20 to 30 minutes. Your position may be lying or sitting, but all parts of your body should be supported, including your head. Wear loose clothing, taking off restrictive items, such as glasses and shoes.

Begin by closing your eyes and clearing your mind. Moving from head to toe, focus on each part or your body and assess the level of tension. Visualize each group of muscles as heavy and relaxed.

Take two or three slow abdominal breaths, pausing briefly between each breath. Imagine the tension flowing from your body.

Each muscle group listed below should be tightened (or tensed isometrically) for 5 to 10 seconds and then abruptly released; visualize this group of muscles as heavy, limp, and relaxed for 15 to 20 seconds before tightening the next group of muscles. There are several methods to tighten each muscle group, and suggestions are provided below. Each muscle group may be tightened two to three times until relaxed. Do not overtighten or strain. You should not experience pain.

- Hands: tighten by making fists
- Biceps: tighten by drawing forearms up and "making a muscle"
- Triceps: extend forearms straight, locking elbows
- Face: grimace, tightly shutting mouth and eyes
- Face: open mouth wide and raise eyebrows
- Neck: pull head forward to chest and tighten neck muscles
- Shoulders: raise shoulders toward ears
- Shoulders: push shoulders back as if touching them together
- Chest: take a deep breath and hold for 10 seconds
- Stomach: suck in your abdominal muscles
- Buttocks: pull buttocks together
- Thighs: straighten legs and squeeze muscles in thighs and hips
- Leg calves: pull toes carefully toward you, avoid cramps
- Feet: curl toes downward and point toes away from your body

Finally, repeat several deep abdominal breaths and mentally check your body for tension. Rest comfortably for several minutes, breathing normally, and visualize your body as warm and relaxed. Get up slowly when you are finished.

Pharmacologic Interventions

Antidepressants (selective serotonin reuptake inhibitors [SSRIs], serotonin–norepinephrine reuptake inhibitors [SNRIs], tricyclic antidepressants [TCAs], and monoamine oxidase inhibitors [MAOIs]) and antianxiety medication (benzodiazepines) have been shown to be effective in treating people with panic disorders (see Table 26.3). The use of the TCAs for the treatment of panic disorder is declining significantly, so their use is not discussed in this chapter. The MAOIs are reserved for those who do not respond to the SSRIs or SNRIs. See Chapters 11 and 24 for nursing care for patients taking TCAs and MAOIs.

Selective Serotonin Reuptake Inhibitors

The SSRIs are recommended as the first drug option in the treatment of patients with panic disorder. They have the best safety profile, and if side effects occur, they tend to be present early in treatment before the therapeutic effect takes place. Hence, the SSRIs should be started at low doses and titrated every 5 to 7 days. Antidepressant therapy is recommended for long-term treatment of the disorder and antianxiety as adjunctive treatment (Andrisano, Chiesa, & Serretti, 2013).

The SSRIs produce anxiolytic effects by increasing the transmission of serotonin by blocking serotonin reuptake at the presynaptic cleft. The initial increase in serotonergic activity with SSRIs may cause temporary increases in panic symptoms and even panic attacks. After 4 to 6 weeks of treatment, anxiety subsides, and the antianxiety effect of the medications begins (see Chapter 11). Increased serotonin activity in the brain is believed to decrease norepinephrine activity. This decrease lessens cardiovascular symptoms of tachycardia and increased blood pressure that are associated with panic attacks. See Chapter 24 for administration and monitoring side effects.

> **NCLEXNOTE** Psychopharmacologic treatment is almost always needed. Antidepressants are the medication of choice. Antianxiety medication is used only for short periods of time.

Serotonin–Norepinephrine Reuptake Inhibitors

The SNRIs increase levels of both serotonin and norepinephrine by blocking their reuptake presynaptically. Classified as antidepressants, the SNRIs are also used in anxiety disorders. Venlafaxine (Effexor) is the most commonly used SNRI (see Table 26.3). These medications have been shown to reduce the severity of panic and anticipatory anxiety. Similar to the SSRIs, they should not be abruptly discontinued (see Chapter 11).

Benzodiazepine Therapy

The high-potency benzodiazepines have produced antipanic effects, and their therapeutic onset is much faster (hours, not weeks) than that of antidepressants (see Table 26.3). Therefore, benzodiazepines are tremendously useful in treating intensely distressed patients. Alprazolam (Xanax), lorazepam (Ativan), and clonazepam (Klonopin) are widely used for panic disorder. They are well tolerated but carry the risk for withdrawal symptoms upon discontinuation of use (see Box 26.4). The benzodiazepines are still commonly used for panic disorder even though the SSRIs are recommended for first-line treatment of panic disorder (Stein et al., 2010).

Administering and Monitoring the Benzodiazepines. Treatment may include administering benzodiazepines concurrently with antidepressants for the first 4 weeks and then tapering the benzodiazepine to a maintenance dose. This strategy provides rapid symptom relief but avoids the complications of long-term benzodiazepine

Table 26.3	MEDICATION FOR PANIC DISORDER		
Medication	Starting Dose (mg/day)	Therapeutic Dose	Side Effects
Selective serotonin reuptake inhibitors (SSRIs)			Class effects: nausea, anorexia, tremors, anxiety, sexual dysfunction, jitteriness, insomnia, suicidality
Fluoxetine (Prozac)	10	20–60	Class effects
Sertraline (Zoloft)	25	50–200	Class effects, loose stools
Paroxetine (Paxil)	10	10–60	Class effects, drowsiness, fatigue, weight
Paroxetine (controlled release) (Paxil CR)	12.5	12.5–25	Class effects
Fluvoxamine (Luvox)	50	50–300	Class effects
Citalopram (Celexa)	10	20–60	Class effects
Escitalopram (Lexapro)	10	10–30	Class effects
Serotonin–norepinephrine reuptake inhibitors (SNRIs)			Class effects: nausea, sweating, dry mouth, dizziness, insomnia, somnolence, sexual dysfunction, hypertension
Duloxetine hydrochloride (Cymbalta)	60	60	Suicidality
Venlafaxine (extended release) (Effexor XR)	37.5	75–300	Class effects
Tricyclic Antidepressants (TCAs)			Class effects: sedation, weight gain, dry mouth, urinary hesitancy, constipation, orthostatic hypotension, and slow conduction time through the bundle of His
Imipramine (Tofranil)	10–25	50–300	Class effects
Nortriptyline (Pamelor)	10–25	25–125	Class effects
Desipramine (Norpramin)	10–25	25–300	Class effects
Benzodiazepines			Class effects: sedation, cognitive slowing, physical dependence
Clonazepam (Klonopin)	0.25 tid	0.5–1.5 tid	Class effects
Alprazolam (Xanax)	0.25 tid	0.5–1.5 tid	Class effects
Lorazepam (Ativan)	0.25 tid	0.5–1.5 tid	Class effects

tid, three times a day.

BOX 26.4

Drug Profile: Alprazolam (Xanax)

DRUG CLASS: Antianxiety agent

RECEPTOR AFFINITY: Exact mechanism of action is unknown; believed to increase the effects of γ-aminobutyrate

INDICATIONS: Management of anxiety disorders, short-term relief of anxiety symptoms or depression-related anxiety, panic attacks with or without agoraphobia. Unlabeled uses for school phobia, premenstrual syndrome, and depression.

ROUTES AND DOSAGES: Available in 0.25-, 0.5-, 1-, and 2-mg scored tablets.

Adults: For anxiety: Initially, 0.25 to 0.5 mg PO tid titrated to a maximum daily dose of 4 mg in divided doses. For panic disorder: Initially, 0.5 mg PO tid increased at 3- to 4-d intervals in increments of no more than 1 mg/d. For school phobia: 2 to 8 mg/d PO. For premenstrual syndrome: 0.25 mg PO tid.

Geriatric patients: Initially, 0.25 mg bid to tid, increased gradually as needed and tolerated

HALF-LIFE (PEAK EFFECT): 12 to 15 h (1–2 h)

SELECTED ADVERSE REACTIONS: Transient mild drowsiness, initially; sedation, depression, lethargy, apathy, fatigue, lightheadedness, disorientation, anger,

hostility, restlessness, headache, confusion, crying, constipation, diarrhea, dry mouth, nausea, and possible drug dependence

WARNINGS: Contraindicated in patients with psychosis, acute narrow-angle glaucoma, shock, acute alcoholic intoxication with depressed vital signs, pregnancy, labor and delivery, and breastfeeding. Use cautiously in patients with impaired hepatic or renal function and severe debilitating conditions. Risk for digitalis toxicity if given concurrently with digoxin. Increased CNS depression if taken with alcohol, other CNS depressants, and propoxyphene (Darvon).

SPECIFIC PATIENT AND FAMILY EDUCATION
- Avoid using alcohol, sleep-inducing drugs, and other OTC drugs.
- Take the drug exactly as prescribed and do not stop taking the drug without consulting your health care provider.
- Take the drug with food if gastrointestinal upset occurs.
- Avoid driving a car or performing tasks that require alertness if drowsiness or dizziness occurs.
- Report any signs and symptoms of adverse reactions.
- Notify your health care provider if severe dizziness, weakness, or drowsiness persists or if rash or skin lesions, difficulty voiding, palpitations, or swelling of the extremities occurs.

CNS, central nervous system; OTC, over the counter; PO, oral; tid, three times a day.

use. Benzodiazepines with short half-lives do not accumulate in the body, but benzodiazepines with half-lives of longer than 24 hours tend to accumulate with chronic treatment, are removed more slowly, and produce less intense symptoms on discontinuation of use (see Chapter 11).

Short-acting benzodiazepines, such as alprazolam, are associated with rebound anxiety, or anxiety that increases after the peak effects of the medication have decreased. Medications with short half-lives (alprazolam, lorazepam) should be given in three or four doses spaced throughout the day, with a higher dose at bedtime to allay anxiety-related insomnia. Clonazepam, a longer-acting benzodiazepine, requires less frequent dosing and has a lower risk for rebound anxiety.

Because of their depressive CNS effects, benzodiazepines should not be used to treat patients with comorbid sleep apnea. In fact, these drugs may actually decrease the rate and depth of respirations. Exercise caution in older adult patients for these reasons. Discontinuing medication use requires a slow taper during a period of several weeks to avoid rebound anxiety and serious withdrawal symptoms. Benzodiazepines are not indicated in the chronic treatment of patients with substance abuse but can be useful in quickly treating anxiety symptoms until other medications take effect.

Symptoms associated with withdrawal of benzodiazepine therapy are more likely to occur after high doses and long-term therapy. They can also occur after short-term therapy. Withdrawal symptoms manifest in several ways, including psychological (apprehension, irritability, insomnia, and dysphoria), physiologic (tremor, palpitations, vertigo, sweating, muscle spasm, seizures), and perceptual (sensory hypersensitivity, depersonalization, feelings of motion, metallic taste).

Managing Side Effects. The side effects of benzodiazepine medications generally include headache, confusion, dizziness, disorientation, sedation, and visual disturbances. Sedation should be monitored after beginning medication use or increasing the dose. The patient should avoid operating heavy machinery until the sedative effects are known.

Monitoring for Drug Interactions. Drugs that interact with benzodiazepines include the TCAs and digoxin; interaction may result in increased serum TCA or digoxin levels. Alcohol and other CNS depressants, when used with benzodiazepines, increase CNS depression. Their concomitant use is contraindicated. Histamine-2 blockers (cimetidine) used with benzodiazepines may potentiate sedative effects. Monitor closely for effectiveness in patients who smoke; cigarette smoking may increase the clearance of benzodiazepines.

Teaching Points. Warn patients to avoid alcohol because of the chance of CNS depression. In addition, warn them not to operate heavy machinery until the sedative effects of the medication are known.

Psychological Domain
Assessment

A complete psychological assessment is necessary to determine patterns of panic attacks; characteristic symptoms in attacks; and the patient's emotional, cognitive, or behavioral responses (see Chapter 10). A comprehensive assessment includes overall mental status, suicidal tendencies and thoughts, cognitive thought patterns, and avoidance behavior patterns. Moreover, a complete psychological evaluation provides the health care professional with a picture of the patient's baseline psychiatric condition. The nurse assesses the behavioral responses of the patient during the interview, noting topics that elicit behaviors suggesting the patient is uncomfortable or nervous (twisting hair, leg movements). The patient's self-concept is assessed, and present and past coping strategies are discussed to determine how the patient handles stress. Finally, a risk assessment is performed to determine the risk for developing psychiatric disorders, the threats to the patient's well-being, and the risk for symptom deterioration (see Chapter 10).

Self-Report Scales

Self-evaluation is difficult in panic disorder. Often the memories of the attack and its triggers are irretrievable. Several tools are available to characterize and rate the patient's state of anxiety. Examples of these symptom and behavioral rating scales are provided in Box 26.5. All of these tools are self-report measures and as such are limited by the individual's self-awareness and openness. However, the Hamilton Rating Scale for Anxiety (HAM-A), provided in Table 26.4, is an example of a scale rated by the clinician (Hamilton, 1959). This 14-item scale reflects both psychological and somatic aspects of anxiety.

Mental Status Examination

During a mental status examination, individuals with panic disorder may exhibit anxiety symptoms, including restlessness, irritability, poor concentration, and apprehensive behavior. Disorganized thinking, irrational fears, and a decreased ability to communicate often occur during a panic attack. Assess by direct questioning if the patient is experiencing suicidal thoughts, especially if the person is abusing substances or is taking antidepressant medications.

Assessment of Cognitive Thought Patterns

Catastrophic misinterpretations of trivial physical symptoms can trigger panic symptoms. After they have been identified, these thoughts should serve as a basis for

BOX 26.5

Rating Scales for Assessment of Panic Disorder and Anxiety Disorders

PANIC SYMPTOMS

Panic-Associated Symptom Scale (PASS)
Argyle, N., Delito, J., Allerup, P., et al. (1991). The Panic-Associated Symptom Scale: Measuring the severity of panic disorder. *Acta Psychiatrica Scandinavica, 83,* 20–26.

Acute Panic Inventory
Dillon, D. J., Gorman, J. M., Liebowitz, M. R., et al. (1987). Measurement of lactate-induced panic and anxiety. *Psychiatry Research, 20,* 97–105.

National Institute of Mental Health Panic Questionnaire (NIMH PQ)
Scupi, B. S., Maser, J. D., & Uhde, T. W. (1992). The National Institute of Mental Health Panic Questionnaire: An instrument for assessing clinical characteristics of panic disorder. *Journal of Nervous and Mental Disease, 180,* 566–572.

COGNITIONS

Anxiety Sensitivity Index
Reiss, S., Peterson, R. A., & Gursky, D. M. (1986). Anxiety sensitivity, anxiety frequency, and the prediction of fearfulness. *Behaviour Research and Therapy, 24,* 1–8.

Agoraphobia Cognitions Questionnaire
Chambless, D. L., Caputo, G. C., Bright, P., & Gallagher, R. (1984). Assessment of fear in agoraphobics: The Body Sensations Questionnaire and the Agoraphobic Cognitions Questionnaire. *Journal of Consulting and Clinical Psychology, 52,* 1090–1097.

Body Sensations Questionnaire
Chambless, D. L., Caputo, G. C., Bright, P., & Gallagher, R. (1984). Assessment of fear in agoraphobics: The Body Sensations Questionnaire and the Agoraphobic Cognitions Questionnaire. *Journal of Consulting and Clinical Psychology, 52,* 1090–1097.

PHOBIAS

Mobility Inventory for Agoraphobia
Chambless, D. L., Caputo, G. C., Jasin, S. E., et al. (1985). The mobility inventory for agoraphobia. *Behavior Research and Therapy, 23,* 35–44.

Fear Questionnaire
Marks, I. M., & Matthews, A. M. (1979). Brief standard self-rating for phobic patients. *Behaviour Research and Therapy, 17,* 263–267.

ANXIETY

State-Trait Anxiety Inventory (STAI)
Spielberger, C. D., Gorsuch, R. L., & Luchene, R. E. (1976). *Manual for the State-Trait Anxiety Inventory.* Palo Alto, CA: Consulting Psychologists Press.

Penn State Worry Questionnaire (PSWQ)
16 items developed to assess the trait of worry
Meyer, T., Miller, M., Metzger, R., & Borkovec, T. (1990). Development and validation of the Penn State Worry Questionnaire. *Behaviour Research and Therapy, 28*(6), 487–495.

Beck Anxiety Inventory
21 items rating the severity of symptoms on a 4-point scale
Beck, A., Epstein, N., Brown, G., & Steer, R. (1988). An inventory for measuring clinical anxiety: The Beck Anxiety Inventory. *Journal of Consulting and Clinical Psychology, 56,* 893–897.

---

individualizing patient education to counter such false beliefs. Table 26.5 presents a scale to assess catastrophic misinterpretations of the symptoms of panic.

Several studies have found that individuals who feel a sense of control have less severe panic attacks. Individuals who fear loss of control during a panic attack often make the following type of statements:

- "I feel trapped."
- "I'm afraid others will know or that I'll hurt someone."
- "I feel alone. I can't help myself."
- "I'm losing control."

These individuals also tend to show low self-esteem, feelings of helplessness, demoralization, and overwhelming fears of experiencing panic attacks. They may have difficulty with assertiveness or expressing their feelings.

Nursing Diagnoses for the Psychological Domain

Anxiety is the primary nursing diagnosis applied to patients with any of these disorders, although many diagnoses address the individual areas regarding one's inability to manage the stress of the disorder (Figure 26.1).

Other diagnoses include Risk for Self-Harm, Social Isolation, Powerlessness, and Ineffective Family Coping. Diagnoses specific to physical panic symptoms such as dizziness, hyperventilation, and so forth are likely. These diagnoses may be applied to all the anxiety disorders covered in this chapter. Outcomes vary.

Interventions for the Psychological Domain

Because medications treat only the biologic aspects of anxiety, psychological interventions are used to provide the patient with skills to minimize anxiety. The nurse can assist the patient in identifying triggers to anxiety and countering these triggers with individualized psychological measures. Distraction techniques, positive self-talk, panic control treatment, exposure therapy, implosion therapy, and cognitive behavioral therapy (CBT) can be useful.

Consistent, supportive reassurance should be given to the patient in crisis. Reassure the patient that the panic symptoms are only temporary. After the crisis, the patient should be encouraged to vent his or her feelings. The feedback received from the patient should be used to revise or tailor the care plan.

Table 26.4	HAMILTON RATING SCALE FOR ANXIETY	

Max Hamilton designed this scale to help clinicians gather information about anxiety states. The symptom inventory provides scaled information that classifies anxiety behavior and assists the clinician in targeting behaviors and achieving outcome measures. Provide a rating for each indicator based on the following scale:

0 = None   2 = Moderate   4 = Severe, grossly disabling
1 = Mild   3 = Severe

Item	Symptoms	Rating
Anxious mood	Worries, anticipation of the worst, fearful anticipation, irritability	
Tension	Feelings of tension, fatigability, startle response, moved to tears easily, trembling, feelings of restlessness, inability to relax	
Fear	Of dark, strangers, being left alone, animals, traffic, crowds	
Insomnia	Difficulty in falling asleep, broken sleep, unsatisfying sleep and fatigue on waking, dreams, nightmares, night terrors	
Intellectual (cognitive)	Difficulty concentrating, poor memory	
Depressed mood	Loss of interest, lack of pleasure in hobbies, depression, early waking, diurnal swings	
Somatic (sensory)	Tinnitus, blurring of vision, hot and cold flushes, feelings of weakness, prickly sensation	
Somatic (muscular)	Pains and aches, twitching, stiffness, myoclonic jerks, grinding of teeth, unsteady voice, increased muscular tone	
Cardiovascular symptoms	Tachycardia, palpitations, pain in chest, throbbing of vessels, fainting feelings, missing beat	
Respiratory symptoms	Pressure or constriction in chest, choking feelings, sighing, dyspnea	
Gastrointestinal symptoms	Difficulty in swallowing, wind, abdominal pain, burning sensation, abdominal fullness, nausea, vomiting, looseness of bowels, loss of weight, constipation	
Genitourinary symptoms	Frequency of micturition, urgency of micturition, amenorrhea, menorrhagia, development of frigidity, premature ejaculation, loss of libido, impotence	
Autonomic symptoms	Dry mouth, flushing, pallor, tendency to sweat, giddiness, tension headache, raising of hair	
Behavior at interview	Fidgeting, restlessness or pacing, tremor of hands, furrowed brow, strained face, sighing or rapid respiration, facial pallor, swallowing, belching, brisk tendon jerks, dilated pupils, exophthalmos	

From Hamilton, M. (1959). The assessment of anxiety states by rating. *British Journal of Medical Psychology*, 32, 54.

Peplau (1989) devised general guidelines for nursing interventions that might be successful in treating patients with anxiety. These interventions help the patient attend to and react to input other than the subjective experience of anxiety. They are designed to help the patient focus on other stimuli and cope with anxiety in any form (Table 26.6). These general interventions apply to all anxiety disorders and therefore are not reiterated in subsequent sections. Biopsychosocial interventions are addressed under the pertinent headings in Figure 25.2.

Distraction

After patients can identify the early symptoms of panic, they may learn to implement **distraction** behaviors that take the focus off the physical sensations. Some activities include initiating conversation with a nearby person or engaging in physical activity (e.g., walking, gardening, or house cleaning). Performing simple repetitive activities such as snapping a rubber band against the wrist, counting backward from 100 by threes, or counting objects along the roadway might also deter an attack.

Positive Self-Talk

During states of increased anxiety and panic, individuals can learn to counter fearful or negative thoughts by using planned and rehearsed positive coping statements, called **positive self-talk**. "This is only anxiety, and it will pass," "I can handle these symptoms," and "I'll get through this" are examples of positive self-talk. These types of positive statements can give the individual a focal point and reduce fear when panic symptoms begin. Handheld cards that carry positive statements can be carried in a purse or wallet so the person can retrieve them quickly when panic symptoms are felt (Box 26.6).

Panic Control Treatment

Panic control treatment involves intentional exposure (through exercise) to panic-invoking sensations such as dizziness, hyperventilation, tightness in the chest, and sweating. Identified patterns become targets for treatment. Patients are taught to use breathing training and cognitive restructuring to manage their responses and are

Table 26.5 PANIC ATTACK COGNITIONS QUESTIONNAIRE

Rate each of the following thoughts according to the degree to which you believe each thought contributes to your panic attack.

1 = Not at all   3 = Quite a lot
2 = Somewhat   4 = Very much

1. I'm going to die.	1	2	3	4
2. I'm going insane.	1	2	3	4
3. I'm losing control.	1	2	3	4
4. This will never end.	1	2	3	4
5. I'm really scared.	1	2	3	4
6. I'm having a heart attack.	1	2	3	4
7. I'm going to pass out.	1	2	3	4
8. I don't know what people will think.	1	2	3	4
9. I won't be able to get out of here.	1	2	3	4
10. I don't understand what is happening to me.	1	2	3	4
11. People think I am crazy.	1	2	3	4
12. I'll always be this way.	1	2	3	4
13. I am going to throw up.	1	2	3	4
14. I must have a brain tumor.	1	2	3	4
15. I'll choke to death.	1	2	3	4
16. I'm going to act foolish.	1	2	3	4
17. I'm going blind.	1	2	3	4
18. I'll hurt someone.	1	2	3	4
19. I'm going to have a stroke.	1	2	3	4
20. I'm going to scream.	1	2	3	4
21. I'm going to babble or talk funny.	1	2	3	4
22. I'll be paralyzed by fear.	1	2	3	4
23. Something is physically wrong with me.	1	2	3	4
24. I won't be able to breathe.	1	2	3	4
25. Something terrible will happen.	1	2	3	4
26. I'm going to make a scene.	1	2	3	4

Adapted from Clum, G. A. (1990). Panic attack cognitions questionnaire. *Coping with panic: A drug-free approach to dealing with anxiety attacks.* Pacific Grove, CA: Brooks/Cole.

Table 26.6 NURSING INTERVENTIONS BASED ON DEGREES OF ANXIETY

Degree of Anxiety	Nursing Interventions
Mild	Assist patient to use energy anxiety provides to encourage learning.
Moderate	Encourage patient to talk: to focus on one experience, to describe it fully, and then to formulate the patient's generalizations about that experience.
Severe	Allow relief behaviors to be used but do not ask about them. Encourage the patient to talk: ventilation of random ideas is likely to reduce anxiety to moderate level.
Panic	Stay with the patient. Allow pacing and walk with the patient. No content inputs to the patient's thinking should be made by the nurse. (They burden the patient, who will distort them.) Be direct with the fewest number of words: e.g., "Drink this" (give liquids to replace lost fluids and to relieve dry mouth); "Say what's happening to you," "Talk about yourself," or "Tell what you feel now" (to encourage ventilation and externalization of inner, frightening experience). Pick up on what the patient says, e.g., Patient: "What's happening to me—how did I get here?" Nurse: "Say what you notice." Use short phrases to the point of the patient's comment. Do not touch the patient; patients experiencing panic are very concerned about survival, are experiencing a grave threat to self, and usually distort intentions of all invasions of their personal space.

Adapted from Peplau, H. (1989). Theoretical constructs: Anxiety, self, and hallucinations. In A. O'Toole & S. Welt (Eds.), *Interpersonal theory in nursing practice: Selected works of Hildegarde E. Peplau.* New York: Springer.

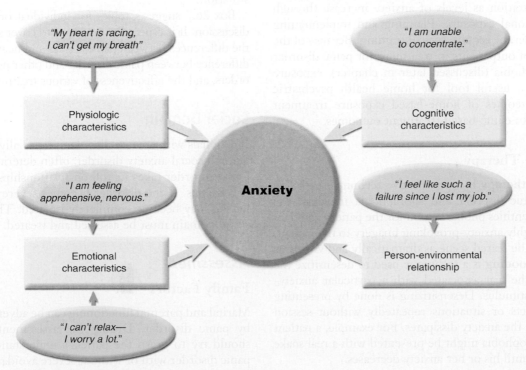

FIGURE 26.1 Nursing diagnosis concept map: anxiety.

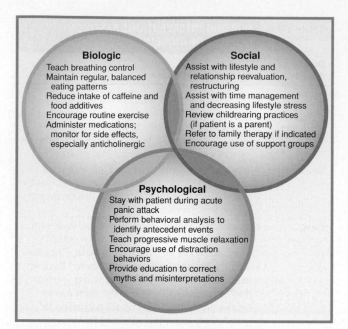

Biologic
Teach breathing control
Maintain regular, balanced
eating patterns
Reduce intake of caffeine and
food additives
Encourage routine exercise
Administer medications;
monitor for side effects,
especially anticholinergic

Social
Assist with lifestyle and
relationship reevaluation,
restructuring
Assist with time management
and decreasing lifestyle stress
Review childrearing practices
(if patient is a parent)
Refer to family therapy if indicated
Encourage use of support groups

Psychological
Stay with patient during acute
panic attack
Perform behavioral analysis to
identify antecedent events
Teach progressive muscle relaxation
Encourage use of distraction
behaviors
Provide education to correct
myths and misinterpretations

FIGURE 26.2 Biopsychosocial interventions for patients with panic disorder.

instructed to practice these techniques between therapy sessions to adapt the skills to other situations.

Systematic Desensitization

Systematic desensitization, another exposure method used to desensitize patients, exposes the patient to a hierarchy of feared situations that the patient has rated from least to most feared. The patient is taught to use muscle relaxation as levels of anxiety increase through multisituational exposure. Planning and implementing exposure therapy require special training. Because of the multitude of outpatients in treatment for panic disorder and agoraphobia (discussed later in chapter), exposure therapy is a useful tool for home health psychiatric nurses. Outcomes of home-based exposure treatment are similar to clinic-based treatment outcomes.

Implosive Therapy

Implosive therapy is a provocative technique useful in treating panic disorder and agoraphobia in which the therapist identifies phobic stimuli for the patient and then presents highly anxiety-provoking imagery to the patient, describing the feared scene as dramatically and vividly as possible. **Flooding** is a technique used to desensitize the patient to the fear associated with a particular anxiety-provoking stimulus. Desensitizing is done by presenting feared objects or situations repeatedly without session breaks until the anxiety dissipates. For example, a patient with ophidiophobia might be presented with a real snake repeatedly until his or her anxiety decreases.

Cognitive Behavioral Therapy

CBT is a highly effective tool for treating individuals with panic disorder. It has been considered the first-line treatment for those with panic and other anxiety disorders and is often used in conjunction with medications, including the SSRIs, in treating those with panic disorder (Ruwaard, Lange, Schrieken, Dolan, & Emmelkamp, 2012). The goals of CBT include helping the patient to manage his or her anxiety and correcting anxiety-provoking thoughts through interventions, including cognitive restructuring, breathing training, and psychoeducation.

> **NCLEXNOTE** Cognitive therapy techniques give patients with anxiety a sense of control over the recurring threats of panic and obsessions.

Psychoeducation

Psychoeducation programs help to educate patients and families about the symptoms of panic. Individuals with panic disorder legitimately fear going crazy, losing control, or dying because of their physical symptoms. Attempting to convince a patient that such fears are groundless only heightens anxiety and impedes communication. Information and physical evidence, such as electrocardiogram results and laboratory test results, should be presented in a caring and open manner that demonstrates acceptance and understanding of their situation.

Box 26.7 suggests topics for individual or small-group discussion. It is especially important to cover such topics as the differences between panic attacks and heart attacks, the difference between panic disorder and other psychiatric disorders, and the effectiveness of various treatment methods.

Social Domain

Individuals with anxiety disorders, especially panic disorder and social anxiety disorder, often deteriorate socially as the disorder takes its toll on relationships with family and friends. If the disorder becomes severe enough, the person may become completely isolated. Therefore, the social domain must be assessed and treated.

Assessment

Family Factors

Marital and parental functioning can be adversely affected by panic disorder. During the assessment, the nurse should try to grasp the patient's understanding of how panic disorder with or without severe avoidance behavior

BOX 26.6 • THERAPEUTIC DIALOGUE • Panic Disorder

Mark, a 55-year-old white man, was admitted 4 days ago to the psychiatric unit with exacerbation of anxiety symptoms and panic attacks during the past 3 weeks. He has a 30-year history of uncontrolled anxiety that is refractory to medications and psychotherapy. On admission, he stated that he feels suicidal at times because he thinks his life is not within his control. He feels embarrassed, angry, and "trapped" by his disorder. During the past 24 hours, Mark is seen crying at times; he also isolates himself in his room. Michelle, Mark's nurse, enters his room to make a supportive contact and to assess his current mental status.

INEFFECTIVE APPROACH

Nurse: Oh. . . . Why are you crying?

Patient: (Looks up, gives a nervous chuckle.) Obviously, because I'm upset. I am tired of living this way. I just want to be normal again. I can't even remember what that feels like.

Nurse: You look normal to me. Everyone has bad days. It'll pass.

Patient: I've felt this way longer than you've been alive. I've tried everything, and nothing works.

Nurse: You're not the first depressed person that I've taken care of. You just need to go to groups and stay out of your room more. You'll start feeling better.

Patient: (Angrily) Oh, it's just that easy. You have no idea what I'm going through! You don't know me! You're just a kid.

Nurse: I can help you if you help yourself. A group starts in 5 minutes, and I'd like to see you there.

Patient: I'm not going to no damn group! I want to be alone so I can think!

Nurse: (Looks about anxiously.) Maybe I should come back after you've calmed down a little.

EFFECTIVE APPROACH

Nurse: Mark, I noticed that you are staying in your room more today. What's troubling you?

Patient: (Looks up) I feel like I've lost complete control of my life. I'm so anxious, and nothing helps. I'm tired of it.

Nurse: I see. That must be difficult. Can you tell me more about what you are feeling right now?

Patient: I feel like I'm going crazy. I worry all the time about having panic attacks. They make me scared I'm going to die. Sometimes I think I'd be better off dead.

Nurse: (Remains silent, continues to give eye contact.)

Patient: Do you know what it's like to be a prisoner to your emotions? I can't even go out of the house sometimes, and when I do, it's terrifying. I don't know what to think anymore.

Nurse: Mark, you have lived with this disorder for a long time. You say that the medications do not work to your liking, but what has helped you in the past?

Patient: Well, I learned in relaxation group that panic symptoms are probably caused by chemicals in my brain that are not working correctly. I learned that medications can help, but they don't work well for me. I tried an exposure plan and relaxation techniques to deal with my fears of leaving the house and my chronic anxiety. That did help some, but it's scary to do.

Nurse: It sounds like you have learned much about your illness, one that can be treated, so that you don't always have to feel this way.

Patient: This is easier to say right now when I'm here and can get help if I need it. It's hard to remember this when I'm in the middle of a panic attack and think I'm dying.

Nurse: It's harder when you're alone?

Patient: Much harder! And I'm alone so much of the time.

Nurse: Let's talk about some ways you can manage your panics when you're alone. Tell me some of the techniques you've learned.

CRITICAL THINKING CHALLENGE

- What tone is established by the nurse's opening question in the first scenario?
- Which therapeutic communication techniques did the nurse use in the second scenario to avoid the pitfalls encountered in the first scenario?
- What information was uncovered in the second scenario that was not touched on in the first?
- What predictions can you make about the interpersonal relationship likely to develop between the nurse and the patient in each scenario?

BOX 26.7

Psychoeducation Checklist: **Panic Disorder**

When caring for the patient with panic disorder, be sure to include the following topic areas in the teaching plan:

- Psychopharmacologic agents (anxiolytics or antidepressants) if ordered, including drug action, dosage, frequency, and possible adverse effects
- Breathing control measures
- Nutrition
- Exercise
- Progressive muscle relaxation
- Distraction behaviors
- Exposure therapy
- Time management
- Positive coping strategies

has affected his or her life along with that of the family. Pertinent questions include the following:

- How has the disorder affected your family's social life?
- What limitations related to travel has the disorder placed on you or your family?
- What coping strategies have you used to manage symptoms?
- How has the disorder affected your family members or others?

Cultural Factors

Cultural competence calls for the understanding of cultural knowledge, cultural awareness, cultural assessment skills, and cultural practice. Therefore, cultural differences must be considered in the assessment of panic disorder. Different cultures interpret sensations, feelings, or understandings differently. For example, symptoms of anxiety might be seen as witchcraft or magic (APA, 2013). Several cultures do not have a word to describe "anxiety" or "anxious" and instead may use words or meanings to suggest physical complaints. In addition, showing anxiety may be a sign of weakness in some cultures (Roberts, 2010). Many Asian OTC herbal remedies contain substances that may induce panic by increasing the heart rate, basal metabolic rate, blood pressure, and sweating (see Chapter 11).

Nursing Diagnoses for the Social Domain

Social Isolation, Impaired Social Interaction, and Risk for Loneliness are usually supported with assessment data. Because the whole family is affected by one member's symptoms, Interrupted Family Processes may also occur.

Interventions for the Social Domain

Individuals with panic disorder, especially those with significant anxiety sensitivity, may need assistance in reevaluating their lifestyle. Time management can be a useful tool. In the workplace or at home, underestimating the time needed to complete a chore or being overly involved in

several activities at once increases stress and anxiety. Procrastination, lack of assertiveness, and difficulties with prioritizing or delegating tasks intensify these problems.

Writing a list of chores to be completed and estimating time to complete them provides concrete feedback to the individual. Crossing out each activity as it is completed helps the patient to regain a sense of control and accomplishment. Large tasks should be broken into a series of smaller tasks to minimize stress and maximize sense of achievement. Rest, relaxation, and family time—frequently omitted from the daily schedule—must be included.

Evaluation and Treatment Outcomes

Patients can be assisted to keep a daily log of the severity of anxiety and the frequency, duration, and severity of panic episodes. This log will be a basic tool for monitoring progress as symptoms decrease. Rating scales may also be helpful to monitor changes in misinterpretations or other symptoms related to panic. Medications alone provide significant short-term improvement for many individuals, but a long-term combination of psychosocial and pharmacologic treatment is usually necessary.

Although many researchers consider panic disorder a chronic, long-term condition, the positive results from outcome studies should be shared with patients to provide encouragement and optimism that patients can learn to manage these symptoms. Outcome studies have demonstrated success with panic control treatment, CBT therapy, exposure therapy, and various medications specific to certain symptoms. Figure 26.3 illustrates a number of examples of biopsychosocial treatment outcomes for individuals with panic disorder.

Continuum of Care

As with any disorder, a continuum of patient care across multiple settings is crucial. Patients are treated in the least restrictive environment that will meet their safety needs. As the patient progresses through treatment, the environment of care changes from an emergency or inpatient setting to outpatient clinics or individual therapy sessions.

Inpatient-Focused Care

Inpatient settings provide control for the stabilization of the acute panic symptoms and initiation of recovery-oriented strategies. Medication use often is initiated here because patients who show initial panic symptoms require in-depth assessment to determine the etiology. The patient is formally introduced to the disorder after the diagnosis is made. As recovery begins, crisis stabilization, medication management, milieu therapy, and psychotherapies are introduced, and outpatient discharge linkage appointments are set. See Nursing Care Plan 26.1.

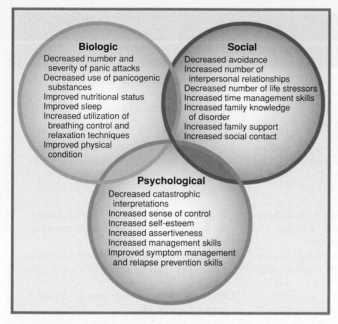

Biologic
Decreased number and severity of panic attacks
Decreased use of panicogenic substances
Improved nutritional status
Improved sleep
Increased utilization of breathing control and relaxation techniques
Improved physical condition

Social
Decreased avoidance
Increased number of interpersonal relationships
Decreased number of life stressors
Increased time management skills
Increased family knowledge of disorder
Increased family support
Increased social contact

Psychological
Decreased catastrophic interpretations
Increased sense of control
Increased self-esteem
Increased assertiveness
Increased management skills
Improved symptom management and relapse prevention skills

FIGURE 26.3 Biopsychosocial outcomes for patients with panic disorder.

Emergency Care

Because individuals with panic disorder are likely to first present for treatment in an emergency department or primary care setting, nurses working in these settings should be involved in early recognition and referral. Consultation with a psychiatrist or mental health professional by the primary care physician can decrease both costs and overall patient symptoms. Unnecessary emergency department visits cause soaring health care costs. Several interventions may be useful in reducing the number of emergency department visits related to panic symptoms. Psychiatric consultation and nursing education can be provided in the emergency department to explore other avenues of treatment. Remembering that the patient experiencing a panic attack is in crisis, nurses can take several measures to help alleviate symptoms, including the following:

- Stay with the patient and maintain a calm demeanor. (Anxiety often produces more anxiety, and a calm presence will help calm the patient.)

NURSING CARE PLAN 26.1

The Patient With Panic Disorder

Douglas is a 50-year-old male who is being evaluated in the emergency room by a nurse from the mental health crisis team. Doug was brought into the emergency department by his wife after experiencing chest pain early in the evening. He arrived in a state of severe level of anxiety and believed that he was having a heart attack. An EKG and laboratory values were normal.

Setting: Day Treatment Program, Adult Psychiatric Services

Baseline Assessment: Doug arrived at the ED trembling, dizzy, pale, experiencing tachycardia, nausea, and feelings of dread. He could not follow directions and responded poorly to redirection. His attention and thoughts are scattered.

Associated Psychiatric Diagnosis	Medications
Panic disorder History of hypertension	Paroxetine CR (Paxil) 12.5 mg every day Lisinopril (Zestril) 20 mg daily Lorazepam (Ativan) 1 mg every 6 hours PRN for extreme anxiety

Nursing Diagnosis 1: Anxiety

Defining Characteristics	Related Factors
Trembling, increased pulse Fearful, irritable, scared, worried Apprehensive	Impending panic attacks Panic attacks

Outcomes

Initial	Long-term
Develop skills to decrease impact of panic attack	Carry out normal daily living and social activities outside of the house

Continued

NURSING CARE PLAN 26.1 *(Continued)*

Interventions

Interventions	Rationale	Ongoing Assessment
Meet daily with Doug to assess if he has had a panic attack within the last 24 hours.	Asking Doug to monitor panic attacks will provide data regarding potential antecedents to attacks.	Determine whether Doug has had a panic attack.
Using a calm, reassuring approach, encourage verbalization of feelings, perceptions, and fears. Identify periods of time when anxiety level is at its highest.	Discussing the experience of anxiety will help the patient notice when his anxiety increases.	Explore the antecedents and determine whether he was able to practice techniques from education programs.
Teach Doug how to perform relaxation techniques.	Having strategies to deal with impending panic attack will decrease the intensity of the experience.	Observe effectiveness of his technique and changes in anxiety/panic episodes.
Teach Doug about the actions and side effects of paroxetine. Explain the purposes of the medication. Track the number of PRN medications that are used for anxiety. Also, monitor for use of alcohol and herbal supplements.	Panic attacks are neurobiologic occurrences that respond to medications.	Determine whether panic attacks decrease over time and whether there are side effects.
		Determine his commitment to living a more normal life.

Evaluation

Outcomes	Revised Outcomes	Interventions
Doug's panic attacks decreased to once a week.	Increase social activity outside of house.	Meet with Doug twice a week to monitor progress.
Attended day treatment program every day.		Continue to reinforce the use of strategies in managing anticipatory anxiety.
Able to go to grocery store.		

- Reassure the patient that you will not leave, that this episode will pass, and that he or she is in a safe place. (The patient often fears dying and cannot see beyond the panic attack.)
- Give clear, concise directions using short sentences. Do not use medical jargon.
- Walk or pace with the patient to an environment with minimal stimulation. (The patient in panic has excessive energy.)
- Administer PRN (as-needed) anxiolytic medications as ordered and appropriate. (Pharmacotherapy is effective in treating those with acute panic.)

After the panic attack has resolved, allow the patient to vent his or her feelings. This often helps the patient in clarifying his or her feelings.

Family Interventions

In addition to learning the symptoms of panic disorder, nurses should have information sheets or pamphlets available concerning the disorder and any medications prescribed. Parents, especially single parents, will need assistance in child rearing and may benefit from services designed to provide some respite. Moreover, the entire family will need support in adjusting to the disorder. A referral for family therapy may be indicated. Involving the entire family in the therapy process is imperative. Families experience the symptoms, treatments, clinical setbacks, and recovery from chronic mental illnesses as a unit. Misunderstandings, misconceptions, false information, and the stigma of mental illness, singly or collectively, impede recovery efforts.

Community Treatment

Most individuals with panic disorder are treated on an outpatient basis. Referral lists of community resources and support groups are useful in this setting. A discussion about the recovery and the importance of the 10 components help healing to begin (see Chapter 2). Nurses are more directly involved in treatment, conducting psychoeducation groups on relaxation and breathing techniques, symptom management, and anger management. Advanced practice nurses conduct CBT and individual and family psychotherapy. In addition, medication monitoring groups reemphasize the role of medications, monitor for side effects, and enhance treatment compliance overall. See Interdisciplinary Treatment/Recovery Plan 26.1.

INTERDISCIPLINARY TREATMENT/RECOVERY PLAN   26.1

The Patient With Panic Disorder   Outpatient Clinic Weekly. A 50-Year-Old Male

Admission Date	Date of This Plan	Type of Plan: Check Appropriate Box					
5/26/15	5/27/15	☐ Initial	☐ Master	☐ 30	☐ 60	☐ 90	☐ Other

Treatment Team Present:
Smith, M., MD; S. Jones, RNC; G. Stevens, LCSW (social worker); V. Bond (Music Therapist), Douglas (patient)

DIAGNOSIS (DSM-5)

Panic disorder
Hypertension
Social problems (unable to leave home)

ASSETS (MEDICAL, PSYCHOLOGICAL, SOCIAL, EDUCATIONAL, VOCATIONAL, RECREATIONAL)

1. No physical illness evident
2. Cognitive abilities intact, wants to get better
3. Has been under stress due to disagreements with employer. Family having financial problems after wife was laid off from her job. Family is supportive, but very stressed. He lives with wife and son who is in high school and experimenting with illegal drugs. Another son is a sophomore in college who is expecting financial help with school expenses. Doug and his wife are having frequent arguments.

MASTER PROBLEM LIST

Prob. No.	Date	Problem	Code	Change Code	Change Date
1	5/25/15	Recurring panic attacks interfere with his ability to engage in social activities and maintain independence			
2					
3					
4					
5					
6					
7					
8					

CODE T = Problem must be addressed in treatment.
N = Problem noted and will be monitored.
X = Problem noted, but deferred/inactive/no action necessary.
O = Problem to be addressed in aftercare/continuing care.
I = Problem incorporated into another problem.
R = Resolved.

INDIVIDUAL TREATMENT PLAN PROBLEM SHEET

#1 Problem/Need	Date Identified	Problem Resolved/Discontinuation Date
Recurring panic attacks interfere with his ability to engage in social activities and maintain independence.	5/26/15	

Objective(s)/Short-Term Goals	Target Date	Achievement Date
1. Patient reports that he experiences no more than two panic attacks per week (down from 2–3 daily)	6/25/15	
2. Patient begins to go places outside of home.	7/25/15	

Continued

| INTERDISCIPLINARY TREATMENT/RECOVERY PLAN | 26.1 *(Continued)* |

The Patient With Panic Disorder   Outpatient Clinic Weekly. A 50-Year-Old Male

Treatment Interventions	Frequency	Person Responsible
Attend group therapy	Weekly	RN monitor attendance
Relaxation group	Weekly	AT
Panic Disorders Education Group	Weekly	SW, RN
Individual counseling for monitoring anxiety and panic attacks	Weekly	RN
Medications for anxiety and prevention of panic attacks	Weekly	MD/RN
Family support group (patient's family)	Weekly	SW

Describe Patient Participation (and/or family, guardian, other agencies, significant others)

Responsible QMHP		Patient or Guardian		Staff Physician	
Signature	Date	Signature	Date	Signature	Date

GENERALIZED ANXIETY DISORDER (GAD)

Generally speaking, patients with GAD feel frustrated, disgusted with life, demoralized, and hopeless. They may state that they cannot remember a time that they did not feel anxious. They experience a sense of ill-being and uneasiness and a fear of imminent disaster. Over time, they may recognize that their chronic tension and anxiety are unreasonable.

Clinical Course

The onset of GAD is insidious. Many patients complain of being chronic worriers. GAD affects individuals of all ages. About half of individuals with GAD report an onset in childhood or adolescence, although onset after 20 years of age is also common. Adults with GAD often worry about matters such as their job, household finances, health of family members, or simple matters (such as household chores or being late for appointments). The intensity of the worry fluctuates, and stress tends to intensify the worry and anxiety symptoms (APA, 2013).

Patients with GAD may exhibit mild depressive symptoms, such as dysphoria. They are also highly somatic, with complaints of multiple clusters of physical symptoms, including muscle aches, soreness, and gastrointestinal ailments. In addition to physical complaints, patients with GAD often experience poor sleep habits, irritability, trembling, twitching, poor concentration, and an exaggerated startle response. People with this disorder often are seen in a primary care setting with somatic symptoms (Kroenke et al., 2013).

Diagnostic Criteria

GAD is characterized by excessive worry and anxiety (apprehensive expectation) for at least 6 months. The anxiety does not usually pertain to a specific situation; rather, it concerns a number of real-life activities or events. Ultimately, the excessive worry and anxiety cause great distress and interfere with the patient's daily personal or social life.

Generalized Anxiety Disorder Across the Life Span

Children and Adolescents

GAD may be overdiagnosed in children because symptoms overlap with those of other psychiatric disorders (APA, 2013). Children with GAD manifest their symptoms through worry about their performance in school or sports and often excel in these areas. Somatic complaints in children with GAD are heightened. Children may also worry about trivial issues, such as what clothes to wear or about their physical appearance or social interactions. Children with the disorder tend to be perfectionistic and conforming, seeking frequent approval from parents or authority figures (Benjamin et al., 2011).

Older Adults

Older adults also experience GAD, although may have fewer symptoms than younger individuals (Miloyan, Byrne, & Pachana, 2014). Nonetheless, many older adults in depression and anxiety studies meet the criteria for GAD or have significant anxiety symptoms (King-Kallimanis et al., 2009).

Epidemiology and Risk Factors

The 12-month prevalence of GAD among adolescents is 0.9% and 2.9% for adults (APA, 2013). GAD is twice as common in women as in men. The lifetime prevalence rate is nearly 5%. Unresolved conflicts, cognitive misinterpretations, and life stressors are examples of potential contributors to the development of the disorder. Patients may have a genetic predisposition to anxiety sensitivity. Behavioral inhibition, characterized by shyness, fear, or becoming withdrawn in unfamiliar situations, may be a risk factor for GAD and other anxiety disorders (Benjamin et al., 2011).

Comorbidity

Patients with GAD often have other psychiatric disorders. Roughly three quarters of patients with GAD have at least one additional current or lifetime psychiatric diagnosis. The most common comorbid disorders are major depressive disorder, social anxiety disorder, specific phobia, panic disorder, and dysthymia (Vesga-Lopez et al., 2008). Substance use is a significant problem associated with GAD because alcohol, anxiolytics, or barbiturates are often used to relieve anxiety symptoms, but this self-medication potentially leads to dependency (Cullen et al., 2013).

Etiology

Biologic Theories

Biologic theories of causation for GAD have not been extensively studied. Nonetheless, the fact that GAD has consistent symptoms, which can be controlled with medication, has led investigators to consider several biologic possibilities.

Neurochemical Theories

Symptoms suggesting activation of the sympathetic nervous system are common in GAD, and studies have found evidence of norepinephrine system dysregulation. Because medications that act on serotonin, such as the SSRIs, are also effective in treating anxiety, serotonin dysfunction may be related to GAD. Although more research is needed to understand the underlying pathophysiology, serotonin and the GABA–benzodiazepine receptor complex appear to be involved.

Genetic Theories

Recent studies have examined genetic and familial factors in the etiology of GAD. Individuals with GAD may have a genetic vulnerability that predisposes them to anxiety sensitivity (Sakolsky, McCracken, & Nurmi, 2012). Biologic foundations involved in the development of anxiety disorders might be the same ones responsible for depression (Molina et al., 2011). The family environment might also play an important role because one may become anxious through learned behavior.

Psychological Theories

Cognitive behavioral theory regarding the etiology of GAD proposes that the disorder results from inaccurate assessment of perceived environmental dangers. These inaccuracies result from selective focus on negative details, distorted information processing, and an overly pessimistic view of one's coping ability. Psychoanalytic theory postulates that anxiety represents unresolved unconscious conflicts. Sources of anxiety change in different developmental stages and include such conflicts as fear of separation or fear of loss of love.

Sociologic Theories

Although no specific sociocultural theories are related to the development of GAD, a high-stress lifestyle and multiple stressful life events may be contributors. Kindling results from overstimulation or repeated stimulation of nerve cells by environmental stressors. Individuals with GAD are hypersensitive to stress and anxiety-provoking events.

NURSING MANAGEMENT: Human Response to Generalized Anxiety Disorder

Nursing assessment and intervention for individuals with GAD include many of the same biopsychosocial considerations that apply to panic disorder. Assessment of the patient's anxiety symptoms should include the following questions; answers are used to tailor individual approaches:

* How do you experience anxiety symptoms?
* Are your symptoms primarily physical, psychological, or both?
* Are you aware when you are becoming anxious?
* Are you aware that anxiety induces the physical symptoms?
* What coping mechanisms do you routinely use to deal with anxiety?
* What life stressors add to these symptoms? What changes can you make to reduce these stressors?

Biologic Domain

Assessment

Diet and Nutrition

Some ordinary food stimulants, such as caffeine, are known to induce anxiety symptoms, and patients with GAD may be hypersensitive to them. Many OTC medications can alter mood and may increase anxiety symptoms. A concrete step that patients with GAD can take to reduce anxiety is to eliminate caffeine from their diets. Nurses can help patients achieve a caffeine-free state through education and dietary management while assisting with pain relief for the headache that often accompanies caffeine withdrawal. Additional substances that can provoke anxiety are diet pills, amphetamines, ginseng, and ma huang (see Chapter 11).

Sleep Patterns

Sleep disturbance is a common symptom for individuals with GAD, so the patient's sleep pattern should be assessed closely. Alcohol should be avoided because it disturbs the sleep cycle. Help the patient with measures that promote sleep, such as eating the last meal of the day in the early evening, avoiding fluids after 8:00 PM, and taking a warm bath before bedtime.

Nursing Diagnosis for the Biologic Domain

Several nursing diagnosis that could be generated from this domain. Insomnia, spiritual distress, and role conflict are examples.

Interventions for the Biologic Domain

Pharmacologic Interventions

The physical symptoms of anxiety and the neurotransmitter systems involved suggest that several medications can be effective in treating GAD. Benzodiazepines are most commonly used, but antidepressants (paroxetine, imipramine, and venlafaxine), buspirone, and β-blockers have all proved effective.

Administering and Monitoring Medications

Although widely used in patients with GAD, benzodiazepine treatment remains somewhat controversial. If the patient self-medicates, benzodiazepines may complicate treatment because of their addictive qualities. However, many people with GAD are reluctant to take prescribed medications, and most do not seek treatment until their level of suffering is substantial. Benzodiazepines offer quick relief from anxiety symptoms until the antidepressant therapeutic effects are felt, which may take a few weeks.

Buspirone. Buspirone is an anxiolytic that acts by inhibiting spontaneous firing of serotonergic neurons in the dorsal raphe and by antagonism of 5-HT1A receptors in the dorsal raphe, hippocampus, and parts of the frontal cortex. Buspirone does not interact with benzodiazepine receptors and may increase brain noradrenergic and dopaminergic activity (see Chapter 11 for additional information). Buspirone must be taken for 3 to 4 weeks before its anxiolytic effects are felt. This delay may be difficult for patients to tolerate, particularly if they have used

benzodiazepines in the past and are familiar with their rapid onset of action. Although buspirone effectively treats anxiety symptoms, patients may discontinue the treatment because of the lag in therapeutic effect.

Antidepressants. Venlafaxine, paroxetine, and imipramine have proven effective in treating patients with GAD. They have serotonergic and noradrenergic effects, which are believed to reduce anxiety symptoms (Ravindran & Stein, 2010).

Managing Side Effects

TCAs (imipramine) and benzodiazepines cause significant side effects and drug interactions that require ongoing monitoring. (See the discussion of these medications in the section on treatment of panic disorder on pages 455–458.)

Buspirone side effects include dizziness, insomnia, drowsiness, and nervousness. Dry mouth, blurred vision, and abdominal distress can occur but are uncommon.

Venlafaxine has a relatively benign side effect profile. Anticholinergic effects, including dry mouth and constipation, are common. This drug also causes dizziness, nervousness, and insomnia. Transient hypertension occurs in some patients; therefore, blood pressure should be monitored. Gastrointestinal effects (nausea and vomiting) can occur as well.

Monitoring for Drug Interactions

Venlafaxine and buspirone both interact with the MAOIs, and neither should be initiated within 14 days of treatment of each other. Although buspirone does not increase alcohol-induced impairment, it is prudent to avoid use of alcohol because it depresses the CNS.

Teaching Points

Teaching points for venlafaxine and buspirone include informing the patient that the anxiolytic effects of the medication will not be felt for several weeks. Warn patients against operating heavy machinery until they know the effects of the medication. If benzodiazepine therapy is being tapered and buspirone therapy started, instructions to the patient should include a warning not to discontinue use of the benzodiazepine suddenly because of the risks of withdrawal, including rebound anxiety and seizures.

Psychological and Social Domains

Psychological and social assessment and intervention strategies for GAD are similar to those for panic disorder; refer to the section on panic disorder on pages 458–462.

Nursing diagnoses that apply to GAD are the same as for panic disorder, including Anxiety; Powerlessness; Sleep Pattern; Low Self-Esteem; and Disturbed, Ineffective Family Coping. Interventions are individualized and are focused on the patient and the family in controlling or coping with the anxiety. Interventions for panic disorder apply to controlling the symptoms of GAD. Cognitive and behavioral therapies, effective treatments for GAD, are generally underused. Outcome studies indicate that cognitive treatment achieves significant reductions in the severity of somatic and anxiety symptoms, with many patients regaining normal function. Combining relaxation, supportive, and cognitive therapies may potentiate therapeutic effects.

Evaluation and Treatment Outcomes

Treatment outcomes for patients with GAD include reducing the frequency and intensity of anxiety and controlling the factors that stimulate or provoke this uncomfortable state. Specifically, evaluation can focus on the individual's ability and skills in using techniques that control anxiety, such as relaxation, positive self-talk, and stress management. Reducing personal and environmental stress; eliminating certain foods and drinks, such as caffeine, in the diet; and developing strategies to deal with stressful family situations are outcome successes.

Continuum of Care

Similar to patients with panic disorder, patients with GAD often seek treatment in emergency departments or from medical internists, cardiologists, or neurologists because of the physical symptoms associated with the illness. Nurses in these settings must be aware of the disorder and able to provide necessary assessment and intervention. Nurses in home health settings have an excellent opportunity to identify symptoms of undiagnosed GAD and make appropriate referrals.

Inpatient and outpatient management of patients with GAD is similar to the treatments detailed in the section on panic disorder. Because anxiety produces more anxiety, a calm, reassuring, and nonjudgmental approach is necessary. Whether treatment is home or clinic based, both the patient and the provider must actively participate in monitoring and managing environmental stress levels. Patients need a relaxing and nonstimulating environment. Reducing noise and lowering lights induces relaxation; methods such as breathing control exercises, progressive muscle relaxation, and other interventions discussed previously in this chapter may also be helpful (Box 26.8).

OTHER ANXIETY DISORDERS

Other disorders exist that have anxiety as their defining feature. These include generalized phobia, agoraphobia, specific phobias, and social anxiety disorder.

> **BOX 26.8**
>
> *Psychoeducation Checklist:* **Generalized Anxiety Disorder**
>
> When caring for the patient with generalized anxiety disorder, be sure to include the following topic areas in the teaching plan:
> - Psychopharmacologic agents (benzodiazepines, antidepressants, nonbenzodiazepine anxiolytics, β-blockers) if ordered, including drug action, dosage, frequency, and possible adverse effects
> - Breathing control
> - Nutrition and diet restriction
> - Sleep measures
> - Progressive muscle relaxation
> - Time management
> - Positive coping strategies

Agoraphobia

Agoraphobia is fear or anxiety triggered by about two or more situations such as using public transportation, being in open spaces, being in enclosed places, standing in line, being in a crowd, or being outside of the home alone (APA, 2013). When these situations occur, the individual believes that something terrible might happen and that escape may be difficult. The individual may experience panic-like symptoms or other embarrassing symptoms such as vomiting, or diarrhea (APA, 2013). Agoraphobia leads to avoidance behaviors. Such avoidance interferes with routine functioning and eventually renders the person afraid to leave the safety of home. Some affected individuals continue to face feared situations but with significant trepidation (i.e., going in public only to pay bills or to take children to school). Agoraphobia may occur with panic disorder, but is considered a separate disorder.

Specific Phobia

Specific phobia is a disorder marked by persistent fear of clearly discernible, circumscribed objects or situations, which often leads to avoidance behaviors. Phobic objects can include animals (spiders, snakes), natural environment (heights, storms), blood injection injury (fear of blood, injections), and situational (elevators, enclosed spaces) (APA, 2013). The lifetime prevalence rates range from 7% to 9%, and the disorder generally affects women twice as much as men. It has a bimodal distribution, peaking in childhood and then again in the 20s. The focus of the fear in specific phobia may result from the anticipation of being harmed by the phobic object. For example, dogs are feared because of the chance of being bitten or automobiles are feared because of the potential of crashing. The focus of fear may likewise be associated with concerns about losing control, panicking, or fainting on exposure to the phobic object.

BOX 26.9

Common Phobias

Acrophobia: fear of heights
Agoraphobia: fear of open spaces
Ailurophobia: fear of cats
Algophobia: fear of pain
Arachnophobia: fear of spiders
Brontophobia: fear of thunder
Claustrophobia: fear of closed spaces
Cynophobia: fear of dogs
Entomophobia: fear of insects
Hematophobia: fear of blood
Microphobia: fear of germs
Nyctophobia: fear of night or dark places
Ophidiophobia: fear of snakes
Phonophobia: fear of loud noises
Photophobia: fear of light
Pyrophobia: fear of fire
Topophobia: stage fright
Xenophobia: fear of strangers
Zoophobia: fear of animal or animals

Anxiety is usually felt immediately on exposure to the phobic object, and the level of anxiety is usually related to both the proximity of the object and the degree to which escape is possible. For example, anxiety heightens as a cat approaches a person who fears cats and lessens when the cat moves away. At times, the level of anxiety escalates to a full panic attack, particularly when the person must remain in a situation from which escape is deemed to be impossible. Fear of specific objects is fairly common, and the diagnosis of specific phobia is not made unless the fear significantly interferes with functioning or causes marked distress. Assessment differentiates simple phobia from other diagnoses with overlapping symptoms. Box 26.9 lists a number of specific phobias. Among adult patients who are seen in clinical settings, the most to least common phobias are situational phobias, natural environment phobias, blood injection, injury phobia, and animal phobias (APA, 2013).

Blood injection injury phobia merits special consideration because the phobia surrounds medical treatments. The physiologic processes that are exhibited during phobic exposure include a strong vasovagal response, which significantly increases blood pressure and pulse, followed by deceleration of the pulse and lowering of blood pressure in the patient. Monitor closely when giving required injections or medical treatments.

About 75% of patients with blood injection injury phobia report fainting on exposure. Factors that may predispose individuals to specific phobias may include traumatic events; unexpected panic attacks in the presence of the phobic object or situation; observation of others experiencing a trauma; or repeated exposure to information warning of dangers, such as parents repeatedly warning young children that dogs bite.

Phobic content must be evaluated from an ethnic or cultural background. In many cultures, fears of spirits or

magic are common. They should be considered part of a disorder only if the fear is excessive in the context of the culture, causes the individual significant distress, or impairs the ability to function.

Psychotropic drugs have not been effective in the treatment of specific phobia. Anxiolytics may give short-term relief of phobic anxiety, but there is no evidence that they affect the course of the disorder. The treatment of choice for specific phobia is exposure therapy. Patients who are highly motivated can experience success with treatment (Peñalba, McGuire, & Leite, 2008).

Exposure Therapy

Many of the treatment approaches used for panic disorder is effective for phobias. **Exposure therapy** is the treatment of choice for phobias. The patient is repeatedly exposed to real or simulated anxiety-provoking situations until he or she becomes desensitized and anxiety subsides.

Social Anxiety Disorder (Social Phobia)

Social anxiety disorder involves a persistent fear of social or performance situations in which embarrassment may occur. Exposure to a feared social or performance situation nearly always provokes immediate anxiety and may trigger panic attacks. People with social anxiety disorder fear that others will scrutinize their behavior and judge them negatively. They often do not speak up in crowds out of fear of embarrassment. They go to great lengths to avoid feared situations. If avoidance is not possible, they suffer through the situation with visible anxiety (APA, 2013).

People with social anxiety disorder appear to be highly sensitive to disapproval or criticism, tend to evaluate themselves negatively, and have poor self-esteem and a distorted view of their personal strengths and weaknesses. They may magnify their personal flaws and underrate any talents. They often believe others would act with more assertiveness in a given social situation. Men and women with social anxiety disorder tend to have difficulties with dating and with sexual relationships (Xu et al., 2012). Children tend to underachieve in school because of test-taking anxiety. This is an important area that should be assessed in all patients.

Generalized social anxiety disorder is diagnosed when the individual experiences fears related to most social situations, including public performances and social interactions. These individuals are likely to demonstrate deficiencies in social skills, and their phobias interfere with their ability to function (MacKenzie & Fowler, 2013). Generalized social anxiety disorder may be linked to low dopamine receptor binding, as suggested by recent research (Cervenka et al., 2012).

People with social anxiety disorder fear and avoid only one or two social situations. Classic examples of such situations are eating, writing, or speaking in public or using public bathrooms. The most common fears for individuals with social anxiety disorder are public speaking, fear of meeting strangers, eating in public, writing in public, using public restrooms, and being stared at or being the center of attention.

Pharmacotherapy is a relatively new area of research in treating patients with social anxiety disorder. SSRIs are used to treat those with social anxiety disorder because they significantly reduce social anxiety and phobic avoidance. Benzodiazepines are also used to reduce anxiety caused by phobias. Providing referrals for appropriate psychiatric treatment is a critical nursing intervention.

OBSESSIVE-COMPULSIVE DISORDER AND RELATED DISORDERS

Obsessions and compulsions are not necessarily signs of a psychiatric disorder if they are short lived and do not persistently interfere with a person's ability to function. However, if obsessions are so consuming that they interfere with a person's judgment and daily activities, they may be symptoms of OCD or one of the related disorders. See Table 26.1 on page 448.

OBSESSIVE-COMPULSIVE DISORDER

In OCD, affected patients have both obsessions and compulsions and believe that they have no control over them, which results in devastating consequences for the individuals.

> **KEYCONCEPT   Obsessions** are excessive, unwanted, intrusive, and persistent thoughts, impulses, or images that cause anxiety and distress. Obsessions are not under the patient's control and are incongruent with the patient's usual thought patterns. **Compulsions** are behaviors that are performed repeatedly in a ritualistic fashion with the goal of preventing or relieving anxiety and distress caused by obsessions.

Common obsessions include fears of contamination, pathologic doubt, the need for symmetry and completion, thoughts of hurting someone, and thoughts of sexual images. Common compulsions include hand washing, excessive cleaning, checking, arranging things, counting, ordering, and hoarding. Because of the nature of the disorder, nurses who work in settings other than psychiatric settings or in home health care may be among the first to identify a patient's symptoms as OCD and make the appropriate referrals.

Clinical Course

The average age of onset of OCD is 19 years, but can occur into the 20s to mid-30s (NIMH, 2014). Although

symptoms of OCD often begin in childhood, many patients receive treatment only after the disorder has significantly affected their lives. The astute parent may notice that the child spends great amounts of time on trivial tasks or has falling grades because of poor concentration. Symptom onset of the disorder is gradual, with some individuals showing a progressive decline in social and occupational functioning (APA, 2013). Men are affected more often as children and are most commonly affected by obsessions. Women have a higher incidence of checking and cleaning rituals, with onset typically in the early 20s. This chronic disorder is characterized by episodes of symptom amelioration and exacerbation (APA, 2013).

Diagnostic Criteria

OCD is characterized by recurrent obsessions or compulsion. Some individuals recognize that these obsessions or compulsions are excessive and unrealistic; others have limited insight and are unsure whether the obsessive thoughts are true, but continue to have the thoughts and feel compelled to perform the actions. There is another group of individuals who are convinced that their obsessive thoughts are true. These thoughts and compulsive behaviors are stressful and interfere with normal daily routines (APA, 2013).

Some patients have obsessions surrounding aggressive acts of hurting someone or themselves. After hitting a bump in the road, for example, these patients may obsess for hours over whether or not they hit a person. Parents may have recurrent intrusive thoughts that they may hurt their child. Others obsess over the meaning of sins and whether they have followed the letter of the law. They tend to be hypermoral and have the need to confess. Their obsessions are seen as a form of religious suffering. These patients are often resistant to treatment. Religious obsessions are most common where severe religious restrictions exist. Diagnosis is not made unless the thoughts or rituals clearly exceed cultural or religious norms, occur at inappropriate times as described by members of the same religion or culture, or interfere with social obligations (APA, 2013).

Rituals are common compulsions where objects must be in a certain order, motor activities are performed in a rigid fashion, or things are arranged in perfect symmetry. A ritual consumes a great deal of time to complete even the simplest task. Some patients experience discontent, rather than anxiety, when things are not symmetrical or perfect. Others think magically and perform compulsive rituals to ward off an imagined disaster such as repeatedly turning on and off the alarm clock to prevent disaster. Those who hoard are compelled to check their belongings repeatedly to see that all is accounted for and check the garbage to make sure that nothing of value was discarded.

Obsessive-Compulsive Disorder Across the Life Span

OCD affects people of all ages. Identification, diagnosis, and treatment of OCD are necessary for recovery and optimal functioning.

Children and Adolescents

OCD affects between 1% and 3% or more of children and adolescents (Jacob & Storch, 2013). Because children subscribe to myths, superstition, and magical thinking, obsessive and ritualistic behaviors may go unnoticed. Behaviors such as touching every third tree, avoiding cracks in the sidewalk, or consistently verbalizing fears of losing a parent in an accident may have some underlying pathology but are common behaviors in childhood. Typically, parents notice that a child's grades begin to fall as a result of decreased concentration and great amounts of time spent performing rituals.

Older Adults

OCD typically manifests in childhood and the second decade of life and can be a lifelong illness, lasting more than 30 years (Lochner & Steing, 2010). One large population survey of older adults found a 1-year prevalence rate of 1.5% (Grenier, Preville, Boyer, & O'Connor, 2009). Late onset is more likely to occur in females with a history of subclinical obsessive-compulsive symptoms, co-occurrence of PTSD after age 40, and a history of recent pregnancy in self or significant others (Frydman et al., 2014). Predictors of poor outcomes during lifelong treatment include initial symptom onset during childhood, low social functioning, and the presence of both obsessions and compulsions (Ruscio, Stein, Chiu, & Kessler, 2010).

Epidemiology and Risk Factors

OCD has a lifetime prevalence rate of 1.2% with females having a slightly higher rate than males (APA, 2013). First-degree relatives of people with OCD have a higher prevalence rate than the general population. Early-onset OCD increases the chances of OCD in relatives and predicts poorer treatment outcomes (Ruscio et al., 2010).

Studies provide some support for a link between infection with β-hemolytic streptococci and OCD (Hachiya et al., 2013). High rates of OCD are found among individuals who are young, divorced or separated, and unemployed. OCD appears to be less common among African Americans than among non-Hispanic whites.

Comorbidity

It is estimated that one third of patients with OCD experience depression because of OCD's effects on their lifestyle. Bipolar, cyclothymic, panic, mood, eating, and impulse control disorders also commonly occur in those with OCD. A significant number of older depressed patients have OCD. Tourette's syndrome and OCD frequently occur together (Grados, 2010).

Many patients self-medicate to relieve the anxiety produced by obsessive thoughts. About one third experience substance abuse or dependence in their lifetime. In addition, some patients may abuse benzodiazepines and other prescription medication. Personality disorders are also prevalent in those with OCD, occurring in more than 80% of patients. Dependent personality disorder most frequently coexists with OCD and is diagnosed in about half of patients (see Chapters 27 and 28).

People with OCD are highly somatic and frequently seek medical treatment for physical symptoms, often just to get reassurance. Acquired immunodeficiency syndrome, cancer, heart attacks, and sexually transmitted infections are some of the most common obsessional fears.

Etiology

During the 1990s, research evidence from neuroimaging studies, neurochemical studies, and treatment advances substantiated a predominantly neurobiologic basis for OCD. The following sections provide a brief overview of these findings and evidence pointing to genetic vulnerability. Psychological factors are also discussed because of their contributions to the disorder. Because no one explanation accounts for all aspects of OCD, a combination of factors will probably be found to produce the disorder.

Biologic Theories

Genetic, neuropathologic, and biochemical research, reviewed in this section, suggests that OCD has a biologic basis involving several neuroanatomic structures.

Genetic Factors

OCD occurs more often in people who have first-degree relatives with OCD or with Tourette's disorder than it does in the general population. Some studies show an increased prevalence of anxiety and mood disorders in relatives of individuals who have OCD. Twin studies indicate that OCD occurs more frequently in siblings of twins. Further studies implicate specific genes and associate them with OCD (Shaw et al., 2014). These discoveries may lead to breakthroughs in pharmacologic treatments of OCD.

Neuropathologic Theories

Recent neuroimaging studies of patients with OCD show hyperactivity in the orbitofrontal cortex, anterior cingulated cortex, and caudate nucleus, suggesting a causal role in the etiology of OCD (Shaw et al., 2014).

Increased cerebral glucose metabolism is identified in a variety of studies. The most replicated results demonstrate increased glucose metabolism in the caudate nuclei (part of the basal ganglia), the orbitofrontal gyri (the gyri directly above the orbit of the eye), and the cingulate gyri (considered to be part of the limbic system). Studies measuring cerebral blood flow and glucose metabolism in patients with OCD during exposure to feared stimuli and during relaxation further implicate these regions of the brain (Shaw et al., 2014).

Biochemical Theories

Serotonin plays a role in OCD. It has been studied through challenge tests in which serotonin agonists were administered to patients with OCD and control subjects. The most convincing evidence for serotonin's role is that serotonin-specific antidepressants relieve the symptoms of OCD for most patients. A single neurotransmitter is unlikely to be entirely responsible for OCD, but to date, serotonin is the only neurotransmitter to have been implicated. Conventional and novel antipsychotic medications and mood stabilizers are used in conjunction with serotonin-targeting medications to treat refractory symptoms, indicating that other biochemical processes exist (Ravindran & Stein, 2010).

Psychological Theories

Although psychological theories of OCD have not been scientifically tested, the rich literature describing clinical examples and case histories help us understand the symptoms and behaviors related to OCD. In addition, behavioral treatment of individuals with severe compulsions improves symptoms.

Psychodynamic Factors

The psychodynamic theory hypothesizes that OCD symptoms and character traits arise from three unconscious defense mechanisms: isolation (separation of affect from a thought or impulse), undoing (an act performed with the goal of preventing consequences of a thought or impulse), and reaction formation (behavior and consciously stated attitudes that oppose underlying impulses). Classic psychoanalytic theory describes OCD as regression from the oedipal phase to the anal phase of development, which includes preoccupations with anger and dirt (see Chapter 7). This regression occurs when the patient becomes anxious about retaliation or loss of love.

Behavioral Factors

Behavioral explanations for OCD stem from learning theory. From this viewpoint, obsessions are seen as conditioned stimuli. Through being associated with noxious events, stimuli that are usually considered neutral become anxiety provoking. The individual then engages in activities to escape or avoid the anxiety. Compulsions develop as the individual discovers behaviors that successfully reduce the obsessional anxiety. As the principles of operant conditioning indicate, the more the behaviors decrease the anxiety, the more likely the individual is to continue using them. However, the rituals or behaviors preserve the fear response because the person avoids the initial stimuli and thus never extinguishes the compulsion. Interrupting this cycle is the focus of behavioral therapy in treating an individual with OCD.

Family Response to Disorder

Marital status appears to be affected by OCD. Patients with OCD tend to remain single more often than do people without the disorder. They also have higher rates of celibacy, possibly because they fear being dirty or becoming contaminated. The divorce rate is lower than would be expected, given the stress of living with this disorder, and patients with OCD are able to draw their families gradually into accommodating abnormal behavior. For example, the families of patients with cleaning compulsions may forego normal family and social activities to "help" the patient complete compulsive cleaning of the family home and decrease the anxiety level in the household.

Family assessment will reveal the amount of education and support needed and will begin the partnership among the patient, family, and treatment team. Evaluate the family's understanding of the disorder and of proposed treatments. Are they able and willing to help the patient practice cognitive and behavioral techniques? Are they knowledgeable about prescribed medicines? These questions offer a wonderful opportunity for patient and family education.

Family members offer a perspective on the severity of the patient's illness. Family members are experts in the patient's rituals and may observe subtle changes. Evaluate the family's response to changes in the patient's behavior as treatment progresses. You may have to discuss how the family will manage the changes brought about by a decrease in rituals. If obsessions and compulsions make it difficult for the individual to leave the home or function at work, financial difficulties may result. These factors should be assessed and appropriate assistance obtained through social services when necessary.

Interdisciplinary Treatment

Patients with OCD can be difficult to treat because their obsessions and compulsions consistently interfere with recovery efforts. Staff may have differing opinions about

Clinical Vignette

BOX 26.10
OBSESSIVE-COMPULSIVE DISORDER

Robert, a 32-year-old man, is a new patient at a local psychiatric unit. He admitted himself to have his medicines evaluated because his obsessive thoughts and depression have worsened since his recent divorce. While in the hospital, he has quickly become viewed as a "problem patient" because he hoards linens and demands a new bar of soap for each of his five daily showers. He is compelled to open and close his door five times when he leaves or enters his room but does not know why. This behavior has led to arguments with his roommate. In an effort to "help him," the psychiatric technicians locked his bathroom door to prevent him from showering so frequently. He tried to enter his bathroom to shower and panicked when the technicians refused to allow him to shower, telling him, "You can live without it." After receiving PRN medication for extreme anxiety, Robert signed out of the hospital against medical advice because of embarrassment and anger toward the nursing staff.

What Do You Think?
- How could the technicians have handled the situation differently so as to not disrupt Robert's or the unit's clinical care?
- What nursing interventions might be appropriate in providing Robert's care?

the amount of control the patient has over the behavior, but these differences of opinion must be resolved, and all staff must be consistent in their expectations and acceptance of the patient's behaviors, to keep these patients from becoming frustrated or confused regarding expectations during treatment (Box 26.10).

Priority Care Issues

As with any patient with a psychiatric disorder, a suicide assessment must be completed. Although patients with OCD do not usually become suicidal as a direct result of anxiety, the disorder greatly distresses the patient, who realizes the pointlessness and absurdity of the behaviors. Often, the patient has tolerated symptoms for quite some time before seeking treatment. The patient may feel a sense of hopelessness and helplessness and may contemplate suicide to end the suffering. An additional risk for suicide is created by the high probability of major depression, which often accompanies OCD. Patients may feel a need to punish themselves for their intrusive thoughts (e.g., religious coupled with sexual obsessions). Some patients have aggressive obsessions, and external limits may have to be imposed for the protection of others.

NURSING MANAGEMENT: Human Response to Obsessive-Compulsive Disorder

Obsessions create tremendous anxiety, and patients perform compulsions to relieve the anxiety temporarily. If the compensatory ritual is not performed, the person feels increased anxiety and distress. Compulsions are necessary, not pleasurable. They are often recognized as odd or strange to the patient. Initially, there are attempts to resist the compulsive behavior, but eventually, resistance fails, and the repetitive behaviors are incorporated into daily routines.

The most common obsession is fear of contamination and results in compulsive hand washing. Fear of contamination usually focuses on dirt or germs, but other materials may be feared as well, such as toxic chemicals, poison, radiation, and heavy metals. Patients with contamination obsessions report anxiety as their most common effect, but shame and disgust, linked with embarrassment and guilt, also are experienced.

Patients with OCD may become incapacitated by their symptoms and may spend most of their waking hours locked in a cycle of obsessions and compulsions. They may even become unable to complete a task as simple as walking through a door without performing rituals. Interpersonal relationships suffer, and the patient may actively isolate him- or herself. Patients with OCD may use dissociation as a defense mechanism.

Biologic Domain
Assessment

Patients with OCD do not have a higher prevalence of physical disease. However, they may complain of multiple physical symptoms. With late-onset OCD (after 35 years of age) and with symptoms that occur with a febrile illness, cerebral pathology should be considered. Each patient with OCD should be assessed for dermatologic lesions caused by repetitive hand washing, excessive cleaning with caustic agents, or bathing. Osteoarthritic joint damage secondary to cleaning rituals may also be observed.

Nursing Diagnoses for the Biologic Domain

Patients with OCD may present with various symptoms, depending on the particular obsession and the compulsions that have evolved to cope with that obsession. As a result, the nursing diagnoses applied to patients with this disorder can run the gamut from the primary diagnosis of Anxiety to other physiologic disturbances of the compulsion, such as Impaired Skin Integrity, which may result from continuous hand washing. Outcomes depend on the nursing diagnoses and treatments selected.

Interventions for the Biologic Domain

Maintaining Skin Integrity

For the patient with cleaning or hand-washing compulsions, attention to skin condition is necessary. Encourage the patient to use tepid water when his or her washing and hand cream after washing. Remove harsh, abrasive soaps and replace them with moisturizing soaps. Attempt to decrease the frequency of washing by agreeing on a time schedule and time-limited washing.

Psychopharmacologic Interventions

The SSRIs and TCAs are considered to be the most effective treatment agents used for patients with OCD. Clomipramine was the first drug to produce significant advances in treating OCD. Other medications, including sertraline, fluoxetine, fluvoxamine, and paroxetine, have proved effective.

Administering and Monitoring Medications

Antidepressants used to treat patients with OCD are often given in higher doses than those normally used to treat those with depression. Aggressive treatment may be indicated to bring the symptoms under control. Thus, medication effects must be closely monitored, including signs of toxicity, to provide safe and adequate care. These medications often take several weeks or months to relieve compulsions and even longer to decrease obsessions.

Clomipramine. Clomipramine pharmacotherapy should begin at 25 mg daily, taken at night, with gradual titration during a period of 2 weeks to 150 mg to 250 mg daily, in divided doses. The maximum dose for children is 200 mg daily. This drug is not approved for children younger than 10 years.

Sertraline and Fluvoxamine. Sertraline and fluvoxamine are indicated for OCD and should be initiated at 50 mg daily (25 mg daily in children). Sertraline can be titrated to a maximum dose of 200 mg daily but incrementally increased no less frequently than once a week. Fluvoxamine can be titrated by 50 mg daily every 4 to 7 days to a maximum daily dose of 300 mg. Doses greater than 100 mg should be divided. For children ages 8 to 11 years, start at 25 mg daily and increase by 25 mg every 4 to 7 days to a maximum daily dose of 200 mg. For children older than 11 years, 300 mg is the maximum daily dose.

Paroxetine or Fluoxetine. Paroxetine or fluoxetine should be started at 20 mg daily, usually in the morning. Paroxetine can be titrated by 10 mg per week to a maximum of 60 mg daily. Fluoxetine dosage is titrated according to patient response to a maximum of 80 mg daily. The usual effective dose is 20 to 40 mg daily. Neither paroxetine nor fluoxetine is approved for the treatment of OCD in children.

Managing Side Effects

Side effects pose a particular problem for some individuals who are preoccupied with somatic concerns. Unwanted physical symptoms from the medications can become the focus of obsessions. These individuals particularly need frequent reassurance that they are not becoming physically ill and that the side effects are a common response to medication. To ignore or minimize these concerns will only heighten the patient's anxiety and potentially interfere with the desire to continue treatment.

Common side effects of clomipramine include significant sedation, anticholinergic side effects, and an increased risk for seizures. Dizziness, tremulousness, and headache are frequent complaints. Administration at night minimizes complaints of sedation and fatigue.

SSRIs all cause sedation, dizziness, somnolence, and headache. In addition, sexual dysfunction is a common complaint in patients being treated with fluvoxamine, sertraline, paroxetine, or fluoxetine. The SSRIs can cause excitability when first started. Monitor patients for insomnia and adjust the dosing time if needed. Weight gain can occur with SSRIs but is relatively rare.

Monitoring for Drug Interactions

All antidepressant medications interact with the MAOIs, causing hypertensive crises; interaction with tryptophan may cause serotonin syndrome. Therefore, concomitant use should be avoided. Fluoxetine also interacts with thioridazine, the TCAs, and lithium. Paroxetine interacts with thioridazine, histamine-2 blockers (cimetidine), phenytoin, digoxin, and warfarin. The use of thioridazine, cisapride, diazepam, and pimozide is contraindicated with fluvoxamine.

Because of the extensive list of drug–drug interactions associated with these medications, a prudent nurse will consult a drug reference handbook before administering medications. Quick recognition of signs and symptoms of interactions or toxic symptoms is imperative for safe care.

Teaching Points

Nurses play an important interdisciplinary role in managing medication for patients with OCD, which includes educating patients and families about medications. Because patients may become discontented with a perceived lack of effect, they should be informed that these medications may take several weeks before their effects are felt. All patients should be warned not to abruptly stop taking prescribed medications.

Patients should be instructed to avoid alcohol and not to operate heavy machinery while taking these medications until the sedative effects are known. Instruct patients to inform their providers about any OTC medications they are taking because some will interact with these medications.

Electroconvulsive Therapy

The effect of electroconvulsive therapy (ECT) on decreasing obsessions and compulsions has not been extensively studied. However, it may be helpful in treating symptoms that occur with depression. It also may be used to treat depressive symptoms in patients who have not experienced response to other treatments and who are at risk for suicide. Nursing's role in caring for the patient undergoing ECT is outlined in Chapter 11.

Psychosurgery

Psychosurgery has been used to treat extremely severe OCD that has not responded to prolonged and intensive drug treatment, behavioral therapy, or a combination of the two. Modern stereotactic surgical techniques that produce lesions of the cingulum bundle (a bundle of connective tissue) or anterior limb of the internal capsule (a region near the thalamus and part of the circuit connecting to the cortex) may bring about substantial clinical benefit in some patients without causing significant morbidity (Csigó, Harsányi, Demeter, Rajkai, Németh, & Racacsmány, 2010). Other treatment options include radiotherapy and deep brain stimulation in which electrical current is applied through an electrode inserted into the brain (Robinson, Taghva, Liu, & Apuzzo, 2013).

Psychological Domain

Assessment

The nurse should assess the type and severity of the patient's obsessions and compulsions. If the assessment occurs in a hospital, remember that some patients with OCD experience a transient decrease in symptoms when admitted to a hospital; therefore, enough time must be allowed for an accurate assessment. If time is unavailable, family members or significant others may provide an important source of information, with the patient's permission.

Most individuals will appear neatly dressed and groomed, cooperative, and eager to answer questions. Orientation and memory are not usually impaired, but patients may be distracted by obsessional thoughts. Individuals with severe symptoms may be preoccupied with fears or with discussing their obsessions, but in most instances, direct questions must be asked to reveal symptoms. For example, the nurse may begin indirectly by asking how long it takes the individual to dress in the morning or leave the house, but usually follow-up questions are needed, such as: Do you find yourself frequently returning to the house to make sure that you have turned off the lights or the stove, even when you know that you have already checked these things? Does this happen every day? Are you ever late for work or for important appointments?

> **BOX 26.11**
>
> **Rating Scales for Assessing Obsessive-Compulsive Symptoms**
>
> **YALE-BROWN OBSESSIVE COMPULSIVE SCALE (Y-BOCS)**
> Goodman, W., Price, L., Rasmussen, S., Mazure, C., Fleischmann, R. L., Hill, C. L., et al. (1989). The Yale-Brown Obsessive Compulsive Scale (Y-BOCS): Part I. Development, use and reliability. *Archives of General Psychiatry, 46,* 1006–1011.
>
> **THE MAUDSLEY OBSESSIONAL-COMPULSIVE INVENTORY (MOC)**
> Rachman, S. & Hodgson, R. (1980). *Obsessions and compulsions.* New York: Prentice-Hall.
>
> **THE LEYTON OBSESSIONAL INVENTORY**
> Cooper, J. (1970). The Leyton Obsessional Inventory. *Psychiatric Medicine, 1,* 48.

Speech will be of normal rate and volume, but often, individuals with an obsessional style of thinking exhibit circumferential speech. This speech is loaded with irrelevant details but eventually addresses the question. Listening may be frustrating and require considerable patience, but you must remember that such speech is part of the disorder and may be beyond the patient's awareness. Continually interrupting and redirecting them can interfere with establishing a therapeutic relationship, especially in the initial assessment. Redirection should be done in a gentle and noncritical manner to allow the patient to refocus.

Identifying the degree to which the OCD symptoms interfere with the patient's daily functioning is important. Several rating scales can be used to identify symptoms and monitor improvement. Examples of these scales are provided in Box 26.11. Some of these scales are to be used by the nurse; others are self-rating scales. The Yale-Brown Obsessive Compulsive Scale (Y-BOCS) is a popular, clinician-rated 16-item scale that obtains separate subtotals for severity of obsessions and compulsions. The Maudsley Obsessive-Compulsive Inventory is a 30-item, true–false, self-assessment tool that may help the individual to recognize individual symptoms.

Nursing Diagnosis for the Psychological Domain

Several nursing diagnosis that could be generated from this domain. For example, Hopelessness, Loneliness, Powerlessness, and Self-Concept are areas to consider for generating a nursing diagnosis.

Interventions for the Psychological Domain

The nurse's interpersonal skills are crucial to successful intervention with the patient who has OCD. Nurses must control their own anxiety. The nurse should interact with the patient in a calm, nonauthoritarian fashion

BOX 26.12
Using Reflection

DEVELOPING SELF-AWARENESS

INCIDENT • An energetic, excitable nurse told a patient who has obsessive-compulsive disorder (OCD) to hurry up and get dressed in order to get to the cafeteria for lunch. A few minutes later, the patient is found sorting his clothes, making no progress toward getting dressed.

REFLECTION • The nurse reflected on her interaction with the patient. Although the nurse knew that interacting with a patient with OCD affected the level of anxiety the patient would feel, she was direct, hurried, and too autocratic in her approach to the patient. A calm, nonconfrontational approach would have been better.

without exhibiting any disapproval of the patient or the patient's behaviors while demonstrating empathy about the distress that the disorder has caused (Box 26.12). This approach is one of the most effective means available for communicating appreciation for the individual as separate from the illness.

Response Prevention

An effective behavioral intervention for patients with OCD who perform rituals is exposure with response prevention. The patient is exposed to situations or objects that are known to induce anxiety but is asked to refrain from performing the ritualistic behaviors. One goal of this procedure is to help the patient understand that resisting the rituals while exposed to the object of anxiety is less stressful and time consuming than performing the rituals. Another goal is to confound the expectation of distressing outcomes and eventually extinguish the compulsive behaviors. Most patients improve with exposure and response prevention, but few become completely symptom free.

Thought Stopping

Thought stopping is used with patients who have obsessional thoughts. The patient is taught to interrupt obsessional thoughts by saying, "Stop!" either aloud or subvocally. This activity interrupts and delays the uncontrollable spiral of obsessional thoughts. Research supporting this technique is scant; however, practitioners have found it useful in multimodal treatment with exposure and response prevention, relaxation, and cognitive restructuring.

Relaxation Techniques

Patients with OCD experience insomnia because of their heightened anxiety levels. Relaxation exercises may be helpful in improving sleep patterns. These exercises do not affect OCD symptoms, but they may be used to decrease anxiety. The nurse may also teach the patient other relaxation measures, such as deep breathing, taking warm baths, meditation, music therapy, or other quiet activities.

Cognitive Restructuring

Cognitive restructuring is a method of teaching the patient to restructure dysfunctional thought processes by defining and testing them (Beck & Emery, 1985). Its goal is to alter the patient's immediate, dysfunctional appraisal of a situation and perception of long-term consequences. The patient is taught to monitor automatic thoughts and then to recognize the connection between thoughts, emotional response, and behaviors. The distorted thoughts are examined and tested by for-or-against evidence presented by the therapist, which helps the patient to realistically assess the likelihood that the feared event will happen if the compulsive behavior is not performed. The patient begins to analyze his or her thoughts as incongruent with reality. For example, even if the alarm clock is not checked 30 times before going to bed, it will still go off in the morning, and the patient will not be disciplined for tardiness at work. Maybe it needs to be checked only once or twice.

Cue Cards

Cue cards are tools used to help the patient restructure thought patterns. They contain statements that are positively oriented and pertain to the patient's specific obsessions and compulsions. Cue cards use information from the patient's symptom hierarchy, an organizational system that breaks down the obsessions and compulsions from least to most anxiety provoking. These cards can help reinforce the belief that the patient is safe and can tolerate the anxiety caused by delaying or controlling compulsive rituals. Examples of cue cards are in Box 26.13.

Psychoeducation

Psychoeducation is a crucial nursing intervention for the patient with OCD. Knowledge is power, and the more the patient knows about his or her disorder, the more control he or she will have over symptoms. The patient should be instructed not only about the biologic components of OCD but also about its treatments and disease course. Treatment is a shared responsibility between the patient and the provider, and the patient should be included in the medication and treatment decision-making processes. If local support groups are available, the patient should be referred to reduce feelings of uniqueness and embarrassment about the disease. Family education is also important

---

BOX 26.13

Examples of Cue Card Statements

- It's the OCD, not me.
- These are only OC thoughts. OC thoughts don't mean action; I will not act on the thoughts.
- My anxiety level goes up but will always go down.
- I never sat with the anxiety long enough to see that it would not harm me.
- Trust myself.
- I did it right the first time.
- Checking the locks again won't keep me safe. I am really safe in the world.

---

so the patient will have help in practicing behavioral homework (Box 26.14).

Social Domain

Assessment

Nurses must consider sociocultural factors when evaluating OCD. At times, cultural or religious beliefs may be misunderstood and mistaken for obsessions or compulsions. These beliefs and actions must be evaluated in the context of the individual's culture. If these beliefs are consistent with the patient's social or cultural environment, are not harmful to the individual or others, and do not interfere with individual functioning in that environment, they are not considered symptoms of OCD.

Nursing Diagnosis for the Social Domain

Several nursing diagnosis could be generated from this domain. For example, role conflict, sedentary lifestyle, or social interaction should be considered for generating a nursing diagnosis.

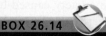

BOX 26.14

Psychoeducation Checklist: Obsessive-Compulsive Disorder

When caring for the patient with obsessive-compulsive disorder, be sure to include the patient's caregiver, if appropriate, and address the following topic areas in the teaching plan:

- Psychopharmacologic agents (SSRIs, MAOIs, lithium, or anxiolytics) if ordered, including drug action, dosage, frequency, and possible adverse effects
- Skin care measures
- Ritualistic behaviors and alternative activities
- Thought stopping
- Relaxation techniques
- Cognitive restructuring
- Recovery strategies
- Community resources

MAOI, monoamine oxidase inhibitor; SSRI, selective serotonin reuptake inhibitor.

Interventions for the Social Domain

- For the hospitalized patient, unit routines must be carefully and clearly explained to decrease fear of the unknown.
- At least initially, do not prevent the patient from engaging in rituals because the patient's anxiety level will increase.
- Recognize the significance of the rituals to the person and empathize with the patient's need to perform them.
- Assist the patient in arranging a schedule of activities that incorporates some private time but also integrates the patient into normal unit activities.

Evaluation and Treatment Outcomes

Several methods can be used to measure the response to treatment, including nursing care: changes in Y-BOCS scores or other rating scales, remission of presenting symptoms, and the ability to complete activities of daily living. The patient should be able to participate in social or group activities with a degree of comfort and without self-harming or aggressive intent. He or she should also be able to demonstrate common knowledge of OCD by describing its symptoms, biologic basis, and treatments.

Continuum of Care

The symptoms of OCD can become debilitating. The symptoms wax and wane throughout treatment. As the focus of treatment shifts from inpatient to outpatient environments, patients must be assessed continually to ensure favorable patient outcomes through early intervention if symptoms resurface.

Inpatient-Focused Care

In an inpatient setting, the presence of a patient with severe OCD may present a nursing management challenge. These patients require a significant amount of staff time. They may monopolize bathrooms or showers or have disruptive rituals involving eating. Nurses play an integral role in treating the patient with OCD. The nurse should help the patient perform activities of daily living to ensure that they are completed. Monitoring medication effects, teaching psychoeducation groups, ensuring adequate caloric intake, and providing individual patient counseling are additional inpatient interventions.

Emergency Care

Individuals with OCD frequently use medical services long before they seek psychiatric treatment. Therefore, early recognition of symptoms and referral are important concerns for nurses working in primary care and other medical settings. After individuals are referred, most psychiatric treatment of OCD occurs on an outpatient basis. Although only individuals with severely debilitating symptoms or self-harming thoughts and actions are hospitalized, patients may experience intense anxiety symptoms to the point of panic. In such an emergency, benzodiazepines and other anxiolytics can be used.

Family Interventions

The families of patients with OCD need to be educated about the etiology of the disorder. Understanding the biologic basis of the disorder should decrease some of the stigma and embarrassment they may feel about the bizarre nature of the patient's obsessions and compulsions. Education about both biologic and psychological treatment approaches should be provided.

Family assistance in monitoring symptom remission and medication side effects is invaluable. Family members can also assist the patient with behavioral and cognitive interventions.

When caring for the patient with OCD, be sure to include the patient's caregiver, if appropriate, and address the following topic areas in the teaching plan:

- Medications, including drug action, dosage, frequency, and possible adverse effects
- Skin care measures
- Ritualistic behaviors and alternative activities
- Thought stopping
- Relaxation techniques
- Cognitive restructuring
- Community resources

Community Treatment

Partial hospitalization programs and day treatment programs help individuals in the quest for recovery. These programs can support independence while patients begin medications and behavioral therapies. Some patients require outpatient treatment daily when symptoms are increased. Maintenance outpatient therapy may be scheduled weekly or twice weekly for several weeks until the symptoms are well controlled. Community agency visits are recommended to monitor medication.

TRICHOTILLOMANIA AND EXCORIATION DISORDER

Trichotillomania is chronic, self-destructive hair pulling that results in noticeable hair loss, usually in the crown, occipital, or parietal areas, although sometimes of the eye-

brows and eyelashes. The patient has an increase in tension immediately before pulling out the hair or when attempting to resist the behavior. After the hair is pulled, the person feels a sense of relief. Some would classify this disorder as one of self-mutilation. It becomes a problem when there is a significant distress or impairment in other areas of function. A hair-pulling session can last several hours, and the individual may ritualistically eat the hairs or discard them. Hair ingestion may result in the development of a hair ball, which can lead to anorexia, stomach pain, anemia, obstruction, and peritonitis. Other medical complications include infection at the hair-pulling site. Hair pulling is done alone, and usually patients deny it. Instead of pain, these persons experience pleasure and tension release (Duke, Keeley, Geffken, & Storch, 2010).

The onset of trichotillomania occur among children before the age of 5 years and in adolescence. For the young child, distraction or redirection may successfully eliminate the behavior. The behavior in adolescents may begin a chronic course that may last well into adulthood.

This disorder is poorly understood. An etiologic relationship to OCD has not been established, but there is support for a familial connection (Keuthen, Altenburger, & Pauls, 2014). The prevalence of trichotillomania is estimated at 1% to 2% of the population (APA, 2013). No particular medication class demonstrates effectiveness in treatment. Studies of individual medications including olanzapine (antipsychotic) and clomipramine (tricyclic antidepressant) show treatment effectiveness (Rothbart et al., 2013). Cognitive behavior therapy and habit reversal training, a behavioral intervention, can improve the symptoms (Duke et al., 2010; Rogers et al., 2014).

The assessment includes a review of current problems, developmental history (especially school conflicts and learning difficulties), family history, and social history, identification of support systems, previous psychiatric treatment, and health history. The cultural context in which the trichotillomania occurs must be taken into consideration because in some cultures, this behavior is viewed as socially acceptable. The hair-pulling history and pattern are also solicited to determine the duration and severity of the disorder. The typical nursing diagnoses include Self-mutilation, Low Self-esteem, Hopelessness, Impaired Skin Integrity, and Ineffective Denial. Within the therapeutic relationship, a cognitive behavioral approach can be used to help the patient identify when hair pulling occurs, the precipitating events, and the details of the episode.

Individuals with trichotillomania report that anxiety, loneliness, anger, fatigue, guilt, frustration, and boredom can all trigger the hair-pulling behaviors. Current research also showed that persons with chronic hair pulling typically avoid social activities and events. In addition, the economic impact of trichotillomania can be significant in relation to lost work or school days. Teaching about the disorder will help patients understand that they are not alone and that others have also had this problem. The goal of treatment is to help the patient learn to substitute positive behaviors for the hair-pulling behavior through self-monitoring of events that precipitate the episodes.

EXCORIATION (SKIN-PICKING) DISEASE

Repetitive and compulsive picking of skin causing tissue damage characterizes **excoriation or skin-picking disease** (APA, 2013). Face, arms, or hands are the most common sites for picking, but it can occur at other body sites. Most pick with their fingers, but tweezers or pins are sometimes used. Similar to other disorders, skin picking causes significant distress to individuals. Prevalence is estimated at 1.4% and it occurs more frequently in persons with OCD. Treatment data are limited, but lamotrigine (mood stabilizer/anticonvulsant agent) has been shown to be successful in one study (Grant, Odluag, Chamberlain, & Kim, 2010). Nursing care is similar to caring for a person with trichotillomania.

BODY DYSMORPHIC DISORDER

Individuals with **body dysmorphic disorder** (BDD) focus on real (but slight) or imagined defects in appearance, such as a large nose, thinning hair, or small genitals. Preoccupation with the defect causes significant distress and interferes with their ability to function socially. They feel so self-conscious that they avoid work or public situations. Some fear that their "ugly" body part will malfunction. Surgical correction of the problem by a plastic surgeon or a dermatologist does not correct their preoccupation and distress. BDD is an extremely debilitating disorder and can significantly impair an individual's quality of life. BDD usually begins in adolescence and continues throughout adulthood. These individuals are not usually seen in psychiatric settings unless they have a coexisting psychiatric disorder or a family member insists on psychiatric attention.

This disorder occurs in men and women, with a prevalence of 2.4% in the United States (APA, 2013). Sixty percent of the persons with BDD also have an anxiety disorder (Mufaddel, Osman, Almugaddam, & Jafferany, 2013). The risk of depression, suicide ideation, and suicide is high. The lifetime suicide attempt rate is estimated at 22% to 24% (Bjornsson, Didie, & Phillips, 2010). There is no one theory that explains the cause of BDD. Unrealistic cultural expectations, and genetic predisposition most likely underlie this disorder. See Box 26.15.

HOARDING DISORDER

Difficulty parting with or discarding possessions, regardless of actual value characterizes a **hoarding disorder**.

Clinical Vignette

BOX 26.15
BODY DYSMORPHIC DISORDER

K, a 16-year-old girl, for about 6 months has believed that her pubic bone is becoming increasingly dislocated and prominent. She believes that everyone stares at and talks about it. She does not remember a particular event related to the appearance of the symptom but is absolutely convinced that she can be helped only by a surgical correction of her pubic bone.

She was treated recently for anorexia nervosa with marginal success. Although her weight is nearly normal, she continues to be preoccupied with the looks of her body. She spends almost the entire day in her bedroom, wearing excessively large pajamas, and she refuses to leave the house. Once or twice a day, she lowers herself to the ground and measures, with her fingers, the distance between her pelvic girdle and the ground in order to check the position of the pubic bone.

In desperation, her parents called the clinic for help.

The family was referred to a home health agency and a psychiatric home health nurse who arranged for an assessment visit.

What Do You Think?
- How should the nurse approach K? Should an assessment begin immediately?
- From the vignette, identify nursing diagnoses, outcomes, and interventions.

Adapted from Sobanski, E. & Schmidt, M. H. (2000). "Everybody looks at my pubic bone"—a case report of an adolescent patient with body dysmorphic disorder. *Acta Psychiatrica Scandinavica, 101,* 80–82.

Individuals with this disorder have a need to save items and experience distress if their items are discarded. Most of the individuals with hoarding disorder also have excessive acquisition (excessive purchasing of items or collecting free items).

The prevalence of this disorder is estimated 2% to 6% (APA, 2013). Hoarding can begin in childhood with an increase in severity throughout their lifespan. This disorder tends to be familial and present in different generations. Being Native American, being born in the United States, over the age of 45 years, high school educated, widowed, separated or divorced, and living in a rural community increases the likelihood of having difficulty discarding items. Being African American, Asian, and Hispanic, and earning more than $35,000 per year, and never married decrease the likelihood of having difficulty discarding items (Rodriguez, Simpson, Liu, Levinson, & Blanco, 2013). These individuals seek out mental health care with depression being the most common reason (Hall, Tolin, Frost, & Steketee, 2013).

Hoarding poses public health and safety risks for individuals, families, and communities (Fleury, Gaudette, &

BOX 26.16

Research for Best Practice: **Compulsive Hoarding Syndrome**

Singh, S. & Jones, C. (2013). Compulsive hoarding syndrome: Engaging the patients in treatment. Mental Health Practice, 17(4), 16–20.

THE QUESTION: How can persons with hoarding disorder be engaged in treatment?

METHODS: A CBT treatment approach is described that has been adapted to include visual methods (photographs, videos) and imagery. The group approach encourages the individuals to be "in the moment" and experience the discomfort of their difficulties. Participants photographed cluttered areas in their home and used five questions based on the acronym HOARD. This exercise helped them recognize the problem and what to do about it. Psychoeducation is included in the group and is based on themes that emerge in the session.

FINDINGS: Using group processes described by Yalom, the group members became supportive of each other when undertaking changes. The group developed a buddy system when members supported each other outside the group. Through using the visual methods, the individuals were able to distance themselves from the problem and decrease the feeling of being overwhelmed. They were able to be more objective and develop an action plan.

IMPLICATIONS FOR NURSING: Helping individuals with this disorder will require creative, eclectic approaches using a combination of modalities.

Moran, 2012). Excessive collection of items not only clutters living areas, but can lead to being trapped in an inaccessible environment and one that is high risk for fire. Home health nurses are often the first providers that recognize the problem and are a valuable resource in determining the safety hazards and helping the individual become aware of the problem and seek treatment. The nurse can also contact community agencies (Sorrell, 2012). Currently, treatment outcomes with medication and CBT are limited. More research is needed to understand the disorder and treatment (Singh & Jones, 2013). See Box 26.16.

TRAUMA- AND STRESSOR-RELATED DISORDERS

Exposure to a traumatic or stressful event can lead to a trauma- and stressor-related disorder such as reactive attachment disorder, disinhibited social engagement disorder, posttraumatic disorder, acute stress disorder, and adjustment disorder. See Table 26.1. This section highlights **posttraumatic disorder**, one of the most severe mental disorders with long-term consequences for the individual and family.

Posttraumatic Stress Disorder

Posttraumatic Stress Disorder (PTSD) can occur following exposure to an actual or threatened traumatic event such as death, serious injury, or sexual violence (APA, 2013).

> **KEYCONCEPT** Traumatic events include those that are directly experienced, witnessed, learned about from others, or repeated exposure to aversive events. Examples of traumatic events are violent personal assault, rape, military combat, natural disasters, terrorist attacks, being taken hostage, incarceration as a prisoner of war, torture, an automobile accident, or being diagnosed with a life-threatening illness.

Clinical Course

Responses to traumatic events vary with some individuals never experiencing PTSD and others having severe physical and emotional reactions. Most people who experience a traumatic event do not develop PTSD. However, for those who do, the symptoms often develop 3 to 6 months after the event. About one-third of the persons diagnosed with PTSD develop chronic symptoms. For these individuals, symptoms fluctuate in intensity with time and usually are worse during periods of stress.

Diagnostic Criteria

PTSD is diagnosed following exposure to a traumatic event when the individual manifests symptoms in four general areas: intrusive symptoms, avoidance of person, places or objects that are a reminder of the traumatic event, negative mood and cognitions or negative thoughts associated with the event, and hyperarousal characterized by aggressive, reckless or self-destructive behavior, sleep disturbances or hypervigilance for at least 1 month (APA, 2013).

Intrusion

In PTSD, thoughts, memories, or dreams of traumatic events occur involuntarily, especially when there are cues that symbolize or resemble the events, causing psychological and sometimes physiologic distress. At times images, thoughts, or perceptions are re-experienced and nightmares are common. Intrusive symptoms also include dissociative reactions (feeling or acting as if the event is re-occurring). Flashbacks and nightmares, which the survivor experiences with terrifying immediacy, are vivid and often include fragments of traumatic events exactly as they happened. A wide variety of stimuli associated with the trauma can elicit flashbacks and dreams. Sleeping is difficult. Consequently, these individuals avoid such stimuli (Heir, Piatigorsky, & Weisaeth, 2010).

Avoidance and Numbing (Dissociative Symptoms)

Individuals with PTSD avoid reminders of the event including people, places, or activities associated with the event (e.g., fireworks may bring back memories of war). Many persons suffering with this disorder escape situations by altering their state of consciousness, that is, by dissociating. **Dissociation** is a disruption in the normally occurring linkages among subjective awareness, feelings, thoughts, behavior, and memories (APA, 2000). A person who dissociates is making him- or herself "disappear." That is, the person has the feeling of leaving his or her body and observing what happens to him or her from a distance. During trauma, dissociation enables a person to observe the event while experiencing no pain or only limited pain and to protect him- or herself from awareness of the full impact of the traumatic event. Examples of dissociation include (1) **derealization** (feelings of unreality) and **depersonalization** (the experience of self or the environment as strange or unreal); (2) periods of disengagement from the immediate environment during stress, such as "spacing out"; (3) alterations in bodily perceptions; (4) emotional numbing; (5) out-of-body experiences; and (6) amnesia for abuse-related memories.

Mood and Cognitions

After a traumatic event, moods often becomes more irritable with episodes of explosive anger, fear, guilt, or shame. Individuals with PTSD often have difficulty experiencing positive emotions such as happiness or love. Consequently, they become estranged from loved ones who become frustrated with their family member's unpredictable moods and lack of emotional connection. In PTSD the thought process becomes distorted with exaggerated negative beliefs or expectations about oneself, others, and the world. They may believe that no one can be trusted or that they are terrible people (APA, 2013).

Hyperarousal

After a traumatic experience, the stress system seems to go on permanent alert, as if the danger might return at any time. In this state of physiologic **hyperarousal**, the traumatized person is hypervigilant for signs of danger, startles easily, reacts irritably to small annoyances, and sleeps poorly. These symptoms are characteristic of increased noradrenergic function, particularly in the locus ceruleus and limbic system (hypothalamus, hippocampus, and amygdala), and of increased dopamine activity, particularly in the prefrontal cortical dopamine system (Jovanovic & Ressler, 2010). The state of hyperarousal causes other problems for family members. The individual is irritable and overreacts to others which

cause others to avoid the person who in turn maintains a state of continual arousal (Lanius et al., 2010).

Behavioral sensitization may be one mechanism underlying the hyperarousal seen in PTSD. This phenomenon, sometimes referred to as **kindling**, occurs after exposure to severe, uncontrollable stressors. The sensitized person reacts with a magnified stress response to later, milder stressors (Heim & Nemeroff, 2009). Research shows that a single or repeated exposure to a severe stressor potentiates the capacity of a subsequent stressor to increase synaptic levels of norepinephrine and dopamine in the forebrain. This finding would account for the fact that some individuals with PTSD experience intense fear, anxiety, and panic in response to minor stimuli. One example of behavioral sensitization is that PTSD after combat exposure is more likely to develop in veterans who are survivors of childhood abuse than in those who have not experienced prior trauma (Jovanic & Ressler, 2010; Heim & Nemeroff, 2009).

Epidemiology and Risk Factors

PTSD affects approximately 8% of men and 20% of women who are exposed to traumatic events, but is variable among different groups (Warner, Warner, Appenzeller, & Hogue, 2013). Risk factors for PTSD include a prior diagnosis of acute stress disorder; the extent, duration, and intensity of trauma involved; and environmental factors. High levels of anxiety, low self-esteem, and existing personality difficulties may increase the likelihood that PTSD will develop.

PTSD varies among the genders. Women are approximately twice as likely as men to experience PTSD, and the median time from onset to remission for women is 4 years compared with 1 year for men. Several factors may contribute to these differences. Men and women experience different types of traumatic events. More men report exposure to events such as fires or disasters, life-threatening accidents, physical assault, combat, being threatened with a weapon, and being held captive. More women report anxiety and depressive disorders, child abuse, sexual molestation, sexual assault, and traumatic events before the age of 18 years. Sexual violence is associated with a high risk for the development of PTSD (Masho & Ahmed, 2007; Roth, Geisser, & Bates, 2008).

PTSD symptoms in women who were sexually assaulted were found to vary based on their age at the time of the first sexual assault. In one study, the prevalence among women who had never experienced sexual assault was 8%, but rates for those who were sexually assaulted ranged from 30% (older than 18 years of age) to 35% (younger than 18 years of age) (Masho & Ahmed, 2007). Women who experienced intimate partner violence had a rate of 74% to 92% compared to 6% to 13% among non-abused women (Scott-Tilley, Tilton, & Sandel, 2010).

Childhood cancer survivors have been found to have four times the risk of developing PTSD as their siblings (Stuber et al., 2010). In another study of childhood cancer survivors, nearly 16% had PTSD (Rourke, Hobbie, Schwartz, & Katz, 2007). Similarly, high rates of PTSD have been reported among patients with alcohol and drug dependence who have experienced childhood abuse (Driessen et al., 2008; Moselhy, 2009).

However, high rates of PTSD in returning veterans from Iraq and Afghanistan are unprecedented in modern times. Approximately 27% of women and 35% of men have been diagnosed with PTSD. These veterans have more medical conditions than those without mental disorders (Kimerling, 2010).

Etiology

There is a growing body of research postulating that biologic factors, including neurobiology and genetics, interact with environmental factors, such as childhood experiences, and the severity and extent of the traumatic exposure, to influence susceptibility to PTSD. The amygdala and hippocampus also appear to be important players in fear conditioning along with the thalamus, locus ceruleus, and sensory cortex. Interaction between the cortex and the amygdala may be necessary for specific stimuli to elicit traumatic memories (Lanius et al., 2010).

Several neurochemical systems are involved in regulating fear conditioning, including norepinephrine, dopamine, opiate, and corticotropin-releasing systems. In addition, N-methyl-D-aspartate (NMDA), one of the major excitatory neurotransmitters in the brain, appears necessary for this type of learning to occur. NMDA antagonists applied to the amygdala prevent the development of fear-conditioned responses (Heim & Nemeroff, 2009; Jovanovic & Ressler, 2010; Lanius et al., 2010).

Interdisciplinary Treatment

Major approaches to the treatment of PTSD include pharmacotherapy and psychotherapy. The SSRIs, benzodiazepines, and β-blockers have been shown to be effective in reducing the symptoms of PTSD (Bastien, 2010). When prescribed in conjunction with psychotherapy, pharmacotherapy can minimize the excessive fear and anxiety of PTSD (Ellen, Olver, Norman, & Burrows, 2008). Psychotherapeutic approaches to the treatment of patients with PTSD include psychodynamic psychotherapy; CBT; and eye movement, desensitization, and reprocessing (EMDR).

Nursing Management of PTSD

The nursing assessment of persons with PTSD should focus on the patient's responses to the traumatic event or events. Specifically, the consequences of intrusive thoughts, irritable moods, negative thoughts, avoidance behaviors, and arousal behaviors should be determined. These individuals are at high risk for substance abuse and suicide. A suicide risk assessment should be included in the nursing assessment. A family assessment focusing on any changes in family dynamics that has occurred since the traumatic event should also be included.

Nursing interventions include counseling, medication administration, and education. While there is not one medication for PTSD, medications will be used to target various symptoms such as depression (antidepressants), mood dysregulation (mood stabilizers or antipsychotic), stress, and hyperarousal (antianxiety medications). Teaching stress management, including relaxation techniques and meditation, can help the patient learn effective ways to cope with the symptoms of PTSD. Although few studies have explored the neurobiologic effects of psychotherapy, growing evidence indicates that psychotherapeutic approaches, such as CBT and meditation, improve the synaptic links with the amygdala, and thus effect the processing of emotion and anxiety (Mayo, 2010).

Some clinicians use exposure techniques, in which the patient is guided through images of the trauma, allowing for progressive desensitization. EMDR is a recent approach that has been successful in minimizing the fear response and avoidance pattern of those with PTSD. Under deep relaxation, the patient maintains an image of the traumatic event while focusing on the lateral movement of the clinician's finger. Patients and clinicians report success with EMDR (Beevers, Lee, Wells, Ellis, & Telch, 2011).

Group therapy and family therapy should also be considered in the treatment of those with PTSD. Sharing the traumatic experiences with family or with others who have experienced trauma can be both supportive and therapeutic. PTSD disrupts both the life of the patient and his or her significant others. Social support is a protective factor in the development of the disorder, and patients who have PTSD can benefit from tangible social support they receive from spouses, family, and friends (Pietrzak & Southwick, 2011).

OTHER TRAUMA- AND STRESSOR-RELATED DISORDERS

Acute stress disorder is similar to PTSD except that it is resolved within 1 month of the traumatic event. Acute stress disorder can develop into PTSD if the symptoms last more than 1 month. Two trauma- and stressor-related disorders typically occur in childhood. *Reactive attachment disorder* is characterized by inhibited, emotionally withdrawn behavior toward an adult caregiver. These children rarely seek or respond to comfort when distressed. This disorder usually occurs when there are frequent changes in the primary caregiver. In *disinhibited social engagement disorder*, the child is overly familiar with others that is uncharacteristic of the cultural norms. The child does not hesitate to go with an unfamiliar adult.

One of the most common diagnoses for hospitalized persons is adjustment disorder (APA, 2013). These disorders occur within 3 months of the stressor. The individuals experience distress that is out of proportion to the severity of the stressor. The person may be unable to function socially. Once the situation is resolved, the symptoms subside.

DISSOCIATIVE DISORDERS

Dissociative disorders are thought to be responses to extreme external or internal events or stressors. Prevalence is higher among people who experience childhood physical or sexual abuse than among others. The onset of these disorders may be sudden or occur gradually, and the course of each may be long term or transient.

Dissociation, or a splitting from the self, may occur as a form of coping with severe anxiety. The essential feature of the disorders in this class involves a failure to integrate identity, memory, and consciousness. This class of disorders includes dissociative amnesia (the inability to recall important yet stressful information), depersonalization/derealization disorder (the feeling of being detached from one's mental processes), dissociative identity disorder (formerly multiple personality disorder), and dissociative disorder not otherwise specified. Assessment findings in patients with dissociative identity disorder reveal two distinct personality or identity states. Persons with dissociative disorders may also have comorbid substance abuse, mood disorders, personality disorders, or PTSD (APA, 2013).

Treatment options include the use of antidepressants to treat the patient's underlying mood and anxiety. Psychotherapy options include hypnotherapy, CBT, and psychoanalytic psychotherapy to discover the triggers that lead to heightened anxiety and dissociation.

SUMMARY OF KEY POINTS

- Anxiety-related disorders are the most common of all psychiatric disorders and comprise a wide range of disorders, including panic disorder, OCD, GAD, phobias, acute stress disorder, PTSD, and dissociative disorder.

- The anxiety disorders share the common symptom of recurring anxiety but differ in symptom profiles. Panic attacks occur in many of the disorders.

- Those experiencing anxiety disorders have a high level of physical and emotional illness and often experience dual diagnoses with other anxiety disorders, substance abuse, or depression. These disorders often render individuals unable to function effectively at home or at a job.

- Patients with panic disorder are often seen in a number of health care settings, frequently in hospital emergency departments or clinics, presenting with a confusing array of physical and emotional symptoms. Skillful assessment is required to eliminate possible life-threatening causes.

- Treatment approaches for all anxiety-related disorders are somewhat similar, including pharmacotherapy, psychological treatments, or often a combination of both.

- Persons with OCD experience extreme anxiety if their compulsions are interrupted. Most common obsession is the fear of contamination. Medications can help them through episodes and reduce the compulsive behavior. Nursing care focuses on motivating the patient for change and supporting the new behaviors.

- PTSD occurs following a traumatic event and is characterized by involuntary intrusive thoughts, avoidance and numbing, negative moods and thoughts, and hyperarousal. Nursing care focuses on counseling interventions, administration of medication, psychoeducation, and family support.

CRITICAL THINKING CHALLENGES

1. How does the patient's culture affect the assessment of anxiety?
2. How might one differentiate shyness from social anxiety disorder?
3. How might the etiology of depression and anxiety be similar because antidepressant medications are used to treat both?
4. What are some of the barriers in assessing pathologic anxiety in children? Are anxiety disorders under- or overdiagnosed in children? Explain.
5. What role might parents, aside from genetics, play in contributing to the development of anxiety disorders in their offspring?
6. What are the risks and benefits of treating anxiety disorders with benzodiazepine medications in persons with substance abuse?
7. How should a nurse approach a military veteran who is having intrusive thoughts, nightmares, and is unable to sleep?

![MOVIES] ***Dirty Filthy Love:*** 2004. Mark Furness (played by Michael Sheen) is an architect whose marriage and career are threatened by his OCD and Tourette's syndrome. The story is about his divorce; his best friend's matchmaking efforts; and a woman who introduces him to therapy, a healthy relationship, and unconditional love. This film depicts several realistic symptoms of OCD and Tourette's syndrome and the emotional turmoil these individuals undergo.

Viewing Points: Differentiate Mark's response to his Tourette's syndrome and OCD. Which disorder is ultimately more problematic? If Mark were your patient, what medication would you expect to be prescribed? Identify teaching needs related to medication and the obsessions and compulsions. Explain the dynamics of the relationship of Mark and Charlotte. Can you identify Charlotte's mental disorder?

A related Psychiatric-Mental Health Nursing video on the topic of anxiety is available at: http://thePoint.lww.com/Boyd5eUpdate.

References

American Psychiatric Association. (2013). *Diagnostic and statistical manual of mental disorders DSM-5* (5th ed.). Arlington, VA: Author.

Andrisano, C., Chiesa, A., & Serretti, A. (2013). Newer antidepressants and panic disorder: A meta-analysis. (Review). *International Clinical Psychopharmacology, 28*(1), 33–45.

Asnaani, A., Gutner, C., Hinton, D., & Hofmann, S. (2009). Panic disorder, panic attacks and panic attack symptoms across race-ethnic groups: Results of the collaborative psychiatric epidemiology studies. *CNS Neuroscience & Therapeutics, 15*(3), 249–254.

Ayazi, T., Lien, L., Eide, A., Swartz, L., & Hauff, E. (2014). Association between exposure to traumatic events and anxiety disorders in a post-conflict setting: A cross-sectional community study in South Sudan. *BMC Psychiatry, 14*, 6. doi:10.1186/1471-244X-14-16

Bastien, D. (2010). Pharmacological treatment of combat-induced PTSD: A literature review. *British Journal of Nursing, 19*(5), 318–321.

Beck, A. & Emery, G. (1985). *Anxiety disorders and phobias: A cognitive perspective*. New York: Basic Books.

Beevers, C. G., Lee, H., Wells, T. T., Ellis, A. J., & Telch, M. J. (2011). Association of predeployment gaze bias for emotion stimuli with later symptoms of PTSD and depression in soldiers deployed in Iraq. *American Journal of Psychiatry, 168*:735–741. doi:10.1176/appi.ajp.2011.10091309

Benjamin, C. L., Beidas, R. S., Comer, J. S., Puliafico, A. C., & Kendall, P. C. (2011). Generalized anxiety disorder in youth: Diagnostic considerations. *Depression and Anxiety, 28*(2), 173–182.

Bjornsson, A. S., Didie, E. R., & Phillips, K. A. (2010). Body dysmorphic disorder. *Dialogues in Clinical Neuroscience, 12*(2), 221–232.

Centers for Disease control and Prevention. (2013). Mental health surveillance among children–United States, 2005–2011. *Morbidity and Mortality Weekly Report, 62*(suppl 2), 1–35.

Cervenka, S., Hedman, E., Ikoma, Y., Djurfeldt, D. R., Rück, C., Halldin, C., et al. (2012). Changes in dopamine D2-receptor binding are associated to symptom reduction after psychotherapy in social anxiety disorder. *Translational Psychiatry, 2*, e120. doi:10.1038/tp.2012.40

Clum, G. A. (1990). Panic attack cognitions questionnaire. *Coping with panic: A drug-free approach to dealing with anxiety attacks*. Pacific Grove, CA: Brooks/Cole.

Cooper, J. (1970). The Leyton obsessional inventory. *Psychological Medicine, 1*, 48–64.

Csigó, K., Harsányi, A., Demeter, G., Rajkai, C., Németh, A., & Racacsmány, M. (2010). Long-term follow-up of patients with obsessive-compulsive disorder treated by anterior capsulotomy: A neuropsychological study. *Journal of Affective Disorders, 126*(1–2), 198–205.

Cullen, B. A., La Flair, L. N., Storr, C. L., Green, K. M., Alvanzo, A. A., Mojtabai, R., et al. (2013). Association of comorbid generalized anxiety disorder and alcohol use disorders symptoms with health-related quality of life: Results from the National Epidemiological Survey on Alcohol and Related Conditions. *Journal of Addiction Medicine, 7*(6), 394–400.

Del Casale, A., Serata, D., Rapinesi, C., Kotzalidis, G. D., Angeletti, G., Tatarelli, R., et al. (2013). Structural neuroimaging in patients with panic disorder: Findings and limitations of recent studies. *Psychiatria Danubina, 25*(2), 108–114.

Driessen, M., Schulte, S., Luedecke, C., Schaefer, I., Sutmann, F., Ohlmeier, M., et al. (2008). Trauma and PTSD in patients with alcohol, drug, or dual dependence: A multi-center study. *Alcoholism, Clinical & Experimental Research, 32*(3), 481–488.

Duke, D. C., Keeley, J. L., Geffken, G. R., & Storch, E. A. (2010). Trichotillomania: A current review. *Clinical Psychology Review, 30*(2), 181–93.

Ellen, S., Olver, J., Norman, T., & Burrows, G. (2008). The neurobiology of benzodiazepine receptors in panic disorder and post-traumatic stress disorder. *Stress and Health, 24*, 13–21.

Fleury, G., Gaudette, L., & Moran, P. (2012). Compulsive hoarding: Overview and implications for community health nurses. *Journal of Community Health Nursing, 29*(3), 154–162.

Frydman, I., do Brasil, P. E., Torres, A. R., Shavitt, R. G., Ferrão, Y. A., Rosário, M. C., et al. (2014). Late-onset obsessive-compulsive disorder: Risk factors and correlates. *Journal of Psychiatric Research, 49*, 68–74. doi:10.1016/j.jpsychres.2013.10.021

Goodman, W., Price, L., Rasmussen, S., Mazure, C., Fleischmann, R. L., Hill, C. L., et al. (1989). The Yale-Brown Obsessive Compulsive Scale (Y-BOCS): Part 1. Development, use and reliability. *Archives of General Psychiatry, 46*, 1006–1011.

Grados, M. A. (2010). The genetics of obsessive-compulsive disorder and Tourette syndrome: An epidemiological and pathway-based approach for gene discovery. *Journal of the American Academy of Child and Adolescent Psychiatry, 49*(8), 810–819.

Grant, B. F., Hasin, D. S., Stinson, F. S., Dawson, D. A., Goldstein, R. B., Smith, S., et al. (2006). The epidemiology of DSM-IV panic disorder and agoraphobia in the United States: Results from the National Epidemiologic Survey on Alcohol and Related Conditions. *The Journal of Clinical Psychiatry, 67*(3), 363–374.

Grant, J. E., Odlaug, B. L., Chamberlain, M. D., & Kim, S. W. (2010). A double-blind, placebo-controlled trial of lamotrigine for pathologic skin picking: Treatment efficacy and neurocognitive predictors of response. *Journal of Clinical Psychopharmacology, 30*(4), 396–403.

Grenier, S., Preville, M., Boyer, R. & O'Connor, K. (2009). Prevalence and correlates of obsessive-compulsive disorder among older adults living in the community. *Journal of Anxiety Disorders, 23*(7), 858–865.

Hachiya, Y., Miyata, R., Tanuma, N., Hongou, K., Tanaka, K., Shimoda, K., et al. (2013). Autoimmune neurological disorders associated with group-A beta-hemolytic streptococcal infection. *Brain & Development, 35*(7), 670–674.

Hall, B. J., Tolin, D. F., Frost, R. O., & Steketee, F. (2013). An exploration of comorbid symptoms and clinical correlates of clinically significant hoarding symptoms. *Depression & Anxiety, 30*(1), 67–76.

Hamilton, M. (1959). The assessment of anxiety states by rating. *British Journal of Medical Psychology, 32*, 54.

Heim, C., & Nemeroff, C. (2009). Neurobiology of posttraumatic stress disorder. *International Journal of Neuropsychiatric Medicine, 14*(1 suppl 1), 13–14.

Heir, T., Piatigorsky, A., & Weisaeth, L. (2010). Posttraumatic stress symptoms clusters associations with psychopathology and functional impairment. *Journal of Anxiety Disorders, 24*(8), 936–940.

Jacob, M. L., & Storch, E. A. (2013). Pediatric obsessive-compulsive disorder: A review for nursing professionals. *Journal of Child and Adolescent Psychiatric Nursing, 26*, 138–148.

Jovanovic, T., & Ressler, K. (2010). How the neurocircuitry and genetics of fear inhibition may inform our understanding of PTSD. *American Journal of Psychiatry, 167*(6), 648–662.

Jovanovic, T., Smith, A., Kamkwalala, A., Poole, J., Samples, T., Norrholm, S. D., et al. (2011). Physiological markers of anxiety are increased in children of abused mothers. *Journal of Child Psychology and Psychiatry, and allied disciplines*.

Katz, C., Yaseen, Z. S., Mojtabai, R., Cohen, L. J., & Galynker II. (2011). Panic an independent risk factor for suicide attempt in depressive illness: Findings from the National Epidemiological survey on Alcohol and Related Conditions (NESARC). *Journal of Clinical Psychiatry, 72*(12), 1628–1635.

Kessler, R. C., Avenevoli, S., Costello, E. J., Georgiades, K., Green, J. G., Gruber, M. J., et al. (2012a). Prevalence, persistence, and sociodemographic correlates of DSM-IV disorders in the national Comorbidity survey Replication Adolescent Supplement. *Archives of General Psychiatry, 69*(4), 372–380.

Kessler, R. C., Avenevoli, S., Costello, J., Green, J. G., Gruber, M. J., McLaughlin, K. A., et al. (2012b). Severity of 12-month *DSM-IV* disorders in the National Comorbidity Survey Replication Adolescent Supplement. *Archives of General Psychiatry, 69*(4), 381–389.

Keuthen, N. J., Altenburger, E. M., & Pauls, D. (2014). A family study of trichotillomania and chronic hair pulling. *American Journal of Medical Genetics. Part B: Neuropsychiatric Genetics, 165*(2), 167–174.

Kimerling, R. (2010). *Gender and medical needs of OEF/OIF veterans with PTSD II. HSR&D study.* Retrieved from http://www.hsrd.research.va.gov

King-Kallimanis, B., Gum, A., & Kohn, R. (2009). Comorbidity of depressive and anxiety disorders for older Americans in the national comorbidity survey replication. *American Journal of Geriatric Psychiatry, 17*(9), 782–792.

Konishi, Y., Tanii, H., Otowa, T., Sasaki, T., Tochigi, M., Umekage, T., et al. (2014). GeneXgeneXgender interaction of BDNF and COMT genotypes associated with panic disorder. *Progress in Neuro-Psychopharmcology & Biological psychiatry.* doi:10.1016/j.pnpbp.2014.01.020

Korczak, D., Goldstein, B., & Levitt, A. (2007). Panic disorder, cardiac diagnosis and emergency department utilization in an epidemiologic community sample. *General Hospital Psychiatry, 29*(4), 335–339.

Kroenke, K., Outcalt, S., Krebs, E., Bair, M. J., Wu, J., Chumbler, N., et al. (2013). Association between anxiety, health-related quality of life and functional impairment in primary care patients with chronic pain. *General Hospital Psychiatry, 35*(4), 359–365.

Lanius, R. A., Vermetten, E., Loewenstein, R. J., Brand, B., Schmal, C., Bremner, J. D., et al. (2010). Emotion modulation in PTSD: Clinical and neurobiological evidence for a dissociative subtype. *The American Journal of Psychiatry, 167*(6), 640–647.

Lochner, C., & Stein, D. J. (2010). Obsessive-compulsive spectrum disorders in obsessive-compulsive disorder and other anxiety disorders. *Psychopathology, 43*(6), 389–396.

MacKenzie, M. B., & Fowler, K. F. (2013). Social anxiety disorder in the Canadian population: Exploring gender differences in sociodemographic profile. *Journal of Anxiety Disorders, 27*(4), 427–434.

Masho, S., & Ahmed, G. (2007). Age at sexual assault and posttraumatic stress disorder among women: Prevalence, correlates, and implications for prevention. *Journal of Women's Health, 16*(2), 262–267.

Mayo, K. (2010). Support from neurobiology for spiritual techniques for anxiety: A brief review. *Journal of Healthcare Chaplaincy, 16*(1–2), 53–57.

Miloyan, B., Byrne, G. F., & Pachana, N. A. (2014). Age-related changes in generalized anxiety disorder symptoms. *International Psychogeriatrics,* doi:10.1017/S1041610213002470

Molina, E., Cervilla, J., Rivera M., Torres, F., Bellón, J. A., Moreno, B., et al. (2011). Polymorphic variation at the serotonin 1-A receptor gene is associated with comorbid depression and generalized anxiety. *Psychiatric Genetics, 21*(4), 195–201.

Moselhy, H. (2009). Co-morbid post-traumatic stress disorder and opioid dependence syndrome. *Journal of Dual Diagnosis, 5,* 30–40.

Mufaddel, A., Osman, O. T., Almugaddam, F., & Jafferany, M. (2013). A review of body dysmorphic disorder and its presentation in different clinical settings. *Primary Care Companion for CNS Disorders, 15*(4). doi:10.4088/PCC.12r1464

National Institute of Mental Health. (2014). Obsessive compulsive disorder among adults. www.nimh.nih.gov/statistics/locd_adult.shtml

Pace, T. W., & Heim, C. M. (2011). A short review on the psychoneuroimmunology of posttraumatic stress disorder: From risk factors to medical comorbidities. *Brain Behavior and Immunity, 25*(1), 6–13.

Peñalba, V., McGuire, H., & Leite, J. R. (2008). Psychosocial interventions for prevention of psychological disorders in law enforcement officers. *The Cochrane Database of Systematic Reviews,* (3), CD005601.

Peplau, H. (1989). Theoretic constructs: Anxiety, self, and hallucinations. In A. O'. Toole & S. Welt (Eds.), *Interpersonal theory in nursing practice: Selected works of Hildegarde E. Peplau.* New York: Springer.

Pietrzak, R. H. & Southwick, S. M. (2011). Psychological resilience in OEF-OIF Veterans: Application of a novel classification approach and examination of demographic and psychosocial correlates. *Journal of Affective Disorders, 133*(3), 560—568.

Pilecki, B., Arentoft, A., & McKay, D. (2011). An evidence-based causal model of panic disorder. *Journal of Anxiety Disorders, 25*(3), 381–388.

Rachman, S. & Hodgson, R. (1980). *Obsessions and compulsions.* New York: Prentice-Hall.

Ravindran, L. N. & Stein, M. B. (2010). The pharmacologic treatment of anxiety disorders: A review of progress. *Journal of Clinical Psychiatry, 71*(7), 839–854.

Roberts, L. W. (2010). Stigma, hope, and challenge in psychiatry: Trainee perspectives from five countries on four continents. *Academic Psychiatry, 34*(1), 1–4.

Rodriguez, C. I., Simpson, H. B., Liu, S. Levinson, A. & Blanco, C. (2013). Prevalence and correlates of difficulty discarding: Results from a national sample of the US population. *The Journal of Nervous and Mental Disease, 201*(9), 795–801.

Robinson, R. A., Taghva, A., Liu, C. Y., & Apuzzo, M. L. (2013). Surgery of the mind, mood, and conscious state: An idea in evolution. *World Neurosurgery, 80*(3), S2–S26.

Rogers, K., Banis, M., Falkenstein, M. F., Malloy, E. J., McDonough, L, Nelson, S. O., et al. (2014). Stepped care in the treatment of trichotillomania. *Journal of Consulting and Clinical Psychology, 82*(2), 361–367.

Roth, R., Geisser, M., & Bates, R. (2008). The relation of post-traumatic stress symptoms to depression and pain in patients with accident-related chronic pain. *Journal of Pain, 9*(7), 588–596.

Rothbart, R., Amos, T., Siegfried, N., Ipser, J. C., Fineberg, N., Chamberlain, S. R., et al. (2013). Pharmacotherapy for trichotillomania. *The Cochrane Database of Systematic Reviews.* doi:10.1002/14651858. CD007662.pub2.

Rourke, M., Hobbie, W., Schwartz, L., & Kazak, A. (2007). Posttraumatic stress disorder (PTSD) in young adult survivors of childhood cancer. *Pediatric Blood and Cancer, 49*(2), 177–182.

Ruscio, A. M., Stein, D. J., Chiu, W. T., & Kessler, R. C. (2010). The epidemiology of obsessive-compulsive disorder in the National Comorbidity Survey Replication. *Molecular Psychiatry, 15*(1), 53–63.

Ruwaard, J., Lange, A., Schrieken, B., Dolan, C. V., & Emmelkamp, P. (2012). The effectiveness of online cognitive behavioral treatment in routine clinical practice. *PLoS One, 7*(7), e40089.

Sakolsky, D. J., McCracken, J. T., & Nurmi, E. L. (2012). Genetics of pediatric anxiety disorders. *Child & Adolescent Psychiatric Clinics of North America, 21,* 479–500.

Scott-Tilley, D., Tilton, A., & Sandel, M. (2010). Biologic correlates to the development of post-traumatic stress disorder in female victims of intimate partner violence: Implications for practice. *Perspectives in Psychiatric Care, 46*(1), 26–31.

Shaw, P., Sharp, W., Sudre, G., Wharton, A., Greenstein, D., Raznahan, A., et al. (2014). Subcortical and cortical morphological anomalies as an endophenotype in obsessive-compulsive disorder. *Molecular Psychiatry.* doi:10.1038/mp.2014.3

Singh, S. & Jones, C. (2013). Compulsive hoarding syndrome: Engaging the patients in treatment. *Mental Health Practice, 17*(4), 16–20.

Sorrell, J. M. (2012). Understanding hoarding in older adults. *Journal of Psychosocial Nursing & Mental Health Services, 50*(3), 17–21.

Stein, D. J., Aquilar-Gaxiola, S., Alonso, J., Bruffaerts, R., de Jonge, P., Liu, Z., et al. (2014). Associations between mental disorders and subsequent onset of hypertension. *General Hospital Psychiatry, 36*(2), 142–149. doi:10.1016/j.genhosppsych.2013.11.002

Stein, M., Steckler, T., Lightfoot, J. D., Hay, E., & Goddard, A. W. (2010). Pharmacologic treatment of panic disorder. *Current Topics in Behavioral Neurosciences, 2,* 469–485.

Stuber, M., Meeske, K. A., Krull, K. R., Leisenring, W., Stratton, K., Kazak, A. E., et al. (2010). Prevalence and predictors of posttraumatic stress disorder in adult survivors of childhood cancer. *Pediatrics, 125*(5), e1124–e1134.

Torres, A. R., Ferrão, Y. A., Shavitt, R. G., Diniz, J. B., Costa, D. L., do Rosário, M. C, et al. (2014). Panic Disorder and Agoraphobia, in OCD patients: Clinical profile and possible treatment implications. *Comprehensive Psychiatry, 55*(3), 588–97.doi:10.1016/j.comppsych.2013.11.017

Tully, P. J., & Baune, B. T. (2014). Comorbid anxiety disorders alter the association between cardiovascular diseases and depression: The German National Health Interview and Examination Survey. *Social Psychiatry and Psychiatric Epidemiology, 49*(5), 683–691. doi:10.1007/s00127-013-0784-x

Vesga-Lopez, O., Schneier, F. R., Wang, S., Heimberg, R. G., Liu, S. M., et al. (2008). Gender differences in generalized anxiety disorder: Results from the National Epidemiologic Survey on Alcohol and Related Conditions (NESARC). *The Journal of Clinical Psychiatry, 69*(10), 1606–1616.

Warner, C. H., Warner, C. M., Appenzeller, G. N., & Hoge, C. W. (2013). Identifying and managing posttraumatic stress disorder. *American Family Physician, 88*(12), 827–834.

Xu, Y., Schneier, F., Heimberg, R. G., Princisvalle, K., Liebowitz, M. R., Wang, S., et al. (2012). Gender differences in social anxiety disorder: Results from the national epidemiologic sample on alcohol and related conditions. *Journal of Anxiety Disorders, 26*(1), 12–19.

Zwanzger, P., Domschke, K., & Bradwejn, J. (2012). Neuronal network of panic disorder: The role of the neuropeptide cholecystokinin. (Review). *Depression & Anxiety, 29*(9), 762–774.

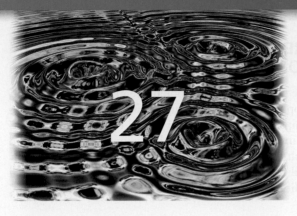

27 Borderline Personality Disorder
Management of Emotional Dysregulation and Self-Harm

Ann R. Bland, Deborah McNeil Whitehouse, and Mary Ann Boyd

KEY CONCEPTS

- borderline personality disorder
- emotional dysregulation
- personality
- personality disorder
- self harm

LEARNING OBJECTIVES

After studying this chapter, you will be able to:

1. Describe the prevalence and incidence of personality disorders.

2. Delineate the clinical symptoms of borderline personality disorder (BPD) with emphasis on emotional dysregulation and self-harm.

3. Analyze the biopsychosocial theories explaining BPD, emotional dysregulation, and self-harm.

4. Identify evidence-based interventions for patients diagnosed with BPDs.

5. Develop recovery-oriented strategies that address the needs of persons diagnosed with BPD, emotional dysregulation, and self-harm.

6. Analyze communication issues within the nurse–patient relationship for those with emotional dysregulation.

KEY TERMS

- affective instability • cognitive schemas • communication triad • dialectical behavior therapy (DBT)
- dichotomous thinking • dissociation • emotional vulnerability • identity diffusion • impulsivity • inhibited grieving • interpersonal functioning • invalidating environment • parasuicidal behavior • personality traits
- projective identification • self-identity • separation-individuation • skills groups • splitting • thought stopping

The concept of personality seems deceivingly simple but is very complex. Historically, the term *personality* was derived from the Greek word *persona*, the theatrical mask used by dramatic players that had the connotation of a projected pretense or allusion. With time, the connotation changed from being an external surface representation to the internal traits of the individual.

KEYCONCEPT   **Personality** is a complex pattern of characteristics, largely outside of the person's awareness, that comprise the individual's distinctive pattern of perceiving, feeling, thinking, coping, and behaving.

Personality traits are prominent aspects of personality that are exhibited in a wide range of social and personal contexts. Intrinsic and pervasive, personality traits emerge from a complicated interaction of biologic dispositions, psychological experiences, and environmental situations that ultimately comprise a distinctive personality (Millon, 2011).

No sharp division exists between normal and abnormal personality functioning. Instead, personalities are viewed on a continuum from normal at one end to abnormal at the other. Many of the same processes involved in the development of a "normal" personality are responsible for the development of a personality disorder.

This chapter provides an overview of personality disorders and discusses borderline personality disorder (BPD). Additional personality disorders are discussed in Chapter 28.

OVERVIEW OF PERSONALITY DISORDERS

A personality disorder is "an enduring pattern of inner experience and behavior that deviates markedly from the expectations of the individual's culture, is pervasive and inflexible, has an onset in adolescence or early adulthood, is stable over time, and leads to distress or impairment" (American Psychiatric Association [APA], 2013, p. 646).

> **KEYCONCEPT**   A **personality disorder** diagnosis is based on abnormal, inflexible behavior patterns of long duration, traced to adolescence or early adulthood that deviate from acceptable cultural norms.

Estimates of the prevalence of personality disorders vary from 4.4% to 13.4% with a median of 9.6% (Samuels, 2011). This rate results in public health significance because of the extreme social dysfunction and high health care utilization of persons with personality disorders. Many others do not seek treatment for the distress or impairment related to their personality disorder because they do not perceive themselves as having a problem. However, they frequently seek help for co-occurring medical or mental health disorders.

Currently, 10 personality disorders are recognized in the *DSM-5* within three clusters. Cluster A disorders are characterized by odd or eccentric behavior; Cluster B are characterized by dramatic, emotional, or erratic behavior; in Cluster C disorders individuals appear anxious or fearful (see Box 27.1).

The *DSM-5* describes an alternative diagnostic approach that reformulates these disorders according to personality functioning and traits. This text will discuss the currently recognized 10 *DSM-5* personality disorders.

BOX 27.1

DSM-5 Personality Disorders

CLUSTER A	CLUSTER B	CLUSTER C
Paranoid	Antisocial	Avoidant
Schizoid	Borderline	Dependent
Schizotypal	Histrionic	Obsessive-Compulsive
	Narcissistic	

BORDERLINE PERSONALITY DISORDER

People with BPD have problems regulating their moods, developing a self-identity, maintaining interpersonal relationships, maintaining reality-based thinking, and avoiding impulsive or destructive behavior. The severity and difficulty in treating the disorder leads to enormous public health costs from health care utilization and functional disability (Gunderson et al., 2011).

> **KEYCONCEPT**   **Borderline personality disorder** is characterized by a disruptive pattern of instability related to self-identity, interpersonal relationships, and affects combined with marked impulsivity and destructive behavior.

Clinical Course

Individuals with BPD appear more competent than they actually are and often set unrealistically high expectations for themselves. When these expectations are not met, they experience intense shame, self-hate, and self-directed anger. Their lives are like soap operas—one crisis after another. Some of the crises are caused by the individual's dysfunctional lifestyle or inadequate social milieu, but many are caused by fate—the death of a spouse or a diagnosis of an illness. They react emotionally with minimal coping skills. The intensity of their emotions often frightens them and others. Friends, family members, and coworkers limit their contact with the person, which furthers their sense of aloneness, abandonment, and self-hatred. It also diminishes opportunities for learning self-corrective measures.

Remissions from the acute symptoms (self-injurious behaviors and suicide attempts or threats) are fairly common and the relapse rate relatively low compared to other disorders. However, psychosocial functioning does not necessarily improve as symptoms decrease. Younger age and more education predicts better functioning (Gunderson et al., 2011).

Diagnostic Criteria

BPD is a "pervasive pattern of instability of interpersonal relationships, self-image, and affects, and marked impulsivity beginning by early adulthood and present in a variety of contexts" (APA, 2013, p. 663). See Key Diagnostic Characteristics 27.1. Individuals with BPD also exhibit related cognitive and behavioral dysfunctions.

Lady Diana Frances Spencer
Princess Diana (1961–1997)

PUBLIC PERSONA

Lady Diana was reared in the British upper class and lived her short life in privilege and wealth. She came onto the world stage as the fairytale princess, when at 21 years of age, she married Prince Charles, age 33 years, in a royal wedding in front of 3,500 guests and an international television audience. Her startling beauty and charm enchanted the world. Publicly, Princess Diana projected grace, kindness, charisma, and vulnerability. Her charitable works related to landmines and AIDS issues brought world attention and understanding to these poignant social problems, creating a legacy. She was frequently photographed around the world as she greeted the public and engaged in charitable works, often including her two young sons in these.

PERSONAL REALITIES

Parental divorce resulted in the departure of her mother and emotional withdrawal of her father early in her life. Friends described her low self-esteem and identity confusion. Diana's brother referred to her deep feelings of unworthiness. She looked to the press, the public, and those around her to define her identity. "Diana brought a ferocious intensity to her relationships, pleading for attention and time, and demanding intense loyalty" (Smith, 1999, p. 446). She fluctuated between total intensity to withdrawal with intimate relationships and frequently experienced mercurial moods. Privately, she had episodes of self-mutilation by cutting, but she talked openly of her bouts with bulimia and feelings of emptiness. She admitted to adultery and multiple affairs (Smith, 1999). In tapes broadcast by NBC that were released after her death, Princess Diana talked of her relationship with Prince Charles and her suicide attempts.

Source: Smith, S. B. (1999). *Diana in search of herself: Portrait of a troubled princess.* New York: Times Books/Crown Publishing.

Unstable Interpersonal Relationships

People with BPD have an extreme fear of abandonment as well as a history of unstable, insecure attachments (Miano, Fertuck, Arntz, & Stanley, 2013). Most never experienced a consistently secure, nurturing relationship and are constantly seeking reassurance and validation. In an attempt to meet their interpersonal needs, they idealize others and establish intense relationships that violate others' interpersonal boundaries, which lead to rejection. When these relationships do not live up to their expectations, they devalue the person. Continually disappointed in relationships, these individuals, who already are intensely emotional and have a poor sense of self, feel estranged from others and inadequate in the face of perceived social standards. Intense shame and self-hate follow. These feelings often result in self-injurious behaviors, such as wrist cutting, self-burnings, or head banging.

In social situations, people with BPD use elaborate strategies to structure interactions. That is, they restrict their relationships to ones in which they feel in control. They distance themselves from groups when feeling anxious (which is most of the time) and rarely use their social support system. Even if they are married or have a supportive extended family, they are reluctant to share their feelings. They do not want to burden anyone; they fear rejection and assume that people are tired of hearing them repeat the same issues (Miano et al., 2013).

Unstable Self-Image

Identity diffusion occurs when a person lacks aspects of personal identity or when personal identity is poorly developed (Erikson, 1968). Four factors of identity are most commonly disturbed: role absorption (narrowly defining

---

KEY DIAGNOSTIC CHARACTERISTICS 27.1 • BORDERLINE PERSONALITY DISORDER 301.83

Diagnostic Criteria

A pervasive pattern of instability of interpersonal relationships, self-image, and affects, and marked impulsivity, beginning by early adulthood and present in a variety of contexts, as indicated by five (or more) of the following:

1. Frantic efforts to avoid real or imagined abandonment. (**Note:** Do not include suicidal or self-mutilating behavior covered in Criterion 5.)
2. A pattern of unstable and intense interpersonal relationships characterized by alternating between extremes of idealization and devaluation.
3. Identity disturbance: markedly and persistently unstable self-image or sense of self.
4. Impulsivity in at least two areas that are potentially self-damaging (e.g., spending, sex, substance abuse, reckless driving, binge eating). (**Note:** Do not include suicidal or self-mutilating behavior covered in Criterion 5.)
5. Recurrent suicidal behavior, gestures, or threats, or self-mutilating behavior.
6. Affective instability due to a marked reactivity of mood (e.g., intense episodic dysphoria, irritability, or anxiety usually lasting a few hours and only rarely more than a few days).
7. Chronic feelings of emptiness.
8. Inappropriate, intense anger or difficulty controlling anger (e.g., frequent displays of temper, constant anger, recurrent physical fights).
9. Transient, stress-related paranoid ideation or severe dissociative symptoms.

Associated Behavioral Findings

- Pattern of undermining self at the moment a goal is to be realized
- Possible psychotic-like symptoms during times of stress
- Recurrent job losses, interrupted education, and broken marriages
- History of physical and sexual abuse, neglect, hostile conflict, and early parental loss or separation

Reprinted with permission from the *Diagnostic and Statistical Manual of Mental Disorders,* Fifth Edition (Copyright ©2013). American Psychiatric Association. All Rights Reserved.

self within a single role), painful incoherence (distressed sense of internal disharmony), inconsistency (lack of coherence in thoughts, feelings, and actions), and lack of commitment (Westen, Betan, & Defife, 2011). Other factors of the personality identity (religious ideology, moral value systems, sexual attitudes) appear to be less important in identity diffusion. Clinically, these patients appear to have no sense of their own identity and direction; this becomes a source of great distress to these patients and is often manifested by chronic feelings of emptiness and boredom. It is not unusual for people with BPD to direct their actions in accord with the wishes of other people. For example, one woman with BPD describes herself: "I am a singer because my mother wanted me to be. I live in the city because my manager thought that I should. I become whatever anyone tells me to be. Whenever someone recommends a song, I wonder why I didn't think of that. My boyfriend tells me what to wear."

Unstable Affects

Affective instability (rapid and extreme shift in mood) is a core characteristic of BPD and is evidenced by erratic emotional responses to situations and intense sensitivity to criticism or perceived slights. For example, a person may greet a casual acquaintance with intense affection yet later be aloof with the same acquaintance. Friends describe individuals with BPD as moody, irresponsible, or intense. These individuals often fail to recognize their own emotional responses, thoughts, beliefs, and behaviors and have difficulty recognizing facial affects of others. In this disorder recognizing emotions in others is altered (Mitchell, Dickens, & Picchioni, 2014). Clinically, when a stressful situation is encountered, these individuals react with shifts in emotions. They seem to have a limited ability to develop emotional buffers to stressful situations and may subjectively magnify a subtle negative affect (Daros, Uliaszek, & Ruocco, 2014).

Cognitive Dysfunctions

People with BPD have **dichotomous thinking**. Cognitively, they evaluate experiences, people, and objects in terms of mutually exclusive categories (e.g., good or bad, success or failure, trustworthy or deceitful), which informs extreme interpretations of events that would normally be viewed as including both positive and negative aspects. There are also times when their thinking becomes disorganized. Irrelevant, bizarre notions and vague or scattered thought connections are sometimes present, as well as delusions and hallucinations.

Another cognitive dysfunction common in BPD is **dissociation**, or times when thinking, feeling, or behaviors occur outside a person's awareness (van Dijke, van der Hart, Ford, van Son, van der Heijden, & Bühring, 2010).

Dissociation can be conceptualized on a continuum from minor dissociations of daily life, such as daydreaming, to a breakdown in the integrated functions of consciousness, memory, perception of self or the environment, and sensory-motor behavior. For example, in driving familiar roads, people often get lost in their thoughts or dissociate and suddenly do not remember what happened during that part of the trip. Environmental stimuli are ignored, and there are changes in the perception of reality. The individual is physically present but mentally in another place. Dissociation serves a useful purpose; in the case of driving a familiar road, dissociation alleviates the boredom of driving. It is also a coping strategy for avoiding disturbing events. In dissociating, the person does not have to be aware of or remember traumatic events.

Behavioral Dysfunctions

Impaired Problem Solving

In BPD, there is often failure to engage in active problem solving. Instead, problem solving is attempted by soliciting help from others in a helpless, hopeless manner. Suggestions are rarely taken.

Impulsivity

Impulsivity is also characteristic of people with BPD. Because impulse-driven people have difficulty delaying gratification or thinking through the consequences before acting on their feelings, their actions are often unpredictable. Essentially, they act in the moment and clean up the mess afterward. Gambling, spending money irresponsibly, binge eating, engaging in unsafe sex, and abusing substances are typical of these individuals. They can also be physically or verbally aggressive. Job losses, interrupted education, and unsuccessful relationships are common.

Self-Harm Behaviors

The turmoil and unsuccessful interpersonal relationships and social experiences associated with BPD may lead the person to undermine him- or herself when a goal is about to be reached. The most serious consequences are a suicide attempt or **parasuicidal behavior** (deliberate self-injury with intent to harm oneself).

> **KEYCONCEPT** **Self-harm** is deliberate self-injurious behavior with the intent to hurt oneself.

Self-harm behavior can be compulsive (e.g., hair pulling), episodic, or repetitive (cutting wrists, arms, or other body parts) and is more likely to occur when the individual with

BPD is depressed; has highly unstable interpersonal relationships, especially problems with intimacy and sociability; and is paranoid, hypervigilant (alert, watchful), and resentful. All self-harm behavior should be considered potentially life threatening and taken seriously.

Borderline Personality Disorder Across the Life Span

Many children and adolescents show symptoms similar to those of BPD, such as moodiness, self-destruction, impulsiveness, lack of temper control, and rejection sensitivity. If a family member has BPD, the adolescent should be carefully assessed for this disorder. Because symptoms of BPD begin in adolescence, it makes sense that some of the children and adolescents would meet the criteria for BPD even though it is not diagnosed before young adulthood. More likely, some personality traits, such as impulsivity and mood instability, in many adolescents should be recognized and treated whether or not BPD actually develops.

Epidemiology and Risk Factors

The estimated prevalence of BPD in the general population ranges from 0.5% to 2.7%, with a median rate of 1.6%. In clinical populations, BPD is one of the most frequently diagnosed personality disorders with a higher proportion of women (Sansone & Sansone, 2011). One explanation for more women is that it is more socially acceptable for women than men to seek help from the health care system. Another reason is that childhood sexual abuse, which more commonly affects girls, is one of the strongest risk factors for BPD. Gender bias in diagnosing may have a role. Still, another explanation is that eating disorders are more common in women with borderline personality disorder and they have a greater likelihood of also having a mood, anxiety, or posttraumatic stress disorder. Men with BPD are more likely to have a substance use issue and intermittent explosive disorder. Women are more likely to seek treatment than men (Sansone & Sansone, 2011)

Various studies show that physical and sexual abuse appears to be significant risk factors for BPD (Zanarini, Laudate, Frankenburg, Reich, & Fitzmaurice, 2011). Other studies cite parental loss and separation (Steele & Siever, 2010). Clearly, more studies are needed to identify risk factors for the development of BPD.

Comorbidity

Ample clinical reports show the coexistence of personality disorders with Axis I disorders (mood, substance abuse, eating, dissociative, and anxiety disorders) and other personality disorders (Gunderson et al., 2011). The coexistence of BPD with other disorders presents clinicians with the difficult choice of which disorder receives treatment priority. Symptoms associated with this disorder often provoke negative reactions on the part of clinicians, which interfere with clinicians' ability to provide effective care (Fielding, 2013).

Etiology

Evidence supports a biopsychosocial etiology. Recent studies demonstrate differences in brain functioning between those with and without BPD but also provide evidence that psychological and social factors contribute to the development of the disorder. The following discussion highlights the leading explanations for BPD.

Biologic Theories

There is now clear evidence of central nervous system dysfunction in BPD, including possible structural changes (Koenigsberg et al., 2014). Biologic abnormalities are associated with three BPD characteristics: affective instability; transient psychotic episodes; and impulsive, aggressive, and suicidal behavior. Associated brain dysfunction occurs in the limbic system and frontal lobe and increases the behaviors of impulsiveness, parasuicide, and mood disturbance (Stone, 2013).

It has also been hypothesized that an increase in dopamine may be responsible for transient psychotic states. These dysfunctions could be caused by a number of events, including trauma, epilepsy, and attention deficit hyperactivity disorder. People with BPD manifest psychotic-like symptoms, including paranoid thinking, dissociation, depersonalization, and derealization. These symptoms seem to be associated with intense anxiety.

Psychological Theories

Psychoanalytic Theories

The psychoanalytic views of BPD focus on two important psychoanalytic concepts: separation-individuation and projective identification. A person with BPD has not achieved the normal and healthy developmental stage of **separation-individuation**, during which a child develops a sense of self, a permanent sense of significant others (object constancy), and integration of seeing both bad and good components of oneself (Clarkin & De Panfilis, 2013). Those with BPD lack the ability to separate from the primary caregiver and develop a separate and distinct personality or self-identity. Psychoanalytic theory suggests that these separation difficulties occur because the primary caregivers' behaviors have been inconsistent or insensitive to the needs of the child. The child develops ambivalent feelings regarding interpersonal relationships and therefore has no basis for establishing trusting and secure relationships in the future. Children experience feelings of intense fear and anger in separating themselves from others. This problem continues into adulthood, and they continue to experience difficulties in maintaining personal boundaries and in interpersonal interactions and relationships. Often, these patients falsely attribute to others their own unacceptable feelings, impulses, or thoughts, termed **projective identification**. Projective identification is believed to play an important role in the development of BPD and is a defense mechanism by which people with BPD protect their fragile self-image. For example, when overwhelmed by anxiety or anger at being disregarded by another, they defend against the intensity of these feelings by unconsciously blaming others for what happens to them. They project their feelings onto a significant other with the unconscious hope that that person knows how to deal with it. Projective identification becomes a defensive way of interacting with the world, which leads to more rejection.

Maladaptive Cognitive Processes

Cognitive schemas are patterns of thoughts that determine how a person interprets events. Each person's cognitive schema screen, code, and evaluate incoming stimuli. In personality disorders, maladaptive cognitive schemas cause misinterpretation of other people's actions or reactions and of events that result in dysfunctional ways of responding. Cognitive schemas are important in understanding BPD (and antisocial personality disorder as well).

Individuals with BPD develop dysfunctional beliefs and maladaptive schemas early in life, leading them to misinterpret environmental stimuli continuously, which in turn leads to rigid and inflexible behavior patterns in response to new situations and people (Lawrence, Allen, & Chanen, 2011). Because those with BPD have been conditioned to anticipate rejection and disappointment in the past, they become entrenched in a pattern of fear and anxiety regarding encountering new people or situations. They have fears that disaster is going to strike any minute. The work of cognitive therapists is to challenge distortions in thinking patterns and replace them with realistic ones.

Social Theories: Biosocial Theories

The biosocial viewpoint proposed by Marsha Linehan and colleagues sees BPD as a multifaceted problem, a combination of innate **emotional vulnerability** (sensitivity and reactivity to environmental stress), emotional dysregulation (inability to control emotions in social interactions), and the environment (Linehan, 1993) (Box 27.2).

BOX 27.2

Behavioral Patterns in Borderline Personality Disorder

1. *Emotional vulnerability.* Person experiences a pattern of pervasive difficulties in regulating negative emotions, including high sensitivity to negative emotional stimuli, high emotional intensity, and slow return to emotional baseline.
2. *Self-invalidation.* Person fails to recognize one's own emotional responses, thoughts, beliefs, and behaviors and sets unrealistically high standards and expectations for self. May include intense shame, self-hate, and self-directed anger. Person has no personal awareness and tends to blame social environment for unrealistic expectations and demands.
3. *Unrelenting crises.* Person experiences pattern of frequent, stressful, negative environmental events, disruptions, and roadblocks—some caused by the individual's dysfunctional lifestyle, others by an inadequate social milieu, and many by fate or chance.
4. *Inhibited grieving.* Person tries to inhibit and overcontrol negative emotional responses, especially those associated with grief and loss, including sadness, anger, guilt, shame, anxiety, and panic.
5. *Active passivity.* Person fails to engage actively in solving of own life problems but will actively seek problem solving from others in the environment; learned helplessness, hopelessness.
6. *Apparent competence.* Tendency for the individual to appear deceptively more competent than he or she actually is; usually because of failure of competencies to generalize across expected moods, situations, and time and failure to display adequate nonverbal cues of emotional distress.

Adapted from Linehan, M. (1993). *Cognitive-behavioral treatment of borderline personality disorder* (p. 10). New York: Guilford Press.

KEYCONCEPT **Emotional dysregulation** is the inability to control emotions in social interactions and includes an instability of mood, marked shifts from or to depression, stress-related and transient mood crashes, rejection sensitivity, and inappropriate and intense outbursts of anger.

The emotional dysregulation and aggressive impulsivity entail both social learning and biologic regulation. Much of the neurobiologic research is directed at corticolimbic function and other circuitry (Stone, 2013). In fact, restoring balance in these systems permits more consistent neural firing between the limbic system and the frontal and prefrontal cortex. When these circuits are functional, the person has a greater capacity to think about his or her emotions and modulate behavior more responsibly.

According to the biosocial approach, the ability to control emotion is partly learned from private experiences and encounters with the social environment. BPD is believed to develop when emotionally vulnerable individuals interact with an **invalidating environment**, a social situation that negates private emotional responses and communication. When core emotional responses and communications are continuously dismissed, trivialized, devalued, punished, and discredited (invalidated) by respected or valued persons, the vulnerable individual becomes unsure about his or her feelings. A minor example of an invalidating environment or response follows: The parents of Emily, a 4-year-old girl, tell her that the family is going to grandmother's house for a family meal. The child responds, "I am not going to Gramma's. I hate Stevie (cousin)." The parents reply, "You don't hate Stevie. He is a wonderful child. He is your cousin, and only a spoiled, selfish little girl would say such a thing." The parents have devalued Emily's feelings and discredited her comments, thereby invalidating her feelings and sense of personal worth.

The most severe form of invalidation occurs in situations of child sexual abuse. Often, the abusing adult has told the child that this is a "special secret" between them. The child experiences feelings of fear, pain, and sadness, yet this trusted adult continuously dismisses the child's true feelings and tells the child what he or she should feel.

Family Response to Disorder

Individuals with BPD are typically part of a chaotic family system, but they usually add to the chaos. Family members often feel captive to these patients. Family members are afraid to disagree with them or refuse to meet their multiple needs, fearing that self-destructive behavior will follow. During the course of the disorder, family members often get "burned out" and withdraw from the patient, only adding to the patient's fear of abandonment (Miano et al., 2013).

Interdisciplinary Treatment and Recovery

BPD is a very complex disorder that requires collaboration of treatment by the whole mental health care team. Because BPD patients view the world in absolutes, nurses and other treatment team members are alternately categorized as all good or all bad. This defense is called **splitting** and presents clinicians with a challenge to work openly with each other as well as the patient until the issue can be resolved through team meetings and clinical supervision. Several types of medications are usually needed, including mood stabilizers, antidepressants, and anxiolytics; careful medication monitoring is necessary.

Psychotherapy is needed to help the individual with BPD manage the dysfunctional moods, impulsive behavior, and self-injurious behaviors. Specially trained

---

BOX 27.3

Response Patterns of Persons With Borderline Personality Disorder

Affective (mood) dysregulation
Mood lability
Problems with anger
Interpersonal dysregulation
Chaotic relationships
Fears of abandonment
Self-dysregulation
Identity disturbance or difficulties with sense of self
Sense of emptiness
Behavioral dysregulation
Parasuicidal behavior or threats
Impulsive behavior
Cognitive dysregulation
Dissociative responses
Paranoid ideation

Courtesy of M. Linehan, Department of Psychology, Box 351525, University of Washington, Seattle, WA 98195-1525, 1993.

---

therapists who are comfortable with the many demands of these patients are needed. These therapists represent a variety of mental health disciplines, including psychology, social work, and advanced practice nursing. This is a lifelong disorder requiring ongoing treatment as the individual copes with multiple interpersonal crises.

Priority Care Issues

Persons with BPD can be extremely volatile emotionally. Because they experience emotions so intensely, they are high risk for self-harm and suicide. Self-harm threats should be taken very seriously.

NURSING MANAGEMENT: Human Response to Borderline Personality Disorder

Persons with BPD may enter the mental health system early (young adulthood or before) because of their chaotic lifestyles. There are unstable moods, problems with interpersonal relationships, low self-esteem, and self-identity issues. Thinking and behavior are dysregulated (Box 27.3). They have problems in daily living, including maintaining intimate relationships, keeping a job, and living within the law (Box 27.4).

They drop in and out of treatment as it suits their mood and usually do not remain with one clinician for long-term treatment. They do not receive consistent treatment and usually seek help from health care workers because of consequences of their numerous life crises, medical conditions, and other psychiatric disorders (e.g., depression) or for physical treatment of self-injury. Thus, other problems usually may need attention before the patient's underlying personality disorder can be addressed. Sometimes the

BOX 27.4
BORDERLINE PERSONALITY DISORDER

JS is a 22-year-old single woman who was recently fired from her job as a data entry clerk. She is living with her mother and stepfather, who brought her to the emergency department after finding her crouched in a fetal position in the bathroom, her wrists bleeding. She seemed to be in a daze. This is her first psychiatric admission although her mother and stepfather have suspected that she has "needed help" for a long time. In high school, she received brief treatment for a potential eating disorder. She remains very thin but is able to eat at least one meal per day. During periods of stress, she will go for days without eating. Joanne is the second of three children. Her parents divorced when she was 3 years old. She has not seen her father since he left. Although she has pleasant memories of her father, her mother has told her that he beat Joanne and her sisters when he was drinking. When Joanne was 6 years old, her older sister died after an automobile accident. Joanne was in the car but was uninjured. As a child, Joanne was seen as a potential singing star. Her natural musical talent attracted her teachers' support, which encouraged her to develop her talent. She received singing lessons and entered statewide competitions in high school. Although she enjoyed the attention, she was never really comfortable

in the limelight and felt "guilty" about having a talent that she sometimes resented. She was able to make friends but found that she was unable to keep them. They described her as "too intense" and emotional. She had one boyfriend in high school, but she was very uncomfortable with any physical closeness. After ending the relationship with the boyfriend, she concentrated on dieting to have a "perfect body." When her dieting attracted her parents' attention, she vowed to eat just enough to keep them "off her back about it." She spent much of her leisure time with her grandmother. She attended college briefly but was unable to concentrate. It was during college and after her grandmother's death that Joanne began cutting her wrists during periods of stress. It seemed to calm her.

After leaving college, Joanne returned home. She had several jobs and short-lived friendships. She was usually fired from her job because of "moodiness," and it took her several months before she would again find another. She spent days in her room listening to music. Her recent episode occurred after she was fired from work and spent 3 days in her bedroom.

What Do You Think?
- How would you describe Joanne's mood?
- Are Joanne's losses (father, sister) really severe enough to affect her ability to relate to others now? Do the losses seem to relate to the self-injury?
- What behaviors indicate that there are problems with self-esteem and self-identity?

---

nurse will not know that the person has BPD. However, during an assessment, it becomes clear that these individuals let things bother them more than do others or have an inflexible view of the world. They also seem to have great difficulty changing behavior, no matter the consequences. Because they see the world differently from the average person, they have difficulty in successfully relating to other people and living a satisfying life.

Biologic Domain

Assessment

People with BPD are usually able to maintain personal hygiene and physical functioning. Because of the comorbidity of BPD and eating disorders and substance abuse, a nutritional assessment may be needed. The assessment should also include the use of caffeinated beverages, such as coffee, tea, soda, and alcohol. With patients who engage in binging or purging, assessment should include examining the teeth for pitting and discoloration, as well as the hands and fingers for redness and calluses caused by inducing vomiting. The patient should be queried about physi-

ologic responses of emotion. Sleep patterns also should be assessed because sleep alterations may suggest coexisting depression or mania.

Physical Indicators of Self-Injurious Behaviors

Patients with BPD should be assessed for self-injurious behavior or suicide attempts. It is important to ask the patient about specific self-abusive behaviors, such as cutting, scratching, or swallowing. The patient may wear long sleeves to hide injury on the arms. Specifically, asking about thoughts of hurting oneself when experiencing a major upset provides an opportunity for prevention and for coaching the patient toward alternative self-soothing measures.

Pharmacologic Assessment

Patients with BPD may be taking several medications. For example, one patient may be taking a small dose of an antipsychotic and a mood stabilizer. Another may be taking a selective serotonin reuptake inhibitor (SSRI). Initially, patients may be reluctant to disclose all of the medications they are taking because, for many, there has been a period of trial and error. They are fearful of having medication taken away from them. Development of rapport with special attention to a nonjudgmental approach is especially important when eliciting current medication practices. The effectiveness of the medication in relieving the target symptom needs to be determined. Use of alcohol, over-the-counter (OTC) medications, and street drugs should be carefully assessed to determine drug interactions.

Nursing Diagnoses for the Biologic Domain

Nursing diagnoses focusing on the biologic domain include Insomnia, Imbalanced Nutrition, Self-mutilation or Risk for Self-mutilation, and Ineffective Therapeutic Regimen Management.

Interventions for the Biologic Domain

The interventions for the biologic domain may address a whole spectrum of problems. Usually, the patients are managing hydration, self-care, and pain well. This section focuses on those areas that are most likely to be problematic.

Teaching Sleep Enhancement

Facilitation of regular sleep–wake cycles may be needed because of disturbed sleep patterns. Conservative approaches should be exhausted before recommending medication. Establishing a regular bedtime routine, monitoring bedtime snacks and drinks, and avoiding foods and drinks that interfere with sleep should be tried. If relaxation exercises are used, they should be adapted to the tolerance of the individual. Moderate exercises (e.g., brisk walking) 3 to 4 hours before bedtime activates serotonin and endorphins, thereby enhancing calmness and a sense of well-being before bedtime. For patients who have difficulty falling asleep and experience interrupted sleep, it helps to establish some basic sleeping routines. The bedroom should be reserved for only two activities: sleeping and sex. Therefore, the patient should remove the television, computer, and exercise equipment from the bedroom. If the patient is not asleep within 15 minutes, he or she should get out of bed and go to another room to read, watch television, or listen to soft music. The patient should return to bed when sleepy. If the patient is not asleep in 15 minutes, the same process should be repeated.

Special consideration must be made for patients who have been physically and sexually abused and who may be unable to put themselves in a vulnerable position (such as lying down in a room with other people or closing their eyes). These patients may need additional safeguards to help them sleep, such as a night light or repositioning of furniture to afford an easy exit.

Teaching Nutritional Balance

The nutritional status of the person with BPD can quickly become a priority, particularly if the patient has coexisting eating disorders, mood disorders, schizophrenia, or substance abuse. Eating is often a response to stress, and patients can quickly become overweight. This is especially a problem when the patient has also been taking medications that promote weight gain, such as antipsychotics, antidepressants, or mood stabilizers. Helping the patient learn the basics of nutrition, make reasonable choices, and develop other coping strategies are useful interventions. If patients are engaging in purging or severe dieting practices, teaching the patient about the dangers of both of these practices is important (see Chapter 30). Referral to an eating disorders specialist may be needed. In addition, a dietary consult can be recommended to explore the possibility of an omega-3 diet because some research indicates a beneficial effect with comorbid disorders that these patients usually experience (Ripoll, 2012; Stoffers, Völlm, Rücker, Timmer, Huband, & Lieb, 2010).

Preventing and Treating Self-Harm

Patients with BPD are usually admitted to the inpatient setting because of threats of self-harm. Observing for antecedents of self-injurious behavior and intervening before an episode are important safety interventions. Patients can learn to identify situations leading to self-destructive behavior and develop preventive strategies.

> **EMERGENCY CARE ALERT !** Because patients with BPD are impulsive and may respond to stress by harming themselves, observation of the patient's interactions and assessment of mood, level of distress, and agitation are important indicators of impending self-injury.

Remembering that self-harm is an effort to self-soothe by activating endogenous endorphins, the nurse can assist the patient to find more productive and enduring ways to find comfort. Linehan (1993) suggests using the Five Senses Exercise:

- Vision (e.g., go outside and look at the stars or flowers or autumn leaves)
- Hearing (e.g., listen to beautiful or invigorating music or the sounds of nature)
- Smell (e.g., light a scented candle, boil a cinnamon stick in water)

- Taste (e.g., drink a soothing, warm, nonalcoholic beverage)
- Touch (e.g., take a hot bubble bath, pet your dog or cat, get a massage)

Pharmacologic Interventions

Less medication is better for people with BPD. Patients should take medications only for target symptoms for a short time (e.g., an antidepressant for a bout with depression) because they may be taking many medications, particularly if they have a comorbid disorder, such as a mood disorder or substance abuse. Pharmacotherapy is used to control emotional dysregulation, impulsive aggression, cognitive disturbances, and anxiety as an adjunct to psychotherapy, but limited studies support the treatment of BPD with medication. Available evidence shows some benefit from atypical antipsychotics and mood stabilizers but little support for the use of antidepressants (Ripoll, 2012; Stoffers et al., 2010).

Administering and Monitoring Medications

In inpatient settings, it is relatively easy to control medications; in other settings, patients must be aware that it is their responsibility to take their medication and monitor the number and type of drugs being taken. Patients who rely on medication to help them deal with stress and those who are periodically suicidal are at high risk for abuse of medications. Patients who have unusual side effects are also at high risk for noncompliance. The nurse determines whether the patient is actually taking medication, whether the medication is being taken as prescribed, the effect on target symptoms, and the use of any OTC drugs (such as antihistamines or sleeping pills).

Managing Side Effects

Patients with BPD appear to be sensitive to many medications, and the dose may need to be adjusted based on the side effects they experience. Listen carefully to the patient's description of the side effects. Any unusual side effects should be accurately documented and reported to the prescriber.

Teaching Points

The patient cannot rely just on the medication. Assuming responsibility for taking the medication regularly, understanding the effects of the medication, and augmenting the medication with other strategies is the most effective approach. The nurse helps the patient assume this responsibility and provides guidance that supports self-efficacy and competence. It is also important for the nurse to emphasize that the medications provide the physiologic balance, but the patient's effort and skills provide the social and behavioral balance. By stressing this, the patient does not overinvest in the medication and feels more confident in her or his own skills.

Patients should be educated about the medications and their interactions with other drugs and substances. Interventions include teaching patients about the medication and how and where it acts in the brain and body, helping establish a routine for taking prescribed medication, reporting side effects, and facilitating the development of positive coping strategies to deal with daily stresses rather than relying on medications. Eliciting the patient's partnership in care improves adherence and thereby outcomes.

Psychological Domain
Assessment

People with BPD have usually experienced significant losses in their lives that shape their view of the world. They experience **inhibited grieving**, "a pattern of repetitive, significant trauma and loss, together with an inability to fully experience and personally integrate or resolve these events" (Linehan, 1993). They have unresolved grief that can last for years and avoid situations that evoke those feelings of separation and loss. During the assessment, the nurse can identify the losses (real or perceived) and explore the patient's experience during these losses, paying particular attention to whether the patient has reached resolution. A history of physical or sexual abuse and early separation from significant caregivers may provide important clues to the severity of the disturbances (Box 27.5).

Mood fluctuations are common and can be assessed by any number of the depression and anxiety screening scales or by asking the following questions:

- What things or events bother you and make you feel happy, sad, or angry?
- Do these things or events trouble you more than they trouble other people?
- Do friends and family tell you that you are moody?
- Do you get angry easily?
- Do you have trouble with your temper?
- Do you think you were born with these feelings or did something happen to make you feel this way?

Appearance and activity level generally reflect the person's mood and psychomotor activity. Many of those with BPD have been physically or sexually abused and thus should be assessed for depression. A disheveled appearance can reflect depression or an agitated state. When feeling good, these patients can be very engaging; they tend to be dramatic in their style of dress and attract attention, such as by wearing an unusual hairstyle or heavy makeup. Because physical appearance reflects identity, patients may experiment with their appearance and seek affirmation and acceptance from others. Body piercing, tattoos, and other adornments provide a mechanism to define self.

Impulsivity

Impulsivity can be identified by asking the patient if he or she does things impulsively or spur of the moment. For example: "Have there been times when you were hurt by your actions or were sorry later that you acted in the way you did?" Direct questions about gambling, choices in sexual partners, sexual activities, fights, arguments, arrests, and alcohol drinking habits can also help in identifying areas of impulsive behavior.

From a neurophysiologic perspective, impulsively acting before thinking seems to be mediated by rapid nerve firing in the mesolimbic area. This activates psychomotor responses before pathways reaching the prefrontal cortex (Wolf et al., 2011). Teaching the patient strategies to slow down automatic responses (e.g., deep breathing, counting to 10) buys time to think before acting.

Cognitive Disturbances

The mental status examination of those with BPD usually reveals normal thought processes that are not disor-ganized or confused except during periods of stress. Those with BPD usually exhibit dichotomous thinking, or a tendency to view things as absolute, either black or white, good or bad, with no perception of compromise. Dichotomous thinking can be assessed by asking patients how they view other people. Evidence of dichotomous thinking is indicated with responses of "good" or "bad," "wonderful" or "terrible."

Dissociation and Transient Psychotic Episodes

With BPD, there may be periods of dissociation and transient psychotic episodes. Dissociation can be assessed by asking if there is ever a time when the patient does not remember events or has the feeling of being separate from his or her body. Some patients refer to this as "spacing out." By asking specific information about how often, how long, and when dissociation first was used, the nurse can get an idea of how important dissociation is as a coping skill. It is important to ask the person what is happening in the environment when dissociation occurs. Frequent dissociation indicates a highly habitual coping mechanism that is difficult to change. Because transient psychotic states occur, it is also important to elicit data regarding the presence of hallucinations or delusions and their frequency and circumstances.

Risk Assessment: Suicide or Self-Injury

It is critical that patients with BPD be assessed for suicidal and self-damaging behavior, including alcohol and drug abuse (see Chapter 21). An assessment should include direct questions, asking if the patient thinks about or engages in self-injurious behaviors. If so, the nurse should continue to explore the behaviors: what is done, how it is done, its frequency, and the circumstances surrounding the self-injurious behavior. It is helpful to explain briefly to the patient that sometimes people cut, scratch, or pick at themselves as a way of bringing some relief and comfort. Although the behavior brings temporary relief, it also places the person at risk for infection. Approaching the assessment in this way conveys a sense of understanding and is more likely to invite the patient to disclose honestly.

Nursing Diagnoses for the Psychological Domain

One of the first diagnoses to consider is Risk for Self-mutilation because protection of the patient from self-injury is always a priority. If cognitive changes are present (dissociation and transient psychosis), two other diagnoses may be appropriate: Disturbed Thought Process and Ineffective Coping. The Disturbed Thought Process diagnosis is used if dissociative and psychotic

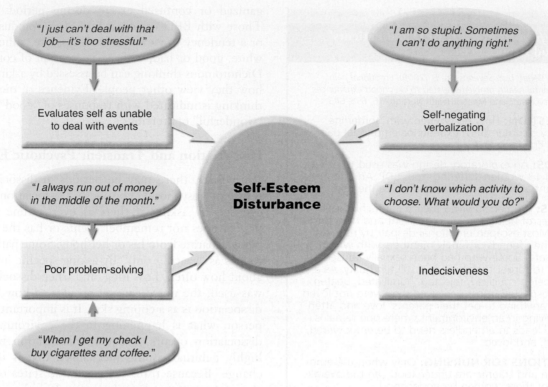

"I just can't deal with that job—it's too stressful."

Evaluates self as unable to deal with events

"I always run out of money in the middle of the month."

Poor problem-solving

"When I get my check I buy cigarettes and coffee."

Self-Esteem Disturbance

"I am so stupid. Sometimes I can't do anything right."

Self-negating verbalization

"I don't know which activity to choose. What would you do?"

Indecisiveness

FIGURE 27.1 Nursing diagnosis concept map: chronic low self-esteem.

episodes actually interfere with daily living. For example, a secretary could not complete processing letters because she was unable to differentiate whether the voices on the dictating machine were being transmitted by the machine or her hallucinations.

If the individual copes with stressful situations by dissociating or hallucinating, the diagnosis Ineffective Coping is used. The outcome in this instance would be the substitution of positive coping skills for the dissociations or hallucinations.

Other nursing diagnoses that are typically supported by assessment data include Personal Identity Disturbance, Anxiety, Grieving, Chronic Low Self-esteem, Powerlessness, Post-trauma Response, Defensive Coping, and Spiritual Distress. The identification of outcomes depends on the nursing diagnoses (Figure 27.1).

Interventions for the Psychological Domain

The challenge of working with people with BPD is engaging the patient in a therapeutic relationship that will survive its emotional ups and downs. The patient needs to understand that the nurse is there to coach her or him to develop self-modulation skills. A relationship based on mutual respect and consistency is crucial for helping the patient with those skills. Self-awareness skills are needed by the nurse along with access to clinical supervision

(Norrie, Davidson, Tata, & Gumley, 2013; Wright & Jones, 2012). Because patients with BPD are frequently hospitalized, even nurses in acute care settings have an opportunity to develop a long-term relationship (Figure 27.2).

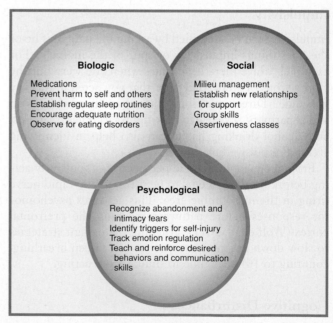

Biologic

Medications
Prevent harm to self and others
Establish regular sleep routines
Encourage adequate nutrition
Observe for eating disorders

Social

Milieu management
Establish new relationships
 for support
Group skills
Assertiveness classes

Psychological

Recognize abandonment and
 intimacy fears
Identify triggers for self-injury
Track emotion regulation
Teach and reinforce desired
 behaviors and communication
 skills

FIGURE 27.2 Biopsychosocial interventions for patients with borderline personality disorder.

> ## BOX 27.6 • THERAPEUTIC DIALOGUE • Borderline Personality Disorder

INEFFECTIVE APPROACH

Patient: Hey, you know what? You are my favorite nurse. That night nurse sure doesn't understand me the way you do.

Nurse: Oh, I'm glad you are comfortable with me. Which night nurse?

Patient: You know, Sue.

Nurse: Did you have problems with her?

Patient: She is terrible. She sleeps all night or she is on the telephone.

Nurse: Oh, that doesn't sound very professional to me. Anything else?

Patient: Yeah, she said that you didn't know what you were doing. She said that you couldn't nurse your way out of a paper bag (smiling).

Nurse: She did, did she? (Getting angry.) She should talk.

Patient: Well, I gotta go to group. Where will you be? I feel so much better if I know where you are. I don't know how I can possibly be discharged tomorrow.

EFFECTIVE APPROACH

Patient: Hey, you know what? You are my favorite nurse. That night nurse sure doesn't understand me the way you do.

Nurse: I really like you, Sara. Tomorrow you will be discharged, and I'm glad that you will be able to return home. (Nurse avoided responding to "favorite nurse" statement. Redirected interaction to impending discharge.)

Patient: That night nurse slept all night.

Nurse: What was your night like? (Redirecting the interaction to Sara's experience.)

Patient: It was terrible. Couldn't sleep all night. I'm not sure that I'm ready to go home.

Nurse: Oh, so you are not quite sure about discharge? (reflection)

Patient: I get so, so lonely. Then, I want to hurt myself.

Nurse: Lonely feelings have started that chain of events that led to cutting, haven't they? (validation)

Patient: Yes, I'm very scared. I haven't cut myself for 1 week now.

Nurse: Do you have a plan for dealing with your lonely feelings when they occur?

Patient: I'm supposed to start thinking about something that is pleasant—like spring flowers in the meadow.

Nurse: Does that work for you?

Patient: Yes, sometimes.

CRITICAL THINKING CHALLENGE

- How did the nurse in the first scenario get sidetracked?

- How was the nurse in the second scenario able to keep the patient focused on herself and her impending discharge?

Psychiatric-mental health registered nurses do not function as the patient's primary therapists, but they do need to establish a therapeutic relationship that strengthens the patient's coping skills and self-esteem and supports individual psychotherapy. The therapeutic relationship helps the patient to experience a model of healthy interaction with consistency, limit setting, caring, and respect for others (both self-respect and respect for the patient). Patients who have low self-esteem need help in recognizing genuine respect from others and reciprocating with respect for others. In the therapeutic relationship, the nurse models self-respect by observing personal limits, being assertive, and clearly communicating expectations (Box 27.6).

Using Dialectical Behavior Therapy

Dialectical behavior therapy (DBT) combines cognitive and behavior therapy strategies. Clinicians partner with patients and focus on the many interconnected behaviors (e.g., parasuicidal and substance abuse). Patients learn to understand their disorder by actively participating in establishing treatment goals, collecting data about their own behavior, identifying treatment targets, and working with the therapists in changing the problematic behaviors. When used on an inpatient basis with total staff commitment and reinforcement, improvement in depression, anxiety, and dissociation symptoms and a decrease in parasuicidal behavior occur (Bloom, Woodward, Susmaras, & Pantalone, 2012). Staff must maintain a positive approach and assume a skills coach role with patients. DBT is more often incorporated into a long-term partial hospitalization and outpatient treatment approach because the greatest effectiveness occurs when skills are reinforced over time and practiced in a variety of daily living settings.

Core interventions include problem solving, exposure techniques (gradual exposure to cues that set off aversive emotions), skill training, contingency management (reinforcement of positive behavior), and cognitive modification. **Skills groups** are an integral part of DBT and are taught in group settings in which patients practice emotional regulation, interpersonal effectiveness, distress tolerance, core mindfulness, and self-management skills.

Emotion regulation skills are taught to manage intense, labile moods and involve helping the patient label and analyze the context of the emotion and develop strategies to reduce emotional vulnerability. Teaching individuals to observe and describe emotions without judging them or blocking them helps patients experience emotions without stimulating secondary feelings that cause more distress. For example, describing the emotion of anger without judging it as being "bad" can eliminate feelings of guilt that lead to self-injury.

Interpersonal effectiveness skills include the development of assertiveness and problem-solving skills within an interpersonal context. *Mindfulness skills* are the psychological and behavioral versions of meditation skills usually taught in Eastern spiritual practice and are used to help the person improve observation, description, and participation skills by learning to focus the mind and awareness on the current moment's activity.

Distress tolerance skills involve helping the individual tolerate and accept distress as a part of normal life. *Self-management skills* focus on helping patients learn how to control, manage, or change behavior, thoughts, or emotional responses to events (Dimeff, Woodcock, Harned, & Beadnell, 2011; Linehan, 1993).

Addressing Abandonment and Intimacy Fears

A key to helping patients with BPD is recognizing their fears of both abandonment and intimacy, including as they relate to the nurse–patient relationship. Informing the patient of the length of this relationship as much as possible allows the patient to engage in and prepare for termination with the least pain of abandonment. If the patient's hospitalization is time limited, it is important to overtly acknowledge the limit and remind the patient with each contact how many sessions remain.

In day treatment and outpatient settings, the duration of treatment may be indeterminate, but the nurse may not be available that entire time. The termination process cannot be casual; this would stimulate abandonment fears. However, some patients end prematurely when the nurse informs them of the impending end as a way to leave before being rejected. The best approach is to explore these anticipated feelings with the patient. After careful planning, the nurse and patient discuss how to cope with anticipated feelings, including the wish to run away, review the progress the patient has made, and summarize what the patient has learned from the relationship that can be generalized to future encounters.

Establishing Personal Boundaries and Limitations

Personal boundaries are highly context specific; for example, stroking the hair of a stranger on the bus would be inappropriate, but stroking the hair and face of one's intimate partner while sitting together would be appropriate. Our personal physical space needs (boundaries) are distinct from behavioral and emotional limits we have. These concepts apply both to the patient and the nurse. Furthermore, limits may be temporary (e.g., "I can't talk with you right now, but after the change of shift, I can be available for 30 minutes").

Testing limits is a natural way of identifying where the boundaries are and how strong they are. Therefore, it is necessary to state clearly the enduring limits (e.g., the written rules or contract) and the consequences of violating them. The limits must then be consistently maintained. Clarifying limits requires making explicit what is usually implicit. Despite the clinical setting (e.g., hospital, day treatment setting, outpatient clinic), the nurse must clearly state the day, time, and duration of each contact with the patient and remain consistent in those expectations. This may mean having a standing appointment in day treatment or the mental health clinic or noting the time during each shift the nurse will talk individually with the hospitalized patient. The nurse should refrain from offering personal information, which is frequently confusing to the person with BPD. At times, the person may present in a somewhat arrogant and entitled way. It is important for the nurse to recognize such a presentation as reflective of internal confusion and dissonance. Responding in a very neutral manner avoids confrontation and a power struggle, which might also unwittingly reinforce the patient's internal sense of inferiority.

Some additional strategies for establishing the boundaries of the relationship include the following:

- Documenting in the patient chart the agreed-on appointment expectations

- Sharing the treatment plan with the patient
- Confronting violations of the agreement in a nonpunitive way
- Discussing the purpose of limits in the therapeutic relationship and applicability to other relationships

When patients violate boundaries, it is important to respond right away but without taking the behavior personally. For example, if a patient is flirtatious, simply say something like, "X, I feel uncomfortable with your overly friendly behavior. It seems out of place because we have a professional relationship. That would be more fitting for an intimate relationship that we will never have."

Using Behavioral Interventions

The goal of behavioral interventions is to replace dysfunctional behaviors with positive ones using the behavioral models discussed in Chapters 7 and 10. The nurse has an important role in helping patients control emotions and behaviors by acknowledging and validating desired behaviors and ignoring or confronting undesired behaviors. Patients often test the nurse for a response, and nurses must decide how to respond to particular behaviors. This can be tricky because even negative responses can be viewed as positive reinforcement for the patient. In some instances, if the behavior is irritating but not harmful or demeaning, it is best to ignore rather than focus on it. However, grossly inappropriate and disrespectful behaviors require confrontation. If a patient throws a glass of water on an assistant because she is angry at the treatment team for refusing to increase her hospital privileges, an appropriate intervention would include confronting the patient with her behavior and issuing the consequences, such as losing her privileges and apologizing to the assistant.

However, this incident can be used to help the patient understand why such behavior is inappropriate and how it can be changed. The nurse should explore with the patient what happened, what events led up to the behavior, what the consequences were, and what feelings were aroused. Advanced practice nurses or other therapists explore the origins of the patient's behaviors and responses, but the generalist nurse needs to help the patient explore ways to change behaviors involved in the current situation. The laboriousness of this analytical process may be a sufficient incentive for the patient to abandon the dysfunctional behavior.

Challenging Dysfunctional Thinking

The nurse can often challenge the patient's dysfunctional ways of thinking and encourage the person to think about the event in a different way. When a patient engages in catastrophic thinking, the nurse can chal-

---

BOX 27.7

Challenging Dysfunctional Thinking

Ms. S had worked for the same company for 20 years with a good job record. After an accident, she made some minor mistakes in her work that she quickly corrected. She informed her company nurse that her work was "really slipping" and that she was fearful of her coworkers' disapproval and getting fired from her job. The nurse asked her to keep a journal of coworkers' comments for the next week. At the next visit, the following dialogue occurred:

Nurse: I noticed that you received several compliments on your work. Even a close friend of your boss expressed appreciation for your work.

Ms. S: It was a light week at work. I really don't believe they meant what they said.

Nurse: I can see how you can believe that one or two comments are not genuine, but how do you account for four and five good reports on your work?

Ms. S: Well, I don't know.

Nurse: It looks like your beliefs are not supported by your journal entries. Now, what makes you think that your boss wants to fire you after 20 years of service?

---

lenge by asking, "What is the worst that could happen?" and "How likely would that be to occur?" Or in dichotomous thinking, when the patient fixates on one extreme perception or alternates between the extremes only, the nurse can ask the patient to think about any examples of exceptions to the extreme. The point of the challenge is not to debate or argue with the patient but to provide different perspectives to consider. Encouraging patients to keep journals of real interactions to process with the nurse or therapist is another effective way of testing the reality of their thinking and anticipations, affording more choices and flexibility (Box 27.7).

In problem solving, the nurse might encourage the patient to debate both sides of the problem and then search for common ground. Practicing communication and negotiation skills through role-playing helps the patient make mistakes and correct them without harm to her or his self-esteem. The nurse also encourages patients to use these skills in their everyday lives and report back on the results, asking patients how they feel applying the skills and how doing so affects their self-perceptions. Success, even partial success, builds a sense of competence and self-esteem (Table 27.1).

Providing Patient Education

Patient education within the context of a therapeutic relationship is one of the most important, empowering interventions for the generalist psychiatric–mental health nurse to use. Teaching patients skills to resist parasuicidal urges, improve emotional regulation, enhance interpersonal relationships, tolerate stress,

Table 27.1	THOUGHT DISTORTIONS AND CORRECTIVE STATEMENTS	
Thought Distortion		**Corrective Statement**
Catastrophizing		
"This is the most awful thing that has ever happened to me"		"This is a sad thing but not the most awful."
"If I fail this course, my life is over."		"If you fail the course, you can take the course again. You can change your major."
Dichotomizing		
"No one ever listens to me."		"Your husband listened to you last night when you told him . . ."
"I never get what I want."		"You didn't get the promotion this year, but you did get a merit raise."
"I can't understand why everyone is so kind at first and then always dumps me when I need them the most."		"It is hard to remember those kind things and times when your friends have stayed with you when you needed them."
Self-Attribution Errors		
"If I had just found the right thing to say, she wouldn't have left me."		"There is not a single right thing to say, and she left you because she chose to."
"If I had not made him mad, he wouldn't have hit me."		"He has a lot of choices in how to respond, and he chose hitting. You are responsible for your feelings and actions."

and enhance overall quality of life provides the foundation for long-term behavioral changes. These skills can be taught in any treatment setting as a part of the overall facility program (Box 27.8). If nurses are practicing in a facility where DBT is the treatment model, they can be trained in DBT and can serve as group skills leaders.

Managing Dissociative States

The desired outcome for someone who dissociates is to reduce or eliminate the dissociative experiences. The natural tendency is to want to "fix it." Unfortunately, there are limited medications for dissociation, but because the SSRIs, dopamine antagonists, and sero-tonin–dopamine antagonists affect other target symptoms, the dissociative experiences decrease. Because dissociation occurs during periods of stress, the best approach is to help the patient develop other strategies to deal with stress.

The nurse can teach the patient how to identify when he or she is dissociating and then to use some grounding strategies in the moment. Basic to grounding is planting both feet firmly on the floor or ground and then taking a deep abdominal breath to the count of 4, holding it to the count of 4, exhaling to the count of 4, and then holding it to the count of 4. This is called the four-square method of breathing. The benefit of this approach is to bring about a deep, slow breath that activates the calming mechanisms of the parasympathetic system.

After the grounding exercise, the patient uses one or more senses to make contact with the environment, such as touching the fabric of a nearby chair or listening to the traffic noise. As the patient improves in self-esteem and ability to relate to others, the frequency of dissociation should decrease.

Emotional Regulation

A major goal of cognitive therapeutic interventions is emotional regulation—recognizing and controlling the expression of feelings. Patients often fail even to recognize their feelings; instead, they respond quickly without thinking about the consequences. Remember, the time needed for taking action is shorter than the time needed for thinking before acting. Pausing makes up for the momentary lag between the limbic and autonomic response and the prefrontal response.

The nurse can help the patient identify feelings and gain control over expressions such as anger,

BOX 27.8

Psychoeducation Checklist: **Borderline Personality Disorder**

When caring for the patient with borderline personality disorder, be sure to include the following topic areas in the teaching plan:

- Management of medication, if used, including drug action, dosage, frequency, and possible adverse effects
- Regular sleep routines
- Nutrition
- Safety measures
- Functional versus dysfunctional behaviors
- Cognitive strategies (distraction, communication skills, thought stopping)
- Structure and limit setting
- Social relationships
- Recovery strategies
- Community resources

disappointment, or frustration. The goal is for patients to tolerate their feelings without feeling compelled to act out those feelings on another person or on themselves.

A helpful technique for managing feelings is known as the **communication triad**. The triad provides a specific syntax and order for patients to identify and express their feelings and seek relief. The "sentence" consists of three parts:

- An "I" statement to identify the prevailing feeling
- A nonjudgmental statement of the emotional trigger
- What the patient would like differently or what would restore comfort to the situation

The nurse must emphasize with patients that they begin with the "I" statement and the identification of feelings although many want to begin with the condition. If the patient begins with the condition, the statement becomes accusatory and likely to evoke defensiveness (e.g., "When you interrupt me, I get mad."). Beginning with "I" allows the patient to identify and express the feeling first and take full ownership. For example, the patient who is angry with another patient in the group might say, "Joe, I feel angry ("I" statement with ownership of feeling) when you interrupt me (the trigger or conditions of the emotion), and I would like you to apologize and try not to do that with me (what the patient wants and the remedy)." This simple skill is easy to teach, is easy to reinforce and to encourage others to reinforce, and is a surprisingly effective way of moderating the emotional tone.

Another element of emotional regulation is learning to delay gratification. When the patient wants something that is not immediately available, the nurse can teach patients to distract themselves, find alternate ways of meeting the need, and think about what would happen if they have to wait to meet the need.

The practice of **thought stopping** might also help the patient to control the inappropriate expression of feelings. In thought stopping, the person identifies what feelings and thoughts exist together. For example, when the person is ruminating about a perceived hurt, the individual might say, "Stop that" (referring to the ruminative thought) and engage in a distracting activity. Three activities associated with thought stopping are effective:

- Taking a quick deep breath when the behavior is noted (this also stimulates relaxation)
- Visualizing a stop sign or saying, "Stop" when possible (this allows the person to hear externally and internally)
- Deliberately replacing the undesired behavior with a positive alternative (e.g., instead of ruminating about an angry situation, think about a neutral or positive self-affirmation). The sequencing and combining of the steps puts the person back in control.

Managing Transient Psychotic Episodes

During psychotic episodes with auditory hallucinations, the patient should be protected from harming him- or herself or others. In an inpatient setting, the patient should be monitored closely and a determination made as to whether the voices are telling the patient to engage in self-harm (command hallucinations). The patient may be observed more closely and begin taking antipsychotic medication. In the community setting, the nurse should help the patient develop a plan for managing the voices. For example, if the voices return, the patient contacts the clinic and returns for evaluation. There may be a friend or relative who should be contacted or a case manager who can help the patient get the necessary protection if it is needed. In some instances, hearing the voices is a prelude to self-injury. Another person can help the patient resist the voices. After other aspects of the disorder are managed, the episodes of psychosis decrease or disappear.

Teaching and practicing distress tolerance skills help the patient have power over the voices and control intense emotions. When not experiencing hallucinations, the patient can practice deep abdominal breathing, which calms the autonomic nervous system. Using brainstorming techniques, the patient identifies early internal cues of rising distress while the nurse writes them on an index card for the patient to refer to later. Next, the nurse teaches some skills for tolerating painful feelings or events. To help the patient remember, suggest the mnemonic "A wise mind ACCEPTS" with the following actions:

- **A**ctivities to distract from stress
- **C**ontributing to others, such as volunteering or visiting a sick neighbor
- **C**omparing yourself with people less fortunate than you
- **E**motions that are opposite what you are experiencing
- **P**ushing away from the situation for a while
- **T**houghts other than those you are currently experiencing
- **S**ensations that are intense, such as holding ice in your hand (Linehan, 1993)

Social Domain

Assessment

Some individuals with BPD can function very well except during periods when symptoms erupt. They hold jobs, are active in communities, and can perform well. During periods of stress, symptoms often appear. On the other hand, some individuals with severe BPD function poorly; they are always in a crisis, which they have often created.

Social Support Systems

Identification of social supports, such as family, friends, and religious organizations, is the purpose in assessing resources. Knowing how the patient obtains social support is important in understanding the quality of interpersonal relationships. For example, some patients consider their "best friends" nurses, physicians, and other health care personnel. Because these are false friendships (i.e., not reciprocal), they inevitably lead to frustration and disappointment. However, helping the patient find ways to meet other people and encouraging the patient's efforts are more realistic.

Interpersonal Skills

Assessment of the person's ability to relate to others is important because interpersonal problems are linked to dissociation and self-injurious behavior. Information about friendships, frequency of contact, and intimate relationships provide data about the person's ability to relate to others. Patients with BPD often are sexually active and may have numerous sexual partners. Their need for closeness clouds their judgment about sexual partners, and it is not unusual to find these patients in abusive, destructive relationships with people with antisocial personality disorder. During assessment, nurses should use their own self-awareness skills to examine their personal response to the patient. How the nurse responds to the patient can often be a clue to how others perceive and respond to the person. For example, if the nurse feels irritated or impatient during the interview that is a sign that others respond to this person in the same way; on the other hand, if the nurse feels empathy or closeness, chances are this patient can evoke these same feelings in others.

Self-Esteem and Coping Skills

Coping with stressful situations is one of the major problems of people with BPD. Assessment of their coping skills and their ability to deal with stressful situations is important. Because the patient's self-esteem is usually very low, assessment of self-esteem can be done with a self-esteem assessment tool or by interviewing the patient and analyzing the assessment data for evidence of personal self-worth and confidence. Self-esteem is highly related to identifying with health care workers. Patients with BPD perceive their families and friends as being weary of their numerous crises and their seeming unwillingness to break the vicious self-destructive cycle. Feeling rejected by their natural support system, these indi-

viduals create one within the health system. During periods of crisis or affective instability, especially during the late evening, early morning, or on weekends, they call or visit various psychiatric units asking to speak to specific personnel who formerly cared for them. They even know different nurses' scheduled days off and make the rounds to several hospitals and clinics. Sometimes they bring gifts to nurses or call them at home. Because their newly created social support system cannot provide the support that is needed, the patient continues to feel rejected. One of the treatment goals is to help the individual establish a natural support network.

Family Assessment

Family members may or may not be involved with the patient. These individuals are often estranged from their families. In other instances, they are dependent on them, and this is also a source of stress. Childhood abuse is common in these families, and the perpetrator may be a family member. Ideally, family members are interviewed for their perspectives on the patient's problem. Assessment of any mental disorder in the patient's family and of the current level of functioning is useful in understanding the patient and identifying potential resources for support.

Nursing Diagnoses for the Social Domain

Defensive coping, Chronic Low Self-esteem, and impaired Social Interaction are nursing diagnoses that address the social problems faced by patients with BPD.

Interventions for the Social Domain

Environmental management becomes critical in caring for a patient with BPD. Because the unit can be structured to represent a microcosm of the patient's community, patients have an opportunity to identify relationship problems, boundary violations, and stressful situations. When these situations occur, the nurse can help the patient cope by finding alternative explanations for the situation and practicing new skills. Individual sessions help the patient to try out some skills, such as putting feelings into words without actions. Role-playing may help patients experience different degrees of effectively relating feelings without the burden of hurting someone they care about. Day treatment and group settings are excellent places for patients to learn more effective feeling management and to practice these techniques with each other. The group helps members develop empathy and diffuses attachment to any one person or therapist.

Building Social Skills and Self-Esteem

In the hospital, the nurse can use groups to discuss feelings and ways to cope with them. Women with BPD benefit from assertiveness classes and women's health issues classes. Many of the women are involved in abusive relationships and lack the ability to resolve these relationships because of their extreme anxiety regarding separating from those they love and their extreme need to feel connected. These women verbalize desires to leave, but they do not have the strength and self-confidence needed to leave. Exposing them to a different style of interaction as well as validation from other people increases their self-esteem and ability to separate from negative influences.

Implementing Interventions for Family Members

The family often serves as an informal case manager and is subject to all the stresses and challenges as the clinicians, usually without the specialized training and support of a treatment team. Few interventions are directed specifically at the family of the patient with BPD even though family therapy and multiple-family group therapy is helpful to families of these patients (Hoffman, Fruzzetti, & Buteau, 2007; Schuppert, Albers, Minderaa, Emmelkamp, & Nauta, 2012; Stobie & Tromski Klingshirn, 2009). Dependency on family members is a problem for many people with BPD. In some families, a patient's positive progress may be met with negative responses, and patients in these situations need help in maintaining a separate identity while staying connected to family members for social support. Usually, the nurse helps the patient explore family and new relationships that can provide additional social contacts and support.

Teaching Effective Ways to Communicate

An important area of patient education is teaching communication skills. Patients lack interpersonal skill in relating because they often had inadequate modeling and few opportunities to practice. The goals of relationship skill development are to identify problematic behavior that interferes with relationships and to use appropriate behaviors in improving relationships. The starting point is with communication. The nurse teaches the patient basic communication approaches, such as making "I" statements, paraphrasing what the other party says before responding, checking the accuracy of perceptions with others, compromising and seeking common ground, listening actively, and offering and accepting reactions. Besides modeling the behaviors, the nurse guides patients in practicing a variety of communication approaches for common situations. When role-playing, the nurse needs to discuss not only what the skills are and how to perform them but also the feelings patients have before, during, and after the role-play.

In day treatment and outpatient settings, the nurse can give the patient homework, such as keeping a journal, applying role-playing skills to actual situations, and observing behaviors in others. In the hospital, the patient can experience the same process, and the nurse is available to offer immediate feedback. Whatever the setting or even the specific problems addressed, the nurse must keep in mind and remind the patient that change occurs slowly. Thus, working on the problems occurs gradually, with severity of symptoms as the guide to deciding how fast and how much change to expect.

Evaluation and Treatment Outcomes

Evaluation and treatment outcomes vary depending on the severity of the disorder, the presence of comorbid disorders, and the availability of resources. For a patient with severe symptoms or continual self-injury, keeping the patient safe and alive may be a realistic outcome. Helping the patient resist parasuicidal urges may take years. In contrast, individuals who rarely need hospitalization and have adequate resources can expect to recover from the self-destructive impulses and learn positive interaction skills that promote a quality lifestyle. Most patients fall somewhere in between, with periods of symptom exacerbation and remission. In these patients, increasing the symptom-free time may be the best indicator of outcomes.

Continuum of Care

Treatment and recovery involves long-term therapy. Hospitalization is sometimes necessary during acute episodes involving parasuicidal behavior, but after this behavior is controlled, patients are discharged. It is important for these individuals to continue with treatment in the outpatient or day treatment setting. They often appear more competent and in control than they are, and nurses must not be deceived by these outward appearances. These individuals need continued follow-up and long-term therapy, including individual therapy, psychoeducation, and positive role models (see Nursing Care Plan 27.1).

(text continues on page 510)

NURSING CARE PLAN 27.1

The Patient With Borderline Personality Disorder

YJ, a 28-year-old, single woman, was brought to the emergency department of a hospital by police officers after finding her in a Burger Chef with superficial self-inflicted lacerations on both forearms. She pleaded with the police not to take her to the hospital. The police report noted that she fluctuated between intense crying and pleading to fighting physically and using foul language. By the time she arrived in the emergency department, however, she was calm, cooperative, pleasant, and charming. When asked why she cut herself, YJ reported she wasn't sure but added that her therapist was leaving today for a 4-week trip to Europe. YJ specifically asked the staff not to call her therapist because "she will be angry with me."

After the emergency physician examined YJ, the advanced practice mental health nurse assessed her developmental and psychiatric history and a summary of recent events, before she reached a provisional diagnosis of borderline personality disorder with a primary nursing diagnosis of risk for self-mutilation related to abandonment anticipation. YJ had several previous self-destructive episodes with minor injuries, only one requiring sutures, and two hospitalizations. She lives with her boyfriend, who is currently on a business trip, and works part time at a bookstore. Her invalid mother lives with her younger sister. There are no other relatives. YJ's father died traumatically in an automobile accident when she was 3 years old. YJ was in the car when it crashed; she received minor injuries.

Because YJ refused to agree not to harm herself, the nurse admitted YJ to the psychiatric unit with suicide precautions. Once on the unit, YJ was assessed by a staff nurse as having a basically normal mental status examination except that her mood was very tearful at times but charming and joking at other times. She said, "Don't mind me, I cry at the drop of a hat sometimes." Toward the middle of the interview she said, "I feel safer here than I ever felt before. It must be you. Are you sure you're just a staff nurse?" YJ agreed to a contract for safety just for today, but added, "Are you going to be my nurse tomorrow? I feel safest with you." When the nurse had completed her assessment, she showed YJ around the unit. As the nurse left her in the day room, YJ said, "My therapist doesn't understand me very well. I don't care if she is going out of town. After 4 years, she hasn't helped. If I had you as a therapist, I wouldn't be here now."

Setting: Inpatient Psychiatric Unit in a General Hospital

Baseline Assessment: YJ, a 28-year-old woman, came into the emergency department with superficial self-inflicted wounds on both forearms. There was a marked discrepancy in her behavior at the scene of the incident reported by emergency medical technicians from her presentation in the emergency department and now on the inpatient unit. She was admitted this time because she refused to agree not to harm herself further if released. She is angry and sad that her therapist is leaving for 4 weeks for a vacation and doesn't know how she will cope while the therapist is gone. She fears the therapist will not return.

Psychiatric Diagnosis	Medications
Borderline personality disorder	Sertraline (Zoloft) 150 mg daily for anxiety and depression

Nursing Diagnosis 1: Self-Mutilation

Defining Characteristics	Related Factors
Cuts and scratches on body Self-inflicted wounds	Fears of abandonment secondary to therapist's vacation Inability to handle stress

Outcomes

Initial	Discharge
1. Remain safe and not harm herself. 2. Identify feelings before and after cutting herself. 3. Agree not to harm herself over the next 24 h. 4. Identify ways of dealing with self-harming impulses if they return.	5. Verbalize alternate thinking with more realistic base. 6. Identify community resources to provide structure and support while therapist is gone.

Continued

NURSING CARE PLAN 27.1 *(Continued)*

Interventions

Interventions	Rationale	Ongoing Assessment
Monitor patient for changes in mood or behavior that might lead to selfinjurious behavior.	Close observation establishes safety and protection of patient from self-harm and impulsive behaviors.	Document according to facility policy. Continue to observe for mood and behavior changes.
Discuss with patient need for close observation and rationale to keep her safe.	Explanation to patient for purpose of nursing interventions helps her cooperate with the nursing activity.	Assess her response to increasing level of observation.
Administer medication as prescribed and evaluate medication effectiveness in reducing depression, anxiety, and cognitive disorganization.	Allows for adjustment of medication dosage based on target behaviors and outcomes.	Observe for side effects.
After 6–8 h, present written agreement to not harm herself.	Permits patient time to return to more thoughtful ways of responding rather than her previous reactive response. Also permits her to save face and avoid embarrassment of a losing power struggle if presented much earlier.	Observe for her willingness to agree to not harm herself.
Communicate information about patient's risk to other nursing staff.	The close observation should be continued throughout all shifts until patient agrees to resist self-harm urges.	Review documentation of close observation for all shifts.

Evaluation

Outcomes	Revised Outcomes	Interventions
Remained safe without further harming self. Identified fears of abandonment before cutting herself and relief of anxiety afterward.	Use hotlines or call friends if fears to harm self return.	Give patient hotline number and ask her to record friends' numbers in an accessible place.
She identified friends to call when fears return and hotlines to use if necessary.		
Agreed to not harm herself over the next 3 d.	Does not harm self for 3 d.	Remind her to call someone if urges return.
Enrolled in a day hospital program for 4 wk.	Attend day hospital program.	Follow-up on enrollment.

Nursing Diagnosis 2: Risk for Loneliness

Defining Characteristics	Related Factors
Social isolation	Fear of abandonment secondary to therapist's impending vacation

Outcomes

Initial	Discharge
1. Discuss being lonely. 2. Identify previous ways of coping with loneliness.	3. Identify strategies to deal with loneliness while therapist is away.

Continued

NURSING CARE PLAN 27.1 *(Continued)*

Interventions

Interventions	Rationale	Ongoing Assessment
Develop a therapeutic relationship.	People with BPD are able to examine loneliness within the structure of a therapeutic relationship.	Assess her ability to relate and nurse's response to the relationship.
Discuss past experience with therapist being gone with emphasis on how she was able to survive it.	She has survived therapist's absences before. By identifying the strategies she used, she can build on those strengths.	Assess her ability to assume any responsibility for "living through it." This will become a strength.
Acknowledge that it is normal to feel angry when the therapist is gone, but there are other strategies that may help the patient deal with the loneliness besides cutting.	Acknowledging feelings is important. Helping patient focus on the possibility of other strategies for dealing with the anger helps her regain a sense of control over her behavior.	Assess whether she is willing to acknowledge that there are other behavioral strategies of handling anger.
Begin immediate disposition planning with focus on day hospitalization or day treatment for skills training and management of loneliness.	While patient is in hospital, she is out of stressful environment in which she can learn more effective behaviors and use the therapy. Moving out of the hospital and back into outpatient therapy decreases possibility of regression and lost learning (Linehan, 1993).	Assess her willingness to learn new skills within a day treatment setting.
Teach her about stress management techniques. Assign her to anger management group while she is in the hospital.	Learning about ways of dealing with feelings and stressful situations helps the patient with BPD choose positive strategies rather than self-destructive ones.	Monitor whether she actually attends the groups. She should be encouraged to attend.

Evaluation

Outcomes	Revised Outcomes	Interventions
YJ was able to verbalize her anger about her therapist leaving and fears of abandonment. The last two times her therapist went on vacation, the patient became self injurious and was hospitalized for 2 wk.	None	
YJ was willing to be discharged the next day if she could attend day treatment while her therapist was gone.	Identify other strategies of dealing with therapist vacations besides cutting.	Attend stress management, communication, and self-comforting classes.

SUMMARY OF KEY POINTS

- A personality is a complex pattern of characteristics, largely outside of the person's awareness, that comprise the individual's distinctive pattern of perceiving, feeling, thinking, coping, and behaving.

- Personality disorder is an enduring pattern of inner experience and behavior that deviates markedly from the expectations of the individual's culture, is pervasive and inflexible, has an onset in adolescence or early adulthood, is stable over time, and leads to distress or impairment.

- People with borderline personality disorder have difficulties regulating emotion and have extreme fears of abandonment, leading to dysfunctional relationships; they often engage in self-injury.

- Medications, including mood stabilizers, antidepressants, and antipsychotics, are useful in regulating the symptoms. They should, however, only be taken for target symptoms for a short time because patients may already be taking other medications, particularly for a comorbid disorder.

- During hospitalizations, keeping the patients safe by preventing self-harm is priority. Open communication and use of dialectical behavior therapy techniques are important interventions.

- Recovery-oriented approaches are grounded in cognitive behavioral therapy. The interdisciplinary treatment or recovery team needs to maintain open communication to work effectively with a person with BPD.

CRITICAL THINKING CHALLENGES

1. Define the concepts *personality* and *personality disorder*. When does a normal personality become a personality disorder?

2. Karen, a 36-year-old woman receiving inpatient care, was admitted for depression; she also has a diagnosis of borderline personality disorder. After a telephone argument with her husband, she approaches the nurse's station with her wrist dripping with blood from cutting. What nursing diagnosis best fits this behavior? What interventions should the nurse use with the patient after the self-injury is treated?

3. A 22-year-old man with borderline personality disorder is being discharged from the mental health unit after a severe suicide attempt. As his primary psychiatric nurse, you have been able to establish a therapeutic relationship with him but are now terminating the relationship. He asks you to meet with him "for just a few sessions" after his discharge because his therapist will be on vacation. What are the issues underlying this request? What should you do? Explain and justify.

4. Compare the biologic theory with the psychoanalytic and Linehan's biosocial theory. What are the primary differences between these theories?

Fatal Attraction: 1987. This award-winning film portrays the relationship between a married attorney, Dan Gallagher (played by Michael Douglas), and Alex Forest, a single woman (played by Glenn Close). Their one-night affair turns into a nightmare for the attorney and his family as Alex becomes increasingly possessive and aggressive, demonstrating behaviors characteristic of borderline personality disorder, including anger, impulsivity, emotional lability, fear of rejection and abandonment, vacillation between adoration and disgust, and self-mutilation.

VIEWING POINTS: Identify the behaviors of Alex that are characteristics of borderline personality disorder. Identify the feelings that are generated by the movie. With which characters do you identify? For which characters do you feel sympathy? If Alex had lived and been admitted to your hospital, what would be your first priority?

M**O**VIE viewing**GUIDES** related to this chapter are available at http://thePoint.lww.com/Boyd5eUpdate.

A related Psychiatric-Mental Health Nursing video on the topic of Borderline Personality Disorder is available at http://thePoint.lww.com/Boyd5eUpdate.

References

American Psychiatric Association. (2013). *Diagnostic and statistical manual of mental disorders* (5th ed.) Arlington, VA: American Psychiatric Association.

Bloom, J. M., Woodward, E. N., Susmaras, T., & Pantalone, D. W. (2012). Use of dialectical behavior therapy in inpatient treatment of borderline personality disorder: A systematic review. *Psychiatric Services, 63*(9), 881–888.

Clarkin, J. F., & De Panfilis, C. (2013). Developing conceptualization of borderline personality disorder. *The Journal of Nervous and Mental Disease, 201*(2), 88–93.

Daros, A. R., Uliaszek, A. A., & Ruocco, A. C. (2014). Perceptual biases in facial emotion recognition in borderline personality disorder. *Personality Disorders, 5*(1), 79–87.

Dimeff, L. A., Woodcock, F. A., Harned, M. S., & Beadnell, B. (2011). Can dialectical behavior therapy be learned in highly structured learning environments? Results from a randomized controlled dissemination trial. *Behavior Therapy, 42*(2), 263–275.

Erikson, E. H. (1968). *Identity: Youth and crisis.* New York: Norton.

Fielding, P. (2013). The stigma of diagnosis. *Mental Health Practice, 17*(3), 11.

Gunderson, J. G., Stout, R. L., McGlashan, T. H., Shea, M. T., Morey, L. C., Gril, C. M., et al. (2011). Ten-year course of borderline personality disorder: Psychopathology and function from the collaborative longitudinal personality disorders study. *Archives of General Psychiatry, 68*(8), 827–837.

Hoffman, P. D., Fruzzetti, A. E., & Buteau, E. (2007). Understanding and engaging families: An education, skills and support program for relatives impacted by borderline personality disorder. *Journal of Mental Health, 16*(1), 69–82.

Koenigsberg, H. W., Denny, B. T., Fan, J., Liu, X., Guerreri, S., Mayson, S. J., et al. (2014). The neural correlates of anomalous habituation to negative emotional pictures in borderline and avoidant personality disorder patients. *American Journal of Psychiatry, 17*(1), 82–90.

Lawrence, K., Allen, J., & Channen, A. (2011). A study of maladaptive schemas and borderline personality disorder in young people. *Cognitive Therapy & Research, 35*(1), 30–39.

Linehan, M. (1993). *Cognitive-behavioral treatment of borderline personality disorder.* New York: Guilford Press.

Miano, A., Fertuck, E. A., Arntz, A., & Stanley, B. (2013). Rejection sensitivity is a mediator between borderline personality disorder features and facial trust appraisal. *Journal of Personality Disorders, 27*(4), 442–446.

Millon, T. (2011). *Disorders of Personality: Introducing a DSM/ICD Spectrum from Normal to Abnormal* (3rd ed.). Hoboken: John Wiley & Sons.

Mitchell, A. E., Dickens, G. L., & Picchioni, M. M. (2014). Facial emotion processing in borderline personality disorder: A systematic review and meta-analysis. *Neuropsychological Review, 24*(2):166–184. *doi:10.1007/s1106-014-9254-9*

Norrie, J., Davidson, K., Tata, P., & Gumley, A. (2013). Influence of therapist competence and quantity of cognitive behavioural therapy on suicidal behavior and inpatient hospitalisation in a randomized controlled trial in borderline personality disorder: Further analyses of treatment effects in the BOSCOT study. *Psychology and Psychotherapy, 86*(3), 280–293.

Ripoll, L. H. (2012). Clinical psychopharmacology of borderline personality disorder: an update on the available evidence in light of the Diagnostic and Statistical Manual of Mental Disorders-5. *Current Opinion in Psychiatry, 25*(1), 52–58.

Samuels, J. (2011). Personality disorders: Epidemiology and public health issues. *International Review of Psychiatry, 23*(3), 223–233.

Sansone, R. A. & Sansone, L. A. (2011). Gender patterns in borderline personality disorder. *Innovations in Clinical Neuroscience, 8*(5), 16–20.

Schuppert, H. M., Albers, C. J., Minderaa, R. B., Emmelkamp, P. M., & Nauta, M. H. (2012). Parental rearing and psychopathology in mothers of adolescents with and without borderline personality symptoms. *Child and Adolescent Psychiatry and Mental Health, 6,* 29. http://www.capmh.com/content/6/1/29.

Steele, H., & Siever, L. (2010). An attachment perspective on borderline personality disorder: in gene-environment considerations. *Current Psychiatry Reports, 12*(1), 61–67.

Stobie, M. R., & Tromski-Klingshirn, D. M. (2009). Borderline personality disorder, divorce and family therapy: The need for family crisis intervention strategies. *The American Journal of Family Therapy, 37*(5), 414–432.

Stoffers, J., Völlm, B. A., Rücker, G., Timmer, A., Huband, N., & Lieb, K. (2010). Pharmacological interventions for people with borderline personality disorder. *Cochrane Database of Systematic Reviews,* (1), CD005653.

Stone, M. H. (2013). The brain in overdrive: A new look at borderline and related disorders. (2013) *Current Psychiatry Reports, 15*(10), 1–8.

van Dijke, A., van der Hart, O., Ford, J. D., van Son, M., van der Heijden, P., & Bühring, M. (2010). Affect dysregulation and dissociation in borderline personality disorder and somatoform disorder: Differentiating inhibitory and excitatory experiencing states, *Journal of Trauma & Dissociation, 11*(4), 424–443.

Westen, D., Betan, E., & Defife, J. A. (2011). Identity disturbance in adolescence: Associations with borderline personality disorder. *Development and Psychopathology, 23*(1), 305–313.

Wolf, R. C., Sambataro, F., Vasic, N., Schmid, M., Thomann, P. A., Bienentreu, S. D., et al. (2011). Aberrant connectivity of resting-state networks in borderline personality disorder. *Journal of Psychiatry & Neuroscience, 36*(2), 402–411. doi:10.1503/jpn.100150

Wright, K., & Jones, F. (2012). Therapeutic alliances in people with borderline personality disorder. *Mental Health Practice, 16*(2), 31–35.

Zanarini, M. C., Laudate, C. S., Frankenburg, F. R., Reich, D. B., & Fitzmaurice, G. (2011). Predictors of self-mutilation in patients with borderline personality disorder: A 10-year follow-up study. *Journal of Psychiatric Research, 45*(6):823–828.

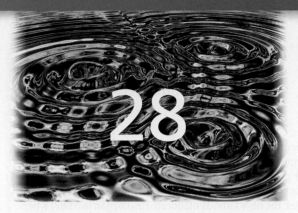

28

Antisocial Personality and Other Personality and Impulse-Control Disorders
Management of Personality Responses

Kimberlee Hansen and Mary Ann Boyd

KEY CONCEPTS

- antisocial personality disorder
- difficult temperament
- impulse-control disorders
- temperament
- impulsivity

LEARNING OBJECTIVES

After studying this chapter, you will be able to:

1. Describe the prevalence and incidence of personality disorders.
2. Delineate the clinical symptoms of antisocial personality with emphasis on temperament and impulsivity.
3. Analyze the theories explaining personality disorders, temperament, and impulsivity.
4. Identify evidence-based interventions for patients with personality disorders.
5. Develop recovery-oriented strategies that address the needs of persons with personality disorders.
6. Compare and contrast the disruptive, impulse-control disorders.

KEY TERMS

- attachment • avoidant personality disorder • conduct disorder • dependent personality • histrionic personality • intermittent explosive disorder • kleptomania • narcissistic personality • obsessive-compulsive personality disorder • oppositional defiant disorder • paranoid personality • psychopath • pyromania • schizoid personality • schizotypy • schizotypal personality disorder • sociopath

The concepts of personality and personality disorders were introduced in Chapter 27 along with the discussion of borderline personality disorder. This chapter highlights antisocial personality disorder (ASPD) along with the other personality disorders. Disruptive, impulse-control and conduct disorders, a closely related group of disorders, are also covered here.

ANTISOCIAL PERSONALITY DISORDER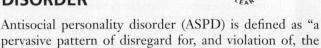

Antisocial personality disorder (ASPD) is defined as "a pervasive pattern of disregard for, and violation of, the rights of others occurring since age 15 years" (American Psychiatric Association [APA], 2013, p. 659). This diagnosis is given to individuals 18 years of age or older who fail to follow society's rules—that is, they do not believe that society's rules are made for them and are consistently irresponsible. For many, there is evidence of a conduct disorder (introduced later in the chapter) before the age of 15 years. The term **psychopath**, or **sociopath**, a person with a tendency toward antisocial and criminal behavior with little regard for others, is often used in describing the behaviors of people with ASPD.

> **KEYCONCEPT**   **Antisocial personality disorder** is characterized by a pervasive pattern of disregard for and violation of the rights of others.

Clinical Course and Diagnostic Criteria

ASPD has a chronic course, but the antisocial behaviors tend to diminish later in life, particularly after the age of 40 years (APA, 2013). Individuals with ASPD are arrogant and self-centered and feel privileged and entitled. They are self-serving, and they exploit and seek power over others. They can be interpersonally engaging and charming, which is often mistaken for a genuine sense of concern for other people. In reality, they lack empathy; are unable to express human compassion; and tend to be insensitive, callous, and contemptuous of others. Deceit and manipulation for personal profit or pleasure are central features associated with this disorder. They are behaviorally impulsive and interpersonally irresponsible. Many with this disorder repeatedly perform acts that are grounds for arrest (whether they are arrested or not), such as destroying property, harassing others, or stealing or pursuing other illegal occupations. They act hastily and spontaneously, are temperamentally aggressive and shortsighted, and fail to plan ahead or consider alternatives. They fail to adapt to the ethical and social standards of the community.

BOX 28.1
Using Reflection

WHO IS RESPONSIBLE?

INCIDENT • An adult patient with ASPD told the nurse that he had been arrested because his parents and wife would not pay his parking tickets. He further explained that his former boss was responsible for a shortage of funds that caused the patient to be fired. The nurse empathized with the patient and wondered how so many bad things could happen to one person. When family members arrived, they expressed sincere regret for not paying the parking tickets. His wife wondered what she had done wrong.

REFLECTION • Upon reflection, the nurse realized that the patient was not assuming responsibility for his own actions. The patient was blaming others for his poor judgment.

FAME & FORTUNE

David Hampton (1964–2003)
Socialite Imposter

PUBLIC PERSONA
Although his name might not be familiar, his story is. David Hampton was the teenager who gained infamy in the 1980s after conning New York's wealthy elite out of thousands of dollars by convincing them he was the son of actor Sidney Poitier. His now famous elaborate ruse began in 1983, when he and a friend were trying to get into Studio 54. Unable to gain entry, Hampton's friend decided to pose as Gregory Peck's son, while Hampton assumed the persona of "David Poitier" and touted himself as Sidney Poitier's son.

PERSONAL REALITIES
The cost of his deceit and swindling of New York's affluent ultimately ended formal charge of attempted burglary, for which he received 21 months in prison. His story became the inspiration for the play and later the movie titled *Six Degrees of Separation.* Attempting to turn the play's success to his own advantage, David Hampton gave interviews to the press; gate crashed producers' party; and began a campaign of harassment against the playwright John Guare, which included calls and death threats, prompting Guare to apply for a restraining order against Hampton. Believing others were profiting from his hoax, Hampton filed a $100 million lawsuit, claiming that the play had stolen the copyright on his persona and his story. The lawsuit was eventually dismissed.

Continuing to dupe others for money, attention, and entrée into New York society, Hampton met men in bars, dazzled them with his good looks and intellect, dropped celebrity tidbits, and then fleeced them, often using other alias names. Hampton's name appeared more often in crime reports than society pages for such crimes as fare beating, credit card theft, and threats of violence.

David Hampton's pursuit of a fabulous Manhattan life ended in July 2003 when he died alone of AIDS-related complications in Manhattan hospital.

Source: Barry, D. (2003, July 19). About New York: He conned the society crowd but died alone. *The New York Times.* Retrieved from http://www.nytimes.com/2003/07/19/nyregion/about-new-york-he-conned-the-society-crowd-but-died-alone.html.

They lack a sense of personal obligation to fulfill social and financial responsibilities, including those involved with being a spouse, parent, employee, friend, or member of the community (Box 28.1). They lack remorse for transgressions (APA, 2013).

Some of these individuals openly and flagrantly violate laws, ending up in jail (see Fame & Fortune). But most people with ASPD never come in conflict with the law and instead find a niche in society, such as in business, the military, or politics that rewards their competitive, tough behavior. Although ASPD is characterized by continual antisocial acts, the disorder is not

Diagnostic Criteria

A. A pervasive pattern of disregard for and violation of the rights of others, occurring since age 15 years, as indicated by three (or more) of the following:
1. Failure to conform to social norms with respect to lawful behaviors, as indicated by repeatedly performing acts that are grounds for arrest.
2. Deceitfulness, as indicated by repeated lying, use of aliases, or conning others for personal profit or pleasure.
3. Impulsivity or failure to plan ahead.
4. Irritability and aggressiveness, as indicated by repeated physical fights or assaults.
5. Reckless disregard for safety of self or others.
6. Consistent irresponsibility, as indicated by repeated failure to sustain consistent work behavior or honor financial obligations.
7. Lack of remorse, as indicated by being indifferent to or rationalizing having hurt, mistreated, or stolen from another.

B. The individual is at least age 18 years.
C. There is evidence of conduct disorder with onset before age 15 years.
D. The occurrence of antisocial behavior is not exclusively during the course of schizophrenia or bipolar disorder.

Associated Findings
• Lacking empathy
• Callous, cynical, and contemptuous of the feelings, rights, and suffering of others
• Inflated and arrogant self-appraisal
• Excessively opinionated, self-assured, or cocky
• Glib, superficial charm; impressive verbal ability
• Irresponsible and exploitative in sexual relationships; history of multiple sexual partners and lack of a sustained monogamous relationship
• Possible dysphoria, including complaints of tension, inability to tolerate boredom, and depressed mood

Reprinted with permission from the *Diagnostic and Statistical Manual of Mental Disorders*, Fifth Edition (Copyright ©2013). American Psychiatric Association. All Rights Reserved.

synonymous with criminality. See Key Diagnostic Characteristics 28.1.

Epidemiology and Risk Factors

Twelve-month prevalence rates of ASPD are estimated between 0.2% and 3.3% (APA, 2013). Males with alcohol use disorder and those from substance abuse clinics, prisons, or other forensic settings have the highest rates. Adverse socioeconomic (i.e., poverty) or sociocultural (i.e., migration) factors also are associated with higher prevalence (APA, 2013). Gender differences also exist in how symptoms manifest (Box 28.2).

Age of Onset

To be diagnosed with ASPD, the individual must be at least 18 years old and must have exhibited one or more childhood behavioral characteristics of conduct disorder before the age of 15 years, such as aggression to people or animals, destruction of property, deceitfulness or theft, or serious violation of rules. There is an increased likelihood of developing adult ASPD if there was an early onset of conduct disorder (before age 10 years) as well as an accompanying childhood attention deficit hyperactivity disorder (ADHD) diagnosis (APA, 2013).

Ethnicity and Culture

People with ASPD or psychopathic personalities are found in many cultures, including industrialized and non-industrialized societies. In a classic analysis of the Inuit of Northwest Alaska, individuals who knowingly break the rules when they are known are called *kunlangeta*, meaning "his mind knows what to do, but he does not do it" (Murphy, 1976, p. 1026). This term is used for someone who repeatedly lies, cheats, and steals. He is described as someone who does not go hunting and, when the other men are out of the village, takes sexual advantage of the women. In another culture in rural southwest Nigeria, the Yorubas use the word *arankan* to mean a "person who always goes his own way regardless of others, who is uncooperative, full of malice and bullheaded" (Murphy, 1976, p. 1026). In both cultures, the healers and shamans do not consider these people treatable.

In the United States, there are prevalence differences found among some of the cultural groups. In the 2001 to 2002 National Epidemiologic Survey on Alcohol and Related Conditions (*n* = 43,093), the odds of ASPD were greater among Native Americans and lower among Asians compared with whites (Grant et al., 2004).

Comorbidity

ASPD is associated with several other psychiatric disorders, including mood, anxiety, and other personality disorders. ASPD is strongly associated with alcohol and drug abuse (Black, Gunter, Loveless, Allen, & Sieleni, 2010). However, a diagnosis of ASPD is not warranted if the antisocial behavior occurs only in the context of substance abuse. For example, some people who misuse substances sometimes engage in criminal behavior, such as stealing or prostitution, only when in pursuit of drugs. Therefore, it is crucial to assess whether the person with possible ASPD has engaged in illegal activities at times other than when pursuing or using substances.

Clinical Vignette

BOX 28.2
ANTISOCIAL PERSONALITY DISORDER: MALE VERSUS FEMALE

Stasia (female) and Jackson (male) are fraternal twins, 22 years old, who received diagnoses of antisocial personality disorder. The following are their clinical profiles.

Jackson

Jackson is currently in the county jail for the third time. Although his juvenile records begin at age 9 years and include misdemeanors and class B felonies, his burglary conviction is his first adult crime. His school teachers thought Jackson was very bright but that he had significant difficulty with peers and authority figures. He fought regularly, was described as a bully, and seemed always to be scamming. At age 16 years, Jackson dropped out of school and joined a gang.

Jackson's juvenile probation officer explained that Jackson came from a very violent family and neighborhood and described the situation by saying, "If gangs hadn't gotten him, his father would have." His lawyer described him as "a likeable guy, but I wouldn't turn my back on him."

The jail nurse described Jackson as "a real charmer, but nothing is ever his fault." Oddly, he is the only person in the jail with an adequate supply of cigarettes and CDs. "We get along fine," the nurse says. "I don't understand why guards

have such difficulty with him." Sometimes the guards send Jackson to the dispensary for injuries, and Jackson plaintively explains to the nurse, "Those guards beat me up again; I don't know why."

Stasia

Stasia was recently hospitalized for the sixth time when one of her male friends beat her. She has been working as a prostitute for 5 years. Her physical examination noted not only multiple bruises but also tattoos that cover 50% of her body. In addition, she has piercings of her tongue, ears, eyebrow, lips, and nipples. She is emotionally volatile, manipulative, and angry. Stasia has many acquaintances and sexual partners, but none are truly intimate. She has periods when she uses drugs regularly.

Stasia and Jackson's mother was jailed when the twins were 18 months old and did not return until they were 6 years old. They were raised mostly by their paternal grandmother, who hated their mother and reminded Stasia frequently of how much she looked like her mother. Their father, when present, was violent toward Jackson and sexually abused Stasia.

What Do You Think?

- How might gender influence the development of symptoms?
- How might culture influence early recognition of problems and provision of early intervention to prevent future serious mental disorders?

- What are some possible outcomes in this situation?
- How does this case demonstrate the interaction between socialization, biology, and culture?

Etiology

Biologic Theories

Perhaps more than any other personality disorder, there exists an extensive number of biologically oriented studies that explore the genetic bases, neuropsychological factors, and arousal levels among this group of pathologies (Millon, 2011). Many of these studies show changes associated with personality disorders or characteristics, but we do not have evidence that these changes caused the disorder. These studies often overlap with studies of aggression, temperament, and substance use (Alcorn, Gowin, Green, Swann, Moeller, & Lane, 2013; Jovev, Whittle, Yücel, Simmons, Allen, & Chanen, 2014).

Early MRI studies showed that persons with ASPD failed to activate the limbic-prefrontal circuit (amygdala, orbitofrontal cortex, insula, and anterior cingulate) during fearful situations (Birbaumer et al., 2005). These findings support the neural basis of fearlessness in these individuals. Impairment in moral judgment is associated with dysfunction of the prefrontal cortex (Taber-Thomas, Asp, Koenigs, Sutterer, Anderson, & Tranel, 2014). Emotional distance, aggression, and impulsivity are consistently associated with neural dysfunction (Millon, 2011).

Psychological Theories

Scientists believe temperament is neurobiologically determined, and many believe that it is central to understanding personality disorders. A temperament, the natural predisposition to express feelings and actions, is evident during the first few months of life and remains stable through development. For example, whereas some infants are more relaxed or calm and sleep a lot, others are extremely alert, startled by the slightest noise, cry more, and sleep less.

Difficult temperaments are common in ASPD and are often at the basis of their aggression and impulsivity.

> **KEYCONCEPT** **Temperament** is a person's characteristic intensity, rhythmicity, adaptability, energy expenditure, and mood. A **difficult temperament** is characterized by withdrawal from stimuli, low adaptability, and intense emotional reactions. Four key behaviors are present in a difficult temperament: aggression, inattention, hyperactivity, and impulsivity.

Temperaments consist of two behavioral dimensions that interact with each other. The activity spectrum varies from intense to passive. The adaptability spectrum varies from having a positive attitude about new stimuli with high flexibility to withdrawal from new stimuli and minimal flexibility in response to change. There is a strong relationship between difficult temperament and ASPD behaviors (Lennox & Dolan, 2014).

One of the leading explanations of ASPD is that unsatisfactory attachments in early relationships lead to antisocial behavior in later life. **Attachment**, attaining and retaining interpersonal connection to a significant person, begins at birth. In a secure attachment, a child feels safe, loved, and valued and develops the self-confidence to interact with the rest of the world. Experiences within the context of secure relationships enable the child to develop trust in others. Strong attachments between parents and child may lower the risk of delinquency, assault, and other offenses that are characteristic of those who develop antisocial behavior (Sousa et al., 2011).

In individuals with ASPD, a failure to make or sustain stable attachments in early childhood can lead to avoidance of future attachments. Risk factors for developing dysfunctional attachments include parental abandonment or neglect, loss of a parent or primary caregiver, and physical or sexual abuse. Parents who lacked secure attachment relationships in their own childhoods may be unable to form secure attachment relationships with their own children.

Social Theories

In many cases, individuals with ASPD come from chaotic families in which alcoholism and violence are the norm. Individuals who have been victims of abuse or neglect, live in a foster home, or had several primary caregivers are more likely to be victimized by antisocial behaviors, especially aggression (Gao, Raine, Chan, Veneables, & Mednick, 2010). Child abuse and growing up in a home with domestic violence increases risk of antisocial behavior (Sousa et al., 2011). However, it is difficult to separate the influence of social factors on the development of the disorder because the symptoms of ASPD are expressed as social manifestations, including unemployment, divorces and separations, and violence.

Family Response to Disorder

If family members are present in a patient's life, they have probably been abused, mistreated, or intimidated by these patients. For example, one patient sold his mother's possessions while she was at work. Another abused his wife after drinking. However, family members may be fiercely loyal to the patient and blame themselves for his or her shortcomings.

Interdisciplinary Treatment

People rarely seek mental health care for ASPD but rather for treatment of depression, substance abuse, uncontrolled anger, or forensic-related problems. Patients with psychiatric disorders who are admitted through the courts often have a comorbid diagnosis of ASPD. Antisocial personality disordered patients usually present for treatment as a result of an ultimatum. Treatment is often a choice between losing a job, being expelled from school, ending a marriage or relationship with children, or giving up on a chance at probation and psychological treatment. Under these circumstances treatment is usually forced on them; most prisons and other correctional facilities require inmates to attend psychotherapy sessions. In either case working with people with ASPD is likely to be a frustrating and exasperating experience for the nurse due to the patient's clear lack of insight and/or motivation to change. People with ASPD do not regard their behavior to be problematic for themselves and its consequences for others, who are judged to be potentially unreliable and disloyal, is not a concern of theirs. The patients attitude toward nurse involved in their care typically take one of two forms. Either the person with ASPD will try to enlist the nurse as an ally against those individuals who forced them to enter therapy or, alternatively, will try to con the nurse into being impressed with his or her insight and reform in an effort to secure advantage with some legal institution (Millon, 2011). Treatment is difficult and involves helping the patient alter his or her cognitive schema. The overall treatment goals are to develop a nurturing sense of attachment and empathy for other people and situations and to live within the norms of society.

Priority Care Issues

Patients with ASPD are often very persuasive and engage staff with complimentary, but divisive statements such as "You are the only one who understands me." "How can you stand to work here with all these jerks, I swear you are the only nice nurse on the whole floor." If the nurse engages and supports this type of interaction, the nurse may inadvertently set up dysfunctional group dynamics with staff members that lead to trust and communication problems. The nurse should remain objective in interacting and avoid compromising situations such as granting special favors or privileges. Persons with ASPD use charm, cunningness, and even seduction to impress and manipulate others for their own purposes, and to gain the nurse's favor.

Although they can be interpersonally charming, these patients can become verbally and physically abusive if their expectations are not met. Protection of other patients and staff is a priority.

NURSING MANAGEMENT: Antisocial Personality Disorder

Biologic Domain

Assessment

ASPD does not significantly impair physical functioning unless there is coexisting substance use disorder or another psychiatric diagnosis involved. Because substance abuse is a major problem with this population, the physical effects of chronic use of addictive substances must be considered. Conversely, someone who has health problems secondary to chronic substance misuse should also be assessed for co-occurring personality disorders.

Nursing Diagnoses for the Biologic Domain

A common nursing diagnosis in ASPD is Dysfunctional Family Processes.

Interventions for Biologic Domain

In instances in which there are co-occurring disorders, the personality disorder may actually interfere with interventions aimed at improving physical functioning. For example, a patient with schizophrenia and ASPD may not develop enough trust within a relationship to examine his or her delusional thoughts or other aspects of dysfunction, such as alcohol or drug abuse.

Psychological Domain

Assessment

Many patients with ASPD are committed to mental health care by the court system. Assessment generally involves using basic psychological assessment tools to evaluate aberrant behaviors.

Nursing Diagnoses for the Psychological Domain

Because so many patients with ASPD have dysfunctional thinking patterns, a common nursing diagnosis is Risk for Other Directed Violence.

Interventions for the Psychological Domain

Therapeutic relationships are difficult to establish because these individuals do not attach to others and are often unable to use the relationship to change behavior. The goal of the therapeutic relationship is to identify dysfunctional thinking patterns and develop new problem-solving

behaviors. After the first few meetings with these patients, the nurse may believe that the relationship has a good start, but in reality, a superficial alliance is usually formed. Additional sessions reveal the lack of patient commitment to the relationship. These patients begin to revisit topics discussed in previous sessions or lose interest in trying to work on problems. By using self-awareness skills and accessing supervision regularly, the nurse can identify blocks in the development of a therapeutic relationship (or lack of) and his or her response to the relationship. See Nursing Care Plan 28.1.

Facilitating Self-Responsibility

Facilitating self-responsibility (encouraging a patient to assume more responsibility for personal behavior) is an important intervention. The nursing activities that are particularly helpful include holding the patient responsible for his or her behavior, monitoring the extent that self-responsibility is assumed, and discussing the consequences of not dealing with responsibilities. The nurse needs to refrain from arguing or bargaining about the unit rules, such as time for meals, use of the television room, and smoking. Instead, positive feedback is given to the patient for accepting additional responsibility or changing behavior.

Enhancing Self-Awareness

Enhancing self-awareness (exploring and understanding personal thoughts, feelings, motivation, and behaviors) is another nursing intervention that is helpful in developing an understanding about relating peacefully to the rest of the world. Encouraging patients to recognize and discuss their thoughts and feelings helps the nurse understand how the patient views the world. Some evidence indicates that substance misuse can be improved through cognitive behavioral treatment, but there is little evidence that the core problems of this disorders (aggression, reconviction, global functioning, and social functioning) are improved with psychological interventions (Gibbon et al., 2010).

Teaching Points

Patient education efforts have to be creative and thought provoking. In teaching a person with ASPD, a direct approach is best, but the nurse must avoid "lecturing," which the patient will resent. In teaching the patient about positive health care practices, impulse control, and anger management, the best approach is to engage the patient in a discussion about the issue and then direct the topic to the major teaching points. These patients often take great delight in arguing or showing how the rules of life do not apply to them. A sense of humor is important, as are clear teaching goals and avoiding being sidetracked (see Box 28.3).

NURSING CARE PLAN 28.1

The Patient With Antisocial Personality Disorder

Danny, a 28-year-old man, was brought to the emergency department of the psychiatric hospital by the local police after threatening suicide. He was arrested and jailed after physically assaulting his girlfriend with whom he lives after she called the police. "I hit her because she nags me. I went to jail because my girlfriend called the police." Danny is now homeless after his girlfriend obtained a restraining order. Danny was diagnosed with conduct disorder at age 10, has a history of being aggressive toward animal and people, often tormented small animals and younger children, and was expelled from high school after repeated conflicts with authority figures. He has not held a job more than a few months and has never been able to independently support himself. He is easily bored and behaves irresponsibly.

Setting: Inpatient Psychiatric Unit in a General Hospital

Baseline Assessment: Danny is a 28-year-old male with a quick walk and an engaging smile. He appears confident. After his arrest, he attempted to commit suicide by hanging in his cell. He currently denies any suicidal ideation. His family reports that he has been in trouble all his life, most recently for selling drugs. Danny believes that he has to put his own needs above others and that he can exploit others because they will eventually take advantage of him. His father is currently in prison for murder.

Associated Psychiatric Diagnoses	Medications
Antisocial personality disorder	None

Nursing Diagnosis 1: Risk for Suicide

Defining Characteristics	Related Factors
Threatened to commit suicide	Has no real friends Arrested for assaulting girlfriend History of numerous arrests

Outcomes

Initial	Discharge
1. Remain safe and not harm himself. 2. Agree not to harm himself over the next 24 h.	3. Identify ways of dealing with stress instead of suicide threats. 4. Verbalize alternate thinking with a more realistic base.

Interventions

Interventions	Rationale	Ongoing Assessment
Monitor patient for changes in mood or behavior that might lead to self-injurious behavior. Discuss with the patient the need for close observation and rationale to keep him safe.	Close observation establishes safety and protection of patient from self-harm and impulsive behaviors. Close observation should be continued throughout all shifts until the patient agrees to resist self-harm urge.	Document according to facility policy. Continue to observe for mood and behavior changes. Communicate information about the patient's risk to other nursing staff. Review documentation of close observation for all shifts.

Evaluation

Outcomes	Revised Outcomes	Interventions
Remained safe without further harming self	None	

Continued

NURSING CARE PLAN 28.1 *(Continued)*

Nursing Diagnosis 2: Ineffective Role Performance

Defining Characteristics	Related Factors
Violence, harassment Inadequate coping Inadequate self-management System conflict	Inadequate role preparation Lack of education Unrealistic role expectations

Outcomes

Initial	Discharge
1. Identify need to learn new coping skills. 2. Begin to assume responsibility for actions. 3. Seek substance abuse treatment.	4. Develop a plan to finish high school. 5. Seek additional help in developing empathy for others.

Interventions

Interventions	Rationale	Ongoing Assessment
Discuss the importance of looking at lifestyle and relationship with others.	People with antisocial personality disorder often blame others for their misfortune. Focusing on lifestyle and relationships initiates a dialogue.	Observe the willingness of Danny to assume responsibility for own choices.

Evaluation

Outcomes	Revised Outcomes	Interventions
Expressed interest in changing lifestyle only if nurse agreed to maintain contact after discharge.	Continue to discuss lifestyle and developing positive relationships. None	Set boundary limits with Danny. Emphasize the importance of personal responsibility for behavior change.

Social Domain

Assessment

Eliciting social data from persons with ASPD may be difficult because of their basic mistrust toward authority figures.

BOX 28.3

Psychoeducation Checklist: **Antisocial Personality Disorder**

When caring for the patient with antisocial personality disorder, be sure to include the following topic areas in the teaching plan:

- Positive health care practices, including substance abuse control
- Effective communication and interaction skills
- Impulse control
- Anger management
- Group experience to help develop self-awareness and impact of behavior on others
- Analyzing an issue from the other person's viewpoint
- Maintenance of employment
- Interpersonal relationships and social interactions

They may not give an accurate history or may embellish aspects to project themselves in a more positive light. They often deny any criminal activity even if they are admitted in police custody. Key areas of assessment are determining the quality of relationships, impulsivity, and the extent of aggression. These individuals do not assume responsibility for their own actions and often blame others for their misfortune. Their disregard for others is manifested in their interactions. For example, one patient with human immunodeficiency virus was engaging in unprotected sex with several different women because he wanted to "have fun as long as I can." He was completely unconcerned about the possibility of transmitting the virus. These individuals often make good first impressions. Self-awareness is especially important for the nurse because of the initial charming quality of many of these individuals. When these patients realize that the nurse cannot be used or manipulated, they lose interest in the nurse and revert to their normal, egocentric behaviors.

Nursing Diagnoses for the Social Domain

Nursing diagnoses for patients with ASPD are related to their interpersonal detachment, lack of awareness of

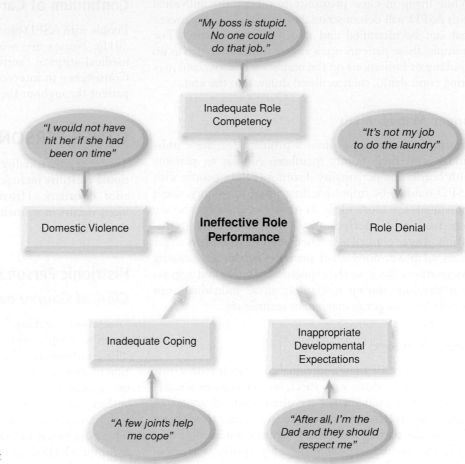

FIGURE 28.1   Nursing diagnosis concept map: Ineffective Role Performance.

others, avoidance of feelings, impulsiveness, and discrepancy between their perception of themselves and others' perception of them. Typical diagnoses are Ineffective Role Performance (unemployment) (Fig. 28.1), Ineffective Individual Coping, Impaired Communication, Impaired Social Interactions, Low Self-esteem, and Risk for Violence. Outcomes should be short term and relevant to a specific problem. For example, if a patient has been chronically unemployed, a reasonable short-term outcome is to set up job interviews rather than obtain a job.

Interventions for the Social Domain

These patients have a long-standing history of difficulty in interpersonal relationships. In an inpatient unit, interventions can be more intense and focus on helping the patient develop positive interaction skills and experience a consistent environment. For example, the focus of nursing interventions may be the patient's continual disregard of the rights of others. On one unit, a patient continually placed orders for pizzas in the name of another patient who had limited intelligence and was genuinely afraid of the person with ASPD. The victimized patient always paid for the pizza. When the nursing staff realized

what was happening, they confronted the patient with ASPD about the behavior and revoked his unit privileges.

Group Interventions

Group interventions are more effective than individual modalities because other patients and staff can validate or challenge the patient's view of a situation. Problem-solving groups that focus on identifying a problem and developing a variety of alternative solutions are particularly helpful because patient self-responsibility is reinforced when patients remind each other of the better alternatives. Patients are likely to confront each other with dysfunctional schemas or thinking patterns. Teaching patients with ASPD the same communication techniques as those with borderline personality disorder will also encourage self-responsibility. These patients often attend groups that focus on the development of empathy.

Milieu Interventions

Milieu interventions, such as providing a structured environment with rules that are consistently applied to patients who are responsible for their own behavior, are important.

While living in close proximity to others, the individual with ASPD will demonstrate dysfunctional social patterns that can be identified and targeted for correction. For example, these patients often violate ward rules, such as no smoking or limitations on the number of visitors, and may bring contraband, such as illegal drugs, into the unit.

Anger Management

Aggressive behavior is often a problem for these individuals and their family members. Similar to patients with borderline personality disorder (BPD), people with ASPD tend to be impulsive. Instead of self-injury, these individuals are more likely to strike out at those who are perceived to be interfering with their immediate gratification. Anger control assistance (helping to express anger in an adaptive, nonviolent manner) becomes a priority intervention. Because the expression of anger and aggression develops during a lifetime, these individuals can benefit from anger management techniques.

Social Support

Social support for these individuals is often minimal, just as it is for individuals with BPD, but the reasons are different. These individuals have often taken advantage of friends and relatives who, in turn, no longer trust them. Helping the patient build a new support system after new skills are learned is usually the only option. For these individuals to develop friends and re-engage family members, they must learn to interact in new ways, develop empathy, and risk an attachment. For many, this never truly becomes a reality.

Interventions for Family Members

Family members of patients with ASPD usually need help in establishing boundaries. Because there is a long-term pattern of interaction in which family members feel responsible for the patient's antisocial behavior, these patterns need to be interrupted. Families need help in recognizing the patient's responsibility for his or her actions.

Evaluation and Treatment Outcomes

The outcomes of interventions for patients with ASPD need to be evaluated in terms of management of specific problems, such as maintaining employment or developing a meaningful interpersonal relationship. The nurse will most likely see these patients for other health care problems, so adherence to treatment recommendations and development of health care practices (e.g., reduce smoking and alcohol consumption) can also be factored into the evaluation of outcomes.

Continuum of Care

People with ASPD rarely seek mental health care (Millon, 2011). Nurses are most likely to see these patients in medical–surgical settings for comorbid conditions. Consistency in interventions is necessary in treating the patient throughout the continuum of care.

OTHER PERSONALITY DISORDERS

Two other personality disorders characterized by emotional volatility include histrionic and narcissistic personality disorders. Histrionic personality disorder more likely occurs in women and narcissistic personality disorder in men.

Histrionic Personality Disorder

Clinical Course and Diagnostic Criteria

"Attention seeking," "excitable," and "emotional" describe people with **histrionic personality** disorder. These individuals are lively and dramatic and draw attention to themselves by their enthusiasm, dress, and apparent openness. They are the "life of the party" and, on the surface, seem interested in others. Their insatiable need for attention and approval quickly becomes obvious. There are two main ways their need to be "center stage" is exhibited: (1) their interests and topics of conversation focus on their own desires and activities, and (2) their behavior, including their speech, continually calls attention to themselves. These needs are inflexible and persistent even after others attempt to meet them. Persons with histrionic personality disorders are quick to form new friendships and just as quick to become demanding. Because they are trusting and easily influenced by other opinions, their behavior often appears inconsistent. Their strong dependency need makes them overly trusting and gullible. They are moody and often experience a sense of helplessness when others are disinterested in them. They are sexually seductive in their attempts to gain attention and often are uncomfortable within a single relationship. Their appearance is provocative and their speech dramatic. They express strong opinions without supporting facts. Loyalty and fidelity are lacking (APA, 2013).

Gender influences the manifestations of this disorder. Women dress seductively, may express dependency on selected men, and may "play" a submissive role. Men may dress in a very masculine manner and seek attention by bragging about athletic skills or successes in their jobs. Individuals with this disorder have difficulty achieving any true intimacy in interpersonal relationships. They seem to possess an innate sensitivity to the moods and thoughts of those they wish to please. This hyperalertness enables them to maneuver quickly to gain their attention. Then they attempt to control relationships by their seductiveness at one level but become extremely dependent on their friends at another level. Their demand for constant attention quickly alienates their friends. They become depressed when they are not the center of attention.

Epidemiology and Risk Factors

The prevalence of histrionic personality disorder is estimated at 1.8% of the general population (Grant et al., 2004). There are no gender differences in the occurrence of this disorder; however, this diagnosis is seen more frequently in women than men in the clinical setting. There is a greater risk of occurrence of this disorder among African Americans than whites. Low-income groups and less educated persons are also at higher risk for occurrence of histrionic personality disorder. Widowed, separated, divorced, or never married people are at greater risk than married ones. This disorder co-occurs with other mental disorders; anxiety disorder, obsessive-compulsive syndromes, somatoform syndromes, substance use disorder, and mood disorders in which they overplay their feelings of dysthymia by expressing them through dramatic and eye-catching gestures (Millon, 2011).

Etiology

Research related to this personality disorder is minimal. Some speculate that there is a biologic component and that heredity may play a role but that the biologic influence is less than in some of the previously discussed personality problems. In infancy and early childhood, these individuals are extremely alert and emotionally responsive. The tendencies for sensory alertness may be traced to responses of the limbic and reticular systems. They demonstrate a high degree of dependence on others and a type of dissociation in which they have reduced awareness of their behavior in relation to others (Millon, 2011).

It is believed that these highly alert and responsive infants seek more gratification from external stimulation during their first few months of life. Depending on the responsiveness of caregivers to them, they develop behavior patterns in response to their caregivers. It is believed that these children experience brief, highly charged, and irregular reinforcement from multiple caregivers (parents, siblings, grandparents, foster parents) who are unable to provide consistent experiences.

Parental behavior and role modeling are also believed to contribute to the development of histrionic personality disorder. Many of the women with this disorder reported that they are just like their mother, who is emotionally labile, bored with the routines of home life, flirtatious with men, and clever in dealing with people. It is believed that through role modeling, these children learn and mimic the behaviors observed in caregivers or adults (Millon, 2011).

Nursing Management

The ultimate treatment goal for patients with histrionic personality disorder is to correct the tendency to expect others to fulfill all of their needs. When these individuals seek mental health care, they have usually experienced a period of social disapproval or deprivation. Their hope is that the mental health providers will help fulfill their needs. Specific goals are needed to protect the person from becoming dependent on a mental health system. In the nursing assessment, the nurse focuses on the quality of the individual's interpersonal relationships. It is common that the person is dissatisfied with his or her partner, and sexual relations may be nonexistent.

During the assessment, the patient will make statements that indicate low self-esteem. Because these individuals believe that they are incapable of handling life's demands and have been waiting for a truly competent person to take care of them, they have not developed a positive self-concept or adequate problem-solving abilities.

Nursing diagnoses that are usually generated include Chronic Low Self-esteem, Ineffective Individual Coping, and Ineffective Sexual Patterns. Outcomes focus on helping the patient develop autonomy, a positive self-concept, and mature problem-solving skills.

A variety of interventions support the outcomes. A nurse–patient relationship that allows the patient to explore positive personality characteristics and develop independent decision-making skills forms the basis of the interventions. Reinforcing personal strengths, conveying confidence in the patient's ability to handle situations, and examining the patient's negative perceptions of him- or herself can be done within the therapeutic relationship. Encouraging the patient to act autonomously can also improve the individual's sense of self-worth. Attending assertiveness groups can help increase the individual's self-confidence and improve self-esteem.

Continuum of Care

Patients with histrionic personality disorder do not seek mental health care unless they have a coexisting medical or mental disorder. They are likely to be treated within the community for most of their lives, with the exception of short hospitalizations for nonpsychiatric problems.

Narcissistic Personality

Clinical Course and Diagnostic Criteria

People with **narcissistic personality** disorder are grandiose, have an inexhaustible need for admiration, and lack empathy. Beginning in childhood, these individuals believe that they are superior, special, or unique and that others should recognize them in this way (APA, 2013). They are often preoccupied with fantasies of unlimited success, power, beauty, or ideal love. They overvalue their personal worth, direct their affections toward themselves, and expect others to hold them in high esteem. They define the world through their own self-centered view. Their sense of entitlement is striking. People with narcissistic personality disorder are benignly arrogant and feel themselves above the conventions of their cultural group. They handle criticism poorly and may become enraged if someone dares to criticize them or else they may appear totally indifferent to criticism. They believe they are entitled to be served and that it is their inalienable right to receive special considerations. People with this disorder want to have their own way and are frequently ambitious to achieve fame and fortune. These individuals are often successful in their jobs but may alienate their significant others, who grow tired of their narcissism. They cannot show empathy, and they feign sympathy only for their own benefit to achieve their selfish ends. Clinically, those with narcissistic personality disorder show overlapping characteristics of BPD and ASPD.

Epidemiology

The prevalence of narcissistic personality is 6.2% of the general population with rates greater for men (7.7%) than for women (4.8%) according to a recent national epidemiologic survey (Stinson et al., 2008). Narcissistic personality disorder can be found in professionals who are highly respected such as law, medicine, and science and those associated with celebrity status. Persons with this disorder may impart an unrealistic sense of omnipotence, grandiosity, beauty, and talent to their children; therefore, children of parents with a narcissistic personality disorder have a higher than usual risk of developing the disorder themselves. It also commonly occurs in only children and among first-born boys in cultural groups in which males have special privileges (Millon, 2011).

Etiology

There is little evidence of any biologic factors that contribute to the development of this disorder. One notion about its development is that it is the result of parents' overvaluation and overindulgence of a child. These children are overly pampered and indulged, with every whim catered to. They learn to view themselves as special beings and to expect special treatment and subservience from others. They do not learn how to cooperate, share, or consider others' desires and interests. An alternate explanation is that the child never truly separated emotionally from his or her primary caregiver and therefore cannot envision functioning independently. According to another set of theories, these individual try to avoid or reduce intense feelings of shame and engage in a variety of strategies to divert attention from themselves (Roepke & Vater, 2014).

Nursing Management

The nurse usually encounters persons with narcissism in medical settings and in psychiatric settings with a coexisting psychiatric disorder. They are difficult patients who often appear snobbish, condescending, and patronizing in their attitudes. It is unlikely that these individuals are motivated to develop sensitivity to others and socially cooperative attitudes and behaviors. Building a therapeutic relationship is a slow process because they avoid self-reflection and often reject the clinician's approaches. Nurses need to use their self-awareness skills in interacting with these patients. The nursing process focuses on the coexisting responses to other health care problems (Ronningstam & Weinberg, 2013).

Continuum of Care

Similar to patients with histrionic disorder, those with narcissistic personality disorder do not seek mental health care unless they have a coexisting medical or mental disorder. They are likely to be treated within the community for most of their lives, with the exception of short hospitalizations for nonpsychiatric problems.

PARANOID, SCHIZOID, AND SCHIZOTYPAL PERSONALITY DISORDERS

The disorders discussed in this section include paranoid, schizoid, and schizotypal personality disorders. All are characterized with behavior that is odd or eccentric.

Paranoid Personality Disorder

Clinical Course and Diagnostic Criteria

Paranoid personality disorder is characterized by a long-standing suspiciousness and mistrust of persons in general. Individuals with these traits refuse to assume personal responsibility for their own feelings, assign responsibility to others, and avoid relationships in which they are not in control or lose power. These individuals are suspicious, guarded, and hostile. They are consistently mistrustful of others' motives, even relatives and close friends. Actions of others are often misinterpreted as deception, deprecation, and betrayal, especially regarding loyalty or trustworthiness of friends and associates (APA, 2013).

People with paranoid personality disorder are unforgiving and hold grudges; their typical emotional responses are anger and hostility. They distance themselves from others and are outwardly argumentative and abrasive; internally, they feel powerlessness, fearful, and vulnerable. Other hallmark features of paranoid personality disorder are persistent ideas of self-importance and the tendency to be rigid and controlled. Blind to their own unattractive behaviors and characteristics, they often attribute these traits to others. Their outward demeanor often seems cold, sullen, and humorless. They want to appear controlled and objective, yet often they react emotionally, displaying signs of nervousness, anger, envy, and jealousy. Orderly by nature, they are hypervigilant to any environmental changes that may loosen their control on the world. Occupational problems are common. They do not seek mental health care until they decompensate into a psychosis.

Epidemiology and Risk Factors

A prevalence estimate for paranoid personality based on a probability subsample from Part II of the National Comorbidity Survey Replication suggests a prevalence of 2.3%, while the National Epidemiologic Survey on Alcohol and Related Conditions data suggest a prevalence of paranoid personality disorder of 4.4% (APA, 2013).

Etiology

The etiologic factors of paranoid personality are unclear, but there may be a genetic predisposition for an irregular maturation. An underlying excess in limbic and sympathetic system reactivity or a neurochemical acceleration of synaptic transmission may exist. These dysfunctions can give rise to the hypersensitivity, cognitive autism, and social isolation that characterize these patients. As children, these individuals tend to be active and intrusive, difficult to manage, hyperactive, irritable, and have frequent temper outbursts.

Nursing Management

Nurses most likely see these patients for other health problems but formulate nursing diagnoses based on the patient's underlying suspiciousness. Assessment of these individuals reveals disturbed or illogical thoughts that demonstrate misinterpretation of environmental stimuli. For example, a man was convinced that his wife was having an affair with the neighbor because his wife and the neighbor left their homes for work at the same time each morning. Although the man's beliefs were illogical, he never once considered that he was wrong. He frequently followed them but never caught them together. He

continued to believe they were having an affair. The nursing diagnosis of Disturbed Thought Processes is usually supported by the assessment data.

Because of their inability to develop relationships, these patients are often socially isolated and lack social support systems. However, the nursing diagnosis of Social Isolation is not appropriate for the person with paranoid personality disorder because the person does not meet the defining characteristics of feelings of aloneness, rejection, desire for contact with people, and insecurity in social situations.

Nursing interventions based on the establishment of a nurse–patient relationship are difficult to implement because of the patient's mistrust. If a trusting relationship is established, the nurse helps the patient identify problematic areas, such as getting along with others or keeping a job. Through therapeutic techniques such as acceptance, confrontation, and reflection, the nurse and patient examine a problematic area to gain another view of the situation. Changing thought patterns takes time. Patient outcomes are evaluated in terms of small changes in thinking and behavior.

Continuum of Care

Individuals with paranoid personalities are unlikely to participate in treatment or recovery plans. If they have other comorbid disorders and are forced to seek treatment (loss of job or court ordered), they may seek help for depression or psychosis.

Schizoid Personality

Clinical Course and Diagnostic Criteria

People with **schizoid personality** disorder are characterized as being expressively impassive and interpersonally unengaged (Millon, 2011). They tend to be unable to experience the joyful and pleasurable aspects of life. They are introverted and reclusive and clinically appear distant, aloof, apathetic, and emotionally detached. Typically lifelong loners, they have difficulty making friends, seem uninterested in social activities, and appear to gain little satisfaction in personal relationships. In fact, they appear to be incapable of forming social relationships. Their interests are directed at objects, things, and abstractions. They may do well at solitary jobs other people might find difficult to tolerate. Often people with schizoid personality disorders may daydream excessively and become attached to animals, and they frequently do not marry or even form long-lasting romantic relationships. As children, they engage primarily in solitary activities, such as stamp collecting, computer games, electronic equipment, or academic pursuits such as mathematics or engineering. In addition, they seem to have a cognitive deficit characterized by obscure thought processes, particularly about social matters. Communication with others is confused and lacks focus. These individuals reveal minimum introspection and self-awareness, and interpersonal experiences are described in a very mechanical way.

Epidemiology

Schizoid personality disorder is rarely diagnosed in clinical settings. It is estimated that the prevalence is 3.1% (APA, 2013).

Etiology

The etiologic processes are speculative. There may be defects in either the limbic or reticular regions of the brain that may result in the development of the schizoid pattern (Millon, 2011). The defects of this personality may stem from an adrenergic–cholinergic imbalance in which the parasympathetic division of the autonomic nervous system is functionally dominant. Excesses or deficiencies in acetylcholine and norepinephrine may result in the proliferation and scattering of neural impulses that may be responsible for the cognitive "slippage" or affective deficits.

Nursing Management

Impaired Social Interactions and Chronic Low Self-esteem are typical diagnoses of patients with schizoid personality disorder. Major treatment goals are to enhance the experience of pleasure, prevent social isolation, and increase emotional responsiveness to others. Because these individuals often lack customary social skills, social skills training is useful in enhancing their ability to relate in interpersonal situations. The primary focus is to increase the patient's ability to feel pleasure. The nurse balances interventions between encouraging enough social activity that prevents the individual from retreating to a fantasy world and too much social activity that becomes intolerable.

The nurse may find working with these individuals unrewarding and become frustrated, feel helpless, or feel bored during the interactions. It is difficult to establish a therapeutic relationship with these individuals because they tend to shy away from interactions and are rarely motivated for treatment. Evaluation of outcomes should be in terms of increasing the patient's feelings of satisfaction with solitary activities.

Continuum of Care

People with schizoid personalities are rarely hospitalized unless they have a comorbid disorder. Family members may seek treatment for them in an outpatient setting.

Schizotypal Personality Disorder

Clinical Course and Diagnostic Criteria

Schizotypal personality disorder is characterized by a pattern of social and interpersonal deficits. The term **schizotypy** refers to traits that are similar to the symptoms of schizophrenia but are less severe. Cognitive perceptual symptoms are a primary characteristic and include magical beliefs (similar to delusions) and perceptual aberrations (similar to hallucinations). Other common symptoms include referential thinking (interpreting insignificant events as personally relevant) and paranoia (suspicious of others).

Schizotypal personality disordered persons are more dramatically eccentric than those with schizoid personality disorder who are characteristically flat, colorless, and dull (Millon, 2011). These individuals are perceived as strikingly odd or strange in appearance and behavior, even to laypersons. They may have unusual mannerisms, an unkempt manner of dress that does not quite "fit together," and inattention to usual social conventions (e.g., avoiding eye contact, wearing clothes that are stained or ill fitting, and being unable to join in the give-and-take banter of coworkers). Void of any close friends other than first-degree relatives, their mood is constricted or inappropriate, with excessive social anxieties. They usually exhibit an avoidant behavior pattern.

Persons with schizotypal personality disorder can respond to stress with transient psychotic episodes (lasting minutes to hours). Because of their short duration, the symptoms mirror but fall short of features that would justify the diagnosis of schizophrenia. Many individuals (30% to 50%) with schizotypal personality disorder also have a co-occurring major depressive disorder diagnosis when admitted to a hospital (APA, 2013; Cicero & Kerns, 2010). Schizotypal personality disorders may be slightly more common in males (APA, 2013).

Epidemiology and Risk Factors

The lifetime prevalence of schizotypal personality disorder is 3.9% with greater rates among men (4.2%) than women. There is cultural variation with black women and low-income individuals having a greater risk than others (Pulay et al., 2009).

Etiology

MRI studies of individuals with schizotypal personality disorder show smaller gray matter volume which are correlated with negative symptoms. This pattern of gray matter loss is similar to schizophrenia, there does not appear to be the progression of volume reduction present in schizophrenia. These individuals may be spared from psychosis and severe social and cognitive deterioration of chronic schizophrenia by the genetic or environmental factors that promote greater frontal capacity and reduced striatal dopaminergic reactivity (Asami et al., 2013; Rapp et al., 2010).

Nursing Management

Depending on the amount of decompensation (deterioration of functioning and exacerbation of symptoms), the assessment of a patient with a schizotypal personality disorder can generate a range of nursing diagnoses. If a person has severe symptoms, such as delusional thinking or perceptual disturbances, the nursing diagnoses are similar to those for a person with schizophrenia (see Chapter 22). If symptoms are mild, the typical nursing diagnoses include Social Isolation, Ineffective Coping, Low Self-esteem, and Impaired Social Interactions.

People with schizotypal personality disorder need help in developing recovery-oriented strategies to increase their sense of self-worth and recognize their positive attributes. They can benefit from social skills training and environmental management that increases their psychosocial functioning. Their odd, eccentric thoughts and behaviors alienate them from others. Reinforcing socially appropriate dress and behavior can improve their overall appearance and ability to relate in the environment. Because they have a hard time generalizing from one situation to another, attention to cognitive skills is important.

Continuum of Care

Quality of life for a patient with schizotypal personality disorder can be improved with supportive psychotherapy, but their suspiciousness, lack of trust, or impaired social interactions make it difficult to establish a therapeutic relationship. These individuals do not usually seek treatment unless more serious symptoms appear, such as depression or anxiety. Medications are not generally used unless the individual has coexisting anxiety or depression.

Nursing care is often provided in a home or clinic setting, with the personality disorder being secondary to the purpose of the care. This means that nurses are focusing on other aspects of patient care and may miss the underlying psychiatric disorder. A psychiatric nursing consult may be needed for these patients to help identify the disorder.

AVOIDANT, DEPENDENT, AND OBSESSIVE-COMPULSIVE PERSONALITY DISORDER

The disorders discussed in this section include avoidant, dependent, and obsessive-compulsive personality disorders. Individuals with these disorders appear anxious or fearful.

Avoidant Personality Disorder
Clinical Course and Diagnostic Criteria

Avoidant personality disorder is characterized by avoiding social situations in which there is interpersonal contact with others. Individuals appear timid, shy, and hesitant, and they fear criticism and feel inadequate. These individuals are extremely sensitive to negative comments and disapproval and appraise situations more negatively than others do. The behavior becomes problematic when they restrict their social activities and work opportunities because of their extreme fear of rejection.

In childhood, they are shy, but instead of growing out of the shyness, it becomes worse in adulthood. They perceive themselves as socially inept, inadequate, and inferior, which in turn justifies their isolation and rejection by others. Vocationally, people with avoidant personality disorder often take jobs on the sidelines, rarely obtaining personal advancement or exercising much authority, but to employers, they seem shy and eager to please. They are reluctant to enter relationships unless they are given strong assurance of uncritical acceptances, so they consequently often have no close friends or confidants (Millon, 2011).

Epidemiology and Risk Factors

The prevalence of avoidant personality disorder is 2.4% in the general population (APA, 2013), but it has been reported in 10% of outpatients in mental health clinics (Grant et al., 2004). The problem with examining the epidemiology of avoidant personality disorder is its potential overlap with generalized social phobia. Several studies found that a significant portion of the patients with diagnoses of social phobia also met criteria for avoidant personality disorder (Carter & Wu, 2010; Cox, Pagura, Stein, & Sareen, 2009). More research is needed to clarify the relationship between personality and anxiety disorders.

Etiology

Experts speculate that individuals with avoidant personality disorder experience aversive stimuli more intensely and more frequently than do others because they may possess an overabundance of neurons in the aversive center of the limbic system (Millon, 2011).

Nursing Management

Assessment of these individuals reveals a lack of social contacts, a fear of being criticized, and evidence of chronic low self-esteem. The nursing diagnoses Chronic Low Self-esteem, Social Isolation, and Ineffective Coping can be used. The establishment of a therapeutic relationship is necessary to be able to help these individuals meet their treatment outcomes. The development of the nurse–patient relationship is a slow process and requires an extreme amount of patience on the part of the nurse. These individuals may not have had positive interpersonal relationships and need time to be able to trust that the nurse will not criticize and demean them. Interventions should focus on refraining from any negative criticism, assisting the patient to identify positive responses from others, exploring previous achievements of success, and exploring reasons for self-criticism. The patient's social dimension should be examined for activities that increase self-esteem and interventions focused on increasing these self-esteem–enhancing activities. Social skills training may help reduce symptoms.

Continuum of Care

Long-term therapy is ideal for patients with avoidant personality disorder because it takes time to make the changes. Mental health nurses may see these individuals for other health problems. Encouraging the patient to continue with therapy and contacting the therapist when necessary are important in maintaining continuity of care. These patients are hospitalized only for a coexisting disorder.

Dependent Personality

Clinical Course and Diagnostic Criteria

People with **dependent personality** disorder cling to others in a desperate attempt to keep them close. Their need to be taken care of is so great that it leads to doing anything to maintain the closeness, including total submission and disregard for themselves.

Decision making is difficult or nil. They adapt their behavior to please those to whom they are attached. They lean on others to guide their lives. They ingratiate themselves to others and denigrate themselves and their accomplishments. Their self-esteem is determined by others. Behaviorally, they withdraw from adult responsibilities by acting helpless and seeking nurturance from others. In interpersonal relationships, they need excessive advice and reassurance. They are compliant, conciliatory, and placating. They rarely disagree with others and are easily persuaded. Friends describe them as gullible. They are warm, tender, and noncompetitive. They timidly avoid social tension and interpersonal conflicts (APA, 2013). However, these individuals are at risk for suicide and parasuicide, perpetration of child abuse, perpetration of domestic violence (in men), and victimization by a partner (in women) (Bornstein, 2012).

Epidemiology and Risk Factors

A recent study estimates the prevalence at 0.49% (APA, 2013). The diagnosis is made more frequently in women than in men. This gender difference may represent a sex bias by clinicians because when standardized instruments are used, men and women receive diagnoses at equal rates. The risk of dependent personality disorder is greater for the least educated and widowed, divorced, separated, and never married women (Disney, 2013).

Etiology

It is likely that there is a biologic predisposition to develop the dependency attachments of this disorder. However, no research studies support a biologic hypothesis. Dependent personality most often is explained as a result of parents' genuine affection, extreme attachment, and overprotection. Children then learn to rely on others to meet their basic needs and do not learn the necessary skills for autonomous behavior. Persons with chronic physical illnesses in childhood may be prone to developing this disorder.

Nursing Management

Nurses can determine the extent of dependency by assessment of self-worth, interpersonal relationships, and social behavior. They should determine whether there is currently someone on whom the person relies (parent, spouse) or if there has been a separation from a significant relationship by death or divorce.

Nursing diagnoses that are usually generated from the assessment data are Ineffective Individual Coping, Low Self-esteem, Impaired Social Interaction, and Impaired Home Maintenance Management. Home management skills may be a problem if the patient does not have the useful skills and now has to make decisions related to finances, shopping, cooking, and cleaning. The challenge of caring for these patients is to help them recognize their dependent patterns; motivate them to want to change; and teach them adult skills that have not been developed, such as balancing a checkbook, planning a weekly menu, and paying bills. Occasionally, if a patient is extremely fatigued, lethargic, or anxious and the disorder interferes with efforts at developing more independence, antidepressants or antianxiety agents may be used.

These patients readily engage in a nurse–patient relationship and initially look to the nurse to make all decisions. The nurse can support patients to make their own decisions by resisting the urge to tell them what to do. Ideally, these patients are in individual psychotherapy and working toward long-term personality changes. The nurse can encourage patients to stay in therapy and to practice the new skills that are being learned. Assertiveness training is helpful.

Continuum of Care

Individuals with dependent personality readily seek out therapy and are likely to spend years seeking therapy.

Hospitalization occurs for comorbid conditions such as depression.

Obsessive-Compulsive Personality Disorder

Clinical Course and Diagnostic Criteria

Obsessive-compulsive personality disorder (OCPD) stands out because it bears close resemblance to obsessive-compulsive disorder (OCD), and is closely related to anxiety disorder. Although these disorders have similar names, the clinical manifestations are quite different. A distinguishing difference is that those with the OCD tend to use obsessive thoughts and compulsions when anxious but less so when anxiety decreases. Persons with OCPD do not demonstrate obsessions and compulsions but rather a pervasive pattern of preoccupation with orderliness, perfectionism, and control. They also have the capacity to delay rewards; whereas those with OCD do not (Pinto, Steinglass, Greene, Weber, & Simpson, 2013). Individuals with this disorder attempt to maintain control by careful attention to rules, trivial details, procedures, and lists (APA, 2013). They may be completely devoted to work, which typically has a rigid character, such as maintaining financial records or tracking inventory. They are uncomfortable with unstructured leisure time, especially vacations. Their leisure activities are likely to be formalized (season tickets to sports, organized tour groups). Hobbies are approached seriously.

Behaviorally, individuals with OCPD are perfectionists, maintaining a regulated, highly structured, strictly organized life. A need to control others and situations is common in their personal and work lives. They are prone to repetition and have difficulty making decisions and completing tasks because they become so involved in the details. They can be overly conscientious about morality and ethics and value polite, formal, and correct interpersonal relationships. They also tend to be rigid, stubborn, and indecisive and are unable to accept new ideas and customs. Their mood is tense and joyless. Warm feelings are restrained, and they tightly control the expression of emotions (APA, 2013).

Epidemiology and Risk Factors

Obsessive-compulsive personality disorder is one of the most prevalent personality disorders in the general population, with estimated prevalence ranging from 2.1% to 7.9% (APA, 2013). This disorder is associated with higher education, employment, and marriage. Subjects with the disorder had a higher income than did those without the disorder.

Etiology

As with some of the other personality disorders, there is little evidence for a biologic formulation. The basis of the compulsive patterns that characterize OCPD is parental overcontrol and overprotection that is consistently restrictive and sets distinct limits on the child's behavior. Parents teach these children a deep sense of responsibility to others and to feel guilty when these responsibilities are not met. Play is viewed as shameful, sinful, and irresponsible, leading to dire consequences. They are encouraged to resist the natural inclinations toward play and impulse gratification, and parents try to impose guilt on the child to control behavior.

Nursing Management

These individuals seek mental health care when they have attacks of anxiety, spells of immobilization, sexual impotence, and excessive fatigue. The nursing assessment focuses on the patient's physical symptoms (sleep, eating, sexual), interpersonal relationships, and social problems. Typical nursing diagnoses include Anxiety, Risk for Loneliness, Decisional Conflict, Sexual Dysfunction, Insomnia, and Impaired Social Interactions. People with OCPD realize that they can improve their quality of life, but they find it extremely anxiety provoking to make the necessary changes. To change the compulsive pattern, psychotherapy is needed. There may be short-term pharmacologic intervention with an antidepressant or anxiolytic as an adjunct. A supportive nurse–patient relationship based on acceptance of the patient's need for order and rigidity will help the person have enough confidence to try new behaviors. Examining the patient's belief that underlies the dysfunctional behaviors can set the stage for challenging the childhood thinking. Because the compulsive pattern was established in childhood, it will take a long time to modify the behavior.

Continuum of Care

People with OCPD are treated primarily in the community. If there is a coexisting disorder or the person experiences periods of depression, hospitalization may be useful for a short period of time.

DISRUPTIVE, IMPULSE-CONTROL AND CONDUCT DISORDERS

Disruptive, impulse-control disorders and conduct disorders are a group of mental disorders that have the essential feature of irresistible impulsivity. Behaviors associated with these disorders violate the rights of others and/or are in conflict with societal norms (APA, 2013). Disorders discussed include oppositional defiant disorder, conduct disorder, intermittent explosive disorder, kleptomania, and pyromania. ASPD was discussed earlier in this chapter.

> **KEYCONCEPT** **Impulsivity,** acting without considering consequences or alternative actions, results when neurobiologic overactivity is stimulated by psychological, personality, or social factors related to personal needs of the individual (Tansey, 2010).

> **KEYCONCEPT** **Impulse-control disorders** often coexist with other disorders and are characterized by an inability to resist an impulse or temptation to complete an activity that is considered harmful to oneself or others.

There is an increase in tension before the individual commits the act and excitement or gratification at the time the act is committed. The release of tension is perceived as pleasurable, but remorse and regret usually follow the act. The disruptive behavior disorders, which include oppositional defiant disorder and conduct disorder, are a group of syndromes marked by significant problems of conduct.

Oppositional defiant disorder is characterized by a persistent pattern of disobedience, argumentativeness, angry outbursts, low tolerance for frustration, and tendency to blame others for misfortunes, large and small. Children with oppositional defiant disorder have trouble making friends and often find themselves in conflict with adults.

Conduct disorder is characterized by more serious violations of social norms, including aggressive behavior, destruction of property, and cruelty to animals. Children and adolescents with conduct disorder often lie to achieve short-term ends, may be truant from school, may run away from home, and may engage in petty larceny or even mugging (Box 28.4).

Epidemiology

Disruptive behavior disorders are more common in boys and are associated with lower socioeconomic status and urban living (Rowe et al., 2010). These disorders are relatively common in school-aged children and are frequently presenting complaints in child psychiatric treatment settings.

The prevalence of conduct disorder estimates range from 2% up to 10% with a median of 4%. The disorder appears to be fairly consistent across various countries that differ in race and ethnicity. Prevalence rates rise from childhood to adolescence and are higher among males than among females. Males with conduct disorder frequently exhibit fighting, stealing, vandalism, and school disciplinary problems. Females with the diagnosis are more likely to exhibit lying, truancy, running away, substance use, and prostitution. Whereas males tend to exhibit both physical aggression and relational aggression (behaviors that harm social relations of others), females tend to exhibit relatively more relational aggression

Clinical Vignette

BOX 28.4
LEON (CONDUCT DISORDER)

Leon, a 14-year-old Hispanic boy, was admitted to the child psychiatric inpatient service from the emergency department (ED) after a fight with his mother. His mother reported that she and Leon had argued earlier in the evening and that he stormed out of the house screaming and vowing he would never return. Several hours later, Leon came back, yelling and demanding entry into the apartment. Leon's father was working. While his mother was getting up to open the door, Leon continued to yell and scream, waking the neighbors. This led to further arguing between Leon and his mother. Before long, the police were called, and Leon was taken to the ED.

The admission interview revealed that Leon had run away on several occasions and had even stayed away overnight. Although he strongly denied drug use, he had gotten drunk on several occasions. He had also been in several fights, the latest of which resulted in an expulsion from school. Three months before admission, he was caught trying to steal a CD from a music store. More recently, he boasted that he and his friends had snatched a purse at an outdoor concert and had broken into a car to steal its contents. Leon's school performance has been declining; he was truant on several occasions and will probably have to repeat ninth grade.

Leon was born in Puerto Rico and is the oldest of three children. His family moved to the mainland shortly after his birth, and the primary language at home is Spanish. His father is employed as a janitor and speaks very little English. His mother works as a secretary and has achieved fairly good command of English. He has received no treatment except for consultation with the school social worker.

What Do You Think?
- When conducting a nursing assessment, what would you want to learn about Leon's school performance?
- What information could you provide Leon's parents about pharmacotherapy? About behavior management?

(APA, 2013). Conduct disorder is one of the most frequently diagnosed disorders in children in mental health facilities. Individuals with conduct disorder are at greater risk for experiencing mood or anxiety disorders and substance-related disorders (APA, 2013).

Etiology

The etiologies of oppositional defiant disorder and conduct disorder are complex. More attention has been paid to conduct disorder, probably because it is the more serious of the two. Models used to understand aggressiveness (see Chapter 19) are useful in examining these childhood disorders, which appear to have both genetic and environmental components. See Figure 28.2.

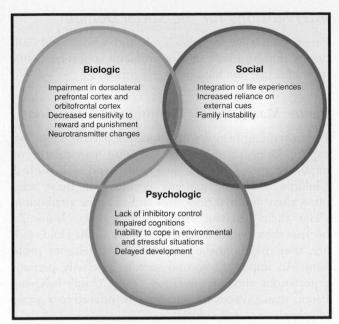

Biologic

Impairment in dorsolateral prefrontal cortex and orbitofrontal cortex
Decreased sensitivity to reward and punishment
Neurotransmitter changes

Social

Integration of life experiences
Increased reliance on external cues
Family instability

Psychologic

Lack of inhibitory control
Impaired cognitions
Inability to cope in environmental and stressful situations
Delayed development

FIGURE 28.2 Biopsychosocial etiology for patients with impulsivity.

NURSING MANAGEMENT: Oppositional Defiant and Conduct Disorders

Biologic Domain

Assessment

The nurse gathers data from multiple sources. Adolescents with these disorders are at high risk for physical injury as a result of fighting and impulsive behavior. Sexual promiscuity is common, resulting in an increased frequency of pregnancy and sexually transmitted diseases.

An important aspect of assessment is to rule out comorbid conditions that may partially explain or complicate the person's lack of behavioral control. These conditions include ADHD, learning disabilities, chemical dependency, depression, bipolar illness, or generalized anxiety. Young people who are chronically depressed may be irritable and easily frustrated. Given the tendency of adolescents to act out their frustration, chronic depression may exacerbate their behavior. Conduct problems can also elevate the risk for depression because young people who regularly elicit negative attention from parents and teachers and are constantly at odds with their environment may become despondent.

Nursing Diagnoses for the Biologic Domain

Typical nursing diagnoses in the biologic domain are Risk for Other Directed Violence, Risk for Self-directed Violence, and Impaired Verbal Communication. Although the outcomes are individualized for each patient, some outcomes for these patients are as follows:

- Maintenance of physical safety in the milieu (or other treatment setting)
- Decreased frequency of verbal and physical aggressive episodes

Interventions for the Biologic Domain

Children with oppositional defiant disorder or conduct disorder who also have specific neurodevelopmental disorders should be placed in appropriate programs for remediation. If a diagnosis of ADHD or depression emerges from the evaluation, appropriate pharmacotherapy should be considered (see previous discussion of ADHD and after the discussion regarding depression).

Psychological Domain

Assessment

Adolescents with conduct problems are usually brought or coerced into the mental health system by family, school, or the court system because of fighting, truancy, speeding tickets, car accidents, petty crimes, substance abuse, or suicide attempts. These young people may be hostile, sarcastic, defensive, and provocative. At the same time, they may appear calm, outgoing, and engaging. Inconsistencies, distortions, and misrepresentations of the truth are common when interviewing these children, so obtaining a clear history may be difficult. Therefore, instead of asking if an event or behavior occurred, it may be better to ask when it occurred. These adolescents are adept at changing the subject and diverting discussions from sensitive issues. They often use denial, projection, and externalization of anger as defense mechanisms when asked for self-disclosure. The assessment, which may take several sessions, should be conducted in a nonjudgmental fashion.

Nursing Diagnoses for the Psychological Domain

In the psychological domain, a typical nursing diagnosis is Ineffective Coping. Outcomes are individualized for each patient but can include the following:

- Increased personal responsibility for behavior
- Increased use of problem-solving skills as evidenced by decreased interpersonal conflicts
- Decreased rule violations and conflicts with authority figures

Interventions for the Psychological Domain

In planning interventions for patients with oppositional defiant disorder or conduct disorder, the focus is on problem behaviors. Therapeutic progress may be slow, at least partly because these patients often lack trust in authority figures.

Social Skills Training

The nurse should communicate behavioral expectations clearly and enforce them consistently. Consequences of appropriate and inappropriate actions also should be clear. Specific approaches for improving social and problem-solving skills are fundamental features for school-aged children and adolescents. Insofar as children and adolescents with conduct problems fail to recognize the adverse effects of their verbal and nonverbal behavior, their deficit can be formulated as an interpersonal problem. Social skills training teaches adolescents with these behavior disorders to recognize the ways in which their actions affect others. Training involves techniques such as role-playing, modeling by the therapist, and giving positive reinforcement to improve interpersonal relationships and enhance social outcomes.

Problem-Solving Therapy

In contrast to social skills training, which proposes that problems of conduct are the result of poor interpersonal skills, problem-solving therapy conceptualizes conduct problems as the result of deficiencies in cognitive processes. These processes include assessment of situations, interpretation of events, and expectations of others that are congruent with behavior. These children often misinterpret the intentions of others and may perceive hostility with little or no cause. Problem-solving skills training teaches these children to generate alternative solutions to social situations, sharpen thinking concerning the consequences of those choices, and evaluate responses after interpersonal conflicts.

Social Domain

Assessment

High levels of marital conflict, parental substance abuse, and parental antisocial behavior often mark family history.

Nursing Diagnoses for the Social Domain

In the social domain, nursing diagnoses include Compromised Family Coping and Impaired Social Interaction. Some outcomes for these patients are as follows:

- Increased use of problem-solving skills as evidenced by decreased interpersonal conflicts
- Decreased rule violations and conflicts with authority figures

Interventions for the Social Domain

Parent education for preschool- and school-aged children with disruptive behavior problems appears to be the most effective psychosocial intervention.

Parent Management Training and Education

Parent training begins with educating parents about disruptive behavior disorders, focusing particularly on impulsiveness, impaired judgment, and self-control. Children with long-standing problems in these areas often elicit punitive responses and negative attributions about their behavior from their parents. Ironically, because these parental responses focus on the child's failure, they may contribute to the child's behavior problems. An important second step is to clarify parental expectations and interpretation of the child's behavior. Parent management training may be offered to a group of parents or to individuals.

The aims of education are to provide parents with new ways of understanding their child's behavior and to promote improved interactions between parent and child. The most commonly presented techniques include the importance of positive reinforcement (praise and tangible rewards) for adaptive behavior, clear limits for unacceptable behavior, and use of mild punishment (e.g., a time out) (Box 28.5).

BOX 28.5

Time-Out Procedure

- *Labeling behavior:* Identify the behavior that the child is expected to perform or cease. The aim of this statement is to make clear what is required of the child. It typically takes the form of a simple declarative sentence: "Threatening is not acceptable."
- *Warning:* In this step, the child is informed that if he or she does not perform the expected behavior or stop the unacceptable behavior, he or she will be given a "time out." "This is a warning: if you continue threatening to hit people, you'll have a time out."
- *Time out:* If the child does not heed the warning, he or she is told to take a time out in simple straightforward terms: "Take a time out."
- *Duration:* The usual duration for a time out is 5 minutes for children 5 years of age or older.
- *Location:* The child sits in a designated time-out chair without toys and without talking. The chair should be located away from general activity but within view. A kitchen timer can be used to mark the time, but the clock does not start until the child sits quietly in the designated spot.
- *Follow-up:* The child is asked to recount why he or she was given the time out. The explanation need not be detailed, and no further discussion of the matter is required. Indeed, long discourse about the child's behavior is not helpful and should be avoided.

Referral to Family Therapy

Family therapy is directed at assisting the family with altering maladaptive patterns of interaction or improving adjustment to stressors, such as changes in membership or losses. Multisystem family therapy, which considers the child in the context of multiple family and community systems, has shown promise in the treatment of adolescents with conduct disorder.

Evaluation and Treatment Outcomes

The nurse can review treatment goals and objectives to assess the child's progress with respect to verbal and physical aggression, socially appropriate resolution of conflicts, compliance with rules and expectations, and better management of frustration. As is true for the initial assessment, evaluation of treatment outcomes relies on input from parents, teachers, and other team members.

Continuum of Care

Children and adolescents with disorders of conduct may be involved in many different agencies in the community, such as child welfare services, school authorities, and the legal system. Mental health services are requested when a child or adolescent's behavior is out of control or a comorbid disorder is suspected. Helping the patient and family negotiate their way through this maze of services may be an essential part of the treatment plan.

Intermittent Explosive Disorder

Episodes of aggressiveness that result in assault or destruction of property characterize people with **intermittent explosive disorder**. The severity of aggressiveness is out of proportion to the provocation. The episodes can have serious psychosocial consequences, including job loss, interpersonal relationship problems, school expulsion, divorce, automobile accidents, or jail. This diagnosis is given only after all other disorders with aggressive components (delirium, dementia, head injury, borderline personality disorder, ASPD, substance abuse) have been excluded. Little is known about this disorder, but it is a more common condition than previously thought. The prevalence of intermittent explosive disorder in the United States is about 2.7%. The onset is most common in childhood or adolescence and rarely begins for the first time after the age 40 years. The mean age at onset is 14 years. It is more prevalent in individuals with a high school education or less (APA, 2013). The anger experience and expression contribute to suicidality (Hawkins & Cougle, 2013).

The treatment of this disorder is multifaceted. Psychopharmacologic agents are sometimes used as an adjunct to psychotherapeutic, behavioral, and social interventions. Serotonergic antidepressants and GABA-ergic mood stabilizers have been used. Anxiolytics are used for obsessive patients who experience tension states and explosive outbursts. Medication alone is insufficient, and anger management should be included in the treatment plan.

Kleptomania

In **kleptomania**, individuals cannot resist the urge to steal, and they independently steal items that they could easily afford. These items are not particularly useful or wanted. The underlying issue is the act of stealing. The term *kleptomania* was first used in 1838 to describe the behavior of several kings who stole worthless objects. These individuals experience an increase in tension and then pleasure and relief at the time of the theft. Kleptomania occurs in about 4% to 24% of individuals arrested for shoplifting. Its prevalence in the general population however is very rare, at approximately 0.3% to 0.6%. Females outnumber males at a ratio of 3:1 (APA, 2013). Because it is considered a "secret" disorder, there is little information about it, but it is believed to last for years despite numerous convictions for shoplifting. It appears that kleptomania often has its onset during adolescence (Grant & Kim, 2005).

Some shoplifting appears to be related to anxiety and stress in that it serves to relieve symptoms. In a few instances, brain damage has been associated with kleptomania. Depression is the most common symptom identified in a compulsive shoplifter.

Kleptomania is difficult to detect and treat. There are few accounts of treatment. It appears that behavior therapy is frequently used. Antidepressant medication that helps relieve the depression has been successful in some cases. More investigation is needed (Ravindran, Da Siva, Ravindran, Richter, & Rector, 2009).

Pyromania

Irresistible impulses to start fires characterize **pyromania**, repeated fire setting with tension or arousal before setting fires; fascination or attraction to the fires; and gratification when setting, witnessing, or participating in the aftermath of fire. These individuals often are regular "fire watchers" or even firefighters. They are not motivated by aggression, anger, suicidal ideation, or political ideology. Little is known about this disorder because only a small number of deliberate fire starters are apprehended, and of those individuals, only a few undergo a psychiatric evaluation. The prevalence of fire setting in the general population is about 1%, but most fire setting is not done by people with pyromania, which occurs infrequently, mostly in men. However, those with a history of fire setting are most likely male, young, and never married and are more likely to have other psychiatric issues such as ASPD, substance use, and impulsivity (Blanco et al.,

2010). Prevalence rates are lower among African Americans and Hispanics (Vaughn et al., 2010).

Early research demonstrated low serotonin and norepinephrine levels associated with arson. Little is known about treatment, and as with the other impulse-control disorders, no approach is uniformly effective. Historically, fire starters generally possess poor interpersonal skills, exhibit low self-esteem, battle depression, and have difficulty managing anger. Education, parenting training, behavior contracting with token reinforcement, problem-solving skills training, and relaxation exercises may all be used in the management of the patient's responses (Blanco et al., 2010).

Continuum of Care for Disruptive, Impulse-Control Disorders

Impulse-control disorders require long-term treatment, usually in an outpatient setting. Group therapy is often a facet of treatment because patients can talk in a community where people share common experiences. Hospitalization is rare except when patients have comorbid psychiatric or medical disorders.

SUMMARY OF KEY POINTS

- Antisocial personality disorder, often synonymous with psychopathy, includes people who have no regard for and refuse to conform to social rules.

- For many patients with personality disorders, maintaining a therapeutic nurse–patient relationship can be one of the most helpful interventions. Through this therapeutic relationship, the patient experiences a model of healthy interaction, establishing trust, consistency, caring, boundaries, and limitations that help to build the patient's self-esteem and respect for self and others. In some personality disorders, nurses will find it more difficult to engage the patient in a true therapeutic relationship because of the patient's avoidance of interpersonal and emotional attachment (i.e., antisocial personality disorder or paranoid personality disorder).

- Patients with personality disorders are rarely treated in an inpatient facility except during periods of destructive behavior or self-injury. Treatment is delivered in the community and over time. Continuity of care is important in helping the individual change lifelong personality patterns.

- The primary characteristic of disruptive, impulse-control disorders is impulsivity, which leads to inappropriate social behaviors that are considered harmful to oneself or others and that give the patient excitement or gratification at the time the act is committed.

CRITICAL THINKING CHALLENGES

1. Compare the characteristics, epidemiology, and etiologic theories of antisocial and borderline personality disorders (see Chapter 27).

2. Discuss the differences between histrionic and obsessive-compulsive personality disorder.

3. Compare and contrast antisocial personality disorder with narcissistic personality trait.

4. Define and summarize personality disorders. Compare the following among the five disorders:
   a. Defining characteristics
   b. Epidemiology
   c. Biologic, psychological, and social theories
   d. Key nursing assessment data
   e. Nursing diagnoses and outcomes
   f. Specific issues related to a therapeutic relationship
   g. Interventions

5. Define and summarize the five personality trait profiles. Compare the following among the traits:
   a. Defining characteristics
   b. Epidemiology
   c. Biologic, psychological, and social theories
   d. Key nursing assessment data
   e. Nursing diagnoses and outcomes
   f. Specific issues related to a therapeutic relationship
   g. Interventions

6. Define and summarize the impulse-control disorders. Compare the following among the disorders:
   a. Defining characteristics
   b. Epidemiology
   c. Biologic, psychological, and social theories
   d. Key nursing assessment data
   e. Nursing diagnoses and outcomes
   f. Interventions

 Grey Gardens: 1975. This documentary by Albert and David Maysles is the unbelievable true story of Mrs. Edith Bouvier Beale and her daughter Edie, who are the aunt and first cousin of Jacqueline Kennedy Onassis. The film depicts mother and daughter, known as "Big Edie" and "Little Edie," who have descended into a strange life of dependence and eccentricity.

Living in a world of their own in a decaying 28 room East Hampton mansion, their living conditions—infested by fleas, inhabited by numerous cats and raccoons, deprived of running water, and filled with garbage—give viewers a glimpse into schizotypal personality disorder.

VIEWING POINTS: Identify the behaviors of Big Edie and Little Edie that are characteristic of schizotypal personality disorder. Do "Big Edie" and "Little Edie" exhibit a folie à deux (a shared psychotic disorder)? Why or why not?

MVIE viewing **GUIDES** related to this chapter are available at http://thePoint.lww.com/Boyd5eUpdate.

A related Psychiatric-Mental Health Nursing video on the topic of Antisocial Personality Disorder is available at: http://thePoint.lww.com/Boyd5eUpdate.

References

Alcorn, J. L., Gowin, J. L., Green, C. E., Swann, A. C., Moeller, F. G., & Lane, S. D. (2013). Aggression, impulsivity, and psychopathic traits in combined antisocial personality disorder and substance use disorder. *Journal of Neuropsychiatry and Clinical Neurosciences, 25*(3), 229–232.

American Psychiatric Association. (2013). *Diagnostic and statistical manual of mental disorders* (5th ed.). Arlington, VA: Author.

Asami, T., Whitford, T. J., Bouix, S., Dickey, C. C., Niznikiewicz, M., Shenton, M. E., et al. (2013). Globally and locally reduced MRI gray matter volumes in neuroleptic-naïve men with schizotypal personality disorder: Association with negative symptoms. *Journal of the American Medical Association Psychiatry, 70*(4), 361–372.

Birbaumer, N., Veit, R., Lotze, M., Erb, M., Hermann, C., Grodd, W., et al. (2005). Deficient fear conditioning in psychopathy: A functional magnetic resonance imaging study. *Archives of General Psychiatry, 62*(7), 799–805.

Black, D. W., Gunter, T., Loveless, P., Allen, J., & Sieleni, B. (2010). Antisocial personality disorder in incarcerated offenders: Psychiatric comorbidity and quality of life. *Annals of Clinical Psychiatry, 22*(2), 113–120.

Blanco, C., Alergria, A. A., Petry, N. M., Grant, J. E., Simpson, B., Liu, S., et al. (2010). Prevalence and correlates of fire-setting in the United States: Results from the National Epidemiologic Surveys on Alcohol and Related Conditions (NESARC). *Journal of Clinical Psychiatry, 71*(9), 1218–1225.

Bornstein, R. F. (2012). Illuminating a neglected clinical issue: Societal costs of interpersonal dependency and dependent personality disorder. *Journal of Clinical Psychology, 68*(7), 766–781.

Carter, S. A., & Wu, K. D. (2010). Relations among symptoms of social phobia subtypes, avoidant personality disorder, panic, and depression. *Behavior Therapy, 41*(1), 2–13.

Cicero, D. C., & Kerns, J. G. (2010). Multidimensional factor structure of positive schizotypy. *Journal of Personality Disorders, 24*(3), 327–343.

Cox, B. J., Pagura, J., Stein, M. B., & Sareen, J. (2009). The relationship between generalized social phobia and avoidant personality disorder in a national mental health survey. *Depression and Anxiety, 26*(4), 354–362.

Disney, K. L. (2013). Dependent personality disorder: A critical review. *Clinical Psychology Review, 33*, 1184–1196.

Gao, Y., Raine, A., Chan, F., Veneables, P. H., & Mednick, S. A. (2010). Early maternal and paternal bonding, childhood physical abuse and adult psychopathic personality. *Psychological Medicine, 40*(6), 1007–1016.

Gibbon, S., Duggan, C., Stoffers, J., Huband, N., Völlm, B. A., Ferriter, M., et al. (2010). Psychological interventions for antisocial personality disorders. *Cochrane Database of Systematic Reviews*, (6):CD007668.

Grant, B. F., Hasin, D. S., Stinson, F. D., Dawson, D. A., Chou, S. P., Ruan, W. J., et al. (2004). Prevalence, correlates, and disability of personality disorders in the United States: Results from the National epidemiologic survey on alcohol and related conditions. *Journal of Clinical Psychiatry, 65*(7), 948–995.

Grant, J. E., & Kim, S. W. (2005). Quality of life in kleptomania and pathological gambling. *Comprehensive Psychiatry, 46*(1), 34–37.

Hawkins, K. A. & Cougle, J. R. (2013). A test of the unique and interactive roles of anger experience and expression in suicidality. *The Journal of Nervous and Mental Disease. 201*(11), 959–963.

Jovev, M., Whittle, S., Yücel, M., Simmons, J. G., Allen, N. B., & Chanen, A. M. (2014). The relationship between hippocampal asymmetry and temperament in adolescent borderline and antisocial personality pathology.*Development and Psychopathology, 26*(1), 275–285.

Lennox, C., & Dolan, M. (2014). Temperament and character and psychopathy in male conduct disordered offenders. *Psychiatry Research, 215*(3), 706–710.

Millon, T. (2011). *Disorders of personality: Introducing a DSM/ICD spectrum from normal to abnormal* (3rd ed.). Hoboken, NJ: John Wiley & Sons, Inc.

Murphy, J. (1976). Psychiatric labeling in cross-cultural perspective: Similar kinds of disturbed behavior appear to be labeled abnormal in diverse cultures. *Science, 191*(4231), 1019–1028.

Pinto, A., Steinglass, J. E., Greene, A. L., Weber, E. U., & Simpson, H. B. (2013). Capacity to delay reward differentiates obsessive-compulsive disorder and obsessive compulsive personality disorder. *Biological Psychiatry, 75*(8):653–659. doi:10.10.1016/jbiopsych.2013.09.007

Pulay, A. J., Stinson, F. S., Dawson, D. A., Goldstein, R. B., Chou, S. P., Huang, B., et al. (2009). Prevalence, correlates, disability, and comorbidity of DSM-IV schizotypal personality disorder: Results from the Wave 2 National Epidemiologic Survey on Alcohol and Related Conditions. *Journal of Clinical Psychiatry, 11*(2), 53–67.

Rapp, A. M., Mutschler, D. E., Wild, B., Erb, M., Lengsfeld, I., Saur, R., et al. (2010). Neural correlates of irony comprehension: The role of schizotypal personality traits. *Brain and Language, 113*, 1–12.

Ravindran, A. V., Da Siva, T. L., Ravindran, L. H., Richter, N. A., & Rector, N. A. (2009). Obsessive-compulsive spectrum disorders: A review of the evidence-based treatments. *Canadian Journal of Psychiatry, 54*(5), 331–342.

Roepke, S., & Vater, A. (2014). Narcissistic personality disorder: An integrative review of recent empirical data and current definitions. *Current Psychiatry Reports, 16*(5), 445–453.

Ronningstam, E., & Weinberg, I. (2013). Narcissistic personality disorder: Progress in recognition and treatment. *Focus, 11*(2), 167–177.

Rowe, R., Costello, E. J., Angold, A., Copeland, W. E., & Maughan, B. (2010). Developmental pathways in oppositional defiant disorder and conduct disorder. *Journal of Abnormal Psychology, 119*(4), 728–736.

Sousa, C., Herrenkohl, T. I., Moylan, C. A., Tajima, E. A., Klika, J. B., Herrenkohl, R. C., et al. (2011). Longitudinal study on the effects of child abuse and children's exposure to domestic violence, parent-child attachments, and antisocial behavior in adolescence. *Journal of Interpersonal Violence, 26*(1), 111–136.

Stinson, F. S., Dawson, D. A., Goldstein, R. B., Chou, S. P., Huang, B., Smith, S. M., et al. (2008). Prevalence, correlates, disability, and comorbidity of DSM-IV narcissistic personality disorder: Results from the Wave 2 National Epidemiologic Survey on Alcohol and Related Conditions. *Journal of Clinical Psychiatry, 69*(7), 1033–1045.

Taber-Thomas, B. C., Asp, E. W., Koenigs, M., Sutterer, M. Anderson, S. W., & Tranel, D. (2014). Arrested development: Early prefrontal lesions impair the maturation of moral judgement. *Brain, 137*(pt 4), 1254–1261.

Tansey, T. N. (2010). Impulsivity: An overview of a biopsychosocial model. *Journal of Rehabilitation, 76*(3), 3–9.

Vaughn, M. G., Fu, Q., Delisi, M., Wright, J. P, Beaver, K. M., Perron, B. E., et al. (2010). Prevalence and correlates of fire-setting in the United States: Results from the national epidemiological survey on alcohol and related conditions. *Comprehensive Psychiatry, 51*(3), 217–223.

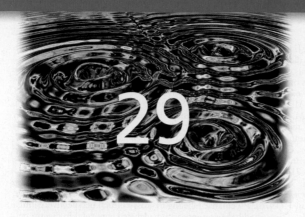

29

Somatic Symptom and Related Disorders
Management of the Consequences of Somatization

Mary Ann Boyd and Victoria Soltis-Jarrett

KEY CONCEPT

- somatization

LEARNING OBJECTIVES

After studying this chapter, you will be able to:

1. Explain the concept of somatization and the occurrence of somatic symptom and related disorders in people with mental health problems.

2. Analyze the prevailing biopsychosocial theories related to somatic symptom and related disorders.

3. Analyze the human response to somatic symptom and related disorders with an emphasis on somatization and cognitive distortions.

4. Formulate nursing diagnoses based on a biopsychosocial assessment of people with somatic symptom and related disorders.

5. Develop recovery-oriented nursing interventions for patients with somatic symptom and related disorders.

6. Analyze the implementation and evaluation of psychotherapeutic drugs used by people with somatic symptom and related disorders and their impact on nursing care planning and intervening.

7. Analyze special concerns within the nurse–patient relationship common to caring for those with somatic symptom and related disorders.

8. Identify expected outcomes and their evaluation for patients with somatic symptom disorders.

KEY TERMS

- alexithymia • somatic symptom disorder (SSD) • conversion disorder • factitious disorder • factitious disorder imposed on another • illness anxiety disorder • hypochondriasis • malingering • Münchausen's syndrome • pseudologia fantastica • psychosomatic • somatic symptom disorder

---

The connection between the "mind" and "body" has been hypothesized and described for centuries. The term **psychosomatic** has been traditionally used to describe, explain, and predict the psychological origins of illness and disease. Unfortunately, this notion perpetuates the stigma that certain disorders are purely "psychological" in nature and thus that they are not real or valid. For example, it was once believed that people with asthma were behaviorally "acting out" their anger, fear, or emotional pain and were seeking attention rather than experiencing an alteration in their respiratory status.

In contrast, the concept of *somatization* acknowledges and respects that bodily sensations and functional changes are expressions of health and illness, and even though they may be unexplained, they are not imaginary or "all in the head" (Boutros & Peters, 2012).

> **KEYCONCEPT** **Somatization** (from *soma*, meaning body) is the manifestation of psychological distress as physical symptoms that may result in functional changes, somatic descriptions, or both.

Whereas some evidence suggests that somatization is a result of abnormally high levels of physiologic response (Boutros & Peters, 2012), other evidence supports the idea that somatization is the physical expression of personal problems or the internalization and expression of stress through physical symptoms. For example, a woman quits her job complaining of chronic fatigue rather than recognizing that she is emotionally stressed from the constant harassment of a coworker.

Historically, the concept of somatization was linked to women and was related to a woman's body, mind, or even her soul. For example, the term *hysteria*, frequently associated with somatization, actually comes from ancient times when it was believed that women's unfounded physical symptoms were related to their "wandering or discontented uterus." Because *hystera* is the Greek word for uterus, the terms *hysteria* and *hysterical* were used to describe a woman whose physical or emotional symptoms could not be substantiated by physicians at that time.

Today we understand that somatization is not linked to the uterus nor is it just a problem for women. Men also are affected by somatization. There is still much research that is needed in this area to be able to make any valid and reliable conclusions about gender and somatization. Somatization also crosses all cultures and is recognized in almost every society (Woolfolk, Allen, & Tiu, 2007). In many cultures, the expression of physical discomfort is more acceptable than acknowledging psychological distress. The disruption of routine body cycles, such as digestion, menstruation, or sleep, is more socially acceptable than having emotional responses related to interpersonal relationships, economic crises, adjustment to marriage, infertility, or the death of a spouse.

This chapter explores the holistic, evidenced-based nursing care for people experiencing the *DSM-5* group of disorders with the prominent symptom of somatization. Somatic symptom disorder (SSD) is highlighted and, illness anxiety disorder, conversion disorder, and factitious disorders are discussed.

SOMATIC SYMPTOM DISORDER

Nurses in primary care and medical–surgical settings are more likely than mental health nurses to encounter persons with these problems. Note: the term *somatoform* is no longer used in the *DSM-5* to describe these disorders.

Clinical Course

Somatic Symptom Disorder (SSD) is one of the most difficult disorders to manage because the symptoms tend to change, are diffuse and complex, and vary and move from one body system to another. For example, initially there may be gastrointestinal (nausea, vomiting, diarrhea) and neurologic (headache, backache) symptoms that change to musculoskeletal (aching legs) and sexual issues (pain in the abdomen, pain during intercourse). The physical symptoms may last for 6 to 9 months.

Individuals with SSD perceive themselves as being "sicker than the sick" and report all aspects of their health as poor. Many eventually become disabled and cannot work. They typically visit health care providers multiple times per month and quickly become frustrated because their primary health care providers do not appreciate their level of suffering and are unable to validate that a particular problem accounts for their extreme discomfort. Consequently, individuals with SSD tend to "provider shop," moving from one to another until they find one who will give them new medication, hospitalize them, or perform surgery. Because the source of worrisome physical symptoms cannot be found through medical or laboratory tests, medical or psychiatric interviews or medical imaging, they repeatedly seek a medical reason for discomfort and ask for relief from suffering. Depending on the severity, these individuals undergo multiple surgeries and even develop iatrogenic illnesses. People with SSD often evoke negative subjective responses in health care providers, who usually wish that the patient would go to someone else.

When individuals are fearful of developing a serious illness based on their misinterpretation of body sensations, the term **hypochondriasis** can be used to describe this preoccupation. The fear of having an illness continues despite medical reassurance and interferes with psychosocial functioning. They spend time and money on repeated examinations looking for feared illnesses. For example, an occasional cough or the appearance of a small sore results in the person making an appointment with an oncologist. Hypochondriasis sometimes appears if the patient had a serious childhood illness or if a family member has a serious illness. See Fame and Fortune.

> **NCLEXNOTE**   Patients with SSD seek health care from multiple providers but avoid mental health specialists.

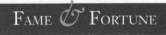

FAME & FORTUNE

Leo Tolstoy (1828–1910)
Russian Novelist

PUBLIC PERSONA

Count Leo Tolstoy was one of the giants of 19th century literature. He was raised in wealth and privilege in Czarist Russia. Among the most famous works authored by Tolstoy are the novels *War and Peace* and *Anna Karenina*. Experts believe that his fiction portrays his own inner character. For example, in *War and Peace*, Pierre Bezukhov reflects the life of the author.

PERSONAL REALITIES

In *Confessions*, Tolstoy describes his own experiences with depression, hypochondriasis, and alcoholism.

Diagnostic Criteria

The diagnostic criteria were updated in the *DSM-5* and include one or more symptoms that cause persistent distress or significant disruption in daily lives for at least 6 months, and excessive thoughts about the seriousness of the symptoms, feelings (such as anxiety about the symptoms or health), or behaviors related to the symptoms or health concerns (such as spending excessive time and energy focusing on these symptoms or health) (American Psychiatric Association [APA], 2013). These symptoms can be explained or unexplained by medical evidence. The expression of the symptoms varies from population to population.

Somatic Symptom Disorder Across the Life Span

This disorder is found in most populations and cultures even though its expression may vary from population to population. In cultures that highly stigmatize mental illness, somatic symptoms are more likely to appear (Dere et al., 2013; Zaroff, Davis, Chio, & Madhaven, 2012).

Children and Adolescents

Although many children have somatic symptoms, SSD disorder is not usually diagnosed until adolescence. However, when children have medical symptoms, further evaluation is needed, and they are often referred to specialists to rule out physical, sexual, or emotional abuse or a comorbid psychiatric illness such as depression or anxiety. In children, the most common symptoms are frequent abdominal pain, headache, fatigue, and nausea. Expression of somatic symptoms in children tends to be overlooked or minimized when it needs to be identified as a risk factor for follow-up (Schulte & Peterman, 2011). In adolescents, initial symptoms are typically menstrual difficulties, pelvic, or abdominal pain. Risk factors for both children and adolescents need to be taken seriously. Research has shown a link between childhood sexual abuse and somatization, substance use, and depression in adults (Zink, Klesges, Stevens, & Decker, 2009).

Older Adults

SSD can be a lifelong pattern of symptoms that persists into old age. The SSD symptoms, however, are often unrecognized by health care providers who tend to accept and minimize them as a part of the natural aging process after no medical cause is found.

Epidemiology

The estimated prevalence of SSD ranges from 5% to 7% (APA, 2013). Millions of dollars of lost revenue and the increased use of short- and long-term disability have prompted employers to study this unique population of employees. In reality, about 20% of persons seeking primary care fall in this group (Fabião, Silva, Fleming, & Barbosa, 2010).

Age of Onset

The SSD usually begins before the age of 30 years with the first symptom often appearing during adolescence. Rarely diagnosed until several years later, seeking help can last for many years with the individual frequently going from one health care provider to another to no avail. Most studies report that somatization is more common in middle-aged and older adults (Woolfolk et al., 2007).

Gender, Ethnic, and Cultural Differences

Epidemiologic studies have reported that SSD occurs primarily in nonwhite, less educated women, particularly those with a lower socioeconomic status and high emotional distress (Woolfolk et al., 2007). Men are less likely to be diagnosed with SSD, partly because of stereotypic male traits, such as a disinclination to admit discomfort or seek help for their symptoms (APA, 2013).

Risk Factors

SSD tends to run in families, and children of mothers with multiple unexplained somatic complaints are more likely to have somatic problems. Individuals with a tendency toward heightened physiologic arousal and a tendency to amplify somatosensory information have a greater risk of developing this disorder. Adults are also at higher risk for unexplained medical symptoms if they experienced them as children or if their parents were in poor health when the patient was about 15 years old. Recent data have also confirmed a strong association between sexual trauma exposure and somatic symptoms, illness attitudes, and healthcare utilization in women (Woolfolk et al., 2007).

Comorbidity

SSD frequently coexists with other psychiatric disorders, most commonly depression and anxiety. Others include panic disorder, mania, social phobia, obsessive-compulsive disorder (OCD), psychotic disorders, and personality disorders (van Dijke, Ford, van der Hart, van Son, van der Heijden, & Bühring, 2010). Older adults are particularly high for comorbid depression (Spangenberg, Forkmann, Brahler, & Glaesmer, 2011).

Ultimately, numerous unexplained medical problems also coexist with this disorder because many patients have received medical and surgical treatments, often unnecessarily, and are plagued with side effects. A disproportionately high number of women who eventually receive diagnoses of SSD have been treated for irritable bowel syndrome, polycystic ovary disease, and chronic pain.

Etiology

The cause of SSD is unknown. There is general agreement that somatization has a biopsychosocial basis with the possibility of biologic dysfunction common in depression and chronic fatigue syndrome (Anderson, Maes, & Berk, 2012).

Biologic Theories

In the biologic domain, there is a decrease in neuroactivity in certain brain areas, such as the caudate nuclei, left putamen, and right precentral gyrus, indicating hypometabolism, prolonged disinhibition of the prefrontal cortex, or both. There is also chronic activation of the hypothalamus–pituitary–adrenal axis indicating a hyperarousal condition from chronic stress (see Chapter 18). One hypothesis proposes that there is a failure in sensory gating mechanism. Normally, we do not feel our internal organs because their sensations are filtered or "gated" out. If there is a failure in the gating mechanism, visceral sensations will reach consciousness and can be falsely interpreted as pathology of the organ (Boutros & Peters, 2012). That is, a minor headache becomes extremely painful when the person believes a brain tumor is the cause.

Although SSD has been shown to run in families, the exact transmission mechanism is unclear. Strong evidence suggests an increased risk for SSD in first-degree relatives, indicating a familial or genetic effect. Because many individuals with SSD live in chaotic families, the high prevalence in first-degree relatives could be explained by environmental influence. Some boys and men in these families show a high risk for antisocial personality disorder and substance abuse (Rief & Broadbent, 2007).

Psychological Theories

Somatization has been explained as a form of social or emotional communication, meaning that the bodily symptoms express an emotion that cannot be verbalized by the individual. An adolescent who experiences severe abdominal pain after her parents' argument or a wife who receives nurturing from her husband only when she has back pain are two examples. From this perspective, somatization may be a way of communicating and maintaining relationships. Following this line of reasoning, an individual's physical problems may also become a way of controlling relationships, so somatization becomes a learned behavior pattern. With time, physical symptoms develop automatically in response to

perceived threats. Finally, SSD develops when somatizing becomes a way of life.

Consistent with a communication explanation, cognitive behaviorists explain somatization symptoms as an interaction of cognitive (negative views) with physical factors (pain, discomfort). In this model, individuals have a heightened response based on their experiences with a stressor, especially if the stressor was uncontrollable and unpredictable. Over time, their exaggerated responses become an automatic pattern, resulting in "sick role" behavior, which in turn provokes either a negative or positive response in others (Dumont & Olson, 2012; Mik-Meyer & Obling, 2012).

Another theoretical explanation for somatization is the personality trait **alexithymia**, which is associated with somatic symptoms disorders. Individuals with alexithymia have difficulty identifying and expressing their emotions. They have a preoccupation with external events and are described as concrete externally oriented thinkers (Deng, Ma, & Tang, 2013; Pedrosa et al., 2009).

Social Theories

SSDs have been reported globally even though its conceptualization is primarily Western. The symptoms may vary from culture to culture. For example, studies in China have identified and discussed the notion of somatization as a moral issue rather than a medical problem. Somatization is a more socially acceptable way to express behavior in lieu of being diagnosed as depressed because in China, mental illness is perceived as a character flaw. In many non-Western societies, where the mind–body distinction is not made and symptoms have different meanings and explanations, these physical manifestations are not labeled as a psychiatric disorder (Box 29.1). In Latin American countries, depression is more likely described in somatic symptoms, such as headaches, gastrointestinal disturbances, or complaints of "nerves," rather than sadness or guilt (Yusim et al., 2010).

Family Response to Disorder

Family dynamics are shaped by all members, including the person with SSD. When one member has a number of ongoing chronic issues, family members' activities and interactions are affected. The physical symptoms of the individual become the focus of family life, and activities are planned around that person. Because so much time and so many resources are used trying to discover an underlying illness, there are reduced resources to other family members. Because the person is always sick, expressing anger toward the situation is difficult. The family members needs support as they learn to understand the seriousness and difficulty of having a SSD (Krishnan, Sood, & Chadda, 2013).

BOX 29.1

Somatization in Chinese Culture

In Chinese tradition, the health of the individual reflects a balance between positive and negative forces within the body. Five elements at work in nature and in the body control conditions (fire, water, wood, earth, metal), five viscera (liver, heart, spleen, kidneys, lungs), five emotions (anger, joy, worry, sorrow, fear), and five climatic conditions (wind, heat, humidity, dryness, cold). All illness is explained by imbalances among these elements. Because emotion is related to the circulation of vital air within the body, anger is believed to result from an adverse current of vital air to the liver. Emotional outbursts are seen as results of imbalances among the natural elements rather than the results of behavior of the person.

The stigma of mental illness in the Chinese culture is so great that it can have an adverse effect on a family for many generations. If problems can be attributed to natural causes, the individual and family are less responsible, and stigma is minimized. The Chinese have a culturally acceptable term for symptoms of mental distress—the closest translation of which would be *neurasthenia*—that comprises somatic complaints of headaches, insomnia, dizziness, aches and pains, poor memory, anxiety, weakness, and loss of energy.

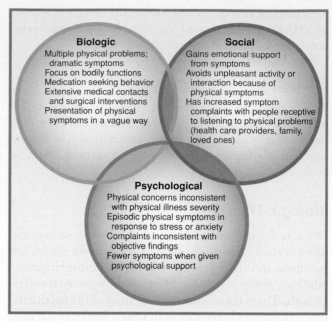

FIGURE 29.1 Biopsychosocial characteristics of patients with somatic symptom disorder.

Interdisciplinary Treatment

The care of patients with SSD involves three approaches:

- Providing long-term general management of the chronic condition
- Conservatively treating symptoms of comorbid psychiatric and physical problems
- Providing care in special settings, including individual and group treatment and the use of complementary and alternative medicine (Moreno et al., 2013; Woolfolk et al., 2007).

The cornerstone of management is trust and believing. Ideally, the patient should see only one health care provider at regularly scheduled visits. During each primary care visit, the provider should conduct a partial physical examination of the organ system in which the patient has complaints. Physical symptoms are treated conservatively using the least intrusive approach. In the mental health setting, the use of cognitive behavior therapy (CBT) is effective (Moreno et al., 2013).

NURSING MANAGEMENT: Human Response to Somatic Symptom Disorder

Somatization is the primary response to this disorder. The defining characteristics, depicted in the biopsychosocial model (Figure 29.1), are so well integrated that separating the psychological and social dimension ns is difficult. The most common characteristics are:

- Reporting the same symptoms repeatedly

- Receiving support from the environment that otherwise might not be forthcoming (such as gaining a spouse's attention because of severe back pain)
- Expressing concern about the physical problems inconsistent with the severity of the illness (being "sicker than the sick")

Biologic Domain

During the assessment interview, the nurse should allow enough time for the patient to explain all medical problems; a hurried assessment interview blocks communication.

Assessment

Psychiatric–mental health nurses typically see these patients for problems related to a coexisting psychiatric disorder, such as depression, not because of the SSD. While taking the patient's history, the nurse may discover that the individual has had multiple surgeries or medical problems, making SSD a strong possibility. If the patient has not already received a diagnosis of SSD, the nurse should screen for it by determining the presence of the most commonly reported problems associated with this disorder, which includes dysmenorrhea, a lump in the throat, vomiting, shortness of breath, burning in the sex organs, painful extremities, and amnesia. If the patient has these symptoms, he or she should be seen by a mental health provider qualified to make the diagnosis. Box 29.2 presents the Health Attitude Survey, which can be used as a screening test for somatization.

BOX 29.2

Health Attitude Survey

On a scale of 1 to 5, please indicate the extent to which you agree (5) or disagree (1).

DISSATISFACTION WITH CARE
1. I have been satisfied with the medical care I have received. (R)
2. Doctors have done the best they could to diagnose and treat my health problems. (R)
3. Doctors have taken my health problems seriously.
4. My health problems have been thoroughly evaluated. (R)
5. Doctors do not seem to know much about the health problems I have had.
6. My health problems have been completely explained. (R)
7. Doctors seem to think I am exaggerating my health problems.
8. My response to treatment has not been satisfactory.
9. My response to treatment is usually excellent. (R)

FRUSTRATION WITH ILL HEALTH
10. I am tired of feeling sick and would like to get to the bottom of my health problems.
11. I have felt ill for quite a while now.
12. I am going to keep searching for an answer to my health problems.
13. I do not think there is anything seriously wrong with my body. (R)

HIGH UTILIZATION OF CARE
14. I have seen many different doctors over the years.
15. I have taken a lot of medicine recently.
16. I do not go to the doctor often. (R)
17. I have had relatively good health over the years.

EXCESSIVE HEALTH WORRY
18. I sometimes worry too much about my health.
19. I often fear the worst when I develop symptoms.
20. I have trouble getting my mind off my health.

PSYCHOLOGICAL DISTRESS
21. Sometimes I feel depressed and cannot seem to shake it off.
22. I have sought help for emotional or stress-related problems.
23. It is easy to relax and stay calm. (R)
24. I believe the stress I am under may be affecting my health.

DISCORDANT COMMUNICATION OF DISTRESS
25. Some people think that I am capable of more work than I feel able to do.
26. Some people think that I have been sick just to gain attention.
27. It is difficult for me to find the right words for my feelings.

(R) indicates items reversed for scoring purposes. Scoring—The higher the score, the more likely somatization is a problem.
From Noyes, R. Jr., Langbehn, D., Happel, R., Sieren, L., & Muller, B. (1999). Health Attitude Survey: A scale for assessing somatizing patients. *Psychosomatics, 40*(6), 470–478.

Review of Systems

Although these patients' symptoms have usually received considerable attention from the medical community, a careful review of systems is important because the appearance of physical problems is usually related to psychosocial problems. Even as the patient continues to be seen for mental health problems, an ongoing awareness of biologic symptoms is important, particularly because these symptoms are de-emphasized in the overall management.

Pain is the most common problem in people with this disorder. Because the pain is usually related to symptoms of all the major body systems, it is unlikely that a somatic intervention such as an analgesic will be effective on a long-term basis. Remember that although there is no medical explanation for the pain, the patient's pain is real and has serious psychosocial implications. A careful assessment should include the following questions:

- What is the pain like?
- What is the extent of the pain?
- What helps the pain get better?
- When is the pain at its worst?
- What has worked in the past to relieve the pain?

Physical Functioning

The actual physical functioning of these individuals is often marginal. They usually have problems with sleep, fatigue, activity, and sexual functioning. Assessment of these areas generates data to be used in establishing a nursing diagnosis. The amount and quality of sleep are important, as are the times when the individual sleeps. For example, an individual may sleep a total of 6 hours each diurnal cycle but only from 2:00 to 6:00 AM plus an afternoon nap.

Fatigue is a constant problem for many people with SSD, and a variety of physical problems interfere with normal activity. These patients report an overwhelming lack of energy, which makes maintaining usual routines or accomplishing daily tasks impossible. Fatigue is accompanied by the inability to concentrate on simple functions, leading to decreased performance and disinterest in surroundings. Patients tend to be lethargic and listless and often have little energy (Box 29.3).

Female patients with this disorder usually have had multiple gynecologic problems, and the physical manifestations of SSD often lead to altered sexual behavior. The reason is not known, but symptoms of dysmenorrhea, painful intercourse, and pain in the "sex organs" suggest involvement of the hypothalamic–pituitary–gonadal axis. Physiologic indicators, such as those produced by laboratory tests, are not available. However, a careful assessment of the patient's menstrual history, gynecologic problems, and sexual functioning is important. It is also important to assess if there is a past or current history of abuse, whether it is sexual, physical, or emotional.

BOX 29.3
SOMATIC SYMPTOM DISORDER AND STRESS

Ms. J, age 42 years, has been coming to the mental health clinic for 2 years for her nerves. She has seen only the physician for medication but now has been referred to the nurse's new stress management group because she is experiencing side effects to all the medications that have been tried. The psychiatrist has diagnosed SSD and wants her to learn to manage her "nerves" without medication.

At the first meeting with the nurse, Ms. J was preoccupied with chest pain and bloating that had lasted for the past 6 months. Her chest pain is constant and sharp at times. The pain does not prevent her from going to her job as a waitress but does interfere with meal preparation at night for her family and her ability to have sexual intercourse. She has numerous other physical problems, including allergies to certain perfumes, dysmenorrhea, ovarian polycystic disease (ovarian cysts), chronic urinary tract infections, and rashes. She is constantly fatigued and has frequent leg cramps. She states that she is too tired to fix dinner for her family. On days off from work, she takes a nap in the afternoon, sleeping until evening. She is unable to fall asleep at night.

She believes that she will soon have to have her gallbladder removed because of occasional referred pain to her back and nausea that occurs a couple hours after eating. She is not enthusiastic about a stress management group and does not believe it will help her problems. However, she has agreed to consider it as long as the psychiatrist will continue prescribing diazepam (Valium).

What Do You Think?
- How would you prioritize Ms. J's physical symptoms?
- What are some possible explanations for Ms. J's fatigue?

Pharmacologic Assessment

A psychopharmacologic assessment of these patients is challenging. Patients with SSD frequently provider shop, perhaps seeing seven or eight different providers within a year. Because they often receive medications from each provider, they are usually taking a large number of drugs. They tend to protect their sources and may not be truthful in identifying the actual number of medications they are ingesting. A pharmacologic assessment is needed not only because of the number of medications but also because these individuals frequently have unusual side effects or they report that they are "sensitive" to medications. Because of their somatic sensitivity, they often overreact to medication.

These patients spend much of their life trying to find out what is wrong with them. When one provider after another can find little if any explanation for their symptoms, many become anxious. To alleviate their anxiety, they either self-medicate with over-the-counter (OTC) medications and

substances of abuse (e.g., alcohol, marijuana) or find a provider who prescribes an anxiolytic. Because the anxiety of their disorder cannot be treated within a few weeks with an anxiolytic, they become dependent on medication that should not have been prescribed in the first place.

Although anxiolytics have a place in therapeutics, they are not recommended for long-term use and only complicate the treatment of individuals with SSD. These medications should also be avoided because of their addictive qualities. Unfortunately, by the time these individuals see a mental health provider, they have already begun taking an anxiolytic for anxiety, usually a benzodiazepine. Many times, they only agree to see a mental health provider because the last provider would no longer prescribe an anxiolytic without a psychiatric evaluation.

Nursing Diagnoses for the Biologic Domain

Because SSD is a chronic illness, patients could have almost any one of the nursing diagnoses at some time in their lives. At least one nursing diagnosis likely will be related to the individual's physical state. Fatigue, Pain, and Insomnia are usually supported by the assessment data. The challenge in devising outcomes for these problems is to avoid focusing on the biologic aspects and instead help the patient overcome the fatigue, pain, or sleep problem through biopsychosocial approaches.

Interventions for the Biologic Domain

Nursing interventions that focus on the biologic dimension become especially important because medical treatment must be conservative, and aggressive pharmacologic treatment must be avoided. Each time a nurse sees the patient, a limited time should be spent respectfully discussing physical complaints. During the discussion, it is important to project the belief that the patient is truly experiencing the problems. Several biologic interventions, including pain management, activity enhancement, nutrition regulation, relaxation, and pharmacologic interventions, may be useful in caring for patients with SSD.

Pain Management

In pain management, a single approach rarely works. Pain is a primary issue and was once considered a separate disorder. Nursing care focuses on helping patients identify strategies to relieve pain and to examine stressors in their lives. After a careful assessment of the pain, nonpharmacologic strategies should be developed to reduce it. If gastrointestinal pain is frequent, eating and bowel habits should be explored and modified. For back pain, exercises and consultation from a physical therapist may be useful. Headaches are a challenge. Self-monitoring and tracking them engages the patient in the therapeutic process and helps to identify psychosocial triggers. Also, suggesting or referring the individual for a variety of complementary and alternative treatments has been shown to be very useful (Woolfolk et al., 2007). Relaxation techniques, identifying thoughts and feelings about their pain or discomfort, and including family members in the intervention have been shown to be useful.

Activity Enhancement

Helping the patient establish a daily routine may alleviate some of the difficulty with sleeping, but doing so may be difficult because most of these patients do not work. Encouraging the patient to get up in the morning and go to bed at night at specific times can help the patient to establish a routine. These patients should engage in regular exercise to improve their overall physical state, but they often have numerous reasons why they cannot. This is where the nurse's patience is tested; the nurse ultimately needs to remember that the patient's symptoms are an expression of their suffering. Agreeing that daily exercise is difficult but continuing to emphasize the importance of exercise can counter some of the reluctance to exercise.

Nutrition Regulation

Patients with SSD often have gastrointestinal problems and may have special nutritional needs. The nurse should discuss the nutritional value of foods with the patient. Because these individuals often take medications that promote weight gain, weight control strategies may be discussed. For overweight individuals, suggest healthy, low-calorie food choices. Teach patients about balancing dietary intake with activity levels to increase their awareness of food choices.

Relaxation

Patients taking anxiety-relieving medication can be taught relaxation techniques to alleviate stress. It is a challenge to help these patients really use these strategies. The nurse should consider a variety of techniques, including simple relaxation techniques, distraction, and guided imagery (see Chapter 10).

Psychopharmacologic Interventions

No medication is specifically recommended for patients with SSD; however, psychiatric symptoms of comorbid disorders, such as depression and anxiety, are treated pharmacologically as appropriate. Usually, the patients who are depressed or anxious are taking an antidepressant to treat their symptoms (see Chapter 24).

Phenelzine (Nardil) is one of the monoamine oxidase inhibitors (MAOIs) that has been effective in treating not just depression but also the chronic pain and headaches common in people with SSD. Food–drug interactions are the most serious side effects of MAOIs (Box 29.4). While taking these agents, patients should avoid foods high in tyramine (e.g., aged cheese, sausage, smoked fish, beer) and certain medications for colds and coughs (see Chapter 11).

Patients with anxiety are treated pharmacologically, similar to those with depression. The first line of treatment for all anxiety disorders is with a selective serotonin reuptake inhibitor (SSRI). Doses for SSD are usually higher than those prescribed for depression to relieve and manage the symptoms of the anxiety disorders, including panic, social phobia, generalized anxiety, OCD, and posttraumatic stress disorder.

Nonpharmacologic approaches such as biofeedback and relaxation are also quite useful in conjunction with pharmacologic treatment. Benzodiazepines may be used initially in the treatment of those with anxiety but should be slowly decreased and discontinued because of the psychological and physiologic dependence associated with these medications. Buspirone (BuSpar), a nonbenzodiazepine, does not lead to tolerance or withdrawal and may be useful for relief of anxiety. If panic disorder is present, it should be treated aggressively.

Pain medication should be prescribed conservatively. If mood disorders are also present, mood stabilizers not only treat the depression but also may treat the pain (Leiknes, Finset, & Moum, 2010).

Administering and Monitoring Medications

In SSD, patients are usually treated in the community, where they commonly self-medicate. Carefully question patients about self-administered medicine and determine which medicines they are currently taking (including OTC and herbal supplements). Also listen carefully to determine any effects the patient attributes to the medication. This information should be documented and reported to the rest of the team. The patient should be encouraged to continue taking only prescribed medication and to seek approval before taking any additional OTC or prescribed medications.

Managing Side Effects

These individuals often have atypical reactions to their medications. Side effects should be assessed, but the patient should be encouraged to compare the benefits of the medication with any problems related to side effects. Patients should also be encouraged to give the medications enough time to be effective because many medications require up to 6 weeks before the patient has a response or a relief of symptoms.

BOX 29.4

Drug Profile: **Phenelzine (Nardil)**

DRUG CLASS: Monoamine oxidase inhibitor (MAOI)

RECEPTOR AFFINITY: Inhibits MAO, an enzyme responsible for breaking down biogenic amines, such as epinephrine, norepinephrine, and serotonin, allowing them to accumulate in neuronal storage sites throughout the central and peripheral nervous systems

INDICATIONS: Treatment of depression characterized as "atypical," "nonendogenous," or "neurotic" or nonresponsive to other antidepressant therapy or in situations in which other antidepressant therapy is contraindicated

ROUTE AND DOSAGE: Available as 15-mg tablets

Adults: Initially, 15 mg PO tid, increasing to at least 60 mg/d at a fairly rapid pace consistent with patient tolerance. Therapy at 60 mg/d may be necessary for at least 4 weeks before response occurs. After maximum benefit has been achieved, the dosage is reduced gradually over several weeks. The maintenance dose may be 15 mg/d or every other day.

Geriatric: Adjust dosage accordingly because patients older than 60 years of age are more prone to develop adverse effects.

Pediatric: Not recommended for children younger than 16 years of age

HALF-LIFE (PEAK EFEECTS): Unknown (48–96 h)

SELECTED ADVERSE REACTIONS: Dizziness, vertigo, headache, overactivity, hyperreflexia, tremors, muscle twitching, mania, hypomania, jitteriness, confusion, memory impairment, insomnia, weakness, fatigue, overstimulation, restlessness, increased anxiety, agitation, blurred vision, sweating, constipation, diarrhea, nausea, abdominal pain, edema, dry mouth, anorexia, weight changes, hypertensive crisis, orthostatic hypotension, and disturbed cardiac rate and rhythm

BOXED WARNING: Suicidality in children and adolescents

WARNINGS: Contraindicated in patients with pheochromocytoma, congestive heart failure, hepatic dysfunction, severe renal impairment, cardiovascular disease, history of headache, and myelography within previous 24 h or scheduled within next 48 h. Use cautiously in patients with seizure disorders, hyperthyroidism, pregnancy, lactation, and those scheduled for elective surgery. Possible hypertensive crisis, coma, and severe convulsions may occur if administered with tricyclic antidepressants; possible hypertensive crisis when taken with foods containing tyramine. Increased risk for adverse interaction is possible when given with meperidine. Additive hypoglycemic effect can occur when taken with insulin and oral sulfonylureas.

SPECIFIC PATIENT/FAMILY EDUCATION

- Take drug exactly as prescribed; do not stop taking it abruptly or without consulting your health care provider.
- Families and caregivers of patients should be advised to observe for the emergence of anxiety, agitation, panic attacks, insomnia, irritability, hostility, aggressiveness, impulsivity, akathisia (psychomotor restlessness), hypomania, mania, other unusual changes in behavior, worsening of depression, and suicidal ideation. Such symptoms should be reported to the patient's prescriber or health professional, especially if they are severe, abrupt in onset, or were not part of the patient's presenting symptoms.
- Avoid consuming any foods containing tyramine while taking this drug and for 2 weeks afterward.
- Avoid alcohol, sleep-inducing drugs, over-the-counter drugs such as cold and hay fever remedies, and appetite suppressants, all of which may cause serious or life-threatening problems.
- Report any signs and symptoms of adverse reactions.
- Maintain appointments for follow-up blood tests.
- Report any complaints of unusual or severe headache or yellowing of your eyes or skin.
- Avoid driving a car or performing any activities that require alertness.
- Change position slowly when going from a lying to sitting or standing position to minimize dizziness or weakness.

Monitoring for Drug Interactions

In working with patients with SSD, always be on the lookout for drug–drug interactions. Medications these patients take for physical problems could interact with psychiatric medications. Patients may be taking alternative medicines, such as herbal supplements, but they usually willingly disclose their experiments. The patient should be encouraged to use the same pharmacy for filling all prescriptions so possible reactions can be checked and monitored.

Psychological Domain

The mental status of individuals with SSD can be within normal limits although most patients report frustration, depression, and hopelessness about their situation. What is most noticeable is their intense focus on their body and the physical symptoms that are causing them distress and disability.

Assessment

Generally, cognition is not impaired in people with SSD, but it may be distorted, such as believing the pain means a life-threatening condition. These individuals seem preoccupied with the signs and symptoms of their illnesses and may even keep a record of their experiences. Living with illness, diseases, and suffering truly becomes a way of life.

Some individuals with SSD have intense emotional reactions to life stressors and have led or are leading traumatic or chaotic lives. These patients usually have had a series of personal crises beginning at an early age. Examples include severe sexual and physical abuse and psychological trauma. Typically, a new symptom or medical problem develops during times of emotional stress as well as during anniversaries of losses or traumas that occurred in the patient's lifetime. It is critical that the link between the physical assessment data and the patient's psychological and social history are considered. A thorough history of major psychological events should be compared with the chronology of physical problems. Special attention should be paid to any history of sexual abuse or trauma in the patient's younger years. Early sexual abuse also may prevent the individual from being able to perform sexually or to have chronic abdominal pain or discomfort during sexual relations.

The individual's mood is usually labile, often shifting from extremely excited or anxious to being depressed and hopeless. Response to physical symptoms is usually magnified, such as interpreting a simple cold as pneumonia or a brief chest pain as a heart attack. Family members may not believe the physical symptoms are real and may view them as attention-getting behavior because symptoms often improve when the patient receives attention. For example, a woman who has been in bed for 3 weeks with severe back pain may suddenly feel much better when her children visit her.

> **NCLEXNOTE** Encourage and allow patients with SSD to discuss their physical problems before focusing on psychosocial issues.

Nursing Diagnoses for the Psychological Domain

Nursing diagnoses that target responses to SSD typical of the psychological domain include Anxiety, Ineffective

Sexuality Patterns, Impaired Social Interactions, Ineffective Coping, and Ineffective Therapeutic Regimen Management (Figure 29.2).

Interventions for the Psychological Domain

The choice of psychological intervention depends on the specific problem the patient is experiencing. The most important and ongoing intervention is the maintenance of a therapeutic relationship.

Development of a Therapeutic Relationship

The most difficult aspect of nursing care is developing a sound, positive nurse–patient relationship, yet this relationship is crucial. Without it, the nurse is just one more provider who fails to meet the patient's expectations. Developing this relationship requires time and patience. Therapeutic communication techniques should be used to refocus the patient on psychosocial problems related to the physical manifestations (Box 29.5).

During periods when symptoms of other psychiatric disorders surface, additional interventions are needed. For example, if depression occurs, additional supportive or cognitive approaches may be needed.

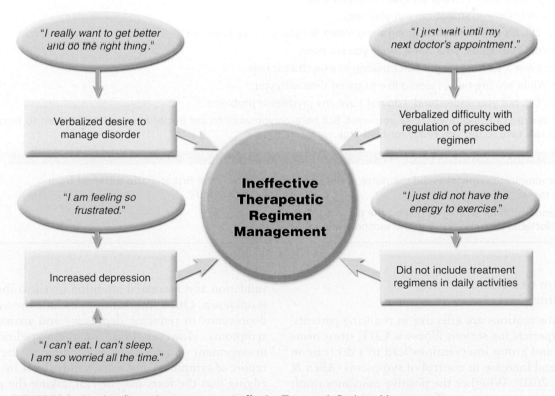

FIGURE 29.2 Nursing diagnosis concept map: Ineffective Therapeutic Regimen Management.

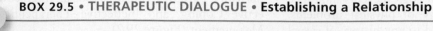

BOX 29.5 • THERAPEUTIC DIALOGUE • Establishing a Relationship

INEFFECTIVE APPROACH

Nurse: Good morning, Ms. C.

Patient: I'm in so much pain. Take that breakfast away.

Nurse: You don't want your breakfast?

Patient: Can't you see? I hurt! When I hurt, I can't eat!

Nurse: If you don't eat now, you probably won't be able to have anything until lunch.

Patient: Who cares? I have no intention of being here at lunchtime. I don't belong here.

Nurse: Ms. C, I don't think that your doctor would have admitted you unless there is a problem. I would like to talk to you about why you are here.

Patient: Nurse, I'm just here. It's none of your business.

Nurse: Oh.

Patient: Please leave me alone.

Nurse: Sure, I will see you later.

EFFECTIVE APPROACH

Nurse: Good morning, Ms. C.

Patient: I'm in so much pain. Take that breakfast away.

Nurse: (Silently removes tray. Pulls up chair and sits down.)

Patient: My back hurts.

Nurse: Oh, when did the back pain start?

Patient: Last night. It's this bed. I couldn't get comfortable.

Nurse: These beds can be pretty uncomfortable.

Patient: My back pain is shooting down my leg.

Nurse: Does anything help it?

Patient: Sometimes if I straighten out my leg it helps.

Nurse: Can I help you straighten out your leg?

Patient: Oh, it's OK. The pain is going away. What did you say your name is?

Nurse: I'm Susan Miller, your nurse while you are here.

Patient: I won't be here long. I don't belong in a psychiatric unit.

Nurse: While you are here, I would like to spend time with you.

Patient: OK, but you understand, I do not have any psychiatric problems.

Nurse: We can talk about whatever you want. But because you want to get out of here, we might want to focus on what it will take to get you ready for discharge.

CRITICAL THINKING CHALLENGE

- What communication mistakes did the nurse in the first scenario make?

- What communication strategies helped the patient feel comfortable with the nurse in the second scenario?

- How is the first scenario different from the second?

Reduction of Patient Anxiety About Illness

Several interventions are effective in reducing patients' fears of experiencing serious illnesses. CBT, stress management, and group interventions lead to a decrease in intensity and increase in control of symptoms (Allen & Woolfolk, 2010). Whether the positive outcomes result from the intervention itself or from the symptom validation and increased attention given to the patient, is unknown. Other interventions include the use of antidepressants in reducing depressive and anxiety-related symptoms. However, based on these studies, nursing management should include listening to the patient's report of symptoms and fears, validating it by acknowledging that the fears may be real, asking the patient to monitor symptoms in a journal, and encouraging the patient to bring the journal to the next visit. By actually seeing the symptom pattern, it is possible to continue to educate the patient and assess for significant symptoms. The outcome of this approach should be a decrease in fears and better control of the symptoms.

Counseling

Counseling with a focus on problem solving is needed from time to time. These patients have chaotic lives and need support through the multitude of crises. Although they may appear fascinating and at times self-assured, they can easily irritate others because of their constant complaints. The consequences of their impaired social interaction with others must be examined within a counseling framework. It will become evident that the patient's problem-solving and decision-making skills could be improved. Identifying stresses and strengthening positive coping responses helps the patient deal with a chaotic lifestyle.

Patient Education: Health

Health teaching is useful throughout the nurse–patient relationship. These patients have many questions about illnesses, symptoms, and treatments. Emphasize positive health care practices and minimize the effects of serious illness. Because of problems in managing medications and treatment, the therapeutic regimen needs constant monitoring, resulting in ample opportunities for teaching. One area that might require special health teaching is impaired sexuality. Because of their long history of physical problems related to the reproductive tract, these patients may have difficulty carrying out normal sexual activity, such as intercourse, reaching orgasm, and so forth. Basic teaching about normal sexual function is often needed (Box 29.6).

BOX 29.6

Psychoeducation Checklist: Somatic Symptom Disorder

When caring for a patient with SSD, be sure to include the following topic areas in the teaching plan:

- Psychopharmacologic agents (anxiolytics) if ordered, including drug, action, dosage, frequency, and possible adverse effects
- Nonpharmacologic pain relief measures
- Exercise
- Nutrition
- Social interaction
- Appropriate health care practices
- Problem solving
- Relaxation and anxiety-reduction techniques
- Sexual functioning

Social Domain

People with this disorder spend excessive time seeking medical care and treating their multiple illnesses. Many are unemployed, and frequently these individuals have changed jobs, had multiple positions over their lifetimes or careers, or have had absences or gaps in employment (Sharma & Manjula, 2013).

Because they believe themselves to be very sick, they also believe that they are disabled and cannot work. Because their symptoms are often inconsistent with any identifiable medical diagnosis, these individuals are rarely satisfied with health care providers, who can find nothing wrong. However, their social network often consists of a series of providers, rather than peers or family members, who can also become weary of the individual's constant complaints of physical problems. Identifying a support network requires sorting out the health care providers from family and friends.

Assessment

Individuals with SSD sometimes live in chaotic families with multiple problems. In assessing the family structure, other members with psychiatric disorders must be identified. Women may be married to abusive men who have antisocial personality disorders; alcoholism is common. Identifying the positive and negative relationships within the family is important.

SSD is particularly problematic because it disrupts the family's social life. Changes in routine or major life events often precipitate the appearance of a symptom. For example, a patient may be planning a vacation with the family but at the last minute decides she cannot go because her back pain has returned and she will not be able to sit in the car. These family disruptions are common. In addition, as already noted, employment history for the person with SSD may be erratic.

Nursing Diagnoses for the Social Domain

Some of the nursing diagnoses related to the social domain that are typical of people with SSD include Risk for Caregiver Role Strain, Ineffective Community Coping, Disabled Family Coping, and Social Isolation.

Interventions for the Social Domain

Patients with SSD are usually isolated from their families and communities. Strengthening social relationships and activities often becomes the focus of the nursing care. The nurse should help the patient identify individuals with whom contact is desired, ask for a commitment to contact them, and encourage them to reinitiate

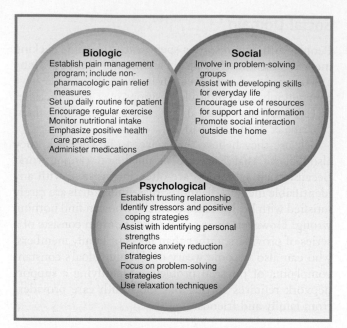

FIGURE 29.3 Biopsychosocial interventions for patients with somatic symptom disorder.

a relationship. The nurse should counsel patients about talking too much about their symptoms with these individuals and emphasize that medical information should be shared with the nurse instead. The nurse must also ensure that patient know when their next appointments are scheduled.

Group Interventions

Although these patients may not be candidates for insight group psychotherapy, they do benefit from cognitive behavioral groups that focus on developing coping skills for everyday life (Allen & Woolfolk, 2010). Because most of the patients are women, participation in groups that address feminist issues should be encouraged to strengthen their assertiveness skills and improve their generally low self-esteem (Figure 29.3).

When leading a group that has members with this disorder, redirection can keep the group from giving too much attention to a person's illness. However, these individuals need reassurance and support while in a group. They may verbalize that they do not fit in or belong in the group. In reality, they are feeling insecure and threatened in the situation. The group leader needs to show patience and understanding to engage the individual effectively in meaningful group interaction.

Family Interventions

The results of a family assessment often reveal that families of these individuals need education about the disorder, helpful strategies for dealing with the multiple

complaints of the patient, and usually help in developing more effective communication patterns. Because of the chaotic nature of some of the families and the lack of healthy problem solving, physical, sexual, and psychological abuse may be evident. It is important to be particularly sensitive to any evidence of current physical or sexual abuse because this may lead to a need for additional interventions (see Chapter 40).

Evaluation and Treatment Outcomes

Recovery outcomes for patients with SSD should be realistic. Because this is a lifelong disorder, small successes should be expected. Specific outcomes should be identified, such as gradually increasing social contact. Over time, there should be a gradual reduction in the number of health care providers the individual contacts and a slight improvement in the ability to cope with stresses (Figure 29.4).

Continuum of Care

Inpatient Care

Ideally, individuals with SSD spend minimal time in the hospital for treatment of their medical or comorbid mental disorders. While an inpatient, the patient should have consistency in providers who care or oversees all of the nursing care. Therapeutic interactions and relationships are very important and can help move the individual toward recovery.

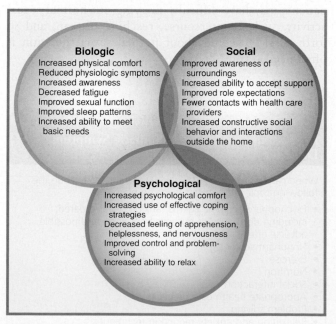

FIGURE 29.4 Biopsychosocial outcomes for patients with somatic symptom disorder.

Emergency Care

The emergencies these individuals experience may be physical (e.g., chest pain, back pain, gastrointestinal symptoms) or stress responses related to a psychosocial crisis. Occasionally, these individuals become suicidal and require an intensive level of care. Generally speaking, nonpharmacologic interventions should be tried first, with very conservative use of antianxiety medications. All attempts should be made to retrieve records from other facilities.

Community Treatment

These patients can spend a lifetime in the health care system and still have little continuity of care. Switching from provider to provider is detrimental to their long-term care. Most are outpatients. When they are hospitalized, it is usually for evaluation of medical problems or to receive care for comorbid disorders. See Nursing Care Plan 29.1.

Mental Health Promotion

Patients with SSD should focus on "staying healthy" instead of focusing on their illnesses. For these individuals, approaching the topic of health promotion usually has to be within the context of preventing further problems. Setting aside time for themselves and identifying activities that meet their psychological and spiritual needs, such as going to church or synagogue, are important in maintaining a healthy balance.

ILLNESS-RELATED DISORDER

Illness-related disorder is a new classification in the *DSM-5*. Previously, the term hypochondriasis was used to classify this disorder. Most of the persons with hypochondriasis were also diagnosed with somatic symptom disorder. However, there are some individuals who either do not have somatic symptoms or have very mild symptoms, but are still preoccupied with having or developing a medical illness (APA, 2013). These individuals would receive the diagnosis of illness-related disorder and would be encouraged to seek mental health treatment for their anxiety and preoccupation.

CONVERSION DISORDER (FUNCTIONAL NEUROLOGIC SYMPTOM DISORDER)

Conversion disorder is a psychiatric condition in which severe emotional distress or unconscious conflict is expressed through physical symptoms (APA, 2013). Patients with conversion disorder have neurologic symptoms that include impaired coordination or balance, paralysis, aphonia (inability to produce sound), difficulty swallowing or a sensation of a lump in the throat, and urinary retention. They also may have loss of touch, vision problems, blindness, deafness, and hallucinations. In some instances, they may have seizures (Nielsen, Stone, & Edwards, 2013). However, laboratory, electroencephalographic, and neurologic test results are typically negative. The symptoms, different than those with an organic basis, do not follow a neurologic course but rather follow the person's own perceived conceptualization of the problem. For example, if the arm is paralyzed and will not move, there still may be reflexes and muscle tone.

There is evidence that there are neurobiologic changes in the brains of people with this disorder that may be responsible for the loss of sensation or control of movement. Stress also may be a contributing factor. There are reports that childhood trauma (such as sexual abuse) is associated with the later development of conversion disorder (Kaplan et al., 2013).

It is important to understand that the lack of physical sensation and movement is real for the patient. In approaching this patient, the nurse treats the conversion symptom as real symptoms that may have distressing psychological aspects. Acknowledging the symptoms helps the patient deal with them. As trust develops within the nurse–patient relationship, the nurse can help the patient develop problem-solving approaches to everyday problems.

FACTITIOUS DISORDERS

Persons with **factitious disorders** intentionally cause an illness or injury to receive the attention of health care workers. These individuals are motivated solely by the desire to become a patient and develop a dependent relationship with a health care provider. There are two types of factitious disorders: factitious disorder and factitious disorder by proxy.

Factitious Disorder

Although feigned illnesses have been described for centuries, it was not until 1951 that the term **Münchausen's syndrome** was used to describe the most severe form of this disorder, which was characterized by fabricating a physical illness, having recurrent hospitalizations, and going from one provider to another (Asher, 1951). Today, this disorder is called *factitious disorder* and is differentiated from **malingering**, in which the individual who intentionally produces illness symptoms is motivated by another specific self-serving goal, such as being classified as disabled or avoiding work.

(text continues on page 552)

NURSING CARE PLAN 29.1

The Patient With Somatic Symptom Disorder

SC is a 48-year-old woman who is making her weekly visit to her primary care physician for unexplained multiple somatic problems. This week, her concern is reoccurring abdominal pain that fits no symptom pattern. Upon physical examination, a cause for her abdominal pain could not be found. She is requesting a refill of alprazolam (Xanax) which is the only medication that relieves her pain. She is in the process of applying for disability income because of being completely disabled by neck and shoulder pain. The physician and office staff avoid her whenever possible. The physician will not refill the prescription until SC is evaluated by the consulting mental health team that provides weekly evaluations and services.

Setting: Primary Care Office

Baseline Assessment: 48-year-old Caucasian, obese woman who appears very angry. She resents being forced to see a psychiatric clinician for the only medication that works. She denies any psychiatric problems or emotional distress. SC is wearing a short, black top and slacks that are too tight. Her hair is in curlers and she says that it is too much trouble to comb her hair. Her mental status is normal, but she admits to being slightly depressed and takes the alprazolam for her nerves. She says she has nothing to live for, but denies any thoughts of suicide. She is dependent on her children for everything and feels very guilty about it. She spends most of her waking hours going to various doctors and taking combinations of medications to relieve her pains. She has no friends or nonfamily social contacts because they would not be able to stand her.

Associated Psychiatric Diagnosis	Medications
R/O depression; SSD	Premarin, 0.625 mg every day
S/P hysterectomy	Alprazolam (Xanax), 25 mg tid
S/P gastric bypass	Ranitidine HCL (Zantac), 150 mg with meals
S/P carpel tunnel release	Simethicone, 125 mg qid with meals
Chronic shoulder, neck pain, vertigo	Calcium carbonate, 1,200 mg every day
	Multiple vitamin, every day
	Zolpidem tartrate (Ambien), 10 mg at bedtime PRN
	Ibuprofen, 600 mg q4h PRN pain
	Maalox, PRN
	Preparation H suppositories

Nursing Diagnosis 1: Chronic Low Self-Esteem

Defining Characteristics	Related Factors
Self-negating verbalizations (long-standing)	Feeling unimportant to family
Hesitant to try new things	Feeling rejected by husband
Expresses guilt	Constant physical problems interfering with normal social activities
Evaluates self as being unable to deal with events	

Outcomes

Initial	Long-term
Identify need to increase self-esteem	Participate in individual or group therapy for esteem building

Interventions

Interventions	Rationale	Ongoing Assessment
Establish rapport with patient	Individuals with low self-esteem are reluctant to discuss true feelings	Self-exam feelings provoked by patient (discuss with supervisor if interfering with care). Determine if patient is beginning to engage in a relationship.

Continued

NURSING CARE PLAN 29.1 *(Continued)*

Interventions	Rationale	Ongoing Assessment
Encourage patient to spend time dressing and grooming appropriately.	Confidence and self-esteem improve when a person looks well-groomed.	Monitor response to suggestions.
Encourage patient to discuss various somatic problems but allow some time to discuss psychological and interpersonal issues.	Patients with SSD need time to express their physical problems. It helps them feel valued. The best way to build a relationship is to acknowledge physical symptoms.	Monitor time that patient spends explaining physical symptoms.
Explore opportunities for SC to meet other people with similar, nonmedical interests.	Focusing SC on meeting others will improve the possibilities of increasing contacts.	Observe willingness to identify other interests besides physical problems.

Evaluation

Outcomes	Revised Outcomes	Interventions
SC admitted to having low self-esteem but was very reluctant to consider meeting new people.	Focus on building self-esteem.	Identify activities that will enhance personal self-esteem.

Nursing Diagnosis 2: Ineffective Therapeutic Regimen Management

Defining Characteristics	Related Factors
Choices of daily living ineffective for meeting health care goal. Verbalizes difficulty with prescribed regimens.	Inappropriate use of benzodiazepines for nerves.

Outcomes

Initial	Long-term
Honestly discuss the use of medications.	Use nonpharmacologic means for stress reduction, especially antianxiety medications.

Interventions

Interventions	Rationale	Ongoing Assessment
Clarify the frequency and purpose of taking alprazolam.	Unsupervised polypharmacy is very common with these patients. Further clarification is usually needed.	Carefully track self-report of medication use; determine if patient is disclosing the use of all medications.
Educate patient about the effects of combining medications, emphasizing negative effects.	Education about combining medication is the beginning of helping patient become effective in medication regimen.	Observe patient's ability and willingness to consider negative effects.
Recommend that patient gradually reduce number of medications and problem-solve other means of managing physical symptoms.	Giving patients clear directions about managing health care regimens needs to be followed up with specific strategies to change behavior.	Evaluate patient's ability to problem solve.

Evaluation

Outcomes	Revised Outcomes	Interventions
Patient disclosed use of medications but was unwilling to consider changing ineffective use of medication.	Identify next step if primary care physician does not refill prescription.	Discuss the possibility of not being able to obtain alprazolam. Refer patient to mental health clinic for further evaluation.

Clinical Course and Diagnostic Criteria

Unlike people with borderline personality disorder, who typically injure themselves overtly and readily admit to self-harm, patients with factitious disorder injure themselves covertly. The illnesses are produced in such a manner that the health care provider is tricked into believing that a true physical or psychiatric disorder is present (McDermott, Leamon, Feldman, & Scott, 2010).

The self-produced physical symptoms appear as medical illnesses and cut across all body systems. They include seizure disorders, wound-healing disorders, the abscess processes (introduction of infectious material below the skin surface), and feigned fever (rubbing the thermometer). These patients are extremely creative in simulating illnesses, and they tell fascinating but false stories of personal triumph. These tales are referred to as **pseudologia fantastica** and are a core symptom of the disorder. Pseudologia fantastica are stories that are not entirely improbable and often contain a matrix of truth and falsehood. These patients falsify blood, urine, and other samples by contaminating them with protein or fecal material. They self-inject anticoagulants to receive diagnoses of "bleeding of undetermined origin" or ingest thyroid hormones to produce thyrotoxicosis. They also inflict injury on themselves by inserting objects or feces into body orifices, such as the urinary tract, open wounds, or even intravenous tubing. They produce their own surgical scars, especially abdominal, and when treated surgically, they delay wound healing through scratching, rubbing, or manipulating the wound and introducing bacteria into the wound. These patients put themselves in life-threatening situations through actions such as ingesting allergens known to produce an anaphylactic reaction.

Patients who manifest primarily psychological symptoms produce psychotic symptoms such as hallucinations and delusions, cognitive deficits such as memory loss, dissociative symptoms such as amnesia, and conversion symptoms such as pseudoblindness or pseudoparalysis. These individuals often become psychotic, depressed, or suicidal after an unconfirmed tragedy. When questioned about details, they become defensive and uncooperative. Sometimes these individuals have a combination of both physical and psychiatric symptoms.

Epidemiology and Risk Factors

The prevalence of factitious disorder is unknown because diagnosing it and obtaining reliable data are difficult. The prevalence was reported to be high when researchers were actually looking for the disorder in specific populations. Within large general hospitals, factitious disorders are diagnosed in about 1% of patients with whom mental health professionals consult. The age range of patients with the disorder is between 19 and 64 years. The median age

of onset is the early 20s. Once thought to occur predominantly in men, this disorder is now reported predominantly in women. No genetic pattern has been identified, but it does seem to run in families. The presence of comorbid psychiatric disorders, such as mood disorders, personality disorders, and substance-related disorders, is common (McDermott, Leamon, Feldman, & Scott, 2010).

Etiology

Many people with factitious disorder have experienced severe sexual or marital distress before the development of the disorder. The psychodynamic explanation is that these individuals, who were often abused as children, received nurturance only during times of illness; thus, they try to recreate illness or injury in a desperate attempt to receive love and attention. During the actual self-injury, the individual is reported to be in a trancelike, dissociative state. Many patients report having an intimate relationship with a health care provider, either as a child or as an adult, and then experiencing rejection when the relationship ended. The self-injury and subsequent attention is an attempt by the individual to re-enact those experiences and gain control over the situation and the other person. Often, the patients exhibit aggression after being discovered, allowing them to express revenge on their perceived tormenter (Feldman, Eisendrath, & Tyerman, 2008).

These patients are usually discovered in medical–surgical settings. They are hostile and distance themselves from others. Their network is void of friends and family and usually consists only of health care providers, who change at regular intervals. In factitious disorder, the patient fabricates a detailed and exaggerated medical history. When the interventions do not work and the fabrication is discovered, the health care team feels manipulated and angry. When the patient is confronted with the evidence, he or she becomes enraged and often leaves that health care system, only to enter another. Eventually, the person is referred for mental health treatment. The course of the disorder usually consists of intermittent episodes (McDermott, Leamon, Feldman, & Scott, 2010).

NURSING MANAGEMENT: Human Response to Factitious Disorder

The overall goal of treatment for a patient with factitious disorder is to replace the dysfunctional, attention-seeking behaviors with positive behaviors. To begin treatment, the patient must acknowledge the deception. Because the pattern of self-injury is well established and meets overwhelming psychological needs, giving up the behaviors is difficult. The treatment is long-term psychotherapy. The psychiatric–mental health nurse will most likely care for the patient during or after periods of feigned illnesses.

Assessment

A nursing assessment should focus on obtaining a history of medical and psychological illnesses. Physical disabilities should be identified. Early childhood experiences, particularly instances of abuse, neglect, or abandonment, should be identified to understand the underlying psychological dynamics of the individual and the role of self-injury. Family assessment is important because family relationships become strained as the members become aware of the self-inflicted nature of this disorder.

Nursing Diagnoses

The nursing diagnoses could include almost any diagnosis, including Risk for Trauma, Risk for Self-Mutilation, Ineffective Individual Coping, or Low Self-Esteem.

Desired outcomes include decreased self-injurious behavior and increased positive coping behaviors. Any nursing intervention must be implemented within the context of a strong nurse–patient relationship.

Nursing Interventions

The fabrications and deceits of patients with factitious disorder provoke anger and a sense of betrayal in many nurses. To be effective with these patients, it is important to be aware of these feelings and resolve them by developing a better understanding of the underlying psychodynamic issues (Box 29.7). Confronting the patient has been reported effective if the patient feels supported and accepted and if there is clear communication among the patient, the mental health care team, and family members. All care should be centralized within one facility,

and the patient should see providers regularly even when not in active crisis. Offering the patient a face-saving way of giving up the behaviors is often crucial. Behavioral techniques that shape new behaviors help the patient move forward toward a new life.

A team that knows the patient, agrees on a treatment approach and follows through is crucial to the patient's eventual recovery. For this to happen, the medical, psychiatric, inpatient, and outpatient teams need to communicate with each other on a regular basis. Family members must also be aware of the need for consistent treatment.

Factitious Disorder Imposed on Another

A rare but dramatic disorder, **factitious disorder imposed on another** (previously factitious disorder by proxy or Münchausen's by proxy), involves a person who inflicts injury on another person. It is commonly a mother, who inflicts injuries on her child to gain the attention of the health care provider through her child's injuries. These actions include inducing seizures, poisoning, or smothering. This most severe form of child abuse is usually identified in the emergency department. The mother rarely admits injuring the child and thus is not amenable to treatment; the child is removed from the mother's care. This form of child abuse is distinguished from other forms by the routine, unwitting involvement of health care workers, who subject the child to physical harm and emotional distress through tests, procedures, and medication trials. Some researchers suspect that children who are abused in this way may later experience factitious disorder themselves (McDermott, Leamon, Feldman, & Scott, 2010).

BOX 29.7

Using Reflection

ETHICAL DILEMMA

INCIDENT • Walking into a patient's room, the nurse observes a patient purposefully tearing open her sutures. The nurse yells at her to stop and asks her why she is doing that. The patient screams at her to get out and leave her alone. The nurse is upset and tries to understand what she just witnessed. She keeps asking, "How could she do that when she just went through a major surgery to repair her problem?"

REFLECTION • Upon reflecting, the nurse realized that her own values were in conflict and that she was very angry with the patient for purposefully traumatizing herself. She then focused on trying to understand the patient's need to carry out such painful self-abuse. She resolved to discuss the behavior with the patient using a nonjudgmental approach to help her develop new ways of dealing with the underlying need for self-mutilation.

SUMMARY OF KEY POINTS

- Somatization is affected by sociocultural and gender factors. It occurs more frequently in women than men and in those who are less educated. It also has been strongly associated with individuals who have been sexually abused as children.

- SSD is a chronic relapsing condition characterized by multiple physical symptoms of unknown origin that develop during times of emotional distress.

- Conversion disorder is a condition of neurologic symptoms (impaired voluntary muscles or sensory stimulation) that is associated with severe emotional distress.

- Factitious disorders include two types, factitious disorder and factitious disorder imposed on another. In factitious disorder, physical or psychological symptoms (or both) are fabricated to assume the sick role. In factitious disorder imposed on another, the intentional production of symptoms is in others, usually children.

■ Identifying somatic symptom disorders is very complex because patients with these disorders refuse to accept any psychiatric basis to their problems and often go for years moving from one health care provider to another to receive medical attention and avoid psychiatric assessment.

■ These patients are often seen on the medical–surgical units of hospitals and go years without receiving a correct diagnosis. In most cases, they finally receive mental health treatment because of comorbid conditions, such as depression, anxiety, and panic disorder.

■ The development of the nurse–patient relationship is crucial to assessing these patients and identifying appropriate nursing diagnoses and interventions. Because these patients deny any psychiatric basis to their problem and continue to focus on their symptoms as being medically based, the nurse must take a flexible, relaxed, and nonjudgmental approach that acknowledges the symptoms but focuses on new ways of coping with stress and avoiding recurrence of symptoms.

■ Health teaching is important in helping the individual develop positive lifestyle changes in place of somatization responses. Identifying personal strengths and supporting the development of positive skills improve self-esteem and personal confidence. Teaching the use of stress management provides the patient with positive coping skills.

CRITICAL THINKING CHALLENGES

1. A depressed young woman is admitted to a psychiatric unit in a state of agitation. She reports extreme abdominal pain. Her admitting provider tells you that she has a classic case of and to de-emphasize her physical symptoms. Under no circumstances is she to have any pain medication. Conceptualize the assessment process and how you would approach this patient.

2. Develop a continuum of "self-injury" for patients with borderline personality disorder, SSD, factitious disorder, and factitious disorder by proxy.

3. Develop a teaching plan for an individual who has a long history of somatization but who recently received a diagnosis of breast cancer. How will the patient be able to differentiate the physical symptoms of somatization from those associated with the treatment of her breast cancer?

4. A Chinese American patient was admitted for panic attacks and numerous somatic problems, ranging from dysmenorrhea to painful joints. The results of all medical examinations have been negative. She truly believes that her panic attacks are caused by a weak heart. What approaches should the nurse use in providing culturally sensitive nursing care?

5. A person with depression is started on a regimen of Nardil, 15 mg tid. She believes that she is allergic to most foods but insists on having wine in the evenings because it helps digest her food. Develop a teaching plan that provides the knowledge that she needs to prevent a hypertensive crisis caused by excessive tyramine but that is sensitive to the patient's food preferences.

MOVIE

Safe: 1995. This is a story of Carol White (Julianne Moore), a married, stay-at-home mother who appears to have everything. She begins having headaches that lead to a grand-mal seizure. As the movie unfolds, she becomes sicker and sicker as she reports she is allergic to environmental toxins. She seeks help from an allergist and psychiatrists. She eventually leaves her husband for a retreat that is actually a scam.

SIGNIFICANCE: The film depicts the pain and suffering that is characteristic of somatization and its impact on the family. It also shows how desperate a person can be to seek out relief of symptoms.

VIEWING POINTS: Identify the mistakes in recognizing and treating the somatic disorder.

References

Allen, L. A., & Woolfolk, R. L. (2010). Cognitive behavioral therapy for somatoform disorders. *Psychiatric Clinics of North America, 33*(3), 579–593.

American Psychiatric Association (APA). (2013). *Diagnostic and statistical manual of mental disorders (5th ed)*. Arlington, VA: American Psychiatric Association.

Anderson, G., Maes, M., & Berk, M. (2012). Biological underpinnings of the commonalties in depression, somatization, and Chronic Fatigue Syndrome. *Medical Hypotheses, 78*(6), 752–756.

Asher, R. (1951). Münchausen's syndrome. *Lancet, 1*, 339–341.

Boutros, N. N., & Peters, R. (2012). Internal gating and somatization disorders: Proposing a yet un-described neural system. *Medical Hypotheses. 78*(1), 174–178.

Deng, Y., Ma, X., & Tang, Q. (2013). Brain response during visual emotional processing: An fMRI study of alexithymia. *Psychiatry Research, 213*(3), 225–229.

Dere, J., Sun, J., Zhao, Y., Persson, T., Zhu, X., Yao, S., et al. (2013). Beyond 'somatization' and "psychologization": Symptom-level variation in depressed Han Chinese and Euro-Canadian outpatients. *Frontiers in Psychology, 4*, 377, doi:10.3389/fpsyg.2013.00377.

Dumont, I. P., & Olson, A. L. (2012). Primary care, expression, and anxiety: Exploring somatic and emotional predictors of mental health status in adolescents. *Journal of the American Board of Family Medicine, 25*(3), 291–299.

Fabião, C., Silva, M. C., Fleming, M., & Barbosa, A. (2010). Somatoform disorders: A revision of the epidemiology in primary health care. *Acta Medica Portuguesa, 23*(5), 865–872.

Feldman, M. D., Eisendrath, S. J., & Tyerman, M. (2008). Psychiatric and behavioral correlates of factitious blindness. *Comprehensive Psychiatry, 49*(2), 159–162.

Leiknes, K. A., Finset, A., & Moum, T. (2010). Commonalities and differences between the diagnostic groups: Current somatoform disorders, anxiety and/or depression, and musculoskeletal disorders. *Journal of Psychosomatic Research, 68*(5), 439–446.

Kaplan, M. M., Dwivedi, A. K., Privitera, M. D., Isaacs, K., Hughes, C., & Bowman, M. (2013). Comparisons of childhood trauma, alexithymia, and defensive styles in patients with psychogenic non-epileptic seizures vs. epilepsy: Implications for the etiology of conversion disorder. *Journal of Psychosomatic Research, 75*(2), 142–146.

Krishnan, V., Sood, M., & Chadda, R. K. (2013). Caregiver burden and disability in somatization disorder. *Journal of Psychosomatic Research, 75*(4), 376–380.

McDermott, B. E., Leamon, M. H., Feldman, M. D., & Scott, C. L. (2010). Factitious disorder and malingering. In R. E. Hales, S. C. Yudofsky, & G. O Gabbard (Eds.). *The American Psychiatric Publishing textbook of clinical psychiatry* (5th ed.). Arlington, VA: American Psychiatric Publishing.

Mik-Meyer, N., & Obling, A. R. (2012). The negotiation of the sick role: General practitioners; classification of patients with medically unexplained symptoms. *Sociology of Health & Illness, 34*(7), 1025–1038.

Moreno, S., Gili, M., Magallón, R., Bauzá, N., Rocal, M., Hoyo, Y. L., et al. (2013). Effectiveness of group versus individual cognitive-behavioral therapy in patients with abridged somatization disorder: A randomized controlled trial. *Psychosomatic Medicine, 75*(6), 600–608.

Nielsen, G., Stone, J., & Edwards, J.J. (2012). Physiotherapy for functional (psychogenic) motor symptoms: A systematic review. *Journal of Psychosomatic Research, 75*(2), 93–102.

Noyes, R. Jr., Langbehn, D., Happel, R., Sieren, L., & Muller, B. (1999). Health Attitude Survey: A scale for assessing somatizing patients. *Psychosomatics, 40*(6), 470–478.

Pedrosa, G. F., Ridout, N., Kessler, H., Neuffer, M., Schoechlin, C., Traue, H. C., et al. (2009). Facial emotion recognition and alexithymia in adults with somatoform disorders. *Depression and Anxiety, 26*(1), e26–e33.

Rief, W., & Broadbent, E. (2007). Explaining medically unexplained symptoms-models and mechanisms. *Clinical Psychology Review, 27*(7), 821–841.

Schulte, I. E., & Petermann, F. (2011). Somatoform disorders: 30 years of debate about criteria! What about children and adolescents? *Journal of Psychosomatic Research, 70*(3), 218–228.

Sharma, M. P., & Manjula, M. (2013). Behavioural and psychological management of somatic symptom disorders: An overview. *International Review of Psychiatry, 25*(1), 116–124

Spangenberg, L., Forkmann, T., Brahler, E., Glaesmer, H. (2011). The association of depression and multimorbidity in the elderly: Implications for the assessment of depression. *Psychogeriatrics, 11*(4), 227–234.

van Dijke, A., Ford, J. D., van der Hart, O., van Son, M., van der Heijden, P., & Bühring, M. (2010). Affect dysregulation in borderline personality disorder and somatoform disorder: Differentiating under-and over regulation. *Journal of Personality Disorders, 24*(3), 296–311.

Woolfolk, R. L., Allen, L. A., & Tiu, J. E. (2007). New directions in the treatment of somatization. *Psychiatric Clinics of North America, 30*(4), 21–44.

Yusim, A., Anbarasan, D., Hall, B., Goetz, R., Neugebauer, R., Stewart, T., et al. (2010). Sociocultural domains of depression among indigenous populations in Latin America. *International Review of Psychiatry, 22*(4), 370–377.

Zaroff, C. M., Davis, J. M., Chio, P. H., & Madhavan, D. (2012). Somatic presentations of distress in China. *Australian and New Zealand Journal of Psychiatry, 46*(11), 1053–1057.

Zink, T., Klesges, L., Stevens, S., & Decker, P. (2009). The development of a sexual abuse severity score: Characteristics of childhood sexual abuse associated with trauma symptomatology, somatization, and alcohol abuse. *Journal of Interpersonal Violence, 24*(3), 395–405.

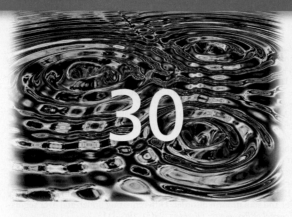

30 Eating Disorders
Management of Eating and Weight

Jane H. White

KEY CONCEPTS

- body dissatisfaction
- body image distortion
- dietary restraint
- drive for thinness
- interoceptive awareness
- perfectionism

LEARNING OBJECTIVES

After studying this chapter, you will be able to:

1. Distinguish the signs and symptoms of anorexia nervosa from those of bulimia nervosa.

2. Describe theories explaining anorexia nervosa and bulimia nervosa.

3. Differentiate binge eating disorder from anorexia nervosa and bulimia nervosa.

4. Describe the risk factors and protective factors associated with the development of eating disorders.

5. Explain the importance of body image, body dissatisfaction, and gender identity in developmental theories that explain etiology of eating disorders.

6. Explain the impact of sociocultural norms on the development of eating disorders.

7. Formulate the nursing diagnoses for individuals with eating disorders.

8. Analyze special concerns within the nurse–patient relationship for the nursing care of individuals with eating disorders.

9. Develop recovery-oriented nursing interventions for individuals with anorexia nervosa and bulimia nervosa.

10. Identify strategies for prevention and early detection of eating disorders.

KEY TERMS

- anorexia nervosa • binge eating • binge eating disorder (BED) • body image • bulimia nervosa
- cue elimination • enmeshment • self-monitoring

Only since the 1970s have eating disorders received national attention, primarily because several high-profile personalities and athletes with these disorders have received front-page news coverage. Since the 1960s, the increased incidence of anorexia nervosa and bulimia nervosa has prompted mental health professionals to address their causes and devise effective treatments. Moreover, there has been a concomitant increase in research studies addressing this intense obsession with being thin and the dissatisfaction with one's body that underlie these potentially life-threatening disorders. Thus, mental health professionals are committed to prevention, early diagnosis, and treatment of individuals with both anorexia nervosa and bulimia nervosa.

This chapter focuses on anorexia nervosa and bulimia nervosa and briefly discusses binge eating disorder (BED).

Eating disorders differ in definition, clinical course, etiologies, and interventions and are presented separately in this chapter. However, symptoms of these disorders, such as dieting, binge eating, and preoccupation with weight and shape overlap significantly. Viewing the symptoms along a continuum from less to more severe eating behaviors helps with this conceptualization, as shown in Figure 30.1 (Dennard & Richards, 2013). There are also common psychological characteristics of people with eating disorders (Box 30.1). Subclinical cases, also called partial syndromes, are usually diagnosed as Eating Disorder Not Otherwise Specified (EDNOS). These individuals still need treatment despite not meeting criteria for anorexia nervosa or bulimia nervosa.

> **BOX 30.1**
>
> ### Psychological Characteristics Related to Eating Disorders
>
> **ANOREXIA NERVOSA**
> Decreased interoceptive awareness
> Sexuality conflict or fears
> Maturity fears
> Ritualistic behaviors
>
> **BULIMIA NERVOSA**
> Impulsivity
> Boundary problems
> Limit-setting difficulties
>
> **ANOREXIA NERVOSA AND BULIMIA NERVOSA**
> Difficulty expressing anger
> Low self-esteem
> Body dissatisfaction
> Powerlessness
> Ineffectiveness
> Perfectionism
> Dietary restraint
> Obsessiveness
> Compulsiveness
> Nonassertiveness
> Cognitive distortions

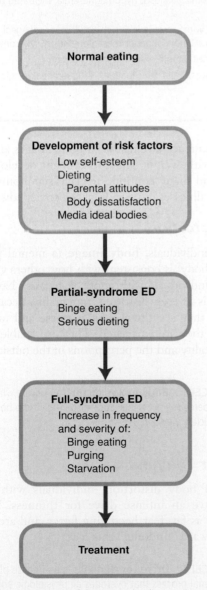

FIGURE 30.1 Progression of symptoms leading to an eating disorder.

ANOREXIA NERVOSA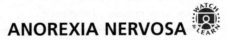

Anorexia nervosa is a mixture of biopsychosocial symptoms that include significantly low body weight, intense fear of gaining weight or becoming fat, and a disturbance in experiencing body weight or shape (undue influence or distorted self-evaluation of body weight or shape or lack of recognition of the seriousness of low body weight).

Anorexia nervosa is further categorized into two major types: *restricting* (dieting and exercising with no binge eating or misuse of laxatives, diuretics, or enemas) and *binge eating and purging* (binge eating and misuse of laxatives, diuretics, or enemas). Malnutrition and semi-starvation result in a preoccupation with food, binge eating, depression, obsession, and apathy, as well as compromising several body systems, leading to medical complications and, in some instances, death (American Psychiatric Association, 2013). See Table 30.1 for a list of complications from eating disorders.

Clinical Course

The onset of anorexia nervosa usually occurs in early adolescence. The onset can be slow with serious dieting occurring before an emaciated body—the result of starvation—is noticed. This discovery often prompts diagnosis. Because the incidence of subclinical or partial-syndrome cases, in which the symptoms are not severe enough to use an anorexia nervosa diagnosis, is higher than that of anorexia nervosa, many young women may not receive early treatment for their symptoms, or in some cases, they

Table 30.1	COMPLICATIONS OF EATING DISORDERS
Body System	**Symptoms**
From Starvation to Weight Loss	
Musculoskeletal	Loss of muscle mass, loss of fat (emaciation), osteoporosis
Metabolic	Hypothyroidism (symptoms include lack of energy, weakness, intolerance to cold, and bradycardia), hypoglycemia, decreased insulin sensitivity
Cardiac	Bradycardia; hypotension; loss of cardiac muscle; small heart; cardiac arrhythmias, including atrial and ventricular premature contractions, prolonged QT interval, ventricular tachycardia, sudden death
Gastrointestinal	Delayed gastric emptying, bloating, constipation, abdominal pain, gas, diarrhea
Reproductive	Amenorrhea, low levels of luteinizing hormone and follicle-stimulating hormone, irregular periods
Dermatologic	Dry, cracking skin and brittle nails caused by dehydration, lanugo (fine, baby-like hair over the body), edema, acrocyanosis (bluish hands and feet), thinning hair
Hematologic	Leukopenia, anemia, thrombocytopenia, hypercholesterolemia, hypercarotenemia
Neuropsychiatric	Abnormal taste sensation (possible zinc deficiency)
	Apathetic depression, mild organic mental symptoms, sleep disturbances, fatigue
Related to Purging (Vomiting and Laxative Abuse)	
Metabolic	Electrolyte abnormalities, particularly hypokalemia, hypochloremic alkalosis; hypomagnesemia; increased blood urea nitrogen
Gastrointestinal	Salivary gland and pancreatic inflammation and enlargement with increase in serum amylase, esophageal and gastric erosion (esophagitis) rupture, dysfunctional bowel with dilation, superior mesenteric artery syndrome
Dental	Erosion of dental enamel (perimylolysis), particularly of the frontal teeth, with decreased decay
Neuropsychiatric	Seizures (related to large fluid shifts and electrolyte disturbances), mild neuropathies, fatigue, weakness, mild organic mental symptoms
Cardiac	Ipecac cardiomyopathy arrhythmias

receive no treatment. The individual's refusal to maintain a normal weight because of a distorted body image and an intense fear of becoming fat make individuals with this disorder difficult to identify and treat.

It can be a chronic condition with relapses that are usually characterized by significant weight loss. Reporting conclusive outcomes for anorexia nervosa is difficult because of the variety of definitions used to determine recovery. Although patients considered to have recovered have restored normal weight, menses, and eating behaviors,

some continue to have distorted body images and be preoccupied with weight and food; many develop bulimia nervosa; and many continue to have symptoms of other psychiatric illnesses, especially of the anxiety disorders.

Body Distortion

For most individuals, **body image** (a mental picture of one's own body) is consistent with how others view them. However, individuals with anorexia nervosa have a body image that is severely distorted from reality. Because of this distortion, they see themselves as obese and undesirable even when they are emaciated. They are unable to accept objective reality and the perceptions of the outside world.

> **KEYCONCEPT** **Body image distortion** occurs when the individual perceives his or her body disparately from how the world or society views it.

Drive for Thinness

Because of body distortion, individuals with anorexia nervosa have an intense drive for thinness. They see themselves as fat, fear becoming fatter, and are "driven" to work toward "undoing" this fear.

> **KEYCONCEPT** **Drive for thinness** is an intense physical and emotional process that overrides all physiologic body cues.

FAME & FORTUNE

Karen Carpenter (1950–1983)

An American Musician

PUBLIC PERSONA

Karen Carpenter and her brother were the top best-selling American recording artists and performing musicians of the 1970s. In the United States alone, the Carpenters had eight gold albums, five platinum albums, and 10 gold single recordings—all proof of significant professional success.

PERSONAL REALITIES

In everyday life, however, Karen Carpenter battled with anorexia nervosa for 7 years—starving herself, using laxatives, drinking water, taking dozens of thyroid pills, and purging. Just as she was beginning to overcome the disorder, she died of complications at 32 years of age.

The individual with anorexia nervosa ignores body cues, such as hunger and weakness, and concentrates all efforts on controlling food intake. The entire mental focus of the young patient with anorexia nervosa narrows to only one goal: weight loss. Typical thought patterns are: "If I gain a pound, I'll keep gaining." This all-or-nothing thinking keeps these patients on rigid regimens for weight loss.

The behavior of patients with anorexia nervosa becomes organized around food-related activities, such as preparing food, counting calories, and reading cookbooks. Much behavior concerning what, when, and how they eat is ritualistic. Food combinations and the order in which foods may be eaten, and under which circumstances, can seem bizarre. One patient, for example, would eat only cantaloupe, carrying it with her to all meals outside of her home and consuming it only if it were cut in smaller than bite-sized pieces and only if she could use chopsticks, which she also carried with her.

Interoceptive Awareness

Feelings of inadequacy and a fear of maturity are also characteristic of individuals with anorexia nervosa. Weight loss becomes a way for these individuals to experience some sense of control and combat feelings of inadequacy and ineffectiveness. Every lost pound is viewed as a success, and weight loss often confers a feeling of virtuousness. Because these individuals feel inadequate, they fear emotional maturation and the unknown challenges the next developmental stages will bring. For some, remaining physically small is believed to symbolize remaining childlike. Patients with anorexia nervosa also have difficulty defining their feelings because they are confused about or unsure of emotions and visceral cues, such as hunger. This uncertainty is called a lack of interoceptive awareness.

KEYCONCEPT **Interoceptive awareness** is a term used to describe the sensory response to emotional and visceral cues, such as hunger.

Patients with anorexia nervosa are confused about sensations; therefore, their responses to cues are inaccurate and inappropriate. Often they cannot name the feelings they are experiencing, such as anxiety. This profound lack of interoceptive awareness is thought to be partially responsible for developing and maintaining this disorder and some instances of bulimia nervosa.

Perfectionism

Perfectionistic behavior, such as making sure that everything is symmetrical or that objects are placed the same distance from each other, is a typical significant symptom of anorexia nervosa and bulimia nervosa and is hypothesized to develop long before eating symptoms occur.

Perfectionism has been highlighted as a significant personality symptom risk factor in eating disorders (Kaye, Wierenga, Bailer, Simmons, & Bischoff-Greffe, 2013a).

KEYCONCEPT **Perfectionism** consists of personal standards (the extent to which the individual sets and tries to achieve high standards for oneself) and concern over mistakes and their consequences for their self-worth and others' opinions.

It is now accepted that perfectionism precedes the development of weight and shape concerns. The more severe the disorder, the more perfectionistic (Kaye et al., 2013b). As symptoms are resolved, perfectionism decreases (Bardone-Cone, Strum, Lawson, Robinson, & Smith, 2010).

Guilt and Anger

Patients with anorexia nervosa tend to avoid conflict and have difficulty expressing negative emotions, especially anger (Manuel & Wade, 2013). They have an overwhelming sense of guilt and anger, which leads to conflict avoidance, common in these families. Because of the ritualistic behaviors, an all-encompassing focus on food and weight, and feelings of inadequacy, social contacts are gradually reduced, and the patient becomes isolated. With more severe weight loss comes other symptoms, such as apathy, depression, and even mistrust of others.

Outcomes

Short-term outcomes for individuals with anorexia nervosa after hospitalization are poor. About 30% usually have a good outcome, 9% a more intermediate outcome, and 55% a poor outcome (Salbach-Andrae et al., 2009). Poor outcomes are related to a low body mass index (BMI) at the beginning of treatment, premorbid depression, comorbidity, and purging (vomiting and laxative use) (Berner, Shaw, Witt, & Lowe, 2013; Keski-Rahkonen et al., 2014). Readiness to change and the rate of weight restoration are associated with a positive outcome for inpatient treatment (Lund, Hernandez, Yates, Mitchell, & McKee, 2009).

Long-term outcomes are more positive than short-term outcomes, probably because of increased awareness of the disorder, early detection, and outpatient treatment after hospitalization. Approximately 70% of individuals with anorexia nervosa are said to have recovered 5 years after diagnosis (Keski-Rahkonen et al., 2007).

Diagnostic Criteria

The diagnosis of anorexia is made when there is a restriction of intake leading to significantly low body weight. The BMI is used as a measure of severity. Other criteria include an intense fear of gaining weight or becoming fat, and body image issues including an undue influence of body weight on self-concept and lack of recognition of seriousness of low body weight (APA, 2103). See Key Diagnostic Characteristics 30.1 for an overview of diagnostic criteria and associated findings. Amenorrhea was a criterion in previous diagnostic taxonomies, but is not included as a diagnostic criterion in the *DSM-5*. Some women with anorexia nervosa report menstrual activity and this criterion cannot be applied to premenarchal and postmenopausal women, men, or women taking oral contraceptives.

Epidemiology

In the United States, the lifetime prevalence of anorexia nervosa is reported to be from 0.5% to 1%. Despite pre-vention and early intervention efforts, the incidence (new cases) for anorexia nervosa has remained the same during the past decade at about 270 per 100,000 (Keski-Rahkonen et al., 2007). These findings lend support to hypothesis that there is a biologic or genetic predisposition for the development of anorexia nervosa.

Age of Onset

The age of onset is typically between 14 and 16 years but can occur much earlier. Adolescents are vulnerable because of stressors associated with their development, especially concerns about body image, autonomy, and peer pressure, and their susceptibility to such influences

---

KEY DIAGNOSTIC CHARACTERISTICS 30.1 • ANOREXIA NERVOSA

Diagnostic Criteria

A. Restriction of energy intake relative to requirements, leading to a significantly low body weight in the context of age, sex, developmental trajectory, and physical health. *Significantly low weight* is defined as a weight that is less than minimally normal or, for children and adolescents, less than that minimally expected.
B. Intense fear of gaining weight or of becoming fat, or persistent behavior that interferes with weight gain, even though at a significantly low weight.
C. Disturbance in the way in which one's body weight or shape is experienced, undue influence of body weight or shape on self-evaluation, or persistent lack of recognition of the seriousness of the current low body weight.

Specify whether:
• **Restricting type:** During the last 3 months, the individual has not engaged in recurrent episodes of binge eating or purging behavior (i.e., self-induced vomiting or the misuse of laxatives, diuretics, or enemas). This subtype describes presentations in which weight loss is accomplished primarily through dieting, fasting, and/or excessive exercise.
• (**Binge-eating/purging type:** During the last 3 months, the individual has engaged in recurrent episodes of binge eating or purging behavior (i.e., self-induced vomiting or the misuse of laxatives, diuretics, or enemas).

Specify if:
• **In partial remission:** After full criteria for anorexia nervosa were previously met, Criterion A (low body weight) has not been met for a sustained period, but either Criterion B (intense fear of gaining weight or becoming fat or behavior that interferes with weight gain) or Criterion C (disturbances in self-perception of weight and shape) is still met.
• **In full remission:** After full criteria for anorexia nervosa were previously met, none of the criteria have been met for a sustained period of time.

Specify current severity:
The minimum level of severity is based, for adults, on current body mass index (BMI) (see below) or, for children and adolescents, on BMI percentile. The ranges below are derived from World Health Organization categories for thinness in adults; for children and adolescents, corresponding BMI percentiles should be used. The level of severity may be increased to reflect clinical symptoms, the degree of functional disability, and the need for supervision.
• **Mild:** BMI ≥ 17 kg/m^2
• **Moderate:** BMI 16–16.99 kg/m^2
• **Severe:** BMI 15–15.99 kg/m^2
• **Extreme:** BMI < 15 kg/m^2

Target Symptoms and Associated Findings
• Depressive symptoms such as depressed mood, social withdrawal, irritability, insomnia, and diminished interest in sex
• Obsessive-compulsive features related and unrelated to food
• Preoccupation with thought of food
• Concerns about eating in public
• Feelings of ineffectiveness
• Strong need to control one's environment
• Inflexible thinking
• Limited social spontaneity and overly restrained initiative and emotional expression

Associated Physical Examination Findings
• Complaints of constipation, abdominal pain
• Cold intolerance
• Lethargy and excess energy
• Emaciation
• Significant hypotension, hypothermia, and skin dryness
• Bradycardia and possible peripheral edema
• Hypertrophy of salivary glands, particularly the parotid gland
• Dental enamel erosion related to induced vomiting
• Scars or calluses on dorsum of hand from contact with teeth for inducing vomiting

Associated Laboratory Findings
• Leukopenia and mild anemia
• Elevated blood urea nitrogen
• Hypercholesterolemia
• Elevated liver function studies
• Electrolyte imbalances, metabolic alkalosis, or metabolic acidosis
• Low normal serum thyroxine levels; decreased serum-triiodothyronine levels
• Low serum estrogen levels
• Sinus bradycardia
• Metabolic encephalopathy
• Significantly reduced resting energy expenditure
• Increased ventricular/brain ratio secondary to starvation

as the media, which extols an ideal body type. An important predictor of anorexia nervosa is early-onset menses, as early as 10 or 11 years of age (Favaro, Caregaro, Tenconi, Bosello, & Santonastaso, 2009).

Gender

Females are 10 times more likely than males to develop anorexia nervosa. This disparity has been attributed to society's influence on females to achieve an ideal body type (Zhao & Encinosa, 2009). Box 30.2 highlights some of the findings about eating disorders in males.

Ethnicity and Culture

In the United States, eating disorders occur in all ethnic and racial groups, but are slightly more common among Hispanic and white populations and less common among African Americans and Asians (Rhea & Thatcher, 2013). Since the 1990s, the incidence among various ethnic groups, especially ethnic minority groups, has increased. Contextual variables that may influence eating disorders in women of color are level of acculturation, socioeconomic status, level of education, peer socialization, family structure, and immigration status (Gordon, Castro, Sitnikov, & Holm-Denoma, 2010).

Comorbidity

Depression is common in individuals with anorexia nervosa, and these individuals are at risk to attempt suicide (Preti, Rocchi, Sisti, Camboni, & Miotto, 2011). However, anxiety disorders such as obsessive-compulsive disorder

(OCD), phobias, and panic disorder are even more strongly associated with anorexia nervosa. In many individuals with anorexia nervosa, OCD symptoms predate the anorexia nervosa diagnosis by about 5 years, leading many researchers to consider OCD a causative or risk factor for anorexia nervosa (Brady, 2014). In fact, perfectionism is an aspect of both OCD and anorexia nervosa and is considered a risk factor for anorexia nervosa (Kaye et al., 2013a). These comorbid conditions often resolve when anorexia nervosa has been treated successfully.

Etiology

Some of the risk factors (discussed later) and the etiologic factors for eating disorders overlap. For example, dieting is a risk factor for the development of anorexia nervosa, but it is also a biologic etiologic factor, and in its most serious form—starving—it is also a symptom. This overlap of risk factors, causes, and symptoms must be kept in mind. Most experts agree that anorexia nervosa (as well as bulimia nervosa) is multidimensional and multidetermined. Figure 30.2 depicts the biopsychosocial etiologic factors for anorexia nervosa.

Biologic Theories

Brain structure in the medial orbitofrontal cortex, insula (a segment of the cerebral cortex associated with diverse functions usually linked to emotions), and striatum is altered in eating disorders suggesting there is also altered brain circuitry. In the presence of food, neuroreceptor dynamics, regional blood flow (cingulate, frontal, temporal, and parietal regions), and cerebral glucose metabolism are activated resulting in body image distortions (Frank, 2011). Pleasantness in taste and sensitivity to

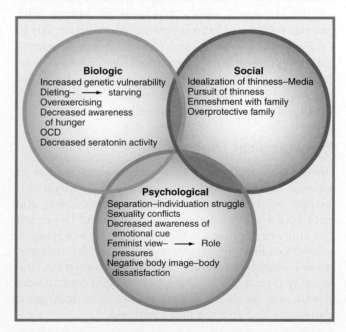

FIGURE 30.2 Biopsychosocial etiologies for patients with anorexia nervosa.

reward in individuals with anorexia nervosa are also associated with alterations in brain structures (Frank, Shott, Hagman, & Mittal, 2013).

Genetic Theories

First-degree relatives of people with anorexia nervosa have higher rates of this disorder. Rates of partial-syndrome or subthreshold cases among female family members of individuals with anorexia nervosa are even higher (Kay et al., 2013). Female relatives also have high rates of depression, leading researchers to hypothesize that a shared genetic factor may influence development of both disorders.

Genetic research shows that there is a genetic vulnerability to anorexia nervosa, especially in females (Baker, Maes, Lissner, Aggen, Lichtenstein, & Kendler, 2009; Kay et al., 2013). Genetic heritability accounts for an estimated 50% to 80% of the risk of developing an eating disorder (Kay et al., 2013a). Separating genetic influences from environmental influences is difficult when twins share a similar family environment.

Neuroendocrine and Neurotransmitter Changes

Several neurobiologic changes occur in an eating disorder. An increase in endogenous opioids (through exercise) contributes to denial of hunger. Malnutrition leads to a decrease in thyroid function. Serotonergic functioning is also blunted in low-weight patients (Frank, 2011). A study of women with both anorexia nervosa and bulimia nervosa demonstrated significantly reduced brain-derived neurotrophic factor (BDNF), which plays a role in memory formation, compared with healthy women. All of these individuals were malnourished; BDNF reduction may represent an adaptive change to counteract the decreased caloric ingestion of women with anorexia nervosa or bulimia nervosa (Monteleone, 2011). Until more definitive research is done, these neurochemical neurotransmitter changes should be viewed as indicating a vulnerability in some individuals, who under certain psychological and environmental conditions, such as cultural pressures, starve themselves.

Psychological Theories

Historically, the most widely accepted explanation of anorexia nervosa was the psychoanalytic paradigm that focused on conflicts of separation–individuation and autonomy. Usually diagnosed between 14 and 18 years of age, anorexia nervosa was thought to occur as a result of a developmental arrest of normal adolescent struggles around identity and role, body image formation, and sexuality (Bruch, 1973). Dieting and weight control were viewed as a means to defend against these feelings of inadequacy and growing into adulthood.

The psychoanalytic paradigm explained the disparity in the prevalence of eating disorders between boys and girls as being related to the development of self-esteem in adolescent girls. It was believed that the normal adolescent increase in self-doubt was linked to naturally occurring pubertal weight gain, which in turn resulted in confusion about one's identity. Unfortunately, this psychoanalytic perspective tended to blame parents, especially mothers, for the development of their child's illness. Today, the psychoanalytic theory is used in some psychotherapies, but it is no longer a competing theory of causation.

Internalization of Peer Pressure

Some adolescents have reported that dieting, binge eating, and purging were learned behaviors, resulting from peer pressure and a need to conform. Peers and friends, as well as peers in the larger school system, influence unhealthy weight-control behaviors among pre-adolescent and adolescent girls (Cave, 2009; Wilkosz, Chen, Kenndey, & Rankin, 2011).

Body Dissatisfaction

Once the body is considered all important, the individual begins to compare her body with others, such as those of celebrities. Images from television and fashion magazines are particularly powerful for young girls and adolescents struggling with the tasks of identity and body image formation. Body dissatisfaction resulting from this comparison, in which one's own body is perceived to fall short of an ideal, may be dissatisfaction about one's weight, shape, size, or even a certain body part. Even in the absence of overweight, most adolescents surveyed in numerous studies were dissatisfied with their bodies (van den Berg, Mond, Eisenberg, Ackard, & Neumark-Sztainer, 2010).

> **KEYCONCEPT** **Body dissatisfaction** occurs when the body becomes overvalued as a way of determining one's worth. Body dissatisfaction is strongly related to low self-esteem (van den Berg et al., 2010).

Many adolescents attempt to overcome this dissatisfaction through dieting and overexercising. Recently, a study on body dissatisfaction demonstrated that high BMIs and body dissatisfaction were more likely to occur in adolescents who later developed eating disorder symptoms (Napolitano & Himes, 2011).

Social Theories

More than with any other psychiatric condition, society plays a significant role in the development of eating disorders with conflicting messages that young women receive from society about their roles in life. Young girls may interpret expectations about how they should look, what roles they should perform, and what they should achieve in society as pressures to achieve "all."

The media, the fashion industry, and peer pressure are significant social influences. Magazines, television, videos, and the Internet depict young girls and adolescents, with thin and often emaciated bodies, as glamorous, successful, popular, and powerful. Girls diet because they want to be similar to these models both in character and appearance. Two of the most common adolescent dieting methods—restricting calories and taking diet pills—have been shown to be influenced by women's beauty and fashion magazines (Luff & Gray, 2009).

Preoccupation with body image and weight is also influenced by public awareness of the obesity epidemic (Cave, 2009). Pre-adolescent children are extreme susceptible to the message to reduce intake and increase exercise as a way to lose weight and maintain health. Coupled with Internet videos that sanction self-starvation, emerging adolescents are already dissatisfied with their bodies and have the tools to lose weight through dieting and exercise.

Feminists have focused on the role of this pressure as one part of an explanation for the significant increase in eating disorders and for the greater prevalence in females.

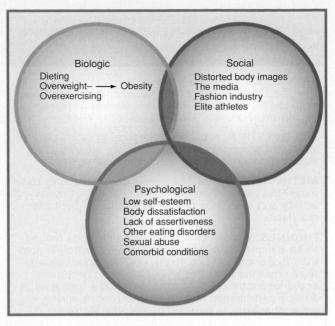

FIGURE 30.3 Biopsychosocial risk factors for anorexia and bulimia nervosa.

Box 30.3 outlines some feminist assumptions regarding role, feminism, and the development of eating disorders.

Risk Factors

Risk factors for eating disorders are multidimensional and can be depicted within the biopsychosocial model (Fig. 30.3). Puberty is a risk period for the development of anorexia nervosa, especially in girls (Klump, 2013). Girls often begin to diet at an early age because of body dissatisfaction, a need for control, a prepubertal weight increase. Restricting food can lead to starvation, binge eating, and purging.

Low self-esteem, body dissatisfaction, and feelings of ineffectiveness also put individuals at risk for an eating disorder. Much of the recent research on these factors has demonstrated that resilience or protective factors, such as healthy eating attitudes; an accepting attitude toward body size; and positive self-evaluation, especially toward physical and psychological characteristics, can mediate these risk factors and prevent development of an eating disorder (Gustafsson, Edlund, Kjellin, & Norring, 2009).

Athletes are at greater risk for developing eating disorders. For athletes, self-esteem, attractiveness, and improving appearance are related to disordered eating. Elite (leanness sports such as running and gymnastics) and non-elite athletes (non-leanness sports such as soccer) experience triad symptoms (disordered eating, menstrual dysfunction, and osteoporosis). See Box 30.4. Athletes involved in lean sports are at the highest risk (Javed, Tebben, Fischer, & Lteif, 2013).

BOX 30.3
Feminist Ideology and Eating Disorders

Since the 1970s, proponents of the feminist cultural model of eating disorders have advanced a position to explain the higher prevalence of these disorders in women. Feminists believe there is a struggle women have today similar to ones they believe women have had in history. They believe that during the Victorian era, "hysteria," a well-known emotional illness, developed as a result of oppression when women were not allowed to express their feelings and opinions and were "silenced" by a male-dominated society. Feminist scholars today have advanced the feminist relational model to understand the development of eating disorders. They view a major issue in development that causes conflict for young girls as the need to be connected versus society's view of the importance of separation. This confusion can be a stress that may be converted into disordered eating. Often at the base of symptoms such as severe food restriction is the gaining of power lost possibly because of this confusion in one's development (Kinsaul, Curtin, Bazzini, & Martz, 2014).

Feminists have taken issue with what they call the biomedical model of explanation for the development of eating disorders, seeing it as limiting and patriarchal. The recovery of society must take place to decrease the prevalence of eating disorders. Feminists believe that this will occur only when women are emancipated, given a voice, and socialized differently. They call for more research in which women are co-researchers as well as "subjects," helping to provide the investigators with their own stories and perspectives. Feminists underscore the need for research, especially on prevention, and the need to consider society and culture as well as individual risk factors such as internalization of thinness and a negative body image (Piran, 2010).

BOX 30.4

Research for Best Practice: **Eating Disorders and Women Athletes**

Holm-Denoma, J. M., Scaringi, V., Gordon K. H., Van Orden, K. A., & Joiner, T. E. (2009). Eating disorder symptoms among undergraduate varsity athletes, club athletes, independent exercisers, and nonexercisers. International Journal of Eating Disorders, 42(1), 47–53.

THE QUESTION: Are there differences in eating disorder symptoms among undergraduate varsity athletes, club athletes, independent exercisers, and nonexercisers?

METHODS: A total of 274 female undergraduates completed the eating disorders inventory and the physical activity and sport anxiety scale and reported their exercise habits.

FINDINGS: Women who participated in sports tended to have higher levels of eating disorder symptomatology than those who did not. Higher levels of sports anxiety were predictive of higher levels of bulimic symptoms and drive for thinness. Athletes who had a high level of athletic participation and experienced sports anxiety were more likely to have eating disorder symptoms.

IMPLICATIONS FOR NURSING: Nurses should be aware that athletes have higher rates of disordered eating and should be assessed for eating disorders. Nurses can teach parents and adolescents about the value of healthy athletic competition and the need to maintain healthy eating habits. An accurate assessment of each young woman is important.

Family Response to Disorder

Historically, the family of the patient with anorexia was labeled as overprotective, enmeshed, being unable to resolve conflicts, and being rigid regarding boundaries. Although an uninformed family can delay and complicate treatment, there is no evidence that family interactions are the primary cause of eating disorders (le Grange, Lock, Loeb, & Nicholls, 2010). Some family interactions can be problematic for the adolescent with an eating disorder. For example, when conflict erupts between two family members and direct communication is blocked, interaction patterns are changed that may result in a dysfunction relay of messages through other family members.

Enmeshment refers to an extreme form of intensity in family interactions and represents low individual autonomy in a family. In an enmeshed family, the individual gets lost in the system. The boundaries that define individual autonomy are weak. This excessive togetherness intrudes on privacy (Minuchin, Rossman, & Baker, 1978).

Overprotectiveness is defined as a high degree of concern for one another and can be detrimental to children at high risk for anorexia nervosa. The parents' overprotectiveness retards the child's development of autonomy and competence (Minuchin, Rossman, & Baker, 1978). *Rigidity* refers to families that are heavily committed to maintaining the status quo and find change difficult.

Conflict is avoided, and a strong ethical code or religious orientation is usually the rationale.

The family, often unwittingly, can transmit unrealistic attitudes about weight, shape, and size. Adolescents are particularly sensitive to comments about their bodies because this is the stage for body image formation. Parental attitudes about weight have been found to influence body dissatisfaction and dieting; parental comments about weight or shape or even parents' worrying about their own weight can influence adolescents in much the same way as the media does (Box 30.5). Children of mothers with eating disorders are at risk for developing such disorders, but the degree of risk depends on environmental factors and specific difficulties, such as the child's temperament. Maladaptive paternal behavior, such as low affection, communication, and time spent with a child, has recently been associated with the development of eating disorders (McElwen & Flouri, 2009).

Interdisciplinary Treatment and Recovery

Treatment for the patient with anorexia nervosa focuses on initiating nutritional rehabilitation to restore the individual to a healthy weight, resolving psychological conflicts around body image disturbance, increasing effective coping, addressing the underlying conflicts related to maturity fears and role conflict, and assisting the family

---

BOX 30.5

Research for Best Practice: **Family Influence on Disordered Eating**

Kluck, A. S. (2010). Family influence on disordered eating: The role of body image dissatisfaction. Body Image, 7(1), 8–14.

THE QUESTION: Does family culture that emphasizes appearance and thinness increase disorder eating and body image dissatisfaction? Do parent comments related to daughter's weight relate to the development of disorder eating?

METHODS: A sample of 268 never-married college women, ranging in age from 16–24 were recruited to participate in a study. Participants' mean weight was 136.57 pounds; height (65.32 in). Sample included 82.8% Caucasian; 6.3% Hispanic; 4.9% African American; 2.6% Asian American; 3% other racial background. Subjects completed the Body Shape questionnaire and Family Influence Scale.

FINDINGS: The findings support that family focus on appearance and specific types of comments (criticism from mother and teasing from father) that parents make about weight and size were associated with increased difficulties with behaviors associated with disordered eating.

IMPLICATIONS FOR NURSING: Families should be cautioned about the negative impact of emphasizing appearance and made aware that specific comments can lead to their daughter's body dissatisfaction.

BOX 30.6
Criteria for Hospitalization of Patients With Eating Disorders

MEDICAL
- Acute weight loss, <85% below ideal
- Heart rate near 40 beats/min
- Temperature, <36.1°C
- Blood pressure, <80/50 mm Hg
- Hypokalemia
- Hypophosphatemia
- Hypomagnesemia
- Poor motivation to recover

PSYCHIATRIC
- Risk for suicide
- Severe depression
- Failure to comply with treatment
- Inadequate response to treatment at another level of care (outpatient)

Adapted from American Psychiatric Association (2006). Treatment of patients with eating disorders, third edition. *American Journal of Psychiatry, 163*(7 suppl), 4–54.

with healthy functioning and communication. Several methods are used to accomplish these goals during the stages of illness and recovery.

When collaborating with the patient and family regarding the best approach to treatment (i.e., inpatient or outpatient), clinicians share evidence-based criteria in order to select the best treatment. Typically, the medical complications presented in Table 30.1 influence the decision to hospitalize an individual with an eating disorder. Suicidality is another reason for hospitalization. The criteria for hospital admission varies, and there is a lack of evidence-based studies determining when adolescents with anorexia nervosa should be hospitalized. The APA criteria are outlined in Box 30.6.

In many instances, a patient with anorexia nervosa must be hospitalized to restore his or her weight. Patients are admitted to a specialized eating disorder unit or program or to a general psychiatric unit. Because these individuals are often engaging and (with the exception of their emaciated state) appear nonimpaired, the severity of their disorder and distress may be underestimated. Particularly in a busy unit where other patients' symptoms of mental illness may be more overt, the needs of patients with eating disorders are at risk for being secondary to those of others because they may be erroneously perceived as less sick. Thus, it is important to remember the high rates of mortality and medical complications among individuals with eating disorders. If the patient's somatic systems are seriously compromised, a medical unit might be the choice for this initial intensive refeeding phase. In most psychiatric units, all members of the team participate in a weight gain protocol. Dietitians plan this weight-increasing program; physicians, nurses, psychologists, and social workers monitor the refeeding

process and its effects on the patient and establish the intensive therapies that must be instituted after the refeeding phase.

The patient's systems must be monitored closely because at the time of admission, most patients are severely malnourished (see Table 30.1). Patients usually are placed on a privilege-earning program in which privileges, such as having visitors and receiving passes to go outside the hospital, are earned based on weight gain. See Chapter 10.

The hospital course goes smoothly at first because the patient with anorexia nervosa resists losing weight. After an acceptable weight (at least 85% of ideal) is established, the patient is discharged to a partial hospitalization program or an intensive outpatient program. The intensive therapies needed to help patients with their underlying issues (e.g., body distortion and maturity fears) and to help families with communication and enmeshment usually begin after refeeding because concentration is usually impaired in severely undernourished patients with anorexia.

Family therapy typically begins while the patient is still hospitalized. Studies have demonstrated that family therapy does not have as significant an effect as individual therapy on the psychopathology and psychological symptoms for adolescents with anorexia nervosa. It does, however, improve overall communication within the family and helps members understand the disorder (Lask & Roberts, 2013).

Priority Care Issues

Mortality is high among patients with anorexia nervosa; the crude rate has been determined to be between 7% and 10%, and therefore higher than for females without anorexia nervosa in the general population (Franko et al., 2013). Suicide is the leading cause of death for individuals with anorexia nervosa (Suokas, Suvisaari, Grainger, Raevuori, Gissler, & Haukka, 2014). These individuals tend to commit suicide with highly lethal means in which rescue is unlikely. Nurses need to pay special attention to the risk of suicide with these individuals (see Chapter 21).

NURSING MANAGEMENT: Human Response to Anorexia Nervosa Disorder

Establishing a therapeutic relationship with individuals with anorexia nervosa may be difficult initially because they are suspicious and mistrustful (Box 30.7). They often express fear of adults, especially health care professionals, whom they believe want to "make them fat." By the time they are hospitalized, mistrust can almost reach a state of paranoia. Because of their low body weight and starvation, they are often impatient and irritable. A firm,

BOX 30.7 • THERAPEUTIC DIALOGUE • The Patient With an Eating Disorder

INEFFECTIVE APPROACH

Nurse: You haven't eaten your lunch yet.

Patient: I can't. I'm already fat.

Nurse: Look at you—you're skin and bones.

Patient: I'll eat when I go out this afternoon on pass.

Nurse: You can't go on pass. You have to start realizing that you are sick. Because you can't take care of yourself, we are in charge.

Patient: You're trying to control me.

Nurse: We are trying to be responsible.

Patient: I won't eat!

Nurse: We have set up punishments for not eating.

Patient: Then I won't go out! At least I won't get fatter.

EFFECTIVE APPROACH

Nurse: You haven't eaten your lunch.

Patient: I can't. I'm already fat.

Nurse: Seeing yourself as fat is part of your eating disorder. We are here to help you.

Patient: I'll eat when I go out on pass.

Nurse: We wrote your behavioral plan together, and you know you will not be able to go out because your pass is dependent on eating both breakfast and lunch. Here!

Patient: You're trying to control me.

Nurse: We are worried about you. That's why we set up this plan. How can I help you now with this meal?

Patient: What if I eat half?

Nurse: No, you must eat all of it. Why don't I sit here while you eat? Eating is scary for you. We can talk about other choices you have on the unit; tonight you can choose the movie or board games.

Patient: Okay. At least I have some choices.

CRITICAL THINKING CHALLENGE

- What effect did the first interaction have on the patient's behavior? Why?

- In the second interaction, what theories and interventions regarding eating disorders did the nurse use in her approach to the patient?

---

accepting, and patient approach is important in working with these individuals. Providing a rationale for all interventions helps build trust, as does a consistent, nonreactive approach. Power struggles overeating are common, and remaining nonreactive is a challenge. During such power struggles, the nurse should always think about his or her own feelings of frustration and need for control.

Biologic Domain

Assessment

A thorough evaluation of body systems is important because many systems are compromised by starvation. A careful history from both the patient with anorexia nervosa and the family, including the length and duration of symptoms, such as fasting, avoiding meals, and overexercising, is necessary to assess altered nutrition. Nursing

management involves various biopsychosocial assessment and interventions (see Nursing Care Plan 30.1).

Patients with longer durations of these maladaptive behaviors typically have more difficult and prolonged recovery periods.

NCLEXNOTE Eating disorders are serious psychiatric disorders that threaten life. Careful assessment and referral for treatment are important nursing interventions.

The patient's weight is determined using the BMI and a scale. Currently, criteria for discharge require patients to be at least 85% of ideal weight according to height and weight tables. BMI, thought to reflect weight most accurately because exact height is used, is calculated by dividing weight in kilograms by height in meters squared. An acceptable BMI is between about 19 and 25.

NURSING CARE PLAN 30.1

The Patient With Anorexia Nervosa

JS is a 16-year-old girl who appears much younger. She is 5′5″ and weighs 92 pounds. She has been treated unsuccessfully in an outpatient clinic and now is being admitted to stabilize her weight. She does not believe that she is too thin and resents being forced to be hospitalized. Hospitalization precipitated by being asked to leave gymnastics team because of low body weight.

Setting: Inpatient Psychiatric Unit

Baseline assessment: JS appears frail, pale, and dressed in oversized clothes. She is tearful, states that she is depressed and angry and that she has no friends. Physical examination results: bradycardia pulse = 58, hypotension, 88/60, constipation, amenorrhea, dry skin patches, and cold intolerance. Hypokalemia (K+ = 3.5); leukopenia (WBCs <5,000). Dehydration, temperature elevation, 99°F, elevated BUN, abnormal thyroid functioning.

Associated Psychiatric Diagnosis	Medications
Anorexia nervosa: Binge-eating/purging type	Fluoxetine (Prozac), 20 mg in am

Nursing Diagnosis 1: Imbalanced Nutrition: Less Than Body Requirements

Defining Characteristics	Related Factors
Unable to increase food intake Weight more than 20% below ideal weight	Believes she cannot eat most foods Purges by vomiting "occasionally" Exercises 6–8 h daily Sleep pattern disturbed by exercise

Outcomes

Initial	Long-term
Maintains daily intake of 1,200 calories Eliminates exercising while in hospital Ceases purging for 1 week	Gains 1–3 pounds Develops strategies to maintain weight

Interventions

Interventions	Rationale	Ongoing Assessment
Allow patient to verbalize feelings such as anxiety related to food and weight gain—develop a therapeutic relationship.	Through a relationship and examining her feelings, she may be more likely to cooperate with nutritional regimen.	Determine anxiety level when discussing food and weight gain.
Monitor meals and snacks, record amount eaten.	Severe anorexia is life threatening. Aggressive interventions are needed to ensure adequate intake.	Monitor intake. Assess JS' ability to complete meals on time and without supplements.
Do not substitute other foods for food on patient tray. Limit caffeine intake to 1 cup coffee (soda) daily.	People with anorexia usually "play games" with food. By prohibiting substitution, a more positive approach is encouraged. Caffeine is an appetite suppressant and has a diuretic effect.	Determine how willing JS is to follow nutritional regimen.
Monitor 1 h after meals for purging. Weigh daily in hospital gown after patient has voided. Monitor vital signs daily, electrolytes.	Physical signs of impending complications include evidence of purging, decreasing body weight, hypotension, hyperthermia, and hypokalemia.	Monitor vital signs, weight, and electrolytes, especially potassium.

Continued

NURSING CARE PLAN 30.1 *(Continued)*

Evaluation

Evaluation	Revised Outcomes	Interventions
JS gains 5 pounds at the end of 1½ weeks. Has been cooperative with meal regimen. She has begun to acknowledge the seriousness of her illness and the life-threatening aspects of severe dieting and purging.	Ceases binge–purge episodes for 1 week. Continues to increase her weight (1–3 pounds/week). Establish and maintain regular, adequate nutritional eating habits.	Daily weights while on unsupervised meals. Praise her for her successes. Arrange or discharge to outpatient clinic. Participation in relapse-prevention classes.

Nursing Diagnosis 2: Disturbed Body Image

Defining Characteristics	Related Factors
Verbalizes that she is too fat Perceives herself as unattractive Hides body in large, baggy clothing	Inaccurate perceptions of physical appearance secondary to anorexia nervosa Believes that one can never be too rich or too thin Equates physical fitness and attractiveness with thinness

Outcomes

Initial	Long term
Verbalizes feelings related to changing body shape and weight. Identifies beliefs about controlling body size.	Acknowledges negative consequences of too little fat on body. Identifies positive aspects of her body and its ability to function.

Interventions

Interventions	Rationale	Ongoing Assessment
Explore JS' beliefs and feelings about body. Maintain a non-judgmental approach. Assist patient in identifying positive physical characteristics.	To help patient gain a more positive body image, an understanding of her own views is important. In anorexia, the body is viewed negatively. By focusing on parts of the body that are positive, such as eyes or hands, the patient can begin to experience a positive image of her body.	Monitor for statements that identify perceptions of her body. Is her view *distorted* or *dissatisfied*? Observe for patient's reaction to her body. Which areas are viewed positively? Observe for negative statements related to body size and self-esteem.
Clarify patient's views about an ideal body.	Many societal cues idealize an unrealistically thin female body.	Monitor for statements indicating external pressures to lose weight, experiences of teasing about body changes, or evidence of sexual abuse from others.
Provide education related to normal growth of women's bodies, role of fat in protection of body.	Providing education will help in reinforcing a broader view of the importance of a healthy body.	Assess patient's willingness to learn information.

Evaluation

Outcomes	Revised Outcomes	Interventions
JS revealed that she believes that she is too fat but does have positive physical traits—eyes. She believes that those who are overweight have lost control of their lives. She knows some models who are 6′ and weigh barely 100 pounds. Willing to read information about normal body functioning.	Accept alternative beliefs related to her own body. Accept a new view of body functioning as a complex phenomenon.	Gradually, focus on other positive physical aspects of JS' body. Discuss grooming that encourages a more attractive look. Challenge her beliefs about body weights of models. Discuss the biologic aspect of the development of body weight. Emphasize multiple factors determine body weight.

Menses history also must be explored. Most patients with anorexia nervosa have reached menarche but have experienced amenorrhea for some months because of starvation. A return to regular menses after treatment signifies substantial body fat restoration.

Nursing Diagnoses for the Biologic Domain

A primary nursing diagnosis is Imbalanced Nutrition: Less Than Body Requirements.

Interventions for the Biologic Domain

Refeeding

Refeeding, the most important intervention during the hospital or initial stage of treatment (Fig. 30.4), is also the most challenging. The nurse will encounter resistance to weight gain and refusal to eat and must monitor and record all intake carefully as part of the weight gain protocol.

The refeeding protocol typically starts with 1,500 calories a day and is increased slowly until the patient is consuming about 3,500 calories a day in several meals. The usual plan for patients with very low weights is a weight gain of between 1 to 2 pounds a week.

Weight-increasing protocols usually take the form of a behavioral plan using positive reinforcements (i.e., excursion passes) and negative reinforcements (i.e., returning to bed rest) to encourage weight gain. The nurse should help patients to understand that these actions are not punitive. When all staff members agree on a clear protocol for behaviors related to eating and weight gain, reactivity of the staff to the patient is greatly reduced. These protocols provide ready-made, consistent responses to food-refusal behaviors and should be carried out in a caring and supportive context. On rare occasions when the patient is unable to recognize or accept her illness (denial), nasogastric tube feedings may be necessary.

Electrolytes may be completely depleted in anorexia nervosa, so nursing care involves stabilizing electrolyte balance. Potassium depletion usually results from use of diuretics, diarrhea, and vomiting. Calcium depletion is related to large intake of dietary fiber, which decreases calcium absorption. During hospitalization, these electrolytes are replaced through oral or intravenous therapy.

Promotion of Sleep

Sleep disturbance is also common, and these individuals are viewed as hyperkinetic. They sleep little, but they usually awaken in an energized state. A structured, healthy sleep routine must be established immediately to conserve energy and calorie expenditure because of low weight. To further conserve energy, patients are often relegated to bed rest until a certain amount of weight is regained. Exercise is generally not permitted during refeeding and only with caution after this phase. Inpatients must be closely supervised because they are often found exercising in their rooms, running in place and doing calisthenics.

Pharmacologic Interventions

The selective serotonin reuptake inhibitor (SSRI) fluoxetine (Prozac) is approved by the Food and Drug Administration for the treatment of anorexia nervosa. Of course, comorbid conditions such as depression or OCD should be treated with appropriate medication. The nurse may be responsible for administering medications or providing patient and family teaching.

Psychological Domain

Assessment

The psychological symptoms that patients with anorexia experience are listed in Box 30.1. The classic symptoms of body distortion—fear of weight gain, unrealistic expectations and thinking, and ritualistic behaviors—are easily noted during a clinical interview. Often, people with anorexia nervosa avoid conflict and have difficulty expressing negative emotions, such as anger. Other conflicts, such as sexuality fears and feelings of ineffectiveness, may underlie this disorder. These symptoms may not be apparent during a clinical interview; however, a variety of instruments is available to clinicians and researchers for determining their presence and severity.

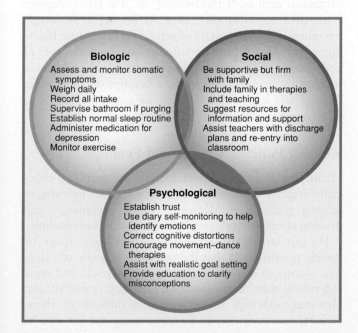

FIGURE 30.4 Biopsychosocial interventions for patients with anorexia nervosa.

BOX 30.8

Assessment Instruments

TESTS FOR DISORDERED EATING (SYMPTOMS)
Compulsive Eating Scale
Dunn, P. K., & Ondercin, P. (1981). Personality variables related to compulsive eating in college women. *Journal of Clinical Psychology, 31,* 43–49.

Eating Attitudes Test
Garner, D. M., & Garfinkel, P. E. (1979). The Eating Attitudes Test: An index of the symptoms of anorexia nervosa. *Psychosomatic Medicine, 10,* 647–656.

Children's Eating Attitude Test (CHEAT)
Maloney, M., McGuire, J., & Daniels, S. R. (1988). Reliability testing of a children's version of the Eating Attitude Test. *Journal of the American Academy of Child and Adolescent Psychiatry, 27,* 541–543.

Eating Disorder Examination—Questionnaire (EDE-Q)
Carolyn Black, Rutgers University Eating Disorders Clinic, 41C Gordon Road, Piscataway, NJ 08854.

Eating Disorder Inventory—2 (EDI-2) and EDI-2 Symptom Checklist (EDI-2-SC)
Psychological Assessment Resources, PO Box 998, Odessa, FL 33556 (800–331–8378).

Eating Habits Questionnaire (Restraint Scale)
Herman, C. P., & Mack, D. (1975). Restrained and unrestrained eating. *Journal of Personality, 43,* 647–660.

Yale-Brown-Cornell Eating Disorder Scale (YBC-EDS)
Mazure, C. M., Halmi, K. A., Sunday, S. R., Romano, S. J., & Einhorn, A. M. (1994). Yale-Brown-Cornell Eating Disorder Scale: Development, use, reliability, and validity. *Journal of Psychiatric Research, 28,* 425–445.

TESTS OF BODY DISSATISFACTION/BODY IMAGE
Body Shape Questionnaire (BSQ)
Cooper, P., Taylor, M., Cooper, Z., & Fairburn, C. (1987). The development and validation of the BSQ. *International Journal of Eating Disorders, 6,* 485–494.

Color-a-Person Test
Wooley, S. C., & Kearney-Cooke, A. (1986). Intensive treatment of bulimia and body image disturbance. In K. D. Brownell & J. P. Foreyt (Eds.), *Handbook of eating disorders: Physiology, psychology and treatment of obesity, anorexia, and bulimia* (pp. 476–502). New York: Basic Books.

TESTS OF EMOTIONAL AND COGNITIVE COMPONENTS
Cognitive Behavioral Dieting Scale
Martz, D. M., Sturgis, E. T., & Gustafson, S. B. (1996). Development and preliminary validation of the Cognitive Behavioral Dieting Scale. *International Journal of Eating Disorders, 19,* 297–309.

Emotional Eating Scale
Arrow, B., Kenardy, J., & Agras, W. S. (1995). The emotional eating scale: The development of a measure to assess coping with negative affect by eating. *International Journal of Eating Disorders, 18,* 79–90.

RISK FACTOR IDENTIFICATION
The McKnight Risk Factor Survey (versions available for younger and older children)
Shisslak, C. M., Renger, R., Sharpe, T., Crago, M., McKnight, K. M, Gray, N., et al. (1999). Development and evaluation of the McKnight Risk Factor Survey for assessing potential risk and protective factors for disordered eating in preadolescent and adolescent girls. *International Journal of Eating Disorders, 25,* 195–214.

Box 30.8 lists well-known instruments used to assess psychological symptoms associated with eating disorders. The Eating Attitudes Test is frequently used in community and clinical samples (Box 30.9). There is also a child version of this test, the CHEAT. The results of these paper-and-pencil tests can help identify the most significant symptoms for an individual patient and indicate a focus for interventions, especially therapy.

Nursing Diagnosis for the Psychological Domain

Two common nursing diagnoses in anorexia nervosa are Anxiety and Disturbed Body Image. See Figure 30.5.

Interventions for the Psychological Domain

Addressing Interoceptive Awareness

For interoceptive awareness problems (inability to experience visceral cues and emotions), the nurse can encourage patients to keep a journal. Most patients use a somatic

complaint such as, "I feel bloated" or "I'm fat" to replace a negative emotion such as guilt or anger. Although refeeding following a state of starvation may cause bloating in some cases, bloating often is imagined and part of body image distortion. Help patients to identify these feelings by having them write a description of the "fat feeling" and list possible underlying emotions and troublesome situations next to this description.

Helping Patients Understand Feelings

Identifying feelings, such as anxiety and fear, and especially negative emotions, such as anger, is the first step in helping patients to decrease conflict avoidance and develop effective strategies for coping with these feelings.

Do not attempt to change distorted body image by merely pointing out that the patient is actually too thin. This symptom is often the last to resolve itself, and some individuals may take years to see their bodies realistically. However, although this symptom is difficult to abate, patients can continue to fear becoming fat but not be driven to act on the distortion by starving. The fear of becoming fat eventually lessens with time.

BOX 30.9

Eating Attitudes Test

Please place an (x) under the column that applies best to each of the numbered statements. All of the results will be strictly confidential. Most of the questions relate to food or eating, although other types of questions have been included. Please answer each question carefully. Thank you.

	ALWAYS	VERY OFTEN	OFTEN	SOMETIMES	RARELY	NEVER
1. Like eating with other people	—	—	—	—	—	×
2. Prepare foods for others but do not eat what I cook	×	—	—	—	—	—
3. Become anxious before eating	×	—	—	—	—	—
4. Am terrified about being overweight	×	—	—	—	—	—
5. Avoid eating when I am hungry	×	—	—	—	—	—
6. Find myself preoccupied with food	×	—	—	—	—	—
7. Have gone on eating binges in which I feel that I may not be able to stop	×	—	—	—	—	—
8. Cut my food into small pieces	×	—	—	—	—	—
9. Am aware of the calorie content of foods that I eat	×	—	—	—	—	—
10. Particularly avoid foods with a high carbohydrate content (e.g., bread, potatoes, rice)	×	—	—	—	—	—
11. Feel bloated after meals	×	—	—	—	—	—
12. Feel that others would prefer I ate more	×	—	—	—	—	—
13. Vomit after I have eaten	×	—	—	—	—	—
14. Feel extremely guilty after eating	×	—	—	—	—	—
15. Am preoccupied with a desire to be thinner	×	—	—	—	—	—
16. Exercise strenuously to burn off calories	×	—	—	—	—	—
17. Weigh myself several times a day	×	—	—	—	—	—
18. Like my clothes to fit tightly	—	—	—	—	—	×
19. Enjoy eating meat	—	—	—	—	—	×
20. Wake up early in the morning	×	—	—	—	—	—
21. Eat the same foods day after day	×	—	—	—	—	—
22. Think about burning up calories when I exercise	×	—	—	—	—	—
23. Have regular menstrual periods	—	—	—	—	—	×
24. Am aware that other people think I am too thin	×	—	—	—	—	—
25. Am preoccupied with the thought of having fat on my body	×	—	—	—	—	—
26. Take longer than others to eat	×	—	—	—	—	—
27. Enjoy eating at restaurants	—	—	—	—	—	×
28. Take laxatives	×	—	—	—	—	—
29. Avoid foods with sugar in them	×	—	—	—	—	—
30. Eat diet foods	×	—	—	—	—	—
31. Feel that food controls my life	×	—	—	—	—	—
32. Display self-control around food	×	—	—	—	—	—
33. Feel that others pressure me to eat	×	—	—	—	—	—
34. Give too much time and thought to food	×	—	—	—	—	—
35. Suffer from constipation	—	×	—	—	—	—
36. Feel uncomfortable after eating sweets	×	—	—	—	—	—
37. Engage in dieting behavior	×	—	—	—	—	—
38. Like my stomach to be empty	×	—	—	—	—	—
39. Enjoy trying new rich foods	—	—	—	—	—	×
40. Have the impulse to vomit after meals	×	—	—	—	—	—

Scoring: The patient is given the questionnaire without the X's, just blank. 3 points are assigned to endorsements that coincide with the X's; the adjacent alternatives are weighted as 2 points and 1 point, respectively. A total score of more than 30 indicates significant concerns with eating behavior.

The nurse can help individuals with cognitive distortions and unrealistic assumptions to restructure the way they view the world, especially relative to food, eating, weight, and shape. Faulty ways of viewing these situations result in ineffective coping. Table 30.2 lists some distortions commonly experienced by individuals with eating disorders and some typical restructuring responses or statements that challenge the distortion, which the nurse can present as more realistic ways of perceiving situations. Other therapies, such as movement and dance therapy, can help the patient experience pleasure from his or her body, although dance should be used cautiously during refeeding because of energy-expenditure concerns. Imagery and relaxation are often used to overcome distortions and to decrease anxiety stemming from a distorted body image. While in the hospital, patients usually are evaluated for discharge to

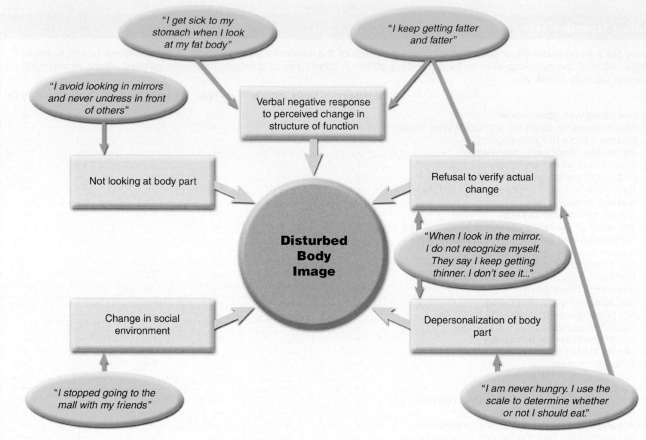

FIGURE 30.5 Nursing diagnosis concept map: Disturbed Body Image.

partial hospitalization or to intensive outpatient therapy, depending on the resources available, the extent of family support, and comorbidity. In both instances, the patient and family participate in a combination of individual and family therapy.

Initiating Interpersonal Therapy

Interpersonal therapy (IPT) is a type of treatment that focuses on uncovering and resolving the developmental and psychological issues underlying the disorder. Nurses

Table 30.2	COGNITIVE DISTORTIONS TYPICAL OF PATIENTS WITH EATING DISORDERS, WITH RESTRUCTURING STATEMENTS
Distortion	**Clarification or Restructuring**
Dichotomous or all-or-nothing thinking "I've gained 2 pounds, so I'll be up by 100 pounds soon."	"You have never gained 100 pounds, but I understand that gaining 2 pounds is scary."
Magnification "I binged last night, so I can't go out with anyone."	"Feeling bad and guilty about a binge are difficult feelings, but you are in treatment, and you have been monitoring and changing your eating."
Selective Abstraction "I can only be happy 10 pounds lighter."	"When you were 10 pounds lighter, you were hospitalized. You can choose to be happy about many things in your life."
Overgeneralization "I didn't eat anything yesterday and did okay, so I don't think not eating for a week or two will harm me."	"Any starvation harms the body, whether or not outward signs were apparent to you. The more you starve, the more problems your body will encounter."
Catastrophizing "I purged last night for the first time in 4 months—I'll never recover."	"Recovery includes up and downs, and it is expected you will still have some mild but infrequent symptoms."

play an important role in IPT by maintaining an empathic, therapeutic relationship with the patient and family and also by encouraging patients to participate in the therapy. Role transitions and negative social evaluations typically are the focus (Rieger, Van Buren, Bishop, Tanofsky-Kraff, Welch, & Wilfley, 2010). Family therapy is usually initiated in the hospital and continued more intensively after discharge.

Providing Patient and Family Education

When weight is restored and concentration is improved, patients with anorexia nervosa can benefit from psycho-education. Although these individuals have a wealth of knowledge about food and calories, they also have misinformation that needs clarifying. For example, they are often unclear about the role of "fats" in a healthy diet and try to be as "fat free" as possible. A thorough assessment of their knowledge is important because they seem to be "walking calorie books" with little information on the role of all of the nutrients and the importance of including them in a healthy diet.

> **NCLEXNOTE** Setting realistic eating goals is one of the most helpful interventions for patients with eating disorders. Because individuals with anorexia nervosa are often perfectionistic, they often set unrealistic goals.

One of the most helpful skills the nurse can teach is to set realistic goals around food and around other activities or tasks. Because of perfectionism, patients with anorexia often set unrealistic goals and end up frustrated. The nurse can help them establish smaller, more realistic, attainable goals (Box 30.10).

Families and friends are eager to help the patient with anorexia but often need direction. Box 30.11 provides a list of strategies that may assist them.

BOX 30.10

Psychoeducation Checklist: **Anorexia Nervosa**

When caring for a patient with anorexia nervosa, be sure to include the following topic areas in the teaching plan:

- Psychopharmacologic agents, if used, including drug, action, dosage, frequency, and possible adverse effects
- Nutrition and eating patterns
- Effect of restrictive eating or dieting
- Weight monitoring
- Safety and comfort measures
- Avoidance of triggers
- Self-monitoring techniques
- Trust
- Realistic goal setting
- Resources

BOX 30.11

What Family and Friends Can Do to Help Those With Eating Disorders

- Tell the person you are concerned, you care, and you would like to help. Suggest that the person seek professional help from a physician or therapist.
- If the person refuses to seek professional help, encourage reaching out to an adult, such as a teacher, school nurse, or counselor.
- Do not discuss weight, the number of calories being consumed, or particular eating habits.
- Do try to talk about things other than food, weight, counting calories, and exercise.
- Avoid making comments about a person's appearance. Concern about weight loss may be interpreted as a compliment; comments regarding weight gain may be felt as criticism.
- It will not help to become involved in a power struggle. You cannot force the person to eat.
- You can offer support. Ultimately, however, the responsibility and the decision to accept help and to change rest with the person.
- Read and educate yourself regarding these disorders.

Social Domain

Assessment

The social assessment of the person with anorexia nervosa should focus on the family interaction, influence, and peer relationships. The role of the patient in the family and community should be considered, as well as the person's ability to cope in social situations. For adolescents who are attending school, a conference with the teacher or counselor provides information regarding the amount and frequency of social contacts.

Nursing Diagnosis for the Social Domain

Ineffective Coping is a predominant nursing diagnosis with regard to the social domain.

Interventions for the Social Domain

Younger patients with anorexia nervosa may have lost some school time because of hospitalization. Integrating back into a school and classroom setting is difficult for most. Shame and guilt about having an eating disorder and being hospitalized must be addressed. Because these patients typically have isolated themselves before hospitalization and treatment, renewing friendships and relationships with peers may provoke anxiety. Involving school nurses and teachers in the reentry process may help.

Denial, guilt, and subsequent greater overprotectiveness are common reactions of the family, especially when hospitalization has been necessary. Family therapy is important if the patient still lives with his or her parents.

Skilled therapists are able to help family members with their feelings, increase effective communication, decrease protectiveness, and resolve guilt. Often, siblings become resentful of the patient with an eating disorder because of the significant amount of attention they get from their parents. Having siblings attend family sessions discuss these feelings and the effect the illness has had on them is helpful.

Evaluation and Treatment Outcomes

Several factors influence the outcome of treatment for individuals with anorexia nervosa. Particularly long duration of symptoms and low weight when treatment begins predict poor outcomes, but family support and involvement generally improve outcomes. Comorbid conditions and their severity also influence recovery. Although patients are discharged from the hospital when their weight has reached 85% of what is considered ideal, restoration of healthy eating and changes in maladaptive thinking may not have yet occurred. Individuals often continue to restrict foods. Therefore, without intensive outpatient treatment, including nutritional counseling and support, they are unlikely to recover fully. Distorted thinking and eating patterns can set the stage for a relapse and later for the possible development of bulimia nervosa. Many of the instruments used to assess eating disorder symptoms can be used throughout the patient's treatment to evaluate attitudes and thinking processes that continue to prevent full recovery (see Box 30.8).

Continuum of Care

Hospitalization

Hospitalization is required based on criteria noted in Box 30.6. Because of its life-threatening nature, anorexia nervosa in its very acute stage is unlikely to be manageable in outpatient settings.

Emergency Care

Emergency care is not usually needed for individuals with anorexia nervosa. Family members and peers usually notice the weight loss and emaciation before patients' systems are compromised to the degree that they require emergency treatment. If systems are compromised enough to warrant emergency treatment, patients usually are admitted immediately for inpatient care.

Family Assessment and Intervention

The family of the person with anorexia will need extensive treatment and follow-up. The therapist, psychologist, advanced practice nurse, or social worker meets regularly, at least once a week, with the individual and the family. Family therapy focuses on such issues as separation–individuation, autonomy, ineffective communication, and practical issues (such as how parents can effectively monitor food intake). Family therapy models facilitate communication and help families negotiate differences of opinion and attitudes, recognizing that rigidity of behavior and emotionality are a part of the disorder (le Grange, Lock, Loeb, & Nicholls, 2010).

Outpatient Treatment

After refeeding, treatment of anorexia nervosa takes place on an outpatient basis and involves individual and family therapy, nutrition counseling to reinforce healthy eating patterns and attitudes, and physician visits to monitor weight and evaluate somatic recovery. Support groups, which are often suggested, should not be substituted for therapy. In fact, some self-directed support groups that lack professional leadership can actually delay or prevent needed professional treatment. However, after full recovery, support groups are useful in maintaining recovery.

Prevention

Eating disorders are among the most preventable mental disorders. Instruments such as the McKnight Risk Factor Survey (Shisslak et al., 1999), which measure the presence and degree of risk factors, can be used to plan prevention or treatment after early detection (see Box 30.8). National eating disorder awareness and advocacy groups work toward educating the general public; those at risk; and those who work with groups at risk, such as teachers and coaches. They also monitor the media and work to remove unhealthy advertisements and articles that appear in magazines appealing to young girls.

Prevention and early detection strategies for parents and schoolteachers are often the focus of school nurses and mental health nurses who work in the community. Some of these strategies appear in Box 30.12 and are based on the research on risk factors and protective factors.

BULIMIA NERVOSA

Bulimia nervosa is a relatively newly identified disorder: Until about 25 years ago, it was thought to be a type of anorexia nervosa. However, findings from extensive investigations have identified its characteristics as a separate entity. It is more prevalent than anorexia nervosa. Individuals with bulimia nervosa are usually older at onset than are those with anorexia nervosa. The disorder generally is not as life threatening as anorexia nervosa. The usual treatment is outpatient therapy. Outcomes are better for bulimia nervosa than for anorexia nervosa, and mortality rates are lower.

Clinical Course

Few outward signs are associated with bulimia nervosa. Individuals binge and purge in secret and are typically of normal weight; therefore, it does not come to the attention of parents and peers as readily as does anorexia nervosa. Treatment consequently can be delayed for years as individuals attempt on their own to get their eating under control. Patients usually initiate their own treatment when control of their eating becomes impossible. When treatment is undertaken and completed, patients typically recover completely, except in cases in which personality disorders and comorbid serious depression are also present.

Patients with bulimia nervosa present as overwhelmed and overly committed individuals, "social butterflies" who have difficulty with setting limits and establishing appropriate boundaries. They have an enormous number of rules regarding food and food restriction, and they feel shame, guilt, and disgust about their binge eating and purging. They may also be impulsive in other areas of their lives, such as spending.

Diagnostic Criteria

Bulimia nervosa involves eating a large amount of food within a discrete period of time (e.g., 2 hours) and engaging in recurrent episodes of binge eating and compensatory purging in various forms such as vomiting or using laxatives, diuretics, or emetics or in nonpurging compen-satory behaviors, such as fasting or overexercising in order to avoid weight gain. These episodes must occur at least once a week for a period of at least 3 months to meet the *DSM-5* criteria. Self-evaluation is excessively and inappropriately influenced by body weight and shape. Unlike anorexia nervosa, there is little or no weight loss. See Box 30.1 for characteristics related to bulimia nervosa.

Binge eating is defined as rapid, episodic, impulsive, and uncontrollable ingestion of a large amount of food during a short period of time, usually 1 to 2 hours. Eating is followed by feelings of guilt, remorse, and often self-contempt, leading to purging. To assuage the out-of-control feeling, severe dieting is instituted, and these restrictions, referred to as *dietary restraint*, precipitate the next binge. The restrictions are viewed as "rules," such as no sweets, no fats, and so forth. Each binge seems to influence stricter and stricter rules about what cannot be consumed, leading to more frequent binge eating. This cycle has prompted clinicians to focus treatment primarily on interventions related to dietary restraint. When dietary restraint is resolved, binge eating is decreased, and generally the purging that follows binge eating also is decreased.

> **KEYCONCEPT** **Dietary restraint** has been described by researchers in the field of eating disorders as a way to explain the relationship between dieting and binge eating.

Dieters' deprivation, or restraint, whether real or imagined, contributes to overeating and binging. Genetic predisposition for binge eating and deprivation may make dieters more prone to feel distress over their dietary "failures," especially if dieting has become a way to overcome body dissatisfaction and to compensate for distress through dietary restraint that leads to overeating (Racine, Burt, Iacono, McGue, & Klump, 2011). Whether the eating is influenced by the attraction of forbidden foods or by internal needs to assuage failure, there is significant evidence that restraining one's intake is a precondition for bouts of overeating.

Bulimia Nervosa Across the Lifespan

Bulimia nervosa occurs in all age groups. It is not as common in children as in adolescents and adults; children appear more likely to have BED, discussed later. This finding has only recently been reported, and more data are needed to substantiate this theory.

Epidemiology

The lifetime prevalence of bulimia nervosa is reported to be from 1% to 2.3%, depending on whether clinical or community populations are sampled, but it is estimated that less than one-third of the cases have been detected

(Smink, van Hocken, & Hoek, 2012). Stricter criteria are used when clinical groups are studied, making the prevalence rate lower. The occurrence is more common than that of anorexia nervosa. The incidence of bulimia nervosa has been decreasing over the past decade; this decrease is not attributable to changes in service utilization, thereby suggesting a change in sociocultural factors is involved in its development (Smink et al., 2012).

Age of Onset

Typically, the age of onset is between 15 and 24 years. Some women older than the typical age of onset have developed bulimia nervosa and symptom cases have been identified as subsequent to life stressors such as a loss (Smink et al., 2012).

Gender

As with anorexia nervosa, females are 10 times more likely than males to experience bulimia nervosa. Box 30.2 highlights differences in males with eating disorders.

Ethnicity and Culture

Bulimia nervosa is related to culture in the same way as anorexia nervosa. In Western cultures and those becoming westernized in their norms, the focus on achieving a thin body ideal underlies the dieting and dietary restraint that sets up the trajectory toward a diagnosable eating disorder. Hispanic and white women have higher rates than do Asian and African American women. The difference as noted earlier in the chapter has much to do with how women from specific cultural backgrounds internalize the thin ideal (Murphy, Straebler, Cooper, & Fairburn, 2010).

Comorbidity

The most common comorbid conditions are substance abuse, depression, and OCD. In one study, women continued having OCD after remission of their bulimic symptoms, underlining the notion that some comorbid conditions may occur before the eating disorder, are trait-related features, and may actually have a role in precipitating the disorder (APA, 2013). Borderline personality disorder and avoidant personality disorder combined with child sexual abuse are also found frequently in these individuals, and many women with bulimia nervosa who have had anorexia nervosa previously (Vrabel, Hofart, Ro, Martinson, & Rosenvinge, 2010).

Etiology

Some of the predisposing or risk factors for anorexia nervosa and bulimia nervosa overlap with theories of causality

(see Fig. 30.3). For example, dieting puts an individual at risk for the development of bulimia nervosa. The dieting can turn into dietary restraint, a symptom that leads to binge eating and purging. However, not all individuals who diet experience bulimia nervosa. The interplay of other risk factors (e.g., body dissatisfaction and separation individuation issues) most likely explains the development of this disorder.

Biologic Theories

Some progress has been made in understanding the biologic changes in bulimia nervosa. Dieting and binging can affect brain function. Dieting is believed to affect serotonergic regulation and binging affects the dopamine (DA), acetylcholine (ACh), and opioid reward-related systems. These alterations occur in response to binge eating palatable foods (Avena & Bocarsly, 2012).

The changes noted in the brain by magnetic resonance imaging of persons with bulimia nervosa are the result of eating dysregulation rather than the cause. As with anorexia nervosa, these changes often disappear when symptoms such as dietary restraint, binge eating, and purging remit.

Genetic and Familial Predispositions

A specific gene responsible for bulimia nervosa has not been conclusively identified (Boraska et al., 2014). Recently, twin studies have been reviewed to determine the role genetics might play in the development of bulimia nervosa. Whereas it has been widely recognized that environment also plays a role, in several twin studies, genetic influences outweighed environmental ones (Thornton, Mazzeo, & Bulik, 2011).

Biochemical Factors

The most frequently studied biochemical theory in bulimia nervosa relates to lowered brain serotonin neurotransmission. People with bulimia nervosa are believed to have altered modulation of central serotonin neuronal systems (Poisinelli, Levitan, & DeLuca, 2012). Recent studies also target the dopamine system in women with bulimia nervosa who experienced childhood abuse (Groleau et al., 2012).

Chronic depletion of plasma tryptophan is thought to be one of the major mechanisms whereby persistent dieting can lead to the development of eating disorders in vulnerable individuals. Studies show that depletion of tryptophan, an amino acid and serotonin precursor, leads to a depressed mood, a desire to binge, and an increase in weight and shape concerns in those who were in the acute state of their illness (Bruce, Steiger, Young, Kin, Israël, & Lévesque, 2009).

Psychological and Social Theories

Psychological factors in the etiology of bulimia nervosa have been studied extensively, and most experts believe that these factors converge with environmental or sociocultural factors within individuals with a biologic predisposition, causing symptoms to develop. Because the age of onset for bulimia nervosa is late adolescence—going away to college, for example—may represent the first physical separation for some adolescents, who are unprepared for the emotional separation. In addition, an inability to set limits and develop healthy boundaries leads to a sense of being overwhelmed and "drained." Overwhelming feelings often lead to binge eating, either to avoid or to distract oneself from feelings such as resentment, or binge eating can serve to assuage emptiness or to fill up a "drained" self with food.

Cognitive Theory

Many experts view cognitive theory as explaining eating disorder symptoms, such as distorted thinking. This explanation is similar for depression, in which a particular thought pattern is learned (see Chapter 24). Many experts view bulimia nervosa as a disorder of thinking in that distortions are the basis of behaviors such as binge eating and purging. Psychological triggering mechanism models explain that cues such as stress, negative emotions, and even environmental cues (e.g., the presence of attractive food) play a role in etiology. However, today these cognitive and triggering theories are viewed as an explanation for maintaining the binge eating after it has been established rather than an explanation of causality.

The same sociocultural factors that underlie anorexia nervosa play a significant role in the development of bulimia nervosa.

Family Factors

The families of individuals who experience bulimia nervosa are reported to be chaotic, with few rules and unclear boundaries. Often, there is an overly close or enmeshed relationship between the daughter and mother. Daughters may relate that their mother is their "best friend." The boundaries are blurred in that the mother may interact with the daughter as a confidante, and this unhealthy relation further impedes the separation–individuation process. The daughters often feel guilty about separation and responsible for their mother's happiness and emotional well-being. Some research on families of individuals with bulimia nervosa has found them to be unempathic and unavailable.

In summary, as with anorexia nervosa, theories do not individually explain the development of bulimia nervosa. Rather, the convergence of many of these factors at a vulnerable stage of individual development best explains causality.

Risk Factors

The risk or predisposing factors for bulimia nervosa are similar to those for anorexia nervosa (see Fig. 30.3). Society's influences, such as the media and peer pressure, underlie the desire to achieve an ideal thin body type. Comparing oneself to these ideal body types leads to body dissatisfaction. These factors influence behaviors such as dietary restraint and overexercising. Dietary restraint leads to binge eating, and purging ensues because of a fear of becoming fat.

Sexual Abuse

There have been conflicting findings from studies of the relationship between eating disorders and sexual abuse. Childhood sexual abuse has often been suggested as a risk factor for eating disorders. However, it has been noted that although childhood sexual abuse has occurred in a larger percentage of women with bulimia nervosa than in the general population, this percentage may not be larger than the percentage of women with other psychiatric disorders who have experienced such abuse. Bulimia is often a comorbid condition with borderline personality disorder and substance abuse disorders. Therefore, recent studies were undertaken to determine if childhood sexual abuse was a predictor of an eating disorder compared with those with other psychiatric disorders. Women with anorexia nervosa reported greater severity and significantly higher rates of negative mood; perfectionism; and family discord, parental mood and substance disorder, and physical and sexual abuse than women with no psychiatric disorder. The sequelae from sexual abuse sets one up to develop an eating disorder and such symptoms as body dissatisfaction or revulsion results from the trauma and this leads to body shape and weight concerns. It is unclear how other symptomatology or environmental conditions interact with eating disorder symptoms after abuse. Assessing a concurrent history of sexual abuse and other factors, such as the development of depression, must be considered to clarify the nature of this relationship (Badura, Huefner, & Handwerk, 2012).

Interdisciplinary Treatment and Recovery

Individuals with bulimia nervosa benefit from a comprehensive multifaceted treatment approach. The goals for treatment for individuals with bulimia nervosa focus on stabilizing and then normalizing eating, which means stopping the binge–purge cycles; restructuring dysfunctional thought patterns and attitudes, especially about eating, weight, and shape; teaching healthy boundary setting; and resolving conflicts about separation–individuation. Treatment usually takes place in an outpatient setting except when the patient is suicidal or when past outpatient treatment has failed (see Box 30.6).

In addition to intensive psychotherapy, usually cognitive behavioral therapy (CBT) or interpersonal psychotherapy and pharmacologic interventions are also necessary. Antidepressants demonstrate effectiveness in treating binge eating and purging even without comorbid depression. Nutrition counseling is an important part of outpatient treatment to stabilize and normalize eating. Some mental health professionals, psychologists, advanced practice psychiatric nurses, and social workers specialize in treating eating disorders, often working with nutritionists who also have expertise in working with this population. Group psychotherapy and support groups are also used. Family therapy is not usually a part of the treatment because many people with bulimia nervosa live on college campuses away from home or are older and on their own. Usually, treatment becomes less intensive as symptoms remit. Therapy focuses on psychological issues, such as boundary setting and separation–individuation conflicts and on changing problematic behaviors and dysfunctional thinking using CBT.

> **NCLEXNOTE** Therapeutic relationships and cognitive interventions are a priority in the nursing care of patients with eating disorders.

Priority Care Issues

Bulimia nervosa is associated with a high risk of suicide independent of other comorbid disorders (Bodell, Joiner, & Keel, 2013). They are also often at risk for self-mutilation. Because they display high levels of impulsivity, shoplifting, and overspending, financial and legal difficulties have been associated with bulimia nervosa.

NURSING MANAGEMENT: Human Response to Bulimia Nervosa Disorder

Establishing a therapeutic relationship precedes biopsychosocial assessment and interventions. Individuals with bulimia nervosa experience a great deal of shame and guilt. They also often have an intense need to please and be liked and may approach the nurse–patient relationship in a superficial manner. They are too ashamed to discuss their symptoms but do not want to disappoint others, so they may discuss more social or unrelated issues in an attempt to engage the nurse (Box 30.13). A nonjudgmental, accepting approach, stressing the importance of the relationship and outlining its purpose, is important at the outset. Explaining the nature of the relationship and the goals of therapy will help clarify the boundaries.

BOX 30.13
Using Reflection

UNDERSTANDING THE "NEED TO PLEASE"

INCIDENT • A nurse became very angry upon discovering that her patient with bulimia had been reporting to the nurse that she was no longer purging. The nurse had worked closely with the patient who disclosed many other psychological issues. The nurse felt that the patient had manipulated her.

REFLECTION • Upon reflection, the nurse began to see the situation differently. The patient was very connected to the nurse, who had made it clear that purging was unacceptable. Fearful of rejection, the patient did not want to disappoint the nurse and focused on other issues.

Biologic Domain

Even though most individuals with bulimia nervosa maintain normal weights, the physical ramifications of this disorder may be similar to those of anorexia nervosa. Hypokalemia can contribute to muscle weakness and fatigability, as well as to the development of cardiac arrhythmias, palpitations, and cardiac conduction defects. Patients who purge risk fluid and electrolyte abnormalities that can further compromise cardiac status. Neuropsychiatric disturbances, such as poor concentration and attention, and sleep disturbances are common.

Assessment

The nurse should assess current eating patterns, determine the number of times a day the individual binges and purges, and note dietary restraint practices. Sleep patterns and exercise habits are also important.

Nursing Diagnoses for the Biologic Domain

Imbalanced Nutrition: Less Than Body Requirements and Disturbed Sleep Pattern are typical nursing diagnoses for the biologic domain.

Interventions for the Biologic Domain

If the patient is admitted to the hospital, meals and all food intake must be strictly monitored to normalize eating. Bathroom visits should also be supervised to prevent purging. Outpatients are asked to record their intake, binges, and purges to form a foundation for changing behaviors with CBT. Because individuals with bulimia nervosa have chaotic lifestyles and are often overcommitted, sleep may be a low priority. Sleep-deprived individuals may assume that food would be helpful, and they begin to eat, triggering a binge. To encourage regular sleep patterns, patients should go to bed and rise at about the same time every day.

Pharmacologic Interventions: Monitoring and Administering Medication

Whereas pharmacologic intervention is effective for symptom remission in bulimia nervosa, experts continue to agree that the combination of CBT and medication has had the best results (Murphy, Straebler, Cooper, & Fairburn, 2010). Fluoxetine (Prozac) has been the most studied for bulimia nervosa in clinical trials (Box 30.14). Effective doses are usually 60 mg per day, a higher dosage than that used to treat individuals with depression. Other SSRIs are also used. The most important concern in using these medications is decreased appetite and weight loss during the first few weeks of administration. Weight should be monitored, especially during this period.

The intake of medication must be monitored for possible purging after administration. The effect of the medication depends on whether it has had time to absorb.

Teaching Points

Patients should be instructed to take medication as prescribed. SSRIs must be taken in the morning because they can cause insomnia. Patients should be informed that any weight loss they initially experience is temporary and is usually regained after a few weeks when the medication dosage has stabilized.

Psychosocial Domain

Assessment

For the individual with bulimia nervosa, psychological assessment focuses on cognitive distortions—cues or stimuli that lead to dysfunctional behavior affecting symptom development—and knowledge deficits. The psychological characteristics typical of patients with bulimia nervosa are presented in Box 30.1.

Individuals with bulimia nervosa display a significant number of cognitive distortions, examples of which are found in Table 30.2. These thought patterns form the basis for "rules" and lead the way to destructive eating patterns. During routine history taking, patients relate many of these erroneous assumptions. Situations that produce feelings of being overwhelmed and powerless need to be explored, as does the patient's ability to set boundaries, control impulsivity, and maintain quality relationships. These underlying issues precipitate binge eating. Body dissatisfaction should be openly explored. Several assessment tools are available to gauge such characteristics as body dissatisfaction and impulsivity (see Box 30.8). Mood

is an important area for evaluation because many people with bulimia nervosa also have depression. Symptoms of depression, especially the vegetative signs, should be thoroughly explored (see Chapter 24).

Nursing Diagnoses for the Psychosocial Domain

Deficient Knowledge, Disturbed Thought Processes, and Powerlessness are among the common diagnoses for the social domain.

BOX 30.14

Drug Profile: **Fluoxetine Hydrochloride (Prozac)**

DRUG CLASS: Selective serotonin reuptake inhibitor

RECEPTOR AFFINITY: Inhibits central nervous system neuronal uptake of serotonin with little effect on norepinephrine; thought to antagonize muscarinic, histaminergic, and α-adrenergic receptors

INDICATIONS: Treatment of depressive disorders, obsessive-compulsive disorder, bulimia nervosa, and panic disorder

ROUTES AND DOSAGE: Available in 10- and 20-mg capsules and 20-mg/5-mL oral solution

Adults: 20 mg/d in the morning, not to exceed 80 mg/d. Full antidepressant effect may not be seen for up to 4 weeks. If no improvement, dosage is increased after several weeks. Dosages greater than 20 mg/d are administered twice daily. For eating disorders: typically 40 mg to 60 mg/d is recommended

Geriatric: Administer at lower or less frequent doses; monitor responses to guide dosage

Children: Safety and efficacy have not been established

HALF-LIFE (PEAK EFFECT): 2 to 3 d (6–8 h)

SELECTED ADVERSE REACTIONS: Headache, nervousness, insomnia, drowsiness, anxiety, tremors, dizziness, lightheadedness, nausea, vomiting, diarrhea, dry mouth, anorexia, dyspepsia, constipation, taste changes, upper respiratory infections, pharyngitis, painful menstruation, sexual dysfunction, urinary frequency, sweating, rash, pruritus, weight loss, asthenia, and fever

BOXED WARNING: Increased risk of suicidal thoughts and behaviors in children, adolescents, and young adults.

WARNINGS: Avoid use in pregnancy and while breastfeeding. Use with caution in patients with impaired hepatic or renal function and diabetes mellitus. Possible risk for toxicity if taken with tricyclic antidepressants.

SPECIAL PATIENT AND FAMILY EDUCATION:
- Be aware that the drug may take up to 4 weeks to get a full antidepressant effect.
- Take the drug in the morning or in divided doses, if necessary.
- Families and caregivers of pediatric patients being treated with antidepressants should monitor patient for agitation, irritation, and unusual changes in behavior.
- Report any adverse reactions.
- Avoid driving a car or performing hazardous activities because the drug may cause drowsiness or dizziness.
- Eat small, frequent meals to help with complaints of nausea and vomiting.

Interventions for the Psychosocial Domain

Both CBT and IPT have been used for individuals with bulimia nervosa. The combination of CBT and pharmacologic interventions is best for producing an initial decrease in symptoms (Murphy, Straebler, Cooper, & Fairburn, 2010).

Behavioral therapy alone has not been as effective as CBT. IPT has had positive outcomes but may take longer to change binge eating and purging symptoms. Although binge eating may persist, little work can be done on underlying interpersonal issues, such as boundary setting, because the patient is intent on feeling out of control with eating. Therefore, cognitive therapy is begun first to address the distorted thinking processes influencing dietary restraint, binge eating, and purging. Decreasing these symptoms will eliminate the out-of-control feelings.

CBT is usually conducted in a group with one or two sessions a week. A series of sessions is instituted to change dysfunctional thinking, rigid rules about eating, and impulsive behaviors. The cognitive interventions focus on distorted or dysfunctional thought patterns.

Promoting Behavioral Techniques

The behavioral techniques, such as **cue elimination** and response prevention, require self-monitoring to individualize the therapy. **Self-monitoring** is accomplished using a diary in which the patient records binges and purges and precipitating emotions and environmental cues. Emotional and environmental cues are identified, and alternative responses are suggested, tried, and reinforced. When a cue or stimulus leads to a dysfunctional or unhealthy response, the response can be eliminated or an alternate, healthier response to the cue can be substituted, tried, and then reinforced. Figure 30.6 gives two examples of behavioral interventions. In example 1, for the patient with anorexia nervosa, the response is modified or altered to a healthier one; in example 2, for the patient with bulimia nervosa, the cue is changed to produce a different, healthier response. Other techniques, such as postponing binges and purges through distraction, a technique to interrupt the cycle, are also effective.

Providing Psychoeducation

In addition to cognitive and behavioral techniques, educational strategies are also incorporated into CBT during weekly sessions. For individuals with bulimia nervosa, psychoeducation focuses on setting boundaries and healthy limits, developing assertiveness, learning nutritional concepts related to healthy eating, and clarifying misconceptions about food. Rules that result from dichotomous thinking also must be addressed because of their role in dietary restraint and resulting binge eating.

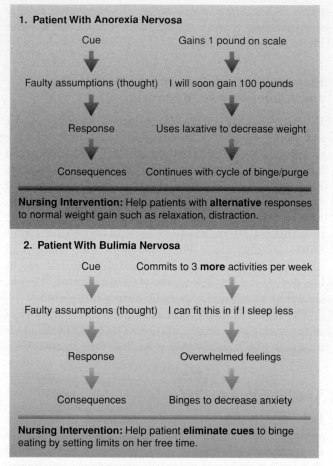

1. Patient With Anorexia Nervosa

Cue → Faulty assumptions (thought) → Response → Consequences

Gains 1 pound on scale → I will soon gain 100 pounds → Uses laxative to decrease weight → Continues with cycle of binge/purge

Nursing Intervention: Help patients with **alternative** responses to normal weight gain such as relaxation, distraction.

2. Patient With Bulimia Nervosa

Cue → Faulty assumptions (thought) → Response → Consequences

Commits to 3 **more** activities per week → I can fit this in if I sleep less → Overwhelmed feelings → Binges to decrease anxiety

Nursing Intervention: Help patient **eliminate cues** to binge eating by setting limits on her free time.

FIGURE 30.6 Examples of the relationship of cues, thoughts, responses, and behavioral interventions.

The nurse can assist patients to understand the binge–purge cycle and the role of rigid rules in contributing to this cycle. The value of eating meals regularly to ward off hunger and reduce the possibility of a binge is also important. Patients who abuse laxatives must be taught that although these drugs produce water-weight loss, they are ineffective for true, lasting weight loss. Patients also need information about potassium depletion, electrolyte imbalances, dehydration, and the medical consequences of binge eating and purging. Other topics for psychoeducation are included in Box 30.15.

Facilitating Group Interventions

Group interventions are cost effective and increase learning more effectively than does individual treatment because patients learn from each other as well as from the nurse, therapist, or leader. Some experts have recommended 12-step programs for treating bulimia nervosa. However, many clinicians who work in this specialty have noted that these programs, with their strict rules, can be counterproductive for patients with bulimia nervosa, who already have rigid rules and are "abstinent" in many ways

Psychoeducation Checklist: Bulimia Nervosa

When caring for the patient with bulimia nervosa, be sure to include the following topic areas in the teaching plan:

- Psychopharmacologic agents, if used, including drug, action, dosage, frequency, and possible adverse effects
- Binge–purge cycle and effects on the body
- Nutrition and eating patterns
- Hydration
- Avoidance of cues
- Cognitive distortions
- Limit setting
- Appropriate boundary setting
- Assertiveness
- Resources
- Self-monitoring and behavioral interventions
- Realistic goal setting

that lead to binge eating. Broad parameters regarding food choices (e.g., all foods allowed in moderation) in combination with knowledge about healthy eating should be encouraged instead.

After symptoms subside, patients can concentrate on interpersonal issues in therapy, such as a fused relationship with their mothers or feelings of inadequacy and low self-esteem, which often underlie their lack of assertiveness.

Evaluation and Treatment Outcomes

Patients with bulimia nervosa have better recovery outcomes than do those with anorexia nervosa. Outcomes have improved since the early 1990s, partially because of earlier detection, research on what treatments are most effective, and neuropharmacologic research and advances such as CBT. Experts in the field of eating disorders report a 55% recovery at 5 years (Keski-Rahkonen et al., 2009), and in a recent study, 83% of women recovered with CBT that included exposure and response prevention techniques (McIntosh, Carter, Bulik, Framptom, & Joyce, 2011). Because CBT requires a specialist's care, current treatment research is exploring the use of self-help models, including manuals that can be combined with psychopharmacology (Murphy, Straebler, Cooper, & Fairburn, 2010).

Continuum of Care

Although patients with bulimia nervosa are less likely than those with anorexia nervosa to require hospitalization, those with extreme dehydration and electrolyte imbalance, depression and suicidality, or symptoms that have not remitted with outpatient treatment need hospitalization.

However, most treatment takes place in outpatient settings. After treatment, referrals to recovery groups and

support groups are important to prevent relapse. Rarely do patients with bulimia nervosa require emergency care.

Prevention

As with anorexia nervosa, preventing bulimia nervosa requires effort on the part of teachers, school nurses, parents, and society as a whole. Because many of the risk factors are seen early in children attending elementary school, educating school nurses and teachers is an important focus for psychiatric–mental health nurses working in the community. Protective factors that mediate between risk factors and the development of an eating disorder must be emphasized and developed. Box 30.12 covers important prevention strategies for parents and their children or adolescents.

Society has begun to engage in an effort to help young girls. The federal government has developed a website called *girlshealth* that is devoted to areas such as body changes, body image, relationships, and self-confidence.

BINGE EATING DISORDER

Another type of disordered eating, **binge eating disorder (BED)**, is now a separate eating disorder in the *DSM-5* (APA, 2013). This disorder is seen in a number of studies that have uncovered a group of individuals who binge in the same way as those with bulimia nervosa but who do not purge or compensate for binges through other behaviors. Individuals with BED also differ from those with other eating disorders in that most of them are obese. In addition, investigators have shown that individuals with BED have lower dietary restraint and are higher in weight than those with bulimia nervosa. It has been estimated that 10% to 30% of obese individuals have BED. Some have reported that they binged without purging for several years beginning as young as fifth grade (Combs, Pearson, & Smith, 2011).

The diagnostic criteria for BED consist of binge eating, which includes both the ingestion of a large amount of food in a short period of time and a sense of loss of control during the binge, distress regarding the binge; eating until uncomfortably full, and feelings of guilt or depression after the binge. As mentioned, purging or other compensatory behavior does not follow the binge. The prevalence of BED is estimated to be 1.6% for females and 0.8% for males in the United States (APA, 2013).

Because this is a newly recognized disorder, additional research is needed to clarify its symptoms, etiology, and treatment. Its etiology is believed to be similar to that of bulimia nervosa. The treatment of individuals with BED is still in the investigative stages, and most experts use interventions similar to those used for bulimia nervosa.

SUMMARY OF KEY POINTS

■ Anorexia nervosa and bulimia nervosa have some common symptoms but are classified as discrete disorders.

■ Eating disorders are best viewed along a continuum that includes subclinical or partial-syndrome disorders; because these disorders occur more frequently than full syndromes, they are often overlooked but, after they are identified, they can be prevented from worsening.

■ Similar factors predispose individuals to the development of anorexia nervosa and bulimia nervosa, and these factors represent a biopsychosocial model of risk. These disorders are preventable, and identifying risk factors assists with prevention strategies.

■ Etiologic factors contribute in combination to the development of eating disorders; no one factor provides an explanation.

■ Treatment of anorexia nervosa frequently includes hospitalization for refeeding; bulimia nervosa is treated primarily on an outpatient basis.

■ Cognitive behavioral therapy and medication improve the symptoms. Individual and group interpersonal psychotherapy are also effective in self-evaluation and communication.

■ The outcomes for bulimia nervosa are better than those for anorexia nervosa. The type and severity of comorbid conditions and the length of the illness influence outcomes.

■ Binge eating disorder is characterized by periods of binge eating not followed by purging or any other compensating behaviors.

CRITICAL THINKING CHALLENGES

1. Discuss the potential difficulties and risks in attempting to treat a patient with anorexia nervosa in an outpatient setting.

2. Parents are often in need of support and suggestions for how to help prevent eating disorders. Develop a teaching program and include the topics and rationale for suggestions chosen.

3. Identify the important nursing management components of a refeeding program for a hospitalized patient with anorexia nervosa.

4. Bulimia nervosa is often described as a closet disorder with secretive binge eating and purging. Identify the signs and symptoms of each system involved for someone with this disorder.

5. Positive outcomes for the recovery of bulimia nervosa and anorexia nervosa depend on many factors. Identify the factors that promote positive outcomes and those related to poorer outcomes and prognosis.

MOVIE viewing GUIDES related to this chapter are available at http://thePoint.lww.com/Boyd5eUpdate.

A related Psychiatric-Mental Health Nursing video on the topic of Eating Disorders is available at: http://thePoint.lww.com/Boyd5eUpdate.

References

American Psychiatric Association. (2013). *Diagnostic and statistical manual of mental disorders* (5th ed.). Arlington, VA: American Psychiatric Association.

Arrow, B., Kenardy, J., & Agras, W. S. (1995). The Emotional Eating Scale: The development of a measure to assess coping with negative affect by eating. *International Journal of Eating Disorders, 18,* 79–90.

Avena, N. M., & Bocarsly, M. E. (2012). Dysregulation of brain reward systems in eating disorders: Neurochemical information from animal models of binge eating, bulimia nervosa, and anorexia nervosa. *Neuropharmacology, 63*(7), 87–96.

Badura, B. A., Huefner, J. C., & Handwerk, M. L. (2012). The impact of abuse and gender on psychopathology, behavioral disturbance, and psychotropic medication count for youth in residential treatment. *American Journal of Orthopsychiatry, 82*(4), 562–572.

Baker, J. H., Maes, H. H., Lissner, L., Aggen, S. H., Lichtenstein, P., & Kendler, K. S. (2009). Genetic risk factors for disordered eating in adolescent males and females. *Journal of Abnormal Psychology, 118*(3), 576–586.

Bardone-Cone, A. M., Strum, K., Lawson, M. A., Robinson, D. P., & Smith R. (2010). Perfectionism across stages of recovery from eating disorders. *International Journal of Eating Disorders, 43*(2), 139–148.

Berner, L. A., Shaw, J. A., Witt, A. A., & Lowe, M. R. (2013). The relation of weight suppression and body mass index to symptomatology and treatment response in anorexia nervosa. *Journal of Abnormal Psychology, 122*(3), 694–708.

Bodell, L. P., Joiner, T. E., & Keel, P. K. (2013). Comorbidity-independent risk for suicidality increases with bulimia nervosa but not with anorexia nervosa. *Journal of Psychiatric Research, 47*(5), 617–621.

Boraska, V., Franklin, C. S., Floyd, J. A., Thornton, L. M., Huckins, L. M., Southam, L., et al. (2014). A genome-wide association study of anorexia nervosa. *Molecular Psychiatry.* doi: 10.1038/mp.2013.187

Brady, C. F. (2014). Obsessive-compulsive disorder and common comorbidities. *Journal of Clinical Psychiatry, 75*(1), e02. doi:10.4088/JCP.13023tx1c

Bruce, K. R., Steiger, H., Young, S. N., Kin, N. M., Israël, M., & Lévesque, M. (2009). Impact of acute tryptophan depletion on mood and eating-related urges in bulimic and nonbulimic women. *Journal of Psychiatry and Neuroscience, 34*(5), 376–382.

Bruch, H. (1973). *Eating disorders: Obesity, anorexia nervosa and the person within.* New York: Basic Books.

Cave, K. E. (2009). Influences of disordered eating in prepubescent children. *Journal of Psychosocial Nursing, 47*(2), 21–24.

Combs, J. L., Pearson, C. M., & Smith, G. T. (2011). A risk model for preadolescent disordered eating. *International Journal of Eating Disorders, 44*(7), 599–604.

Cooper, P., Taylor, M., Cooper, Z., & Fairburn, C. (1987). The development and validation of the BSQ. *International Journal of Eating Disorders, 6,* 485–494.

Dennard, E. E. & Richards, C. S. (2013). Depression and coping in subtreshold eating disorders. *Eating Behaviors, 14*(3), 325–329.

Dunn, P. K. & Ondercin, P. (1981). Personality variables related to compulsive eating in college women. *Journal of Clinical Psychology, 31,* 43–49.

Favaro, A., Caregaro, L., Tenconi, E., Bosello, R., & Santonastaso, P. (2009). Time trends in age at onset of anorexia nervosa and bulimia nervosa. *Journal of Clinical Psychiatry, 70*(12), 1715–1721.

Frank, G. K. (2011). Reward and neurocomputational processes. *Current Topics in Behavioral Neuroscience, 6,* 95–110.

Frank, G. K., Shott, M. E., Hagman, J. O., & Mittal, V. A. (2013). Alterations in brain structures related to taste reward circuitry in ill and recovered anorexia nervosa and in bulimia nervosa. *American Journal of Psychiatry, 170*(10), 1152–1160.

Franko, D. L., Keshaviah, A., Eddy, K. T., Krishna, M., Davis, M. C., Keel, P. K., et al. (2013). A longitudinal investigation of mortality in anorexia nervosa and bulimia nervosa. *American Journal of Psychiatry*, 170(8), 917–925.

Garner, D. M. & Garfinkel, P. E. (1979). The Eating Attitudes Test: An index of the symptoms of anorexia nervosa. *Psychosomatic Medicine*, 10, 647–656.

Gordon, K. H., Castro, Y., Sitnikov, L., & Holm-Denoma, J. M. (2010). Cultural body shape ideals and eating disorder symptoms among white, Latina, and Black college women. *Cultural diversity and Ethnic Minority Psychology*, 16(2), 135–143.

Groleau, P., Steiger, H., Joober, R., Bruce, K.R., Israel, M., Badawi, G., et al. (2012). Dopamine-system genes, childhood abuse, and clinical manifestations in women with Bulimia-spectrum Disorders. *Journal of Psychiatric Research*, 46(9), 1139–1146.

Gustafsson, A., Edlund, S., Kjellin, B., & Norring, C. (2009). Risk and protective factors for disturbed eating in adolescent girls—Aspects of perfectionism and attitudes to eating and weight. *European Eating Disorders Review*, 17(5), 380–389.

Javed, A., Tebben, P. J., Fischer, P. R., & Lteif, A. N. (2013). Female athlete triad and its components: Toward improved screening and management. *Mayo Clinic Proceedings*, 88(9), 996–1009.

Herman, C. P. & Mack, D. (1975). Restrained and unrestrained eating. *Journal of Personality*, 43, 647–660.

Holm-Denoma, J. M., Scaringi, V., Gordon K. H., Van Orden, K. A., & Joiner, T. E. (2009). Eating disorder symptoms among undergraduate varsity athletes, club athletes, independent exercisers, and nonexercisers. *International Journal of Eating Disorders*, 42(1), 47–53.

Kaye, W. H., Wierenga, C. E., Bailer, U. R., Simmons, A. N., & Bischoff-Grethe, A. (2013a). Nothing tastes as good as skinny feels: The neurobiology of anorexia nervosa. *Trends in Neurosciences*, 36(2), 110–120.

Kaye, W. H., Wierenga, C. E., Bailer, U. F., Simmons, A. N., Wagner, A., & Bischoff-Grethe, A. (2013b). Does a shared neurobiology for foods and drugs of abuse contribute to extremes of food ingestion in anorexia and bulimia nervosa? *Biological Psychiatry*, 73(9), 836–842.

Keski-Rahkonen, A., Hoek, H. W., Susser, E. S., Linna, M. S., Sihvola, E., Raevuori, A., et al. (2007). Epidemiology and course of anorexia nervosa in the community. *American Journal of Psychiatry*, 164(8), 1259–1265.

Keski-Rahkonen, A., Hoek, H. W., Susser, E. S., Linna, M. S., Shivola, E., Raevuori A., et al. (2009). Epidemiology and course of anorexia nervosa in the community. *American Journal of Psychiatry*, 164(8), 1259–1265.

Keski-Rahkonen, A., Raevuori, A., Bulik, C.M., Hoek, H.W., Rissanen, A., & Kaprio, J. (2014). Factors associated with recovery from anorexia nervosa: A population-based study. *International Journal of Eating Disorders*, 47(2), 117–23.

Kinsaul, J. A., Curtin, L., Bazzini, D., & Martz, D. (2014). Empowerment, feminism, and self-efficacy: Relationships to body image and disordered eating. *Body Image*, 11(1), 63–67.

Kluck, A. S. (2010). Family influence on disordered eating: The role of body image dissatisfaction. *Body Image*, 7(1), 8–14.

Klump, K. L. (2013). Puberty as a critical risk period for eating disorders: A review of human and animal studies. *Hormones and Behavior*, 64(2), 399–410.

Lask, B. & Roberts, A. (2013). Family cognitive remediation therapy for anorexia nervosa. *Clinical Child Psychology and Psychiatry*. doi:*10.1177/1359104513504313*

le Grange, D., Lock, J., Loeb, K., & Nicholls, D. (2010). Academy for Eating Disorders Position Paper: The role of the family in eating disorders. *International Journal of Eating Disorders*, 43(1), 1–5.

Luff, G. M., & Gray, J.J. (2009). Complex messages regarding a thin ideal appearing in teenage girls' magazines from 1956 to 2005, *Body Image*, 6(2), 133–136.

Lund, B. C., Hernandez, E. R., Yates, W. R., Mitchell, J. R., & McKee, P. A. (2009). Rate of inpatient weight restoration predicts outcome in anorexia nervosa. *International Journal of Eating Disorders*, 42(4), 301–305.

Maloney, M., McGuire, J., & Daniels, S. R. (1988). Reliability testing of a children's version of the Eating Attitude Test. *Journal of the American Academy of Child and Adolescent Psychiatry*, 27, 541–543.

Mangweth-Matzek, C. I., Rupp, A., Hausman, S., Gusmerotti, G., Kemmler, G., & Biebl, W. (2010). Eating disorders in men: Current features and childhood factors. *Eating and Weight Disorders*, 15(1–2), 15–22.

Manuel, A., & Wade, T. D. (2013). Emotion regulation in broadly defined anorexia nervosa: Association with negative affective memory bias. *Behavior Research and Therapy*, 51(8), 417–424.

Martz, D. M., Sturgis, E. T., & Gustafson, S. B. (1996). Development and preliminary validation of the Cognitive Behavioral Dieting Scale. *International Journal of Eating Disorders*, 19, 297–309.

Mazure, C. M., Halmi, K. A., Sunday, S. R., Romano, S. J., & Einhorn, A. M. (1994). Yale-Brown-Cornell Eating Disorder Scale: Development, use, reliability, and validity. *Journal of Psychiatric Research*, 28, 425–445.

McElwen, C. & Flouri, E. (2009). Fathers, parenting, adverse life events and adolescents' emotional and eating disorder symptoms: The role of emotion regulation. *European Child and Adolescent Psychiatry*, 18(4), 206–216.

McIntosh, W., Carter, F. A., Bulik, C. M., Framptom, C. M., & Joyce, P. R. (2011). Five year outcome of cognitive behavioral therapy and exposure with response prevention for bulimia nervosa. *Psychological Medicine*, 41(5), 1061–1071.

Minuchin, S., Rossman, B. L., & Baker, L. (1978). *Psychosomatic families*. Cambridge, MA: Harvard University Press.

Monteleone, P. (2011). New frontiers in endocrinology of eating disorders. *Current Topics Behavioral Neuroscience*, 6, 189–208.

Murphy, R., Straebler, S., Cooper, Z., & Fairburn, C. G. (2010). Cognitive behavioral therapy for eating disorders. *Psychiatric Clinics of North America*, 33(3), 611–627.

Napolitano, M. A. & Himes, S. (2011). Race, weight, and correlates of binge eating in female students. *Eating Behaviors*, 12(1), 29–36.

Piran, N. (2010). A feminist perspective on risk factor research and on the prevention of eating disorders. *Eating Disorders*, 18(3), 183–198.

Preti, A., Rocchi, M. B., Sisti, D., Camboni, M. V., & Miotto, P. (2011). A comprehensive meta-analysis of the risk of suicide in eating disorders. *Acta Psychiatrica Scandinavica*, 124(1), 6–17.

Poisinelli, G. N., Levitan, R. N., & DeLuca, V. (2012). 5-HTTLPR polymorphism in bulimia nervosa: A multiple-model meta-analysis. *Psychiatric Genetics*, 22(5), 219–225.

Racine, S. E., Burt, S. A., Iacono, W. G., McGue, M., & Klump, K. L. (2011). Dietary restraint moderates genetic risk for binge eating. *Journal of Abnormal Psychology*, 120(1), 119–128.

Rieger, E., Van Buren, D. J., Bishop, M., Tanofsky-Kraff, M., Welch, R., & Wilfley, E. D. (2010). An eating disorder-specific model of interpersonal psychotherapy (IPT-ED): Causal pathways and treatment implications. *Clinical Psychology Review*, 30, 400–410.

Rhea, D. J. & Thatcher, W. G. (2013). Ethnicity, ethnic identity, self-esteem and at-risk eating disorders behavior differences of urban adolescent females. *Eating Disorders*, 21(3), 223–237.

Sabel, A. L., Rosen, E., & Mehler, P. S. (2014). Severe anorexia nervosa in males: Clinical presentations and medical treatment. *Eating disorders*, 22(3), 209–220.

Salbach-Andrae, H., Schneider, N., Seifert, K., Pfeiffer, E., Lenz K, Lehmkuhl. U., et al. (2009). Short term outcome of anorexia nervosa in adolescents after inpatient treatment: A prospective study. *European Child and Adolescent Psychiatry*, 18(11), 701–704.

Shisslak, C., Renger, R., Sharpe, T., Crago, M., McKnight, K. M, Gray, N., et al. (1999). Development and evaluation of the McKnight Risk Factor Survey for assessing potential risk and protective factors for disordered eating in preadolescent and adolescent girls. *International Journal of Eating Disorders*, 25, 195–214.

Smink, F. R., van Hocken, D., & Hoek, H. W. (2012). Epidemiology of eating disorders: Incidence, prevalence, and mortality rates. *Current Psychiatry Reports*, 14(4), 404–414.

Suokas, J. R., Suvisaari, J. M., Grainger, M., Raevuori, A., Gissler, M., & Haukka, J. (2014). Suicide attempts and mortality in eating disorders: A follow-up study of eating disorder patients. *General Hospital Psychiatry*, 36(3), 355–357. http://dx.doi.org/10.1016/j.genhosppsych.2014.002.

Thornton, L. M., Mazzeo, S. E., & Bulik, C. M. (2011). The heritability of eating disorders: Methods and current findings. *Current Topics in Behavioral Neurosciences*, 6, 141–156.

van den Berg, P. A., Mond, J., Eisenberg, M., Ackard, D., & Neumark-Sztainer, D. (2010). The link between body dissatisfaction and self-esteem in adolescents: Similarities across gender, age, weight status, race/ethnicity, and socioeconomic status. *Journal of Adolescent Health*, 47(3), 290–296.

Vrabel, K. R., Hofart, A., Ro, Y., Martinson, E. W., & Rosenvinge, J. H. (2010). Co-occurrence of avoidant personality disorder and child sexual abuse predicts poor outcome in long standing eating disorders. *Journal of Abnormal Psychology*, 119(3), 623–629.

Wilkosz, M. E., Chen, J., Kenndey, C., & Rankin, S. (2011). Body dissatisfaction in California adolescents. *Journal of the American Academy of Nurse Practitioners*, 23(2), 101–109.

Wooley, S. C., & Kearney-Cooke, A. (1986). Intensive treatment of bulimia and body image disturbance. In K. D. Brownell & J. P. Foreyt (Eds.), *Handbook of eating disorders: Physiology, psychology and treatment of obesity, anorexia, and bulimia* (pp. 476–502). New York: Basic Books.

Zhao, Y., & Encinosa, W. (2009). *Hospitalizations for eating disorders from 1999–2006. HCUP statistical brief #70*. Rockville, MD: Agency for Healthcare Research and Quality, Retrieved from http://www.hcup-us.ahrq.gov/reports/statbriefs/sb70.pdf.

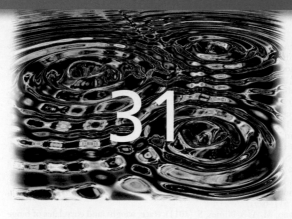

31

Addiction and Substance-Related Disorders
Management of Alcohol and Drug Use

Mary Ann Boyd

KEY CONCEPTS

- addiction
- denial
- motivation

LEARNING OBJECTIVES

After studying this chapter, you will be able to:

1. Describe the actions, effects, and withdrawal symptoms of alcohol, marijuana, stimulants, tobacco, hallucinogens, opioids, inhalants, and gambling disorder.

2. Discuss the evidence that serves as a basis of care and treatment of persons with substance-related and non–substance-related disorders.

3. Formulate nursing diagnoses based on a biopsychosocial assessment of people with substance-related disorders.

4. Compare intervention approaches of substance-related and non–substance-related disorders.

5. Implement treatment interventions for patients with substance-related and non–substance-related disorders.

KEY TERMS

- abuse • Alcoholics Anonymous (AA) • alcohol withdrawal syndrome • blood alcohol level • brief interventions • codependence • confabulation • confrontation • craving • delirium tremens • dependence • detoxification • gambling disorder • hallucinogen • harm reduction • inhalants • Korsakoff's amnestic syndrome • methadone maintenance • motivational interviewing • opioid • peer assistance programs • relapse • substance-induced disorders • substance use disorders • sudden sniffing death • tolerance • use • Wernicke-Korsakoff syndrome • Wernicke's encephalopathy • withdrawal

The human use and abuse of alcohol and other drugs has been around since the beginning of history; so too have the subsequent social and emotional problems that accompany substance use. This chapter reviews the concept of addiction, types of substance use, biologic and psychological effects, current theories of substance-related disorders, and interventions. Gambling disorder is a non–substance-related disorder and will be discussed in this chapter. Gambling behaviors and their consequences have similar characteristics to the behaviors associated with substance disorders. The nurse's role in helping persons with these disorders recover is discussed within the biopsychosocial nursing model. Professional issues related to chemical dependency within the nursing profession are also examined.

OVERVIEW OF SUBSTANCE USE AND ABUSE

Alcohol, tobacco, marijuana, and illegal prescription drug use have reached epidemic proportions in the United States, with the incidence rising in younger age groups, particularly among adolescents and young adults. One of the goals of *Healthy People 2020* is "to reduce substance abuse to protect the health, safety, and quality of life for all, especially children" (U.S. Department of Health and Human Services, 2010). The overriding concern about using mind-altering substances is that these substances will compromise health and continued use will lead to addiction.

> KEYCONCEPT **Addiction** is a condition of continued use of substances (or reward-seeking behaviors) despite adverse consequences.

Many mind-altering substances are physiologically addicting and easily can lead to severe health and legal problems. **Use** (ingestion, smoking, sniffing, or injection) of some mind-altering substances such as alcohol, pain medication, tobacco, or caffeine is legal for adults. Other substances such as cocaine and heroin are illegal in the United States. **Abuse** occurs when a person uses alcohol or drugs for the purpose of intoxication or, in the case of prescription drugs, for purposes beyond their intended use. The substance-related disorders involve substances that are commonly abused.

Physiological **dependence** can develop with many different types of medications such as beta-blockers, antidepressants, opioids, anti-anxiety agents, and others. As long as medications are used for their intended purposes and under the supervision of qualified health care providers, physiological dependence is a part of treatment. That is, dependence can be a normal response to some medications (American Psychiatric Association [APA], 2013).

Diagnostic Criteria

The *Diagnostic and Statistical Manual of Mental Disorders, 5th Edition* (*DSM-5*) organizes substance-related disor-

ders into two categories: substance use disorders and substance-induced disorders. **Substance-induced disorders** occur when medications used for other health problems or medical/mental health disorders causes intoxication, withdrawal, or other health-related problems. A **substance use disorder** occurs when an individual continues using substances despite cognitive, behavioral, and physiological symptoms. The *DSM-5* identifies 10 diagnostic categories of substances including alcohol, caffeine, cannabis (marijuana), hallucinogens, inhalants, opioids, sedative–hypnotics, stimulants, tobacco, and others (American Psychiatric Association, 2013). Gambling disorder is included within the substance use disorder category because gambling behaviors can activate the brain's reward system similar to the substance use disorders.

A substance use disorder occurs when there is an underlying change in brain circuitry that may persist after **detoxification**, the process of safely and effectively withdrawing a person from an addictive substance, usually under medical supervision. These brain changes lead to pathological behaviors that occur with repeated relapses and intense drug cravings when exposed to the drug-related cues (e.g., party, emotional experiences) (APA, 2013). See Box 31.1.

Epidemiology
Age of Onset

In the United States, alcohol is the most abused substance followed by marijuana. Alcohol use is at historically low levels for adolescents. In 2013, 3.5% of 8th graders, 12.8% of 10th graders, and 26% of 12th graders reported getting drunk in the past month. In 2013, 22.1% of high school seniors reported binge drinking – a drop of almost one third since the late 1990s – but illicit drug use among adolescents is on the rise. In 2013, 7% of 8th

---

BOX 31.1

Substance Use Disorders: Diagnostic Characteristics

KEY DIAGNOSTIC CRITERIA
- Impaired control over substance use
  - Taking substance in larger amounts or over a longer period than was intended
  - Persistent desire to cut down or regulate substance use (may have unsuccessful attempts)
  - A great deal of time spent obtaining, using, or recovering from its effects
  - Craving occurs (an intense desire or urge)
- Social impairment
  - Recurrent use results in failure of work, school, or home obligations
  - Continues to use despite persistent or recurrent social or interpersonal problems caused by substance

- Give up or reduce important social, occupational, or recreational activities because of the substance use
  - May withdraw from family activities
- Risky use of substance and failure to abstain despite difficulty
  - Recurrent use in situations that are physically hazardous
  - Continue to use substance despite knowledge of having physical or psychological problems that are likely caused by the use of the substance
- Pharmacological effects
  - Tolerance develops – needing more of the substance to achieve desired effect
  - Withdrawal syndrome occurs when blood or tissue concentration of a substance declines (may not occur for all substances)

Adapted from American Psychiatric Association. (2013). *Diagnostic and Statistical Manual of Mental Disorders* (5th ed.). Arlington, VA: Author.

graders, 18% of 10th graders, and 22.7% of 12th graders used marijuana within the last 12 months. The rising marijuana use reflects a change in attitude and perception that marijuana is a safe drug, especially in light of recent legalization of marijuana in some states (National Institute of Drug Abuse [NIDA], 2014a).

The nonmedical use of prescription and over-the-counter (OTC) medicines continues to be a significant part of the adolescent drug problems. In 2013, 15% of high school seniors used a prescription drug nonmedically in the past year. Adderall, a stimulant used to treat attention deficit hyperactivity disorder (see Chapter 35) was used by 7.4% of seniors for nonmedical reasons. Fewer teens smoke cigarettes (9.6%) than smoke marijuana (15.6%). The use of other forms of tobacco are increasing with 21.4% of 12th graders smoking Hookah water pipes at some point during the past year—an increase from 18.3% in 2012 (USDHHS, 2014a).

Ethnicity and Culture

The use of illicit and legal substances among Asians is consistently lower than the other ethnic groups. In 2012, current illicit drug use was 3.7% among Asians, 7.8% among Native Hawaiians or Other Pacific Islanders, 8.3% among Hispanics, 9.2% among whites, 11.3% among blacks or African Americans, 12.7% among American Indians or Alaska Natives, and 14.8% among persons of two or more races. These statistics have been relatively stable since 2002 except for whites (from 8.5% to 9.2%) and African Americans (from 9.7% to 11.3%) (Substance Abuse and Mental Health Services Administration, 2013).

The highest use of alcohol was among whites (57.4%) and persons reporting two or more races (51.9%) followed by African Americans (43.2%), Hispanics (41.8%), American Indians or Alaska Natives (41.7%), and Asians (36.9%). The highest tobacco use was reported among the American Indians or Alaska Natives (48.4%) followed by persons reporting two or more races (37.3%), whites (29.2%), African Americans (27.2%), Hispanics (19.2%), and Asians (10.8%) (SAMSHA, 2013).

Comorbidity

Many people who abuse substances have comorbid mental disorders. Some disorders are in part a byproduct of long-term substance use; others predispose the individual to alcohol or drug abuse. Whatever the reason, nurses should be aware that patients who abuse substances often have psychotic, anxiety, or mood disorders (Pope, Joober, & Malla, 2013). Other coexisting mental disorders include attention deficit hyperactivity disorder (ADHD) (Nogueira et al., 2014) and personality disorders (Gonzalez, 2014). See Chapter 39.

Individuals who abuse substances are at high risk for death from drug overdoses and are at increased risk for death from other causes, including homicide, suicide, and opportunistic infections (such as HIV) secondary to drug injection. Earlier studies have documented the connection between alcohol abuse and increased risk for diabetes mellitus, gastrointestinal problems, hypertension, liver disease, and stroke (Kottke & Pronk, 2010).

Etiology

Substance abuse encompasses the body, the mind, and society's influences (Bowen et al., 2014; Cadet, Bisagno, & Milroy, 2014). From the biologic perspective, human and animal studies confirm a genetic predisposition for drinking behaviors and self-administering mind-altering drugs, yet no precise genetic marker has been established. From a psychosocial perspective, temperament and feelings about self, age, motivation for change, social consequences for problematic behaviors, and environmental factors such as parental and family relationships and peer pressure all contribute to expression of substance abuse—a chronic and progressive disorder. See Figure 31.1 for depiction of the biopsychosocial etiologies.

Family Responses to Substance Use and Abuse

Abuse of substances by one or more members has devastating effects on families, their functioning, and the community. Fetal alcohol syndrome occurs as a result of drinking alcohol during pregnancy. Addictions lead to loss of jobs and family relationships. Use of illegal substances can lead to arrest and prison.

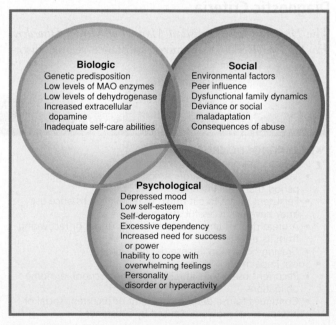

FIGURE 31.1 Biopsychosocial etiologies for patients with substance abuse.

Many families try to help their family member learn to abstain or reduce the use of substances. Support groups provide education and help in understanding the addiction. On the other hand, some persons who recover from substance abuse find that they must distance themselves from families that are actively using and abusing alcohol and drugs.

Treatment and Recovery

The goal for persons abusing substances is to recover from the abuse. Recovery involves a partnership between health care providers and the individual and family. For many of the individuals, a period of intense treatment is necessary to safely manage the physical and psychological **withdrawal** symptoms that occur when a substance is no longer used. Specific withdrawal symptoms depend on the addictive substance and are explained as the substances are discussed. The withdrawal process usually involves **detoxification**. After a person is safely withdrawn from the substance of abuse, the real work toward recovery can begin. A primary concern is **relapse**, the recurrence of alcohol- or drug-dependent behavior in an individual who has previously achieved and maintained abstinence for a significant time beyond the period of detoxification.

TYPES OF SUBSTANCES AND RELATED DISORDERS

Table 31.1 provides a summary of the effects of abused substances.

Alcohol

Alcohol (or ethanol) found in various proportions in liquor, wine, and beer relaxes inhibitions and heightens emotions. Mood swings can range from bouts of gaiety to angry outbursts, and cognitive impairments can vary from reduced concentration or attention span to impaired judgment and memory. Alcohol ultimately produces a sedative effect by depressing the central nervous system (CNS). Depending on the amount of alcohol ingested, the effects can range from feelings of mild sedation and relaxation to confusion and serious impairment of motor functions and speech to severe intoxication that can result in coma, respiratory failure, and death.

All patients should be screened not only for alcohol use disorders but also for drinking patterns or behaviors that may place them at increased risk for experiencing adverse health effects or alcoholism. A frequently used screening tool is the CAGE Questionnaire. This tool consists of four self-report responses to questions about respondents' beliefs of cutting down on their drinking, their experience of others criticizing their drinking, the presence of guilt

about drinking, and early morning drinking (Ewing, 1984). People who abuse alcohol exhibit various patterns of use. Some engage in heavy drinking on a regular or daily basis, others may abstain from drinking during the week and engage in heavy drinking on the weekends, and still others experience longer periods of sobriety interspersed with bouts of binge drinking (several days of intoxication). Risky (binge) drinkers who have not yet become addicted to alcohol often can be screened and receive initial counseling within a primary care setting, but there is little evidence to suggest that permanent behavior change will occur within the primary care setting (Moyer et al., 2013; Butler et al., 2013).

The level of CNS impairment while under the influence of alcohol depends on how much is consumed in a given period of time and how rapidly the body metabolizes it. Intoxication is determined by the level of alcohol in the blood, called **blood alcohol level** (BAL). The body can metabolize 1 oz of liquor, a 5-oz glass of wine, or a 12-oz can of beer per hour without intoxication. Table 31.2 lists behavioral responses at various BALs.

Effects of Long-Term Abuse

People who use alcohol regularly usually develop alcohol **tolerance**, the ability to ingest an increasing amount of alcohol before they experience a "high" and show cognitive and motor effects. The locus ceruleus, which normally inhibits the action of ethanol, is believed to be instrumental in the development of alcohol tolerance. Even though these individuals do not appear intoxicated, their BALs reflect the increase amount of alcohol and are affecting their bodies as described in Table 31.1. Excessive or long-term abuse of alcohol can adversely affect all body systems, and the effects can be serious and permanent. Box 31.2 lists the major physical complications of alcohol abuse for the major organ systems.

Years of alcohol abuse can cause cerebellar degeneration from increased levels of acetaldehyde, a toxic byproduct of alcohol metabolism, and can result in impaired coordination, a broad-based unsteady gait, and fine tremors. Long-term effects also include disturbances in rapid eye movement (REM) sleep and chronic sleep disorders.

Alcohol-Induced Amnestic Disorders

Although certain alcohol-related cognitive impairments are reversible with abstinence, long-term alcohol abuse can cause specific neurologic complications that lead to organic brain disorders, known as alcohol-induced amnestic disorders. Alcohol is directly toxic to the brain, causing atrophy of the frontal cortex and eventually chronic brain syndrome. Patients with alcohol-induced amnestic disorders usually have a history of many years of heavy alcohol use and are generally older than 40 years.

Table 31.1	SUMMARY OF EFFECTS OF ABUSED SUBSTANCES, OVERDOSE, WITHDRAWAL SYNDROMES, AND PROLONGED USE			
Substance	**Route**	**Effects (E) and Overdose (O)**	**Withdrawal Syndrome**	**Prolonged Use**
Alcohol	PO	E: Sedation, decreased inhibitions, relaxation, decreased coordination, slurred speech, nausea O: Respiratory depression, cardiac arrest	Tremors; seizures, increased temperature, pulse, and blood pressure; delirium tremens	Affects all systems of the body. Can lead to other dependencies
Stimulants (amphetamines, cocaine)	PO, IV, inhalation, smoking	E: Euphoria, initial CNS stimulation and then depression, wakefulness, decreased appetite, insomnia, paranoia, aggressiveness, dilated pupils, tremors O: Cardiac arrhythmias or arrest, increased or lowered blood pressure, respiratory depression, chest pain, vomiting, seizures, psychosis, confusion, seizures, dyskinesias, dystonias, coma	Depression: psychomotor retardation at first and then agitation; fatigue and then insomnia; severe dysphoria and anxiety; cravings, vivid, unpleasant dreams; increased appetite. Amphetamine withdrawal is not as pronounced as cocaine withdrawal.	Is often alternated with depressants. Weight loss and resulting malnutrition and increased susceptibility to infectious diseases. May produce schizophrenia-like syndrome with paranoid ideation, thought disturbance, hallucinations, and stereotyped movements
Cannabis (marijuana, hashish, THC)	Smoking, PO	E: Euphoria or dysphoria, relaxation and drowsiness, heightened perception of color and sound, poor coordination, spatial perception and time distortion, unusual body sensations (weightlessness, tingling), dry mouth, dysarthria, and food cravings O: Increased heart rate, reddened eyes, dysphoria, lability, disorientation		Can decrease motivation and cause cognitive deficits (inability to concentrate, memory impairment)
Hallucinogens (LSD, MDMA)	PO	E: Euphoria or dysphoria, altered body image, distorted or sharpened visual and auditory perception, depersonalization, bizarre behavior, confusion, incoordination, impaired judgment and memory, signs of sympathetic and parasympathetic stimulation, palpitations (blurred vision, dilated pupils, sweating) O: Paranoia, ideas of reference, fear of losing one's mind, depersonalization, derealization, illusions, hallucinations, synesthesia, self-destructive or aggressive behavior, tremors	"Flashbacks" or HPPD may occur after termination of use.	
PCP	PO, inhalation, smoking	E: Feeling superhuman, decreased awareness of and detachment from the environment, stimulation of the respiratory and cardiovascular systems, ataxia, dysarthria, decreased pain perception O: Hallucinations, paranoia, psychosis, aggression, adrenergic crisis (cardiac failure, CVA, malignant hyperthermia, status epilepticus, severe muscle contractions)		"Flashbacks," HPPD, organic brain syndromes with recurrent psychotic behavior, which can last up to 6 months after not using the drug, numerous psychiatric hospitalizations and police arrests
Opioids (heroin, codeine)	PO, injection, smoking	E: Euphoria, sedation, reduced libido, memory and concentration difficulties, analgesia, constipation, constricted pupils O: Respiratory depression, stupor, coma	Abdominal cramps, rhinorrhea, watery eyes, dilated pupils, yawning, "goose flesh," diaphoresis, nausea, diarrhea, anorexia, insomnia, fever (see Table 31.4)	Can lead to criminal behavior to get money for drugs, risk for infection-related to needle use (e.g., HIV, endocarditis, hepatitis).

(Continued)

Table 31.1	**SUMMARY OF EFFECTS OF ABUSED SUBSTANCES, OVERDOSE, WITHDRAWAL SYNDROMES, AND PROLONGED USE** (*Continued*)			
Substance	**Route**	**Effects (E) and Overdose (O)**	**Withdrawal Syndrome**	**Prolonged Use**
Sedatives, hypnotics, anxiolytics	PO, injection	E: Euphoria, sedation, reduced libido, emotional lability, impaired judgment O: Respiratory depression, cardiac arrest	Anxiety rebound and agitation, hypertension, tachycardia, sweating, hyperpyrexia, sensory excitement, motor excitation, insomnia, possible tonic-clonic convulsions, nightmares, delirium, depersonalization, hallucinations	Often alternated with stimulants, use with alcohol enhances chance of overdose, risk for infection related to needle use
Inhalants (glue, lighter fluid)	Inhalation	E: Euphoria, giddiness, excitation O: CNS depression: ataxia, nystagmus, dysarthria, coma and convulsions	Similar to alcohol but milder, with anxiety, tremors, hallucinations, and sleep disturbance as the primary symptoms	Long-term use can lead to liver and renal failure, blood dyscrasias, damage to the lungs; CNS damage (OBS, peripheral neuropathies, cerebral and optic atrophy, parkinsonism)
Nicotine	Smoking	E: Stimulation, enhanced performance and alertness, and appetite suppression O: Anxiety	Mood changes (craving, anxiety) and physiologic changes (poor concentration, sleep disturbances, headaches, gastric distress, and increased appetite)	Increased chance for cardiac disease and lung disease
Caffeine	PO	E: Stimulation, increased mental acuity, inexhaustibility O: Restlessness, nervousness, excitement, insomnia, flushing, diuresis, gastrointestinal distress, muscle twitching, rambling flow of thought and speech, tachycardia or cardiac arrhythmia, agitation	Headache, drowsiness, fatigue, craving, impaired psychomotor performance, difficulty concentrating, yawning, nausea	Physical consequences are under investigation

CNS, central nervous system; CVA, cerebrovascular accident; HIV, human immunodeficiency virus; HPPD, hallucinogen persisting perceptual disorder; LSD, ᴅ-lysergic acid diethylamide; MDMA, (3-4 methylenedioxymethamphetamine); OBS, organic brain syndrome; PO, oral; PCP, phencyclidine; THC, D-9-tetrahydrocannabinol.

Table 31.2	**BLOOD ALCOHOL LEVELS AND BEHAVIOR**	
Number of Drinks	**Blood Alcohol Levels (mg%)**	**Behavior**
1–2	0.05	Impaired judgment, giddiness, mood changes
5–6	0.10	Difficulty driving and coordinating movements
10–12	0.20	Motor functions severely impaired, resulting in ataxia; emotional lability
15–20	0.30	Stupor, disorientation, and confusion
20–24	0.40	Coma
25	0.50	Respiratory failure, death

Wernicke's encephalopathy, a degenerative brain disorder caused by thiamine deficiency, is characterized by vision impairment, ataxia, hypotension, confusion, and coma. **Korsakoff's amnestic syndrome**, associated with alcoholism, involves the heart, vascular and nervous systems, but the primary problem is acquiring new information and retrieving memories. Symptoms include amnesia, **confabulation**, (telling a plausible but imagined scenario to compensate for memory loss), attention deficit, disorientation, and vision impairment. Although Wernicke's encephalopathy and Korsakoff's amnestic syndrome can appear as two different disorders, they are generally considered to be different stages of the same disorder called **Wernicke-Korsakoff syndrome**, with Wernicke's encephalopathy representing the acute phase and Korsakoff's amnestic syndrome the chronic phase. Early symptoms can be reversed, but without long-term treatment, the prognosis is poor (Day, Bentham, Callaghan, Kuruvilla, & George, 2013).

BOX 31.2

Medical Complications of Alcohol Abuse

- **Cardiovascular system:** Cardiomyopathy, congestive heart failure, hypertension
- **Respiratory system:** Increased rate of pneumonia and other respiratory infections
- **Hematologic system:** Anemias, leukemia, hematomas
- **Nervous system:** Withdrawal symptoms, irritability, depression, anxiety disorders, sleep disorders, phobias, paranoid feelings, diminished brain size and functioning, organic brain disorders, blackouts, cerebellar degeneration, neuropathies, palsies, gait disturbances, visual problems
- **Digestive system** and **nutritional deficiencies:** Liver diseases (fatty liver, alcoholic hepatitis, cirrhosis), pancreatitis, ulcers, other inflammations of the gastrointestinal (GI) tract, ulcers and GI bleeds, esophageal varices, cancers of the upper GI tract, pellagra, alcohol amnestic disorder, dermatitis, stomatitis, cheilosis, scurvy
- **Endocrine and metabolic:** Increased incidence of diabetes, hyperlipidemia, hyperuricemia, and gout
- **Immune system:** Impaired immune functioning, higher incidence of infectious diseases, including tuberculosis and other bacterial infections
- **Integumentary system:** Skin lesions, increased incidence of infection, burns, and other traumatic injury
- **Musculoskeletal system:** Increased incidence of traumatic injury, myopathy
- **Genitourinary system:** Hypogonadism, increased secondary female sexual characteristics in men (hypoandrogenization and hyperestrogenization), erectile dysfunction in men, electrolyte imbalances due to excess urinary secretion of potassium and magnesium

Detoxification

When a patient enters treatment for alcohol addiction, alcohol ingestion is immediately stopped, and detoxification begins. Because of physiological addiction, **alcohol withdrawal syndrome** occurs, with symptoms of increased heart rate and blood pressure, diaphoresis, mild anxiety, restlessness, and hand tremors (Table 31.3). The severity of withdrawal symptoms ranges from mild to severe, depending on the length and amount of alcohol use. In patients with alcoholism and in chronic drinkers, the alcohol withdrawal syndrome usually begins within 12 hours after abrupt discontinuation or attempt to decrease consumption. The most severe symptoms are **delirium tremens** (acute withdrawal syndrome characterized by autonomic hyperarousal, disorientation, hallucinations, and tremors) and grand mal (tonic-clonic) seizures. These symptoms can be life threatening. If seizures occur, they usually do so within the first 48 hours of withdrawal.

> **NCLEXNOTE** Alcohol abuse continues to require nursing assessment and interventions in all settings. Patients who abuse alcohol for long periods of time are at high risk for alcohol withdrawal syndrome. Observing for signs of seizure activity is a priority nursing intervention.

Uncomplicated alcohol withdrawal is usually completed within 48 to 96 hours. Assessing for vital sign changes, nausea, vomiting, tremors, perspiration, agitation, headache, and change in mental status are important nursing interventions. The Clinical Institute Withdrawal Assessment for Alcohol Scale (CIWA-Ar) is frequently used for assessment (Box 31.3). Close monitoring of withdrawal symptoms continues until BAL is reduced.

Several medications are used to prevent physiological complications and provide a gradual withdraw from alcohol. Antianxiety and sedating drugs, such as benzodiazepines, are titrated downwardly over several days as a substitution for the alcohol. Chlordiazepoxide (Librium) and diazepam have longer half-lives and smoother tapers. Lorazepam (Ativan) is better for the older adult and people with liver impairment. Antidepressants are usually initiated to treat mood states, and sleep medication is used to promote a regular sleep pattern. Antipsychotic medications are also used if needed.

Table 31.3	ALCOHOL WITHDRAWAL SYNDROME		
	Stage I: Mild	**Stage II: Moderate**	**Stage III: Severe**
Vital signs	Heart rate elevated, temperature elevated, normal or slightly elevated systolic blood pressure	Heart rate, 100–120 bpm; elevated systolic blood pressure and temperature	Heart rate, 120–140 bpm; elevated systolic and diastolic blood pressures; elevated temperature
Diaphoresis	Slightly	Usually obvious	Marked
Central nervous system	Oriented; no confusion; no hallucinations	Intermittent confusion; transient visual and auditory hallucinations and illusions, mostly at night	Marked disorientation, confusion, disturbing visual and auditory hallucinations, misidentification of objects, delusions related to the hallucinations, delirium tremens, disturbances in consciousness
	Mild anxiety and restlessness		
	Restless sleep		
	Hand tremors; "shakes"; no convulsions	Painful anxiety and motor restlessness	Agitation, extreme restlessness, and panic states
		Insomnia and nightmares	Unable to sleep
		Visible tremulousness, rare convulsions	Gross uncontrollable tremors, convulsions common
Gastrointestinal system	Impaired appetite, nausea	Anorexia, nausea and vomiting	Rejecting all fluid and food

BOX 31.3

Clinical Institute Withdrawal Assessment of Alcohol Scale, Revised (CIWA-Ar)

Patient:_____ Date:_____ Time:_____ (24 hour clock, midnight = 00:00)

Pulse or heart rate, taken for one minute: _____ Blood pressure:_____

NAUSEA AND VOMITING – Ask "Do you feel sick to your stomach? Have you vomited?" Observation.
0 no nausea and no vomiting
1 mild nausea with no vomiting
2
3
4 intermittent nausea with dry heaves
5
6
7 constant nausea, frequent dry heaves and vomiting

TREMOR – Arms extended and fingers spread apart. Observation.
0 no tremor
1 not visible but can be felt fingertip to fingertip
2
3
4 moderate, with patient's arms extended
5
6
7 severe, even with arms not extended

PAROXYSMAL SWEATS – Observation.
0 no sweat visible
1 barely perceptible sweating, palms moist
2
3
4 beads of sweat obvious on forehead
5
6
7 drenching sweats

ANXIETY – Ask "Do you feel nervous?" Observation.
0 no anxiety, at ease
1 mild anxious
2
3
4 moderately anxious, or guarded, so anxiety is inferred
5
6
7 equivalent to acute panic states as seen in severe delirium or acute schizophrenic reactions

AGITATION – Observation.
0 normal activity
1 somewhat more than normal activity
2
3
4 moderately fidgety and restless
5
6
7 paces back and forth during most of the interview, or constantly thrashes about

TACTILE DISTURBANCES – Ask "Have you any itching, pins and needles sensations, any burning, any numbness, or do you feel bugs crawling on or under your skin?" Observation.
0 none
1 very mild itching, pins and needles, burning or numbness
2 mild itching, pins and needles, burning or numbness
3 moderate itching, pins and needles, burning or numbness
4 moderately severe hallucinations
5 severe hallucinations
6 extremely severe hallucinations
7 continuous hallucinations

AUDITORY DISTURBANCES – Ask "Are you more aware of sounds around you? Are they harsh? Do they frighten you? Are you hearing anything that is disturbing to you? Are you hearing things you know are not there?" Observation.
0 not present
1 very mild harshness or ability to frighten
2 mild harshness or ability to frighten
3 moderate harshness or ability to frighten
4 moderately severe hallucinations
5 severe hallucinations
6 extremely severe hallucinations
7 continuous hallucinations

VISUAL DISTURBANCES – Ask "Does the light appear to be too bright? Is its color different? Does it hurt your eyes? Are you seeing anything that is disturbing to you? Are you seeing things you know are not there?" Observation.
0 not present
1 very mild sensitivity
2 mild sensitivity
3 moderate sensitivity
4 moderately severe hallucinations
5 severe hallucinations
6 extremely severe hallucinations
7 continuous hallucinations

HEADACHE, FULLNESS IN HEAD – Ask "Does your head feel different? Does it feel like there is a band around your head?" Do not rate for dizziness or lightheadedness. Otherwise, rate severity.
0 not present
1 very mild
2 mild
3 moderate
4 moderately severe
5 severe
6 very severe
7 extremely severe

ORIENTATION AND CLOUDING OF SENSORIUM – Ask "What day is this? Where are you? Who am I?"
0 oriented and can do serial additions
1 cannot do serial additions or is uncertain about date
2 disoriented for date by no more than 2 calendar days
3 disoriented for date by more than 2 calendar days
4 disoriented for place/or person

Total **CIWA-Ar** Score _____
Rater's Initials _____
Maximum Possible Score 67

The **CIWA-Ar** is not copyrighted and may be reproduced freely. This assessment for monitoring withdrawal symptoms requires approximately 5 minutes to administer. The maximum score is 67 (see instrument). Patients scoring less than 10 do not usually need additional medication for withdrawal.

Sullivan, J.T.; Sykora, K.; Schneiderman, J.; Naranjo, C.A.; and Sellers, E.M. Assessment of alcohol withdrawal: The revised Clinical Institute Withdrawal Assessment for Alcohol scale (**CIWA-Ar**). *British Journal of Addiction* 84:1353–1357, 1989.

BOX 31.4

Drug Profile: **Disulfiram (Antabuse)**

DRUG CLASS: Antialcoholic agent, enzyme inhibitor

RECEPTOR AFFINITY: Inhibits the enzyme aldehyde dehydrogenase, blocking oxidation of alcohol and allowing acetaldehyde to accumulate to concentrations five to 10 times higher than normal in the blood during alcohol metabolism. Believed to inhibit norepinephrine synthesis.

INDICATIONS: Management of selected patients with chronic alcohol use who want to remain in a state of enforced sobriety

ROUTE AND DOSAGE: Available in 250- and 500-mg tablets

Adults: Initially, a maximum dose of 500 mg/d PO in a single dose for 1–2 weeks. Maintenance dosage of 125 to 500 mg/d PO not to exceed 500 mg/d, continued until patient is fully recovered socially and a basis for permanent self-control is established.

HALF-LIFE (PEAK EFFECT): Unclear (12 h)

SELECTED ADVERSE REACTIONS: Drowsiness, fatigue, headache, metallic or garlic-like aftertaste. If taken with alcohol: flushing, throbbing in head and neck, throbbing headaches, respiratory difficulty, nausea, copious vomiting, sweating, thirst, chest pain, palpitations, dyspnea, hyperventilation, tachycardia, hypotension, syncope, weakness, vertigo, blurred vision, confusion; severe reactions may include arrhythmias, cardiovascular collapse, acute congestive heart failure, and unconsciousness.

WARNINGS: Never administer to an intoxicated patient or without the patient's knowledge. Do not administer

until patient has abstained from alcohol for at least 12 hours.

Contraindicated in patients with severe myocardial disease, coronary occlusion, or psychoses and in patients receiving current or recent treatment with metronidazole, paraldehyde, alcohol, or alcohol-containing preparations. Use cautiously in patients with diabetes mellitus, hypothyroidism, epilepsy, cerebral damage, chronic and acute nephritis, hepatic cirrhosis or dysfunction.

POSSIBLE DRUG INTERACTIONS: Concomitant administration of phenytoin, diazepam, or chlordiazepoxide may cause increased serum levels and risk for drug toxicity. Increased prothrombin time caused by disulfiram may lead to a need to adjust dosage of oral anticoagulants.

SPECIFIC PATIENT AND FAMILY EDUCATION
- Take the drug daily; take it at bedtime if it makes you dizzy or tired. Crush or mix tablets with liquid if necessary.
- Do not take any form of alcohol (such as beer, wine, liquor, vinegars, cough mixtures, sauces, aftershave lotions, liniments, or cologne); doing so may cause a severe unpleasant reaction.
- Wear or carry medical identification with you at all times to alert any medical emergency personnel that you are taking this drug.
- Keep appointments for follow-up blood tests.
- Avoid driving or performing tasks that require alertness if drowsiness, fatigue, or blurred vision occur.
- Know that the metallic aftertaste is transient and will disappear after use of the drug is discontinued.

PO, oral.

Prevention of Relapse

Relapse prevention is important in the recovery of people with substance-related disorders, and alcohol addiction is no exception. Psychosocial interventions such as self-help groups, psychoeducation, and cognitive behavioral therapy (CBT) are designed specifically for those with alcohol addictions. These interventions are discussed later in this chapter.

There are also medications that are used for those who are recovering. Disulfiram (Antabuse) is not a treatment or cure for alcoholism, but it can be used as adjunct therapy to help deter some individuals from drinking while using other treatment modalities to teach new coping skills to alter abuse behaviors (Box 31.4). Disulfiram plus even small amounts of alcohol produces adverse effects. In severe reactions, there may be respiratory depression, cardiovascular collapse, arrhythmias, myocardial infarction, acute congestive heart failure, unconsciousness, convulsions, and death.

Naltrexone was originally used as a treatment for heroin abuse, but it is now approved for treatment of alcohol dependence (Box 31.5). Naltrexone is formulated in a once-daily dose in pill form and a monthly injection. The

precise mechanism of action for naltrexone's effect is unknown; however, reports from successfully treated patients suggest three kinds of effects: (1) it can reduce **craving** (the urge or desire to drink despite negative consequences), (2) it can help maintain abstinence, and (3) it can interfere with the tendency to want to drink more if a recovering patient slips and has a drink. Naltrexone may be particularly useful in patients who continue to drink heavily (Franck & Jayaram-Lindström, 2013).

Promotion of Health: Adequate Nutrition and Supplemental Vitamins

Multivitamins and adequate nutrition are essential for patients who are withdrawing from alcohol. Because malnutrition is common, other vitamin replacement may be necessary for certain individuals. Thiamine (vitamin B_1) is initiated during detoxification, given to decrease ataxia and other symptoms of deficiency. It is usually given orally, 100 mg four times daily, but can be given intramuscularly or by intravenous infusion with glucose. Folic acid deficiency is corrected with administration of 1.0 mg orally four times daily. Magnesium deficiency also is found in

BOX 31.5

Drug Profile: **Naltrexone (Trexan)**

DRUG CLASS: Narcotic antagonist

RECEPTOR AFFINITY: Binds to opioid receptors in the CNS and competitively inhibits the action of opioid drugs, including those with mixed narcotic agonist–antagonist properties

INDICATIONS: Adjunctive treatment of alcohol or narcotic dependence as part of a comprehensive treatment program

ROUTE AND DOSAGE: Available in 50-mg tablets

Adults: For alcoholism: 50 mg/d PO; for narcotic dependence: initial dose of 25 mg PO; if no signs or symptoms seen, complete dose with 25 mg. Usual maintenance dose is 50 mg/d PO.

Children: Safety has not been established for use in children younger than 18 y.

HALF-LIFE (PEAK EFFECT): 3.9–12.9 h (60 min)

SELECTED ADVERSE REACTIONS: Difficulty sleeping, anxiety, nervousness, headache, low energy, abdominal pain or cramps, nausea, vomiting, delayed ejaculations, decreased potency, skin rash, chills, increased thirst, joint and muscle pain

WARNINGS: Contraindicated in pregnancy and patients allergic to narcotic antagonists. Use cautiously in narcotic addiction because may produce withdrawal symptoms. Do not administer unless patient has been opioid free for 7 to 10 d. Also, use cautiously in patients with acute hepatitis, liver failure, depression, or suicidal tendencies and those who are breastfeeding. Must make certain patient is opioid free before administering naltrexone. Always give naloxone challenge test before using, except in patients showing clinical signs of opioid withdrawal.

SPECIFIC PATIENT AND FAMILY EDUCATION

- Know that this drug will help facilitate abstinence from alcohol and block the effects of narcotics.
- Wear a medical identification tag to alert emergency personnel that you are taking this drug.
- Avoid use of heroin or other opioid drugs; small doses may have no effect, but large doses can cause death, serious injury, or coma.
- Report any signs and symptoms of adverse effects.
- Notify other health care providers that you are taking this drug.
- Keep appointments for follow-up blood tests and treatment program.

CNS, central nervous system; PO, oral.

those with long-term alcohol dependence. Magnesium sulfate, which enhances the body's response to thiamine and reduces seizures, is given prophylactically for patients with histories of withdrawal seizures. The usual dose is 1.0 g intramuscularly, four times daily for 2 days.

Stimulants

Cocaine

Cocaine (known as Coke, Snow, Nose Candy, Flake, Blow, Big C, Lady, White, or Snowbirds) is made from the leaves of the *Erythroxylon coca* plant into a coca paste that is refined into cocaine hydrochloride, a crystalline form (white powder appearance), which is commonly inhaled or "snorted" in the nose, injected intravenously (with water), or smoked. The smokeable form of cocaine, often called *free-base cocaine*, can be made by mixing the crystalline cocaine with ether or sodium hydroxide. Crack cocaine, often called "crack," is a form of free-base cocaine produced by mixing the crystal with water and baking soda or sodium bicarbonate and boiling it until a rock precipitant remains. The hardened crystal is then broken into pieces ("cracked") and smoked in cigarettes or water pipes. This extremely potent form produces a rapid high with intense euphoria and a dramatic crash. It is extremely addictive because of the intense and rapid onset of euphoric effects, which leave users craving more.

After cocaine is inhaled or injected, the user experiences a sudden burst of mental alertness and energy ("cocaine rush") and feelings of self-confidence, being in control, and sociability, which last 10 to 20 minutes. This high is followed by an intense let-down effect ("cocaine crash") in which the person feels irritable, depressed, and tired and craves more of the drug. Users experience a serious psychological addiction and pattern of abuse. Although cocaine users typically report that the drug enhances their feelings of well-being and reduces anxiety, cocaine also is known to bring on panic attacks in some individuals. Long-term cocaine use leads to increased anxiety. Increased use of cocaine is associated with stress and drug craving (NIDA, 2013a).

Biologic Responses to Cocaine

Cocaine is absorbed rapidly through the blood–brain barrier and is readily absorbed through the skin and mucous membranes. Rapid intoxication occurs when cocaine is injected intravenously or inhaled. Cocaine increases dopaminergic and serotonergic activity by attaching to transport proteins and in turn blocking neurotransmitter reuptake. Increased dopamine causes euphoria and psychotic symptoms. Cocaine increases norepinephrine levels in the blood, causing tachycardia, hypertension, dilated pupils, and rising body temperatures. Serotonin excess contributes to sleep disturbances and anorexia. With prolonged cocaine use, neurotransmitters are eventually depleted.

Cocaine Intoxication

Intoxication causes CNS stimulation, the length of which depends on the dose and route of administration. With steadily increasing doses, restlessness proceeds to tremors and agitation followed by convulsions and CNS depression. In lethal overdose, death generally results from respiratory failure. A toxic psychosis is also possible and may be accompanied by physical signs of CNS stimulation (tachycardia, hypertension, cardiac arrhythmias, sweating, hyperpyrexia, and convulsions).

There is a potential dangerous interaction between cocaine and alcohol. Taken in combination, the two drugs are converted by the body to cocaethylene, which has a longer duration of action in the brain and is more toxic than either drug alone. Notably, this mixture of cocaine and alcohol is a common two-drug combination that results in drug-related death (Pilgrim, Woodford, & Drummer, 2013; Snipes & Benotsch, 2013).

Cocaine Withdrawal

Severe anxiety, along with restlessness and agitation, is among the major symptoms of cocaine withdrawal. Users quickly seek more cocaine or other drugs, such as alcohol, marijuana, or sleeping pills, to rid themselves of the terrible effects of crashing. Withdrawal causes intense depression, craving (a strong desire to use cocaine despite negative consequences), and drug-seeking behavior that may last for weeks. Individuals who discontinue cocaine use often relapse.

Long-term cocaine use depletes norepinephrine, resulting in a "crash" when use of the drug is discontinued and causing the user to sleep 12 to 18 hours. Upon awakening, withdrawal symptoms may occur, characterized by sleep disturbances with rebound REM sleep, anergia (lack of energy), and decreased libido, depression with possible suicidality, anhedonia, poor concentration, and cocaine craving. Treating individuals with cocaine addiction is complex and involves assessing the psychobiologic, social, and pharmacologic aspects of abuse.

> **NCLEXNOTE** In cocaine withdrawal, patients are excessively sleepy because of the norepinephrine depletion. Recovery is difficult because of the intense cravings. Nursing interventions should focus on helping patients solve problems related to managing these cravings.

Amphetamines

Amphetamines, known on the street as Speed, Uppers, Ups, Black beauties, Pep pills, or Co-pilots, were first synthesized for medical use in the 1880s. Amphetamines (Biphetamine, Delcobese, Dexedrine, Obetrol) and other stimulants, such as phenmetrazine (Preludin) and methylphenidate (Ritalin), act on the CNS and peripheral nervous system. They are used to treat ADHD in children, narcolepsy, depression, and obesity (on a short-term basis). Some people abuse these drugs to achieve the effects of alertness, increased concentration, a sense of increased energy, euphoria, and appetite suppression. Amphetamines are indirect catecholamine agonists and cause the release of newly synthesized norepinephrine.

Similar to cocaine, they block the reuptake of norepinephrine and dopamine, but they do not affect the serotonergic system as strongly. They also affect the peripheral nervous system and are powerful sympathomimetics, stimulating both α and β receptors. This stimulation results in tachycardia, arrhythmias, increased systolic and diastolic blood pressures, and peripheral hyperthermia. The effects of amphetamine use and the clinical course of an overdose are similar to those of cocaine.

Methamphetamine

Methamphetamine, also known as Meth, Speed, Ice, Chalk, Crank, Fire, Glass, and Crystal, is an illegal, potent CNS stimulant that releases excess dopamine responsible for the drug's toxic effects, including damage to nerve terminals. Highly addictive, it comes in many forms and can be smoked, snorted, orally ingested, or injected. A brief, intense sensation, or rush, is reported by those who smoke or inject methamphetamine. Oral ingestion or snorting produces a long-lasting high instead of a rush, which can continue for as long as half a day. This illegal substance is cheap and easy to make and has devastating consequences.

High doses can elevate body temperature and stimulate seizures. Methamphetamine has a longer duration of action than cocaine and leads to prolonged stimulant effects. Long-term effects include dependence and addiction psychosis (paranoia, hallucinations), mood disturbances, repetitive motor activity, stroke, weight loss, and extensive tooth decay (NIDA, 2013b) (Figure 31.2). Methamphetamine is often used in a "binge and crash" pattern. Tolerance occurs within minutes, and the pleasurable effect disappears even before the drug concentration in the blood falls significantly. After being assessed, referral to a drug treatment program is necessary.

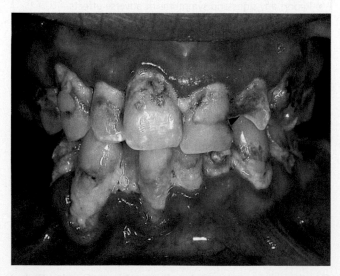

FIGURE 31.2 Severe tooth decay caused by abuse of methamphetamine.

MDMA and Other Club Drugs

MDMA (3-4 methylenedioxymethamphetamine), or Ecstasy or Molly, is known as a "club drug" because it is used by teens and young adults as part of the nightclub, bar, and rave scenes. MDMA, similar in structure to methamphetamine, causes serotonin to be released from neurons in greater amounts than normal. Once released, this serotonin can excessively activate serotonin receptors. Scientists have also shown that MDMA causes excess dopamine to be released from dopamine-containing neurons. Alarmingly, research in animals has demonstrated that MDMA can damage and destroy serotonin-containing neurons. MDMA can cause hallucinations, confusion, depression, sleep problems, drug craving, severe anxiety, and paranoia. In high doses, MDMA can cause a sharp increase in body temperature (malignant hyperthermia), leading to muscle breakdown, kidney and cardiovascular failure, and death (NIDA, 2013c).

Rohypnol, GHB (gamma-hydroxybutyrate), and ketamine are predominately CNS depressants but are also considered "club drugs." Often colorless, tasteless, and odorless, the drugs can be ingested unknowingly. Known also as "date rape" drugs when mixed with alcohol, they can be incapacitating, causing a euphoric, sedative-like effect and producing an "anterograde amnesia," which means that individuals may not remember events they experience while under the influence of these drugs. Ketamine is associated with an increased heart rate and blood pressure, impaired motor function, memory loss, numbness, and vomiting. At high doses, delirium, depression, respiratory depression, and cardiac arrest can occur (NIDA, 2014c).

Nicotine

Nicotine, the addictive chemical mainly responsible for the high prevalence of tobacco use, is the primary reason tobacco is named a public health menace. Smoking is more prevalent among people with alcoholism, polysubstance users, and psychiatric patients than among the general population. Smoking prevalence among persons with any mental disorders is 36.1% compared to 19.9% adults without mental disorders (Centers for Disease Control [CDC], 2013).

Biologic Response to Nicotine

Nicotine stimulates the central, peripheral, and autonomic nervous systems, causing increased alertness, concentration, attention, and appetite suppression. It is readily absorbed and is carried in the bloodstream to the liver where it is partially metabolized. It is also metabolized by the kidneys and is excreted in the urine (NIDA, 2012a).

Nicotine acts as an agonist of the nicotinic cholinergic receptor sites and stimulates autonomic ganglia in both the parasympathetic and sympathetic nervous systems, resulting in increased release of norepinephrine or acetylcholine. The release of epinephrine by nicotine from the adrenal medulla increases fatty acids, glycerol, and lactate levels in the blood, thereby increasing the risk for atherosclerosis and cardiac muscle pathology.

Other medical complications of nicotine use are numerous. Smoking either cigarettes or cigars can cause respiratory problems, lung cancer, emphysema, heart problems, and peripheral vascular disease. In fact, smoking is the largest preventable cause of premature death and disability. Cigarette smoking kills at least 440,000 people in the United States each year and makes countless others ill. The use of smokeless tobacco is also associated with serious health problems (CDC, 2013).

Repeated use of nicotine produces both tolerance and addiction. Recent research has shown that nicotine addiction is extremely powerful and is at least as strong as addictions to other drugs, such as heroin and cocaine; most of those who quit relapse within 1 year (NIDA, 2013d).

Nicotine Withdrawal and Smoking Cessation

Nicotine withdrawal is marked by mood changes (craving, anxiety, irritability, depression) and physiologic changes (difficulty in concentrating, sleep disturbances, headaches, gastric distress, and increased appetite). Nicotine replacements such as transdermal patches, nicotine gum, nasal spray, and inhalers have been used successfully to assist in withdrawal by reducing the craving for tobacco. Patches are rotated on skin sites and help maintain a steady blood level of nicotine. Products such as Habitrol, NicoDerm, and ProStep are used daily, with the decrease in strength of nicotine occurring during a period of 6 to 12 weeks.

Successful smoking cessation usually requires more than one type of intervention, including social support and education. However, studies do show that even giving a brief instruction to patients about quitting smoking can be effective. (See Box 31.6). Medications are often used as a smoking cessation strategy. The antidepressant bupropion (Wellbutrin) is marketed as Zyban to help people quit smoking. Another medication, varenicline tartrate (Chantix) reduces the craving and rewarding effects of nicotine by preventing nicotine from accessing one of the acetylcholine receptor sites involved with nicotine dependence, but it can cause depression and related psychiatric symptoms in some people. This side effect limits its usefulness for people with psychiatric disorders (Faessel, Obach, Rollema, Ravva, Williams, & Burstein, 2010; Tranel, McNutt, & Bechara, 2012).

Auricular therapy, or ear acupressure, is being studied as a potential adjunctive treatment for nicotine addiction. Acupressure is based on the principles of an ancient Chinese system of medicine with a goal of returning the body to a harmonized, balanced state. Through stimulating

BOX 31.6

Research for Best Practices: **Nursing Interventions for Smoking Cessation**

Rice, V. H., Hartmann-Boyce, J., & Stead, L. F. (2013). Nursing interventions for smoking cessation (Review). The Cochrane Database of systematic Reviews, 8. Art. No.: CD001188. doi:10.1002/14651848. CD001188.pub4

QUESTION: Which nursing-delivered smoking cessation interventions are effective?

METHODS: Review of 49 studies that were randomized trials of smoking cessation interventions delivered by nurses or health visitors with follow-up of at least 6 months. The main outcome measure was abstinence from smoking. Participants were adult smokers, 18 years and older, of either gender. Primary intervention was advice defined as verbal instruction to stop smoking. This intervention was further categorized into low intensity advice (verbal instruction only) and high intensity (verbal instruction for more than 10 minutes usually with additional materials such as pamphlets).

FINDINGS: Comparing the nursing intervention groups to control groups or to usual care, the studies showed the intervention increased the likelihood of the participants quitting. There was limited indirect evidence that interventions were more effective for hospital inpatients with cardiovascular disease than for inpatients with other conditions. Interventions in nonhospitalized adults also showed evidence of benefit.

IMPLICATIONS FOR NURING: Even brief instructions to patients regarding the importance of quitting can have a positive effect in changing their smoking behavior.

acupoints on the ear, endogenous endorphin levels and regulation of the sympathetic nervous system changes the taste for tobacco, suppressing nicotine addiction, decreasing nicotine withdrawal symptoms, reducing the desire to smoke, and promoting cessation for a short period of time. The research of this therapy has not yet shown significant effectiveness in smoking cessation (Leung, Neufel, & Marin, 2012; White, Rampes, Liu, Stead, & Campbell, 2014).

Electronic cigarettes (e-cigarettes) were recently introduced as smoking cessation aids. They are smokeless, battery-operated devices designed to deliver nicotine with flavorings or other chemicals to the lungs without burning tobacco. They resemble regular tobacco cigarettes, cigars, or pipes. There are more than 250 e-cigarette brands on the market. E-cigarettes are designed to simulate the act of tobacco smoking without the toxic chemicals produced by burning tobacco leaves. Their safety and effectiveness in smoking cessation are being questioned because e-cigarettes deliver highly addictive nicotine into the lungs and the vapor of some of them contain known carcinogens and toxic chemicals. Additionally, adolescents are increasingly using e-cigarettes believing they are safe, but instead, they may serve as a gateway to try other tobacco products (NIDA, 2013e).

Caffeine

Caffeine is a stimulant found in many drinks (coffee, tea, cocoa, soft drinks); chocolate; and OTC medications, including analgesics, stimulants, appetite suppressants, and cold relief preparations. Metabolism of caffeine is very complicated, involving more than 25 metabolites, and varies among different populations (Weldy, 2010). Recently, high energy drinks, consisting of alcohol and caffeine are being marketed to reduce the impairment caused by ingestion of alcohol. The reality is that these energy drinks give a false sense of physical and mental competence and decrease the awareness of impairment. There have been deaths associated with these drinks (Wolk, Ganetsky, & Babu, 2012).

Symptoms of caffeine intoxication can include five or more of the following: restlessness, nervousness, excitement, insomnia, flushed face, diuresis, gastrointestinal disturbance, muscle twitching, rambling flow of thought and speech, tachycardia or cardiac arrhythmia, periods of inexhaustibility, and psychomotor agitation (Echeverri, Montes, Cabrera, Galán, & Prieto, 2010).

Caffeine withdrawal syndrome has been described as headache, drowsiness, and fatigue, sometimes with impaired psychomotor performance; difficulty concentrating; craving; and psychophysiologic complaints, such as yawning or nausea. Patients with caffeine dependence can be supported in their efforts at withdrawal by learning about the caffeine content of beverages and medication, using decaffeinated beverages, and managing individual withdrawal symptoms.

Cannabis (Marijuana)

Marijuana is the common name for the plant *Cannabis sativa*, also known as hemp. Marijuana's active ingredient is D-9-tetrahydrocannabinol (THC). Hashish, the resin found in flowers of the mature *C. sativa* plant, is its strongest form, containing 10% to 30% THC.

Marijuana is fat soluble and is absorbed rapidly after being smoked or taken orally. After ingestion, THC binds with an opioid receptor in the brain—the μ receptor. This action engages endogenous brain opioid receptors, which are associated with enhanced dopamine activity because THC blocks dopamine reuptake. THC can be stored for weeks in fat tissue and in the brain and is released extremely slowly. Long-term use leads to the accumulation of cannabinoids in the body, primarily the frontal cortex, the limbic areas, and the brain's auditory and visual perception centers. In other areas of the brain, it exerts cardiovascular effects, results in ataxia, and causes increased psychotropic effects. Marijuana use impairs the ability to form memories, recall events, and shift attention from one thing to another. It disrupts coordination of movement, balance, and reaction time. Contrary to popular belief, marijuana is addictive, is an irritant to the lungs and can produce the same respiratory problems experienced by tobacco users (daily cough, phlegm). People who smoke marijuana miss work more than those who do not smoke, but it is not yet known whether marijuana smoke contributes to the risk of lung cancer (NIDA, 2014b).

Marijuana is usually smoked and causes relaxation, euphoria, at times dyscoria (abnormal pupillary reaction or shape), spatial misperception, time distortion, and food cravings. It causes relaxation and drowsiness, unlike other hallucinogens, and is often associated with decreased motivation after long-term use. Effects begin immediately after the drug enters the brain and last from 1 to 3 hours.

Two FDA-approved drugs, dronabinol and nabilone contain THC and are used to treat nausea caused by chemotherapy. The known safety issues related to marijuana include impairment of short-term memory, altered judgment and decision making, anxiety, paranoia or psychosis especially in high dose (NIDA, 2014b). Marijuana is legal as a recreational drug in some states in the United States.

"Spice" a term used for synthetic cannabinoid compounds found in a variety of herbal mixtures that produces an experience similar to marijuana. These spice mixtures are illegal to sell in the United States because of their addictive properties. Some of these compounds bind more strongly to the same receptors as THC and could produce a more powerful and unpredictable effect. Spice products are popular among young people and are second only to marijuana among illegal drugs used mostly by high school seniors (NIDA, 2012b).

Hallucinogens

The term **hallucinogen** refers to drugs that produce euphoria or dysphoria, altered body image, distorted or sharpened visual and auditory perception, confusion, incoordination, and impaired judgment and memory. Severe reactions may cause paranoia, fear of losing one's mind, depersonalization, illusions, delusions, and hallucinations. Hallucinogens typically affect the autonomic and regulatory nervous systems first, increasing heart rate and body temperature and slightly elevating blood pressure. The individual may experience a dry mouth, dizziness, and subjective feelings of being hot or cold. Gradually, these physiologic changes fade, but then perceptual distortions and hallucinations may become prominent. Intense mood and sexual behavior changes may occur; the user may feel unusually close to others or distant and isolated. The true content of hallucinogenic drugs purchased on the street is always in doubt; are often misidentified or adulterated with other drugs. There are more than 100 different hallucinogens with substantially different molecular structures. Psilocybin (mushroom), D-lysergic acid diethylamide (LSD), phencyclidine (PCP), mescaline, and numerous amphetamine derivatives are just a few hallucinogens (NIDA, 2014c).

Patients in acute states of intoxication or in dissociated states may be combative. During the acute state, the primary intervention goals are to reduce stimuli, maintain a safe environment for the patient and others, manage behavior, and observe the patient carefully for medical and psychiatric complications. Instructions to the patient should be clear, short, and simple and delivered in a firm but nonthreatening tone.

Prescription and Over-the-Counter Drugs

Use of prescription drugs for nonmedical purposes has escalated since 2002 with more than 15.2 million Americans taking a pain reliever, tranquilizer, stimulants, or sedative for nonmedical purposes. Abuse of prescription and OTC drugs occurs when one of the following criteria are met:

- Taking a medication that has been prescribed for someone else
- Taking a drug in higher quantity or in another manner than prescribed
- Taking a drug for another purpose than prescribed (NIDA, 2013f)

The opioids (oxycodone, hydrocodone, morphine, fentanyl, and codeine) prescribed for pain are some of the most commonly abused prescription medications. The most commonly abused CNS depressants are the barbiturates (pentobarbital (Nembutal) and benzodiazepines (diazepam, alprazolam, clonazepam, and lorazepam), which are prescribed for anxiety and sleep. The *DSM-5* diagnosis, *sedative, hypnotic, or anxiolytic use disorder* would be given when these drugs are abused. Amphetamines (Adderall, Dexedrine) and methylphenidate (Concerta, Ritalin) are examples of stimulants prescribed for ADHD that are also frequently abused. Often, patients combine these drugs with alcohol, which is extremely dangerous and can put patients at risk for overdose, causing coma or death (NIDA, 2013f).

OTC cough medicine containing dextromethorphan (DXM) can produce the same effects as those of ketamine or PCP, such as impaired motor function, numbness, nausea or vomiting, and increased heart rate and blood pressure. In some cases, severe respiratory depression and hypoxia have occurred (NIDA, 2014f).

Opioids and Morphine Derivatives

The term **opioid** refers to any substance that binds to an opioid receptor in the brain to produce an agonist action. Derived from poppies, opioids are powerful drugs that have been used for centuries to relieve pain. They include opium, heroin, morphine, and codeine. Even centuries after their discovery, opioids are still the most effective pain relievers. They also cause CNS depression and sleep or stupor. Although heroin has no medicinal use, other opioids, such as morphine and codeine, are used to treat pain related to illnesses (e.g., cancer) and medical and dental procedures. When used as directed by a clinician, opioids are safe and generally do not produce addiction. However, opioids also possess very strong reinforcing properties and can quickly trigger addiction when used improperly.

Two important effects produced by opioids are pleasure (or reward) and pain relief. The brain itself also produces substances known as endorphins that activate the opioid receptors. Opioids cause tolerance and physical dependence that appear to be specific for each receptor subtype. Tolerance develops, particularly to the analgesic, respiratory depression, and sedative actions of opioids. Often, a 100% increase in dose is used to achieve the same physical effects when tolerance exists. Physical dependence can develop rapidly. When use of the drug is discontinued, after a period of continuous use, a rebound hyperexcitability withdrawal syndrome usually occurs. Table 31.4 describes the onset, duration, and symptoms of mild, moderate, and severe withdrawal symptoms.

Heroin is an illegal, highly addictive drug that is the most abused and the most rapidly acting of the opioids. Typically sold as a white or brownish powder or as the black sticky substance known as "black tar heroin" on the streets, it is frequently "cut" with other substances, such as sugar, starch, powdered milk, quinine, and strychnine or other poisons. It can be sniffed, snorted, and smoked but is most frequently injected, and this poses risks for transmission of HIV and other diseases from the sharing of needles or other injection equipment.

Naturally occurring neurotransmitters normally bind to the mu-opioid receptors which are involved in pain, hormonal release, and feelings of well being. When heroin enters the brain, it is converted to morphine and immediately binds to the mu-opioid receptors stimulating the release of dopamine causing an intense pleasurable rush. Usually, the individual also experiences a warm flushing of the skin, dry mouth, and a heavy feeling in the extremities. There may be nausea, vomiting, and severe

itching. Following the initial effects, drowsiness, clouded mental function, slowing of the heart, and extreme slowing of breathing can occur (NIDA 2014d).

One of the most detrimental long-term effects of heroin is addiction itself, which causes neurochemical and molecular changes and profoundly alters brain structure and composition. Enlarged ventricular spaces and loss of frontal volume are reported (Cadet et al., 2014). Heroin also produces profound degrees of tolerance and physical dependence, which is powerful motivating factors for compulsive use and abuse. After becoming addicted, heroin users gradually spend more and more time and energy obtaining and using the drug until these activities become their primary purpose in life (NIDA, 2014d).

Opioid Intoxication or Overdose

Emergency treatment of individuals with opioid intoxication is initiated with an assessment of central nervous functioning, specifically arousal and respiratory functioning. Naloxone (Narcan), an opioid antagonist, is given to reverse the respiratory depression, sedation, and hypertension. In the presence of physical dependence on opioids, Narcan produces withdrawal symptoms that are related to the dose of Narcan and the degree and type of opioid dependence. When administered intravenously, the effect is generally apparent within 2 minutes. When administered intramuscularly, the effect is more prolonged.

Initial Opioid Detoxification

Ideally, opioid detoxification is achieved by gradually reducing an opioid dose over several days or weeks. Many treatment programs include administering low doses of a substitute drug, such as methadone that can help satisfy the drug craving without providing the same subjective high. If opioids are abruptly withdrawn ("cold turkey") from someone who is physically dependent on them, severe physical symptoms occur, including body aches,

Table 31.4	SEVERITY OF OPIOID WITHDRAWAL SYNDROME		
Initial Onset and Duration	**Mild Withdrawal**	**Moderate Withdrawal**	**Severe Withdrawal**
Onset: 8–12 h after last use of short-acting opioids. 1–3 d after last use for longer acting opioids, such as methadone	Physical: yawning, rhinorrhea, perspiration, restlessness, lacrimation, sleep disturbance	Physical: dilated pupils, bone and muscle aches, sensation of "goose flesh," hot and cold flashes	Physical nausea; vomiting; stomach cramps; diarrhea; weight loss; insomnia; twitching of muscles and kicking movements of legs; increased blood pressure, pulse, and respirations
Duration: Severe symptoms peak between 48 and 72 h. Symptoms abate in 7–10 d for short-acting opioids. Methadone withdrawal symptoms can last several weeks.	Emotional: increased craving, anxiety, dysphoria	Emotional: irritability, increased anxiety, and craving	Emotional: depression, increased anxiety, dysphoria, subjective sense of feeling "wretched"

diarrhea, tachycardia, fever, runny nose, sneezing, sweating, yawning, nausea or vomiting, nervousness, restlessness or irritability, shivering or trembling, abdominal cramps, weakness, and increased blood pressure.

Maintenance Treatment

Methadone maintenance is the treatment of people with opioid addiction with a daily, stabilized dose of methadone. Methadone is used because of its long half-life of 15 to 30 hours. Methadone is a potent opioid and is physiologically addicting, but it satisfies the opioid craving without producing the subjective high of heroin (Box 31.7).

Detoxification is accomplished by setting the beginning methadone dose and then slowly reducing it during the next 21 days. Treatment programs determine the dose of methadone that will block subjective feelings of craving and will not cause somnolence or intoxication in patients. The initial dose of methadone is determined by the severity of withdrawal symptoms and is usually 20 to 30 mg orally. If symptoms persist after 1 to 2 hours, the dosage can be raised and then should be reevaluated daily during the first few days of treatment. Initial doses of greater than 40 mg can cause severe discomfort as the detoxification proceeds.

Patients receive this dose daily in conjunction with regular drug abuse counseling focused on the elimination of illicit drug use; lifestyle changes, such as finding friends who do not use drugs or achieving stability in one's living situation; strengthening social supports; and structuring time into pursuits that do not involve drug use. After illicit drug use ceases for a period of time, major lifestyle changes have been made, and social supports are in place, patients may gradually detoxify from methadone with continuing support through community support groups, such as Narcotics Anonymous.

The length of methadone treatment varies for each patient. When to begin detoxification from methadone varies widely, depending on the patient's commitment to abstinence, lifestyle changes that have occurred, and strong peer group support, all of which are needed to sustain the patient during methadone detoxification when increased cravings often occur. Methadone treatment combined with behavioral therapy and counseling has been used effectively and safely to treat opioid addiction for more than 40 years. Combined with behavioral therapy and counseling, methadone enables patients to stop using heroin.

Naltrexone has also been used successfully to treat opioid addiction. It binds to opioid receptors in the CNS and competitively inhibits the action of opioid drugs, including those with mixed narcotic agonist–antagonist properties, thereby blocking the intoxicating effects. If an opioid-addicted individual takes naltrexone before he or

---

BOX 31.7

Drug Profile: **Methadone (Dolophine)**

DRUG CLASS. Narcotic agonist, analgesic

RECEPTOR AFFINITY: Binds to opioid receptors in the CNS to produce analgesia, euphoria, sedation; the receptors mediating the effects of the endogenous opioids which are thought to be enkephalins, endorphins

INDICATIONS: Detoxification and temporary maintenance treatment of narcotic addiction; relief of severe pain

ROUTE AND DOSAGE: Available in 5-, 10-, and 40-mg tablets; oral concentrate

Adults: Detoxification: Initially 15 to 30 mg. Increase to suppress withdrawal signs. 40 mg/d in single or divided dose is usually adequate stabilizing dose; continue stabilizing dose for 2 to 3 days; then gradually decrease dosage. Usual maintenance dose is 20 to 120 mg/d in single dosing. Individual dosage as tolerated.

HALF-LIFE (PEAK EFFECT):
PO 90–120 min
IM 1–2 h
SC 1–2 h

SELECTED ADVERSE REACTIONS: Lightheadedness, dizziness, sedation, nausea, vomiting, facial flushing, peripheral circulatory collapse, arrhythmia, palpitations, urethral spasm, urinary retention, respiratory depression, circulatory depression, respiratory arrest, shock, cardiac arrest

WARNINGS: Never administer in the presence of hypersensitivity to narcotics, diarrhea caused by poisoning (before toxins are eliminated), bronchial asthma, or COPD. Use caution in the presence of acute abdominal conditions, cardiovascular disease. Increased effects and toxicity of methadone if taken concurrently with cimetidine, ranitidine. Methadone hydrochloride tablets are for PO administration only and *must not* used for injection. It is recommended that methadone hydrochloride tablets, if dispensed, be packaged in child-resistant containers and kept out of the reach of children to prevent accidental injection.

SPECIFIC PATIENT AND FAMILY EDUCATION
- Take drug exactly as prescribed.
- Avoid use of alcohol.
- Take the drug with food and lying quietly; this should minimize nausea.
- Eat small, frequent meals to treat nausea and loss of appetite.
- If experiencing dizziness and drowsiness, avoid driving a car or performing other tasks that require alertness.
- Administer mild laxative for constipation.
- Report severe nausea, vomiting, constipation, shortness of breath, or difficulty breathing. Methadone products, when used for treatment of narcotic addiction, shall be dispensed only by approved hospital and community pharmacies and maintenance programs approved by the FDA and designated state authority.

CNS, central nervous system; COPD, chronic obstructive pulmonary disease; IM, intramuscular; FDA, Food and Drug Administration; PO, oral; SC, subcutaneous.

she is fully detoxified from opioids, withdrawal symptoms may result (see Table 31.4).

Buprenorphine is a long-acting partial agonist that acts on the same receptors as heroin and morphine, relieving drug cravings without producing the same intense "high" or dangerous side effects. At low doses, buprenorphine produces sufficient agonist effect to enable opioid-addicted individuals to discontinue the misuse of opioids without experiencing withdrawal symptoms. Buprenorphine carries a lower risk of abuse, addiction, and side effects compared with full opioid agonists. Buprenorphine is highly bound to plasma proteins. It is metabolized by the liver via the cytochrome P4503A4 enzyme system into norbuprenorphine and other metabolites. The half-life of buprenorphine is 24 to 60 hours. Buprenorphine has poor oral bioavailability and moderate sublingual bioavailability. Formulations for opioid addiction treatment are in the form of sublingual tablets.

Inhalants

Inhalants are organic solvents, also known as *volatile substances* that are CNS depressants. When inhaled, they cause euphoria, sedation, emotional lability, and impaired judgment. Intoxication can result in respiratory depression, stupor, and coma. Inhalants are typically abused by young children with adolescents using less than younger children. Different inhalants tend to be used by various age groups. New users (ages 12 to 15) are more likely to abuse glue, shoe polish, spray paints, gasoline, and lighter fluids. The 16 to 17 year olds most commonly abuse nitrous oxide or "whippets" and adults a class of nitrites such as amyl nitrites or "poppers" (NIDA 2012c). Addiction is very uncommon, but inhalants can be intermediate between legal and illegal drugs (Sanchez, Ribeiro, Moura, Noto, & Martins, 2013).

Most inhalants are common household or industrial products that give off mind-altering chemical fumes when sniffed. They include the following:

- *Volatile Solvents:* liquids that vaporize at room temperature such as paint thinners or removers, degreasers, dry-cleaning fluids, gasoline, and lighter fluid. Office supply solvents include correction fluids, felt-tip marker fluid, electronic contact cleaners, and glue.
- *Aerosols:* sprays that contain propellant and solvents such as spray paint, hair spray, fabric protector spray, aerosol computer cleaning products, vegetable oil spray, analgesics, asthma sprays, deodorants, air fresheners
- *Gases:* household or commercial products such as butane lighters and propane tanks, whipped cream aerosols or dispenser ("whippets"), and refrigerant gases; medical anesthetics such as ether, chloroform, halothane, and nitrous oxide ("laughing gas").

- *Nitrites:* organic nitrites include cyclohexyl, butyl, and amyl nitrites ("poppers'). When marketed for illicit uses, organic nitrates are sold in small brown bottles labeled "video head cleaner," room odorizer," "leather cleaner," or "room deodorizer" (NIDA, 2012c).

Most inhalants other than nitrites depress the CNS similar to alcohol (slurred speech, lack of coordination, euphoria, and dizziness). They may cause lightheadedness, hallucinations and delusions. The nitrites enhance sexual pleasure by dilating and relaxing blood vessels. They are thought to be antagonistic at the NMDA receptor and may cause neuronal damage in the mesolimbic system (Cousaert, Heylens, & Audenaert, 2013).

Inhalant Intoxication

Inhalants are easily absorbed through the lungs and are widely distributed in the body, reaching the highest concentrations in fat tissue and the nervous system where the most profound effects are exhibited. Mild intoxication occurs within minutes and can last as long as 30 minutes. Often, the drugs are inhaled repeatedly to maintain an intoxicated state for hours. Initially, the person experiences a sense of euphoria, but as the dose increases, confusion, perceptual distortions, and severe CNS depression occurs. Inhalant users are also at risk for **sudden sniffing death**, which can occur when the inhaled fumes take the place of oxygen in the lungs and CNS, causing the user to suffocate. Inhalants can also cause death by disrupting the normal heart rhythm, which can lead to cardiac arrest (NIDA, 2012b).

Long-Term Complications

Chronic neurologic syndromes can result from long-term use. Long-term inhalant use is linked to widespread brain damage and cognitive abnormalities that can range from mild impairment to severe dementia. In recent studies, considerably more inhalant users than cocaine users had brain abnormalities, and their damage was more extensive. Inhalant users also performed significantly worse on tests of working memory and of the ability to focus attention, plan, and solve problems. However, the inhalants can change brain chemistry and may permanently damage the brain and CNS. Magnetic resonance imaging scans of users demonstrate severe changes in cerebral white matter (Cairney et al., 2013).

Steroids

"Anabolic steroids" is the name for synthetic substances related to the male sex hormones (androgens). Developed in the late 1930s to treat hypogonadism, they are also used to treat delayed puberty, some types of impotence, and wasting of the body caused by HIV infection or other diseases. They promote growth of skeletal muscle and the development of male sexual characteristics. There are more than 100 different types; to be used legally, all require a prescription. Some dietary supplements, such as dehydroepiandrosterone (DHEA) and androstenedione (Andro), can be purchased in commercial health stores. They are often used in the belief that large doses can convert into testosterone or a similar compound in the body that promote muscle growth. They can be taken orally or intramuscularly. Some are applied to the skin as a cream or gel. When abused, these preparations are taken at 10 to 100 times higher than used for medical disorders. Although use among men is higher than among women, use among women is growing (NIDA, 2012d).

Case reports and small studies indicate that in high doses, anabolic steroids increase irritability and aggression. Some steroid users report that they have committed aggressive acts, such as physical fighting, armed robbery, using force to obtain something, committing property damage, stealing from stores, or breaking into a house or building, and that they engage in these behaviors more often when they take steroids than when they are drug free. Other behavioral effects include euphoria, increased energy, sexual arousal, mood swings, distractibility, forgetfulness, and confusion.

Anabolic steroids do not trigger a rapid increase in dopamine or cause the "high" associated with other drugs of abuse. However, long-term use can affect neurotransmitter pathways that regulate mood and behavior. With time, anabolic steroid use is associated with an increased risk for heart attacks and strokes, blood clotting, cholesterol changes, hypertension, depressed mood, fatigue, restlessness, loss of appetite, insomnia, reduced libido, muscle and joint pain, and severe liver problems (including hepatic cancer). Males can have reduced sperm production, shrinking of the testes, and difficulty or pain in urinating. There can be undesirable body changes, including breast enlargement in men and masculinization of women's bodies. Both sexes can experience hair loss and acne. Intravenous or intramuscular use of the drug and needle sharing puts users at risk for HIV, hepatitis B and C, and infective endocarditis, as well as bacterial infections at injection sites (NIDA, 2012e).

EMERGING DRUGS AND TRENDS

New drugs and drug use trends rapidly enter our communities. The National Institute of Drug Abuse continuously report on these drugs. Some of the newer drugs include synthetic cathinones (bath salts), Krokodil, (toxic homemade opioid), and synthetic hallucinogens (N-bomb).

Bath salts contain cathinone, an amphetamine-like stimulant naturally found in the Khat plant. Severe intoxication and dangerous health effects are associated with these drugs. These drugs, chemically similar to methamphetamines and MDMA, produce euphoria, increased sociability, and increased sex drive, as well as paranoia, agitation, and hallucinatory delirium. Indication is that they are highly abusive (NIDA, 2012e).

Krokodil, a synthetic form of a heroin-like drug called desomorphine, is made by combining codeine tablets with toxic chemicals such as lighter fluid and industrial cleaners. It is used as a cheap substitute for heroin in poor rural areas of Russia but is making its appearance in the United States. The drug is named Krokodil because a scaly, gray–green dead skin forms at the site of injection (NIDA, 2014e).

Synthetic hallucinogens, the *N-bomb*, are being sold as substitutes for LSD or mescaline. These chemicals, considered more powerful than LSD, act on serotonin receptors and can cause seizures, heart attack, or respiratory arrest and death (NIDA, 2014e).

GAMBLING: A NON–SUBSTANCE–RELATED DISORDER

Social gambling becomes a **gambling disorder** (also referred to as pathologic gambling) when it is persistent and recurrent leading to clinically significant impairment or distress. In the *DSM-5*, this disorder is classified as an addiction and a non–substance-related disorder (APA, 2013). Individuals with this disorder are preoccupied with gambling and experience an aroused, euphoric state during the actual betting. The action of seeking an aroused state is often more important to the pathologic gambler than the desire for money itself. They are drawn to the games and begin making bigger and bigger bets. Characteristically, they relentlessly chase their losses in an attempt to win them back. They are unable to control their gaming and may lie to family, friends, and employers to hide their gambling. They have an intense need to gamble and often turn to gambling when feeling distressed. These individuals are highly competitive, energetic, restless, and easily bored. There is evidence that there are changes in the serotonin system associated with addiction behavior, similar to results reported for nicotine and alcohol dependence (Wilson, da Silva Lobo, Tavares, Gentil, & Vallada, 2013).

One study found a 1% to 3% lifetime prevalence (Grant, Schreiber, Odlaug, & Kim, 2010). According to the *DSM-5*, the lifetime prevalence rate is about 0.4% to 1% (APA, 2013). Individuals with gambling problems are more likely to commit suicide than those who do not have a gambling problem and are less likely to seek mental health treatment (Séquin, Boyd, Lesage, McGirr, Suissa, & Tousignant, 2010).

This disorder is conceptualized as similar to alcohol and other substances of dependence. When substances are used in conjunction with gambling, they cause a deterioration in play and accelerate the progression of the gambling disorder. Other comorbid disorders include depression, ADHD, Tourette's syndrome, and personality disorders (Park et al., 2010). The disorder has four phases: winning, losing, desperation, and hopelessness. Pathologic gambling can be treated by psychotherapists experienced in this disorder; for many, Gamblers Anonymous is sufficient.

Compulsive gamblers feel omnipotent in their ability to win back what was lost. This omnipotence serves as self-deception that leads to denial. Care of these patients involves confronting their omnipotent beliefs. These individuals quickly irritate staff by their self-assurance and overbearing attitude. Staff education about the disorder is important. Family involvement is also crucial. Families often have been dealing with the patient in a dysfunctional manner. Relapse prevention involves learning about specific cues that trigger the gambling behavior.

NURSING MANAGEMENT: HUMAN RESPONSE TO SUBSTANCE-RELATED DISORDERS

In psychiatric and substance-abuse treatment programs, the assessment process is, in part, a treatment intervention. Often, patients are in denial about the severity of the problem and about its emotional, social, legal, vocational, or other consequences.

Assessment Issues

The assessment is crucial to understanding level of use, abuse, or dependence and to determining the patient's denial or acceptance of treatment. Assessment is often detailed and may involve family members and loved ones. Along with the psychiatric nursing interview (see Chapter 10), there are specific areas that should be assessed. Box 31.8 gives examples of typical behaviors exhibited by individuals that are associated with each level of use, abuse, and addiction. The nurse can use the Substance Abuse Assessment as a guide in eliciting a substance use history in the assessment process (Box 31.9).

Usually, nurses encounter individuals during crisis when they seek professional help. These situations offer an opportunity to explore the denial that keeps their addiction thriving. The nurse's approach should be caring, matter-of-fact, gentle, and direct. Approaches that are punitive or attempt to elicit feelings of guilt or shame are destructive to the therapeutic relationship (see Nursing Care Plan 31.1).

Denial of a Problem

Denial can be expressed in a variety of behaviors and attitudes and may not be expressed as an overt denial of the problem. For example, patients may admit to a problem and even thank you for helping them to realize they have

---

BOX 31.8

Behaviors in Substance Use, Abuse, and Addiction

SUBSTANCE USE
- Does not have possible danger or potential legal problems
- Engages in use to enhance social situations and interaction
- Is not intended to result in intoxication
- Has control of the amount and frequency of use
- Exhibits socially acceptable behavior while using

PRESCRIPTION MEDICATION USE
- Use is for the dose, frequency, and indications prescribed
- Use is for the particular episode of the condition for which it was prescribed
- Use is coordinated among prescribing physicians

SUBSTANCE ABUSE
- Use for intoxication or feeling of being "high"
- Use that interferes with normal life functions (e.g., producing sleep when inappropriate, excitability or irritability interfering with social interaction)
- Potential harm to self or others (e.g., driving while intoxicated, use of injection drug equipment)
- Use that has legal consequences (e.g., all use of illicit drugs)
- Use resulting in socially unacceptable behavior (e.g., public drunkenness, verbal or physical abuse)
- Use to alter normal feeling states such as sadness or anxiety

PRESCRIPTION MEDICATION ABUSE
- Use is at a higher dose and greater frequency than prescribed
- Use is for indications other than prescribed or for self-diagnosed condition
- Use results in feeling tired, having a clouded mental state, or feeling "hyperactive" or nervous
- Supplementing medication with alcohol or drugs
- Soliciting more than one physician for the same medication
- Inability to control the amount and frequency of use
- Tolerance to larger amounts of the substance
- Withdrawal symptoms when stopping use
- Severe consequences from alcohol or drug use

SUBSTANCE ADDICTION
- Drug craving
- Compulsive use
- Presence of aberrant drug-related behaviors
- Repeated relapse into drug use after withdrawal

BOX 31.9

Substance Abuse Assessment

DRUG/LAST USE	PATTERN OF USE (AMOUNT, ROUTE, FIRST USE, FREQUENCY, AND LENGTH OF USE)
Alcohol/	
Stimulants/	
Opioids/	
Sedative–hypnotics and anxiolytic agents/	
Hallucinogens/	
Marijuana/	
Inhalants/	
Nicotine/	
Caffeine/	

ABUSE INDICATORS
1. Tolerance (increasing use of drug or alcohol with the same level of intoxication): _____
2. Withdrawal symptoms: a. Shakes? _____ b. Tremors? _____ c. Cramps, diarrhea, or rapid pulse? _____ d. Feeling paranoid, fearful? _____ e. Difficulty sleeping? _____
3. Consequences of use (presenting problems, persistent or recurrent emotional, social, legal, or other problems): _____
4. Loss of control of amount, frequency, or duration of use: _____
5. Desire or efforts to decrease use or control use: _____
6. Preoccupation (increasing focus or time spent on use and obtaining substances): _____
7. Social, vocational, recreational activities affected by use: _____
8. Previous alcohol or drug abuse treatment: _____

NURSING DIAGNOSES: _____

a problem but insist they can overcome the problem on their own and do not need outside help.

> **KEYCONCEPT** **Denial** is the patient's inability to accept his or her loss of control over substance use or the severity of the consequences associated with the substance abuse or addiction.

The following characteristics are typical of a person who has alcoholism and who is in denial:

- Confusion about severity of drinking history: "I went out drinking with friends last week and didn't have any problems; I don't get drunk all the time."
- Difficulty reconciling early positive experiences of alcohol use with current problems: "I used to drink with my buddies after work to unwind. We had a great time. Those were some good times. . . ."
- Confusion regarding the definition of *alcoholic:* "Well, I don't have withdrawal symptoms, so I can't be an alcoholic."
- Relief when they compare themselves with others and find the others in worse condition: "They are the alcoholics, not me!"
- A delusion that drinking can be self-controlled: "If I search hard enough or long enough, I will find a way to control and enjoy drinking."

- Confusion or trouble accepting that behavior is different when intoxicated: "I couldn't have done that; that's just not like me."

This quandary about the nature of the problem has often been met with confrontation by nurses and other professionals in the past. But argumentation, presenting evidence of addiction, and lecturing often fail to elicit admission of a problem or induce behavior change.

Motivation for Change

Motivation is a key predictor of whether individuals will change their substance use behavior (Collins, Malone, & Larimer, 2012).

> **KEYCONCEPT** **Motivation** is a goal-oriented attitude that propels action for change and can help sustain the development of new activities and behaviors.

Ambivalence about substance use is normal and can be resolved by working with the patients' own concerns about their use of alcohol and other drugs. Motivation is fluid and can be modified. Experiences such as increased distress levels, critical life events, a period of evaluation or appraisal of one's life, recognizing negative consequences

(text continues on page 607)

NURSING CARE PLAN 31.1

The Patient With Alcoholism

JG is a 55-year-old veteran with a 25-year history of alcohol dependence. He is the youngest of three children born of "blue-collar" parents who valued hard work. His mother is still living with JG's older sister, but his father died of cirrhosis, a complication of years of alcohol abuse. JG has two children who are married with children, living in other states. He rarely sees them. He has been drinking as much as 1 quart of vodka per day for 3 years since sustaining a work-related back injury. He has a history of binge drinking on weekends. He denies other drug use.

Recently, his wife moved out of the house after 28 years of marriage. An argument about his drinking ended in a physical fight. She was treated in the emergency department (ED) for a broken arm. Their relationship had progressively deteriorated over the years. JG had erectile dysfunction because of excessive drinking, and his wife had moved into the spare bedroom. He was admitted to the hospital ED at a Veteran's Administration medical center with a gash above his right eye from a fall he sustained while intoxicated 2 weeks after his wife left him. His wife returned to care for him.

JG began to have symptoms of alcohol withdrawal and became anxious shortly after admission. He requested hospital admission for alcohol detoxification and was transferred to a detoxification and brief treatment unit.

Setting: Inpatient Detoxification Unit, Veterans Administration Medical Center

Baseline Assessment: First admission, last drink 7 PM. Admission vital signs: T 99.2°F, HR 98, R 20, BP 140/88 on admission to the ED. He has a history of withdrawal seizures and hallucinosis. He had a blood alcohol level of 0.15 mg%, becoming increasingly anxious and restless. He was given diazepam 10 mg PO at that time.

Four hours after admission, vital signs were T 99.8°F, HR 110, R 22, BP 152/100. He continued to be anxious and was tremulous, diaphoretic, and nauseous. Diazepam 20 mg PO stat was given.

Associated Psychiatric Diagnosis	Medications
Alcohol withdrawal	Thiamine Folic acid Multivitamins Diazepam 10 mg q2h for elevated BP, HR, and tremors Haloperidol 5.0 mg IM PRN for hallucinations or agitation

Nursing Diagnosis 1: Risk For Injury

Defining Characteristics	Related Factors
Sensory deficits Balance and equilibrium deficits Lack of awareness of hazards	Altered cerebral function secondary to alcohol withdrawal Potential withdrawal seizures resulting from magnesium deficiency or hypoglycemia Anxiety

Outcomes

Initial	Discharge
1. Prevent falls and other physical injuries.	2. Relate an intent to practice selected prevention measures such as maintaining sobriety, removing loose throw rugs, using adequate lighting.

Interventions

Interventions	Rationale	Ongoing Assessment
Identify stage of alcohol withdrawal and severity of symptoms. Monitor gait and motor coordination, presence of tremors, mental status, electrolyte balance, and seizure activity.	The more severe the reactions, the more likely that disorientation, confusion, and restlessness increase. As the patient moves from stage I to III, he becomes at higher risk for a fall or injury.	Determine whether JG is becoming more disoriented, increasing his risk for injury.

Continued

NURSING CARE PLAN 31.1 *(Continued)*

Interventions	Rationale	Ongoing Assessment
Institute seizure precautions (bed in low position, padded side rails). Orient the patient to his surroundings and call light; maintain a consistent physical environment. Avoid sudden moves, loud noises, discussion of patient at bedside, and lighting that casts shadows downward.	Withdrawal seizures usually occur within 48 hours after last drink. Disorientation often occurs as BAL drops. These symptoms can last several days. Decreased environmental stimulation helps calm the patient, which in turn promotes optimal CNS responses.	Monitor for seizure activity. Determine JG's level of orientation to surroundings. Determine whether he can use a call light. Observe reactions to loud noises and monitor room environment.

Evaluation

Outcomes (at 3 Days)	Revised Outcomes	Interventions
Gait steady; patient hydrated. No seizure activity. Patient oriented.	Maintain current level of orientation.	Continue to monitor for any signs of disorientation.

Nursing Diagnosis 2: Disturbed Thought Process

Defining Characteristics	Related Factors
Hallucinations (auditory, visual, and tactile) Inaccurate interpretation of stimuli Confusion and disorientation	Physiologic changes secondary to alcohol withdrawal

Outcomes

Initial	Discharge
1. Recognize changes in thinking or behavior. 2. Identify situations that occur before hallucinations or delusions.	3. Maintain reality orientation.

Interventions

Interventions	Rationale	Ongoing Assessment
Encourage communication that enhances the development of the nurse–patient relationship and promotes JG's sense of integrity. Assess for the presence of any hallucinations through observation and interview. Administer haloperidol 5.0 mg IM PRN for hallucinations or agitation. JG had one episode of hallucinations. It occurred 8 h after admission with no identifiable precipitating event.	The therapeutic relationship is important to individuals with alcohol withdrawal because of their fear of withdrawal symptoms and need for reassurance and support. Hallucinations can occur when patients are withdrawing from alcohol. If hallucinations are severe, the patient may experience delirium tremens. Administering an antipsychotic eliminates or reduces the occurrence of hallucinations. Continue to maintain reality orientation.	Monitor the development of the nurse–patient relationship. Assess the patient frequently to determine the presence of hallucinations. Observe for hypotension. Instruct the patient to avoid getting out of bed quickly to prevent falling. Continue to monitor for hallucinations.

Continued

NURSING CARE PLAN 31.1 *(Continued)*

Nursing Diagnosis 3: Anxiety

Defining Characteristics	Related Factors
Physiologic: increased heart rate, elevated BP, increased respiratory rate, diaphoresis, trembling, nausea Emotional: apprehension about alcohol withdrawal, nervousness, losing control after back injury Cognitive inability to concentrate; lack of awareness of surroundings	Physiologic changes secondary to alcohol withdrawal

Outcomes

Initial	Discharge
1. Identify an increase in physiologic and psychological comfort. 2. Maintain stable vital signs.	3. Describe anxiety as it relates to fear of detoxification process and use of alcohol.

Interventions

Interventions	Rationale	Ongoing Assessment
Demonstrate an accepting attitude by being calm and informing JG of any treatment.	A calm attitude of the nurse can help relax a patient.	Observe JG's reaction to the explanations and initiation of any treatments.
Include the patient in decision making regarding his care.	Empowering the patient in decision making helps him gain control over his situation.	Monitor decisions in terms of feasibility.
Administer diazepam 10 mg q2h for elevated BP, HR, and tremulousness PRN.	Diazepam can reduce physiologic impact of alcohol withdrawal.	Monitor vital signs, level of anxiety, and patient's sense of control.
Explain that anxiety is a symptom of withdrawal and is usually time limited.	Knowledge that the anxiety will decrease will help the patient deal with the current anxiety.	Monitor whether or not JG understands that his discomfort will disappear.
Observe sleeping behavior.	Sleep is often disturbed. Sleep deprivation contributes to anxiety.	Monitor quality of sleep.

Evaluation

Outcomes	Revised Outcomes	Interventions
JG was able to refocus and redirect attention when exhibiting mild anxiety; sleeping about 6 hours.	None.	None.
Identified an increase in apprehension as his BP increased. Given diazepam as ordered.	Relate an increase in apprehension when it occurs.	Assess patient for apprehension and a change in vital signs.
JG discussed his fears of the detoxification process. Expressed mixed feelings about continuing treatment.	Comply with treatment regimen.	Encourage the patient to follow up with treatment after he is detoxified.

BAL, blood alcohol level; BP, blood pressure; CNS, central nervous system; HR, heart rate; GAF, Global Assessment of Functioning; IM, intramuscular; PO, oral; PRN, as needed; R, respirations; T, temperature.

of use, and positive and negative external incentives for change can all influence a patient's commitment to change.

Techniques that enhance motivation are associated with increased success in treatment, higher rates of abstinence, and successful follow-up treatment (Lozano, LaRowe, Smith, Tuerk, & Roitzsch, 2013). **Motivational interviewing** is a method of therapeutic intervention that seeks to elicit self-motivational statements from patients, supports behavioral change, and creates a discrepancy between the patient's goals and their continued alcohol and other drug use. The acronym FRAMES summarizes elements of brief interventions with patients using motivational interviewing (Box 31.10).

> **NCLEXNOTE** Motivational approaches are priority interventions for patients with substance-related disorders. They help patients recognize a problem and develop change strategies.

Countertransference

Countertransference is the total emotional reaction of the treatment provider to the patient (see Chapter 7). Patients with substance-related disorders can generate strong feelings and reactions in nurses and other health care providers (Table 31.5). These feelings can be generated by overt unpleasant behaviors of the substance-dependent persons, such as lying, deceit, manipulation, or hostility, or these feelings may be more subconscious and stem from past experiences with people with alcoholism or addicts or even from dealing with situations in the care provider's own family.

Codependence

The concept of codependence emerged out of studies of women's relationships with husbands who abused alcohol. Today, the scope of codependency includes both men and women who grew up in any type of dysfunctional family

---

BOX 31.10

FRAMES—Effective Elements of Brief Intervention

FEEDBACK
Provide patients with personal feedback regarding their individual status, such as personal alcohol and other drug consumption relative to norms, information about elevated liver enzyme values, and so forth.

RESPONSIBILITY
Emphasize the individual's freedom of choice and personal responsibility for change. General themes are as follows:

1. It's up to you; you're free to decide to change or not.
2. No one else can decide for you or force you to change.
3. You're the one who has to do it if it's going to happen.

ADVICE
Include a clear recommendation or advice on the need for change, typically in a supportive and concerned, rather than in a judgmental, manner.

MENU
Provide a menu of treatment options from which patients may pick those that seem more suitable or appealing.

EMPATHIC COUNSELING
Show warmth, support, respect, and understanding in communication with patients.

SELF-EFFICACY
Reinforce self-efficacy, or an optimistic feeling that he or she can change.

---

system in which substance abuse may or may not have been a problem. **Codependence** has also been described as "enabling," in which an individual in a relationship with a person who abuses alcohol inadvertently reinforces the drinking behavior of the other person. The codependency label is controversial and is viewed by some as an oversimplification of complex emotions and behaviors of family members. Mental health professionals should be careful not to use it as a catch-all diagnosis and to take special care to assess and plan interventions that address

---

Table 31.5 PATIENT BEHAVIORS AND COUNTERTRANSFERENCE REACTIONS	
Patient Behavior	**Common Nursing Reaction**
Behaves as a victim	Feels a sense of helplessness, increased need to give advice and "fix" the situation and the patient; shows anger toward the patient for not being able to take care of the situation him- or herself
Is intrusive, hostile, belittling	Can be frightened, withdraw from patient, express anger overtly, or be passive-aggressive (i.e., suggesting discharge to the team or ignoring legitimate requests)
Does everything right, is insightful, pleasant, and so forth	Congratulates self on therapeutic interventions; can become bored or complacent
Relapses into drug or alcohol use	Feels angry, personally betrayed; withdraws from other patients; doubts own abilities
Asks personal questions about staff qualifications or prior drug or alcohol abuse	Reveals personal information, resents the intrusion, and may regret divulging information
Is silent or divulges minimal information	Tries harder, doubts own therapeutic ability, is angered by patient's resistance
Tries to "bend" or ignore milieu and group rules	May permit program rule infractions; may feel pressured, angry, or passive-aggressive
Insists that no one can help him or her	Feels pressure to be the one who can help; may feel angry and inept or helpless

Adapted from Imhoff, J. E. (1991). Countertransference issues in alcoholism and drug addiction. *Psychiatric Annals, 21*(5), 292–306.

each person's particular situation, problems, and needs (Mental Health America, 2014).

Nursing Diagnoses

Several nursing diagnoses could be generated for persons using and abusing substances. The type of substance and the patient's addiction will be considered in the formation of the nursing diagnoses. For example, a person who is newly diagnosed with alcoholism will be assessed differently than one who has multiple attempts at treatment for cocaine addiction. One common nursing diagnosis is Ineffective Denial (Figure 31.3).

Nursing Interventions and Treatment Modalities

Several treatment modalities are used in most addiction treatment (pharmacologic modalities were discussed earlier), including 12-step–program-focused, cognitive or psychoeducation, behavioral, group psychotherapy, and individual and family therapy. Discharge planning and relapse prevention are also essential components of successful treatment and are incorporated into most programs. See Table 31.6 for different treatment approaches to chemical addiction and Box 31.11 for Principles of Effective Treatment for Addiction.

Because patients with substance-related disorders differ greatly, no one type of treatment program will work for every individual. Often, several approaches can work together, but others may be inappropriate. Treatment programs usually combine many different interventions to provide a comprehensive approach based on the individual's needs. Nursing interventions vary depending on the nature of the current problems and their severity. For a patient who is being detoxified, physical interventions (e.g., monitoring vital signs and neurologic functioning) are necessary. When the substance use disorder is secondary to other physical or psychiatric problems, education of patient and family may be a priority.

Assessment and interventions should include culturally relevant data such as unique physiological responses to substances, behavioral responses to dependence, and social expectations and sanctions. Staff who are knowledgeable about cultural differences and issues are integral to successful treatment.

Therapeutic Interactions

A variety of nursing interventions are used in the care of persons using substances. It is critical that the nurse establish a therapeutic relationship with these patients (Box 31.12). There are several general guidelines for establishing therapeutic interactions with patients in substance abuse treatment programs:

- Encourage honest expression of feelings.
- Listen to what the individual is really saying.
- Express caring for the individual.
- Hold the individual responsible for his or her behavior.
- Provide consequences for negative behavior that are fair and consistent.

(*text continues on page 611*)

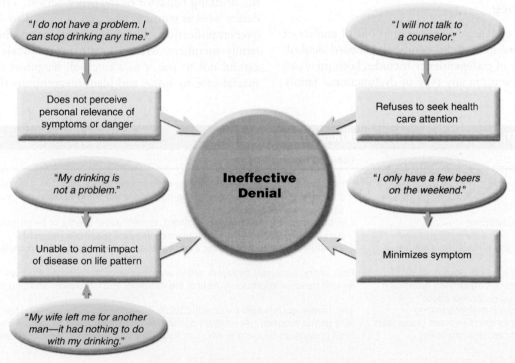

FIGURE 31.3 Nursing diagnosis concept map: Ineffective Denial.

Table 31.6 TREATMENT APPROACHES TO CHEMICAL DEPENDENCE

Approach	Conception of Etiology	Conception of Patient	Conception of Treatment Outcome	Conception of Treatment Process	Advantages of Approach	Disadvantages of Approach
Psychiatric	Symptom of underlying emotional problem	Emotionally disturbed	Emotional conflicts are resolved; there is increased emotional health	Psychotherapy, medication to treat "cause" of substance abuse	Not punitive, treats comorbidity	Focus is only on treatment of mental disorder
Social	Society and environment cause dependence	Victim of circumstance	Improved social functioning or improved environment	Removal of environmental influences and increasing coping responses to it	Stresses social supports and coping skills	Blames "ills of society"—the person not responsible for addiction
Moral	Person is morally weak—can't say "no"	"Hustler," morally deficient	Moral recovery, increased willpower, control, and responsible behavior	"Street addict" behavior and manipulation confronted	Holds person responsible for actions and making amends	Punitive, increases low self-esteem and sense of failure
Learning	Abuse is a learned, reinforced behavior	Has distorted thinking, poor coping skills	Patient learns new ways of thinking and new coping skills	Cognitive therapy techniques and coping skills taught	Not punitive; teaches new coping skills	Places emphasis on control of use
Disease	Probably caused by genetic or biologic factors	Has a chronic progressive disease	Abstinence, arresting disease progression, and beginning of recovery process	Is treated as a primary disease, reinforces patient is an addict and has illness	Not punitive, stresses support and education	Minimizes mental health disorders; discounts return to social use
12-Step	Combination of disease concept and "spiritual bankruptcy"	Has an addiction and is powerless over substances	Abstinence, ongoing spiritual recovery	Use 12 steps, seeking spiritual support, making amends, serving others in need	Widespread success, emphasis is on quality of life and spiritual growth	Self-help group, not a treatment program
Dual diagnosis	Both a primary substance dependence and a mental health disorder	Has both mental and substance abuse disorder	Improvement in both mental health and substance abuse disorders	Concurrent treatment of both disorders	Treats both mental health disorder and dependency, minimizing relapse potential	Not inclusive enough; does not include social or other issues
Biopsychosocial	Biologic basis, with social and psychological influences	Has deficiencies in all three interacting areas	Improvement in mental and physical health, utilization of social supports	Concurrent treatment of all issues	Uses different modalities; is more inclusive	Does not match patient and specific interventions
Multivariant	Many different causes; may be different for each individual	Has multiple issues to be assessed and addressed	Particular issues for individual addressed, and improvement occurs	Treatment strategies are matched with individual patient needs	Treatment matched to individual's needs	Logistical problems can occur in its implementation

BOX 31.11

Principles of Effective Treatment for Addiction

1. Addiction is a complex but treatable disease that affects brain function and behavior.
2. No single treatment is appropriate for everyone.
3. Treatment needs to be readily available.
4. Effective treatment attends to multiple needs of the individual, not just his or her drug use.
5. Remaining in treatment for an adequate period of time is critical.
6. Behavioral therapies—including individual, family, or group counseling – are the most commonly used forms of drug abuse treatment.
7. Medications are an important element of treatment for many patients, especially when combined with counseling and other behavioral therapies.
8. An individual's treatment and service plan must be assessed continually and modified as necessary to ensure that it meets his or her changing needs.
9. Many drug-addicted individuals also have other mental disorders.
10. Medically assisted detoxification is only the first stage of addiction treatment and by itself does little to change long-term drug abuse.
11. Treatment does not need to be voluntary to be effective.
12. Drug use during treatment must be monitored continuously because lapses during treatment do occur.
13. Treatment programs should provide assessment for HIV/AIDS, hepatitis B and C, tuberculosis and other infectious diseases, as well as provide targeted risk-reduction counseling, linking patients to treatment if necessary.

National Institute on Drug Abuse. (2012f). *Principles of drug addiction treatment: A research-based guide* (NIH Publication No. 12-4180) (3rd ed., pp. 3–4). Bethesda: MD: Author.

BOX 31.12 • THERAPEUTIC DIALOGUE • The Patient With Alcoholism

INEFFECTIVE APPROACH

Nurse: I would like to talk with you about your problem with alcoholism.

Patient: Alcoholism! It's not that bad. Everyone gets loaded!

Nurse: You tell me why you were drinking. Your wife left you. You drink a quart of vodka a day. Your blood alcohol level was 0.15% when you were admitted.

Patient: So what! I do have some problems or I wouldn't be here. But, I'm not an alcoholic. (Denial)

Nurse: Do you know what an alcoholic is?

Patient: Sure I do. My father was one. He was a useless bum. I'm not anything like him.

Nurse: It sounds like you are a lot like him.

Patient: I think I need to rest now. My back is killing me. (Avoidance)

EFFECTIVE APPROACH

Nurse: I would like to talk with you about what happens when you drink.

Patient: It's not that bad. Everyone gets loaded!

Nurse: What concerns do you have about your drinking?

Patient: I'm not really concerned. My wife is. She thinks I drink too much. I even quit once for her.

Nurse: What does she tell you about that?

Patient: Well, she nags me a lot and says it costs too much money, but I can stop whenever I want. Her nagging only made me drink again.

Nurse: It sounds as if she is concerned about this, but you have your doubts about how serious it is. Your wife is invited to our family education group, so she can learn about alcohol abuse. Family therapy is also available.

Patient: I have a lot of problems besides alcohol. I never use drugs. I only drink because it relaxes me and makes it easier to deal with stress.

Nurse: Many people drink to help them cope with stress. Sometimes the drinking itself can cause stress. While you are here, do you think it would be useful to look at the stress in your life and how it relates to your drinking?

Patient: Yes. But I only drink when things get too out of hand. My health is pretty good.

Nurse: We can provide information about your health and alcohol use. To evaluate what information may be helpful, I would like to get a little more information about your drinking.

CRITICAL THINKING CHALLENGE

- What effect did the nurse have on the patient in using the word *alcoholism* in the first interaction?

- Discuss what communication approaches the nurse used in the second scenario to engage the patient in disclosing problems with alcohol and his relationship with his wife. How does this nurse's approach vary from the one in the first interaction?

- Talk about specific actions that are objectionable.
- Do not compromise your own values or nursing practice.
- Communicate the treatment plan to the patient and to others on the treatment team.
- Monitor your own reactions to the patient.

Confrontation, or pointing out the inconsistencies in thoughts, feelings, and actions, can promote the person's experience of the natural consequences of one's behavior. Learning from previous behavior and its consequences is how change occurs. Confrontation can be very threatening to patients and should occur within the context of a trusting relationship.

Brief Intervention

Within the alcohol and other drugs field, brief intervention is a highly developed, researched, and accepted approach. A growing body of evidence indicates brief interventions are more effective than no treatment, and there are indications that they are as effective as more intensive interventions (Cole et al., 2012).

Screening and brief intervention are two separate skills that can be used together to reduce risky substance use. Screening involves asking questions about alcohol or drug use. A **brief intervention** is a negotiated conversation between the professional and patient designed to reduce alcohol and drug use.

Not everyone who is screened will need a brief intervention, and not everyone who needs a brief intervention will require treatment. In fact, the goals of screening and brief intervention are to reduce risky substance use before people become dependent or addicted.

Brief intervention is effective for a few reasons. Research indicates that brief interventions are an appropriate response to clients presenting at a general health or community setting and who are unlikely to need, seek, or attend specialist treatment. Brief intervention—to be given clear concise information by a professional—may be all the client may want. It is also an important part of the overall approach of harm reduction (discussed later).

Brief intervention is most successful when working with people who:

- Are experiencing few problems with their drug use
- Have low levels of dependence
- Have a short history of drug use
- Have stable backgrounds
- Are unsure or ambivalent about changing their drug use

It is recommended that brief intervention at a minimum include:

- Advising how to reduce client's drug use
- Providing harm reduction information or self-help manuals that are relevant to the client

- Giving the client relevant information about
  - The consequences of a drug conviction on travel and employment
  - Consequences of further or heavier drug charges
- Discussing harm reduction strategies, especially those relating to
  - Overdose
  - Violence
  - Driving under the influence
  - Safe practices (e.g., safe injecting, safe sex)
- Offering and arranging a follow-up visit

Cognitive and Cognitive Behavioral Interventions and Psychoeducation

Cognitive approaches to addiction hypothesize that if a patient can change the way he or she thinks about a situation, both the emotional reaction to it and the behavioral response will change. Psychoeducational materials, groups, and one-on-one interactions with nurses also impart information to reduce knowledge deficits related to alcohol and drug dependence (Box 31.13). CBT is a brief treatment that is structured and focused on immediate problems. It enables patients to examine the thinking process that leads to decisions to use substances, analyze distortions in thinking, and develop rational responses to these distortions (see Chapter 12).

Enhancing Coping Skills

Improving coping skills is thought to be one component of preventing relapse into alcohol and drug use. Coping skills include the ability to use thought, emotion, and action effectively to solve interpersonal and intrapersonal problems and to achieve personal goals. Groups in addiction treatment programs that also have a relapse

---

BOX 31.13

Psychoeducation Checklist: Substance Abuse

When caring for the patient and family with substance abuse, be sure to include the following topic areas in the family's teaching plan:

- Psychopharmacologic agents, if used, including drug action, dosage, frequency, and possible adverse effects
- Manifestations of intoxication, overdose, and withdrawal
- Emergency medical system activation
- Nutrition
- Coping strategies
- Structured planning
- Safety measures
- Available treatment programs
- Family therapy referral
- Self-help groups and other community resources
- Follow-up laboratory testing, if indicated

BOX 31.14

Skills Training Group Topics

INTERPERSONAL
Starting conversations
Giving and receiving compliments
Nonverbal communication
Receiving criticism
Receiving criticism about drinking
Drink and drug refusal skills
Refusing requests
Close and intimate relationships
Enhancing social support networks

INTRAPERSONAL
Managing thoughts about alcohol
Problem solving
Increasing pleasant activities
Relaxation training
Awareness and management of anger
Awareness and management of negative thinking
Planning for emergencies
Coping with persistent problems

---

prevention component look at coping skills that are needed when drug and alcohol cravings are triggered. The skills listed in Box 31.14 are often taught as coping strategies for dealing with alcohol and drug cravings. Patients role-play new behaviors and learn from the feedback they receive from other group members. They also increase their sense of competency to use these skills in real-life situations. A lengthier discussion of relapse prevention groups appears in Chapter 39.

Group Therapy and Early Recovery

Isolation and alienation from friends and family are common themes in patients with substance-related disorders. In addition, thinking that has become distorted is left unchallenged without contact with others; thus, change is difficult. When a patient enters a group that is working with the goals of continuing recovery, numerous healing advantages can occur.

Groups in treatment settings focus on immediate goals of maintaining sobriety and not on childhood issues. The emphasis is on using problem solving and other skills to deal with stressful events that threaten abstinence. This type of support group is also extremely effective in outpatient treatment settings. After a period of successful abstinence, group therapy can focus more on traditional psychotherapy work.

Individual Therapy

Often, individual therapy is helpful, particularly in conjunction with group therapy or family therapy. In addiction treatment settings, counselors meet with individuals to maintain focus on the goals and objectives of their treat-

ment, to review the fears and anxieties that often arise in early recovery, and to devise new and healthy responses and solutions to stressful and difficult situations.

Family Therapy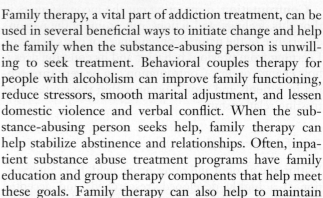

Family therapy, a vital part of addiction treatment, can be used in several beneficial ways to initiate change and help the family when the substance-abusing person is unwilling to seek treatment. Behavioral couples therapy for people with alcoholism can improve family functioning, reduce stressors, smooth marital adjustment, and lessen domestic violence and verbal conflict. When the substance-abusing person seeks help, family therapy can help stabilize abstinence and relationships. Often, inpatient substance abuse treatment programs have family education and group therapy components that help meet these goals. Family therapy can also help to maintain long-term recovery and prevent relapse. Goals of family therapy should be realistic and obtainable. Action plans must be specific and organized into manageable increments. Target dates should be realistic, so pressure is minimal, yet there is motivation to act in a timely manner. Planning for the future is very difficult as long as alcohol or drug abuse continues.

Harm-Reduction Strategies

Harm reduction, a community health intervention designed to reduce the harm of substance use to the individual, the family, and society, has replaced a moral or criminal approach to drug use and addiction. It recognizes that the ideal is abstinence but works with the individual regardless of his or her commitment to reduce use. The goal is to reduce the potential harm of the associated behavior. Harm reduction initiatives range from widely accepted designated driver campaigns to controversial initiatives such as provision of condoms in schools, safe injection rooms, needle exchange programs, and heroin maintenance programs.

Twelve-Step Programs

Alcoholics Anonymous (AA) was the first 12-step, self-help program (see Box 31.15 for a list of these steps). AA is a worldwide fellowship of people with alcoholism who provide support, individually and at meetings, to others who seek help. The program steps include spiritual, cognitive, and behavioral components. Many treatment programs discuss concepts from AA, hold meetings at the treatment facilities, and encourage patients to attend community meetings when appropriate. They also encourage continuing use of AA and other self-help groups as part of an ongoing plan for continued abstinence.

Twelve-step programs do not solicit members, engage in political or religious activities; make medical or psychiatric diagnoses; engage in education about addiction to the general population; or provide mental health, vocational, or legal counseling (Alcoholics Anonymous, 2014). Alternative peer support groups differ from these programs in their approach. Four such groups in the United States are Women for Sobriety, Moderation Management, Men for Sobriety, and S.M.A.R.T. Recovery. For an additional discussion of 12-step programs and mental health patients, see Chapter 39.

Evaluation and Treatment Outcomes

Recovery from alcohol is a journey, often throughout a lifetime. Recovery involves a change in lifestyle and, often, new relationships. Short-term outcomes can be evaluated within the treatment setting. Long-term outcomes are established and evaluated by the patient who often continues to use professional and nonprofessional support as needed.

CHEMICAL DEPENDENCY AND PROFESSIONAL NURSES

Although accurate epidemiologic data specific to nursing is scarce, extrapolations from national data reveal an estimated prevalence that 6% to 8% of nurses use alcohol or drugs to the extent to impair professional practice (National Council of State Boards of Nursing [NCSBN], 2011). A nurse is as susceptible to addiction as is any other individual but has additional risk factors such as access and availability of drugs, training in the administration and injection of drugs, and a familiarity with and a frequency of administering drugs. Difficult working conditions including staffing shortage, increased acuteness and patient ratios, shift rotation, shifts longer than 8 hours and overtime add additional stress to the nurse increasing the risk of substance abuse. Because of the risk of losing a license to practice, nurses are very reluctant to seek help. To protect patients' safety and maintain the standards of the profession, many states have mandatory reporting laws. According to the nurse practice acts, any nurse who knows of any health care provider's incompetent, unethical, or illegal practice must report that information through proper channels (Box 31.16).

In 1982, the ANA House of Delegates adopted a national resolution to provide assistance to impaired nurses. The **peer assistance programs** strive to intervene early, reduce hazards to patients, and increase prospects for the nurse's recovery. The program offers consultation, referral, and monitoring for nurses whose practice is impaired, or potentially impaired, because of the use of drugs or alcohol or a psychological or physiological condition.

A referral can be made confidentially by the employer, Employee Assistance Program, coworker, family member, friend, or the nurse her- or himself. If the nurse is willing to undergo a thorough evaluation to determine the extent of the problem and any treatment needed, all information is kept confidential from the Board of Nursing, and the nurse does not face disciplinary action against his or her nursing license.

BOX 31.16
Using Reflection

AN IMPAIRED NURSE

INCIDENT • A nurse finds her roommate (also a nurse) using a controlled substance that was missing from the hospital. The roommate begs her friend not to turn her in—she is afraid that she will lose her license. The roommate promises to never use illegal substances again. The nurse reports her roommate to the hospital but believes that she has betrayed her friend.

REFLECTION • Reflecting on the incident, the nurse realized that it was very unlikely that her roommate would stop using substances, especially when she has access to the substances. Ultimately, the nurse protected patients from neglect or harm.

Some signs of substance abuse in nurses include mood swings; inappropriate behavior at work; frequent days off for implausible reasons; noncompliance with acceptable policies and procedures; deteriorating appearance; deteriorating job performance; sloppy, illegible charting; errors in charting; alcohol on the breath; forgetfulness; poor judgment and concentration; lying; and volunteering to be the medications nurse.

Other characteristics of nurses with substance abuse include high achievement, both as a student and a nurse; volunteering for overtime and extra duties; no drug use until prescribed after surgery or a chronic illness; and family history of alcoholism or addiction.

SUMMARY OF KEY POINTS

- Substance use disorders are categorized according to the following substances: alcohol, caffeine, cannabis (marijuana), hallucinogens, inhalants, opioids, sedative–hypnotics, stimulants, tobacco, and others.

- Addiction is a condition of continued use of substances despite adverse consequences. Abuse occurs when a person uses alcohol or drugs for the purpose of intoxication or, in the case of prescription drugs, for purposes beyond their use.

- Accurate and comprehensive assessment is crucial in planning addiction treatment interventions. An assessment should consider all substances for pattern of use, including factors of tolerance; withdrawal symptoms; consequences of use; loss of control over amount, frequency, or duration of use; desire or efforts to cease or control use; and social, vocational, and recreational activities affected by use, history of previous addiction treatment, and family and social support systems.

- Denial of a substance use disorder is the individual's attempt to avoid accepting its diagnosis and can be exhibited by attempts to rationalize the substance use, minimize the harmful results, deflect attention from one's own problem to society's or someone else's, or blame childhood experiences.

- Nurses should use a nonconfrontational approach when dealing with patients in denial of their problem. Motivational interviewing approaches are most effective, using empathy and a nonjudgmental approach and helping the patient to realize the discrepancy between life goals and engaging in substance use, thus, motivating patients to change their self-destructive behaviors and make personal choices regarding treatment goals.

- Several effective modalities are used in addiction treatment, and many programs combine several modalities, which can include 12-step programs, social skills groups, psychoeducational groups, group therapy, and individual and family therapies. There is no one best treatment method for all people.

- Substance use disorders have many social and political ramifications. Even the profession of nursing is not immune to substance use disorders among its members.

CRITICAL THINKING CHALLENGES

1. Jeff H, a 35-year-old patient who abuses cocaine, has entered a rehabilitation program. What goals do you believe would be realistic to achieve by the end of his projected 30-day inpatient stay?

2. You are working in an orthopedic unit, and Mary L has been admitted for treatment for a fractured femur. She has been drinking recently and has a blood alcohol level of 0.08%. What further information in the following areas would you need to plan her care?
   a. Medical
   b. Alcohol and drug use related
   c. Other psychosocial issues

3. Normal adolescent behavior is often similar to that associated with substance abuse. How would you differentiate this normal behavior from possible substance abuse or addiction?

4. John M has sought treatment for depression and job stress. He came to your psychiatric assessment unit smelling of alcohol. He believes that he does not have a drinking problem but a job problem. What interventions would you use for possible alcohol abuse or addiction?

5. Sylvia G has been abusing heroin intravenously heavily for 2 years. She has come into the hospital with an abscess on her leg. What symptoms would you expect to observe as she experiences withdrawal? What medications would likely be used to ease these symptoms?

6. After Sylvia G is free of withdrawal symptoms, she expresses interest in obtaining drug treatment. What are her options? How would you describe them to her?

7. Raymond L has been treated for hypertension at your clinic. You notice that he complains of peripheral neuropathy and has an unsteady gait. What other medical signs would corroborate alcoholism?

8. What laboratory test results would help confirm a diagnosis of alcoholism?

Ray: 2004. This award-winning film is based on the life of Ray Charles (played by Jamie Foxx), the musical genius of rhythm and blues. His early childhood experiences included racial discrimination, extreme poverty, an absent father, the traumatic drowning of his younger brother, and the loss of his sight. The film depicts Ray Charles' struggle with his heroin addiction.

VIEWING POINTS: Identify the role of heroin in the development of Ray Charles as a performer, adult, husband, and father. How did denial shape his use of heroin? What was his primary reason for entering treatment? What motivated him to stay clean for the rest of his life?

MOVIE viewing GUIDES related to this chapter are available at http://thePoint.lww.com/Boyd5e Update.

A related Psychiatric-Mental Health Nursing video on the topics of Addiction and Delirium and Alcohol Detoxification are available at: http://thePoint.lww.com/Boyd5eUpdate.

References

Alcoholics Anonymous. (2014). *Alcoholics Anonymous Information on AA.* Retrieved April 12, 2014, from http://www.aa.org.

American Psychiatric Association. (2013). *Diagnostic and Statistical Manual of Mental disorders (5th Ed),* Arlington, VA: American Psychiatric Association.

Bowen, S., Witkiewitz, K., Clifasefi, S. L., Grow, J., Chawla, N., Hsu, S. H., et al. (2014). Relative efficacy of mindfulness-based relapse preventions, standard relapse preventions, and treatment as usual for substance use disorders. *JAMA Psychiatry,* 71(5), 547–556. doi:10.1001/jamapsyciatry.2013.4546

Butler, C. C., Simpson, S. A., Hood, K., Cohen, D., Pickles, T., Spanou, C., et al. (2013). Training practitioners to deliver opportunistic multiple behavior changes counselling in primary care: A cluster randomized trial. *British Medical Journal,* 346, f1191. doi:10.1136/bmj.f1191

Cadet, J. L., Bisagno, V., & Milroy, C. M. (2014). Neuropathology of substance use disorders. Review. *Acta Neuropathology,* 127(1), 91–107

Cairney, S., O'Connor, N., Dingwall, K. M., Maruff, P., Shafiq-Antonacci, R., Currie, J., et al. (2013). A prospective study of neurocognitive changes 15 years after chronic inhalant abuse. *Addiction,* 108(6), 1107–1114.

Centers for Disease Control. (2013). Vital signs: current cigarette smoking among adults aged ≥ 18 years with mental illness-United States, 2009–2011. *Morbidity and Mortality Weekly Report,* 62(5), 81–87.

Cole, B., Clark, D. C., Seale, J. P., Shellenberger, S., Lyme, A., Johnson, J. A., et al. (2012). Reinventing the reel: An innovative approach to resident skill-building in motivational interviewing for brief intervention. *Substance Abuse,* 33(3), 278–281.

Collins, S. E., Malone, D. K., & Larimer, M. E. (2012). Motivation to change and treatment attendance as predictors of alcohol-use outcomes among project-based Housing First residents. *Addictive Behaviors,* 37(9), 931–939.

Cousaert, C., Heylens, G., & Audenaert, K. (2013). Laughing gas abuse is no joke. An overview of the implications for psychiatric practice. *Clinical Neurology and Neurosurgery,* 115(7), 859–862.

Day, E., Bentham, P. W., Callaghan, R., Kuruvilla, T., & George, S. (2013). Thiamine for prevention and treatment of Wernicke-Korsakoff syndrome in people who abuse alcohol (Review). *The Cochran Collaboration,* 7, CD004033. doi:10.1002/14651858.CD004033.pub3

Echeverri, D., Montes, F. R., Cabrera, M., Galán, A., & Prieto, A. (2010). Caffeine's vascular mechanisms of action. *International Journal of Vascular Medicine, 2010,* 834060. doi:10.1135/2010/834060

Ewing, J. A. (1984). Detecting alcoholism. *Journal of the American Medical Association,* 252(14), 1905–1907.

Faessel, H. M., Obach, R. S., Rollema, H., Ravva, P., Williams, K. E., & Burstein, A. H. (2012). A review of the clinical pharmacokinetics and pharmacodynamics of varenicline for smoking cessation. *Clinical Pharmacokinetics,* 49(12), 799–816.

Franck, J. & Jayaram-Lindström, N. (2013). Pharmacotherapy for alcohol dependence: Status of current treatments. *Current Opinion in Neurobiology,* 23(4), 692–699.

Gonzalez, D. (2014). Screening for personality disorder in drug and alcohol dependence. *Psychiatry Research,* 217(1–2):121–123. *doi:10.1016/j.psychres.2014.03.007*

Grant, J. E., Schreiber, L., Odlaug, B. L., & Kim, S. W. (2010). Pathologic gambling and bankruptcy. *Comprehensive Psychiatry,* 51, 115–120.

Kottke, T. & Pronk, N. (2010). Optimal lifestyle adherence and 2-year incidence of chronic conditions. *Clinical Medicine & Research,* 8(3–4), 181–182.

Leung, L., Neufeld, T., & Marin, S. (2012). Effect of self-administered auricular acupressure on smoking cessation-a pilot study. *BMC Complementary and Alternative Medicine,* 12, 11. doi:10.1186/1472-6

Lozano, B. E., LaRowe, S. D., Smith, J. P., Tuerk, P., & Roitzsch, J. (2013). Brief motivational feedback may enhance treatment entry in veterans with comorbid substance use and psychiatric disorders. *American Journal on Addictions,* 22(2), 132–135.

Mental Health America. (2014). Co-dependency. Retrieved April 12, 2014, from http://www.mentalhealthamerica.net/go/codependency.

Moyer, V. A., LeFevre, J. L., Siu, A. L., Peters, J. J., Baumann, L. C., Bibbins-Domingo, K., et al. (2013). Screening and behavioral counseling interventions in primary care to reduce alcohol misuse: U.S. preventive services task force recommendation statement. *Annals of Internal Medicine,* 159(3), 210–218.

National Council of State Boards of Nursing. [NCSBN]. (2011). *Substance use disorders in nursing: A resource manual and guidelines for alternative and disciplinary monitoring programs.* Chicago: National Council of State Boards of Nursing.

National Institute on Drug Abuse. (2012a). Cigarettes and other tobacco products. *Drug Facts.* www.drugabuse.gov.

National Institute on Drug Abuse. (2012b). Spice (Synthetic Marijuana). *Drug Facts.* www.drugabuse.gov.

National Institute on Drug Abuse. (2012c). Inhalants. *Drug Facts.* www.drugabuse.gov.

National Institute on Drug Abuse. (2012d). Anabolic steroids. *Drug Facts.* www.drugabuse.gov.

National Institute on Drug Abuse. (2012e). Synthetic Cathinones ("Bath Salts"). *Drug Facts.* www.drugabuse.gov.

National Institute on Drug Abuse. (2012f). *Principles of drug addiction treatment: A research-based guide* (NIH Publication No. 12-4180) (3rd ed., pp. 3–4). Bethesda, MD: National Institute on Drug Abuse.National Institute on Drug Abuse. (2013a). Cocaine. *Drug Facts.* www.drugabuse.gov.

National Institute on Drug Abuse. (2013b). Methamphetamine. *Research Report Series.* NIH Publication Number 13-4210.

National Institute on Drug Abuse. (2013c), MDMA ("ecstasy" or "Molly"). Drug Facts. www.drugabuse.gov

National Institute on Drug Abuse. (2013d). Tobacco addiction: A research update from the National Institute on Drug Abuse. *Topics in Brief.* www.drugabuse.gov.

National Institute on Drug Abuse. (2013e). Electronic cigarettes (e-Cigarettes). *Drug Facts.* www.drugabuse.gov.

National Institute on Drug Abuse. (2013f). Prescription and over-the-counter medication. *Drug Facts.* www.drugabuse.gov.

National Institute on Drug Abuse. [NIDA]. (2014a). High school and youth trends. *Drug Facts,* www.drugabuse.gov.

National Institute on Drug Abuse. (2014b). Is marijuana medicine? *Drug Facts.* www.durgabuse.gov.

National Institute on Drug Abuse. (2014c). Hallucinogens and dissociative drugs. *Research Report Series.* NIH Publication Number 14-4209. www.drugabuse.gov.

National Institute on Drug Abuse. (2014d). Heroin. *Research Report Series.* NIH Publication Number 14-0165. www.drugabuse.gov.

National Institute of Drug Abuse. (2014e). Emerging Trends. Drugs of Abuse. www.drugabuse.gov/drugs-abuse/emerging-trends.

Nogueira, M., Bosch, R., Valeron, S., Gómez-Barros, N., Palomar, G., Richarte, V., et al. (2014). Early-age clinical and developmental features associated to substance use disorders in attention-deficit/hyperactivity disorder in adults. *Comprehensive Psychiatry,* 55(3), 639–649.

Park, S., Cho, M. J., Jeon, H. J., Lee, H. W., Bae, J. N., Park, J. I., et al. (2010). Prevalence, clinical correlations, comorbidities, and suicidal tendencies in pathological Korean gamblers: Results from the Korean Epidemiologic Catchment Area Study. *Social Psychiatry & Psychiatric Epidemiology,* 45(6), 621–629.

Pilgrim, J. L., Woodford, N., & Drummer, O. H. (2013). Cocaine in sudden and unexpected death: A review of 49 post-mortem cases. *Forensic Science International,* 227(1–3), 52–39.

Pope, M. A., Joober, R., & Malla, A. K. (2013). Diagnostic stability of first-episode psychotic disorders and persistence of comorbid psychiatric disorders over 1 year. *Canadian Journal of Psychiatry,* 58(10), 588–594.

Rice, V. H., Hartmann-Boyce, J., & Stead, L. F. (2013). Nursing interventions for smoking cessation (Review). *The Cochrane Database of systematic Reviews,* 8, CD001188. doi:10.1002/14651848.CD001188.pub4

Sanchez, Z. M., Ribeiro, L. A., Moura, Y. G., Noto, A. R., & Martins, S. S. (2013). Inhalants as intermediate drugs between legal and illegal drugs among middle and high school students. *Journal of Addictive Diseases, 32*(2), 217–226.

Séquin, M., Boyd, R., Lesage, A., McGirr, A., Suissa, A., & Tousignant, M. (2010). Suicide and gambling: Psychopathology and treatment-seeking. *Psychology of Addictive Behaviors, 24*(3), 541–547.

Snipes, D. J. & Benotsch, E. G. (2013). High-risk cocktails and high-risk sex: Examining the relations between alcohol mixed with energy drink consumption, sexual behavior, and drug use in college students. *Addictive Behaviors, 38*(1), 1418–1423.

Strang, J., Metrebian, M., Lintzeris, N., Potts, L., Carnwath, T., & Mayet, S., et al. (2010). Supervised injectable heroin or injectable methadone versus optimised oral methadone as treatment for chronic heroin addicts in England after persistent failure in orthodox treatment (RIOTT): A randomised trial. *The Lancet, 375*(9729), 1885–1895.

Substance Abuse and Mental Health Services Administration. (2013). *Results from the 2012 National Survey on Drug Use and Health: Summary of National Findings.* NSDUH Series H-46, HHS Publication NO. (SMA) 13-4795. Rockville, MD: Substance Abuse and Mental Health Services Administration.

Tranel, D., McNutt, A., & Bechara, A. (2012). Smoking cessation after brain damage does not lead to increased depression: Implications for understanding the psychiatric complications of varenicline. *Cognitive & Behavioral Neurology, 25*(1), 16–24.

U.S. Department of Health and Human Services. (2010). *Healthy people 2020.* Washington, DC: U.S. Government Printing Office. Retrieved from http://www.healthypeople.gov.

Weldy, D. L. (2010). Risks of alcoholic energy drinks for Youth. Risks of alcoholic energy drink for youth. *The Journal of the American Board of Family Medicine, 23*(4), 555–558.

White, A. R., Rampes, H., Liu, J. P., Stead, L. F., & Campbell, J. (2014). Acupuncture and related interventions for smoking cessation. *Cochrane Database System Review, 1,* CD000009 doi:10.1002/14651858.CD00009.pdf

Wilson, D., da Silva Lobo, D. S., Tavares, H., Gentil, V., & Vallada, H. (2013). Family-based association analysis of serotonin genes in pathological gambling disorder: Evidence of vulnerability risk in the 5HT-2A receptor gene. *Journal of Molecular Neuroscience, 49*(3), 550–553.

Wolk, B. J., Ganetsky, M., & Babu, K. M. (2012), Toxicity of energy drinks. *Current Opinion in Pediatrics, 24*(2), 243–251.

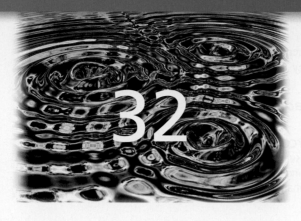

32

Sleep–Wake Disorders
Management of Insomnia and Sleep Problems

Sheri Compton-McBride

KEY CONCEPTS

- sleep–wake cycle
- insomnia
- rhythm

LEARNING OBJECTIVES

After studying this chapter, you will be able to:

1. Describe the major features of sleep.

2. Identify common sleep–wake disorders that co-occur with other mental disorders.

3. Discuss the impact of changes in sleep associated with psychiatric disorders.

4. Perform a sleep history during a patient's assessment.

5. Formulate a model nursing care plan for patients with sleep–wake disorders.

KEY TERMS

- cataplexy • circadian rhythm • chronopharmacotherapy • desynchronized • hypnagogic hallucinations
- imagery rehearsal therapy • luminotherapy • multiple sleep latency test (MSLT) • night terrors • non–rapid eye movement (NREM) sleep • polysomnography • rapid eye movement (REM) sleep • relaxation training • sleep architecture • sleep debt • sleep diary • sleep–wake disorders • sleep efficiency • sleep latency • sleep paralysis • sleep restriction • sleepiness • slow-wave sleep • somnambulism • stimulus control • synchronized

---

Sleep is a recurrent, altered state of consciousness that occupies nearly one third of our lives and occurs for sustained periods. The functions of sleep are important to our development, functioning, and health. Sleep has identifiable cycles, and a variety of cognitive experiences, ranging from memory recall to feeling energetic, that occur as a result of those cycles. The consequences of disturbed sleep are well known and include impaired alertness and performance. Many Americans are severely sleep deprived. Implications for public safety, increased utilization of healthcare services, and morbidity are associated with sleep disturbances (Centers for Disease Control and Prevention [CDC], 2012). The average sleep duration of adults in the United States has plateaued between 6 and 6.5 hours from a high of 8.5 hours in 1960 (Adenekan, Pandey, McKenzie, Zizi,

Casimir, & Jean Louis, 2013). Sleepiness has been responsible for catastrophic disasters such as the Exxon Valdez oil spill, the nuclear meltdown at Chernobyl in the Ukraine, and the Three Mile Island disaster in the United States. Short sleep duration is associated with lower socio-economic groups and the unemployed (Adenekan et al., 2013).

Sleep–wake disorders are diagnosed when an individual is dissatisfied about the quality, timing, and amount of their sleep causing daytime distress and impairment (American Psychiatric Association [APA], 2013). Sleep problems are more common in women, and prevalence increases with age in both genders. Sleep–wake disorders occur independently of the diagnosis of other mental disorders, but they are also seen in people with mental disorders. For example, a core feature of posttraumatic stress disorder (PTSD) is sleep disturbance (Lauterbach, Behnke, & McSweeney, 2011).

Understanding sleep, sleep disturbances, and sleep–wake disorders is crucial for mental health practitioners. Sleep and sleep problems can significantly impact recovery efforts (Glozier et al., 2014; Lauterbach et al., 2011). This chapter presents a discussion of normal sleep rhythms and patterns, sleep–wake disorders that the psychiatric–mental health nurse will most likely encounter in practice, and nursing diagnoses and interventions appropriate for use in patients with sleep problems. Insomnia disorder is highlighted.

OVERVIEW OF SLEEP

Sleep, which is necessary for human survival, can be viewed from both behavioral and physiologic perspectives. Behaviorally, sleep is a state of decreased awareness of environmental stimuli and a relative state of unconsciousness with no memory of the state. Sleep can be disrupted and reversed quite easily, unlike coma. In 2005, a National Institute of Health scientific conference on sleep identified the theoretical concepts associated with sleep including conditioning, hyperarousal, stress response, predisposing personality traits, and attitudes and beliefs about sleep (National Institutes of Health, 2005). Sleep is usually preceded by a period of sleepiness or the urge to fall asleep.

From a physiologic perspective, dopamine, gamma-aminobutyric acid (GABA), adenosine, histamine, hypocretin, melatonin, and cortisol appear to play roles in changing sleep states (Monti, 2013). Wakefulness is maintained by the reticular activating system in the brain. As the cycle of the reticular activating system dwindles, neurotransmitters that promote sleep take over (see Chapter 8).

Pattern of Sleep

Sleep is a patterned activity and is one component of the biphasic 24 hour sleep–wake cycle.

> **KEYCONCEPT** The **sleep–wake cycle** is an endogenously generated rhythm close to 24 to 25 hours synchronized with the day–night cycle. The release of melatonin induces sleep, but its maximum effect is influenced by the circadian phase (Münch & Bromundt, 2012).

Sleep latency is the time period measured from "lights out," or bedtime, to initiation of sleep. **Sleep architecture** is the pattern of non–rapid eye movement (NREM) and rapid eye movement (REM) that are in about a 90- to 110-minute cycle. Sleep occurs in stages, and the timing

of sleep is regulated by circadian rhythms. **Sleep efficiency** is the ratio of total sleep time to time in bed.

Circadian Rhythm

> **KEYCONCEPT** **Rhythm** is movement with a cadence, a measured flow that occurs at regular intervals, with a cycle of coming and going, ebbing and rising, to return at the start point and begin again.

Nearly all physiologic and psychological functions fluctuate in a pattern that repeats itself in a 24-hour cycle, called **circadian rhythm** (Figure 32.1). The biologic clock that regulates our circadian rhythms is located in the *suprachiasmatic nucleus*, an area of the hypothalamus that lies on top of the optic chiasm. Peripheral cells also contribute to the regulation of circadian rhythms. When two or more rhythms reach their peak at the same time, they are **synchronized**; if they reach their peak at different times, they are **desynchronized**.

Most physiologic functions reach their lowest levels during the middle of the sleep period. For example, body temperature follows a predictable pattern from lowest, in the early morning, to highest, in the mid-evening. Manual dexterity, reaction time, and simple recognition appear to coincide with the circadian rhythm of body temperature. Most circadian rhythms continue even when humans are unaware of the time of day. Natural age-related changes in circadian sleep rhythms generally regulate people as they get older toward morning

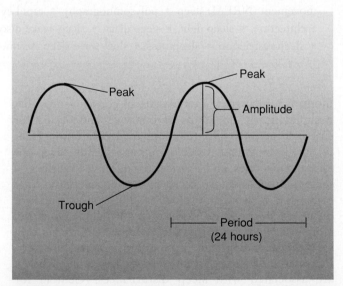

FIGURE 32.1 Circadian rhythms fluctuate in patterns. The *peak* is the point at which the rhythm reaches its maximum, and the *trough* is the point at which the rhythm reaches its minimum. The *period* is the time it takes to complete a cycle. The *amplitude* is the extent of the peak and is half the distance from peak to trough.

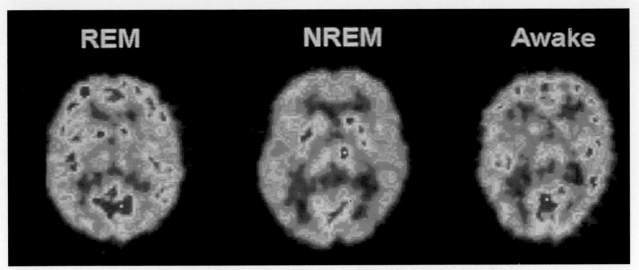

FIGURE 32.2 Brain activity during the sleep–wake cycle. The brain is as active in rapid eye movement (REM) or dreaming sleep as when awake but is metabolically less active in slow-wave or non–rapid eye movement (NREM) sleep. (Courtesy of Monte S. Buchsbaum, MD, the Mount Sinai Medical Center and School of Medicine, New York.)

alertness and productivity and sleepiness at night (Costa, Carvalho, & Fernandes, 2013).

Stages of Sleep

Sleep is biphasic, cycling between NREM and REM (Figure 32.2). During an 8-hour sleep period, the cycle of NREM and REM repeats itself. This duration of the cycles may change as the night progresses. In the first cycle, the amount of REM sleep is brief. With each succeeding cycle, the amount of time spent in REM lengthens. Conversely, NREM is most prominent during the initial cycle but declines as total sleep time progresses (Figure 32.3).

Non–Rapid Eye Movement Sleep

Non–rapid eye movement (NREM) sleep occurs about 90 minutes after falling asleep and consists of four substages. Light sleep is characteristic of stages 1 and 2, in which the person is easily aroused. A person aroused from stage 1 sleep may even deny having been asleep, such as dozing while watching television and awakening minutes later during a loud commercial. Stage 1 accounts for only 2% to 5% of a night's sleep and is a transition between relaxed wakefulness and sleep. Stage 2 comprises about 45% to 55% of sleep. During phase 1 and 2, an electroencephalogram (EEG) shows an alpha rhythm gradually being replaced by a theta rhythm. Sleep spindles or "k complexes" occur in stage 2 (see Figure 32.3).

Slow-wave sleep, or the deepest state of sleep, characterizes stages 3 and 4. Slow-wave sleep is believed to have a restorative function, although the exact mechanism for this is unclear. It may serve to conserve energy because

metabolism and body temperature decrease during this part of sleep. These stages make up 10% to 23% of sleep. EEG findings show high-amplitude waves, slow waves, or delta waves. The difference between stages 3 and 4 is the amount of delta waves seen, with stage 3 demonstrating 20% to 50% of delta waves and stage 4 showing more than 50% of delta waves.

Rapid Eye Movement Sleep

Rapid eye movement (REM) sleep is a state characterized by bursts of rapid eye movements. REM sleep occurs in four to six separate episodes and makes up about 20% to 25% of a night's sleep. Although REM sleep is a deep sleep and muscles seem to be at rest, EEG findings demonstrate an active brain. Brain waves resemble a mixture of wakeful and drowsy patterns. Although vivid dreaming is the outstanding feature reported by adults when awakened out of REM sleep, people also report dreams when they awaken from NREM sleep.

During REM sleep, nerve impulses are blocked within the spinal cord. Muscle tone diminishes to the point of paralysis. Only stronger impulses are relayed, producing muscular twitches, eye movements, and impulses controlling heart rate and respiration. Breathing and heart rate may become irregular.

This type of sleep has a circadian rhythm that closely coincides with the body temperature rhythm. The greatest amount of REM sleep is seen when the body temperature cycle is at its lowest. People do not sweat or shiver during REM sleep because temperature regulation is impaired. Patterns of hormone release, kidney function, and reflexes change. Women have clitoral engorgement and an increase in blood flow to the vagina. Men have penile erections.

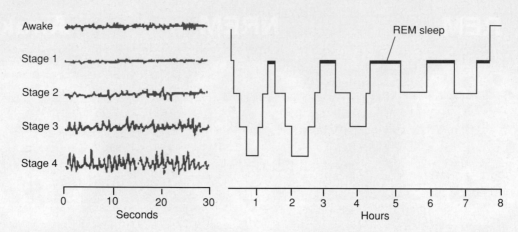

FIGURE 32.3 Brain waves during wakefulness and stages 1, 2, 3, and 4 sleep on the *left* and duration of wakefulness, rapid eye movement (REM), and non–rapid eye movement (NREM) sleep on the *right*. In typical sleep architecture in normal young adults, NREM and REM sleep stages cycle every 90 to 110 minutes through the night. Wakefulness accounts for less than 5% of the night's sleep pattern. Slow-wave sleep dominates the first third of the night during NREM stages 3 and 4. REM sleep occurs in four to six separate episodes throughout the night (20%–25% of sleep) and dominates the last third of the night's sleep. (From Porth, C. M. [2005]. *Pathophysiology: Concepts of altered health states.* Philadelphia: Lippincott Williams & Wilkins.)

Factors Affecting Sleep Pattern and Quality

Gender

Sleep problems and poorer quality sleep are reported more often by women than men. Disturbed sleep and daytime sleepiness have a cumulative effect on mental health (Baker & Colrain, 2010). Women are at greater risk for insomnia and other sleep problems. Sleep in women is influenced by the sex hormones, which vary throughout the life cycle (Soares & Frey, 2010). Socioeconomic factors contribute to poor sleep quality and daytime sleepiness in American women (Baker & Colrain, 2010).

Age

Sleep patterns change dramatically over the course of the life span. Newborns need 17 to 18 hours of sleep each day, which occurs in 3- to 4-hour episodes throughout the day. By age 6 months, 12 hours of sleep at night and two 1- to 2-hour naps each day are needed. After age 5 years, children gradually need less sleep.

Preadolescents need about 10 hours of sleep each night, and napping is rare. A teenager's sleep need is only slightly less, at about 9 hours. During young adulthood, about 8 hours of sleep is needed. The amount of sleep required and sleep architecture typically remain unchanged during the middle-aged years. Poor sleep in women is associated with hormonal changes, such as during the menstrual cycle, pregnancy, and menopause.

For older adults, the need for sleep does not decrease, but the ability to sustain sleep changes. Older people spend more time in bed, sleep less, wake more often during the night, and take longer to fall asleep than younger adults. For some, sleep requirements are met by daytime napping. Furthermore, temperature rhythm in older people peaks earlier; early morning arousals may reflect early rise of body temperature. Older people are at higher risk for sleep disorders (Costa et al., 2013; LeBourgeois et al., 2013).

Environment

Sleep-related problems have multiple factors that make up the clinical picture. Whereas some are external, such as the noise and temperature, others are internal (e.g., stress and pain). A person can be sleepy but may stay awake if in a stimulating environment with bright lights or a lot of activity. In contrast, a sleepy person in a quiet place or engaged in sedentary activity cannot resist the urge to fall asleep. **Sleepiness** is a physiologic state, and although a stimulating environment can temporarily forestall it, when these stimuli are removed, the urge to sleep will persist. Even when someone who is chronically sleep deprived does not feel sleepy, the tendency to fall asleep is much greater and may manifest by causing the person to doze off while sitting in lectures or during the monotonous operation of machinery or driving.

Lifestyles

Many factors can cause disrupted sleep patterns, such as travel across time zones, stress or anxiety, and changes in the sleep–wake pattern because of shift work. When traveling across time zones or working night shifts (and sleeping during the day), one's regular sleepiness–alertness rhythm may persist for several days. Even when daytime sleep is improved with a pharmacologic agent, sleepiness in the early morning hours usually continues for the first 2 to 3 nights. This extreme sleepiness often decreases after a 4- to 6-day reversal of the sleep–wake cycle.

Changes in Normal Sleep

Normal sleep is sensitive to changes, and the body responds when deprived of certain phases of sleep, particularly REM sleep and slow-wave sleep. Certain activities, such as early rising, alcohol intake before bedtime, or consumption of certain medications, can suppress REM sleep. One example is the use of central nervous system (CNS)–acting medications. Fragmented sleep interrupts the restorative function of a good night's sleep. Not only does insufficient sleep cause daytime sleepiness, but disturbed sleep also affects daytime alertness and performance. A **sleep debt** occurs when there is recurrent long-term sleep deprivation.

When individuals are deprived of REM sleep, there is a subsequent "rebound effect," wherein the lost REM sleep is made up during the next sleep period. The body makes up for this lost REM sleep by earlier occurrence of REM sleep during the next night. The presence of REM at sleep onset implies REM deprivation.

Slow-wave sleep does not appear to have a circadian determinant, but it is more sensitive to the amount of previous sleep obtained. When one is deprived of both REM and slow-wave sleep, the body prefers to make up the slow-wave before the REM sleep.

Sleep–Wake Disorders

An occasional change in sleep pattern becomes a sleep disorder when mental and physical health is compromised as a result of problems in the sleep–wake cycle. Sleep–wake disorders include insomnia, hypersomnolence, and narcolepsy. Within the sleep–wake category, the DSM-5 also includes breathing-related sleep disorders (such as obstructive sleep apnea, and circadian rhythm disorders) and parasomnias (APA, 2013). This chapter highlights insomnia disorder with a brief discussion of several of the other disorders.

INSOMNIA DISORDER

> **KEYCONCEPT** **Insomnia**, which is Latin for "no sleep," refers to difficulty falling asleep or maintaining sleep when there are adequate opportunity and circumstances for sleep. Dissatisfaction with sleep quantity or quality is also present (Matthews, Arnedt, McCarthy, Cuddihy, & Aloia, 2013).

Clinical Course

Few studies have described the course of insomnia disorder which can last for short periods in some patients and for decades in others. Limited data show that symptoms are usually of long duration (Mysliwiec, Matsangas, Baxter, McGraw, Bothwell, & Roth, 2014).

Diagnostic Criteria

Insomnia disorder is characterized by dissatisfaction with sleep quantity or quality and difficulty initiating or maintaining sleep, or waking early in the morning, and being unable to return to sleep at least three nights per week for at least 3 months (APA, 2013). The term "primary insomnia" is no longer used to describe this disorder. In insomnia, patients may deny fighting sleep or falling asleep unintentionally during the day.

Epidemiology and Risk Factors

Of all sleep-related problems, insomnia is the most prevalent, with an estimated 23.6% of noninstitutionalized adults; the prevalence of chronic or severe insomnia is estimated to range from 10% to 15% (Kessler et al., 2012; Kraus & Rabin, 2012). Insomnia is one of the most prevalent complaints in primary care (Morin & Benca, 2012). There is a greater prevalence of insomnia among older people and among divorced, separated, and widowed adults.

Increasing age, female sex, and comorbid disorders (medical, mental disorders, and substance use) are all risks of developing insomnia disorder. Individuals at risk often describe themselves as "light sleepers" before persistent sleep problems developed. They have a tendency to be more easily psychologically or physiologically aroused at night. They tend to develop sleep-preventing associations and behaviors (i.e., become obsessive about sleep and have a hard time falling asleep) (Tamanna & Geraci, 2013). Although initially insomnia may be precipitated by stressful situations and tension, this inability to fall asleep and stay asleep persists after the crisis or stressful situation has passed.

Comorbidity

Insomnia is one of the major problems in many other mental disorders and often increases the risk for relapse of the mental disorder. In PTSD, for example, difficulties initiating and falling asleep have been recognized for centuries. Documented comorbid conditions include cardiovascular disorders, diabetes, musculoskeletal disorders (arthritis, chronic back/neck pain), respiratory disorders (COPD, seasonal allergies, chronic bronchitis, emphysema), digestive disorders (gastroesophageal reflux

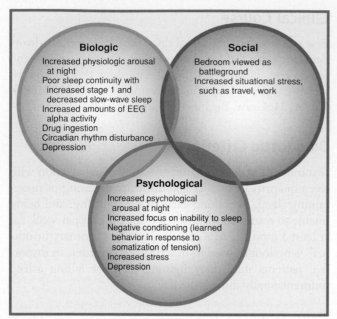

Biologic
Increased physiologic arousal at night
Poor sleep continuity with increased stage 1 and decreased slow-wave sleep
Increased amounts of EEG alpha activity
Drug ingestion
Circadian rhythm disturbance
Depression

Social
Bedroom viewed as battleground
Increased situational stress, such as travel, work

Psychological
Increased psychological arousal at night
Increased focus on inability to sleep
Negative conditioning (learned behavior in response to somatization of tension)
Increased stress
Depression

FIGURE 32.4 Biopsychosocial etiologies of insomnia disorder.

disease, irritable bowel syndrome), pain conditions, and mental disorders including depression, PTSD, and other sleep disorders such as sleep apnea, and restless legs syndrome (RLS) (Kessler et al., 2012).

Etiology

Many factors affect sleep, but there is no one factor that causes insomnia (Figure 32.4). One of the major reasons for insomnia is depression, which accounts for most cases. However, most people with insomnia do not have psychiatric diagnosis (Kraus & Rabin, 2012).

Family Response to Disorder

Living with a family member with insomnia disorder is challenging. Irritability, complaints of sleeplessness, and chronic fatigue interfere with quality interpersonal relationships. Family members become "exhausted" of living with someone who never sleeps.

Interdisciplinary Treatment

Sleep disorders are best treated by clinicians specializing in this area, but primary and mental health care professionals should be able to identify sleep disturbances and provide education and interventions for normalizing sleep. However, because sleep disorders are common in individuals with mental health problems, psychiatric–mental health nurses provide care for those with sleep disorders.

Priority Care Issues

Safety is a priority for people with insomnia disorder. Sleep deprivation can lead to accidents, falls, and injuries, especially in older patients. Sedating medication could potentially increase falls (Kessler et al., 2012).

NURSING MANAGEMENT: Human Response to Insomnia Disorder

Caring for a person with insomnia usually involves a combination of approaches, as illustrated in Figure 32.5.

Biologic Domain
Biologic Assessment

The assessment of a patient's sleep pattern is a part of every psychiatric nursing assessment (see Chapter 10). If a patient has a sleep disorder, a detailed sleep history should be included in the assessment process. During the patient interview, the description, duration (when problem began), stability (every night?), and intensity (how bad is it?) should be determined (Box 32.1). A sleep history includes current sleeping patterns, medical problems, current medications (including over-the-counter [OTC] and supplements), current life events, use of alcohol and caffeine, and emotional and mental status that might be affecting sleep (see Box 32.2 and Box 32.3). A **sleep diary**, a person's written account of the sleep experience, is useful in determining the extent of the sleep problem (Arora, Broglia, Pushpakumar, Lodhi, & Taheri, 2013). The diary

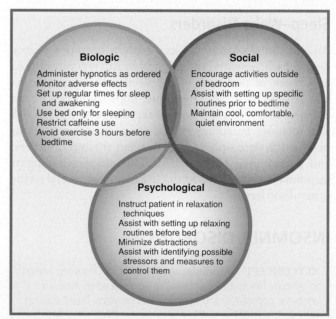

Biologic
Administer hypnotics as ordered
Monitor adverse effects
Set up regular times for sleep and awakening
Use bed only for sleeping
Restrict caffeine use
Avoid exercise 3 hours before bedtime

Social
Encourage activities outside of bedroom
Assist with setting up specific routines prior to bedtime
Maintain cool, comfortable, quiet environment

Psychological
Instruct patient in relaxation techniques
Assist with setting up relaxing routines before bed
Minimize distractions
Assist with identifying possible stressors and measures to control them

FIGURE 32.5 Biopsychosocial interventions for patients with insomnia disorder.

BOX 32.1 • THERAPEUTIC DIALOGUE • Sleep Assessment

INEFFECTIVE APPROACH

Nurse: What time do you go to bed at night?

Patient: Oh, my bedtime varies between 10 PM and 2 AM.

Nurse: What time do you get up?

Patient: I get up anywhere between 6 AM and noon.

Nurse: How do you sleep during the night?

Patient: OK.

Nurse: OK?

Patient: Yeah, no problems sleeping.

EFFECTIVE APPROACH

Nurse: What time do you go to bed at night, and what time do you get up?

Patient: Oh, my bedtime varies between 10 PM and 2 AM. I get up anywhere between 6 AM and noon.

Nurse: Let's be more specific. During a week's time, what time do you go to bed each night?

Patient: Well, this semester I have a morning clinical rotation Monday through Thursday. I'm usually up till 11 or midnight preparing for the next day. On Friday and Saturday nights, I typically go out with my friends and get to bed around 2 AM. On Sunday night, I get in to bed around 10 PM.

Nurse: What time do you get up each day of the week?

Patient: On the mornings that I have clinicals, I have to get up around 6 AM to be at the hospital by 6:45 AM. On Friday, I get up at 8 AM for a 9 o'clock class. Saturday morning, I get up around 8 AM so I can go to my part-time job. On Sunday, I get up by noon.

Nurse: How long do you take to fall asleep?

Patient: That's gotten much better. I fall asleep in 15 minutes or so.

Nurse: Do you take any naps?

Patient: Outside of class, I don't have time to nap. I'm just too busy with my classes, clinical, homework, job, and social life.

Nurse: Before this semester, how much sleep did you get?

Patient: That was last summer; I had an job that started at 1:30 PM, so I could sleep as late as I wanted. I bet I got 8 or even 9 hours of sleep every night. I don't remember being sleepy then.

CRITICAL THINKING CHALLENGE

- Compare the quality and quantity of elicited data in the two scenarios.
- What conclusions could be drawn from the first scenario?

- Are the conclusions different for the second scenario? Explain.

BOX 32.2

Sleep History

Perception of sleep problem
Sleep schedule (bedtime and rise time)
Difficulty falling asleep or maintaining sleep
Quality of sleep
Daytime sleepiness and impact of the sleep disorder on daytime functioning
General emotional and physical problems (e.g., stress)
Sleep hygiene (e.g., consuming caffeine immediately before bed)
Sleep environment (e.g., room temperature, noise, light)

Adapted from Porth, C. M. (Ed.) 2010. Sleep and sleep disorders. *Pathophysiology: Concepts of altered health states* (pp. 1281–1297). Philadelphia: Lippincott Williams & Wilkins.

may cover a few days to several weeks. A simple diary is typically a daily record of the patient's bedtimes, rising times, estimated time to fall asleep, number and length of awakenings, and naps. More complicated sleep diaries involve recording the amount and time of alcohol ingestion, ratings of fatigue, medication, and stressful events.

Nursing Diagnoses for the Biologic Domain

The nursing diagnosis usually applied to the patient with a sleep disorder is Sleep Pattern Disturbance, Insomnia or Sleep Deprivation (Figure 32.6, p. 626). The diagnosis is

BOX 32.3

Medications and Other Substances and Their Effects on Sleep

ALCOHOL
- Increases TST during the first half of the night
- Decreases TST during the second half
- Decreases REM sleep during the first half of the night
- Withdrawal from chronic use of alcohol causes a decrease in TST, increased wakefulness after sleep onset, and REM rebound.

AMPHETAMINES
- Disrupt sleep–wake cycle during acute use
- Decrease TST
- Decrease REM sleep
- Withdrawal may cause REM rebound.

ANTIDEPRESSANTS (TRICYCLICS AND MAOIs)
- Sleep effects vary with sedative potential
- Increase slow-wave sleep
- Decrease REM sleep

BARBITURATES
- Increase TST
- Decrease WASO
- Decrease REM sleep
- Withdrawal may cause a decrease in TST and REM rebound.

BENZODIAZEPINES
- Drugs vary in onset and duration of action.
- Decrease SL
- Increase TST
- Decrease WASO
- Decrease REM sleep
- Daytime sedation may occur with long-acting drugs.

β-ADRENERGIC BLOCKERS
- Decrease REM sleep
- Increase WASO, nightmares
- Daytime sedation may occur

CAFFEINE
- Increases SL
- Decreases TST
- Decreases REM sleep

L-DOPA
- Vivid dreams and nightmares

LITHIUM
- Increases slow-wave sleep
- Decreases REM sleep

OPIOIDS
- Effects vary with specific agents
- Increase WASO
- Decrease REM sleep
- Decrease slow-wave sleep

PHENOTHIAZINES
- Increase TST
- Increase slow-wave sleep

STEROIDS
- Increase WASO

MAOI, monoamine oxidase inhibitor; REM, rapid eye movement; SL, sleep latency; TST, total sleep time; WASO, wake after sleep onset.

BOX 32.4

Sleep Hygiene Tips

Nurses are often involved in helping patients develop and maintain good sleep habits. Teaching tips include the following:

1. The most important healthy sleep habit is to *establish and maintain a regular bedtime and rising time*. Even if you awaken feeling unrefreshed, get up and out of bed at a regular, consistent time. "Sleeping in" can disturb sleep on the subsequent night. For most, time in bed should be limited to 8 hours.
2. Avoid naps.
3. Abstain from alcohol. Although alcohol may assist with sleep onset, there is an alerting effect when it wears off.
4. Refrain from caffeine after midafternoon. Avoid nicotine before bedtime and during the night. Caffeine and nicotine are strong stimulants and fragment sleep.
5. Exercise regularly, avoiding the 3 hours before bedtime. Exercising 6 hours before bedtime tends to strengthen the circadian rhythms of body temperature and sleepiness.
6. Use the bedroom for sleep and sex. Promote the bedroom as a stimulus for sleep, not for studying, watching television, or socializing on the telephone.
7. Set a relaxing routine to prepare for sleep. Avoid frustrating or provoking activities before bedtime.
8. Provide for a comfortable environment. A cool room temperature, minimal light, and limiting noise are suggested.

made when a disruption of sleep time causes discomfort or interferes with lifestyle (see Nursing Care Plan 32.1).

Interventions for the Biologic Domain

Nonpharmacologic health-promoting interventions are the first choice before administering pharmacologic agents (Morin & Benca, 2012). Sleep hygiene strategies can be effective and should be encouraged (Box 32.4). The goal is to normalize sleep patterns to improve well-being.

Activity, Exercise, Nutrition, and Thermoregulation Interventions

Exercise promotes sleep, but regular exercise should be planned for 3 hours before bedtime. Routines are important, especially when preparing your body to sleep. Engaging in quiet, relaxing activity, such as listening to soft music or reading nonstimulating material, is often suggested. Additional interventions include avoiding a heavy meal, alcohol, and caffeine. Patients should be

NURSING CARE PLAN 32.1

The Patient With Insomnia

MT is a 20-year-old student who is majoring in nursing. He presents himself at Student Health Services with a complaint of insomnia. In assessing his problem, the nurse ascertains that MT takes 2 to 3 hours to fall asleep. During this interim of wakefulness, he lies in bed, calm but somewhat restless. He has had no prior difficulty with insomnia. His problem falling asleep occurs 3 nights a week—on Mondays, Wednesdays, and Fridays. He exercises vigorously during his physical education class (7–9 PM) on these three evenings. He denies any sleep problems during spring break, when he took a trip. The patient drinks 1 cup of coffee in the morning and denies the use of other stimulants. He reports that as a consequence, he has had some irritability and difficulty concentrating on the days after a "bad night." He has tried an over-the-counter sleep medication but does not remember the name of it. When he took these sleeping pills, he was able to fall asleep better, but he found the pills to be costly. He would like a prescription for sleeping medication that would be covered by student health insurance.

Setting: Outpatient Student Health Service

Baseline Assessment: A 20-year-old man who presents with difficulty initiating sleep. After vigorous evening exercise, he takes 2–3 hours to fall asleep. Strengths: intelligence, motivated for treatment, adequate insurance coverage, good physical health.

Associated Psychiatric Diagnoses	Medications
Insomnia disorder	None

Nursing Diagnosis 1: Insomnia

Defining Characteristics	Related Factors
Difficulty falling asleep, estimated sleep latency of 2–3 hours three nights a week Mood alterations Poor concentration	Changes in usual sleep environment Poor sleep hygiene

Outcomes

Initial	Discharge
1. Describe factors that prevent or inhibit sleep. 2. Identify strategies to improve sleep hygiene.	3. Report an optimal balance of rest and activity.

Interventions

Interventions	Rationale	Ongoing Assessment
Teach patient good sleep hygiene habits.	Discussion of good sleep hygiene is the first treatment strategy.	Monitor MT's reports of estimated sleep latency.
Instruct the patient to keep a sleep diary for 1 week, including bedtime, sleep latency, rising time, naps, caffeine intake, and time of exercise.	Keeping a sleep diary can give insight into insomnia problems by identifying alerting influences in relation to disturbed sleep.	Exercise before sleep appears to be the primary factor that could be causing insomnia on Mondays, Wednesdays, and Fridays. Monitor other sleep hygiene issues.
Reassure the patient that short-term insomnia will resolve when the factors that caused the problem are eliminated.	Anxiety about insomnia is a predisposing factor to the development of insomnia disorder.	Determine MT's level of anxiety about the insomnia.

Continued

NURSING CARE PLAN 32.1 *(Continued)*

Interventions	Rationale	Ongoing Assessment
Determine whether it is possible for the patient to adjust his schedule so vigorous exercise occurs several hours before sleep.	Physical exercise raises basal metabolism, which may interfere with sleep.	Determine whether it is possible for the patient to adjust his course schedule.
Problem solve with MT how to adjust his sleep schedule to avoid insomnia.	Problem solving allows the patient to learn how to consider alternative strategies.	Evaluate whether strategies are reasonable.

Evaluation

Outcomes	Revised Outcomes	Interventions
After readjustment of exercise schedule, MT was able to resume normal sleep.	None	None

encouraged to evaluate the temperature of the room. Generally, a cooler environment enhances sleep.

Pharmacologic Interventions

Understanding Types of Pharmacologic Agents

Types of drugs used to treat symptoms of insomnia include benzodiazepine receptor agonists, melatonin receptor agonists, sedating antidepressants, and OTC medications and supplements.

Benzodiazepine Receptor Agonists (BzRAs). The BzRA hypnotics have U.S. Food and Drug Administration (FDA) approval for insomnia. They include the benzodiazepines (triazolam, temazepam, estazolam, quazepam, and flurazepam) and the nonbenzodiazepines (zolpidem, zolpidem extended release, zaleplon, and eszopiclone) (Table 32.1). All of these medications bind to benzodiazepine receptors and exert their effects by facilitating GABA effects. GABA, the most common inhibitory neurotransmitter, must be present at the benzodiazepine receptor for the BzRA to

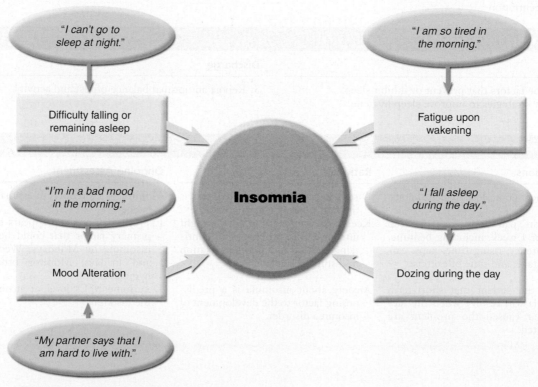

FIGURE 32.6 Nursing diagnosis concept map: Insomnia.

Table 32.1 HYPNOTICS: BENZODIAZEPINE RECEPTOR AGONISTS

	Dosage (mg)	Half-life (h)	CYP Metabolism/Excretion
Estazolam	1–2	10–24	3A/renal
Flurazepam	15–30	48–120	hepatic/renal
Temazepam (Restoril)	15–30	8–20	UGT2B7,2C19, 3A4 /renal
Triazolam (Halcion)	0.125–0.25	2.4	3A4/renal
Quazepam (Doral)	7.5–15	48–120	Hepatic/renal
Zolpidem (Ambien)	5–10	1.4–3.8	3A4, 2C9/renal
Zolpidem ER (Ambien)	6.25–12.5	2.8	3A4, 2C9/renal
Zaleplon (Sonata)	5–20	1	3A4/renal
Eszopiclone (Lunesta)	1–3	6	3A4, 2E1

UGT = uridine 5'-diphosphate glucuronosyltransferase.

exert its effect. All of these medications are absorbed rapidly and reduce sleep latency at recommended doses (Riemann & Perlis, 2009). Benzodiazepines slightly decrease REM sleep but greatly suppress slow-wave sleep. Nonbenzodiazepine hypnotics, which provide immediate relief, are often used for short-term treatment of insomnia. The most common side effects are headache, dizziness, and residual sleepiness (Box 32.5).

BOX 32.5

Drug Profile: Zaleplon (Sonata)

DRUG CLASS: Sedative–hypnotic (pyrazolopyrimidine nonbenzodiazepine hypnotic). It is readily absorbed and metabolized with only about 1% of zaleplon eliminated in the urine.

RECEPTOR AFFINITY: Zaleplon acts at the GABA–benzodiazepine receptor complex.

INDICATION: Treatment of onset or maintenance insomnia

ROUTES AND DOSING: Zaleplon is available in 5- and 10-mg capsules. It should be taken at bedtime or after a nocturnal awakening with difficulty falling back to sleep (but at least 4 hours before the desired rise time).

Adults: The recommended starting dose is 10 mg with a maximum of 20 mg. An initial dose of 5 mg should be considered in adults with low body weight. Doses of over 20 mg have not been sufficiently studied.

Geriatric: Initially, 5 mg is recommended as a starting dose. Older adults should not exceed a 10-mg dose.

HALF-LIFE (PEAK PLASMA CONCENTRATION): 1 hour

SELECTED ADVERSE REACTIONS: Abdominal pain, headache, dizziness, depression, nervousness, difficulty concentrating, back pain, chest pain, migraine, conjunctivitis, bronchitis, pruritus, rash, arthritis, constipation, and dry mouth

WARNINGS: Zaleplon should not be administered to patients with severe hepatic impairment. Zaleplon potentiates the psychomotor impairments of ethanol.

GABA, gamma-aminobutyric acid.

There is agreement among sleep experts that the BzRAs are safe and efficacious. The safety of their long-term use has not been established (Feren, Schweitzer, & Walsh, 2011). The BzRAs are Schedule IV controlled substances by federal regulation, have abuse and dependence potential, and produce withdrawal signs and symptoms after abrupt discontinuation. The risk for residual sedation on the day after using hypnotic medication is determined by the dose and rate of elimination (Riemann & Perlis, 2009). However, the FDA requires that the recommended dose for women using zolpidem (immediate release) be lowered from 10 to 5 mg and zolpidem CR be lowered from 12.5 to 6.25 mg.

Melatonin Receptor Agonist. Melatonin has been shown to shift circadian rhythm, decrease body temperature, alter reproductive rhythm, enhance immune function, and decrease alertness. Normally, levels of melatonin increase with decreasing exposure to light. Ramelteon (Rozerem), indicated for insomnia, is a melatonin receptor agonist with high affinity for melatonin receptors (MT_1 and MT_2). This activity is believed to be related to its sleep-promoting properties (Box 32.6). Ramelteon has a low abuse potential and is not a controlled substance (Feren et al., 2011).

Sedating Antidepressants. Sedating antidepressants have a potent effect on sleep and are used to treat many sleep problems. The most commonly used are trazodone, amitriptyline, and mirtazapine (Remeron, Soltab). The mechanism responsible for the sedating activity has not been identified, but it is unlikely that one mechanism is responsible for all three (Feren et al., 2011).

Over-the-Counter Medications and Supplements. OTC sleeping pills are usually antihistamines. The most common agents are doxylamine (Unisom) and diphenhydramine. These histamine-1 antagonists have a CNS effect that includes sedation, diminished alertness, and slowing of reaction time. These drugs also produce anticholinergic side effects, such as dry mouth, accelerated heart rate,

---

BOX 32.6

Drug Profile: **Ramelteon (Rozerem)**

DRUG CLASS: Sedative–hypnotic. It is readily absorbed and metabolized with median peak concentrations occurring 0.5 to 1.5 hours after fasted oral administration.

RECEPTOR AFFINITY: Ramelteon is a melatonin receptor agonist with high affinity for MT_1 and MT_2. No appreciable affinity for the GABA receptor complex.

INDICATION: Treatment of insomnia characterized by difficulty with sleep onset

ROUTES AND DOSING: The recommended dose is 8 mg. It should be taken at 30 minutes before bedtime. It should not be taken with or immediately after a high-fat meal. Patients should be advised to use caution if they consume alcohol in combination with ramelteon.

Adults: The recommended starting dose is 10 mg, with a maximum of 20 mg. An initial dose of 5 mg should be considered in adults with low body weight. Doses of over 20 mg have not been sufficiently studied.

Geriatric: No differences in safety or efficacy were observed between older and younger adults.

HALF-LIFE (PEAK PLASMA CONCENTRATION): 1 to 2.6 hours

SELECTED ADVERSE REACTIONS: Somnolence, dizziness, nausea, fatigue, headache, and insomnia

WARNINGS: Ramelteon should not be used by patients with severe hepatic impairment. It should not be used in combination with fluvoxamine.

GABA, gamma-aminobutyric acid.

---

urinary retention, and dilated pupils. Drowsiness lasts from 3 to 6 hours after a single dose. Next-morning hangover can be a problem. Diphenhydramine decreases sleep latency and improves quality of sleep for those with occasional sleep problems but is not as effective as benzodiazepines for chronic sleep disturbances (Feren et al., 2011).

Melatonin is a hormone, released from the pineal gland that aids in the regulation of the sleep–wake cycle through activation of MT_1 and MT_2 receptors. Exogenous melatonin has long been available OTC and has been shown to have mild sleep-promoting properties when given outside the period of usual secretion. That is, melatonin can advance the sleep–wake cycle making it easier to fall asleep earlier than usual. There is evidence that in young and older individuals with insomnia, melatonin can be beneficial in ameliorating the symptoms (Cortesi, Giannotti, Sebastiani, Panunzi, & Valente, 2012).

Valerian, a dietary supplement, is used as a medicinal herb in many cultures. The mechanism of action is not fully understood and is believed to inhibit GABA reuptake. Valerian may be useful for sleeplessness, but there is not enough evidence from double-blind studies to confirm this. Mild side effects include headaches, dizziness, upset stomach, and tiredness the morning after its use (National Center for Complementary and Alternative Medicine, 2012).

Administering and Monitoring Medication

Sleeping medications are commonly used in all settings. These medications are usually given nightly for a short period of time to establish a wake–sleep pattern. Rebound insomnia can occur if a drug is abruptly discontinued. This effect can be minimized or prevented by giving the lowest effective dose and tapering before discontinuing. Nurses should assess for confusion, memory problems, excessive sedation, and risk of falls.

Monitoring for Drug-to-Drug Interactions

Sleep medications generally have increased depressive effects when given with other CNS depressants. Because most sleep medications are metabolized by the CYP 3A family, drugs that inhibit or induce these enzymes have the potential to interact. Medications that inhibit 3A include oral contraceptives, isoniazid, fluvoxamine, and verapamil (see Chapter 11). Grapefruit juice should be avoided with these drugs. Ramelteon should not be given with fluvoxamine.

Teaching Points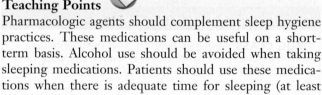

Pharmacologic agents should complement sleep hygiene practices. These medications can be useful on a short-term basis. Alcohol use should be avoided when taking sleeping medications. Patients should use these medications when there is adequate time for sleeping (at least 8 hours). Most sleep-related medications should be taken at bedtime. Patients should be instructed about the safe use of these medications and possible side effects.

Psychosocial Domain
Psychosocial Assessment

The assessment includes evaluating the behavioral and social factors related to sleep problems. Recent changes in relationships, particularly a divorce or death of a loved one, can significantly interfere with sleep. A recent move, travel, and addition of a new family member can impact sleep. Fatigue and stress increase when individuals assume the role of caregiver in their personal lives and in those with occupations as professional health care providers (Box 32.7). Shift work compromises the circadian rhythms and contributes to insomnia.

Nursing Diagnoses for the Psychosocial Domain

The obvious nursing diagnoses are sleep deprivation and Insomnia (as discussed earlier). However, there may be

BOX 32.7

Research For Best Practice: Sleep Quality of Nurses and Rotating Shifts

Chan, M. F. (2009). Factors associated with perceived sleep quality of nurses working on rotating shifts. *Journal of Clinical Nursing, 18(2)* 285–293.

THE QUESTION: Do nurses perceive that rotating shifts contribute to insufficient sleep quality?

METHODS: A cross-sectional study was conducted in two hospitals in Hong Kong. Nurses (*n* = 163) completed a self-reported questionnaire that included information on health status, strain and symptom levels, and perceived sleep quality.

FINDINGS: More than 70% of the nurses reported having insufficient sleep; older age, perceived poor sleep status, gastrointestinal symptoms, and higher strain and symptom levels were risk factors that contributed to insufficient sleep.

IMPLICATIONS FOR NURSING: Nurses, especially older nurses, who rotate shifts are at risk for sleep disorders and other health problems.

other important problem areas such as Social Isolation, Spiritual Distress, Relocation Stress Syndrome, Impaired Parenting, Caregiver Role Strain, and Grieving.

Interventions for the Psychosocial Domain

The nurse can help the patient develop bedtime rituals and good sleep hygiene. Bedtime should be at a regular hour, and the bedroom should be conducive to sleep. Preferably, the bedroom should not be where the individual watches television or does work-related activities. The bedroom should be viewed as a room for resting and sleep (see Box 32.4).

Behavioral Interventions

Behavioral interventions include stimulus control, sleep restriction, and relaxation therapy. **Stimulus control** is a technique used when the bedroom environment no longer provides cues for sleep but has become the cue for wakefulness. Patients are instructed to avoid behaviors in the bedroom incompatible with sleep, including watching television, doing homework, and eating. This allows the bedroom to be reestablished as a stimulus for sleep.

Another behavioral intervention is **sleep restriction**. Patients often increase their time in bed to provide more opportunity for sleep, resulting in fragmented sleep and irregular sleep schedules. Patients are instructed to spend less time in bed and avoid napping.

Relaxation training is used when patients complain of difficulty relaxing, especially if they are physically tense or emotionally distressed. A variety of procedures to reduce somatic arousal can be used, including progressive muscle relaxation, autogenic training, and biofeedback. Imagery training, meditation, and thought stopping are attention-focusing techniques that center on cognitive arousal (see Chapters 10 and 12).

Cognitive Behavioral Therapy

Cognitive behavioral (CBT) therapy is useful in changing negative learned responses that perpetuate the insomnia. This approach is especially helpful for those who also have comorbid depression or anxiety. The objective of CBT is to change the belief system that results in improvement of the self-efficacy of the individual. The objectives are accomplished through (1) identifying maladaptive behaviors and cognition that contribute to insomnia; (2) bringing the cognitive distortions to the patient's attention; (3) using behavioral approaches to extinguish the association between effort to sleep and increased arousal; (4) establishing a regular sleep–wake schedule, healthy sleep habits, and an environment conducive to sleep; and (5) continuing to use other psychological and behavioral techniques that diminish arousal and anxiety about sleep (Morin & Benca, 2012).

Patient Education

Education regarding interventions is crucial for patients with sleep disorders. An explanation of the sleep cycle and the factors that influence sleep are important for these patients. For those with insomnia, teaching about avoiding foods and beverages that interfere with sleep should be highlighted (Box 32.8).

BOX 32.8

Psychoeducation Checklist: Sleep Disorders

When teaching patients with sleep disorders, be sure to include the following topics:

- Maintenance of a sleep log
- Foods to avoid before going to bed
- Importance of developing a bedtime ritual and good sleep habits
- Use of sleep medications as prescribed
- Avoidance of caffeine and rigorous exercise within the 6 hours before bedtime
- Avoidance of cigarette smoking 1 hour before bedtime and during nighttime awakenings
- Allowing for 8 hours of sleep per night
- Maintenance of a regular sleep schedule, specifically a routine rise time
- An occasional "bad night" happens to nearly everyone
- Avoidance of alcohol because it disrupts sleep and is a poor hypnotic
- Daytime sleepiness as a symptom of sleep disorders
- How to do relaxation exercises
- Bedroom rituals
- Appropriate family support

Family Education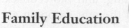

Family and friends should be encouraged to support the new habits the patient is trying to establish. Patients, spouses, and friends must understand that activities engaged in just before sleep can greatly affect sleep patterns and sleep difficulties, such as socializing, alcohol consumption, use of caffeine, and engaging in stimulating activities. Relaxing activities before bedtime are vital contributors to establishing a routine conducive to sleep. Family and friends can help create a positive environment with an emphasis on sleep as a priority.

Evaluation and Treatment Outcomes

The primary treatment outcome is establishing a normal sleep cycle. Changes in diet and behavior (e.g., initiation of an exercise program) should be evaluated for their impact on the individual's sleep. Environmental modifications, such as a change in the level of lighting in the bedroom, decreased stimulation (e.g., turning off cell phone or moving the television out of the bedroom), or modification in room temperature, can be monitored for any changes affecting the sleep cycle.

HYPERSOMNOLENCE DISORDER

The essential characteristic of hypersomnolence disorder is excessive sleepiness at least three times a week for at least 3 months (APA, 2013). Sleepiness occurs on an almost daily basis and causes significant impairment in social and occupational functioning. They have an excessive quantity of sleep, deteriorated quality of wakefulness, and sleep inertia (a period of impaired performance occurring during the sleep–wake transition characterized by confusion, ataxia, or combativeness) (APA, 2013). This diagnosis is reserved for individuals who have no other causes of daytime sleepiness (e.g., narcolepsy, OSA syndrome).

Clinical Course

People with hypersomnolence typically sleep 8 to 12 hours per night. They fall asleep easily and sleep through the night, often having difficulty awakening in the morning. They often have difficulty meeting morning obligations. They exhibit poor concentration and memory. Excessive sleepiness may not be impacted by napping because they may awaken from a nap feeling unrefreshed. They may even describe dangerous situations, such as being sleepy while driving or operating heavy machinery.

Diagnosis

On the day after overnight polysomnography, a multiple sleep latency test (MSLT) may be used. The **multiple sleep latency test (MSLT)** is a standardized procedure that measures sleep variables during a 20-minute period. The process is repeated every 2 hours, occurring approximately five times during the day (Pataka, Yoon, Poddar, & Riha, 2013). The faster a person falls asleep during testing, the greater the physiologic sleep tendency. Polysomnography shows short sleep latency, a normal to long sleep duration, and normal sleep architecture. Subjective symptoms of sleepiness are recognized as heavy eyelids, loss of initiative, reluctance to move, and yawning or slowed speech. Sleepiness is unique to the person and situation, varying from mild to severe.

Nursing Management

Nursing assessment for the patient with hypersomnolence focuses on excessive sleepiness. The following are examples of assessment questions.

- Have you ever nodded off unintentionally?
- When did your sleepiness begin?
- Does anyone in your family experience the same sleepiness symptoms?
- Do you suddenly find yourself awakening feeling refreshed?

Interventions stress the importance of sleep hygiene and helping the patient establish normal sleep patterns. If medications are given, the most commonly prescribed stimulants for treating excessive daytime sleepiness are dextroamphetamine and amphetamine mixtures (Adderall), modafinil (Provigil), methylphenidate (Ritalin, Concerta), and pemoline (Cylert). These agents increase the patient's ability to stay awake and perform. Abuse of these medications should be assessed. In some cases, serotonin antagonists are used off label.

Sleepy people often self-medicate with caffeine. A cup of brewed coffee contains about 100 to 150 mg of caffeine. A 12-oz can of Mountain Dew contains 54 mg of caffeine. Caffeine contents of popular "energy" drinks range from 80 to 300 mg. Peak plasma concentration is reached 30 to 60 minutes after consumption, and the duration of effect is 3 to 5 hours in adults. Caffeine improves psychomotor performance, particularly tasks involving endurance, vigilance, and attention. High doses, especially in people who are not habitual users, may exhibit side effects such as irritability and anxiety.

NARCOLEPSY

The overwhelming urge to sleep is the primary symptom of narcolepsy. This irresistible urge to sleep occurs at any

Clinical Vignette

BOX 32.9

IS IT SLEEPINESS OR NARCOLEPSY?

Jill is a 27-year-old college student and single mother of two young children, ages 5 and 3 years. Jill had difficulty staying awake during school. She attributed this problem to "boring teachers" and dropped out of school when she was a junior. She has recently returned to college. Although she enjoys her studies, she continues to fall asleep during her classes. She gets about 6 hours of sleep each night on average. In the past 2 months, her tendency to nod off is more frequent. She has had a couple of frightening episodes at bedtime, seeing things dance around her bed and not being able to move. She recalls an incident of laughing at a great joke and then feeling as if her face was drooping.

What Do You Think?
- Which symptoms of narcolepsy does Jill have?
- If Jill increases her nighttime sleep, will her symptoms improve?
- What approaches will help Jill with controlling her daytime sleepiness?

time of the day, regardless of the amount of sleep. Falling asleep often occurs in inappropriate situations, such as while driving a car or reading a newspaper. These sleep episodes are usually short, lasting 5 to 20 minutes, but may last up to an hour if sleep is not interrupted. Individuals with narcolepsy may experience sleep attacks and report frequent dreaming. They usually feel alert after a sleep attack, only to fall asleep unintentionally again several hours later (Box 32.9).

Clinical Course

Narcolepsy is a chronic disorder that usually begins in young adulthood between the ages of 15 and 35 years. Excessive sleepiness is the first symptom to appear. The severity of sleepiness may remain stable over the lifetime. Narcolepsy has no cure. Treatment is designed to control symptoms based on clinical presentation and severity. A secondary sleep disorder should be considered if the level of sleepiness changes.

Narcolepsy is distinguished by a group of symptoms, including daytime sleepiness, cataplexy, hypnagogic hallucinations, and sleep paralysis. The symptom of daytime sleepiness is found in all individuals with narcolepsy, but existence of the other three symptoms varies (see Box 32.9).

- **Cataplexy** is the bilateral loss of muscle tone triggered by a strong emotion, such as anger or laughter. This muscle atonia can range from subtle (drooping eyelids) to dramatic (buckling knees). Respiratory muscles are

not affected. Cataplexy usually lasts for seconds. Individuals are fully conscious, oriented, and alert during the episode. Prolonged episodes of cataplexy may lead to unintentional sleep episodes. The frequency and severity of events generally increase when the individual is sleep deprived.

- **Hypnagogic hallucinations** are intense dreamlike images that occur at sleep onset and usually involve the current environment. Hallucinations can be visual or auditory, such as hearing one's name called or a door slammed.

- **Sleep paralysis**, the inability to move or speak when falling asleep or waking up, is often described as terrifying and is accompanied by a sensation of struggling to move or speak. Although the diaphragm is not involved, patients may also complain of not being able to breathe or feeling suffocated. These episodes are typically brief in duration and usually terminate spontaneously or when the individual is touched.

Diagnosis

Excessive daytime sleepiness and the presence of cataplexy are diagnostic of narcolepsy. It is possible to have narcolepsy without cataplexy. The diagnosis should be confirmed by polysomnogram demonstrating at least 6 hours of sleep followed by the MSLT showing a sleep latency of less than or equal to 8 minutes and two or more sleep-onset REM periods. The diagnosis can also be confirmed by a cerebrospinal fluid hypocretin-1 level less than or equal to 110 pg/mL (Ahmed & Thorpy, 2010).

Epidemiology and Etiology

Narcolepsy is found in about one in 2,000 people in the United States (Ahmed & Thorpy, 2010). The cause of narcolepsy involves a deficiency of hypocretin, a hypothalamic peptide that may be linked to chromosome 6 in the class II human leukocyte antigen (Cao & Guilleminault, 2011; Han et al., 2010). Hypocretin neurons are part of the neurologic system that wakes and maintains wakefulness. Injury to the CNS or immunologic factors may also play a part in the development of narcolepsy.

Nursing Management

Nursing assessment is similar to that for insomnia. In general, sleepiness is treated with CNS stimulants. Methylphenidate, dextroamphetamine, modafinil, and pemoline are the most frequently prescribed stimulants. Cataplexy may be treated with tricyclic antidepressants because these drugs suppress REM. Sodium oxybate (Xyrem), classified as a Schedule II drug is indicated for excessive sleepiness and cataplexy. Because of its high abuse potential, patients who are prescribed this medication are closely monitored (Alshaikh, Gucuan, George, Sharif, & Bahamman, 2011).

Patient education focuses on factors that can make symptoms worse, such as sleep deprivation. Patients need to develop strategies to manage symptoms. Naps can be integrated into their daily routines such as during work breaks or before engaging in activities that require sustaining alertness.

BREATHING-RELATED DISORDERS

The *DSM-5* identifies three breathing disorders including obstructive sleep apnea–hypopnea, central sleep apnea, and sleep-related hypoventilation. This section will discuss obstructive sleep apnea–hypopnea disorder (obstructive sleep apnea syndrome) (APA, 2013). The term obstructive sleep apnea (OSA) syndrome is more commonly used in nonpsychiatric areas and will be used in this section instead of the term obstructive apnea–hypopnea disorder. Central sleep apnea and sleep-related hypoventilation will not be discussed.

OBSTRUCTIVE SLEEP APNEA SYNDROME

Obstructive sleep apnea (OSA) syndrome, the most commonly diagnosed breathing-related sleep disorder, may affect up to 20% of the U.S. adults (Santarnecchi et al., 2013). OSA is characterized by snoring during sleep and episodes of sleep apnea (cessation of breathing) that disrupt sleep and contribute to daytime sleepiness. The hallmark symptoms are snoring and daytime sleepiness. Often, snoring is so loud and disturbing that partners choose separate bedrooms for sleeping. Approximately 50% of the U.S. population snores (Ram, Seirawan, Kuma, & Clark, 2009).

Clinical Course

Apneic episodes, which last from 10 seconds up to several minutes, cause restless sleep and abrupt awakenings with feelings of choking or falling out of bed; some people even leap out of bed to restore breathing. The person does not later recall the awakening. These brief awakenings deprive essential sleep, resulting in excessive daytime sleepiness that may reach the same degree of pathologic sleepiness found in narcolepsy. Unlike narcolepsy, naps tend to be unrefreshing.

Esophageal reflux, or heartburn, is a common complaint. Genitourinary symptoms include nocturia (three to seven trips to the bathroom), nocturnal enuresis, and erectile dysfunction. Bradycardia in association with tachycardia is often seen with apneic events. Other cardiac arrhythmias are also seen, including sinus arrest. The onset of

symptoms and sleepiness may coincide with weight gain. About two thirds of apnea patients are overweight or obese (20% over ideal body weight) (American Sleep Apnea Association, 2014).

Diagnosis

Polysomnography, usually performed at night during sleep, monitors many body functions, including brain wave activity, eye movements, muscle activity, heart rhythm, breathing function, and respiratory effort (Figure 32.7). Polysomnography may show poor sleep continuity, increased stage 1 and decreased slow-wave and REM sleep, and an increased amount of EEG alpha wave activity while the individual is asleep. Clinical evaluation includes oral and nasal airflow, respiratory effort, oxyhemoglobin saturation, and electromyogram of limb muscle activity. Typically, patients with OSA demonstrate numerous respiratory events per night during polysomnographic measurement.

Epidemiology and Risk Factors

Incidence of OSA increases with age, especially for those older than 50 years of age (Nasr, Wendt, & Kora, 2010), affecting both men and women. OSA is most common in

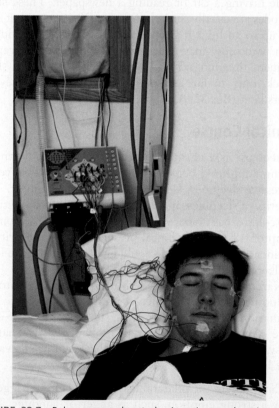

FIGURE 32.7 Polysomnography study. A patient undergoing polysomnography has electrodes affixed or taped to the scalp, face, chest, and legs. (Photo by Hank Morgan/Photo Researchers, Inc.)

middle-aged overweight men. The female-to-male ratio is estimated to be 1:8, with women becoming more likely to develop this syndrome after menopause. Men are twice as likely to snore as women (APA, 2013).

Ethnic and racial differences in sleep disturbances have been suggested. African Americans and Hispanics have an increased frequency of snoring as compared to whites, but the increase may be related to poorer physical health (Baldwin et al., 2010). Individuals who drive and are diagnosed with OSA have an increased risk (two to three times more likely) of involvement in motor vehicle crashes (Tregear, Reston, Schoelles, & Phillips, 2009). OSA is a risk factor for cardiac and cerebrovascular events (Gottlieb et al., 2010). OSA is more prevalent in people with mental health disorders than in the general population. Depression, anxiety, PTSD, and bipolar disorder are associated with OSA. The symptoms of depression such as fatigue, irritability, depressed mood, and poor concentration are similar to the symptoms of OSA. Depressive symptoms have been shown to decrease once OSA is successfully treated (Nasr et al., 2010).

Etiology

An obstruction or collapse of the airway causes apnea, or cessation of breathing. In most cases, the site of obstruction is in the pharyngeal area. Vibrations of the soft, pliable tissues found in the pharyngeal airway cause the snoring sounds that occur during breathing.

Interdisciplinary Treatment

There are nonsurgical and surgical options for the treatment of patients with OSA. Nonsurgical options vary based on the severity of the obstructive breathing. For obese patients with less severe OSA, weight loss may help. For others whose apnea is mild, changing sleeping position from supine to lateral can help control the severity of OSA. There has also been some effort in devising an oral appliance to reduce snoring and the occurrence of apnea. Currently, the most effective nonsurgical treatment is continuous positive airway pressure. This treatment takes place during sleep and involves wearing a nose mask that is connected by a long tube to an air compressor. Airway patency is maintained with air pressure. Although this method of treatment is highly effective, compliance can be a problem (Galetke, Puzzo, Priegnitz, Anduleit, & Randerath, 2011).

The most commonly performed surgical procedure to treat patients with OSA is uvulopalatopharyngoplasty. This procedure involves the removal of redundant soft palate tissue, uvula, and tonsillar pillars. The surgery usually eliminates snoring and is judged to be about 50% effective in reducing the amount of sleep apnea (Schendel, Powell, & Jacobson, 2011).

CIRCADIAN RHYTHM SLEEP DISORDER

The chief feature of a circadian rhythm sleep disorder is the mismatch between the individual's internal sleep–wake circadian rhythm and the timing and duration of sleep (Dodson & Zee, 2010). People with these disorders complain of insomnia at particular times during the day and excessive sleepiness at others. This diagnosis is reserved for those individuals who present with marked sleep disturbance or significant social or occupational impairment (Box 32.10).

BOX 32.10
Clinical Vignette
PSYCHIATRIC MISDIAGNOSIS IN TEENAGER

A 14-year-old adolescent was referred for evaluation for a complaint of daytime sleepiness. Before the referral, this patient had difficulties in functioning for 4 years. Conflicts with parents, teachers, and peers were noted. He was described by a licensed child psychologist as "extremely introverted with severe narcissistic traits, poverty of thought with persecutory content, and self-destruction that led to a paralyzing anxiety, anhedonia, social isolation and withdrawal." An assessment of his learning abilities showed difficulties with written language and poor memory. He also had above-average abilities in verbal comprehension and abstract reasoning. After dropping out of school at age 12 years, he was sent to an inpatient child psychiatry center. After 3 months of evaluation, he was diagnosed as having atypical depressive disorder with possible schizotypal personality.

The patient underwent polysomnography. No primary sleep disorders were found. Three weeks of monitoring with a wrist actigraph (a device that differentiates sleep and waking) suggested a circadian rhythm disorder. Oral temperature and melatonin secretion levels were measured during a 24-hour period and revealed desynchronization of the temperature and melatonin rhythms. Treatment was begun with oral melatonin (5 mg at 8 PM). Follow-up actigraphy after 6 months showed the patient to be fully entrained to the normal 24-hour cycle. The patient returned to school. After one semester, the patient showed excellent grades. His parents reported improvement in his relationship with family and peers. Evaluation by licensed psychiatrists found no evidence of psychopathology; none of the previously described diagnoses were present (Dagan & Ayalon, 2005).

What Do You Think?
- What symptoms of circadian rhythm sleep disorder did the patient experience?
- How did melatonin improve the patient's sleep cycle?

Diagnosis and Clinical Course

The *DSM-5* identifies a broad group of subtypes, including the following (APA, 2013).

- *Delayed sleep phase type:* Individuals with delayed sleep phase type, or "night owls," tend to be unable to fall asleep before 2 to 6 AM; hence, their whole sleep patterns shift, and they have difficulty rising in the morning.
- *Advanced sleep phase type:* Opposite of the night owls, these individuals are "larks" or earlier risers. They are unable to stay awake in the evening and consistently wake up early.
- *Irregular sleep–wake type:* People with this type have a temporarily disorganized sleep pattern that varies in a 24-hour period.
- *Non-24-hour sleep–wake type:* Individuals with this type have an abnormal synchronization between the 24 hour light–dark cycle and their endogenous circadian rhythm which leads to periods of insomnia, excessive sleepiness, or both. This type is most common among blind or visually impaired individuals.
- *Shift work type:* The endogenous sleep–wake cycle is normal but is mismatched to the imposed hours of shift work. Rotating shift schedules are disruptive because any consistent adjustment is prevented. Compared with day and evening shift workers, night and rotating shift workers have a shorter sleep duration and poorer quality of sleep. They may also be sleepier while performing their jobs. This disorder is further exacerbated by insufficient daytime sleep resulting from social and family demands and environmental disturbances (traffic noise, telephone). Because of the job requirements of the profession, nurses often experience this disorder. Furthermore, 20% of the U.S. work force is engaged in shift work and thereby at risk for circadian rhythm disorders.

One of the circadian rhythm sleep–wake disorders not included in the *DSM-5* is the *jet lag type* that occurs after travel across time zones, particularly in coast-to-coast and international travel. The normal endogenous circadian sleep–wake cycle does not match the desired hours of sleep and wakefulness in a new time zone. Individuals traveling eastward are more prone to jet lag because it involves resetting one's circadian clock to an earlier time—it is easier to delay the endogenous clock to a later time period than adjust it to an earlier one.

Epidemiology and Etiology

There are no data regarding the prevalence of circadian rhythm disorders in the general population. The prevalence of circadian rhythm disorders among patients diagnosed at sleep disorder centers accounts for 2% or less of the total patients diagnosed. However, this is a gross underestimate given that jet lag, a circadian rhythm disorder, affects nearly everyone traveling over three time zones.

Circadian rhythm disorders are caused by the dissociation of the internal circadian pacemaker and conventional time. The cause might be intrinsic, such as genetic factors called "clock genes" (Dodson & Zee, 2010), or extrinsic, as in jet lag and shift work. Each results in overwhelming daytime sleepiness and overflowing wakefulness at night.

Interdisciplinary Treatment

The goals of treatment of circadian rhythm disorder are to strengthen timed clues (when to go to sleep), adequately timed bright light (stay awake during the day), and adequately time exogenous melatonin (initiate melatonin secretion at bedtime). Melatonin is often helpful in initiating sleep (Keijzer, Smits, Duffy, & Curgs, 2013). Chronotherapy manipulates the sleep schedule by progressively delaying bedtime until an acceptable bedtime is attained.

Chronopharmacotherapy resets the biologic clock by using short-acting hypnotics to induce sleep. Small amounts of hypnotics can produce high-quality sleep in people who wish to reset their circadian schedules after long transmeridian flights. Conversely, for night shift workers, caffeine taken while working at night improves alertness and performance. However, caffeine should be used judiciously by night shift workers because they become quickly tolerant to the effects after a few nights. **Luminotherapy** (light therapy) is used to manipulate the circadian system. Commercially prepared light boxes produce therapeutic light at 2,500 to 10,000 lux. In contrast, indoor light is about 150 lux.

PARASOMNIAS

Parasomnias are sleep–wake disorders that occur in association with sleep, specific sleep stages, or sleep–wake transitions. They are characterized by abnormal behavioral, experiential, or physiologic events (APA, 2013). Non–rapid eye movement (NREM) sleep arousal disorders including sleepwalking and sleep terror types, usually occur the first third of the major sleep episode. Nightmare disorder is a rapid eye movement (REM) disorder that generally occurs during the second half of the major sleep episode (APA, 2013). RLS is considered a sleep disorder and is classified as a parasomnia.

SLEEP TERRORS AND SLEEPWALKING

In *sleep terrors* (also called night terrors or *pavor nocturnes*), there are episodes of screaming, fear, and panic, causing clinical distress or impairing social, occupational, or other areas of functioning. Sleep terrors usually last 1 to

10 minutes, are frightening to the person and to anyone witnessing them. Often, individuals abruptly sit up in bed screaming; others have been known to jump out of bed and run across the room. Other symptoms include a rapid heart rate and breathing, dilated pupils, and flushed skin. Usually, the person having a sleep terror is inconsolable and difficult to awaken completely. Efforts to awaken the individual may prolong the episode. Once awake, most are unable to recall the dream or event that precipitated such a response. A few report a fragmentary image. Often, the individual does not fully awaken and cannot recall the episode the next morning (Carter, Hathaway, & Lettieri, 2014).

In *sleepwalking* or somnambulism, there are repeated episodes of complex motor behavior during sleep that may involve getting out of bed and walking around. While sleepwalking, people typically have a blank stare and are difficult to awaken. Often, they awaken to find themselves in a different place from where they went to sleep. If awakened during the episode, there is a brief period of confusion.

Clinical Course

Polysomnography shows that these disorders usually begin when slow-wave NREM sleep predominate during the first third of the night. They rarely occur during daytime naps.

Epidemiology and Etiology

The prevalence of sleep terrors is estimated 6.5% in children and 2.2% in adults. Males and females are affected equally. The prevalence of sleepwalking is 17% in children and 4% in adults. Sleepwalking peaks between 8 and 12 years of age and is more common in males. (Carter et al., 2014). Fever, stress, and sleep deprivation can increase the frequency of episodes. There appears to be some genetic predisposition for disorders of arousal, and they tend to run in families.

Interdisciplinary Treatment

Learning about parasomnias and the need for safety precautions for patient and family should be the focus of patient education (Box 32.11). Hypnosis supplemented by psychotherapy may be considered. Treatment might also include medications, such as benzodiazepines. These disorders usually resolve by adolescence.

Nursing Management

Although polysomnography may be used to diagnose or confirm a sleep disorder, the evaluation of a response to a NREM disorder involves a careful sleep history. Episodes

---

BOX 32.11

General Safety Precautions for Sleepwalkers and Their Families

- Ensure adequate sleep. The occurrence of sleepwalking dramatically increases after sleep loss.
- Anticipate sleepwalking when there is a significant sleep loss. Family members should be aware of the likelihood of sleepwalking for the first 2 to 3 hours after the sleepwalker goes to bed.
- Keep a sleep log to assist in identifying how much sleep is needed to prevent a sleepwalking event.
- Consider use of a noise devices on the door of the sleepwalker's room to alert others that the sleepwalker is up.
- Deadbolt locks should be installed on doors leading outside. Windows should be secured to limit their opening.
- When the sleepwalker is spending the night away from home, alert appropriate individuals to the possibility that sleepwalking may occur. Ensure adequate sleep on the preceding nights.

---

of sleep terrors or sleepwalking are often unrealized by the patient but can be described in detail by the parent or partner. Family members may clarify the degree of sleepiness that the patient may want to deny. Sleep diaries should focus on the person's bedtime activities, time of sleep onset and wake up, time to prepare for bed and fall asleep, use of medications, number of awakenings, subjective assessment of quality of sleep, and daytime naps (Porth, 2010).

Nursing interventions range from referring to sleep specialists to patient education about the disorder and strategies in dealing with the disorder. In some instances, nurses care for patients in the inpatient setting who have arousal disorders. In these instances, nurses should develop care plans that address the individual patient's needs. In instances of sleepwalking, staff should be alert to the safety issues and protect the patient from injury.

NIGHTMARE DISORDER

The repeated occurrence of frightening dreams that fully awaken an individual is the essential characteristic of nightmare disorder. Typically, the individual can recall detailed dream content that involves physical danger (e.g., attack or pursuit) or perceived danger (e.g., embarrassment or failure). On awakening, the individual is fully alert and experiences a persisting sense of anxiety or fear. Many people have difficulty returning to sleep. Multiple same-night nightmares may be reported. Some people avoid sleep because of their fear of nightmares. Consequently, people may report that excessive sleepiness, poor concentration, and irritability disrupt their daytime activities. The occurrence of nightmares may be more serious than previously suspected. Nightmares are commonly experienced by military combat personnel who have PTSD (see Chapter 26).

Nightmares are commonly experienced by military combat personnel who have PTSD (see Chapter 26).

Diagnosis and Clinical Course

Nightmares occur in REM sleep almost exclusively. They most often occur during the second half of the night when REM sleep dominates. Polysomnography demonstrates abrupt awakenings from REM sleep. In most cases, the REM sleep episode lasts for at least 10 minutes. Tachycardia and tachypnea may be evident.

Etiology and Epidemiology

The cause and prevalence of nightmares is unknown. Intriguing evidence provokes a debate as to whether nightmares are a symptom or an adaptive reaction to pathophysiologic factors. Negative emotions, primarily fear, are the most common dream emotions. Brain imaging demonstrates increased metabolic activity during REM sleep in the most primitive regions of the brain, the paralimbic and limbic regions. Many classes of drugs trigger nightmares, including catecholaminergic agents, beta-blockers, some antidepressants, barbiturates, and alcohol. Additionally, withdrawal from barbiturates and alcohol causes REM rebound and more vivid dreaming.

Nightmares often begin in children between the ages of 3 and 6 years, and most children outgrow them. In adults, at least 50% of the population reports occasional nightmares. Women are more likely to report nightmares than men.

Interdisciplinary Treatment

If the nightmares cause significant distress, a person will be treated by multiple providers. Traditionally, psychotherapy aimed at conflict resolution has been the treatment of choice. Today CBT is recommended, specifically **imagery rehearsal therapy**, a technique in which patients change the endings of the nightmares while they are awake. After rehearsing new, nonthreatening images and changing the content of the nightmare while awake, a reduction in the frequency of nightmares and associated distress has been shown (Berlin, Means, & Edinger, 2010). Pharmacologically, the best studied and most effective medication to treat nightmares with PTSD is prazosin (Minipress), a centrally active α1-adrenergic antagonist indicated for hypertension (Raskind et al., 2013). It does not have FDA approval for use with nightmares, but prazosin is recommended by the Standards of Practice Committee of the American Academy of Sleep Medicine for PTSD-associated nightmares (Aurora et al., 2010).

Nursing Management

While caring for patients with other disorders, the nurse often is the first health professional to identify nightmares as a problem in a patient. Sleep assessment is vital in every nursing assessment. If nightmares are causing distress, a referral for a sleep evaluation should be made. Sleep hygiene techniques and education about the treatment of nightmares should be included in patient teaching. During hospitalization, the nurse should document that the patient has nightmares and the nurses on the night shift should monitor for them.

RESTLESS LEGS SYNDROME

Restless legs syndrome (RLS) is a sleep–wake disorder characterized by an urge to move the legs which begins or worsens at rest or periods of inactivity, typically in the evening or at night. The urge to move legs is reduced or relieved by movement (APA, 2013).

Diagnostic Criteria and Clinical Course

RLS is a sensorimotor, neurologic disorder described as the intense desire to move legs accompanied by uncomfortable sensations such as creeping, crawling, tingling, burning, or itching (APA, 2013). The diagnosis is made on the basis on self-report. These symptoms can interfere with sleep and cause considerable clinical distress or functional impairment. RLS is usually diagnosed in the second and third decade of life and can get progressively worse later in life.

Epidemiology and Etiology

Prevalence of RLS in the adult general population ranges between 5% to 8% with at least half of the cases reported having infrequent and/or mild RLS. The prevalence is about twice higher in women than in men and increases with age in North America and Europe, but not observed in Asian countries. Comorbid conditions of insomnia, excessive sleepiness, and depressive and/or anxiety symptoms are consistently associated with RLS. RLS is the most common movement disorder occurring during pregnancy, usually developing in the third trimester, but disappearing with the first month after delivery (Ohayon, O'Hara, & Vitiello, 2012).

The etiology of RLS remains unclear, but genetic predisposition, dopaminergic dysfunction, and deficiencies in iron metabolism partially explain the underlying causes. RLS is linked to cardiovascular disease and metabolic syndrome (diabetes, obesity, hypertension, and dyslipidemia) (Innes, Selfe, & Agarwal, 2012). There is emerging evidence that suggests inflammation and/or immunologic disorders have a role in RLS. Recent studies show an increased prevalence of small intestinal bacterial overgrowth, HIV infection, systemic lupus erythematosus, and cases of hepatitis C (Weinstock, Walters, & Paueksakon, 2012).

Interdisciplinary Treatment

The treatment of RLS involves a biopsychosocial approach using pharmacologic and nonpharmacologic treatment options. In cases of mild and intermittent RLS, behavioral therapy, sleep hygiene, and lifestyle interventions (avoiding caffeine, alcohol, heavy meals) help reduce the likelihood of having an episode. For more severe symptoms, medications are prescribed such as L-dopa to increase dopaminergic function. If these medications are not well tolerated or lose their effectiveness, other medication may be substituted such as gabapentin enacarbil, pregabalin, opioids, and benzodiazepines. New medications are currently under development (de Biase, Merlino, Lorenzut, Valente, & Gigli, 2014.)

Nursing Management

A thorough nursing assessment will provide direction for the nursing management of a person with RLS. In many instances there are underlying medical conditions such as diabetes or peripheral neuropathy that contribute to the severity of RLS, particularly for the older adult. If the underlying medical condition is being treated adequately, the patient can be encouraged to engage in moderate regular physical activity 3 days a week or taking a hot bath before going to sleep. If medication is prescribed, the patient and family will benefit from medication education. Sleep hygiene education may be appropriate if RLS is interfering with sleep (Townsend-Roccichelli, Sandford, & VandeWaa, 2010).

SUMMARY OF KEY POINTS

- The normal sleep–wake cycle runs in a pattern called circadian rhythm. Most body systems follow a circadian rhythm and are often associated with the sleep–wake cycle. Hormones, such as melatonin and cortisol, help promote wakefulness during the day and sleepiness at night.
- Polysomnography is clinical testing used to assess for sleep disorders. Results of polysomnography describe a person's sleep architecture (timing and distribution of sleep stages) and any abnormalities occurring during sleep.
- Assessment is key. Information should focus on a comprehensive sleep history, including specific details of the sleep complaint, current sleep patterns, and sleep patterns before sleep difficulties, medical problems, current medications, current life events, and emotional and mental status.
- Nursing interventions for sleep disorders focus on nonpharmacologic approaches such as exercise, nutrition, activity, thermoregulation, and pharmacologic interventions.
- Psychosocial nursing interventions for sleep disorders include educating patients about good sleep habits, instructing patients in relaxation exercises and sleep-promoting activities, providing patients with nutritional suggestions regarding foods and substances to avoid, and educating family members and friends regarding the importance of supporting the need for making quality sleep a priority.
- Insomnia disorder is characterized by difficulty falling asleep or difficulty maintaining sleep. Insomnia is often precipitated by feelings of stress or tension, with associations and behaviors persisting after the crisis or stressful situation has passed.
- Obstructive sleep apnea syndrome is a diagnosed breathing-related sleep disorder characterized by excessive snoring and episodes of apnea (cessation of breathing). These episodes disrupt sleep and may cause daytime sleepiness.
- In circadian rhythm sleep–wake disorders there is a mismatch between the individual's internal sleep–wake circadian rhythm and the timing and duration of sleep.
- Parasomnias occur in association with sleep, specific sleep stages, or sleep–wake transitions and include sleepwalking, sleep terrors, nightmare disorders, and restless legs syndrome. They are characterized by abnormal behavioral, experiential, or physiologic events. The etiology is unknown but appears to be of genetic predisposition. Unrestorative sleep, excessive sleepiness, poor concentration, and irritability are often the result.

CRITICAL THINKING CHALLENGES

1. Discuss the relationship of sleep and circadian rhythm.
2. Identify the stages of sleep and briefly describe each stage.
3. What is sleep architecture, and how does it change as we age?
4. Compare and contrast the experiences of an individual with insomnia and one with hypersomnolence.
5. How does narcolepsy differ from others that experience excessive sleepiness?

6. A 55-year-old truck driver presents reporting excessive daytime sleepiness. Develop a list of assessment questions that could be used to investigate his chief complaint.

7. Outline nursing interventions and educational highlights for the parents of a 12-year-old diagnosed with sleepwalking disorder.

The Cabinet of Dr. Caligari: 1919. This is the first of many movies suggesting that mental health professionals are odd. In this film, the director of an asylum becomes a part of a patient's delusion. The content of the delusion involves Dr. Caligari hypnotizing a sleepwalker, who then murders another man.

VIEWING POINTS: When did you realize that Dr. Caligari was not directing the murders? Is there doubt at the end of the movie as to the innocence of Dr. Caligari? Is it realistic that crimes can be committed during periods of sleepwalking?

Insomnia: 1997. This movie is a compelling thriller that occurs in a state of perpetual light. The setting is north of the Arctic Circle in the middle of summer, where it is daylight 24 hours a day. Jonas Engstrom (Stellan Skarsgard) and Erik Vik (Sverre Anker Ousdal) are cops from Oslo brought into a small town to help with a murder investigation. Things go wrong, and Engstrom finds himself trapped in a web of deceit. His guilty conscience and the never-ending light keep him awake at night, and the lack of sleep makes him increasingly desperate and prone to error.

VIEWING POINTS: How did the lack of sleep impact Engstrom's ability to make sound decisions? If the setting of this movie were in an area that had normal nighttime darkness, would the outcome have been different? If you were conducting a sleep assessment, what nursing diagnosis would be generated from the data?

References

Adenekan, B., Pandey, A., McKenzie, S., Zizi, F., Casimir, G.H., & Jean Louis, G. (2013). Sleep in America: role of racial/ethnic differences. *Sleep Medicine Reviews. 17*(4), 255–262.

Ahmed, I. & Thorpy, M. (2010). Clinical features, diagnosis and treatment of narcolepsy. *Clinics in Chest Medicine, 31*(2), 371–381.

Alshaikh, M. D., Gucuan, D., George, S., Sharif, M., & Bahamman, A. S. (2011). Long-term follow up of patients with narcolepsy-cataplexy treated with sodium oxybate. *Clinical Neurophramacology, 34*(1), 1–4.

American Psychiatric Association. (2013). *Diagnostic and statistical manual of mental disorders* (5th ed.) Arlington, VA: American Psychiatric Association.

American Sleep Apnea Association. (2014). OSA treatment options. www.sleepapnea.org/treat/treatment-options.html.

Arora, T., Broglia, E., Pushpakumar, D., Lodhi, T., & Taheri, S. (2013). An investigation into the strength of the association and agreement levels between subjective and objective sleep duration in adolescents. *PLoS ONE, 8*(8), E72406.

Aurora, R. N., Zak, R. S., Auerbach, S. H., Casey, K. R., Chowdhuri, S., Karippot, A., et al. (2010). Best practice guide for the treatment of nightmare disorder in adults. *Journal of Clinical Sleep Medicine, 6*(4), 389–396.

Baker, F. C. & Colrain, I. M. (2010). Daytime sleepiness, psychomotor performance, waking EEG spectra and evoked potentials in women with severe premenstural syndrome. *Journal of Sleep Research, 19*(1 Pt2), 214–227.

Baldwin, C. M., Ervin, A., Mays, M. Z., Robbins, J., Shafazand, S., Walsleben, J., et al. (2010). Sleep disturbances, quality of life, and ethnicity: The sleep heart health study. *Journal of Clinical Sleep Medicine, 6*(2), 176–183.

Berlin, K. L., Means, M. K., & Edinger, J. D. (2010). Nightmare reduction in a Vietnam veteran using imagery rehearsal therapy. *Journal of Clinical Sleep Medicine, 6*(5), 487–488.

Cao, M. & Guilleminault, D. (2011). Hypocretin and its emerging role as a target for treatment of sleep disorders. *Current Neurology & Neuroscience Reports, 11*(2), 227–234.

Carter, K. A., Hathaway, N. E., & Lettieri, C. F. (2014). Common sleep disorders in children. *American Family Physician, 89*(5), 368–377.

Centers for Disease Control and Prevention. (2012). Short sleep duration among workers–United States, 2010. *Morbidity and Mortality Weekly Report, 61*(16), 281–285.

Cortesi, F., Giannotti, F., Sebastiani, T., Panunzi, S., & Valente, D. (2012). Controlled-released melatonin, singly and combined with cognitive behavioral therapy, for persistent insomnia in children with autism spectrum disorders: A randomized placebo-controlled trial. *Journal of Sleep Research, 21*(6), 700–709.

Costa, I. C., Carvalho, H. N., & Fernandes, L. (2013). Aging, circadian rhythms and depressive disorders: A review. *American Journal of Neurodegenerative Disease, 2*(4), 228–246.

Dagan, Y. & Ayalon, L. (2005). Case study: Psychiatric misdiagnosis of non-24-hours-sleep-wake schedule disorder resolved by melatonin. *Journal of American Academy of Child and Adolescent Psychiatry, 44*(12), 1271–1275.

de Biase, S., Merlino, G., Lorenzut, S., Valent, M., & Gigli, G.L. (2014). Investigational approaches to therapies for restless legs syndrome. *Expert Opinion, 23*(6), 847–856. foi:10.1517/13543784.2014.907793

Dodson, E. R. & Zee, P. C. (2010). Therapeutics for circadian rhythm sleep disorders. *Sleep Medicine Clinics, 5*(4), 701–715.

Feren, S., Schweitzer, P., & Walsh, J. (2011). Pharmacotherapy for insomnia. In P. J. Vinken & G. W. Bruyn (Eds.). *Handbook of clinical neurology* (pp. 747–762).

Galetke, W., Puzzo, L., Priegnitz, C., Anduleit, N., & Randerath, W.J. (2011). Long-term therapy with continuous positive airway pressure in obstructive sleep apnea: Adherence, side effects and predictors of withdrawal - a "real-life" study. *Respiration, 82*(2), 155–61. doi:10.1159/00032283

Glozier, N., O'Dea, B., McGorry, P. D., Pantelis, C., Amminger, G. P., Hermens, D. F., et al. (2014). Delayed sleep onset in depressed young people. *BMC Psychiatry. 14*, 33. www.biomedcentral.com/1471–244X/1433.

Gottlieb, D. J., Yenokyan, G., Newman, A. B., O'Connor, G. T., Punjabi, N. M., Quan, S. F., et al. (2010). Prospective study of obstructive sleep apnea and incident coronary heart disease and heart failure: The sleep heart health study. *Circulation, 122*(4), 352–360.

Han, F., Mignot, E., Wei, Y. C., Dong, S. X., Li, J., Lin, L., et al. (2010). Ventilatory chemoresponsiveness, narcolepsy-cataplexy and human leukocyte antigen DQB1*0602 status. *European Respiratory Journal, 36*(3), 577–583.

Innes, K. E., Selfe, T. K., & Agarwal, P. (2012). Restless legs syndrome and conditions associated with metabolic dysregulation, sympathoadrenal dysfunction, and cardiovascular disease risk: a systematic review. *Sleep Medicine Reviews, 16*(4), 309–339.

Keijzer, H., Smits, M. G., Duffy, J. F., & Curfs, L. M. (2013). Why the dim light melatonin onset (DLMO) should be measured before treatment of patients with circadian rhythm sleep disorders. *Sleep Medicine Reviews, 18*(4), 333–339. http://dx.doi.org/10.1016/j.smrv.2013.12.001

Kessler, R., Berglund, P. A., Coulouvrat, C., Fitzgerald, T., Hajak, G., Roth, T., et al. (2012). Insomnia, comorbidity and risk of injury among insured Americans: results from the America Insomnia survey. *Sleep, 35*(6), 825–834.

Kraus, S. S. & Rabin, L. A. (2012). Sleep America: MANAGING the crisis of adult chronic insomnia and associated conditions. *Journal of Affective Disorders, 138*(3), 192–212.

Lauterbach, D., Behnke, C., & McSweeney, L.B. (2011). Sleep problems among persons with a lifetime history of posttraumatic stress disorder alone and in combination with a lifetime history of other psychiatric disorders: a replication and extension. *Comprehensive Psychiatry. 52*(6), 580–586.

LeBourgeois, M. K., Carskadon, M. A., Akacem, L. D., Simpkin, C. T., Wright, K. P., Achermann, P., et al. (2013). Circadian phase and its relationship to nighttime sleep in toddlers. *Journal of Biological Rhythms, 28*(5), 322–31.

Matthews, E. E., Arnedt, J. R., McCarthy, M. S., Cuddihy, L. J., & Aloia, M. S. (2013). Adherence to cognitive behavioral therapy for insomnia: A systematic review. *Sleep Medicine Reviews, 17*(6), 453–464.

Monti, J. M. (2013). The neurotransmitters of sleep and wake, a physiological review series. *Sleep Medicine Reviews, 17*(4), 313–315.

Morin, C. M. & Benca, R. (2012). Chronic insomnia. *The Lancet, 379*(9821), 1129–1141.

Münch, M. & Bromundt, V. (2012). Light and chronobiology: implications for health and disease. *Dialogues in Clinical Neuroscience, 14*(4), 448–453.

Mysliwiec, F., Matsangas, P., Baxter, T., McGraw, L., Bothwell, N. E., & Roth, B. J. (2014). Comorbid insomnia and obstructive sleep apnea in military personnel: correlation with polysomnographic variables. *Military Medicine, 179*(3), 294–300.

Nasr, S., Wendt, B., & Kora, S. K. (2010). Increased incidence of sleep apnea in psychiatric outpatients. *Annals of Clinical Psychiatry, 22*(1), 29–32.

National Center for Complementary and Alternative Medicine. (2012). *Valerian: Herbs at a glance.* Washington, DC: National Institutes of Health, U.S. Department of Health and Human Services. NCCAM Publication No. D272.

National Institutes of Health. (2005). NIH State-of-the-Science Conference statement on manifestations and management of chronic insomnia in adults. *National Institutes of Health Consensus Scientific Statements, 22*(2), 1–30.

Ohayon, M. M., O'Hara, R., & Vitiello, M. V. (2012). Epidemiology of restless legs syndrome: a synthesis of the literature. *Sleep Medicine Reviews. 16*(4), 283–295.

Pataka, A., Yoon, C., Poddar, A., & Riha, R. L. (2013). Assessment of multiple sleep latency testing in adults in Europe. *Sleep Medicine, 14*(2), 136–139.

Porth, C. M. (Ed.) (2010). Sleep and sleep disorders. *Pathophysiology: Concepts of altered health states* (pp. 1281–1297). Philadelphia, PA: Lippincott Williams & Wilkins.

Ram, S., Seirawan, H., Kuma, S., & Clark, G. (2009). Prevalence and impact of sleep disorders and sleep habits in the United States. *Sleep & Breathing, 14*, 63–70.

Raskind, M. A., Peterson, K., Williams, T., Hoff, D. J., Hart, K., Holmes, H., et al. (2013). A trial of prazosin for combat trauma PTSD with nightmares in active-duty soldiers returned from Iraq and Afghanistan. *American Journal of Psychiatry, 170*(9), 1003–1010.

Riemann, D. & Perlis, M. L. (2009). The treatments of chronic insomnia: A review of benzodiazepine receptor agonists and psychological and behavioral therapies. *Sleep Medicine Review, 13*(3), 204–214.

Santarnecchi, E., Sicilia, I., Richiardi, J., Vatti, G., Polizzotto, N.R., Marina, D., et al. (2013). Altered cortical and subcortical local coherence in obstructive sleep apnea: a functional magnetic resonance imaging study. *Journal of Sleep Research, 22*(3), 337–347.

Schendel, S., Powell, N., & Jacobson, R. (2011). Maxillary, mandibular, and chin advancement: Treatment planning based on airway anatomy in obstructive sleep apnea. *Journal of Oral & Maxillofacial Surgery, 69*(3), 663–676.

Soares, C. M. & Frey, B. N. (2010). Challenges and opportunities to manage depression during the menopausal transition and beyond. *Psychiatric Clinics of North America, 33*(2), 295–308.

Tamanna, S. & Geraci, S. Q. (2013). Major sleep disorders among women: (women's health series). (Review). *Southern Medical Journal, 106*(8), 470–478.

Townsend-Roccichelli, J., Sanford, J. T., & VandeWaa, E. (2010). Managing sleep disorders in the elderly. *The Nurse Practitioner, 35*(5), 31–37.

Tregear, S., Reston, J., Schoelles, K., & Phillips, B. (2009). Obstructive sleep apnea and risk of motor vehicle crash: Systematic review. *Journal of Clinical Sleep Medicine, 15*(5), 573–581.

Weinstock, L. B., Walters, A. S., & Paueksakon, P. (2012). Restless legs syndrome–Theoretical roles of inflammatory and immune mechanisms. *Sleep Medicine Reviews. 16*(4), 341–354.

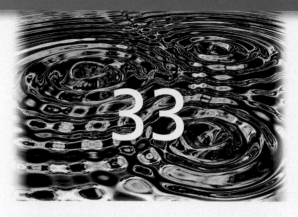

33 Sexual Disorders
Management of Sexual Dysfunction

Mary Ann Boyd

KEY CONCEPTS

- sexual arousal
- sexual disorders
- sexuality

LEARNING OBJECTIVES

After studying this chapter, you will be able to:

1. Discuss the development of sexual behavior.

2. Compare male and female sexual response and theoretical models.

3. Identify human responses to sexual disorders.

4. Develop a nursing care plan for a patient with a sexual disorder.

5. Identify nursing intervention strategies common to treating those with sexual disorders.

KEY TERMS

- anorgasmia • biosexual identity • delayed ejaculation • dyspareunia • erectile dysfunction • excitement • fetishism • frotteurism • gender identity • gender dysphoria • human sexual response cycle • orgasmic disorder • orgasmic phase • paraphilias • pedophilia • plateau • premature ejaculation • resolution • sensate focus • sex role identity • sex therapist • sexual desire • sexual maturation • sexual orientation • vaginismus

---

Sexuality is associated with sensuality, pleasure and pleasuring, intimacy, trust, communication, love and affection, attractiveness, affirmation of one's masculinity and femininity, and reverence for life. Sexuality influences how we view ourselves (self-concept) and consequently how we relate to others.

> **KEYCONCEPT**   **Sexuality** is a life force that encompasses all that is male or female and how these characteristics relate to all that is human.

Sexuality is influenced by a person's emotional and physiologic status, beliefs and values, and morals and laws of society. Barriers to sexual fulfillment can arise from medical problems, such as neurologic, musculoskeletal, cardiovascular, respiratory, renal, hepatic, and cognitive impairments; from pain, weakness, and fatigue; and from sequelae of surgical procedures and drugs. More often, sexual problems are a result of the interplay of multiple causes that can include intrapsychic, interpersonal, and sociocultural factors. This chapter focuses on sexuality and sexual functioning and discusses nursing care for persons experiencing sexual dysfunction, especially those experiencing another co-occurring disorder.

SEXUAL DEVELOPMENT

All of us are sexual beings, whether or not we are sexually active. Sex is what we are, not what we do—the sum total of all of our biologic and experiential influences. **Sexual maturation** encompasses four areas: biosexual identity, gender identity, sex role identity, and sexual orientation. Whereas **biosexual identity** refers to the anatomic and physiologic state of being male or female, **gender identity** is the conviction of belonging to a male or female gender. Both biosexual and gender identities result from genetic and intrauterine hormonal influences, not learned behavior. **Sex role identity** (or gender role) is the outward expression of gender, including behaviors, feelings, and attitudes. **Sexual orientation** refers to a person's sexual attraction to those of the opposite sex (heterosexual), same sex (homosexual), or both sexes (bisexual). Sexual orientation is determined early in development as a result of the influence of genetic factors and the interactions between sex hormones and the developing brain and should not be considered a lifestyle choice. According to the evidence, changing sexual orientation is apparently impossible (Bao & Swaab, 2011).

Genes and Determination of Sex

As a result of the sex-determining genes on the Y chromosome, testosterone is present in male fetuses and, by weeks 6 to 12, is responsible for the formation of the penis, prostate, and scrotum. The formation of ovaries in female fetuses depends on the absence of this male hormone. After the male sex organs are formed, testosterone levels temporarily rise, causing a permanent sexual organization of the brain that is different than that of females. Testosterone is also elevated during the first three months after birth, causing the brain structures and circuits to be fixed for the rest of a boy's life.

These structural differences are thought to be the basis of sex differences that are reflected in behavior from birth. For example, female newborns are more likely to watch human faces, and male infants look more at mobiles. Toy preference (i.e., choosing dolls vs. cars) is obvious at 3 to 8 months (Bao & Swaab, 2011). During puberty, rising hormones stimulate these structures and circuits that were set up many years earlier to further respond in feminine or masculine directions. Since the sexual differentiation of the genitals takes place earlier (first two months of pregnancy) than the sexual differentiation of the brain (second half of pregnancy), these two processes may be influenced differently. In rare cases, transsexuality may occur. For example, people with male sexual organs may experience their identity as female (Bao & Swaab, 2011).

Sexual Behaviors in Children and Adolescents

In infants, sexual behaviors are rare with the exception of hand-to-genital contact. As children become more aware of their body parts and the physical sensations deriving from their genitals, they become more interested in gender differences. For 2- to 5-year-old children, sexual behaviors are varied and more common than in older children, who are aware of the social norms of concealing sexual behaviors. For example, young children observe and comment on body differences, demonstrate interest in bathroom habits and urination, and handle their genitals for pleasure and comfort. Their curiosity leads them to want to look at and touch adult bodies and breasts. Mutual genital exploration or urination among children may be seen at this time along with questions about where babies come from.

Age-appropriate solitary sexual behaviors (touching one's own genitals) are also common. At this early age, these behaviors do not have the sexualized meaning as they do to adults. However, if young children are exposed to sexually explicit material (Internet, movies, observation of parental sexual activities) or if their parents overreact to age-appropriate behaviors, these activities can take on additional, more adult-like, meanings. If preoccupation with the sexual behaviors interferes with the child's ability to grow and function, then the behaviors are problematic. For example, an 8-year-old boy sneaking to the bathroom several times a day to touch his genitals needs help in addressing this behavior.

Sexual behaviors are common and occur in 42% to 73% of children by the time they reach 13 years of age. These behaviors may not be as obvious because as children mature, they become increasingly more covert in their sexual behavior. For example, whereas 6- to 9-year-old boys and girls often touch genitals at home, stand too close to others, and try to look at persons when they are nude, 10- to 12-year-old children, who are actually more interested in and know more about sex, limit their behavior to looking at nudity in magazines, television, and the internet (Kellogg, 2010).

Sexual contact with others occurs at a relatively early age in the United States. In a nationwide survey of 9th through 12th grade students in 50 states, 34.2% were currently sexually active, 46% had had sexual intercourse, and 5.9% of students had sexual intercourse for the first time before age 13 years (Centers for Disease Control and Prevention, 2010). A variety of circumstances lead to this sexual activity. Sex may be engaged in because of peer pressure or because friends or social groups condone sex. The need to be convinced of being in love, wanting to feel loved, and fear of rejection all precipitate risk-taking behavior. Depending on the family environment, stresses, and observation of adult sexual activities, children may exhibit more adult sexual behaviors, which may be considered normal for the environment in which they live. For children and adolescents, sexual behavior (usually involving other people) is considered abnormal when it occurs at a greater frequency or at a much earlier age than would be developmentally or culturally expected.

Sexual Behaviors in Adulthood

Sexual activities occur throughout young adulthood and continue through middle and late adulthood into the 80s and 90s. Although the frequency and types of sexual encounters may change, the quality need not change.

During the fourth to fifth decades of life, physical changes become more obvious, and a number of chronic illnesses, such as hypertension or arthritis, may also develop. As a result of decreased endocrine production, gradual changes to body tissues occur over a 15- to 20-year span. Most of the physical symptoms arise from vasomotor instability, which can include morning fatigue, vague pains, hot flashes, dizziness, chills, sweating, nervousness, crying spells, decreased sexual potency, and palpitations.

In women, estrogen deficiency during menopause affects the sexual system by causing a gradual thinning of the vaginal mucosa, decreasing the elasticity of muscles and orgasmic force, and increasing breast involution (sagging of breast tissue). Vaginal lubrication decreases, which may cause **dyspareunia** (pain during intercourse), often requiring the use of a water-soluble lubricant or saliva. Although many women experience little or no change in sexual function, both decreased and increased sexual activity and interest are possible. In some women, an increase in time is required to lubricate the vulvovaginal areas and to strengthen clitoral response. Orgasmic capacity and breast response remain fairly constant in appropriately stimulated women.

In men, decreasing testosterone production is responsible for sexual changes. The amount and viability of sperm decrease, erections become less firm, and more direct sexual stimulation is needed. The testicles begin to decrease in elasticity and size, ejaculation time increases, and the force of ejaculation decreases. Spermatogenesis decreases, although viable sperm, capable of impregnation, continue to be produced. Seminal fluid is less voluminous and viscous, and ejaculatory force is decreased. Older men, however, are capable of sustaining erection much longer with decreased ejaculatory demand, potentially benefiting older women, who require increased time to reach orgasm. Coupled with women's increased sexual enjoyment in the later years, sexual activity is often perceived as more satisfactory than previously experienced.

Sexual continuity depends to a great extent on good physical health, activity, and regular opportunities for sexual expression and sexual activity in all forms, including masturbation and same-gender behavior. An important influence on sexuality is the attitudes of others, especially attitudes that define specific behaviors as acceptable or unacceptable. This is especially true in later life (Kellogg, 2010). In healthy adults, sexual function, although modified by the aging process, should remain satisfying despite a differently timed sequence. Frequent sexual activity, whether by coitus or masturbation, usually preserves sexual potency.

SEXUAL RESPONSES

Understanding normal sexual responses helps when discussing this very personal but important aspect of being human

with patients. The following section provides an overview of major concepts and theories related to sexual responses.

Sexual Desire and Arousal

Sexual desire is the ability, interest, or willingness to receive or a motivational state to seek sexual stimulation. In healthy adults, the sex drive is integrated through the central nervous system (CNS) with the autonomic nervous system governing extragenital changes (increased respiration and heart rate). The parasympathetic nervous system largely controls arousal, and the sympathetic nervous system largely controls orgasmic discharge. Sexual stimulation brings about a total-body response with dramatic changes seen in the genitals and breasts. Sex hormones, particularly androgen, influence desire in both genders, but less is known about hormonal influence in women. That the higher centers of the brain apparently mediate the lower reflex response centers supports the relationship between cognitive and affective states and sexual function.

During sexual arousal, both men and women experience an increased heart rate, blood pressure, respiration, and myotonia.

> **KEYCONCEPT** **Sexual arousal** is state of mounting sexual tension characterized by vasoconstriction and myotonia.

In men, visual stimulation (i.e., seeing a naked person), fantasies, memories, or physical stimulation of the genitals or other regions (e.g., nipples) causes the parasympathetic system to involuntarily release chemicals that dilate penile arteries. A rapid inflow of arterial blood to the corpora cavernosa, facilitated by high levels of intrapenile nitric oxide, causes stiffening and elongation of the penis. With continued stimulation, an emission of semen and an ejaculation occurs. Dopaminergic activity in the CNS facilitates arousal and ejaculation; serotonergic systems inhibit them (Will, Hull, & Dominguez, 2014).

Fantasies, visual stimuli, and physical stimulation are also important for sexual arousal in women, but physical stimulation seems more important for women and visual stimuli for men. Similar to the case in men, the parasympathetic nervous system brings about an increase in blood flow to the female genitalia, causing a lubrication of the vagina and some enlargement of the breast and clitoris. Estrogens and progestins are involved in female sexual functioning, but androgens are needed by people of both genders to maintain arousal.

Theoretical Models of Sexual Response

In 1966, Masters and Johnson described the classic **human sexual response cycle** as consisting of four phases: excitement, plateau, orgasm, and resolution. In the **excitement** phase, erotic feelings of both genders lead to a penile erection in men and vaginal lubrication in women. Heart rate and respirations also increase. The **plateau** phase is represented by sexual pleasure and increased muscle tension, heart rate, and blood flow to the genitals. For men, the **orgasmic** phase is ejaculation of semen, and for women, it consists of rhythmic contractions of the vaginal muscles. For most men, immediately after orgasm and before resolution, there is a refractory period when no response is possible. **Resolution** is the gradual return of the organs and body systems to the unaroused state. Muscle tension and vasocongestion subside. Breathing and heart rate gradually return to normal rates. Usually, the person feels a sense of relaxation, relief of tension, and satisfaction (Masters & Johnson, 1966, 1970).

After publication of Masters and Johnson's work, Kaplan (1979) proposed a three-phase model of sexual response—desire, excitement, and orgasm—and identified low-desire states as a frequent cause of sexual dysfunction.

This linear approach is criticized as being primarily a biologic model and does not account for nonbiologic experiences such as pleasure, satisfaction, and the context of the relationship. To account for emotional and psychological aspects of sexual response, a circular model focusing on women's sexual responses was developed by Basson (2001). This model proposes that nonsexual interpersonal factors, such as a desire for physical connection and intimacy needs, also motivate women to engage in sexual relations, not just simply sexual release. Arousal and desire appear to be interchangeable and inseparable from one another, with one reinforcing the other. Subjective feelings of interest may follow the sensation of arousal, and sexual satisfaction may be felt without orgasm.

These two models—linear and circular—have been debated for years (Hayes, 2011; Wylie & Mimoun, 2009). Both models are supported empirically as being relevant to sexual responses in women. In one study of 133 women, approximately half of the women reported their sexual experience consistent with the linear model and progressing through stages of desire, arousal, orgasm, and resolution (Sand & Fisher, 2007). In another study of women with and without female sexual dysfunction, those without sexual dysfunction reported that the linear model was an accurate representation of their sexual response; those with a sexual dysfunction were aligned with a circular model (Giles & McCabe, 2009).

Dual-Control Model

Another conceptualization, the dual-control model focuses on individual variability and proposes that sexual responses involve an interaction between sexual excitement and sexual inhibition (Bancroft, Graham, Janssen, & Sanders, 2009). This model assumes that (1) neurobiologic inhibition of sexual response is adaptive and occurs in situations

when sexual activity would be a disadvantage, dangerous, or distracting; (2) individuals vary in their propensity for sexual excitation and inhibition; and (3) the context and cultural meaning attributed to the interaction of the individuals are important stimuli for both excitatory and inhibitory processes. Research shows that gender differences in inhibitory mechanisms are better developed in women than in men; men tend to have stronger excitatory responses. Ultimately, more research is needed to truly understand the human sexual response (Bancroft et al., 2009).

SEXUAL DYSFUNCTIONS AND PROBLEMATIC BEHAVIORS

Sexual dysfunctions are a group of disorders that are characterized by clinically significant disturbances in the person's ability to respond sexually or to experience sexual pleasure (American Psychiatric Association [APA], 2013). The *DSM-5* identifies the following as sexual disorders: delayed ejaculation, erectile disorder, female orgasmic disorder, female sexual interest/arousal disorder, genito-pelvic pain/penetration disorder, male hypoactive sexual desire disorder, and premature ejaculation. These dysfunctions can be lifelong or acquired and are categorized as mild, moderate, or severe. An occasional episode is not considered dysfunctional (APA, 2013). In this chapter, female orgasmic disorder is highlighted because it is among the most commonly occurring sexual disorders in women, and **anorgasmia** (the inability to achieve an orgasm) is a frequent medication side effect.

Other sexually-related behaviors, paraphilias, and gender dysphoria will also be discussed.

> **KEYCONCEPT** **Sexual disorders** are clinical disturbances caused by the inability to respond sexually or to experience sexual pleasure.

Interventions for sexual disorders are summarized in Table 33.1.

FEMALE ORGASMIC DISORDER

A female orgasm is the least understood of all sexual responses, and a universal definition is nonexistent (Bancroft & Graham, 2011). Women's descriptions of the orgasmic experience vary from altered consciousness to focused sensation. Many women require clitoral stimulation to reach orgasm and a minority of women report that they always experience orgasm during intercourse.

According to the *DSM-5*, an **orgasmic disorder** is the inability to reach orgasm by any means, either alone or with a partner and/or markedly reduced intensity of orgasmic sensations for at least 6 months. The inability to experience an orgasm causes clinically significant distress (APA, 2013).

Table 33.1	INTERVENTIONS FOR COMMON SEXUAL DYSFUNCTIONS	
Sexual Dysfunction	**Intervention**	**Goal**
Female orgasmic dysfunction	Medical examination	Rule out organic etiology
	Sensate focus: progressive exercises from nongenital to genital stimulation and intercourse	Decrease pressure to perform Increase awareness of pleasurable sensations Eliminate spectatoring Increase partner awareness of sites and methods of pleasuring
	Masturbation	Teach self-pleasuring, reaching orgasm
	Vibrator	
	Assertiveness training	Teach entitlement to and approach to request pleasurable sexual stimuli
	Facilitative communication	
	Counseling or psychotherapy	Increase awareness of personal, sexual, and relationship issues
	Marital or couples therapy	
	Education	Knowledge of anatomy and physiology of human sexual response
Ejaculatory disorders	Sensate focus	Decrease pressure to perform Increase awareness of ejaculatory inevitability
	Squeeze technique: includes progressive exercises from partner masturbation to controlled intromission and thrusting	Learn new ejaculatory control responses
	Counseling or psychotherapy	Awareness and resolution of personal, sexual, and relationship issues
	Marital or couples therapy	
	Education	Knowledge of arousal–orgasm mechanism
Erectile dysfunction	Medical examination	Rule out penile hemodynamic, neurologic, hormonal, or other organic causes
	Organic etiology: penile implant, vascular surgery, intracavernosal pharmacotherapy, vacuum pump, drugs	Treat, control, or reverse physiologic cause
	Sensate focus	Decrease pressure to perform Eliminate spectatoring
	Counseling or psychotherapy	Relearn new response
	Education	Awareness and resolution of personal, sexual, and relationship issues
	Marital or couples therapy	
Female sexual interest/arousal disorder	Treating factors that contribute to lack of arousal	Identify underlying issues; awareness and resolution of personal sexual and personal relationship issues
	Cognitive behavioral therapy	
Male hypoactive sexual desire	Medical examination	Rule out hormonal imbalance
	Facilitative communication	Awareness and resolution of personal, sexual, and relationship issues
	Psychotherapy	
	Education	
Genito-pelvic pain/penetration disorder	Medical examination	Rule out organic etiology
	Organic etiology: hormone replacement, localized infections or inflammation, and so on	Treat, control, or reverse physiologic cause
	Artificial lubricant, oral stimulation	Teach need for and promote increased lubrication to decrease susceptibility to abrasion
	Education	Teach relationship of sexual response and changes related to age, illness, or emotions
	Assertiveness training	Teach communication skills
	Sensate focus	Decrease performance anxiety; promote relaxation
	Counseling or psychotherapy	Promote self-knowledge; uncover sexual or relationship issues.

Diagnostic Criteria

Female orgasmic disorder is characterized by the inability of a woman to experience orgasm or the intensity of the orgasm is markedly reduced at least 75% of the time. If there are other explanations for the anorgasmia such as substance use, medications, or interpersonal issues, the diagnosis is not used.

Epidemiology and Risk Factors

There is considerable debate around the issue of female orgasms. Estimated prevalence of women's inability to reach orgasm ranges from 9% (in the United States) to 41.2% in Southeast Asia (Bancroft & Graham, 2011).

Poor physical and mental health and relationship issues, especially partner difficulties, are the primary risk factors. Research does not support previously suggested risk factors, such as age and personality characteristics (Graham, 2010).

Etiology

In general, any local genital or pelvic pathology, trauma, or surgery that causes pain on intercourse can produce impaired response to sexual stimulation. Spinal cord damage, endocrine disorders, systemic diseases, chronic pain, and general debility can interfere with sexual responses. CNS depressants (e.g., alcohol, barbiturates, and narcotics), psychiatric disorders, infections, inflammatory disorders, and pregnancy have all been associated with female orgasmic disorder. Additionally, many medications such as antidepressants, antihypertensives, and substances (e.g., alcohol) can also affect the sexual response (Clayton, Croft, & Handiwala, 2014).

Sexual responses can be inhibited by many different emotional and cognitions, including sexual anxiety and guilt, anger or hostility toward one's partner, indifference toward one's partner, depression, or excessive and intrusive thoughts. Misinformation or lack of information contributes to the inhibition. Cultural expectations also play an important role in the sexual experience. Religious prohibitions and cultural taboos often contribute to a woman's view of her sexuality. If a woman believes that sexual relationships are sinful or "a woman's duty," she is not as likely to explore her own sexual potential.

Interdisciplinary Treatment

The treatment of the woman with an orgasmic disorder is best left to clinicians who specialize in this area, but other health care providers can first treat underlying health, mental health, and relationship issues. If the orgasmic problem is not related to any of these areas, she should be referred to a qualified **sex therapist**, who blends education and counseling with psychotherapy and specific sexual exercises. For example, **sensate focus** is a method for partners to learn what each finds arousing and to learn to communicate those preferences. It begins with nongenital contact and gradually includes genital touch and sexual intercourse.

NURSING MANAGEMENT: Human Response to Female Orgasmic Disorder

The psychiatric–mental health nurse has a responsibility to conduct an assessment to determine the presence of any sexual issues or problems. The scope of practice dictates the level of assessment and interventions. The nurse will most likely be seeing the patient for another problem (psychiatric problem, acute or chronic physical health problem) and will discover a sexual problem during a health assessment. Patients are sometimes reluctant to discuss sexual problems, especially those who are socially stigmatized (same-sex couples, developmentally disabled, and seniors). The depth and context of a sexual assessment depend on the patient's life status and condition. See Box 33.1 for a Sexual Assessment Guide.

Attention should be paid to special populations' high risk for sexual problems, such as those with mental illnesses or chronic health problems. For older adults, poor physical health and lack of a partner are common barriers to sexual continuity. Other barriers include a lack of privacy or institutionalization. Lack of knowledge about the impacts of aging or health conditions on sexuality, the normality of continued sexual desire and interest, and the alternatives for sexual gratification may also inhibit sexual activity.

If a sexual dysfunction exists, one of the most important questions is does the individual want to change sexual functioning? Many women may not see a need to pursue therapy even if a sexual problem exits.

Biologic Domain

Assessment

Current sexual functioning, age, physical health, and the presence of any medical or psychiatric and substance use problems as well as factors that contribute to sexual functioning (e.g., rest, nutrition, personal hygiene) are considered in the sexual assessment (Box 33.2). A careful medication history is important because so many medications have a negative effect on sexual performance (see Chapter 11). Adults with chronic medical illnesses and disabilities who have problems with sensation, movement, body structure, fertility, energy, or negative self-image should be asked about the impact of the medical problems on their sexual function. The woman's sexual knowledge should also be determined. Does she understand the sexual responses, effects of medications, hormonal changes that occur during the woman's life cycle (adolescence, menstruation, pregnancy, menopause, aging), and the importance of adequate rest and nutrition?

Nursing Diagnoses for the Biologic Domain

The assessment data usually lead to a nursing diagnosis of either Ineffective Sexuality Patterns or Sexual Dysfunction. Ineffective Sexuality Patterns is used as the nursing diagnosis if the person is at risk for or has already experienced a change in sexual functioning. Sexual Dysfunction refers to problematic sexual function that the individual perceives as unsatisfying, unrewarding, or inadequate and for which nursing can intervene.

Interventions for the Biologic Domain

Nursing interventions include providing counseling, sex education, problem-solving opportunities, or referrals.

BOX 33.1

Sexual Assessment Guide

SEXUAL DEVELOPMENT AND REPRODUCTION
How did you learn about sex and how were your questions answered?
What did you learn from your family, school, or religion?
How did you feel about being a male or female? Problem?
Beliefs about your body; satisfaction with looks or function?
Diet, drugs, anorexia or /bulimia, steroids, fitness or exercise regimen?
Menstruation or menopause experience? Issues? Questions?
Contraceptive practices? Pregnancies? Problems? Questions?
Infertility problems, treatments, outcomes?

HEALTH CONDITIONS AND PRACTICES
Women
Do you practice breast self-examination? Vaginal self-examination?
How often have you had a pelvic examination? Pap smear?

Men
Do you practice testicular self-examination?

Women and Men
Health promotion activities? What type? Frequency?
Have you had any discharge, itching, swelling, or genital surgery?
Any sexually transmitted diseases? Frequency? Treatment? Outcomes?
Medical conditions? Injuries? Medications, prescribed and non-prescribed?
Amount, type, and frequency of alcohol, tobacco, and other drugs?
Psychiatric conditions? Appearance, mood state.

SOCIAL AND SEXUAL ACTIVITY
How would you describe your social life? Often feel lonely? What do you do about these feelings?
Have you ever been sexually active? Currently sexually active?
How would you describe your current sexual activity? Satisfactory or unsatisfactory? What would you change?
Is it a problem for you being sexually active? How so? Or if not sexually active, how have you dealt with this?
At this time, how important is having a sexual relationship?
How have you dealt with your sexual needs since changing your status (i.e., becoming single, unattached, or divorced)?
Do you ever feel guilty or anxious about anything pertaining to your sexual lifestyle or behavior?
What types of sexual practices do you engage in? Penile–vaginal intercourse? Oral–genital sex? Anal sex?
Are you aware of sexual practices that may put you at risk? What do you do to protect yourself?
Have you had a past sexual trauma? Treatment or counseling received?

SEXUAL FUNCTION
Do you believe that you have a sexual problem? For how long? Did you always have this problem? What happens?
Are you interested in having sex? All the time? Some of the time? Never?
Does the thought of sex make you fearful or anxious? Do you avoid it?
Do you ever have difficulty becoming sexually aroused?

Men
Do you ever have difficulty achieving or maintaining an erection?
Have you ever noticed any change in the rigidity, size, or circumference of your penis? Other changes?
Do you feel you ejaculate too quickly? Too slowly? Unable to ejaculate in the vagina? Other?

Women
Do you have difficulty becoming lubricated?
Do you tighten up before intercourse, so that penile insertion is impossible?
Do you have problems reaching orgasm? How often? Under what circumstance?

Women and Men
Do you ever experience pain? On intromission? Thrusting? Orgasm? What happens?
Do you have sexual or other problems with your partner? What are they?
Do you feel your partner has problems? What are they?
Can you communicate your sexual concerns or preference?

ORIENTATION
Have you had or are you in a sexual relationship with someone of your own gender?
Do you consider yourself to be exclusively heterosexual? Bisexual? Exclusively gay or lesbian? Are others aware of your sexual orientation?
How has your sexual orientation affected your life?

GENERAL
Do you have any questions about sexuality or sexual function?
Do you want to speak with someone who specializes in sexual problems? Marital issues? Other?

CUES AND CLUES
Sexual humor, ribald remarks, obscene gestures
Self-depreciation
Genital exposure, public masturbation
Inappropriate touching of care provider or other person
Questions pertaining to sexual relationship of care provider
Statements or questions beginning with "I have a friend who. . . ."
Nervousness related to sexual topic

Several health care practices are also known to promote sexual health such as getting adequate rest, maintaining optimal nutrition, and exercising regularly. Explaining the dynamics of sexual responses is another important nursing action. Individuals who report difficulties with sexual response often benefit from factual information and helpful suggestions and are not in need of sex therapy. However, when long-standing, highly complex problems emerge in the assessment, it is better to refer the individual or couple to a formally trained, certified sex therapist. Nurses should be aware that certain processes, techniques, and adaptive devices can improve

sexual functioning. See Figure 33.1 for biopsychosocial interventions.

Psychosocial Domain

Assessment

The psychosocial assessment focuses on the woman's self-concept and body image and her relationship with her partner. A poor self-concept can prevent a woman from engaging in sexual relationships. Mood states, such as chronic depression and grief, also seriously affect the woman's ability to have an orgasm. The amount of stress

BOX 33.2

Medical Conditions and Substances Affecting Sexual Function

- Cardiovascular conditions and vascular conditions
- Endocrine conditions, particularly diabetes mellitus, that cause gradual impotence in half of men and orgasmic dysfunction in one third of women
- Cancer or cancer treatments, such as radiation
- Surgery, particularly hysterectomy, mastectomy, prostatectomy, and bowel surgery
- Arthritis and neuromuscular disorders
- Spinal cord injury
- Head injury
- Cerebrovascular accident (stroke)
- Organic brain syndrome (senile dementia, Alzheimer's disease)
- Cerebral palsy
- Asthma, emphysema, and chronic obstructive pulmonary disease
- Chronic renal failure
- Obesity
- Localized genital conditions, such as Sjögren's syndrome, balanitis, vulvar ulcers, and psoriasis
- Prescription medications (antihypertensive drugs, anticholinergic drugs, some antidepressants)
- Chronic use of most recreational drugs
- Chronic alcohol abuse

BOX 33.3

Psychoeducation Checklist: Female Orgasmic Disorder

When caring for the patient with female orgasmic disorder, be sure to include the following topics in your teaching plan for the patient and partner:

- Possible etiologic factors
- Anxiety reduction techniques
- Communication skills
- Sexual preferences
- Sexual play
- Sensate focus
- Kegel exercises
- Erotic fantasy
- Group therapy
- Sex therapy

and the ability to relax and focus on her sexuality are important assessment data. An unsatisfactory partner relationship may be at the core of the sexual problem. Cultural and family values play an important role in understanding a patient's response to orgasmic dysfunction and should be considered. Lifestyle disruptions, a birth of a child, a move to another city, or a change in financial or social status may coincide with sexual dysfunction.

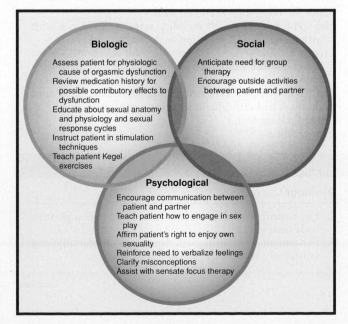

FIGURE 33.1 Biopsychosocial interventions for patients with female orgasmic disorder.

Nursing Diagnoses for the Psychosocial Domain

The assessment data could generate a number of nursing diagnoses such as Low Self-esteem or Stress Overload. If there are relationship issues, additional assessment data may generate other nursing diagnosis such as disabled family coping.

Interventions for the Psychosocial Domain

Unless the nurse has additional preparation in sexual counseling, simply providing factual information and helping patients identify issues related to sexual problems and develop problem-solving skills are the primary psychosocial interventions. Patients often benefit from learning how to communicate their sexual needs better in such areas as type of stimulation desired, positioning, and the amount of time required for maximum sexual pleasure. Resource materials and referral sources can be recommended. Box 33.3 outlines topics for patient education.

Women with orgasmic dysfunction can also benefit from a support group that includes women with similar problems. Group modalities, such as psychoeducation groups, are useful in helping patients decrease their embarrassment and uneasiness about sexual topics and increase their knowledge. Partner support is critical and should be encouraged throughout treatment.

Evaluation and Treatment Outcomes

Outcomes related to improved sexual functioning are developed with the patient and may vary from acquiring knowledge to increasing communication with her partner and to making a decision about a referral for specialized treatment.

Nursing Care Plan 33.1 demonstrates the nursing process in a patient with multiple sclerosis who has developed altered sexual expression and sexual dysfunction.

(text continues on page 652)

NURSING CARE PLAN 33.1

The Patient With Multiple Sclerosis and Sexual Dysfunction

AD is a 35-year-old woman, happily married for 11 years, and the mother of two children. She attended college and earned a master's degree in education. She has been employed as a sixth grade teacher but is currently not working.

AD was diagnosed with multiple sclerosis 3 years ago. She is being seen for a periodic check-up by the nurse practitioner. Some of AD's present symptoms include transitory visual blurring, weakness of the lower extremities, and mood swings. She also has had problems with urinary leakage and occasional bowel incontinence. She admits, with some obvious discomfort, that she is experiencing sexual difficulty and that her sexual activity is far less frequent than before her illness. Although AD claims her husband has remained attentive and affectionate, she feels she is no longer attractive or able to fulfill her functions as a wife. She says she wouldn't blame her husband if he found someone else.

The physical examination has demonstrated decreased sensation and reflexes in the lower extremities, decreased hand grasp, slight delayed blink response and nystagmus, clear speech pattern, nondistended bladder, normal bowel sounds, BP 124/76, P 76, and R 24. The patient wears an absorbent pad for urinary incontinence with a slight odor of urine. She is weepy and wrings her hands, and her eyes are downcast when discussing marital relationship. AD's husband accompanied her to the appointment, holding her hand in the waiting room. He offered to be present during the examination or answer questions if desired.

Setting: Outpatient Clinic

Baseline Assessment: AD is a 35-year-old, happily married woman diagnosed with multiple sclerosis 3 years ago. Present symptoms: visual blurring, weakness of extremities, mood swings, urinary leakage, occasional bowel incontinence. Experiencing decreased sexual enjoyment, low self-esteem, and low body image. Has had difficulty experiencing orgasm for 2 years. Has difficulty communicating needs.

Associated Diagnosis	Medications
Rule out: female orgasmic disorder Multiple sclerosis	Interferon-β (Betaseron) 8 mIU (0.25 mg) subcutaneously every other day Oxybutynin (Ditropan) 5 mg three times a day

Nursing Diagnosis 1: Ineffective Sexuality Patterns

Defining Characteristics	Related Factors
Feels unattractive, can't fulfill roles, would understand husband finding another woman. "How would you feel if you had an 'accident' right before you were supposed to make love?" States husband has remained attentive and considerate but believes it's because he feels pity. States she has moods, ". . . really feeling sorry for myself. I suppose . . . I'm depressed . . . frustrated . . . MS affects you that way."	States she often feels tired and weak. Has some difficulty with mobility, requires assistance with bathing in tub and fastening back buttons and hooks. Frequently has urinary incontinence and occasional loss of bowel control. States she is usually unable to hold urine and sometimes bowels. Satisfactory sexual relationship before onset of illness, although had difficulty verbalizing sexual needs. Altered self-esteem Chronic illness

Outcomes

Initial	Discharge
1. The patient and partner will identify three barriers and three enhancers to effective communication regarding their sexual needs and problems.	2. The patient will adapt to limitations and regain positive body image. 3. The patient and partner will experience comfortable and satisfactory sexual expression.

Continued

NURSING CARE PLAN 33.1 *(Continued)*

Interventions

Interventions	Rationale	Ongoing Assessment
Deficient Knowledge		
Educate the patient and family; provide written materials; encourage questions.	Patients and families need factual information on the trajectory, treatment, and impact of multiple sclerosis.	The patient and partner correctly explain emotional aspects and pathophysiology of multiple sclerosis.
Communication		
Demonstrate empathy for the patient's difficulty in communicating sexual needs.	Talking about sex makes some people embarrassed.	The patient and partner correctly identify factors that promote or impede their communication.
Explain common reasons for experiencing difficulty when discussing sexual issues.	Individuals may not know how to phrase what they mean. They may be afraid of insulting their partner or have religious or cultural taboo.	The couple increase comfort in discussing sexual needs.
Emphasize the importance of being able to tell each other what is personally satisfying.	Clear communication is more successful than "telepathy."	The patient is able to identify her need for more time and foreplay.
Help patients establish effective communication patterns by using role play or teaching assertive communication skills (e.g., beginning statements with "I really like it when you . . .").	Becoming assertive often requires changing male/aggressive and female/passive learned behavior patterns. Use of a fictional situation that can be role-played and analyzed is an instructive, nonthreatening model for learning new behaviors.	The patient and partner report more open communication, which allows more sharing of true feelings and fears.
Encourage the establishment of a consistent, mutually agreeable, relaxed time to talk.	Communication is easier when it is planned and viewed as a value.	The patient and partner report that communication is improved by allotting a half hour for "together time" each evening.
Encourage the use of support or self-help groups.	Communication can be enhanced through sharing thoughts, feelings, and experiences with others.	Has contacted Multiple Sclerosis Society.
Describe sexual concerns commonly identified by partners.	Partner may feel guilt about sexual desire when mate is ill; fear of harming, increasing discomfort, or overburdening mate; difficulty when mate assumes caretaking and lover role, often helped by use of a home health aide.	The couple is beginning to address their issues; express difficulty in adapting to the current and inevitable changes of the disease; express fear of complete loss of function in all aspects of function, not just sexuality.
Disturbed Body Image/Altered Self-concept		
Related to illness and change in function	Common sequelae of chronic illness.	The patient is able to express her thoughts and feelings about the effects of the disease.
Help the patient confront reality but identify positive aspects of her personality.	Allows the patient to focus on health function and inner being.	Sees herself as a good mother, teacher, and wife.
Encourage the patient to maintain good hygiene, dress attractively, use grooming aids such as perfume, and treat herself to manicures.	Optimizing appearance is a mood enhancer.	The patient states she is having a friend take her to hairdresser every other week; bought a new outfit through a catalog.

Continued

NURSING CARE PLAN 33.1 *(Continued)*

Fatigue and Weakness

Identify optimal time for sexual interaction.	Decreases stress; increases relaxation.	Reports using time when children are with grandparents for intimacy.
Do not eat or drink before activity.	Decreases expenditure of energy and potential for incontinence.	Able to cite correct rationale for food and fluid limitations.
Teach use of sidelying or rear entry position during intercourse.	Decreases energy expenditure of patient.	Reports ability to use these positions.
Use pillows to support weakened extremities.	Assists positioning when there is muscle weakness.	Reports increased satisfaction in sexual activity when pillows are used for positioning.
Inform patient of effect of medications being taken.	Some drugs cause impaired sexual response and fatigue.	Not applicable at this time.

Impaired Mobility

Teach active or passive range-of-motion exercises.	Helps to prevent contractures.	Has been evaluated by physical therapist; reports range of motion exercises done twice daily.
Consider use of a waterbed.	Assists with movement.	
Teach possibility and treatment of contractures or adductor spasms.	Antispasmodics may be needed and are effective when taken 10–15 min before sexual activity.	Not applicable at this time.

Bladder Incontinence

For urinary leakage, teach to the patient empty her bladder in accordance with prescribed bladder training program.	To maximize urinary function, bladder training should be initiated as early as possible.	Reports following bladder training program.
Discuss decreasing fluids a few hours before sexual activity and having padding or towels on hand.	These techniques decrease urinary leakage or incontinence; protect bed linens if an accident occurs.	The patient empties her bladder and decreases fluid before attempting sexual intercourse; pads bed. If using an indwelling catheter, tapes the catheter over her abdomen.
Before sexual activity, void on cue or via intermittent catheterization. If using an indwelling catheter, may advise temporary removal or moving the clamp and taping the catheter to one side.	Permits a patient with urinary retention or indwelling catheter to have coitus.	

Bowel Incontinence

Establish a regular bowel program.	Helps decrease the occurrence of accidental bowel elimination; may require use of a suppository or enema.	Reports following a regulated bowel training program.
Cover bed linens with towels.	Helps prepare for accidents.	

Nursing Diagnosis 2: Sexual Dysfunction

Defining Characteristics	**Related Factors**
Verbalizes difficulty with vaginal lubrication occasional discomfort and decreased genital sensations; "weird feelings," during orgasm; frequent inability to achieve orgasm; some loss of desire.	Disease process; knowledge deficit; difficulty verbalizing sexual needs.

Continued

NURSING CARE PLAN 33.1 *(Continued)*

Outcomes

Initial	Discharge
1. The patient and partner will cite at least five effects of multiple sclerosis on sexual function and at least five adaptive methods to promote satisfactory sexual expression.	2. The patient and partner will use methods that minimize the psychological and organic effects of multiple sclerosis on sexual function. 3. The patient and partner will experience comfortable and satisfactory sexual expression.

Interventions

Interventions	Rationale	Ongoing Assessment
Deficient Knowledge Teach sexual effects of multiple sclerosis.	Disease precipitates numerous biopsychosocial effects.	The patient and partner correctly explain the emotional aspects and pathophysiology of the disease and its relationship to sexual dysfunction.
Suggest sexuality handbook from local chapter of Multiple Sclerosis Society and resources for self-help, counseling, and respite.	Resources include MS Toll-Free Information, 800-FIGHT-MS (800-344-4687); Sex Information and Educational Council of the United States (SIECUS), 130 W. 42nd St., Suite 350, New York, NY 10036.	Sexual information requested from the Multiple Sclerosis Society.
Identify local resources, including individual service providers, Planned Parenthood, hospital departments of sexual health care, national organizations offering professional and nonprofessional sexual information.		
Dyspareunia	Multiple sclerosis can cause unusual sensations, but this effect is often transitory.	Able to cite rationale for sensations but finds them distressing.
Rule out or treat infection.	Infectious processes can cause painful intercourse.	No infection noted on examination.
Decreased Lubrication Substitute natural lubrication with water-based lubricant such as K-Y Jelly; benefits of oral sex and lubricating effect of saliva.	Vaginal dryness is a result of disease as well as stress.	Dyspareunia lessened with K-Y Jelly.
Teach need for relaxation.	Sexual function is greatly affected by stress.	Report more relaxation during intimacy when children at grandparents' home.
Teach partner to increase foreplay and stimulation.	When sensations decreased, longer and more direct stimulation is required.	
Secondary Orgasmic Dysfunction Encourage discussion of concerns.	Often fear rejection or abandonment.	Reports communication has improved.
Suggest individual or couples counseling if difficulties cannot be resolved.	If partner is planning to leave, refer patient or family for social and other necessary support services.	Not applicable at this time.
Assess mental status.	Depression may result from organic or psychological factors; may also require medication.	Demonstrates appropriate level of grieving; may need counseling at later time.
Teach experimenting with new erotic areas and techniques such as fantasy and visual aids.	Enhances excitement and orgasmic stages of sexual response.	Have not begun yet.
If sex therapy desired or necessary, refer to a certified sex therapist.	Important to access qualified counselor.	Not desired at this time.

EJACULATORY DYSFUNCTIONS

The ejaculatory response involves sensory receptors and areas, afferent pathways, cerebral sensory areas, cerebral motor centers, spinal motor centers, and efferent pathways. Serontonergic and dopaminergic neuronal activity with secondary involvement of cholinergic, adrenergic, oxytocinergic, and GABA neurons add to the complexity of the ejaculatory response. The ejaculatory process is divided into three phases: *emission* (contractions of seminal vesicles and the prostate with expulsion of sperm and seminal fluid into the posterior urethra), *ejection* (contractions of the pelvic floor muscles with relaxation of the external urinary sphincter), and *orgasm* (cerebral processing of pudendal nerve stimulation from increased pressure in the posterior urethra) (McMahon, Jannini, Waldinger, & Rowland, 2012).

Ejaculatory dysfunction is one of the most common male sexual disorders and ranges from **premature ejaculation (PE)**, inability to control ejaculation before or shortly after penetration to **delayed ejaculation** (DE), delay or absence of ejaculation. These dysfunctions cause negative personal consequences, clinical distress, frustration, and the avoidance of sexual intimacy (McMahon et al., 2012). The dysfunction needs to be present for 6 months in order to be diagnosed as a sexual dysfunction and is not diagnosed in a man whose difficulty is caused by drug or alcohol abuse. In those cases, a substance abuse diagnosis is made, with the sexual disorder generally resolving when the substance abuse is treated (APA, 2013).

Epidemiology

Based on patient self-report, PE is viewed as the most common male sexual dysfunction, with prevalence rates of 20% to 30%. Unlike erectile dysfunction (ED), which has been studied formally and for which most sexual therapy is sought, information on PE has arisen primarily through self-report. It is estimated that about 27% of men seeking treatment report PE as a problem. Most men with PE do not seek treatment (McMahon et al., 2012).

Etiology

The etiology of PE is unknown with little data to support suggested biologic or psychological theories such as anxiety, penile hypersensitivity, and serotonin receptor dysfunction. Age does not seem to an etiologic factor or a risk (McMahon et al., 2012).

Interdisciplinary Treatment

The treatment of PE involves medication and behavioral strategies. Men with PE are usually treated by specialists.

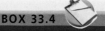

BOX 33.4

Psychoeducation Checklist: **Premature Ejaculation**

When caring for the patient with premature ejaculation, be sure to include the following topics in your teaching plan for the patient and partner:

- Possible etiologic factors
- Pharmacologic agents, if indicated, including drug, dosage, action, frequency, and possible adverse effects
- Measures to decrease anxiety performance
- Communication skills
- Sexual counseling
- Sensate focus
- Sex therapy

Nurses are instrumental in teaching patients about the disorder and potential treatments and facilitating decision making about seeking treatment.

Nursing Management

The problem of PE may become apparent during a health history that includes specific sexual data. Patients need assurance that many men have similar problems and that treatment is possible (Box 33.4). Patients can be referred to specialists for behavioral strategies. Younger men may find that masturbation before anticipation of sexual intercourse may help. Pharmacotherapy with selective serotonin reuptake inhibitors has been shown to be effective, but their use would be off label. Paroxetine (20–40 mg/d), sertraline (25–200 mg/d), and fluoxetine (10–60 mg/d) are commonly used. Ejaculation delay may start a few days after drug intake, but it is more evident in 1 to 2 weeks after its initiation.

ERECTILE DYSFUNCTION

Erectile dysfunction (ED) refers to the inability of a man to achieve or maintain an erection sufficient for satisfactory completion of the sexual activity.

Diagnostic Criteria

Although most men experience an occasional lack of erection, intervention is required when there is consistent (more than 6 months) erectile inefficiency during masturbation, intercourse, or on awakening (APA, 2013; Hatzimouratidis et al., 2010).

Epidemiology

Estimates of ED vary from 5% to 20% of men. ED may occur at any age although the incidence increases with aging. Men with diabetes, cardiovascular disease, or chronic renal failure also have a higher incidence of ED. For those undergoing radical prostatectomy, 25% to 75% experience ED (Hatzimouratidis et al., 2010).

Etiology
Biologic Theories

Common biologic causes of ED include genital trauma, vascular insufficiency, renal disease, hormonal deficiencies, Parkinson's disease, diabetes, multiple sclerosis, surgical procedures, use of antihypertensive and antidepressant drugs, and heavy cigarette smoking. Long-term alcohol or cocaine consumption can affect the erectile response. It is also more common with the aging process (Hatzimouratidis et al., 2010).

Psychological Theories

ED may also have a psychogenic basis. Numerous psychosocial etiologies have been identified. Fear of failure, relationship stress, poor body image, fear of rejection, partner hostility, guilt, cultural taboos, religious proscriptions, lack of knowledge, and negative attitudes are some of the identified etiologic factors. Not surprisingly, one may observe psychological sequelae to biologically based erectile failure, validating the multifactorial basis often identified and the imperative need to pursue a thorough investigation of causes before instituting a treatment regimen (Balon & Segraves, 2014).

Interdisciplinary Treatment

The treatment of men with ED is usually managed in primary care setting except for those with mental disorders, who may seek treatment within the mental health system. Since the introduction of the phosphodiesterase 5 (PDE5) inhibitors, pharmacologic agents such as sildenafil citrate, tadalafil, and vardenafil, many men choose the convenience of medication. For persons with psychiatric disorders, monitoring medications and their potential interaction is important. However, behavioral interventions have also been shown to be useful.

NURSING MANAGEMENT: Human Response to Erectile Dysfunction

ED is present in approximately 10% of men aged 40 to 70 who have severe or complete erectile dysfunction, defined as the total inability to achieve or maintain erections sufficient for sexual performance (Boston University School of Medicine, 2014). An additional 25% of men in this age category have moderate or intermittent erectile

difficulties. Although less common in younger men, erectile dysfunction still affects 5% to 10% of men below the age of 40. Findings from these studies show that erectile dysfunction impacts significantly on mood state, interpersonal functioning, and overall quality of life. Many men with mental disorders attribute their ED to their psychotropic medication. Consequently, these individuals stop taking their medications. Within a few weeks to months, they have a psychiatric elapse.

Biologic Domain
Assessment

Most men are not comfortable discussing sexuality and sexual problems. The assessment should be conducted in an atmosphere of trust and understanding. In many cultures, male self-esteem is related to the ability to perform sexually. When a man has problems with maintaining an erection, it is embarrassing and demeaning to him. Sensitivity to the patient's feelings should be reflected throughout the assessment (Box 33.5).

Nursing Diagnoses for the Biologic Domain

The nursing diagnoses usually generated from the assessment data are similar to those of the female orgasmic disorder—Ineffective Sexuality Patterns or Sexual Dysfunction.

Nursing Interventions for the Biologic Domain
Lifestyle Changes

Promotion of positive health practices that focus on adequate nutrition, rest, and exercise is important in promoting erectile functioning. Weight loss may improve overall health and enhance the strength of the erection. Regular exercise is also related to sexual health. Helping the patient develop a better lifestyle is important in promoting sexual functioning. Reducing alcohol consumption can also improve sexual performance.

Pharmacologic Interventions

PDE5 inhibitors are the treatment of choice. With sexual stimulation, nitric oxide is released into the nerve terminations and endothelial cell, stimulating the production of cyclic guanylate monophosphate (GMPc), a substance that enables the smooth muscle cells of the corpora cavernosa to relax. The PDE enzymes are involved in the breakdown of GMPc. The PDE inhibitors inactivate PDE5, thereby enabling the buildup of GMPc, sustaining relaxation of the corpora cavernosa.

There are several approved PDE5 inhibitors including sildenafil citrate (Viagra), vardenafil chloride (Levitra and Staxyn), tadalafil (Cialis), and avanafil (Stendra). These

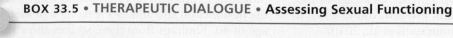

BOX 33.5 • THERAPEUTIC DIALOGUE • Assessing Sexual Functioning

INEFFECTIVE APPROACH

Nurse: Mr. J, are you currently sexually active?

Patient: I'm married. Of course I am.

Nurse: How would you describe your sexual activity?

Patient: OK.

Nurse: What do you mean, OK?

Patient: Just OK. (Getting irritated)

Nurse: Is there a problem?

Patient: Look, I just don't want to talk about it.

EFFECTIVE APPROACH

Nurse: Mr. J, are you currently sexually active?

Patient: I'm married. Of course I am.

Nurse: Well . . . sometimes it can be difficult to maintain a sexual relationship with the same partner over many years.

Patient: Yeah, you got that right.

Nurse: (Silence)

Patient: I wish I were younger. Then, sex was really good.

Nurse: Oh, has it changed?

Patient: Well, yeah.

Nurse: (Silence)

Patient: I just wish I could satisfy my wife.

Nurse: Is there a specific problem, such as becoming aroused, maintaining an erection, or having an ejaculation?

Patient: Yes, I can't keep my erection. It's so frustrating.

Nurse: Are you able to become excited?

Patient: That part's OK. I just wish I could keep an erection long enough to satisfy my wife.

Nurse: Have you talked to her about it?

Patient: Yeah, she wants me to go to that clinic.

Nurse: The male sexuality clinic?

Patient: That's the one. Do you know anything about it?

Nurse: Yes, the staff are all well qualified. I would be happy to make a referral for you.

CRITICAL THINKING CHALLENGE

- Compare the course of the first dialogue with the second one. What did the second nurse do differently to elicit information about the patient's erectile dysfunction?

- What is problematic about the first dialogue?

- The nurse in the second dialogue did not continue to ask questions. Instead, this nurse chose to discuss the general topic of sexual relationships within marriage and then made a referral. Debate whether or not the nurse should have pursued more details about the sexual dysfunction.

medications enhance the effect of nitric oxide, which is released in the corpus cavernosum during sexual stimulation. These medications are rapidly absorbed, with maximum observed plasma concentrations reached within 30 to 120 minutes of oral dosing in the fasted state. Cialis is long acting, up to 36 hours. Although these medications are approved for the treatment of ED in men, they have not been shown to be efficacious in sexual arousal disorders in women.

Before the introduction of PDE5 inhibitors, intracavernosal pharmacotherapy was the treatment of choice for ED. A vascular smooth muscle relaxant such as papaverine hydrochloride, phentolamine mesylate, or prostaglandin is directly injected into the corpus cavernosum by the patient or partner. This increases arterial flow of blood into the corpora and decreases venous outflow. Neurogenic rather than vascular ED appears to respond better. Complications can include excessive bleeding, scarring and priapism, and potential liver involvement. Counseling, strict monitoring, and specific teaching are required (Balon & Segraves, 2014).

Another treatment is the use of alprostadil (prostaglandin) in microsuppository form inserted into the urethra using a special applicator. The system called MUSE causes a rapid absorption of the medication through the urethral mucosa into the corpus spongiosum. It is particularly useful for men who are unable to inject themselves (Balon & Segraves, 2014).

Other Treatments

When erection is determined to be permanently impaired, several options may be considered to facilitate intercourse. An external penile prosthesis can be placed over the flaccid penis although some find this not esthetically pleasing. A pumping device that creates a vacuum can be used for blood entrapment followed by placement of a rubber band at the base of the penis. Surgical techniques for improving vascular sufficiency are also showing promising results.

Surgical implant of a penile prosthesis into each of the corpora has been a popular alternative. Several types exist. Mechanical or nonhydraulic implants may be a pair of semirigid rods that are bent up or down or activated by a switch that shortens a cable and pulls the device into a rigid position. Hydraulic prostheses use pumped fluid to expand hollow cylinders in the corpora.

Multicomponent prostheses require implantation of two penile cylinders, a fluid reservoir implanted within the abdomen, a pump in the scrotum, and connective tubing. This system requires extensive surgery. The potential for complications is lessened with use of a two or one-piece prosthesis. The one-piece or self-contained inflatable prosthesis uses a pump implanted on each side of the coronal ridge that transfers fluid from an outer to an inner cylinder; bending the penis releases a valve, and detumescence occurs.

Psychosocial Domain

Assessment

The psychosocial assessment should include a discussion about the impact of sexual dysfunction on the quality of the relationship with the partner. If a mental disorder, such as depression or posttraumatic stress disorder, is present comparing the timing of the dysfunction with the onset of symptoms and medication can determine whether the ED is related to the disorder and medication.

Nursing Diagnoses for the Psychosocial Domain

A variety of nursing diagnoses could be generated from the assessment data. Anxiety, stress overload, moral distress, and spiritual distress are examples. It is impor-

---

> **BOX 33.6**
>
> *Psychoeducation Checklist:* **Male Erectile Dysfunction**
>
> When caring for the patient with male erectile disorder, be sure to include the following topics in your teaching plan for the patient and partner:
> - Possible etiologic factors
> - Psychopharmacologic agents (e.g., intracavernosal therapy or yohimbine), including drug, action, frequency, administration technique, and possible adverse reactions
> - Alternative methods of sexual expression
> - Prosthesis use
> - Sexual education and counseling
> - Communication skills
> - Sex therapy

---

tant that nurse and patient identify the underlying psychosocial issues.

Interventions for the Psychosocial Domain

Education is important for the patient with erectile disorder. Teaching the patient about positive health practices and treatment options (i.e., mechanical devices, medications, surgical procedures) is usually needed (Box 33.6). The patient's concern about his partner's satisfaction needs to be explored. Many times, men believe that partner satisfaction is related only to penile penetration and their ability to sustain an erection. Encouraging the patient to talk with his partner about her (or his) sexual needs and other aspects of their sexual experience (physical closeness, kissing, hugging, mutual exploration of their bodies) helps him broaden his understanding of the sexual experience.

Evaluation and Treatment Outcomes

The major outcome for ED is improved sexual functioning. Acceptance of change of physical status is an outcome that is difficult to obtain. Improvement in sexual satisfaction may include increasing the ability for erectile functioning. If ED is permanent, exploration of other avenues of sexual expression may indicate a successful outcome. In this disorder, partner satisfaction is usually of prime concern. Improved communication with the man's partner may also be a positive outcome.

FEMALE SEXUAL INTEREST/AROUSAL DISORDER

Female sexual interest/arousal disorder is the lack of or significantly reduced sexual interest/arousal. Women with this disorder rarely initiate sexual activity and are unreceptive of their partner's attempts. They do not experience sexual excitement, which results in personal or interpersonal distress (APA, 2013).

Female sexual interest/arousal disorder may be the least studied of the sexual disorders, but it is more common than most believe, necessitating more accurate assessment and research. Its actual prevalence is unknown (DeRogatis & Burnett, 2008).

A female sexual interest/arousal disorder may occur at any age and may cause relationship difficulties and personal stress along with avoidance of sexual activity and impaired communication. Other etiological factors, such as anxiety, guilt, and history of sexual abuse, and changes in androgen levels during the menstrual cycle have been shown to affect arousal. Aging also affects sexual arousal because vasocongestion develops more slowly in older women, there is decreased vaginal lubrication after menopause, and lower estrogen levels at this life stage may affect sexual arousal.

Intervention focuses on treating factors that contribute to the lack of arousal. Cognitive behavioral therapy is recommended for psychosocial issues. For hormonal changes, a referral to a women's health provider is useful (Balon & Segraves, 2014).

MALE HYPOACTIVE SEXUAL DESIRE DISORDER

Male hypoactive sexual desire disorder is a recurrent deficiency or absence of sexual fantasies and desire for sexual activity. Individuals with this disorder are uninterested in sex, do not or cannot get "turned on," and require no sexual gratification. There may be active avoidance of potential sexual relationships. The prevalence is unknown, but it is believed to affect only a small proportion of men. Often, the disorder develops in adulthood after a period of adequate sexual interest and is associated with psychological distress, stressful life events (e.g., childbirth), or relationship difficulties (Balon & Segraves, 2014).

Therapy for psychological issues related to hypoactive sexual desire aims at helping the patient gain insight into the problem and develop strategies to enhance sexual arousal. Treatment approaches may include individual and couples therapy, sex therapy techniques, clinical hypnosis, cognitive behavioral therapy, guided fantasy exercises, and sexual assertiveness training.

If the problem is related to medication, changing to another classification of medication, giving drug holidays, or lowing the dose may help. Bupropion has been used in both men and women with some success.

GENITO-PELVIC PAIN/PENETRATION DISORDER

Genito-pelvic pain/penetration disorder is characterized by persistent or recurrent difficulties with vaginal pene-

tration during intercourse, marked vulvovaginal or pelvic pain during vaginal intercourse or penetration attempts, or significant fear or anxiety about the vuvovaginal or pelvic pain in anticipation of, during or as a result of vaginal penetration (APA, 2013).

Dyspareunia is a term used to describe the genital pain associated with sexual intercourse which may be caused by vaginismus, spastic, involuntary constriction of the perineal and outer vaginal muscles fostered by imagined, anticipated, or actual attempts at vaginal penetration. This disorder may be related to interpersonal or emotional factors such as sexual dissatisfaction or poor technique leading to inadequate relaxation and lubrication. Biologic etiologies include intact or biperforate hymen, postmenopausal atrophic changes, trauma, malignancy, intestinal disease, or other pelvic disorders (Balon & Segraves, 2014).

PARAPHILIAS

Paraphilias are described as "intense and persistent sexual interest other than sexual interest in genital stimulation or preparatory fondling with phenotypically normal, physically mature, consenting human partners characterized by recurrent, intense sexual urges, fantasies, or behaviors involving unusual objects, activities, or situations" (APA, 2013, p. 685). These interests cause significant distress to the individual or impair social or occupational functioning. The paraphilias include voyeuristic, exhibitionistic, frotteuristic, sexual masochism, sexual sadism, pedophilic, fetishistic, and transvestic disorders (APA, 2013).

Paraphilias are rarely diagnosed and is complicated across cultures because acceptability of sexual practices varies across cultures. Although there are very few studies, there is evidence that comorbid mood disorders are often associated with paraphilia disorders (Becker & Johnson, 2014). These disorders often come to the attention of mental health professionals within the context of illegal sexual activity or sexually violent predators. Treatment of paraphilias is rarely sought by the individual; rather, it is a result of the psychosocial or criminal ramifications.

Certain behaviors and fantasies associated with paraphilias are said to begin in childhood and become more elaborate and better defined during adolescence and early adulthood. The disorders are often found to be chronic and lifelong, with the fantasies and behavior diminishing with old age. Table 33.2 includes the different categories of paraphilias along with their descriptions.

GENDER DYSPHORIA

Gender dysphoria is the term used to describe an incongruence between an individual's experienced/expressed gender and assigned gender (APA, 2013). These individuals have a strong desire to be of the other gender. In boys

Table 33.2   PARAPHILIAS

Paraphilias	Description
Exhibitionism	The behavior involves exposing one's genitals to strangers, with occasional masturbation. There may be an awareness of the desire to shock the individual or the fantasy that the individual will become sexually aroused on observation of the exposure.
Fetishism	An object such as women's undergarments or foot apparel is used for sexual arousal. The individual usually masturbates while holding, rubbing, or smelling the item or it is worn by a partner during sexual activity. Fetishism usually begins in adolescence and continues throughout life.
Frotteurism	Sexually arousing urges, fantasies, and behaviors occur when touching or rubbing one's genitals against the breasts, genitals, or thighs of a nonconsenting person. This paraphilia usually begins in early adolescence or young adulthood and diminishes with age.
Pedophilia	Sexual activity occurs with a child usually 13 years of age or younger by an individual at least 16 years of age or 5 years older than the child. Pedophilic acts include fondling, oral sex, and anal or vaginal intercourse with the penis, fingers, or objects, with varying amounts of force.
Sexual masochism	This behavior involves the act of being humiliated, beaten, bound, or made to suffer. Self-induced masochistic acts include use of electric shock, pin sticking, restraints, and mutilation; partner-induced acts may include bondage, whipping, being urinated or defecated on; and being forced to crawl, bark, or wear diapers. One dangerous form of sexual masochism that may be practiced alone or with a partner is "hypoxyphilia." Oxygen deprivation by means of a noose, plastic bag, chest compression, or drug effect is used during sexual activity to heighten orgasmic sensation. Deaths have occurred as a result of these techniques.
Sexual sadism	Sexual excitement occurs when causing physical or psychological suffering to another individual. Commonly, the individual with sadistic behavior interacts with a masochistic partner. Sadistic behavior includes various forms of physical punishment, use of restraints, rape, burning, stabbing, strangulation, torture, and murder. This is usually a chronic paraphilia that begins as early sexual fantasies and increases in severity over time.
Transvestic fetishism	This behavior applies generally to the heterosexual man who cross-dresses for the purpose of sexual excitement. The fantasies, sexual urges, or behaviors associated with the cross-dressing are recurrent and cause clinically significant distress or impairment in social, occupational, or other important areas of functioning.
Voyeurism	This behavior involves "peeping," for the purpose of sexual excitement, at unsuspecting people who are nude, undressing, or engaged in sexual activity.
Other paraphilias	Sexual fantasies, urges, and activities involving animals (zoophilia), corpses (necrophilia), feces (coprophilia), urine (urophilia), body parts (partialism), and obscene telephone calls (telephone scatalogia).

(assigned gender), there is a strong preference for cross-dressing or simulating female attire. In girls (assigned gender), there is a strong preference for wearing typical masculine clothing and a strong resistance to the wearing of typical female clothing (APA, 2013).

In child clinical samples, there are about four boys for each girl referred with this disorder, but these differences disappear in adolescence (Becker & Perkins, 2014). Gender dysphonia does not necessarily persist into adulthood. Treatment focuses on acceptance, support, and self-esteem enhancement for both children and parents. Treatment goals should be made by the patient and family with the clinician providing the research literature.

SUMMARY OF KEY POINTS

- Sexuality is a basic dimension of every individual's personality.

- Biosexual and gender identities result from genetic and intrauterine hormonal influences and are already established at birth.

- There are at least three models explaining sexual responses, but more research is sorely needed. The human sexual response cycle is a linear model consisting of four phases (excitement, plateau, orgasm, and resolution) and is based on physiological responses. The circular model includes nonsexual interpersonal factors, such as a desire for physical connection and intimacy needs, not just simply sexual release. The dual-control model focuses on excitatory and inhibitory processes.

- Female orgasmic disorder is a common disorder affecting women; erectile dysfunction and premature ejaculation are the most common disorders affecting men.

- Nursing interventions for people experiencing sexual dysfunction include (but are not limited to) counseling, education, and referral to sex therapists.

- Various medical conditions, psychological states, and medications negatively affect the sexual response cycle. Education about medication side effects and sexual experiences is important in maintaining health.

- Paraphilias are rarely diagnosed, but the prevalence may be higher than usually presented.

- Gender dysphoria occurs when the individual is uncomfortable with assigned sex or gender role.

CRITICAL THINKING CHALLENGES

1. Compare the physiologic changes of men and women during the phases of sexual response.

2. A 36-year-old woman was recently diagnosed with depression and treated with a selective serotonin reuptake inhibitor (antidepressant). Her depression is improving, but she has not been interested in sexual relations with her husband. Her lack of sexual interest is beginning to cause problems in her marriage. What could account for the changes in sexual interest? Develop a brief care plan for this patient.

3. A 52-year-old married man who is being successfully treated with lithium carbonate for his bipolar disorder was recently diagnosed with diabetes mellitus. He was told that his diabetes could be controlled by weight loss and diet. His major worry is that the diabetes and lithium are causing his impotence. He casually mentions that he is considering stopping the lithium. What issues should the nurse explore with the patient? What actions could the patient begin that would improve his sexual health?

4. During a nursing assessment, a young adult woman reveals that she is a lesbian and that she is currently living with her partner. She has not yet told her parents about her sexual orientation and is experiencing some anxiety about sharing this part of her life with her family. Her partner is supportive and encourages the young woman to take her time in telling her family members. Is this patient experiencing symptoms of a gender dysphoria? Explain.

5. A man is distressed about his wife's inability to enjoy sexual relations after the birth of their third child. He has never been unfaithful to his wife but is frustrated with their current relationship. He is considering having an affair with one of his coworkers. What would be the best approach for this patient? Is referral to a sex therapist appropriate?

MOVIES ***The Birdcage:*** 1996. In this remake of the 1978 French comedy, *La Cage aux Folles*, Robin Williams stars as Armand Goldman, a gay cabaret owner who lives in Miami's South Beach with his partner Albert, the club's star performer. Armand and Albert must try to disguise their gay relationship when the in-laws of Armand's son, Val, come for dinner.

VIEWING POINTS: Would anyone in the film meet any criteria for having a mental disorder, including a gender dysphoria? Observe your feelings about Armand and Albert's lifestyle.

References

American Psychiatric Association. (2013). *Diagnostic and statistical manual of mental disorders* (5th ed.), Arlington, VA: American Psychiatric Association.
Bancroft, J. & Graham, C. A. (2011). The varied nature of women's sexuality: Unresolved issues and a theoretical approach. *Hormones and Behavior, 59*(5), 717–729.
Bancroft, J., Graham, C. A., Janssen, E., & Sanders, S. A. (2009). The dual control model: Current status and future directions. *Journal of Sex Research, 46*(2–3), 121–142.
Balon, R. & Segraves, R. (2014). Sexual dysfunctions. In R. E. Hales, S. C. Yudofsy, & L.W. Roberts (Eds.). *The American Psychiatric Publishing Textbook of Psychiatry* (6th ed.), Arlington, VA: American Psychiatric Publishing. www.psychiatryonline.org. doi:*10.1176/appi.books.978158625031.682032*
Bao, A. & Swaab, D. F. (2011). Sexual differentiation of the human brain: relation to gender identity, sexual orientation and neuropsychiatric disorders. *Frontiers in Neuroendocrinology, 32*(2), 214–226.
Basson, R. (2001). Female sexual response: The role of drugs in the management of sexual dysfunction. *Obstetrics & Gynecology, 98*(2), 350–353.
Becker, J. & Johnson, B. (2014). Paraphilic disorders. In R. E. Hales, S. C. Yudofsy, & L.W. Roberts (Eds.). *The American Psychiatric Publishing Textbook of Psychiatry* (6th ed.), Arlington, VA: American Psychiatric Publishing. www.psychiatryonline.org. doi:*10.1176/appi.books.978158625031.146239*
Becker, J. & Perkins, A. (2014). Gender dysphoria. In R. E. Hales, S. C. Yudofsy, & L.W. Roberts (Eds.). *The American Psychiatric Publishing Textbook of Psychiatry* (6th ed.), Arlington, VA: American Psychiatric Publishing. www.psychiatryonline.org. doi:*10.1176/appi.books.978158625031.939093*
Boston University School of Medicine. (2014). Epidemiology of ED. www.bumc.bu.ed/sexualmedicine/physicianinformation/epidemiology-of-ed/
Centers for Disease Control and Prevention, Eaton, D. K., Kann, L., Kinchen, S., Shanklin, S., Ross, J., et al. (2010). Youth risk behavior surveillance-United States, 2009. *Morbidity and Mortality Weekly Report, 59*, 1–142.
Clayton, A. H., Croft, H. A., & Handiwala, L. (2014). Antidepressants and sexual dysfunction: mechanisms and clinical implications. *Postgraduate Medicine, 126*(2), 91–99.
DeRogatis, L. R. & Burnett, A. L. (2008). The epidemiology of sexual dysfunctions. *Journal of Sexual Medicine, 5*(2), 289–300.
Giles, K. R. & McCabe, M. P. (2009). Conceptualizing women's sexual function: Linear vs. circular models of sexual response. *Journal of Sexual Medicine, 6*(10), 2761–2771.
Graham, C. A. (2010). The DSM diagnostic criteria for female orgasmic disorder. *Archives of Sexual Behavior, 39*(2), 256–270.
Hatzimouratidis, K., Amar, E., Eardley, I., Giuliano, F., Hatzichristou, D. Montorsi, F., et al. (2010). Guidelines on male sexual dysfunction: Erectile dysfunction and premature ejaculation. *European Urology, 57*(5), 804–814.
Hayes, R. D. (2011). Circular and linear modeling of female sexual desire and arousal. *Journal of Sex Research, 48*(2), 130–141.
Kaplan, H. S. (1979). *Disorders of sexual desire and other concepts and techniques in sex therapy.* New York: Simon & Schuster.
Kellogg, N. D. (2010). Sexual behaviors in children: Evaluation and management. *American Family Physician, 82*(10), 1233–1238.
Masters, W. H. & Johnson, V. E. (1966). *Human sexual response.* Boston, MA: Little, Brown.
Masters, W. H. & Johnson, V. E. (1970). *Human sexual inadequacy.* Boston, MA: Little, Brown.
McMahon, C. G., Jannini, E., Waldinger, M., & Rowland, D. (2013). Standard operating procedures in the disorders of orgasm and ejaculation. *Journal of Sexual Medicine, 10*(1), 204–229.
Sand, M. & Fisher, W. (2007). Women's endorsement of models of female sexual response: The nurses' sexuality study. *Journal of Sexual Medicine, 4*(3), 708–719.
Will, R. F., Hull, E. M., & Dominguez, J. M. (2014). Influences of dopamine and glutamate in the medial preoptic area on male sexual behavior. *Pharmacology Biochemistry, and Behavior, 121*, 115–123. doi:*10.1016/j.pbb.2014.02.005*
Wylie, K. & Mimoun, S. (2009). Sexual response models in women. *Maturitas, 63*(2), 112–115.

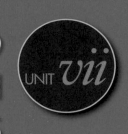

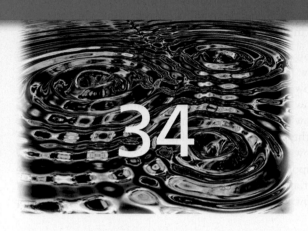

34

Mental Health Assessment of Children and Adolescents

Vanya Hamrin and Catherine Gray Deering

KEY CONCEPTS

- assortative mating
- comprehensive assessment

LEARNING OBJECTIVES

After studying this chapter, you will be able to:

1. Define the assessment process for children and adolescents.

2. Discuss techniques of data collection used with children and adolescents.

3. Delineate important biopsychosocial areas of assessment for children and adolescents.

KEY TERMS

- attachment • attachment disorganization • developmental delays • egocentrism • maturation
- temperament

The mental health assessment of children and adolescents is a specialized process that considers their unique problems and responses within the context of their development. Any nurse who cares for a child should be comfortable with conducting a mental health nursing assessment because the emotional and psychological aspects are central to understanding health needs and behaviors.

The assessment of children and adolescents generally follows the same format as for adults (see Chapter 10), but there are significant differences. Children think in more

concrete terms; thus, the nurse needs to ask more specific and fewer open-ended questions than would typically be asked of adults. The nurse should use simple phrasing because children have a narrower vocabulary than do adults. Examples include saying "sad" instead of "depressed" or "nervous" instead of "anxious." The nurse needs to corroborate information that children offer with more sources (e.g., parents, teachers) than they would for adults. The nurse may want to use artistic and play media (e.g., puppets, family drawings) to engage children and evaluate their perceptions, inner worlds, fine motor skills, and intellectual functions. Children have a less specific sense of time and a less developed memory than do adults. When children are asked about a sequence of events or specific times when events occurred, they may not be able to provide accurate information.

A comprehensive evaluation includes a biopsychosocial history, mental status examination, additional testing (e.g., cognitive or neuropsychological) if necessary, records of the child's school performance and medical–physical history, and information from other agencies that may be providing services (e.g., Department of Child and Family Services [DCF], juvenile court). The nurse may use various assessment tools, including the Child Attention Profile (CAP) and the Devereux Childhood Assessment (DECA), the Behavior Assessment System for Children (BASC), the Child Behavior Checklist (CBCL), or the Children's Depression Inventory (CDI).

> **NCLEXNOTE** Whenever assessing children or adolescents, developmental level will frame the assessment and implementation of the management plan.

TECHNIQUES FOR DATA COLLECTION: THE CLINICAL INTERVIEW

The clinical interview is the primary assessment tool used in child and adolescent psychiatry. A unique set of skills is necessary for interviewing children and adolescents. How the nurse obtains mental health information depends on the developmental level of each child, specifically considering the child's language, cognitive, social, and emotional skills. For example, the nurse should simplify questions for young children or children with **developmental delays** (e.g., intellectual disability, autism spectrum disorder, mood disorder) so these children can understand and respond appropriately.

The assessment interview may be the initial contact between the child and parent or guardian and the nurse. The first step is to establish a treatment alliance, and the second is to assess the interactions between the child and parent.

Establishment of a Treatment Alliance

The nurse can establish rapport by greeting the child or adolescent in a friendly, polite, open manner and putting him or her at ease. Speaking clearly and at a normal volume and using friendly, reassuring tones are essential measures. The nurse can establish a treatment alliance by recognizing the child's individuality and showing respect and concern for the child. The nurse should demonstrate sensitivity, objectivity, and confidentiality. The child will be

more forthcoming if he or she feels that the nurse is listening carefully and is interested in what he or she has to say.

Child and Parent Observation

Because the child's primary environment is with the parent, child–parent interactions provide important data about the child–parent attachment and parenting practices. The nurse's observations focus on both the child alone and the child within the family. The nurse can actually make some of these observations while the family is in the waiting area, including:

* How the child and parent talk to each other, including how frequently each initiates conversation
* How the parent disciplines the child
* How attached the parent and child appear
* How the child and parent separate
* If the parent and child play together
* How the child gets the parent's attention and how responsive the parent is to the child's attention-seeking initiatives
* How the parent and child show affection to each other

Separate Child and Parent Interviews

To get an accurate picture of the child, the nurse should interview the child and parent individually because each can provide unique meaningful information. Research has shown that when parent and child are interviewed separately in a structured interview about the child's psychopathology, they rarely agree on the presence of diagnostic criteria, regardless of the diagnostic type (Frick, Barry, & Kamphaus, 2010). Generally, children provide better information about internalizing symptoms (e.g., mood, sleep, suicide ideation), and parents provide better information about externalizing symptoms (e.g., behavior disturbances, oppositionality, relationship with parents).

Discussion With the Child

After talking with the parent and child together, the nurse should ask to speak with the child alone for awhile. Young children may fear separating from their parents. The nurse can reassure children by showing them where the waiting area is and telling them that if they get scared, the nurse will accompany them to check on their parents. Introducing a toy or game or allowing the child to hold a transitional object may help. Remember that observing how the child separates from the parent is part of the data needed to complete the assessment.

Adolescents may act indifferent or even hostile when the nurse asks to speak with them alone. Teens tend to be skeptical that adults can really understand their experience, suspicious that they will be blamed for their problems, and fearful that their thoughts and feelings are abnormal. The nurse should be patient with adolescents and say something like, "I can see you're pretty angry about being here. What are you particularly angry about? Perhaps there is some way I can help you." Another useful and reassuring question is, "During the last few minutes, you've been quiet. I'm wondering what you are feeling." Or the nurse may ask, "It can be uncomfortable to tell personal information to someone you don't know. Do you feel this way?" (Frick et al., 2010).

To begin the initial assessment of a child, the nurse introduces him- or herself and explains briefly what they will be doing. For children younger than 11 years of age, the nurse should explain that he or she helps worried or upset children by talking, playing, and giving advice to them and their parents. The nurse should then ask about the child's understanding of why he or she is there. This question often helps to identify children's misperceptions (e.g., believing the nurse is going to give them an injection, thinking they have done something bad) that could create barriers to working with them. When conducting the child interview, the nurse needs to get several releases of information from the child's guardian to obtain the corroborating reports, such as the child's physical assessment from the pediatrician or pediatric nurse practitioner; the school's report about the child's academic and behavioral performance, including the child's report card, behavior at school, peer interactions, and adult interactions; and records of diagnosis and treatment from any previous psychiatric provider.

The nurse must adapt communication to the child's age level (Box 34.1). The challenge is to avoid using overly complex vocabulary or talking down to children. Young children often express themselves more easily in the context of play than through adult-like conversation. For example, a child may re-enact a conversation that he had with a sibling or parent using puppets. Children respond well to third-person conversation prompts, such as: "Some kids don't like being compared with their brothers and sisters," or "I know a kid who was so sad when he lost his dog that he thought he would never be happy again."

Early in the interview, the goal is to explain the nurse's purpose, elicit any concerns the child may have about what is happening, and establish rapport with the child by engaging in unthreatening discussion. Many adults rarely ask children about things that truly interest them but expect children to respond readily to adult conversation. The nurse can establish a high degree of credibility simply by taking note of and asking about things that are obviously important to children (e.g., a sport the child participates in, a rock group displayed on a shirt, a toy a child has brought with her). However, children have an uncanny natural "radar" for phony adult behavior. Attempts to establish rapport work only when the nurse is genuinely interested in the child's life.

BOX 34.1

Strategies for Interviewing Children

- Use a simple vocabulary and short sentences tailored to the child's developmental and cognitive levels.
- Be sure that the child understands the questions and that you do not lead the child to give a particular response. Phrase your questions so the child does not receive any hint that one response is more acceptable than another.
- Select the questions for your interview on an individual basis using judgment and discretion and considering the child's age and developmental level.
- Be sure that the manner and tone of your voice do not reveal any personal biases.
- Speak slowly and quietly and try to allow the interview to unfold, using the child's verbalizations and behavior as guides.
- Use simple terms (e.g., "sad" for "depressed") in exploring affective reactions and ask the child to give examples of how he or she behaves or how other people behave when emotionally aroused.
- Assume an accepting and neutral attitude toward the child's communications.
- Learn about children's current interests by looking at Saturday morning television programs, talking with parents, visiting toy stores, looking at children's books, and visiting day care centers and schools to observe children in their natural habitats.

Discussion With the Parents

After meeting alone with the child, the nurse should spend some time alone with the parents and ask for a detailed description of their view of the problem. When alone, parents may feel comfortable discussing their children in depth and sharing frustrations with their behavior. Parents need this opportunity to speak freely without being constrained by concern for the child's feelings. In some cases, it would be detrimental for the child to hear the full force of the parents' complaints and feelings, such as helplessness, anger, or disappointment. Parents need the nurse to allow them to express their feelings without passing judgment. This is the nurse's opportunity to enlist the help of parents as partners in the child's evaluation and treatment. This time is also good for filling in any gaps in the history and clarifying the data obtained from the interview with the child.

Parents need the chance to describe the presenting problem in their own words. The nurse can encourage them by asking general questions, such as, "What brings you here today?" or "How have things been in your family?" The nurse should then reflect his or her understanding of the problem, showing empathy and respect for both the parent and child. Asking any other family members about their view of the problem is always a good idea to clarify discrepant points of view, obtain additional data, and communicate awareness that different family members experience the same problem in different ways.

Development of Rapport

To reduce anxiety about the evaluation, the nurse must develop rapport with the family members. Establishing rapport can be facilitated by maintaining appropriate eye contact; speaking slowly, clearly, and calmly with friendliness and acceptance; using a warm and expressive tone; reacting to communications from interviewees objectively; showing interest in what the interviewees are saying; and making the interview a joint undertaking (Frick et al., 2010). Suggestions for building rapport with children and adolescents are also addressed in each of the developmental sections that follow. The information in Box 34.2 can serve as a guide to asking specific questions during a comprehensive assessment.

> **KEYCONCEPT** A **comprehensive assessment** includes a very detailed, focused interview that elicits all aspects of the biopsychosocial responses and health promotion information that provides direction for care.

Preschool-Aged Children

When interviewing preschool-aged children, the nurse should understand that these children may have difficulty putting their feelings into words and that their thinking is very concrete. For example, a preschool-aged child might assume that a tall container holds more water than a wide container even if both containers hold the same amount of fluid.

The nurse can achieve rapport with preschool-aged children by joining their world of play. Play is an activity by which children transform an experience from real life into a symbolic, nonliteral representation. Play encourages verbalizations, promotes manual strength, teaches rules and problem solving, and helps children master control over their environment (Mendelsohn, Huberman, Berkule, Brockmeyer, Morrow, & Dreyer, 2011). With children younger than 5 years of age, the nurse may conduct the assessment in a playroom. Useful materials are paper, pencils, crayons, paints, paint brushes, easels, clay, blocks, balls, dolls, doll houses, puppets, animals, dress-up clothes, and a water supply. The nurse must inform preschool-aged children about any rules for the play. For example, the nurse must tell the child that the nurse must ensure safety, so there will be no hitting in the playroom.

When observing the child in a free play setting, the nurse should pay attention to initiation of play, energy level, manipulative actions, tempo, body movements, tone, integration, creativity, products, age appropriateness, and attitudes toward adults. In addition, themes of play, expression of emotions, and temperament are important to observe. The nurse must allow children to direct and initiate these

themes. When evaluating a young child's peer relationships through play therapy in a playgroup or school setting, observe play settings and themes, initiation of play, response to peer initiations of play, integration of affect and action during play, resolution of conflicts, responses to suggestions of others during play, and the ability to engage in role taking and role reversals. Play therapy that uses a humanistic approach produces a positive effect over other forms of play therapy (Bratton, Ray, Rhine, & Jones, 2005).

The nurse's roles are to be a good listener; use appropriate vocabulary; tolerate a child's anxious, angry, or sad behavior; and use reflective comments about the child's play. Through play, the nurse can assess the child's sensorimotor skills, cognitive style, adaptability, language functioning, emotional and behavioral responsiveness, social level, moral development, coping styles, problem-solving techniques, and approaches to perceiving and interpreting the surrounding world. Lidz (2003) developed a tool that clinicians can use to assess preschoolers' play (Box 34.3). Analyzing children's perceptions of fairy tales can provide clinicians with clues to culture, problems, solutions, and elements of mental functioning (Turkel, 2002).

Drawings are also used in child assessment to illuminate the child's intellect, creative talents, neuropsychological deficits, body image difficulties, and perceptions of family life (Fig. 34.1). Types of drawings used in child assessments are free drawings; self-portraits; the kinetic family drawing; tree, person, and house drawing; and a picture of someone of the opposite sex (Perets-Dubrovsky, Kaveh, Deutsh-Castel, Cohen, & Tirosh, 2010). The DECA instrument measures protective factors of attachment, self-control, and initiative in children 2 to 5 years of age. The DECA tool is used in the preschool classroom

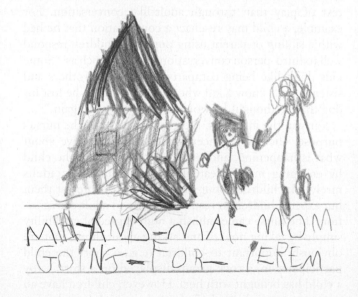

FIGURE 34.1 Me and my mom going for ice cream. Drawing and writing by a 5-year-old girl.

BOX 34.2

Semistructured Interview With School-Aged Children

Precede the questions below with a preliminary greeting, such as the following: "Hi, I am (your name and title). You must be (child's name). Come in."

FOR ALL SCHOOL-AGED CHILDREN
 1. Has anyone told you about why you are here today?
 2. (If yes) Who?
 3. (If yes) What did he (she) tell you?
 4. Tell me why *you* think you are here. (If child mentions a problem, explore it in detail.)
 5. How old are you?
 6. When is your birthday?
 7. Your address is . . . ?
 8. And your telephone number is . . .?

School
 9. Let's talk about school. What grade are you in?
10. What is your teacher's name?
11. What grades are you getting?
12. What subjects do you like the best?
13. And what subjects do you like least?
14. What subjects give you the most trouble?
15. And what subjects give you the least trouble?
16. What activities are you in at school?
17. How do you get along with your classmates?
18. How do you get along with your teachers?
19. Tell me how you spend a usual day at school.

Home
20. Now let's talk about your home. Who lives with you at home?
21. Tell me a little about each of them.
22. What does your father do for work?
23. What does your mother do for work?
24. Tell me what your home is like.
25. Tell me about your room at home.
26. What chores do you do at home?
27. How do you get along with your father?
28. What does he do that you like?
29. What does he do that you don't like?
30. How do you get along with your mother?
31. What does she do that you like?
32. What does she do that you don't like?
33. (When relevant) How do you get along with your brothers and sisters?
34. What do (does) they (he/she) do that you like?
35. What do (does) they (he/she) do that you don't like?
36. Who handles the discipline at home?
37. Tell me about how they (he/she) handle (handles) it.

Interests
38. Now let's talk about you. What hobbies and interests do you have?
39. What do you do in the afternoons after school?
40. Tell me what you usually do on Saturdays and Sundays.

Friends
41. Tell me about your friends.
42. What do you like to do with your friends?

Moods and Feelings
43. Everybody feels happy at times. What things make you feel happiest?
44. What are you most likely to get sad about?
45. What do you do when you are sad?
46. Everybody gets angry at times. What things make you angriest?
47. What do you do when you are angry?

Fears and Worries
48. All children get scared sometimes about some things. What things make you feel scared?
49. What do you do when you are scared?
50. Tell me what you worry about.
51. Any other things?

Self-Concerns
52. What do you like best about yourself?
53. Anything else?
54. What do you like least about yourself?
55. Anything else?
56. Tell me about the best thing that ever happened to you.
57. Tell me about the worst thing that ever happened to you.

Somatic Concerns
58. Do you ever get headaches?
59. (If yes) Tell me about them. (How often? What do you usually do?)
60. Do you get stomach aches?
61. (If yes) Tell me about them. (How often? What do you usually do?)
62. Do you get any other kinds of body pains?
63. (If yes) Tell me about them.

Thought Disorder
64. Do you ever hear things that seem funny or usual?
65. (If yes) Tell me about them. (How often? How do you feel about them? What do you usually do?)
66. Do you ever see things that seem funny or unreal?
67. (If yes) Tell me about them. (How often? How do you feel about them? What do you usually do?)

Memories and Fantasy
68. What is the first thing you can remember from the time you were a very little baby?
69. Tell me about your dreams.
70. Which dreams come back again?
71. Who are your favorite television characters?
72. Tell me about them.
73. What animals do you like best?
74. Tell me about these animals.
75. What animals do you like least?
76. Tell me about these animals.
77. What is your happiest memory?
78. What is your saddest memory?
79. If you could change places with anyone in the whole world, who would it be?
80. Tell me about that.
81. If you could go anywhere you wanted to right now, where would you go?
82. Tell me about that.
83. If you could have three wishes, what would they be?
84. What things do you think you might need to take with you if you were to go to the moon and stay there for 6 months?

Aspirations
85. What do you plan on doing when you become an adult?
86. Do you think you will have any problem doing that?
87. If you could do anything you wanted when you become an adult, what would it be?

Concluding Questions
88. Do you have anything else that you would like to tell me about yourself?
89. Do you have any questions that you would like to ask me?

Continued

BOX 34.2

Semistructured Interview With School-Aged Children (*Continued*)

FOR ADOLESCENTS
These questions can be inserted after number 67.

Sexual Relations
1. Do you have any special girlfriend (boyfriend)?
2. (If yes) Tell me about her (him).
3. What kind of sexual concerns do you have?
4. (If present) Tell me about them.

Drug and Alcohol Use
5. Do your parents drink alcohol?
6. (If yes) Tell me about their drinking. (How much, how frequently, and where?)

7. Do your friends drink alcohol?
8. (If yes) Tell me about their drinking.
9. Do you drink alcohol?
10. (If yes) Tell me about your drinking.
11. Do your parents use drugs?
12. (If yes) Tell me about the drugs they use. (How much, how frequently, and for what reasons?)
13. Do your friends use drugs?
14. (If yes) Tell me about the drugs they use.
15. Do you use drugs?
16. (If yes) Tell me about the drugs you use.

---

setting with the goal of promoting positive resilience in children.

School-Aged Children

Unlike preschool-aged children, school-aged (5–11 years) children can use more constructs, provide longer descriptions and make better inferences of others, and acquire more complete conceptions of various social roles. Children in middle school are more capable of verbal exchange and can tolerate limited periods of direct questioning (Box 34.4). The nurse can establish rapport with school-aged children by using competitive board games, such as checkers and playing cards. A therapeutic game helpful in assessing the child's perceptions, cognition, and emotions and in establishing rapport between a clinician and child is the thinking–feeling–doing game. In this game, the clinician and child take turns drawing cards that pose hypothetical situations and ask what a person might think, feel, or do in such scenarios. For example, one card might say, "A boy has something on his mind that he is afraid to tell his father. What is he scared to talk about?" Another might read, "A girl heard her parents fighting. What were they fighting about? What was the girl thinking while she listened to her parents?"

Adolescents

Adolescents have an increased command of language concepts and have developed the capacity for abstract and formal operations thinking. Their social world is also more complex. Some early adolescents tend to assume that their subjective experiences are real and congruent with objective reality, which can lead to egocentrism. **Egocentrism** includes the concepts of the imaginary audience (others are watching them) and the personal fable (they are special and unique and omnipotent) (Rycek, Stuhr, McDermott, Benker, & Swartz, 1999). Egocentrism is a preoccupation with one's own appearance, behavior, thoughts, and feelings. For example, a preteen may think that he caused his parents to divorce because he fought with his father the day before the parents announced their decision to separate. Because teenagers have a heightened sense of self-consciousness, they may be preoccupied during the interview with applying makeup or other self-grooming tasks.

During early adolescence, cognitive changes include increased self-consciousness, fear of being shamed, and demands for privacy and secrecy. An adolescent's willingness to talk to a nurse will depend partly on his or her perception of the degree of rapport between them. The nurse's ability to communicate respect, cooperation, honesty, and genuineness is important. Rejection by the adolescent, even outright hostility, during the first few interactions is common, especially if the teen is having behavior problems at home, at school, or in the community. The nurse should be patient and avoid jumping to conclusions. Hostility or defiance may be a test of how much

---

BOX 34.3

LIDZ Assessment Tool

Child's Name: _____ Birth Date: _____ Age: ___

Assessor: _____ Date of Assessment: _____

Describe typical play style/sequence.
Describe range of levels of play from lowest to highest level with age estimates and within contexts of independent/facilitated, familiar/unfamiliar, single/multiple toys.
Describe language and evidence of self-talk and internalized speech.
Describe interpersonal interactions with assessor and facilitator (if not assessor).
Describe content of any play themes.
What held the child's attention the longest? (For how long?) And what were the child's toy/play preferences?
Describe the child's affective state during play.
Implications of above for intervention.

From Lidz, C. S. (2003). *Early childhood assessment* (p. 92). Hoboken, NJ: Wiley & Sons, Inc. Copyright 2003, John Wiley & Sons. Used with permission.

BOX 34.4

Biopsychosocial Psychiatric Nursing Assessment of Children and Adolescents

1. Identifying information
Name
Sex
Date of birth
Age
Birth order
Grade
Ethnic background
Religious preference
List of others living in household

2. Major reason for seeking help
Description of presenting problems or symptoms
When did the problems (symptoms) start?
Describe both the child's and the parent's perspective.

3. Psychiatric history
Previous mental health contacts (inpatient and outpatient)
Other mental health problems or psychiatric diagnosis
    (besides those described currently)
Previous medications and compliance
Family history of depression, substance abuse, psychosis,
    etc., and treatment

4. Current and past health status
Medical problems
Current medications
Surgery and hospitalizations
Allergies
Diet and eating habits
Sleeping habits
Height and weight
Hearing and vision
Menstrual history
Immunizations
If sexually active, birth control method used
Date of last physical examination
Pediatrician or nurse practitioner's name and telephone
    number

5. Medications
Prescription (dosage, side effects)
Over-the-counter drugs

6. Neurologic history
Right handed, left handed, or ambidextrous
Headaches, dizziness, fainting
Seizures
Unusual movement (tics, tremors)
Hyperactivity
Episodes of weakness or paralysis
Slurred speech, pronunciation problems
Fine motor skills (eating with utensils, using crayon or
    pencil, fastening buttons and zippers, tying shoes)
Gross motor skills and coordination (walking, running,
    hopping)

7. Responses to mental health problems
What makes problems (symptoms) worse or better?
Feelings about those experiences (what helped and did
    not help)
What interventions have been tried so far?
Major loss or changes in past year
Fears, including punishment

8. Mental status examination
See Box 34.5

9. Developmental assessment
Mother's pregnancy, delivery
Child's Apgar score
Physical maturation
Psychosocial
Language
Developmental milestones: walking, talking, toileting

10. Attachment, temperament or significant behavior patterns
Attachment
Concentration, distractibility
Eating and sleeping patterns
Ability to adjust to new situations and changes in routine
Usual mood and fluctuations
Excitability
Ability to wait, tendency to interrupt
Responses to discipline
Lying, stealing, fighting, cruelty to animals, fire setting

11. Self-concept
Beliefs about self
Body image
Self-esteem
Personal identity

12. Risk assessment
History of suicidal thoughts, previous attempts
Suicide ideation, plan, lethality of plan, accessibility of plan
History of violent, aggressive behavior
Homicidal ideation

13. Family relationships
Relationship with parents
Deaths or losses
Family conflicts (nature and content)
Disciplinary methods
Quality of sibling relationship
Sleeping arrangements
Who does the child relate to or trust in the family?
Relationships with extended family

14. School and peer adjustment
Learning difficulties
Behavior problems at school
School attendance
Relationship with teachers
Special classes
Best friend
Relationships with peers
Dating
Drug and alcohol use
Participation in sports, clubs, other activities
After-school routine

15. Community resources
Professionals or agencies working with child or family
Day care resources

16. Functional status
Global Assessment of Functioning Scale (GAF)

17. Stresses and coping behaviors
Psychosocial stresses
Coping behaviors (strengths)

18. Summary of significant data

the teen can trust the nurse, a defense against anxiety, or a transference phenomenon (see Chapter 7).

Adolescents are likely to be defensive in front of their parents and concerned with confidentiality. At the start of the interview, the nurse should clearly convey to the adolescent what information will and will not be shared with parents. Adolescents generally prefer a straightforward, candid approach to the interview because they often distrust those in authority. Mentioning to adolescents that they do not have to discuss anything that they are not ready to reveal is also a good idea, so they will feel in control while they gradually build trust.

BIOPSYCHOSOCIAL PSYCHIATRIC NURSING ASSESSMENT OF CHILDREN AND ADOLESCENTS

As discussed, the comprehensive assessment of the child or adolescent includes interviews with the child and parents, child alone, and parents alone. After completing these components, the nurse should bring the child and parents back together to summarize his or her view of their concerns and to ask for feedback regarding whether these perceptions agree with theirs. The nurse must give the family a chance to share additional information and ask questions. Then the nurse should thank them for their willingness to talk and give them some idea of the next steps. Use of an assessment tool is helpful in organizing data for mental health planning and intervention.

When interviewing both a child and parents, directly asking the child as many questions as possible is generally the best way to get accurate, first-hand information and to reinforce interest in the child's viewpoint. Asking the child questions about the history of the current problem, previous psychiatric experiences (both good and bad), family psychiatric history, medical problems, developmental history (to get an idea of what the child has been told), school adjustment, peer relationships, and family functioning is particularly important. If necessary, the nurse can ask some or all of these same questions of the parents to verify the accuracy of the data, attain supplemental information, or both. Keep in mind that developmental research shows moderate to low correlation between parent and child reports of family behavior.

Biologic Domain

Nurses should include a thorough history of psychiatric and medical problems in any comprehensive assessment. A physical assessment is necessary to rule out any medical problems that could be mistaken for psychiatric symptoms (e.g., weight loss resulting from diabetes, not depression; drug-induced psychosis). Pharmacologic assessment should include prescription and over-the-counter medications.

Nurses should ask about any allergies to food, medications, or environmental triggers.

Genetic Vulnerability

The line between nature and nurture is not always clear. Characteristics that appear to be inborn may influence parents and teachers to respond differently toward different children, thus creating problems in the family environment. A phenomenon called assortative mating may contribute to the genetic transmission of psychiatric disorders.

> **KEYCONCEPT** **Assortative mating** is the tendency of individuals to select mates who are similar in genetically linked traits such as intelligence and personality style.

Research increasingly shows that major psychiatric disorders (e.g., depression, anxiety disorder, schizophrenia, bipolar disorder, substance abuse) run in families. Thus, having a parent or sibling with a psychiatric disorder usually indicates an increased risk for the same or another closely related disorder in a child or adolescent. In addition, many childhood psychiatric disorders, such as autism, mental retardation, developmental learning disorders, some language disorders (e.g., dyslexia), attention deficit hyperactivity disorder (ADHD), Tourette's syndrome, and enuresis (bed wetting), appear to be genetically transmitted (Pivac et al., 2011; Shreeram, He, Kalaydjian, Brothers, & Merikangas, 2009; Steinberg, King, & Apter, 2010; Williams, Tsang, Clarke, & Kohn, 2010).

Neurologic Examination

A full neurologic evaluation is beyond the scope of practice for a baccalaureate-level or master's-level nurse without specific neuropsychiatric training. However, a screening of neurologic soft signs can help establish a database that will clarify the need for further neurologic consultation. The nurse should ask the brief neurologic screening questions suggested in Box 34.4 directly of the child and should also note any soft signs of neurologic dysfunction, such as slurred speech, unusual movements (e.g., tics, tremors), hyperactivity, and coordination problems. The nurse can ask young children to hop on one foot, skip, or walk from toe to heel to assess their gross motor coordination and to draw with a crayon or pencil or play pick-up sticks or jacks to assess their fine motor coordination.

Psychological Domain

Children can usually identify and discuss what improves or worsens their problems. The assessment may be the first time that someone has asked the child to explain his or her view of the problem. It is also a perfect opportunity to discuss any life changes or losses (e.g., death of grandparents or pets, parental divorce) and fears, especially of punishment.

Mental Status Examination

As discussed in Chapter 10, the mental status examination is an organized systematic approach to assessment of an individual's current psychiatric condition. It is essential in formulating a diagnosis. It can provide initial data that alert the clinician to obtain further cognitive, neurologic, or psychological testing. The mental status examination of children combines observation and direct questioning (Box 34.5). The nurse should note any areas where the child or adolescent is symptomatic or has difficulty with the task. A mental status examination should be obtained on subsequent visits so improvements or changes in the patient's functioning can be noted.

The nurse should note the child's general appearance, including level of attractiveness. Although it perhaps should not be so, social-psychological research shows that the appearance and attractiveness of both children and adults strongly influence their social relationships (Murray et al., 2010). The nurse also should note the following:

- Does he or she seem to have difficulty focusing on the interview, sitting still, refraining from impulsive behavior, and listening without interrupting? (possible signs of ADHD)
- Does the child seem underactive, lethargic, distant, or hopeless? (possible signs of depression)
- Are there problems with speech patterns, such as rate (overly fast or slow), clarity, and volume, or any speech dysfluencies (e.g., stuttering, halting)?
- Are there possible mood disorders (e.g., depression, mania), language disorders, or psychotic processes?

When assessing thought processes, keep in mind that whereas young children are in the concrete operations stage, middle schoolers can begin to use logic and understand conversations. Adolescents should be able to demonstrate abstract thinking and think hypothetically, although they may appear to be self-conscious and introspective. Assessment of preteens and adolescents should address substance use and sexual activity because responses may provide useful information about high-risk behavior or substance abuse. In addition, the nurse should inquire about any obsessions or compulsions (e.g., worries about germs, severe hand washing).

Developmental Assessment

Children respond to life's stresses in different ways and in accord with their developmental level. Knowing the difference between normal child development and psychopathology is crucial in helping parents view their children's behavior realistically and respond appropriately. The key areas for assessment include maturation, psychosocial development, and language.

Maturation

Healthy development of the brain and nervous system during childhood and adolescence provides the foundation for successful functioning throughout life. Such development, called **maturation**, unfolds through sequential and orderly growth processes. These processes are biologically and genetically based but depend on constant interactions with a stimulating and nurturing environment. If trauma or neglect impairs the process of normal biologic maturation, developmental delays and disorders that may not be fully reversible can result. For example, babies born with fetal alcohol syndrome experience permanent brain damage, often resulting in mental retardation, learning disabilities, behavior disorders, and delays in language (Landgren, Svensson, Stromland, & Gronlund, 2010). A pregnant woman's use of crack cocaine deprives the fetus of nutrients and oxygen, leading to developmental delays, speech and language problems, deformities, and behavior disorders (e.g., impulsivity, withdrawal, hyperactivity). The nurse can assess for developmental delays by asking questions from specific sections of the mental status examination:

- *Intellectual functioning:* Evaluate the child's creativity, spontaneity, ability to count money and tell time, academic performance, memory, attention, frustration tolerance, and organization.
- *Gross motor functioning:* Ask the child to hop on one foot, throw a ball, walk up and down the hall, and run.
- *Fine motor functioning:* Ask the child to draw a picture or pick up sticks.
- *Cognition:* The nurse can evaluate the child's general level of cognition by assessing the child's vocabulary, level of comprehension, drawing ability, and responsiveness to questions. Testing, such as the Wechsler Intelligence Scale for Children (WISC-III), provides measures of intelligence quotient (IQ). A psychologist usually performs such tests. The nurse can request cognitive testing if he or she has concerns about a child's developmental delays or learning disabilities.
- *Thinking and perception:* Evaluate level of consciousness; orientation to date, time, and person; thought content; thought process; and judgment.
- *Social interactions and play:* Assess the child's organization, creativity, drawing capacity, and ability to follow rules. Children experiencing developmental delays may remain engaged solely in parallel play instead of moving to reciprocal play. They may consistently play

BOX 34.5

Mental Status Examination

APPEARANCE
Provide a head to toe assessment: describe head shape and size (Down syndrome, fragile X syndrome, Turner's syndrome, fetal alcohol syndrome), eyes (clarity, gaze, glasses, eye contact), height, weight, cleanliness, facial expressions, mannerisms, ears, hearing, skin (bruising could indicate physical abuse), gait, posture, nutritional status (possible eating disorder).

Evaluate dress: Is it appropriate for the weather? Does the child wear shirts with logos or groups? Does the child appear older or younger looking? Inquire about symptoms of physical illness.

MOTOR ACTIVITY
Use the following descriptors to assess motor activity: calm, psychomotor retardation, akathisia, agitated, hyperalertness, tics, muscle spasms, nail biting, hyperactivity, anxiety, restlessness, or compulsions.

SELF-CONCEPT
Ask about play, favorite stories, and three wishes. Ask the child to draw a self-portrait, describe best- and least-liked qualities. Ask what he or she imagines doing for an occupation when grown up. Also evaluate planning ability and sense of a future.

BEHAVIOR
Observe for temper tantrums, attention span, separation from family member, self-care activities, dressing, toileting, feeding, oppositionality, compliance, and so on.

SOCIAL INTERACTION
How does the child relate to the examiner? Is the child wary, submissive, attentive, friendly, manipulative, approval seeking, conforming, hostile, or guarded? Assess the child's relationships with the child's parent or guardian, siblings, and friends.

GENERAL INTELLIGENCE
Assess the child's general vocabulary, fund of knowledge, alertness, orientation, concentration, memory, calculations, organization, abstract reasoning creativity, spontaneity, and frustration tolerance. Ask about school, including regular or special education, grades, and grade retention.

FUND OF KNOWLEDGE
Ask child: How many legs does a dog have? How many pennies in a nickel? Have child identify body parts, draw a person, name colors, count as high as possible, and inquire about letter identification (younger children).

Inquire about the time. How many states are in the United States? Who was George Washington? How many days are in a week? What are the seasons of the year? (middle schoolers) What does the stomach do? Who is Charles Darwin? (teenagers)

ORIENTATION
Ask questions such as: How old are you?
Who is the current president of the United States?
Do you know who was the president before our current president?
What are two major news events in the past month? (older children)
What are the year, seasons, date, day, and month?
Where are we? (country, state, city, clinic)

RECENT MEMORY
Ask the child to repeat a memory phrase; remember three to five objects that you say or show and then recall them in a few minutes. Ask: What school do you currently attend? What did you have for breakfast or lunch today?

REMOTE MEMORY
Ask questions such as: What did you do last weekend? What was your last birthday like? What is your address and telephone number? Who is your first best friend? How old were you when you learned to ride a bike? What was the name of your kindergarten teacher?

ABSTRACT REASONING AND ANALOGIES
Ask what is meant by a stitch in time saves nine; a rolling stone gathers no moss; a bird in the hand is worth two birds in a tree; too many cooks spoil the broth.

Which object does not belong in this group: fish, tree, rock? Why?

Assess the similarity about objects such as peaches and lemons, oceans and lakes, a pencil and typewriter, a bicycle and a bus.

To evaluate comparative ability Complete this sentence: An engine is to an airplane as an oar is to a _____.

ARITHMETIC CALCULATIONS
Provide simple addition and subtraction questions based on the child's age. Ask older children multiplication and division problems. Count backward 20 to 1 for younger children. Ask how many quarters are in $3.50 or if you buy something that cost $2.50 and you have $5, how much change you will receive.

WRITING AND SPELLING ABILITY
Ask a first or second grader to spell cat, hat, bad, old, dog. Ask a third or fourth grader to spell words such as clock, face, house, or flower. Ask older children to write a sentence such as: "The grass is greener on the mountains."

READING
Have the child read a paragraph from an age-appropriate book. Reading begins in first grade. Children should demonstrate basic reading skills by the end of second grade.

GROSS MOTOR SKILLS
Assess level of activity, type of activity, and any unusual gestures or mannerisms and compulsions.

Have the patient walk, jump, hop on one foot, and walk heel to toe, throw a ball, balance and climb stairs.

By age 3 years, a child should walk up stairs with alternating feet, pedal a tricycle, jump in one place, and broad jump.

By age 4 years, a child can balance on one foot for 5 seconds, and catch a bounced ball two of three times.

By age 5 years, a child can do heel-to-toe walking.

By age 6 years, a child should jump, tumble, skip, hop, walk a straight line, skip rope with practice, and ride a bicycle.

By age 7 years, a child should skip and play hopscotch, and run and climb with coordination.

By age 9 years, a child should have highly developed eye–hand coordination.

FINE MOTOR SKILLS
Have the child draw a picture or self-portrait as well as pick up sticks.

Have the child copy a design that you have drawn. Ask the child to draw a circle (age 3 years), an X (age 3 to 4 years), a square (age 5 years), a triangle (age 6 years), a diamond (age 7 years), and connecting diamonds (age 8 years).

At age 3 years, a child should unbutton front buttons, copy a vertical line, copy a circle, and build an eight-block tower.

By age 4 years, a child should copy a cross and button large buttons.

By age 5 years, a child should dress him- or herself with minimal assistance, color within lines, and draw a three-part human.

Continued

BOX 34.5

Mental Status Examination (*Continued*)

By age 6 years, a child should be able to draw a six-part human.

By age 7 years, a child should print well and begin to write script.

By age 8 years, a child should demonstrate mature handwriting skills.

ATTENTION SPAN

Ask the patient to follow a series of short commands. Observe motor activity, attention, concentration, impulsivity, hyperactivity, outbursts, and organization.

Observe the child's ability to stay on task and focus during the course of the interview. Tasks include counting backwards by 7, spelling the word "world" backwards, and saying the letters of the alphabet backward.

INSIGHT AND JUDGMENT

Ask the child to provide a solution to a hypothetical situation such as what would you do if you found a stamped envelope lying on the ground? What would you do if a policeman stopped you for driving your bike through a red light? What would you do if you saw two children fighting on the school ground? Assess the child's ideas about the current problem and the solutions tried so far. Assess if child can make use of assistance. Evaluate how impaired child is in activities of daily living, including attending school, attending recreational activities, making friends, self-care activities, and so on.

COMPREHENSION

Read a few pages or paragraphs from a short book or newspaper article and ask the child to relate what happened in the story.

MOOD AND FEELINGS

Affect is the child's emotional tone. Evaluate the child's range of emotions, intensity and appropriateness.

Assess for any mood swings, crying, anxiety, depression, anger, hostility, hyperalertness, lability, or pressured speech. Assess mood by asking how many times a week do you feel sad and how often do you cry? What makes you sad, angry, anxious, and so on? Risk assessment questions include: Have you ever felt like hurting yourself or someone else? Do you have a plan to hurt yourself? Have you ever done anything to hurt yourself in the past?

THOUGHT PROCESS AND CONTENT

Were there any recurrent themes?

Observe the child's patterns of thinking for appropriateness of sequence, logic, coherence, and relevance to the topics discussed. Does the child talk about age-appropriate topics; is there any thought blocking, or disturbance in the stream of thinking, repetition of words, circumstantial or tangential thinking, perseverations, preoccupations, obsessive thoughts, actions, or compulsive behaviors, any grandiose reasoning, ideas of reference, or paranoia (feelings of being watched or followed, controlled, manipulated, and ritual or checking routines)?

Evaluate the child's perceptions for hallucinations (false perceptions or false impressions or experiences) and delusions (false beliefs that contradict social reality, such as hears voices, sees images or shadowy figures, smells offensive odors, tastes offensive flavors, feels worms crawling on skin). Assess hallucinations in all five senses: auditory, visual, tactile, gustatory, and olfactory. Assess for command hallucinations, which tell the patient to do something.

SPEECH AND LANGUAGE

Note any speech impediments and incongruence between verbal and nonverbal communication. Show a pencil and a watch and ask the patient to name them. Have the patient repeat "no ifs, ands, or buts."

Assess communication skills, including expressive language, vocabulary, and the ability to understand what you are saying (receptive language). Check voice quality, articulation, pronunciation, fluency, rhythm, rate, and ease of expression and volume.

Assess comprehension by giving the child a task. Assess coherence for flight of ideas, loose associations, word salad (meaningless, disconnected word choices), neologisms, clang associations (words that rhyme in a nonsensical way), echolalia (repetition of another person's words), thought blocking, perseveration, irrelevance, and vagueness. Check for aphasia by listening for an omission or addition of letters, syllables, and made-up words or misuse or transposition of words.

---

with toys designed for younger children, draw crude body pictures, or display receptive or expressive language problems.

Psychosocial Development

Assessment of psychosocial development is very important for children with mental health problems. Various theoretical models are available from which to choose; the most commonly used model is Erikson's stages of development. When considering this model, the nurse should examine the child's gender and cultural background for appropriateness. The nurse also may use the Baker Miller's model for girls (see Chapter 7).

Language

At birth, infants can emit sounds of all languages. Maturation of language skills begins with babbling, or the utterance of simple, spontaneous sounds. By the end of the first year, children can make one-word statements, usually naming objects or people in the environment. By age 2 years, they should speak in short, telegraphic sentences consisting of a verb and noun (e.g., "want cookie"). Between ages 2 and 4 years, vocabulary and sentence structure develop rapidly. In fact, a preschooler's ability to produce language often surpasses motor development, sometimes causing temporary stuttering when the child's mind literally works faster than his or her mouth.

Language development depends on the complex interaction of physical maturation of the nerves, development of head and neck musculature, hearing abilities, cognitive abilities, exposure to language, educational stimulation, and emotional well-being. Social needs create a natural inclination toward communication, but children need reinforcement to develop correct pronunciation, vocabulary, and grammar.

Before a diagnosis of a communication disorder (i.e., impairment in language expression, comprehension, or both) can be made, the child must be tested to rule out hearing, visual, or other neurologic problems. Brain damage, especially to the left hemisphere (dominant for language in most individuals), can seriously impair the development of communication abilities in children. Any child who has experienced brain damage from anoxia at birth, congenital trauma, head injury, infection, tumor, or drug exposure should be closely monitored for signs of a communication disorder. Before the age of 5 years, the brain has amazing plasticity, and sometimes other intact areas of the brain can take over functions of damaged areas, especially with immediate speech therapy. Genetically based disorders such as autism cause language delays that are sometimes permanent and severe. Children with language delays need particular encouragement to communicate properly because they tend to compensate by using nonverbal signals (Hudry et al., 2010).

The nurse must recognize normal variations in child development and assess lags in the development of vocabulary and sentence structure during the critical preschool years. Delays in this area can seriously affect other areas, such as cognitive, educational, and social development. Many children who receive psychiatric treatment have speech and language disorders that are sometimes undetected, either leading to or compounding their emotional problems (Redmond, Thompson, & Goldstein, 2011; Rodriguez et al., 2010).

Children's Rating Scales for Psychiatric Disorders

A number of children's rating scales can assist in the assessment of various psychiatric disorders. The BASC, developed by Reynolds and Kamphouse (1998), is a tool used to measure behaviors and emotions in children ages 2 to 18 years. The scales include a teacher rating scale, a parent rating scale, and a 180-item self-report of personality. The scale evaluates several dimensions, including attitude to school, attitude toward teachers, sensation seeking, atypicality, locus of control, somatization, social stress, anxiety, depression, sense of inadequacy, relations with parents, interpersonal relations, self-esteem, and self-reliance. The CBCL, developed by Achenbach and Edelbrock (1983), is a 113-item self-report tool used to identify forms of psychopathology and competencies that occur in children ages 4 to 16 years. This instrument provides scores on internalizing and externalizing behaviors.

Several scales are useful for diagnosing specific problems in children and adolescents. The CDI, developed by John March (1997), is a 27-item self-rated symptom orientation scale for children ages 7 to 17 years that is useful for diagnosing physical symptoms, harm avoidance, social anxiety, and separation and panic disorder.

The pediatric anxiety rating scale (PARS) developed by the Rupp Anxiety Study Group, is a clinician-administered, 50-item semistructured interview used to assess severity of anxiety in children ages 6 to 17 years (Riddle et al., 2001). The Swanson, Nolan, and Pelham Scale, fourth revision (SNAP_IV) is a 90-item teacher and parent rating scale containing items from the Conners questionnaire for measuring inattention and overactivity (Swanson, 1983); it is useful for diagnosing ADHD (inattentive and impulsive types) and oppositional defiant disorder. The Children's Yale-Brown Obsessive Compulsive Scale, developed by Goodman et al. (1989), is a 19-item scale that can help diagnose childhood obsessive-compulsive disorder in children 6 to 17 years of age.

Attachment

Attachment is the emotional bond between an infant and his or her parental figure. Studies of attachment show that the quality of the emotional bond between the infant and parental figures provides the groundwork for future relationships. The need to touch and be close to a parental figure appears biologically driven and has been demonstrated in classic studies of monkeys who bonded with a terry-cloth surrogate mother (Harlow, Harlow, & Suomi, 1971). A secure attachment is based on the caretaker's consistent, appropriate response to the infant's attachment behaviors (e.g., crying, clinging, calling, following, protesting). Children who have developed a secure attachment protest when their parents leave them (beginning at about age 6 to 8 months), seek comfort from their parents in unfamiliar situations, and playfully explore the environment in the parent's presence. Mother–child separation for 1 week or longer within the first 2 years of life has been shown to be related to higher levels of child negativity (at age 3 years) and aggression (at ages 3 to 5 years) (Martin, Berlin, & Brooks-Gunn, 2011).

Secure attachments in early childhood produce cooperative, harmonious parent–child relationships in which the child is responsive to the parents' socialization efforts and likely to adopt the parents' viewpoints, values, and goals. Securely attached young children also socialize competently, are popular with well-acquainted peers during the preschool years, and have warm relationships with important adults in their lives. Securely attached children see themselves and others constructively and have relatively sophisticated emotional and moral understanding (Howard Martin, Berlin, & Brooks-Gunn, 2011).

Although the importance of the parent's responsiveness is unquestionable in determining the development of a secure attachment, the process works both ways. Some babies seem to encourage attachment naturally with their parents by responding positively to holding, cuddling, and comforting behaviors. Others, such as those with developmental delays or autistic disorders, may respond less readily and even reject parental attempts at bonding.

Attachment Theories

Bowlby's early studies (1969) of maternal deprivation formed the initial framework for attachment theory based on the notion that the infant tends to bond to one primary parental figure, usually the mother. Although this pattern is common, recent studies show that children make multiple attachments to parents and other caregivers, but high-quality, intense bonds remain essential for healthy development. Contemporary nursing theories, such as Barnard's parent–child interaction model, have stressed the importance of the interaction between the child's spontaneous behavior and biologic rhythms and the mother's ability to respond to cues that signal distress (Barnard & Brazelton, 1990). Whereas a positive attachment is likely to result in a happy child with a sense of self-worth, insecure attachment is associated with depressive symptoms (Ponizovsky, Levov, Schultz, & Radomislensky, 2011). Although most attachment research has been done with mothers, the father's role in child development has become better understood through research done during the past two decades. Fathers' emotional support tends to enhance the quality of mother–child relationships and facilitates positive adjustment by children. When fathers are unsupportive and marital conflict is high, children suffer (Hohmann-Marriott, 2009).

Fathers play an important role in children's play, which affects the quality of the child's attachment. Playful interactions involving emotional arousal provide an especially good opportunity to learn how to get along with peers by reinforcing turn taking, affect regulation, and acceptable ways of competing. Fathers are important as role models who assist in their sons' identity formation and serve as models of gender-appropriate behavior, particularly around aggressive behavior (Ford, Nalbone, Wechler, & Sutton, 2008). Evidence supports the importance of including the father in the mental health assessment of his child.

Disrupted Attachments

Disrupted attachments may result from deficits in infant attachment behaviors, lack of responsiveness by caregivers to the child's cues, or both and may lead to reactive attachment disorder, feeding disorder, failure to thrive, or anxiety disorder. A reactive attachment disorder is a state in which a child younger than 5 years of age fails to initiate or respond appropriately to social interaction and the caregiver subsequently disregards the child's physical and emotional needs. Attachment disorder behaviors are related to attention and conduct problems (Woodhouse, Ramos-Marcuse, Ehrlich, Warner, & Cassidy, 2010).

Attachment disorganization is a consequence of extreme insecurity that results from feared or actual separation from the attached figure. Disorganized infants appear to be unable to maintain the strategic adjustments in attachment behavior represented by organized avoidant or ambivalent attachment strategies, with the result that both behavioral and physiological dysregulation occurs. Preschoolers with disorganized attachment manifest behaviors of fear, contradictory behavior, or disorientation or disassociation in the caregivers' presence. Attachment disorganization appears moderately stable over time and has been associated with distinct, apparently genetically based, physiologic profiles (Reiner, & Spangler, 2010).

Temperament and Behavior

Temperament is a person's characteristic intensity, activity level, threshold of responsiveness, rhythmicity, adaptability, energy expenditure, and mood. According to research findings, temperamental differences can be observed early in life, suggesting that they are at least partly biologically determined, and patterns of temperament can be correlated with emotional and behavioral problems (Rihmer, Akiskal, Rihmer, Akiskal, 2010). When looking at the cerebral activity in 9-month-old infants, consistent with early development of externalizing behaviors, electroencephalographic activity increased in response to fear rather than love and comfort (Santesso, Schmidt, & Trainor, 2007).

The classic New York Longitudinal Study (Thomas, Chess, & Birch, 1968) identified three main patterns of temperament seen in infancy that often extend into childhood and later life:

- *Easy temperament* characterized by a positive mood, regular patterns of eating and sleeping, positive approach to new situations, and low emotional intensity
- *Difficult temperament* characterized by irregular sleep and eating patterns, negative response to new stimuli, slow adaptation, negative mood, and high emotional intensity
- *Slow-to-warm-up temperament* characterized by a negative, mildly emotional response to new situations that is expressed with intensity and initially slow adaptation but evolves into a positive response

On the positive side, an easy temperament can serve as a protective factor against the development of psychopathology. Children with easy temperaments can adapt to change without intense emotional reactions. Difficult temperament places children at high risk for adjustment problems, such as with adjustment to school or bonding with parents.

Temperament has a major influence on the chances that a child may experience psychological problems; however, temperament is not unchangeable, and environmental influences can change or modify a child's emotional style (Kendler & Myers, 2009). Children who respond positively to the environment continue in this pattern. Children who have other temperaments may develop positive temperaments at a later time.

The concept of temperament provides an excellent example of the interaction between biologic–genetic and environmental factors in producing child psychopathology. Although a child may be born with a particular temperament, longitudinal studies show that the temperament can be influenced by other factors such as parental control (Benson & Johnson, 2009). However, difficult children in particular may evoke negative reactions in parents and teachers, thereby creating environments that exacerbate their biologically based behavior problems, initiating a vicious cycle. Difficult temperament that persists beyond 3 years of age is correlated with the development of child psychopathology (Koenig, Barry, Kochanska, 2010). The nurse can help parents accept biologically based differences in their children and learn to adapt their behavior to each child's needs.

Self-Concept

For young children, eliciting their view of themselves and the world is helpful. One technique is asking them what they would wish for if they had three wishes. Answers can be revealing. Whereas an inability to wish for anything beyond a nice meal or place to live may reflect hopelessness, wishes to conquer the world or put one's teacher in jail may indicate feelings of grandiosity. Another technique is to tell a story and ask the child to make up an ending for it. For example, a baby bird fell out of a nest—what happened to it? The nurse may design stories to elicit particular fears or concerns that may be relevant for the individual child.

Drawings also provide an excellent window into the child's internal world (Fig. 34.2). Asking the child to draw a picture of a person can provide data about the child's self-concept, sexual identity, body image, and developmental level. By age 3 years, children should be able to draw some facial features and limbs, but their drawings may have an "x-ray" quality, in which clothing is transparent and the body can be seen underneath. Older children should produce more sophisticated drawings unless they are resistant to the task. After the child has finished the drawing, the nurse can ask what the person in the drawing is thinking and feeling, using this device to assess the child's mental processes. For example, one adolescent with school phobia drew a person fully dressed, in great detail, but with no feet. When asked about the drawing, he said that the boy could not go anywhere because his mother was afraid to let him leave home.

Other ways to assess children's self-concepts include asking them what they want to do when they grow up, what their best subjects are in school, what things they are really good at, and how well-liked they are at school. Before concluding the individual interview with a child,

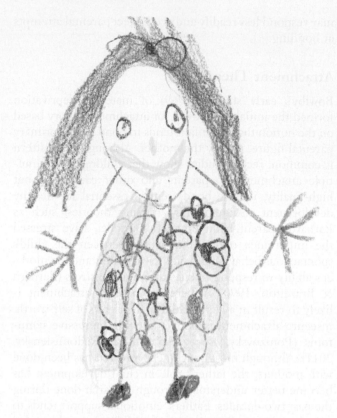

FIGURE 34.2 Self portrait of a girl, age 5 years.

the nurse should always ask if the child has any other information to share and whether he or she has any questions.

Risk Assessment

The nurse must ask the child about any suicidal or violent thoughts. The best way to assess these areas is to ask straightforward questions, such as, "Have you ever thought about hurting yourself? Have you ever thought about hurting someone else? Have you ever acted on these thoughts? Have you thought about how you would do it? What did you think would happen if you hurt yourself? Have you ever done anything to hurt yourself before?" Contrary to popular belief, even young children attempt suicide, and they are capable of violent acts toward other children, adults, and animals. When a child shares the intent to commit a suicidal or violent act, the nurse must remind him or her that they will have to discuss this concern with the parent to keep the child and others safe.

Substance abuse disorders across the life span account for more deaths, illness, and disabilities than any other preventable health condition. Screening for potential use and abuse of substances is becoming a priority in mental health assessment of adolescents. House (2002) developed an interview protocol that can be useful in identifying substance abuse problems in youth (Box 34.6).

BOX 34.6

Practice Note 0.1 An Interview Protocol for Reviewing Chemical Use in Youths

As with other topics, questions about substance use are interactive—the answers given determine to some extent the subsequent questions. However, certain topics and areas should be addressed irrespective of the previous responses. In the sample questions below, those marked with an asterisk should always be asked.

Now I'd like to ask you about your experience with cigarettes, alcohol, and other drugs.

- When was the last time you smoked tobacco?
- Have you ever smoked? Tell me about that.
- How old were you when you first smoked a cigarette?
- How many cigarettes do you smoke a day now?
  - How long have you smoked this much?
- Where do you usually do your smoking?
- Where do you usually get your cigarettes from?
- What kind of problems has smoking caused for you?
  - How do your parents feel about your smoking?
  - Have you gotten into trouble at school for smoking?
  - Have you lost any friends or had problems with friends over smoking?
- What other tobacco products have you used?
- When was the last time you drank any alcohol?
  - How much alcohol did you drink? What kinds of alcohol were you drinking? What happened afterward?
  - Who was with you the last time you were drinking? What happened?
  - How about the time before that? Tell me about that.
- What is the most alcohol you have ever drunk? What happened?
- How do you get alcohol?
- What kinds of problems have drinking caused for you?
  - How do your parents feel about your drinking?
  - Have you ever gotten into problems at school because of drinking?
  - Have you ever gotten into legal problems because of drinking?
  - Have you had problems with your friends because of drinking?

- What is the worst thing that has happened while you were drinking?
- How old were you the first time you drank alcohol? When did most of your friends start drinking? How does your drinking compare with other kids in your classes at school or other kids your age?
- How has your drinking changed over the past year?
- When was the last time you used any marijuana?
  - How old were you when you first tried marijuana?
  - How often have you used marijuana in the past month?
  - What's usually going on when you use marijuana?
- What other drugs have you used?
  - When was the first time you used _____?
  - When was the last time you used _____?
  - How many times have you used _____?
  - Where did you get the _____? How did you know that's what it was?
  - How did _____ affect you?
  - What has been the biggest effect you have gotten using _____?
  - What has been the worst thing about using _____?
- Have you ever 'huffed' or inhaled something to get high? Tell me about that.
- Have you ever used another person's prescription medications? Tell me about that.
- How many people do you regularly do things with— hang out, party with, talk to?
- How many of your friends smoke tobacco occasionally?
- How many of your friends smoke tobacco regularly?
- How many of your friends drink alcohol occasionally?
- How many of your friends drink alcohol regularly?
- How many of your friends smoke marijuana occasionally?
- How many of your friends smoke marijuana regularly?
- What other drugs do your friends use?
- How has drug use affected your friends?

From House, A. (2002). *The first session with children and adolescents: Conducting a comprehensive mental health evaluation* (pp. 202–203). New York: Guilford Press. Used with permission.

Social Domain

Family Relationship

Children depend on adults to create a safe, nurturing, and appropriate environment to support their development. The nurse should assess the quality of the home, including living space, sleeping arrangements, safety, cleanliness, and child care arrangements, either through a home visit or by discussing these issues with the family. When gathering a family history, a genogram and timeline are useful tools to map family members' birth order and medical and psychiatric histories; family roles, norms, boundaries, strengths, and family subgroups; birth dates, deaths, and relationships; stage in the family cycle; and critical events. To understand fully the family's values, goals, and beliefs, the nurse must consider the family's ethnic, cultural, and economic background throughout the assessment. A comprehensive family assessment should be considered (see Chapter 14).

School and Peer Adjustment

The child's adjustment to school is also significant. Often, children are referred for a mental health assessment as a result of changes in behavior at school. Falling grades, loss of interest in normal activities, decreased concentration, or withdrawal from or aggression toward peers may indicate that the child is experiencing emotional problems. It is very important that the nurse obtain signed permission from the parents to talk to the child's teacher for his or her observations of the child. The nurse may want to observe the child in school, if feasible, to see how the child functions there. The parent can request a treatment planning conference in which the teacher, parent, and nurse discuss the child's school performance and plan ways to promote the child's emotional, cognitive, and social functioning in school. Suggestions may range from having the child tested for learning disabilities to designing behavior plans that include rewards for improved functioning, such as computer time at the end of the day.

Peers are an important aspect of child and adolescent social development. Assessment of peer relationships and activities with friends provides a rich source of information about the adolescent. Assessment of victimization by peers in the form of bullying is important because it can have a negative impact on social development and self-esteem.

Community

Youth in healthy communities have been shown to be more likely to attend religious services, to believe their schools were places of caring and encouragement, to be involved in structured activities, and to remain committed to their own learning. Assessing the child's economic status, access to medical care, adequate home environment, exposure to environmental toxins (e.g., lead), neighborhood safety, and exposure to violence is important because these community factors place the child at risk (Pullmann, Vanhooser, Hoffman, & Heflinger, 2010).

Children and adolescents function better if they are linked to community supports, such as churches, recreational programs, park district programming, and after-school programming. The Big Brother/Big Sister program fosters mentoring relationships for children. A parent or child may call the local Big Brother/Big Sister organization to request a mentor for the child. The mentor may perform a wide range of services, from taking a child to community events, helping with homework, or talking about how the child can achieve his or her dreams and goals. Some towns offer community-based juvenile justice programs to rehabilitate children who have had altercations with the legal system. Juvenile justice programs provide support, such as individual and family counseling and prosocial recreational activities; teach children how to make positive choices about spending free time; and closely monitor their behaviors.

Religious and Spiritual Assessment

Spiritual assessment is an integral part of a mental health assessment. There is a growing body of research suggesting that religious and spiritual practices may promote both physical and mental health (Koenig et al., 2010; Maltby, Lewis, Freeman, Day, Cruise, & Breslin, 2010). The Joint Commission requires that each psychiatric evaluation include spiritual assessment questions.

Questioning about a patient's spiritual life should include interviewing strategies that are unbiased and facilitate understanding of the client's spiritual values. Questions can include but are not limited to the child's and family's specific faith background, level of activity with that group, support received from spiritual practices, religious rituals of importance, and religious influences on lifestyle and health choices. During a child interview, appropriate questions include, "Where is God?" or asking if the child could talk to God.

Functional Status

Functional status is evaluated in children and adolescents using the Global Assessment of Functioning (GAF) scale, which tallies behaviors related to school, peers, activity level, mood, speech, family relationships, behavioral problems, self-care skills, and self-concept. The GAF scale ranges from 0 to 100; the lower the score, the higher the level of impairment, indicated by psychiatric symptoms and level of general functioning. For example, a score of 30 may indicate that the child is severely homicidal or suicidal and has made previous attempts, that hallucinations or delusions influence the child's behavior, or that the child has serious impairment in communication or judgment. Moderate impairment scores usually fall in the range of 51 to 69. Indications of moderate impairment include difficulty in one area, such as school phobia, that hinders school attendance or performance, while the child is functioning well within other areas, such as with family and peers. Children in this category are not homicidal or suicidal and usually respond well to outpatient interventions. A score of 70 to 100 usually indicates that the child is functioning well in relation to school, peers, family, and community. The GAF is always measured at the initial assessment so treatment can be evaluated in terms of symptom improvement.

Evaluation of Childhood Sexual Abuse

There are several special considerations in interviewing an abused child. First, the nurse must establish a safe and supportive environment in which to conduct the evaluation. Second, the nurse needs to understand the forensic implications of assessment so that the interview format will be acceptable for disclosure in a court hearing. The American Academy of Pediatrics offers practice guidelines for evaluating children who may have been abused (Kellog & the Committee on Child Abuse and Neglect, 2005). If the child reports abuse, the nurse has a legal responsibility to report the abuse to child protection agencies. The nurse must use the same language and vocabulary that the child uses to describe the abuse or anatomical terms and ask nonleading questions. Nursing professionals who regularly interview children who have been abused may have special training in the use of anatomically correct dolls to obtain information about the abuse. The use of anatomically correct dolls is beneficial because it does not overstimulate or distress the child; assists in identifying and naming specific body parts; increases verbal productivity during the examination; helps to prompt memory; and is useful with immature, language-impaired, and cognitively delayed children (Adi-Japha, Berberixh-Artzi, & Libnawi, 2010).

Stresses and Coping Behaviors

Biologic, behavioral, and personality predispositions; family; and community environment may affect a child's ability to cope with stressful life events. Stressful experiences for children include the death of a loved person or pet, parental divorce, violence, physical illness (especially chronic illness), mental illness, social isolation, racial discrimination, neglect, and physical and sexual abuse.

The number of stressful events that a child experiences, the supports that the child has in place, and the child's developmental stage may also influence his or her ability to cope with stressors. Children who appear to have experienced mild stress may actually manifest posttraumatic stress symptoms (Copeland, Keeler, Angold, & Costello, 2010). It is important to consider a stressful situation within the context of each child's support system and developmental stage.

SUMMARY OF KEY POINTS

- Mental health assessment of children and adolescents includes evaluating the child's biologic, psychological, and social factors, primarily through interviewing and observation.

- Assessment of children and adolescents differs from assessment of adults in that the nurse must consider the child's developmental level, specifically addressing the child's language, cognitive, social, and emotional skills. Establishing a treatment alliance and building rapport are essential to obtaining a good mental health history.

- The mental status examination includes observations and questions about the child's appearance, motor activity, self-concept, behavior, social interaction, general intelligence, fund of knowledge, attention span, insight and judgment, comprehension, mood and feelings, thought process and content, speech and language, orientation, memory, reasoning, writing and spelling, reading, and motor skills. Assessment of the child and caregiver together provides important information regarding child–parent attachment and parenting practices.

- The three main types of temperament include the easy temperament, difficult temperament, and slow-to-warm-up temperament. Temperament can be evaluated by assessing the child's sleep and eating habits, mood, emotional intensity, and responses to new stimuli.

- A child's self-concept can be evaluated using tools such as play, stories, asking three wishes, and asking the child to draw a picture of him- or herself.

- If a child reveals suicidal ideation in the interview, the nurse must determine whether the child has a plan; let the parent know the child is suicidal; and make a plan to keep the child safe, such as inpatient hospitalization.

- If a child reports to the nurse neglect or physical or sexual abuse, the nurse must by law report the child's disclosure to the state's DCF.

CRITICAL THINKING CHALLENGES

1. An adolescent is hostile and refuses to talk in an interview. How would you respond?

2. What are some strategies for building rapport with children?

3. A child reports that he is suicidal. What would be your next question? What measures would you take next?

4. What are some techniques and media for obtaining information about a child's inner world, such as self-concept, sexual identity, body image, and developmental level?

5. Explain why it may be detrimental to interview a child in front of his or her parent. Why may it be detrimental to interview a parent in front of his or her child?

6. Why is obtaining the mental health histories of parents relevant to the child's mental health assessment?

7. What are useful tools in obtaining a family history from the child and parent?

8. Anatomically correct dolls are used in what specific type of child assessment?

9. What types of questions would you ask to inquire about a child's spiritual life?

References

Achenbach, T. M., & Edelbrock, C. (1983). *The child behavior checklist: Manual for the child behavior checklist and revised child behavior profile.* Burlington, VT: Queen City Printers.

Adi-Japha, E., Berberish-Artzi, J., & Libnawi, A. (2010). Cognitive flexibility in drawings of bilingual children. *Child Development, 81*(5), 1356–1366.

Barnard, K. E., & Brazelton, T. B. (1990). *Touch: The foundation of experience.* Madison, CT: International Universities Press.

Benson, J. E., & Johnson, M. K. (2009). Adolescent family context and adult identity formation. *Journal of Family Issues, 30*(9), 1265–1286.

Bowlby, J. (1969). *Attachment* (Vol. 1 of *Attachment and loss*). New York: Basic Books.

Bratton, S., Ray, D., Rhine, T., & Jones, L. (2005). The efficacy of play therapy with children: A meta-analytic review of treatment outcomes. *Professional Psychology: Research and Practice, 36*(4), 376–390.

Copeland, W. E., Keeler, G., Angold, A., Costello, E. J. (2010). Postraumatic stress without trauma in children. *American Journal of Psychiatry, 167*(9), 1059–1065.

Ford, J. J., Nalbone, D. P., Wetchler, J. L., & Sutton, P. M. (2008). Fatherhood: How differentiation and identity status affect attachment to children. *American Journal of Family Therapy, 36*(4), 284–299.

Frick, P. J., Barry, C. T., & Kamphaus, R. W. (2010). *Clinical assessment of child and adolescent personality and behavior* (3rd ed). New York: Springer.

Goodman, W. K., Price, L. H., Rasmussen, S. A., Mazure, J. C., Fleischmann, R. L., Hill, C. L., et al. (1989). The Children's Yale-Brown Obsessive Compulsive Scale (CYBOCS) I. Development, use, and reliability. *Archives of General Psychiatry, 46*, 1006–1011.

Harlow, H. F., Harlow, M. K., & Suomi, S. J. (1971). From thought to therapy: Lessons from a private laboratory. *American Scientist, 59*(5), 538–549.

Hohmann-Marriott, B. E. (2009). Father involvement ideals and the union transitions of unmarried parents. *Journal of Family Issues, 30*(7), 898–920.

House, A. (2002). *The first session with children and adolescents: Conducting a comprehensive mental health evaluation.* New York: Guilford Press.

Howard, K., Martin, A., Berlin, L. J., & Brooks-Gunn, J. (2011). Early mother-child separation, parenting, and child well-being in Early Head Start families. *Attachment & Human Behavior. 13*(1), 5–26.

Hudry, K., Leadbitter, K., Temple, K., et al. (2010). Preschoolers with autism show greater impairment in receptive compared with expressive language abilities. *International Journal of Language & Communication Disorders, 45*(6), 681–690.

Landgren, M., Svensson, L., Stromland, K., & Gronlund, M. A. (2010). Prenatal alcohol exposure and neurodevelopmental disorders in children adopted in Eastern Europe. *Pediatrics, 125*(5), 1178–1185.

Lidz, C. S. (2003). *Early childhood assessment.* Hoboken, NJ: John Wiley & Sons, Ltd.

Kellog, N., & the Committee on Child Abuse and Neglect. (2005). The evaluation of sexual abuse in children. *Pediatrics, 116*(2), 506–512.

Kendler, K. S., & Myers, J. (2009). A developmental twin study of church attendance and alcohol and nicotine consumption: A model for analyzing the changing impact of genes and environment. *American Journal of Psychiatry, 166*(10), 1150–1155.

Koenig, J. L., Barry, R. A., & Kochanska, G. (2010). Rearing difficult children: Parents' personality and children's proneness to anger as predictors of future parenting. *Parenting: Science & Practice, 10*(4), 258–273.

Maltby, J., Lewis, C. A., Freeman, A., Day, L, Cruise, S. M., & Breslin, M. J. (2010). Religion and health: The application of a cognitive-behavioural framework. *Mental Health, Religion & Culture, 13*(7.8), 749–759.

March, J. (1997). *Multidimensional anxiety scale for children.* North Tonawanda, NY: Multi-Health Systems, Inc.

Martin, H. K., Berlin, L. J., & Brooks-Gunn, J. (2011). Early mother-child separation, parenting and child well-being in early head start families. *Attachment & Human Development, 13*(1), 5–26.

Mendelsohn, A. L., Huberman, H. S., Berkule, S. B., Brockmeyer, C. A., Morrow, L. M., & Dreyer, B. P. (2011). Primary care strategies for promoting parent-child interactions and school readiness in at-risk families: The Bellevue Project for early language, literacy and education success. *Archives of Pediatrics & Adolescent Medicine, 165*(1), 33–41.

Murray, L., Arteche, A., Bingley, C., et al. (2010). The effect of cleft lip on socio-emotional functioning in school-aged children. *Journal of Child Psychology & Psychiatry & Allied Disciplines, 51*(1), 94–103.

Perets-Dubrovsky, S., Kaveh, M., Deutsh-Castel, T., Cohen, A., & Tirosh, E. (2010). The human figure drawing as related to attention-deficit hyperactivity disorder (ADHD). *Journal of Child Neurology, 25*(6), 689–693.

Pivac, N., Knezevic, A., Gornik, O., et al. (2011). Human plasma glycome inattention-deficit hyperactivity disorder and autism spectrum disorders. *Molecular & Cellular Proteomic, 10*(1):M110.004200.

Ponizovsky, A. M., Levov, K., Schultz, Y., & Radomislensky, I. (2011). Attachment insecurity and psychological resources associated with adjustment disorders. *American Journal of Orthopsychiatry, 81*(2), 265–276.

Pullmann, M., VanHooser, S., Hoffman, C., & Heflinger, C. (2010). Barriers to and supports of family participating in a rural system of care for children with serious emotional problems. *Community Mental Health Journal, 46*(3), 211–220.

Redmond, S. M., Thompson, H. L., & Goldstein, S. (2011). Psycholinguistic profiling differentiates specific language impairment from typical development and from attention-deficit/hyperactivity disorder. *Journal of Speech, Language & Hearing Research, 54*(1), 99–117.

Reiner, I., & Spangler, G. (2010) Adult attachment and gene polymorphisms of the dopamine D4 receptor and serotonin transporter (5-HTT). *Attachment & Human Development, 12*(3), 209–229.

Reynolds, C. R., & Kamphouse, R. W. (1998). *Behavior assessment system for children (BASC).* Circle Pines, MN: American Guidance Service.

Riddle, M. A., Reeve, E. A., Yaryura-Tobias, J. A., Yang, H. M., Claghorn, J. L., et al. (2001). Fluvoxamine for children and adolescents with obsessive-compulsive disorder: A randomized, controlled, multicenter trial. *Journal of the American Academy of Child and Adolescent Psychiatry, 40*(2), 222–229.

Rihmer, Z., Akiskal, K. K., Rihmer, A., & Akiskal, H. S. (2010). Current research on affective temperaments. *Current Opinion in Psychiatry, 23*(1), 12–18.

Rodriguez, A., Kaakinen, M., Moilanen, T., Taanila, A., McGough, J. J., Loo, S., & Järvelin, M. (2010). Mixed-handedness is linked to mental health problems in children and adolescents. *Pediatrics, 125*(2), 340–348.

Rycek, R., Stuhr, S., McDermott, J., Benker, J., & Swartz, M. (1998). Adolescent egocentrism and cognitive functioning during late adolescence. *Adolescence, 33*(132), 745–749.

Santesso, D. L., Schmidt, L. A., & Trainor, L. J. (2007). Frontal brain electrical activity (EEG) and heart rate in response to affective infant-directed (ID) speech in 9-month-old infants. *Brain & Cognition, 65*(1), 14–21.

Shreeram, S., He, J. P., Kalaydjian, A., Brothers, S., & Merikangas, K. R. (2009). Prevalence of enuresis and its association with attention-deficit/hyperactivity disorder among U.S. children: Results from a nationally representative study. *Journal of the American Academy of Child & Adolescent Psychiatry, 48*(1), 35–41.

Steinberg, T., King, R., & Apter, A. (2010). Tourette's syndrome: A review from a developmental perspective. *Israel Journal of Psychiatry & Related Sciences, 47*(2), 105–109.

Swanson, J. M. (1983). *The SNAP-IV.* Irvine, CA: University of California, Irvine.

Thomas, A., Chess, S., & Birch, H. G. (1968). *Temperament and behavior disorders in childhood.* New York: New York University Press.

Turkel, A. R. (2002). From victim to heroine: Children's stories revisited. *Journal of the American Academy of Psychoanalysis, 30*(1), 71–81.

Williams, L. M., Tsang, T. W., Clarke, S., & Kohn, M. (2010). An "integrative neuroscience" perspective on ADHD: Linking cognition, emotion, brain, and genetic measures with implications for clinical support. *Expert Review of Neurotherapeutics, 10*(10), 1607–1621.

Woodhouse, S. S., Ramos-Marcuse, F., Ehrlich, K. B., Warner, S., & Cassidy, J. (2010). The role of adolescent attachment in moderating and mediating the links between parent and adolescent psychological symptoms. *Journal of Clinical Child and Adolescent Psychology, 39*(1), 51–63.

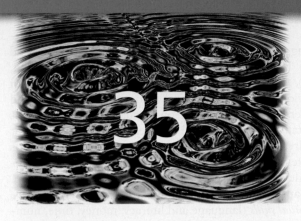

35 Psychiatric Disorders of Childhood and Adolescence

Mary Ann Boyd

KEY CONCEPTS

- attention
- neurodevelopmental delay
- hyperactivity
- impulsiveness
- tics

LEARNING OBJECTIVES

After studying this chapter, you will be able to:

1. Describe mental disorders usually diagnosed in childhood or adolescence.

2. Analyze the prevailing theories relevant to the disorders diagnosed in childhood and adolescence.

3. Discuss the nursing care of children with neurodevelopmental disorders.

4. Analyze the nursing assessment, diagnosis, intervention, and evaluation processes in caring for a child or adolescent with attention-deficit hyperactivity disorder.

5. Discuss the epidemiology, etiology, psychopharmacologic interventions, and nursing care of children with tic disorders.

6. Discuss the nursing care of children and adolescents with separation anxiety and obsessive-compulsive disorders.

7. Discuss the significance of behavioral intervention strategies for children who have elimination disorders.

8. Compare the nursing care of children and adolescents with mood disorders and schizophrenia with that for adults with similar disorders.

KEY TERMS

- adaptive behavior • attention-deficit hyperactivity disorder (ADHD) • autism spectrum disorders
- communication disorders • dyslexia • encopresis • enuresis • externalizing disorders • intellectual disability
- internalizing disorders • learning disorder • motor tics • phonic tics • phonologic processing • school
phobia • separation anxiety disorder • stereotypic behavior • Tourette's disorder

Psychiatric problems are less easily recognized in children than they are in adults. Normal growth and development behaviors of one age group may be a symptom of a disorder in another age group. For example, an imaginary friend is age appropriate for a 4-year-old child but not for an adolescent. Despite the difficulty in diagnosing, about 20% of U.S. youth in their lifetimes are affected by a mental disorder that impairs their ability to function (Merikangas et al., 2010). Only minority of youths with mental disorders receive services for their illnesses (Costello, Jian-ping, Sampson, Kessler, & Merikangas, 2014). Major depressive disorder, schizophrenia, and bipolar disorder are the main causes of disability worldwide among young people ages 10 to 24 years (Gore et al., 2011).

This chapter presents an overview of selected childhood disorders and discusses nursing care for children and their families with these problems. Because it is beyond the scope of this text to present all child psychiatric disorders, this chapter discusses selected ones, including intellectual disability, autism spectrum disorders, tic disorders, separation anxiety disorder, obsessive-compulsive disorder, and elimination disorders. Oppositional defiant and conduct disorders are discussed in Chapter 28. Attention-deficit hyperactivity disorder (ADHD) is highlighted in this chapter.

> **NCLEXNOTE** All of the psychiatric disorders of childhood and adolescence should be viewed within the context of growth and development models. Safety and self-esteem are priority considerations.

Neurodevelopmental Disorders of Childhood

Under the primary influences of genes and environment, neurodevelopment of attention, cognition, language, affect, and social and moral behavior proceeds along several pathways. Developmental pathways and developmental delays are closely interwoven. For example, a language delay can interfere with a child's social development and contribute to behavior problems (Foster-Cohen, Friesen, Champion, & Woodward, 2010). This section discusses neurodevelopmental disorders of childhood that include several conditions that are etiologically unrelated; however, their common feature is a significant delay in one or more lines of development.

> **KEYCONCEPT** **Neurodevelopmental delay** means that the child's development in attention, cognition, language, affect, and social or moral behavior is outside the norm and are manifested by delayed socialization, communication, peculiar mannerisms, and idiosyncratic interests.

INTELLECTUAL DISABILITY

Intellectual disability is defined as limitation in intellectual functioning and adaptive behavior, which covers many social and practical skills (American Association on Intellectual and Developmental Disabilities [AAIDD], 2010). The disability begins before the age of 18 years.

Diagnostic Criteria and Clinical Course

The diagnosis of intellectual disability involves an assessment of *intellectual function* such as reasoning, problem solving, and *adaptive function* in personal independence and social responsibility (American Psychiatric Association, 2013). A diagnosis is made through clinical assessment of behavioral features; historical accounts from parents and teachers; and performance on standardized tests such as the Stanford-Binet or the Wechsler Intelligence Scales for Children. The usual threshold for intellectual disability is an intelligence quotient (IQ) of 70 or less (i.e., two standard deviations below the population mean).

Adaptive behavior is composed of three skill types: *conceptual skills* (language and literacy, money, time, number concepts, and self-direction), *social skills* (interpersonal skills, social responsibility, self-esteem, gullibility, social problem solving, and the ability to follow rules and obey laws and to avoid being victimized), and *practical skills* (activities of daily living, occupational skills, healthcare, travel and transportation, schedules and routines, safety, use of money, use of telephone) (AAIDD, 2011). Impaired adaptive functioning is primarily a clinical judgment based on the child's capacity to manage age-appropriate tasks of daily living. However, standardized assessment instruments are available to assist with determination of the child's capabilities (Lecavalier & Butter, 2010).

An intellectual disability is not necessarily lifelong. Some children may be diagnosed at school age as having an intellectual disability, but with guidance and education, they may no longer meet the criteria as adults.

Epidemiology and Etiology

A large meta-analysis estimated the prevalence of intellectual disabilities to be about 1% in the United States and worldwide (Maulik, Mascarenhas, Mathers, Dua, & Saxena, 2011). There is considerable variability worldwide, with low- and middle-income countries (e.g., Pakistan, Bangladesh) reporting higher rates of disability than high income countries such as the United States (Maulik et al., 2011). The rate of co-occurring psychiatric disorders is estimated between 10% and 39%. In children and adolescents with intellectual disabilities, mental health problems are three to seven times higher than in those without an intellectual disability (Toth & King, 2010).

Intellectual disabilities result from a variety of causes with the most common etiology related to genetic syndromes. Chromosomal changes or defects (e.g., Down syndrome) and exposure to toxins during prenatal development (e.g., fetal alcohol syndrome), heredity, pregnancy and perinatal complications, medication conditions, and environmental influences are all associated with intellectual disabilities. The cause is unknown in about 50% of the cases (Toth & King, 2010).

Nursing Management

The assessment of a child with an intellectual disability focuses on current adaptive skills, intellectual status, and social functioning. A developmental history is a useful way to gather information about past and current capacities (Box 35.1). The nurse compares these data with normal growth and development. Developmentally delayed children who have not had a psychological evaluation should be considered for referral. These children also require evaluation for other comorbid psychiatric disorders, which may be a challenge because of the child's cognitive limitations. Discussions about feelings and behavior may be too complex for these children. If children or adolescents with intellectual disabilities have a comorbid mental disorder or serious behavioral problems, a carefully constructed interdisciplinary behavioral plan will guide care and treatment.

The nurse also assesses the child's support systems (family, school, rehabilitative, and psychiatric) to ensure that the child's special needs have been identified and are being addressed. For example, occupational therapy may be recommended to improve motor coordination, but the family may not have transportation to these services. Availability to alternative services should be explored.

The child and family's response to intellectual disability and other comorbid conditions will determine the nursing diagnoses, planning, and implementation of nursing interventions. Associated nursing diagnoses include Ineffective Coping, Delayed Growth and Development, and Interrupted Family Processes. Nursing interventions include promoting coping skills (interventions directed at building strengths, adapting to change, and maintaining or achieving a higher level of functioning), patient education, and parent education.

Few psychiatric medications are approved for use in children and adolescents, but they are frequently prescribed "off-label" for behaviors that compromise growth and development. Psychostimulants, antidepressants, antipsychotics, and anticonvulsants are the most commonly prescribed psychotropic medications. Before administering these medications or educating parents about them, the nurse should review any new data related to the use of the medications in this population. For example, weight gain can be a major issue for an adolescent taking an antipsychotic.

The overall goals of treatment and nursing care are an optimal level of functioning for the family and eventual independent functioning within a normal social environment for the child. For many children with intellectual disability, achieving independence in adulthood will be delayed but not impossible.

Continuum of Care

Children and families may require varying levels of interventions at different times throughout the life cycle. When a child is young, the family requires special academic support and, for some, residential services. The need for psychiatric intervention varies according to the severity of disability, family functioning, and the existence of other disorders. Feelings of grief and loss in family members (especially parents) related to having a child with a disability may be relieved through family therapy. More specific parent training may be needed to deal with emerging maladaptive behaviors.

AUTISM SPECTRUM DISORDERS

Autism spectrum disorder is characterized by persistent impairment in social communication and social interaction with others (APA, 2103). Children with autism spectrum disorder may or may not have an intellectual disability, but they commonly show an uneven pattern of intellectual strengths and weaknesses. This condition may be a lifelong pattern of being rigid in style, intolerant of change, and prone to behavioral outbursts in response to environmental demands or changes in routine. Two conditions, autism disorder and Asperger syndrome, were previously diagnosed as separate disorders. However, because they have many overlapping symptoms and are difficult to differentiate from each other, the *DSM-5* no longer considers autism and Asperger syndrome as separate disorders, but considers both as **autism spectrum disorder** differentiated by language or intellectual impairment (APA, 2013).

Autism spectrum disorder with restricted, repetitive patterns of behavior such as stereotype or repetitive motor movement, use of objects, inflexible adherence to routine or ritualized patterns, and fascination with lights or movement has been a subject of considerable interest and research effort since its original description more than 50 years ago. Leo Kanner (1943) described the profound isolation of these children and their extreme desire for sameness. These children appear aloof and indifferent to others and often seem to prefer inanimate objects.

The impairment in communication is severe and affects both verbal and nonverbal communication. Children with autism spectrum disorder may manifest delayed and deviant language development, as evidenced by *echolalia* (repetition of words or phrases spoken by others) and a tendency to be extremely concrete in interpretation of language. Pronoun reversals and abnormal intonation are also common. Other common features of autism spectrum disorder are **stereotypic behavior,** self-stimulating, nonfunctional repetitive behaviors, such as repetitive rocking, hand flapping, and an extraordinary insistence on sameness. These children may also engage in self-injurious behavior, such as hitting, head banging, or biting. In some children, their unusual interests may evolve into fascination with specific objects, such as fans or air conditioners, or a particular topic, such as Civil War generals.

A child with autism spectrum disorder may have age-appropriate language and intelligence, but have severe and sustained impairment in social interaction and restricted, repetitive patterns of behavior, interests, and activities. This type of autism spectrum disorder was previously known as Asperger syndrome and appears to be a milder form of autism spectrum disorder. These children have social deficits marked by inappropriate initiation of social interactions, an inability to respond to usual social cues, and a tendency to be concrete in their interpretation of language (APA, 2013). They may also display stereotypic behaviors, such as rocking and hand flapping, and have highly restricted areas of interest, such as train schedules, fans, air conditioners, or dogs. Signs of developmental delay may not be apparent until preschool or school age, when social deficits become evident (Box 35.2).

Epidemiology and Etiology

Autism spectrum disorder is estimated to occur in 2.64% of the general population (Kim et al., 2011). It occurs in boys more often than girls (Brugha et al., 2011). About half of children with autism spectrum disorder have an intellectual disability, and about 25% have seizure disorders. Recent claims that the prevalence of autism is increasing are confounded by improved diagnosis (Pickles, Simonoff, Chandler, Louicas, & Baird, 2011).

Research is accelerating in understanding the etiology of autism spectrum disorder as structural and functional imaging studies provide intriguing leads for future inquiry (Figure 35.1). There are multiple etiological hypotheses related to this disorder. Recent studies support a shared genetic etiology between autism spectrum disorder and schizophrenia (McCarthy et al., 2014). Expression of multiple genes related to the regulation of neurogenesis, brain, and differentiation process are

> **Clinical Vignette**
>
> ### BOX 35.2
> ### FRANK (AUTISM SPECTRUM DISORDER ASPERGER SYNDROME)
>
> *A pediatrician refers Frank, age 5 years, 6 months, for an evaluation because of Frank's unusual preoccupation with ceiling fans and lawn sprinklers. According to his mother, Frank became interested in ceiling fans at age 3 years when he began drawing them, tearing pictures of them out of magazines, and engaging others in discussions about them. In the months before the evaluation, Frank also became fascinated by lawn sprinklers. These preoccupations so dominated Frank's interactions with others that he was practically incapable of discussing any other topics. He remained on the periphery of his kindergarten class and had few friends. Although he tried to make friends, his approaches were inept, and he had trouble reading others.*
>
> *Frank was the product of a full-term uncomplicated pregnancy, labor, and delivery to his then 25-year-old mother. It was her first pregnancy, and both parents eagerly anticipated Frank's birth. As an infant, Frank was healthy but seemed to cry a lot and was difficult to comfort, causing his mother to feel inadequate and depleted. His motor development was also delayed, and at age 3 years, nonfamily members had difficulty understanding his speech. His articulation, however, was within normal limits at the time of consultation. Frank received regular pediatric care and had no history of serious illness or injury. There was no family history of intellectual disability or psychiatric illness; results of genetic testing for chromosomal abnormality were negative.*
>
> *In addition to his unusual preoccupations and social deficits, Frank resisted any change in his routine, was easily frustrated, and was prone to temper tantrums. His parents sharply disagreed about the nature of and appropriate response to his problems.*
>
> **What Do You Think?**
> * What effect do you think Frank's preoccupation may have on his family and their relationships?
> * What kind of teaching program would you develop if you were the nurse assigned to this family?

implicated in autism spectrum disorder (Vaishnavi, Manikandan, & Munirajan, 2014). One line of research is showing defects in the metabolism of cellular antioxidants (Raymond, Deth, & Ralston, 2014). Studies show that higher levels of lead and mercury and lower levels of antioxidants are found in inpatients with autism spectrum disorder when compared to control groups (Alabdali, Al-Ayadhi, & El-Ansary, 2014). Symptoms of gastrointestinal disturbance has focused other research on the role of the GI microbiota and their fermentation products (Wang, Conlon, Christophersen, Sorich, & Angley, 2014). Still, other researchers suggest a role of maternal autoantibodies to the fetal brain in some cases (Elamin & Al-Ayadhi, 2014).

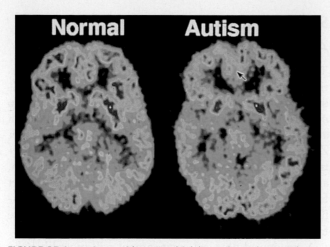

FIGURE 35.1 Patients with autism (*right*) may have decreased metabolic rates in the cingulate gyrus and other associated areas; however, wide heterogeneity in brain metabolic patterns is seen in patients with autism. (Courtesy of Monte S. Buchsbaum, MD, The Mount Sinai Medical Center and School of Medicine, New York.)

Interdisciplinary Treatment and Recovery

Autism spectrum disorders require long-term care at various levels of intensity. Treatment consists of designing academic, interpersonal, and social experiences that support the child's development. Children with autism, even those who are severely affected, may be able to live at home and attend special schools that use behavioral techniques. Other outpatient services may include family counseling, home care, and medication. As the child moves toward adulthood, living at home may become more difficult given the appropriate need for greater independence. The level of structure required depends primarily on IQ and adaptive functioning.

NURSING MANAGEMENT: Human Response to Autism Spectrum Disorders

Biologic Domain

Assessment

The assessment of children with an autism spectrum disorder should follow the mental health assessment discussed in Chapter 34. Biologic assessment should include a review of physical health and neurologic status, giving particular attention to coordination, childhood illnesses, injuries, and hospitalizations. The nurse should assess sleep, appetite, and activity patterns because they may be disturbed in these children. Lack of adequate sleep can increase irritability. Comorbid seizure disorders are common in those with autism, and depression is often seen concurrently when there is no intellectual or language impairment. Thus, the nurse should consider these conditions in the assessment.

Children with additional psychiatric disorders or seizures may be receiving multiple medications and require the care of several clinicians. Therefore, the assessment should include a careful review of current medications and treating clinicians.

Nursing Diagnoses for the Biologic Domain

Assessment data generate a variety of potential nursing diagnoses, including Self-Care Deficits, Delayed Growth and Development, and Disturbed Sleep Pattern. Treatment outcomes need to be individualized to the child, family, and social environment.

Interventions for the Biologic Domain

In teaching self-care skills, the nurse needs to consider the child's current adaptive skills and language limitations. Developing a list of activities for the child to post in his or her bedroom may be effective for some children. Drawings or symbols may be useful for nonverbal children. Physical safety is an important concern for children who are cognitively delayed and may have impaired judgment.

No medication has proved effective at changing the core social and language deficits of autism. However, there are numerous psychiatric medications such as atypical antipsychotics for aggression and irritability and antidepressants to treat anxiety and compulsions. There is minimal evidence that anticonvulsants and traditional mood stabilizers are useful in managing mood lability and aggression. Stimulant and nonstimulant ADHD medication can be helpful in reducing hyperactivity, inattention, and impulsivity (Politte, Henry, & McDougle, 2014; Baribeau & Anagnostou, 2014).

Psychological Domain

Assessment

Communication, behaviors, and flexibility are critical assessment areas. Direct behavioral observation is important to evaluate the child's ability to relate to others, to verify the selection of age-appropriate activities, and to watch for stereotypic behaviors. Assessment of the child with autistic spectrum disorder can be guided by the following categories:

- Communication
  - Verbal and nonverbal
  - Use of picture cards, writing, or drawing
  - Comfortable with eye contact
  - Understand emotional cues
  - Presence of pain
- Behaviors
  - Items of fixation (how does family manage?)
  - Triggers for agitation
  - Early signs that indicate beginning of agitation
  - Interventions that work when child is overstimulated or agitated

- Flexibility or adherence to routine
  - Home schedule
  - What aggravates or irritates the person
  - Early warning signs of agitation
  - When overagitated, what interventions work best (Scarpinato, Bradley, Kurbjun, Bateman, Holtzer, & Ely, 2010).

Inquiry should also include the presence of repetitive behaviors and preoccupation with restricted interests. These odd behaviors may not necessarily cause a problem, but they often interfere with the child's relationships. The nursing assessment is an ongoing process in which attention is given to establishing a positive relationship with the child and the family.

Nursing Diagnoses for the Psychological Domain

Assessment data generate a variety of potential nursing diagnoses, including Anxiety and Disturbed Thought Processes. Because of the long-term nature of these disorders, outcomes may change with time.

Interventions for the Psychological Domain

When working with children with neurodevelopmental disorders, building on their strengths and using positive reinforcement are very important. If they feel that they are constantly criticized or need "fixing," their self-esteem will be eroded, and they will be unlikely to cooperate and learn (Scarpinato et al., 2010).

Children with autism spectrum disorders often need specific behavioral interventions to reduce the frequency of inappropriate or aggressive behavior (Scarpinato et al., 2010). For example, a child may exhibit angry outbursts in response to routine transitions. If the tantrum is dramatic, the consequence may be that the transition does not take place. By structuring the environment and using visual cues to signal the end of one activity and the start of another, it may be possible to reduce the number and intensity of responses to transitions. Safety is always a concern. Self-injury and aggression are sometimes present, and children may need to be protected from hurting themselves and others.

Managing the repetitive behaviors of these children depends on the specific behavior and its effects on others or the environment. If the behavior, such as rocking, has no negative effects, ignoring it may be the best approach. If the behavior, such as head banging, is unacceptable, redirecting the child and using positive reinforcement are recommended. In some cases, especially in severely delayed children, these strategies may not work, and environmental alterations and perhaps protective headgear are needed.

Social Domain
Assessment

The child's behavior, need for structure, and communication style can affect family functioning. Parents of children who are characterized as resilient are better able to manage the adversity associated with care for a child with autism spectrum disorder (Bekhet, Johnson, & Zauszniewski, 2012). Having a child with an autism spectrum disorder is bound to influence family interaction, and responding to the child's needs may adversely affect family functioning. For example, sleep disruption in family members who care for these children may increase family stress. See Chapter 14.

A structured physical environment will most likely be important to a child with a development disorder. Keeping furniture, dishes, and toys in the same place helps ease anxiety and fosters secure feelings. The nurse should identify the child's specific needs for structure in the physical environment and what happens when the physical environment is changed.

Nursing Diagnoses for the Social Domain

Assessment data generate a variety of potential nursing diagnoses, including Social Isolation. The family may be grieving the loss of the child they had expected and are trying to cope with the multitude of problems inherent in raising a child with a disability. Because of the long-term nature of these disorders, the aims of treatment may change with time. However, throughout childhood, the focus should be on the development of age-appropriate adaptive and social skills.

Interventions for the Social Domain

Planning interventions for children with an autism spectrum disorder considers the child; family; and community supports, such as schools, rehabilitation centers, or group homes. First and foremost, the various clinicians involved in the child's treatment should collaborate with the family toward the same general goals. As the number of clinicians and educators involved increases, the chance of fragmentation in treatment planning also increases. The nurse can serve as a case coordinator.

Promoting Interaction

Structuring interventions for social isolation should fit the child's cognitive, linguistic, and developmental levels. Interventions fostering nonverbal social interactions may be more useful than those based on speech. For higher functioning children, activities such as getting the mail, passing out snacks, or taking turns in the context of simple games can engage them in social activities without requiring the use of their limited language skills. Structuring social interactions so that the child shares a task with another, such as carrying a load of books, may help boost confidence in relating to others.

Ensuring Predictability and Safety

When children with autism spectrum disorders are hospitalized, milieu management—a consistent, structured environment with predictable routines for activities, mealtimes, and bedtimes—is necessary for successful treatment. Changes in routine may provoke disorganization in the child, leading to emotional disequilibrium and explosive behavior. The safety of the inpatient unit offers an opportunity to try behavioral strategies, such as rewards for managing transitions. Health care professionals can pass on successful strategies to parents or primary caretakers (Reaven, 2009).

Managing Behavior

Autism spectrum disorders call for extraordinary patience and determination. With help, these children can learn social and communication skills, such as taking turns in conversation and warning the listener before changing the subject in the context of milieu. If aggressive or assaultive behavior is a problem, a brief "time out" followed by prompt reentry into activities is usually effective.

Residential care may be necessary in some cases. After making the decision to place a child into a residential facility, family members may experience guilt, loss, and a sense of failure concerning their inability to care for the child at home.

Supporting Family

Unfortunately, lack of integration of medical, psychiatric, social, and educational services can add to the family's burden. Parents may manifest denial, grief, guilt, and anger at various points as they adjust to their child's disability. The nurse can offer parents the opportunity to express their frustrations and disappointments and can be alert for indications that parents are in need of additional assistance, such as parent support groups or respite care.

Family interventions include support, education, counseling, and referral to self-help groups. Whenever possible, the nurse provides education to help parents determine appropriate expectations for their child and to meet the child's special needs. The following are examples of potentially useful nursing interventions focusing on the family:

- Interpreting the treatment plan for parents and child
- Modeling appropriate behavior modification techniques
- Including the parents as cotherapists for the implementation of the care plan
- Assisting the family in identifying and resolving their sense of loss related to the diagnosis

- Coordinating support systems for parents, siblings, and family members
- Maintaining interdisciplinary collaboration

Evaluation and Treatment Outcomes

Evaluation of patient and family outcomes is an ongoing process. Short-term outcomes might consist of discrete behavioral improvements, such as reducing self-injurious behavior by 50%. The long-term goal is for the patient to achieve the highest level of functioning.

ATTENTION-DEFICIT HYPERACTIVITY DISORDER

Attention-deficit hyperactivity disorder (ADHD) is one of the most commonly diagnosed disorder in school-aged children (CDC, 2013). It is almost certainly a heterogeneous disorder with multiple etiologies. The relatively high frequency of ADHD and associated behavior problems virtually guarantees that nurses will meet these children in all pediatric treatment settings. ADHD is also diagnosed in adults, but it is less common than in children (Kessler et al., 2010).

Clinical Course and Diagnostic Criteria

A persistent pattern of inattention, hyperactivity, and impulsiveness that interferes with functioning characterizes ADHD (APA, 2013). A diagnosis is made based on school behavior, parents' reports, and direct observation of inattention and hyperactivity-impulsivity that are inconsistent with developmental level. Parents and teachers describe children with ADHD as restless, always on the go, highly distractible, unable to wait their turn, heedless, and frequently disruptive. Indeed, it is often disruptive behavior that brings these children into treatment.

> **KEYCONCEPT** **Attention** involves concentrating on one activity to the exclusion of others, as well as the ability to sustain focus.

In ADHD, the person finds it difficult to attend to one task at a time and is easily distracted. For some, the lack of attention is related to being unable to filter incoming information, which leads to being unable to screen and select the important information. That is, all incoming stimuli are treated the same (e.g., directions from a teacher elicits the same importance as noise in the hallway). For others, the distractibility may be related to stimuli-seeking behavior. Given the heterogeneity of ADHD, either of these models explains problems of attention for subgroups of affected children.

Children with ADHD are prone to impulsive, risk-taking behavior and often fail to consider the consequences of their actions (Shaw et al., 2011). They tend to exercise poor judgment and to have more than the usual lumps, bumps, and bruises because of their risk-taking behavior. They often require a high degree of structure and supervision (Davis & Williams, 2011).

> **KEYCONCEPT** **Impulsiveness** is the tendency to act on urges, notions, or desires without adequately considering the consequences.

Although hyperactivity is a characteristic often associated with ADHD, controversy is long-standing about whether attention-deficit can occur without overactivity. In many cases, the hyperactivity prompts the search for treatment. Parents typically report that a child's hyperactivity was manifested early in life and is evident in most situations (APA, 2013). Hyperactivity and impulsivity in childhood are associated with conduct disorder (Chapter 28) and intimate partner violence perpetration in adults (Fang et al., 2010).

> **KEYCONCEPT** **Hyperactivity** is excessive motor activity, as evidenced by restlessness, an inability to remain seated, and high levels of physical motion and verbal output.

ADHD Across the Lifespan

ADHD is a disorder usually diagnosed in childhood and was traditionally viewed as a problem of children. We now understand that ADHD persists into adulthood, and it is sometimes first diagnosed later than childhood. In adults, symptoms of hyperactivity and impulsivity tend to decline with age and deficit of attention persist and become more varied (Kessler et al., 2010). However, the majority of the adults with ADHD are undiagnosed and untreated (Waite & Ramsay, 2010). Many of the adults with ADHD become the parents of children with the same disorder. The parents often do not have the necessary parenting skills to be effective (Mokrova, O'Brien, Calkins, & Keane, 2010).

Epidemiology and Risk Factors

Although prevalence estimates vary depending on the diagnostic criteria used, the sources of data, and the sampling procedure, ADHD in school-aged children is about 6%, with a range of 2% to 14% (Kessler et al., 2010; Syed, Masaud, Nkire, Iro, & Garland, 2010). Boys are twice as likely as girls to be diagnosed with ADHD (Centers for Disease Control and Prevention, 2013). A familial history of ADHD, bipolar disorder, or substance

use (Kessler et al., 2010), early exposure to pesticides (Kuehn, 2011), prenatal tobacco exposure, and high blood lead concentrations (Polanska, Jurewicz, & Hanke, 2012) are associated with increasing the risk for ADHD.

Etiology

There is no one explanation for the occurrence of ADHD; instead, this disorder is viewed as having multiple causes. Genetic factors are implicated in the etiology of ADHD, and they clearly play a fundamental role in the manifestation of the ADHD behavior (Gagne, Saudino, & Asherson, 2011). In some children, ADHD may have developed because of having hypersensitivity to environmental stimuli such as foods (Pelsser, Buitelaar, & Savelkoul, 2009).

Biologic Theories

Although the etiology of ADHD is uncertain, there is a pervasive evidence of neurobiologic dysfunction. Several lines of research have shown that the frontal lobe and functional connections are impacted with specific subcortical structures also dysregulated. One clearly dysfunctional area is the dorsolateral prefrontal cortex, the center of directed attention and the ability to manage emotions or delay emotional reactions (Manos, Tom-Revzon, Bukstein, & Crismon, 2007). Several neurotransmitters (e.g., dopamine, serotonin) are dysregulated (Halmey, Johansson, Winge, McKinney, Knappskog, & Haavik, 2010). Clinically, the hyperactive-impulsive behavior characteristic of ADHD has been shown to be predominantly related to biologic factors, not psychosocial (Freitag, Hänig, Schneider, Switz, Palmason, & Meyer, 2011).

Psychosocial Theories

Although genetic endowment clearly plays a fundamental role in the etiology of ADHD, psychosocial factors are also important risk factors, particularly related to inattention (Freitag et al., 2011). Family stress, marital discord, and parental substance use are also associated with ADHD (Palcic, Jurbergs, & Kelley, 2009). Other implicated psychosocial factors are poverty, overcrowded living conditions, and family dysfunction.

Family Response to ADHD

Living with a child who has ADHD is a challenge for all family members, particularly those members who also have similar issues as the affected child. The family will not only be raising a child who needs a structured environment that helps support focus and attention, but the parents have to partner with their children's school system. For some families, the relationship with the school is positive and supportive. For others, the relationship with the school can be strained and lead to additional stress. It is important that the teachers and parents work together and provide consistent directions to the child.

If parents also have problems related to attention, impulse, and hyperactivity, home chaos and ineffective parenting practices can occur (Mokrova et al., 2010). If the parents also have ADHD, they might not be able to provide a calm, structured environment for the child. Effective parenting requires the ability to resist overreacting emotionally, to focus on the child, to keep track of activities, and to provide consistency in discipline.

Interdisciplinary Treatment and Recovery

Children with ADHD and their families benefit from symptom management, education, and support from a variety of disciplines in order to have a quality life. Successful recovery efforts involve early recognition and treatment. By recognizing the problem early, family members and teachers can structure the child's interactions, develop meaningful discipline strategies, and modify the physical environment so the child can learn coping skills to deal with the impulsivity, distractibility, and hyperactivity. Evidence has accumulated over the years that medication is helpful, especially in the early years, but for long-term effects, a combination of medication management and behavioral approaches results in the best outcomes for the children and their families (Moriyama, Polanczyk, Terzi, Farla, & Rhode, 2013).

ADHD is not an easy disorder to treat or manage. Comorbidity complicates successful recovery. Children with ADHD have more conduct problems (e.g., run-ins with police), depression, and psychiatric admissions (McQuade et al., 2014). There are many other problems that interfere with recovery efforts, such as family disruptions and economic problems, as well as naturally occurring changes such as maturational issues during their adolescent years. Additionally, children from disadvantaged backgrounds fare worse than those children who have socioeconomic and educational support (Law, Sideridis, Prock, & Sheridan, 2014).

Priority Care Issues

Children, adolescents, and adults with ADHD are high risk for moodiness that could lead to risk-taking behavior and suicide ideation or attempts (Balazs, Miklósi, Keresztény, Dallos, & Gádoros, 2014). Mood lability, the presence of depression, and potential for self-harm should be carefully assessed in these individuals.

NURSING MANAGEMENT: Human Response to ADHD

The planning of nursing interventions must be done within the context of the family, treatment setting, and school environment. With the parents, clinical team members, and school personnel, the nurse participates in designing a plan of care that fits the child's and family's needs. Persons with ADHD and their families will benefit from nursing care at many different times in the course of their disorder. Unless hospitalized for a comorbid mental health problem, most treatment will occur outside the mental health system. School nurses often provide most of the nursing care and family education.

Biologic Domain

The nursing assessment for the biologic domain may be initiated either before or after the diagnosis of ADHD is made. In the school setting, the nurse may suspect ADHD and collect assessment data similar to that collected by the nurse in a psychiatric facility.

Assessment

In the school setting, the primary focus of the assessment is the impact of ADHD on classroom behavior and school performance. In the hospital, the nurse tries to determine the contribution of ADHD to the acute psychiatric problem. In both cases, the nurse collects assessment data through direct interview, observation of the child and parent, and teacher ratings. Because children with ADHD may have difficulty sitting through long sessions, interviews are typically brief. Parents and teachers are extremely important sources for assessment data. To this end, the nurse can make use of several standardized instruments (Box 35.3).

As with other psychiatric disorders with onset in childhood, the nursing assessment of children with ADHD begins with identification and exploration of the presenting problem. This typically entails a review of the child's developmental course, the onset and pattern of the current symptoms, factors that have worsened or improved the child's problems, and prior treatment or self-initiated efforts to remedy the situation. Medical history is also essential, consisting of perinatal course, childhood illnesses, hospital admissions, injuries, seizures, tics, physical growth, general health status, and timing of the child's last physical examination.

The behavior of these children is characteristically very active and can often be observed in the office. They cannot sit still. They fidget. Even in sleep, they may be more active than normal children. Thus, a careful assessment of eating, sleeping, and activity patterns is essential. Assessing daily food intake, typical diet, and frequency of eating will help identify any nutrition problems. Caffeinated products can contribute to hyperactivity. Sleep is often disturbed for children with ADHD and consequently the family. A detailed sleep assessment can provide points for interventions and help the interpretation of drug effects.

BOX 35.3

Standardized Tools for ADHD Diagnosis*

CONNERS QUESTIONNAIRES

The Conners Parent Questionnaire is a 48-item scale that a parent completes about his or her child. Each item is a statement that the parent rates on a 4-point scale from 0 (not at all) to 3 (very much). The Conners Teacher Questionnaire is a 28-item questionnaire that the child's teacher completes according to the same 4-point scale as the Parent Questionnaire. Both questionnaires have been standardized by age and gender for a mean of 50 and a standard deviation of 10 (Conners 1989; Goyette et al., 1978).

ADHD RATING SCALE

The ADHD Rating Scale is a recently developed measure that asks parents or teachers to respond directly to 18 items in the *Diagnostic and Statistical Manual of Mental Disorders-IV-TR (DSM-IV-TR)* criteria (The Foundation for Medical Practice Education, 2008). A similar scale called the SNAP-IV is available online for free at www.adhd.net. The SNAP-IV was used as the primary outcome measure in the MTA Cooperative Group Study (Molina et al., 2009).

CHILD BEHAVIOR CHECKLIST

The Child Behavior Checklist (CBCL) is a 118-item questionnaire that a parent completes. In addition to the 118 questions about specific behaviors and psychiatric symptoms, the CBCL also includes questions concerning the child's competence in social and academic spheres as well as age-appropriate activities. Normative data are available, allowing the conversion of raw scores to standard scores for age and gender. There is also a teacher version of this scale.

*Note that the diagnosis of ADHD is not made on the basis of questionnaires alone. Data from these rating scales augment the information gathered through interview and observation. These questionnaires can be especially useful before and after initiating a treatment plan to measure change.

Nursing Diagnoses for the Biologic Domain

Depending on the severity of the responses, family situation, and school environment, several nursing diagnoses could be generated from the assessment data, including Self-Care Deficit, Risk for Imbalanced Nutrition, Risk for Injury, and Disturbed Sleep Pattern. The outcomes should be individualized to the child.

Interventions for the Biologic Domain

Modifying Nutrition

A link between adverse reaction to food (dietary salicylates and artificially added food colors, flavors, and preservatives) and ADHD was suggested many years ago when the Feingold diet was introduced (Feingold, 1975). Over the years, interest in the link between food and behavior continues to spark interest in ADHD as a problem related to food. Study outcomes are mixed. There seems to be agreement that in some children, the behaviors associated with ADHD can be decreased with diet changes (Ghuman, 2011; Pelsser et al., 2011). The

Restricted Elimination Diet has been shown to improve behavior in some children and can be used as an instrument to determine whether ADHD behaviors are induced by food. In this diet, all-natural, chemical-free foods are eaten, and most of the foods that are regularly eaten are removed (Lomangino, 2011). Fruits, vegetables, nuts, nut butters, beans, seeds, gluten-free grains such as rice and quinoa, fish, lamb, wild game meats, organic turkey and large amounts of water are consumed. This diet is very restricted and consequently difficult to follow all of the time (Pelsser et al., 2011).

If patients are adhering to this diet, the nurse should support the patient and family in providing the nutritional information needed for this diet. Additionally, the patient and family will need education regarding those foods that are chemical free. A referral to a dietitian will benefit the patient and family.

A subgroup of children with ADHD show inattention, impulsivity, and hyperactivity following ingestion of foods containing artificial food color (Nigg, Lewis, Edinger, & Falk, 2012; Stevens, Kuczek, Burgess, Stochelski, Arnold, & Galland, 2013). The reason some children seem susceptible to artificial food color is unclear. More research is needed in this area.

Children with ADHD seem to be more susceptible to being overweight and developing obesity (Pauli-Pott, Albayrak, Hebebrand, & Pott, 2010). Because of the impulsivity and inattention characteristic of ADHD, these children may be unable to resist external cues for high-fat foods. The nurse can help the family and patient structure the external environment so the child has healthy choices available.

Promoting Sleep

Sleep can be a problem for children with ADHD for many reasons. The overactivity of the disorder itself and the side effects of the psychostimulants contribute to sleep problems. A sleep history should be taken before medications are prescribed. If problems exist, atomoxetine (Strattera) should be considered before the psychostimulants (see next section). If sleep problems arise while taking medications, sleep diaries should be kept. Sleep hygiene and behavior therapy techniques should be implemented (Graham et al., 2011). See Chapter 32.

Using Pharmacologic Interventions

The first-line recommended medications for ADHD symptoms are the psychostimulants and atomoxetine (Strattera). It is not unusual for two psychostimulants or a psychostimulant and atomoxetine to be prescribed together for maximum response. Second-line medications include bupropion (Wellbutrin) and other antidepressants (tricyclic antidepressants [TCAs]). Then, if symptoms are not improved, alpha agonists (guanfacine or clonidine) are usually used (Hirota, Schwartz, & Correll, 2014).

Psychostimulants

Psychostimulants (see Chapter 11) are by far the most commonly used medications for the treatment of ADHD. These medications enhance dopamine and norepinephrine activity and thereby improve attention and focus, increase inhibition of impulsive actions, and quiet the "noise" associated with distractibility and shifting attention (Moriyama et al., 2013).

Methylphenidate (Ritalin) has a total duration of action of about 4 hours (Box 35.4). Thus, parents or teachers often describe a return of overactivity and distractibility as the first dose of medication wears off. This "rebound effect" can often be managed by moving the second dose of the day slightly closer to the first dose. Longer acting preparations of methylphenidate such as Concerta, Ritalin LA, and Metadate or amphetamine–dextroamphetamine (Adderall) do not require frequent dosing and may be a better fit with a school day schedule.

One of the major concerns with the psychostimulants is the potential for abuse. With the increase in recognition of the ADHD, there has been an increase in psychostimulant prescriptions. There has also been an increase in teen and preteen abuse of amphetamine products. These abused prescription medications most often belong to the adolescents or a friend. Nurses should caution parents about the potential for abuse and prevent their child's medication from being a source of recreational use.

Atomoxetine

Atomoxetine (Strattera), a noradrenergic reuptake inhibitor, is not classified as a stimulant and is effective in the treatment of ADHD, especially when it is used in combination with the psychostimulants. Because it has little risk of abuse or misuse, it is often used for those who have a comorbid substance abuse issue (Murthy & Chand, 2012). It is also helpful in treating comorbid anxiety and inattention (Wagner & Pliszka, 2011). This medication is generally well tolerated in children and adults. Common adverse events include headache, abdominal pain, decreased appetite, vomiting, somnolence, and nausea (Childress & Berry, 2012).

Other Medications for ADHD

Bupropion (Wellbutrin) has both noradrenergic and dopaminergic actions and is sometimes used for ADHD. Before atomoxetine was available, the TCAs (desipramine, imipramine, amitriptyline, and clomipramine) were the primary alternative to psychostimulants, but their use has declined significantly.

Teaching Points

Medication can help the child's hyperactivity, impulsiveness, and inattention; therefore, teaching the parent, child, and school personnel about the importance of the medication in ADHD and the potential side effects is a place to begin. Explaining to the child that the medication

BOX 35.4

Drug Profile: **Methylphenidate (Ritalin)**

DRUG CLASS: Central nervous system stimulant

RECEPTOR AFFINITY: The mechanisms of effect are not completely clear. At low doses, it provides mild cortical stimulation similar to that of amphetamines. This stimulation results from methylphenidate's ability to promote release and interfere with the reuptake of dopamine in the synaptic cleft. Main sites appear to be the cerebral cortex, striatum, and pons.

INDICATIONS: Treatment of narcolepsy, attention-deficit disorders, and hyperkinetic syndrome; unlabeled uses for treatment of depression in elderly patients and patients with cancer or stroke.

ROUTES AND DOSAGE: Available in 5- to 10-mg immediate-release tablets and 20-mg sustained-release tablets (Ritalin-SR). Newer long-acting preparations such as Concerta and Metadate, in various dose strengths, are also available.

Adult Dosage: Must be individualized; range from 10 to 60 mg/d orally in divided doses bid (twice a day) to tid (three times a day), preferably 15 to 30 min before meals. If insomnia is a problem, drug should be administered before 6 PM.

Child Dosage: The immediate-release formulation can be started at 5 mg twice or three times daily on a 4-hour schedule with weekly increases depending on response. Starting doses of the long acting preparations are equivalent to the total tid dose (e.g., 5 tid of short-acting would translate into 18 mg of Concerta). Usually given on a tid schedule, with the last dose being roughly half that of the first and second dose. Daily dosage of more than 60 mg is not recommended. Discontinue after 1 month if no improvement is seen.

PEAK EFFECT: 1 h; half-life: 3–4 h for the immediate-release preparations

SELECT ADVERSE REACTIONS: Nervousness, insomnia, dizziness, headache, dyskinesias (including tics), toxic psychosis, anorexia, nausea, abdominal pain, increased pulse and blood pressure, palpitations, tolerance, psychological dependence

WARNING: The drug is discontinued periodically to assess the patient's condition. Contraindications include marked anxiety, tension and agitation, glaucoma, severe depression, and obsessive-compulsive symptoms. Use cautiously in patients with a personal or family history of tic disorders, seizure disorders, hypertension, drug dependence, alcoholism, or emotional instability.

SPECIFIC PATIENT AND FAMILY EDUCATION
- Do not chew or crush sustained-release tablets; they must be swallowed whole.
- Take the drug exactly as prescribed; if insomnia is a problem, the time and dose may need adjustment. The drug is rarely taken after 5 PM.
- Avoid alcohol and over-the-counter products, including decongestants, cold remedies, and cough syrups; these could accentuate side effects of the stimulant.
- Keep appointments for follow-up, including evaluations for monitoring the child's growth and use of parent and teacher ratings to monitor benefit.
- Note that the prescriber may discontinue the drug periodically to confirm effectiveness of therapy.

improves concentration and the ability to sit still can help strengthen patient motivation.

Many times parents are reluctant to initiate treatment with psychostimulants because of the fear that their use in childhood will increase the risk of using substances in adulthood. Studies show that treatment of ADHD is not associated with a risk of substance use disorders (Humphreys, Eng, & Lee, 2013). Teaching patients and families about the biologic basis of ADHD helps parents understand that these children are not "bad" kids but that they have problems with impulse control and attention. It may be helpful to review the purposes of the medications and assure parents that there is evidence that medications help most children.

Psychological Domain

Assessment

Hyperactivity, impulsivity, and inattention are typically pervasive problems that are evident both at school and at home. Discipline is frequently an issue because parents may have difficulty controlling their child's behavior, which is disruptive and occasionally destructive. These children are at risk for depression and suicidal ideation, especially in adolescence. Girls and those with mothers who experience depression when the child is 4 to 6 years of age are more likely to attempt suicide 5 to 13 years later (Chronis-Tuscano et al., 2010).

Children with ADHD are more likely to have problems with their cognitive process with changing demands of teachers and parents (Mulder et al., 2011; Shaw et al., 2011). Consequently, they may have more difficulty in school with decision making.

Nursing Diagnoses for the Psychological Domain

Assessment of the psychological domain may generate several diagnoses, including Anxiety and Defensive Coping. The outcomes should be individualized to the child.

IInterventions for the Psychological Domain

Behavioral programs based on rewards for positive behavior, such as waiting turns and following directions, can foster new social skills. Behavioral parent training, behavioral classroom management, and behavioral peer interventions are well-established treatments. Specific cognitive behavioral techniques are helpful in which the child learns to "stop, look, and listen" before doing. These approaches have been refined, and several useful treatment manuals are available (Evans, Owens, & Bunford, 2013). In general, interactions with children can be guided by the following:

- Set clear limits with clear consequences. Use few words and simplify instructions.
- Establish and maintain a predictable environment with clear rules and regular routines for eating, sleeping, and playing.
- Promote attention by maintaining a calm environment with few stimuli. These children cannot filter extraneous stimuli and react to all stimuli equally.
- Establish eye contact before giving directions; ask the child to repeat what was heard.
- Encourage the child to do homework in a quiet place outside of a traffic pattern.
- Assist the child to work on one assignment at a time (reward with a break after each completion).

Social Domain

Assessment

Dysfunctional interactions can develop within the family. Reviewing the problem behaviors and the situations in which they occur is a way to identify negative interaction patterns. These children are often behind in their work at school because of poor organization, off-task behavior, and impulsive responses. They can exhaust their parents, aggravate teachers, and annoy siblings with their intrusive and disruptive behavior. Because ADHD often occurs in the context of psychosocial adversity, it is important to review the family situation, including parenting style, stability of household membership, consistency of rules and routines, and life events (e.g., divorce, moves, deaths, job loss). Identification of these factors can be useful in shaping a care plan that builds on potential strengths and mitigates the effects of environmental factors that may perpetuate the child's disruptive behavior. Data regarding school performance, behavior at home, and comorbid psychiatric disorders are essential for developing school interventions and behavior plans and establishing the baseline severity for medication.

Nursing Diagnoses for the Social Domain

Depending on the severity of the child's responses, family situation, and school environment, several nursing diagnoses could be generated from the assessment data, including Impaired Social Interaction, Ineffective Role Performance, and Compromised Family Coping. Short-term outcomes, such as decreasing the number of classroom ejections within a 2-week period, may be useful for one child, but reducing the frequency and amplitude of angry outbursts at home may be relevant to another child.

Interventions for the Social Domain

Family treatment is nearly always a component of cognitive behavioral treatment approaches with the child. This

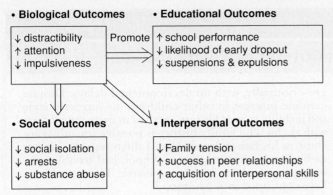

FIGURE 35.2 Long-term outcomes of optimal treatment for patients with attention-deficit hyperactivity disorder.

may involve parent training that focuses on principles of behavior management, such as appropriate limit setting and use of reward systems, as well as revising expectations about the child's behavior. School programming often involves increasing structure in the child's school day to offset the child's tendency to act without forethought and to be easily distracted by extraneous stimuli. Specific remediation is required for the child with comorbid deficits in learning or language. Some children may require small, self-contained classrooms.

Evaluation and Treatment Outcomes

Children may not notice any effects after taking medication, but people in their environment do. Often, within 1 to 2 weeks of initiating therapy, children with ADHD become more attentive, less impulsive, and less active. Parents and teachers are often the first to notice improvement. With time, academic achievement also may improve (Figure 35.2).

Continuum of Care

Treatment of ADHD typically is conducted in outpatient settings. Optimal treatment is multimodal (includes several types of interventions), encompassing four main areas: individual treatment for the child, family treatment, school accommodations, and medication. Parent training and social skills training also help diminish disruptive and defiant behavior. See Nursing Care Plan 35.1.

OTHER NEURODEVELOPMENTAL DISORDERS

Other neurodevelopmental disorders are characterized by a narrower range of deficits. These include specific neurodevelopmental disorders generally classified as learning, communication, and motor skills disorders. This section focuses primarily on learning and communication disorders.

Specific Learning Disorders

Generally, a **learning disorder** (also called learning disability) is defined as a discrepancy between actual achievement and expected achievement based on the person's age and intellectual ability. The definition varies depending on the source and state statute. Learning disorders are typically classified as verbal (reading and spelling) or nonverbal (mathematics).

Reading disability, also called **dyslexia**, has been recognized for more than 100 years. It is defined as a significantly lower score for mental age on standardized tests in reading that is not the result of low intelligence or inadequate schooling. This relatively common problem affects about 5% of school-aged children, with some studies reporting higher prevalence. In clinical samples, dyslexia affects boys more often than girls; however, a large community-based sample of children with reading disorders found no gender difference. This discrepancy suggests that the observed difference in clinic samples may be related to biases in seeking treatment rather than a true gender difference (Ferrer, Shaywitz, Holahan, Marchione, & Shaywitz, 2011; Stoeckel, Colligan, Barbaresi, Weaver, Killian, & Katusci, 2013).

Although it is clear that no single cause will provide a sufficient explanation for reading disability, the underlying problem appears to be a deficit in **phonologic processing**, which involves the discrimination and interpretation of speech sounds. A disturbance in the development of the left hemisphere is believed to cause this deficit. Both genetic and environmental factors have been implicated in the etiology of reading disability. Data from family studies show that reading disability is familial and that shared environmental factors alone cannot explain the high rate of recurrence in affected families (van der Leij, van Bergen, van Zuijen, de Jong, Maurits, & Maassen, 2013).

Less is known about the prevalence of nonverbal learning disorder (mathematics disorder), with estimates of occurrence ranging from 0.1% to 1.0% of school-aged children and no apparent difference between boys and girls. Mathematical ability is moderately inheritable and negatively associated with inattentiveness and hyperactivity-impulsivity symptoms of ADHD (Greven, Kovas, Willcutt, Petrill, & Plomin, 2014).

Communication Disorders

Communication disorders involve speech or language impairments. *Speech* refers to the motor aspects of speaking; *language* consists of higher order aspects of formulating and comprehending verbal communication. Communication disorders are fairly common, and are more common in children with autism spectrum disorders, ADHD, anxiety, and conduct disorders (Mackie &

(text continues on page 692)

NURSING CARE PLAN 35.1

The Patient With Attention-Deficit Hyperactivity Disorder

Jamie, age 6 years, comes to the primary health care clinic with his mother Lillian because of motor restlessness, distractibility, and disruptive behavior in the classroom. According to Lillian, Jamie had a reasonably good year in kindergarten, but early in the first grade, the teacher began to report disruptive behavior. On reflection, Lillian recalls that kindergarten was a half-day program with more activity. By contrast, Jamie is expected to sit in his seat and pay attention for longer periods in first grade.

Jamie's medical history is unremarkable. Lillian's pregnancy with Jamie was her first and was unplanned. Although there were no complications during the pregnancy, the period was marked by significant marital discord, culminating in divorce before Jamie's first birthday. Jamie was born by cesarean section after a long, unproductive labor. He was healthy at birth and grew normally, with no developmental delays. Despite genuine interest in other children, his intrusive style and inability to wait his turn resulted in frequent conflicts with them. The family history is positive for substance abuse in his father. In addition, Lillian reports that her ex-husband was disruptive in school, had trouble concentrating, and was highly impulsive. These problems have continued into adulthood.

During the two evaluation sessions, Jamie is active but cooperative. His speech is fluent and normal in tone and tempo but somewhat loud. His discourse is coherent, but at times, he makes rather abrupt changes in conversation without warning his listeners. Psychological testing done at the school revealed average to above-average intelligence. Parent and teacher questionnaires concurred that Jamie was overactive, impulsive, inattentive, and quarrelsome but not defiant.

Setting: Psychiatric Home Care Agency

Baseline Assessment: Jamie is a 6-year-old boy with prominent hyperactivity and disruptive behavior. He lives with Lillian, his single mother. These problems interfere with his interpersonal relationships and academic progress. Lillian is discouraged and feels unable to manage Jamie's behavior.

Associated Psychiatric Diagnosis	Medications
Attention-deficit hyperactivity disorder (ADHD)	Methylphenidate 7.5 mg at breakfast and lunch (i.e., at 8 AM and 12 noon) and then adding 5 mg at 7 PM.

Nursing Diagnosis 1: Impaired Social Interaction

Defining Characteristics	Related Factors
Cannot establish and maintain developmentally appropriate social relationships	Impulsive behavior
Has interpersonal difficulties at school	Overactive
Is not well accepted by peers	Inattentive
Is easily distracted	Risk-taking behavior (tried to climb out the window to get away from his mother)
Interrupts others	Failure to recognize effects of his behavior on others
Cannot wait his turn in games	
Speaks out of turn in the classroom	

Outcomes

Initial	Discharge
1. Decrease hyperactivity and disruptive behavior.	4. Improve capacity to identify alternative responses in conflicts with peers.
2. Improve attention and decrease distractibility.	5. Improve capacity to interpret behavior of age mates.
3. Decrease frequency of acting without forethought.	

Continued

NURSING CARE PLAN 35.1 (Continued)

Interventions

Intervention	Rationale	Ongoing Assessment
Educate mother and teach about ADHD and use of stimulant medication.	Better understanding helps to ensure adherence; also parents and teachers often miscast children with ADHD as "troublemakers."	Determine the extent to which parent or teacher "blames" Jamie for his problems.
Monitor adherence to medication schedule.	Uneven compliance may contribute to failed trial of medication.	Administer parent and teacher questionnaires; inquire about behavior across entire day.
Ensure that medication is both effective and well tolerated.	Stimulants can affect appetite and sleep.	Administer parent and teacher questionnaires; check height and weight; ask about sleep and appetite.

Evaluation

Outcomes	Revised Outcomes	Interventions
Jamie shows decreased hyperactivity and less disruption in the classroom.	Improve ability to identify disruptive classroom behavior.	Initiate point system to reward appropriate behavior.
Jamie shows improved attention and decreased distractibility.	Improve school performance.	Move to front of classroom as an aid to attention.
Mother and teacher attest to Jamie's decreased impulsive behavior.	Increase Jamie's capacity to recognize the effects of his behavior on others.	Encourage participation in structured activities.
Jamie identifies alternative responses such as walking away until it is his turn.	Increase frequency of acting on these alternative approaches.	Inquire about social skills group at school, if available.
Jamie improves interpretation of motives and behaviors of others.	Improve acceptance by peers.	Encourage participation in community activities.

Nursing Diagnosis 2: Ineffective Coping (Lillian)

Defining Characteristics	Related Factors
Verbalizes discouragement and inability to handle situation with Jamie	Chronicity of ADHD More than average childrearing problems

Outcomes

Initial	Discharge
1. Verbalize frustration at trying to raise a child with ADHD alone. 2. Identify positive methods of interacting and disciplining Jamie that will support the parent–child relationship as well as meet Jamie's development needs.	3. Identify coping patterns that decrease the sense of frustration and increase parental competence. 4. Initiate a collaborative relationship with the schoolteacher. 5. Identify sources of support in the community and begin to access these resources.

Interventions

Intervention	Rationale	Ongoing Assessment
Assess mother's discouragement and feelings about parenting, identifying specific problem areas.	Helping the mother verbalize her feelings and identify problem areas helps in formulating problem-solving strategies.	Assess the severity of the problems with which she is living.
Refer mother to Community Mental Health Center for free parenting class.	Parent training based on clear directives and rewards can be effective for decreasing impulsive and disruptive behavior.	Monitor mother's level of confidence and perceived change in Jamie's behavior.
Refer mother to self-help organization.	Parent groups such as Children and Adults with Attention-deficit Disorder (CHAAD) can be sources of support and information.	Determine whether contact was made and whether it was helpful.
Make contact with school to enhance collaboration with mother.	Assess effectiveness of medication and other interventions; need feedback from teachers.	Determine whether mother has been able to contact teacher.

Continued

NURSING CARE PLAN 35.1 *(Continued)*

Evaluation

Outcomes	Revised Outcomes	Interventions
After four sessions, Lillian expresses her frustrations, but she has begun to identify different ways of relating to Jamie and his developmental needs.	None	None
Through attending the parenting class and joining a support group, Lillian begins to change her coping patterns, decrease her frustrations, and increase her parental competence.	Complete parenting class; attend at least two support group meetings each month.	If necessary, refer for additional parent counseling.
Lillian initiates a collaborative relationship with Jamie's teacher.	Lillian and teacher mutually develop and implement behavior plans for home and school.	Have mother observe in the classroom; have mother visit highly structured classroom.

Law, 2010). As with reading disability, there are undoubtedly multiple causes of speech or language deficit.

A delay in speech or language development can adversely affect the child's socialization and education. For example, peers may rebuff or tease a child with an articulation defect or stutter, contributing to withdrawal and a negative self-image. The resulting isolation could limit opportunities to negotiate rules, take turns, and learn cooperation. These same tasks could also be difficult for children with language delay. Moreover, language appears to play a role in the regulation of behavior and impulses (Mackie & Law, 2010).

Nursing Management

Nursing assessment of children with a known specific developmental disorder includes (1) evidence of interference in daily life, (2) determination of the child's ability (and limitations) to communicate during the interview, (3) assessment of the child's perception about his or her disability, (4) observation for impaired learning and communication, and (5) past and current interventions for the learning or communication deficit with data gathered through direct interview of the child and significant others such as parents. Several nursing diagnoses can be generated from these data, such as Impaired Verbal Communication and Social Isolation.

For the child with learning disabilities, nurses can focus on building self-confidence and helping the family connect with guidance and educational resources that support the child's development into adulthood. For the child with communication disorders, the interventions focus on fostering social and communication skills and making referrals for specific speech or language therapy. Modeling appropriate communication in spontaneous

situations with the child can be a useful intervention for some children. The following is an overview of nursing interventions for the child with specific developmental difficulties:

- Introduce strategies for increasing communication skills (e.g., initiating conversation, taking turns in conversation, facing the listener).
- Identify and develop specific intervention strategies for problems secondary to learning communication disorders, such as low self-esteem.
- Provide parental support for coping with the disorder.
- Maintain interdisciplinary medical, dental, speech therapy, and educational collaboration.
- Refer to learning or speech specialist for evaluation and assistance.

Continuum of Care

Children with learning disabilities obviously require careful psychoeducational and cognitive testing to identify their strengths and deficits. School or clinical psychologists usually perform this type of specialized testing. When a learning disability has been identified, the Education for the Handicapped Act (PL 94-142) mandates that public school systems provide remedial services in the least restrictive educational setting. Families occasionally need help in advocating for these services.

The same is true for children with communication disorders, although the services requested may be different. Speech pathologists conduct the diagnostic assessment of speech and language disorder. Nurses may be involved with formal screening for communication disorders. Services such as speech therapy (directed at the motor aspects of speaking) or social skills groups (directed at the social and interpersonal aspects of language) are often available in school districts and can be obtained if a speech or language disorder has been identified. For some children with communication disorders, the services offered by the school may be insufficient. In such cases, the nurse can help the family locate a facility that can provide these needed services.

Tic Disorders and Tourette's Disorder

Tics are a part of several mental health problems. **Motor tics** are usually quick, jerky movements of the eyes, face, neck, and shoulders, although they may involve other muscle groups as well. Occasionally, tics involve slower, more purposeful, or dystonic movements. **Phonic tics** typically include repetitive throat clearing, grunting, or other noises but may also include more complex sounds, such as words; parts of words; and in a minority of patients, obscenities. Transient tics by definition do not endure over time and appear to be fairly common in school-aged children. *Tic disorder* is a general term encompassing several syndromes that are chiefly characterized by motor tics, phonic tics, or both.

> **KEYCONCEPT** **Tics** are sudden, rapid, repetitive, stereotyped motor movements or vocalizations.

Tourette's disorder, the most severe tic disorder, is defined by multiple motor and phonic tics for at least 1 year. Because no diagnostic tests are used for this disorder, the diagnosis is based on the type and duration of tics present (Jankovic, Gelineau-Kattner, & Davidson, 2010). The typical age of onset for tics is about 7 years, and motor tics generally precede phonic tics. Parents often describe the seeming replacement of one tic with another. In addition to this changing repertoire of motor and phonic tics, Tourette's disorder exhibits a waxing and waning course. The child can suppress the tics for brief periods. Thus, it is not uncommon to hear from parents that their child has more frequent tics at home than at school. Older children and adults may describe an urge or a physical sensation before having a tic. The general trend is for tic symptoms to decline by early adulthood.

Epidemiology and Etiology

The prevalence of Tourette's disorder is estimated to be between one and 3 to 6 per 1,000 in school-aged children, with boys being affected three to six times more often than girls (CDC, 2014). Obsessive-compulsive disorder (OCD) frequently occurs with Tourette's disorder (Matthews & Grados, 2011).

The precise nature of the underlying pathophysiology in this highly inherited disorder is unclear, but the basal ganglia and functionally related cortical areas are presumed to play a central role. Findings from neuroimaging studies are consistent with the presumption that a dysregulation of the cortico–striatal–thalamic circuitry of the brain underlies Tourette's disorder. Additionally, multiple genes on different chromosomes interacting with environmental factors are involved. Several neurochemical systems have been implicated in the etiology of Tourette's disorder, including dopamine systems, noradrenaline, endogenous opioids, and serotonin (Scharf et al., 2013).

Family Response to Disorder

Before evaluation and diagnosis of Tourette's disorder, most families struggle with various explanations for the child's tics. Because tics fluctuate in severity with time and may be more prominent in some settings than in others, family members may have difficulty understanding their involuntary nature. Some parents may be convinced that the tics are deliberate and done to secure attention; others may judge that the tics are "nervous habits" indicative of underlying trouble. Such views require reconciliation with the currently accepted view that tics are involuntary. Some parents may conclude that the child is incapable of controlling any behavior because of Tourette's disorder. They may subsequently feel uncertain about setting limits. In these families, delineating the boundaries of Tourette's disorder can be helpful (Cavanna & Seri, 2014; CDC, 2014).

On learning that this disorder is probably genetic, some parents may harbor guilt for having passed it on to their child. The nurse can assist such families by listening to these concerns and providing information about the natural history of Tourette's disorder—it is not a progressive condition, tics often diminish in adulthood, and it need not restrict what the child can achieve in life.

NURSING MANAGEMENT: Human Response to Tourette's Disorder

Assessment

Nursing assessment of a child with tics includes a review of the onset, course, and current level of the symptoms. The goals of the assessment are to identify the frequency, intensity, complexity, and interference of the tics and their effects on functioning; determine the child's level of adaptive functioning; identify the child's areas of strength and weakness in general and in school; and identify social supports for the child and family.

Another important aspect of the assessment is to determine the effects of the tic symptoms on the child and family. Some children and families adjust well; however, others are embarrassed or devastated and tend to withdraw socially. Some children with Tourette's disorder have ADHD, and a substantial percentage have symptoms of OCD (Matthews & Grados, 2011). Therefore, in addition to inquiring about tics, the nurse should assess the child's overall development, activity level, and capacity to concentrate and persist with a single task, as well as explore repetitive habits and recurring worries.

Nursing Diagnoses

Nursing diagnoses could include Ineffective Coping, Impaired Social Interaction, Anxiety, and Compromised Family Coping. Children with Tourette's disorder typically have normal intelligence, but their tics can interfere with their ability to relate to others and perform in school.

Interventions

The approach to planning nursing interventions depends on the primary source of impairment: tics themselves; OCD symptoms; or the triad of hyperactivity, inattention, and poor impulse control. The nurse can provide counseling and education for the patient, education for the parents, and consultation for the school. Most children and their families need some education about Tourette's disorder. Individual psychotherapy with a mental health specialist (e.g., a psychologist or an advanced practice nurse) may be indicated for some children and adolescents with Tourette's disorder to deal with maladaptive responses to the chronic condition.

Psychopharmacologic Interventions

Two classes of drugs are commonly used in the treatment of tics: antipsychotics and α-adrenergic receptor agonists. The use of atypical antipsychotics such as risperidone and aripiprazole is replacing the use of older antipsychotics, haloperidol, and pimozide (Cavanna & Seri, 2013). These potent dopamine blockers are often effective at low doses. Attempts to eradicate all tics by increasing the dosages of these antipsychotics almost certainly results in diminishing therapeutic returns and additional side effects. The most frequently encountered side effects include drowsiness, dulled thinking, muscle stiffness, akathisia, increased appetite and weight gain, and acute dystonic reactions. Long-term use carries a small risk for tardive dyskinesia.

The α$_2$-adrenergic receptor agonist clonidine (Catapres) has been used in treating Tourette's disorder for more than 30 years. Guanfacine (Tenex) is a newer α$_2$-adrenergic receptor agonist that has only recently been studied in children with Tourette's disorder. Both drugs were originally developed as antihypertensive agents, but their regulatory action on the brain's norepinephrine system led researchers to try these medications in patients with

Tourette's disorder. However, the level of improvement in tic symptoms is generally less than that observed with the antipsychotics (Parraga, Harris, Parraga, Balen, & Cruz, 2010).

Teaching Points

Teachers, guidance counselors, and school nurses may need current information about Tourette's disorder and related problems. Discussions with school personnel often include issues such as how to deal with tic behaviors that are disruptive in the classroom, how to manage teasing from other children, and how to handle medication side effects. A careful discussion of the boundaries of Tourette's disorder and tic symptomatology usually can resolve these matters. Teachers who understand the involuntary nature of tics can often generate creative solutions, such as excusing the child for errands. This strategy allows the child to step out of the classroom briefly to release a bout of tics, thereby reducing stress. In some situations, a brief presentation about Tourette's disorder to the class will reduce teasing and help both teachers and classmates tolerate the tic symptoms (Box 35.5).

Before initiating these interventions with the school personnel, it is essential to identify the child's needs and to pursue these strategies in collaboration with the family and other clinical team members. The Education for the Handicapped Act (Public Law 94–142) ensures that children with conditions such as Tourette's disorder are eligible for special education services even if they do not meet full criteria for having a learning disability. Thus, if evidence shows that Tourette's disorder is hindering academic progress, parents can demand special education services for their child. Nurses can help families negotiate with the school to obtain appropriate services.

Evaluation and Treatment Outcomes

Treatment outcomes will vary over the years and will be influenced by growth and development changes, family interaction and understanding of the disorder, and reduction or elimination of the frequency of the tics. Outcomes should include the improvement of the child's quality of life and ability to learn to manage the symptoms of the disorder.

Separation Anxiety Disorder

Anxiety disorders are the most common mental disorders in children and adolescents (Beesdo, Knappe, & Pine, 2009). Nearly one in three adolescents (31%) meets the criteria for an anxiety disorder. Although some degree of worry and fearfulness is considered normal during the course of childhood, in children and adolescents with anxiety disorders, the level of anxiety is excessive and

BOX 35.5 • THERAPEUTIC DIALOGUE • Tics and Disruptive Behaviors

INEFFECTIVE APPROACH

Teacher: I see the tics. He jerks his head, makes faces, and flicks his hands.

Nurse: What do you do about them?

Teacher: What can I do? If he isn't disrupting the class, I leave him alone. Even when he is throwing spitballs.

Nurse: Spitballs! He shouldn't be allowed to throw spitballs.

Teacher: Oh, I thought that was a part of his problem.

Nurse: Well, throwing spitballs has nothing to do with tics.

EFFECTIVE APPROACH

Teacher: I see the tics. He jerks his head, makes faces, and flicks his hands.

Nurse: He cannot help the tics that you are seeing. Tic disorders can exhibit a wide range of severity, from mild to severe and from simple to complex. Some complex tics may be difficult to distinguish from habits or rituals.

Teacher: What about things like throwing spitballs? When he does things like that, I try to ignore that behavior.

Nurse: Sounds like you give him the benefit of the doubt. (Validation) However, throwing a spitball is not a tic behavior.

Teacher: What should I do?

Nurse: How do you usually handle that type of behavior? (A modification of reflection)

Teacher: I'd ask him to stop and sometimes go into the hall.

Nurse: Disruptive behavior that is voluntary in a student with a tic disorder should be handled as you would handle any other child.

CRITICAL THINKING CHALLENGE

• Compare the responses of the nurse in these scenarios. What made the difference in the teacher's responsiveness to the nurse?

---

hinders daily functioning. This section focuses on separation anxiety, a disorder diagnosed in childhood, and OCD, a disorder that occurs in both adults and children. For a discussion of other anxiety disorders, see Chapter 26.

Separation anxiety is normal for very young children, but typically declines between ages 3 to 5 years of age. When the child's fear and anxiety around separation becomes developmentally inappropriate, **separation anxiety disorder** is diagnosed. Although many children experience some discomfort on separation from their attachment figures, children with separation anxiety disorder suffer great worry or fear when faced with ordinary separations or being away from home, such as when going to school. When separation is about to occur, children often resist by crying or hiding from their parents (Milrod et al., 2014). When asked, most children with separation anxiety disorder will express worry about harm to or permanent loss of their major attachment figure. Other children may express worry about their own safety.

A common manifestation of anxiety is **school phobia**, in which the child refuses to attend school, preferring to stay at home with the primary attachment figure. The term *school phobia* was coined to distinguish it from truancy; whether it is a phobia in the usual sense is a matter of some

debate. However, school phobia is common in other disorders such as general anxiety disorder, social phobia, OCD, depression, and conduct disorder. When another disorder such as depression is identified, it becomes the focus of treatment. In some cases, the school phobia may resolve when the primary disorder is successfully treated.

Epidemiology and Etiology

The prevalence of separation anxiety disorder is estimated at 2% to 8% of school-aged children, with an onset usually between 7 and 9 years of age; thus, it is relatively common (Merikangas et al., 2010). Insecure attachment, difficult temperaments, and genetic factors contribute to the development of separation anxiety disorder. Anxiety disorders run in families, and it appears that both environmental and genetic factors affect the risk for separation anxiety disorder. For example, separation anxiety may emerge after a move, change to a new school, or death of a family member or pet.

There is no one etiological factor, but instead, several risk factors are associated with the onset of the disorder. For example, children of parents with at least one anxiety disorder have an increased risk of also having an anxiety disorder. The risk increases even more when two parents are affected. Parental depression is also associated the anxiety disorders in children (Milrod et al., 2014).

Family Response to Disorder

There is no one family response to a child who is experiencing separation anxiety. Parenting style, life events, and environmental factors vary from family to family. The family dynamics related to the child's behavior have to be carefully assessed. In some instances, the family may be undergoing a separation of a significant family member through death, divorce, or military deployment. In other situations, the arrival of a new family member may precede the child's separation anxiety. A family assessment is important in determining the relationship of the child's fears and anxiety and the family dynamics.

Interdisciplinary Treatment and Recovery

An interdisciplinary approach is needed for the treatment of separation anxiety disorder. Effective treatment includes child and parent psychoeducation, school consultation, cognitive-behavioral therapy, and selective serotonin reuptake inhibitors (SSRIs) (Rapp, Dodds, Walkup, & Rynn, 2013).

Nursing Management

School refusal is often what prompts the family to seek consultation for the child. Because school refusal can be a behavioral manifestation of several different child psychiatric disorders, it requires careful assessment. Issues to consider are whether the parents have been aware that the child is avoiding school (separation versus truancy); what efforts the family has used to return the child to school; the presence of significant subjective distress in the child with anticipation of going to school; and whether the school refusal occurs in the context of other behavioral, social, or emotional problems. The nurse should also review the purpose and dose of current medications.

The child's developmental history and response to new situations and prior separations provide essential background information for understanding the child's current separation anxiety. The assessment should also include a review of recent life events and the methods the family has used to promote the child's return to school. Finally, the family history with respect to anxiety, panic attacks, or phobias is also informative.

Nursing diagnosis and interventions will depend on the role of the nurse (school nurse, acute care, or community practice) and the relationship with the child and family. In some instances, the nurse will be responsible for education of the child and family. If the child is receiving medication, nursing care related to administration of medications and education should be implemented. Nurses will also be involved in educating teachers and

serving as a liaison between treating physicians, family and child, and school.

OBSESSIVE-COMPULSIVE DISORDER

Obsessive-compulsive disorder is characterized by intrusive thoughts that are difficult to dislodge (obsessions) or ritualized behaviors that the child feels driven to perform (compulsions) (see Chapter 26). Children tend to exhibit both multiple obsessions and compulsions that relate to fear of catastrophic family event, contamination, sexual or somatic obsessions, and overly moralistic thoughts. Washing, checking, repeating and ordering are the most commonly reported compulsions (Geller, 2010).

Epidemiology and Etiology

The prevalence rate of OCD is estimated at 1% to 2% with two peaks of incidence across the lifespan, one occurring in pre-adolescent children and later a peak in early adult life (Geller, 2010). More than half of the cases of OCD in youth involve a comorbid disorder such as a tic, mood, or anxiety disorder. The etiology of OCD in children is thought to be similar to that of adults (see Chapter 26). However, there is a subset of children whose OCD behavior that may be related to an immune response to group A beta-hemolytic streptococcus infections that led to inflammation of the basal ganglia (Geller, 2010).

Family Response to Disorder

Parents' responses to their child's obsessions and compulsions depend on their understanding of the thoughts and behaviors. Because OCD is highly familial, if the parents are recovering from their disorder, they may be able to support their child's ability to begin to deal with the symptoms. On the other hand, the parents may find their child's thoughts and behaviors tiring and become easily irritated with the multiple obsessions and compulsions. Parents need education and support to help their child.

Interdisciplinary Treatment and Recovery

Interdisciplinary treatment including school personnel is important for the child and family with OCD. Cognitive behavior therapy (CBT), including psychoeducation, cognitive training, exposure and response preventions, and relapse prevention is the treatment of choice. For greatest efficacy, CBT is combined with medications, usually an SSRI.

Nursing Management

Recurrent worries and ritualistic behavior can occur normally in children at particular stages of development. The first step in the assessment of OCD in children is to distinguish between normal childhood rituals and worries and pathologic rituals and obsessional thoughts. Obsessional thoughts are recurrent, nagging, and bothersome. Although children may describe obsessions as occurring "out of the blue," external events may trigger obsessions. For example, a child may fear contamination whenever he or she is in contact with a certain person or object. Likewise, compulsions waste time, cause distress, and interfere with daily living (Box 35.6).

The severity of the child's and family's response to OCD will determine the appropriate nursing diagnoses. When the obsessions and compulsions emerge, these children or adolescents are in distress because of the disturbing and relentless nature of the symptoms. Ineffective Coping, Compromised Family Coping, and Ineffective Role Performance are likely nursing diagnoses.

Nursing interventions will be guided by the needs of the family and the developmental needs of the child or adolescent. If medication is prescribed, it is important to emphasize safe management of medications. Because the antidepressants have a "black box" warning regarding suicide in the adolescents, the nurse must discuss with the parents and child the importance of monitoring mood and keeping regularly scheduled mental health appointments.

Elimination Disorders

ENURESIS

Enuresis is the involuntary excretion of urine after the age at which the child should have attained bladder control. It usually involves involuntary bedwetting at night, but repeated urination on clothing during waking hours can occur (diurnal enuresis). Enuresis is a self-limiting disorder, with most children experiencing a spontaneous remission.

Epidemiology and Etiology

The prevalence of nocturnal enuresis varies with age and gender, being most common in young boys—an estimated 5% to 10% of 5-year-old boys, and 3% to 5% in 10-year old boys have nocturnal enuresis (Mikkelsen, 2014). The frequency in girls is about half that of boys in each age group. The etiology of enuresis is unknown, with probably no single cause. Most children with nocturnal enuresis are urologically normal. Some evidence has shown that at least some children with nocturnal enuresis secrete decreased amounts of antidiuretic hormone during sleep, which may play a role in enuresis (Mikkelsen, 2014).

Nursing Management

The nursing assessment should include the child's developmental history, the onset and course of enuresis, prior treatment, presence of emotional problems, and medical history. The nurse should also explore the family's home

> **Clinical Vignette**
>
> **BOX 35.6**
> ## KIMBERLY AND OCD
>
> *Kimberly, an 11-year-old fifth grader, comes for evaluation because her mother and teacher have become increasingly concerned about her repetitive behaviors. In retrospect, Kim's mother recalls first noticing repetitive rituals about 2 years before, but she did not become alarmed about these behaviors until recently when they began to interfere with daily living. At the time of referral, Kim exhibits complicated jumping rituals that involve a specific number of jumps and a particular manner of jumping. She also turns light switches off and on and performs complex movements, such as blinking in patterns and thrusting her arms back and forth a certain number of times. Her mother also reports Kim's near-constant request for reassurance about her own safety. In recent months, her incessant demands for reassurance have been more frequent and elaborate. For example, Kim's mother has to answer three times that everything is all right and then say, "I swear to it."*
>
> *At the evaluation, Kim expresses fears that some ill fate, such as catastrophic illness or injury, will befall her. This fear is triggered by contact with any individual who seems sick, chance exposures to foul smells or dirt, and minor scrapes or bumps. When the fear is triggered, she becomes increasingly anxious and consumed with the fear that she will develop an illness and die. Sometimes her fears are specific, such as cancer or AIDS. Other times her fears are more ambiguous, as evidenced by statements such as, "Something bad will happen" if she doesn't complete the ritual. Kim acknowledges that the ritual is probably not related to the feared event, but she is reluctant to take a chance. If the ritual does not reduce her anxiety, she seeks reassurance from her mother.*
>
> *Kim's medical history was negative for serious illness or injury. She was born after an uncomplicated pregnancy, labor, and delivery and achieved developmental milestones at appropriate times. Indeed, her mother could recall no unusual problems in the first few years of life except that Kim was typically anxious in new situations. Kim's mother reports a prior history of panic attacks, but the family history is otherwise negative for anxiety disorders, including obsessive-compulsive disorder.*
>
> ### What Do You Think?
> • What assessment information would you want to elicit from Kim?
> • What additional information should be considered from Kim's mother about her history of panic attacks?
> • What nursing interventions should be considered if Kim were your patient?

environment, family attitudes about the child's enuresis, and the family's medical history. Routine laboratory tests such as urinalysis and a urine culture are used to determine the presence of infection. The nurse should obtain baseline data regarding toileting habits, including daytime incontinence, urinary frequency, and constipation. He or she should refer children with persistent daytime enuresis for consultation with an urologist.

In many cases, limiting fluid intake in the evening and treating constipation (if present) is sufficient to decrease the frequency of bedwetting. One of the most effective methods is the bell and pad. In this approach, the child sleeps on a pad that has wires on it, and when the child voids, a bell sounds, waking up the child. With use, the child either wakes up to urinate or learns to sleep through the night without voiding. A more temporary solution is the use of desmopressin (DDAVP), a synthetic antidiuretic hormone that actually inhibits the production of urine. After medication is withdrawn, the enuresis frequently returns (Mikkelsen, 2014).

ENCOPRESIS

Encopresis involves soiling clothing with feces or depositing feces in inappropriate places. Additional diagnostic criteria include that the child is older than 4 years; that the soiling occurs at least once per month; and that the soiling is not the result of a medical disorder, such as aganglionic megacolon (Hirschsprung's disease). The most common form of encopresis is fecal impaction accompanied by leakage around the hardened mass of stool. Because of the loss of muscle tone in the lower bowel, the child loses the usual urge to defecate and may not feel the leakage. Surprisingly, the child may not detect the smell of the stool because the olfactory apparatus becomes accustomed to the odor. If left untreated, this problem generally resolves independently by middle adolescence. Nonetheless, the social consequences may be substantial (Mikkelsen, 2014).

Epidemiology and Etiology

As with enuresis, encopresis is more common in boys, and the frequency of the condition declines with age. The current estimate of prevalence is 1.5% of school-aged children ages 7 to 8 years old, with boys three times more likely to have encopresis than girls (Mikkelsen, 2014).

The reasons for withholding stool and starting the cycle of fecal impaction are unclear but are usually not the result of physical causes. However, as noted, when the fecal impaction occurs, there is a loss of tone in the bowel and leakage.

Nursing Management

The assessment includes a detailed interview with the child and parent regarding the pattern of the encopresis. A calm, matter-of-fact approach can help to reduce the child's embarrassment. A physical examination is also necessary; thus, collaboration with the child's primary care provider or consulting pediatric specialist is essen-

tial. The presence of encopresis does not necessarily signal severe emotional or behavioral disturbances, but the nurse should inquire about other psychiatric disorders. The diagnosis of encopresis is presumed given a history of intermittent constipation and soiling. Collaboration with primary care consultants often is helpful to rule out rare medical conditions, such as Hirschsprung's disease.

Effective intervention begins with educating the parents and the child about normal bowel function and the self-perpetuating cycle of fecal impaction and leakage of stool around the hardened mass of feces. The short-term goal of this educational effort is to decrease the anger and recrimination that often complicate the picture in these families. Because encopresis often results in a loss of bowel tone, it may help to motivate children by emphasizing the need to strengthen their muscles.

In many cases, cleaning out the bowel is necessary before initiating behavioral treatment. The bowel catharsis is usually followed by administration of mineral oil, which is often continued during the bowel retraining program. A high-fiber diet is often recommended.

The behavioral treatment program involves daily sitting on the toilet after each meal for a predetermined period (e.g., 10 minutes). The child and parents can measure the time with an ordinary kitchen timer, and the parents can encourage the child to read or look at picture books while sitting. They can give the child rewards in the form of stars, stickers, or points for complying with the retraining program and add bonuses for successful defecation. The family can tally stickers or points on a calendar, and the child can "cash in" collected points for small prizes.

Caring for children with encopresis on an inpatient unit is a challenge, and there is very little research providing direction for positive outcomes. Staff can become frustrated with the child's seemingly unwillingness to cooperate. Possible interventions are maintaining discretion, assisting children with the development of age-appropriate social skills and empathy, and providing positive peer pressure (Hardy, 2009).

Other Mental Disorders

MOOD DISORDERS

Mood disorders in children and adolescents are a major public health concern. The prevalence of mood disorder in adolescents is estimated to be 14.3%, with depression representing the largest percentage (11.7%) and bipolar I or II comprising 2.9% (Merikangas et al., 2010). (See Chapters 24 and 25 for a complete discussion of these disorders.) Females are more likely to meet the diagnostic criteria for these disorders. These disorders cause severe impairment in 11% of the adolescents diagnosed.

Children with mood disorders may not spontaneously express feelings (sadness, irritability) and are more likely to show their suffering through their behavior. These children may act out their feelings rather than discuss them. Thus, behavior problems may accompany depression. Reports from parents are important sources of information about changes in sleep patterns, appetite, activity level and interests, and emotional stability.

Nursing diagnoses for children or adolescents who are depressed are similar to those for adults, including Ineffective Coping, Risk for Suicide, Chronic Low Self-Esteem, Disturbed Thought Processes, Self-Care Deficit, Imbalanced Nutrition, and Disturbed Sleep Pattern.

Treatment goals include improving the mood and restoring sleep, appetite, and self-care. Interventions for responses to mood disorders in children and adolescents are also similar to those for adults. The psychiatric nurse develops a therapeutic relationship with the child and provides parent education and support. Developing sensitivity to the influence of environmental events on the child is important for the nurse, parents, and teachers (Box 35.7).

BOX 35.7
Questions, Choices, and Outcomes

Mrs. S has just returned with her son Jared to the child psychiatric inpatient services after an overnight pass. She reports that the visit did not go well because of Jared's anger and defiance. She remarked that this behavior was distressingly similar to his behavior before the hospitalization. She expressed additional concern because of the upcoming discharge from the hospital. After saying goodbye to Jared, she pulled the nurse aside and stated that she had decided to file for divorce.

Mrs. S indicated that she had not told her husband or the family therapist. When asked whether Jared knew about her decision, Mrs. S suddenly realized that he may have overheard her discussing the matter with her sister on the telephone during this home visit.

How should the nurse approach this situation?

Choice	Possible Outcomes
Discuss her hypothesis about Jared's behavior and his uncertainty	Mother can see relationship between Jared's behavior and her plan for divorce Mother ignores the nurse Mother is interested but does not see the connection
Ignore the statement	Child and family did not learn about the connection between Jared's behavior and the events at home
Encourage mother to sort out her problems	The focus is then on mother's problems

ANALYSIS
The best response is focusing on the possible relationship between Jared's recent behavioral deterioration and his uncertainty of his family's future. If the nurse ignores the statement or focuses on the mother's interpretation of Jared's behavior, the mother is less likely to appreciate the connection between pending divorce and Jared's behavior. The nurse should also emphasize the importance of discussing the matter in family therapy.

Children and adolescents may be treated with medication. Antidepressant medications are used for depression, and mood stabilizers or antipsychotics are given for bipolar disorders. These medications may be prescribed off-label; nurses have a responsibility to educate parents and children about the effects of these medications. The controversy surrounding the use of SSRIs in children reminds us that all treatments involve a risk–benefit equation. Given the modest benefit of the SSRIs and the potential for adverse behavioral effects, these medications merit careful monitoring in children and adolescents. Patient monitoring should focus on evidence of benefit and adverse effects, including sleep problems, hyperactivity, sudden changes in mood or behavior, suicidal ideation, or self-injurious behavior.

CHILDHOOD SCHIZOPHRENIA

Childhood (early-onset) schizophrenia is diagnosed by the same criteria as those used in adults (see Chapter 22). The difficulty in diagnosing a psychiatric disorder in children has led to years of debate and controversy regarding whether childhood schizophrenia differs from the adult type or is merely an early manifestation of the same disorder. For many years, it was believed that autism represented the childhood form of schizophrenia. However, today autism and childhood schizophrenia are differentiated (Kuniyoshi & McClellan, 2010). As currently defined, childhood schizophrenia (occurring before the age of 13 years) is very rare, but increases sharply during adolescence, especially in young me. There are reports of children diagnosed with schizophrenia younger than the age of 6 years, but the validity of the diagnosis has not been established (Kuniyoshi & McClellan, 2010).

Childhood schizophrenia is usually characterized by poorer premorbid functioning than later onset schizophrenia. Common premorbid difficulties include social, cognitive, linguistic, attentional, motor, and perceptual delays. Taken together, these findings suggest that early-onset schizophrenia is a more severe form of the disorder.

Nursing care for children with schizophrenia follows an approach similar to that for autism spectrum disorder. Antipsychotic medication is prescribed for symptoms. Although the newer, atypical antipsychotic medications appear to have a lower risk for neurologic effects, other side effects such as weight gain also warrant careful monitoring (see Chapters 11 and 22 for more detailed descriptions of the atypical antipsychotics).

Development of an individualized care plan for children with schizophrenia begins with a nursing assessment to identify functional problems specific to the child. Similarly, the recognition that childhood schizophrenia is a chronic and severe condition should guide the identification of outcomes. Goals should be realistic, and the nurse should pay special attention to the child's support systems. Parent education about the disorder, medications, and long-term management (including use of community resources) is an essential part of the treatment plan. Long-term management also requires monitoring of chronic antipsychotic therapy.

SUMMARY OF KEY POINTS

■ An estimated 20% of American youths are affected by a mental disorder that impairs their ability to function.

■ In addressing intellectual disabilities, the emphasis is on determining adaptive behaviors (conceptual skills, concepts, self-direction), social skills, and practical skills. With guidance and education, many children will no longer have a disability as adults.

■ Children with autism spectrum disorder benefit from structure and specific behavioral interventions.

■ ADHD is defined by the presence of inattention; impulsiveness; and in most cases, hyperactivity. As currently defined, ADHD is the most common disorder of childhood. This heterogeneous disorder affects boys more often than girls. Nursing interventions involve family and child education and support. The family must partner with the school system to help the child receive the best educational experience. Effective treatment of ADHD often involves multiple approaches, including medication and parent education and support.

■ Tourette's disorder is a tic disorder characterized by motor and phonic tics. It is a frustrating disorder that requires patience and understanding. About half of the children with this disorder also have ADHD.

■ Separation anxiety is relatively common in school-aged children. OCD becomes more common in adolescents. Treatment of separation anxiety and OCD may include medication, behavioral therapy, or a combination of these treatments.

■ Elimination disorders include encopresis and enuresis. Behavioral therapy approaches are the most effective treatment for these disorders. Medication may also be used.

■ Major depression in children is believed to be similar to major depression in adults.

■ Childhood schizophrenia is a rare disorder, and other diagnoses should be carefully considered. Nursing care is similar to care of children with autism spectrum disorders.

CRITICAL THINKING CHALLENGES

1. Interview parents of a child with an intellectual disability. Determine their approach to providing support in education and socialization.

2. Examine the differences and similarities between autism spectrum disorder with and without intellectual and language impairment. Determine if there are differences in the nursing care according to the diagnoses. Develop a teaching plan for parents of children who have autism spectrum disorder and are trying to understand the underlying problems related to the disorder.

3. Compare and contrast nursing approaches for a child with ADHD with those used for a child with autism disorder. How are they different? How are they similar?

4. Learning disabilities and communication disorders are more common in children with psychiatric disorders than in the general population. How might a learning disability or a communication disorder complicate a psychiatric illness in a school-aged child?

5. How would you answer these questions from a parent: "What causes ADHD? Is it my fault?"

6. A child is threatening to kill himself. What information is needed in order to keep this child safe?

 Rain Man: 1988. This classic film stars Dustin Hoffman as Raymond Babbitt, a man who has autism (savant). Tom Cruise plays his brother Charlie, a self-centered hustler who believes that he has been cheated out of his inheritance. Discovering Raymond in an institution, Charlie abducts Raymond in a last-ditch effort to get his fair share of the family estate. The story revolves around the relationship that develops as the brothers drive across the country.

Dustin Hoffman brilliantly portrays the behaviors and symptoms of high-functioning autism, such as the monotone speech, insistence on sameness, and repetitive behavior.

Viewing Points: Identify and describe Raymond's ritualistic behaviors. Observe Raymond's language patterns and any distinct abnormalities. What happens when Raymond's rituals are interrupted?

References

Alabdali, A., Al-Ayadhi, L., & El-Ansary, A. (2014). A key role for an impaired detoxification mechanism in the etiology and severity of autism spectrum disorders. *Behavioral and Brain Functions, 10*(1), 14.

American Association on Intellectual and Developmental Disabilities. (2010). *Definition of intellectual disability.* Retrieved on June 5, 2011, from http://www.aamr.org/content_100.cfm?navID=21.

American Psychiatric Association. (2013). *Diagnostic and statistical manual of mental disorders,* (5th ed). Arlington, VA: American Psychiatric Association.

Balazs, J., Miklósi, M., Keresztény, A., Dallos, G., & Gádoros, J. (2014). Attention-deficit hyperactivity disorder and suicidality in a treatment naïve sample of children and adolescents. *Journal of Affective Disorders, 152–154,* 282–287. doi:10.1016/j.jad.2013.09.026

Baribeau, D. A. & Anagnostou, E. (2014). An update on medication management of behavioral disorders in autism. *Current Psychiatry Reports, 16*(3), 437.

Beesdo, K., Knappe, S., & Pine, D. S. (2009). Anxiety and anxiety disorders in children and adolescents: Developmental issues and implications for DSM-V. *Psychiatric Clinics of North America, 32*(3), 483–524.

Bekhet, A. K., Johnson, N. L., & Zauszniewski, J. A. (2012). Resilience in family members of persons with autism spectrum disorder: A review of the literature. *Issues in Mental Health Nursing, 33*(10), 650–656.

Brugha, T. S., McManus, S., Bankart, J., Scott, F., Purdon, S., Bebbington, P., et al. (2011). Epidemiology of autism spectrum disorders in adults in the community in England. *Archives of General Psychiatry, 68*(5), 459–465.

Cavanna, A. E., & Seri, S. (2013). Tourette's syndrome. Clinical Review *BMJ, 347,* f4964. doi:10.1136/bmj.f4964

Centers for Disease Control and Prevention. (2013). *Mental health surveillance among children-United States, 2005–2011. MMWR, 62*(Suppl), 1–35. www.cdc.gov/mmwr/preview/mmwrhtml/su6202a1.htm?s

Centers for Disease Control and Prevention. (2014). Tourette syndrome, Data & statistics. National Center on Birth Defects and Developmental Disabilities. www.cec.gov/NCBDDD/tourette/data.html

Childress, A. C. & Berry, S. A. (2012). Pharmacotherapy of attention-deficit disorder in adolescents. (Review). *Drugs, 72*(3), 309–325.

Chronis-Tuscano, A., Molina, B. S., Pelham, W. E., Applegate, B., Dahlke, A., Overmyer, M., et al. (2010). Very early predictors of adolescent depression and suicide attempt in children with attention-deficit/hyperactivity disorder. *Archives of General Psychiatry, 67*(10), 1044–1051.

Conners, C. K. (1989). *Conners' rating scales manual.* North Tonawanda, NY: Multi-Health Systems.

Costello, E. J., Jian-ping, H., Sampson, N. A., Kessler, R. C., & Merikangas, K. R. (2014). Services for adolescents with psychiatric disorders: 12-month data from the National Comorbidity Survey Adolescent., *Psychiatric services, 65*(3), 359–366.

Davis, D. W. & Williams, P. G. (2011). Attention-deficit hyperactivity disorder in preschool-aged children: Issues and concerns. *Clinical Pediatrics, 50*(2), 144–152.

Elamin, N. E. & Al-Ayadhi, L. Y. (2014). Brain autoantibodies in autism spectrum disorders. *Biomarkers in Medicine, 8*(3), 345–352.

Evans, S. W., Owens, J. S., & Bunford, N. (2013). Evidence-Based Psychosocial Treatments for Children and Adolescents with Attention-Deficit/Hyperactivity Disorder. *Journal of Clinical Child and Adolescent Psychology,* PMID: 24245813.

Fang, X., Massetti, G. M., Ouyan, L., Srosse, S. D., & Mercy, J. A. (2010). Attention-deficit/hyperactivity disorder, conduct disorder and young adult intimate partner violence. *Archives of General Psychiatry, 67*(11), 1179–1186.

Feingold, B. M. (1975). Hyperkinesis and learning disabilities linked to artificial food flavors and colors. *American Journal of Nursing, 75*(5), 797–783.

Ferrer, E., Shaywitz, B. A., Holahan, J. M., Marchione, K., & Shaywitz, S. E. (2010). Uncoupling of reading and IQ over time: Empirical evidence for a definition of dyslexia. *Psychological Science, 21*(1), 93–101.

Foster-Cohen, S. H., Friesen, M. D., Champion, P. R., & Woodward, L. J. (2010). High prevalence/low severity language delay in preschool children born very preterm. *Journal of Developmental & Behavioral Pediatrics, 31*(8), 658–667.

Freitag, C. M., Hänig, S., Schneider, A., Switz, D., Palmason, H., & Meyer, R. W. (2011). Biological and psychosocial environmental risk factors influence symptom severity and psychiatric comorbidity in children with ADHD. *Journal of Neural Transmission,* in press.

Gagne, J. R., Saudino, K. J., & Asherson, P. (2011). The genetic etiology of inhibitory control and behavior problems at 24 months of age. *Journal of Child Psychology & Psychiatry, 52*(11):1155–1163.

Geller, D. (2010). Obsessive-compulsive disorder. In M. K. Dulcan (Ed.), *Dulcan's textbook of child and adolescent psychiatry.* Arlington, VA: American Psychiatric Publishing.

Ghuman, J. K. (2011). Restricted elimination diet for ADHD: The INCA study. *The Lancet, 377*(9764), 446–448.

Gore, F. M., Bloem, P. J., Patton, G. C., Ferguson, J., Joseph, V., Coffey, C., et al. (2011). Global burden of disease in young people aged 10–24 years: A systematic analysis. *The Lancet, 377*(9783), 2093–2102.

Goyette, C. H., Connors, C. K., & Ulrich, R. F. (1978). Normative data on the Connors Parent and Teachers Rating Scales. *Journal of Abnormal Child Psychology, 6*(2), 221–236.

Graham, J., Banaschewski, T., Buitelaar, J., Coghill, D., Danckaerts, M., Dittmann, R. W., et al. (2011). European guidelines on managing adverse effects of medications for ADHD. *European Child & Adolescent Psychiatry, 20*(1), 17–37.

Greven, D. U., Kovas, Y., Willcutt, E., Petrill, S. A., & Plomin, R. (2014). Evidence for shared genetic risk between ADHD symptoms and reduced mathematics ability: A twin study. *Journal of Child Psychology and Psychiatry, 55*(1), 39–48.

Halmey, A., Johansson, S., Winge, I., McKinney, J. A., Knappskog, P. M., & Haavik, J. (2010). Attention-deficit/hyperactivity disorder symptoms in offspring of mothers with impaired serotonin production. *Archives of General Psychiatry, 67*(10), 1033–1043.

Hardy, L. T. (2009). Encopresis: A guide for psychiatric nurses. *Archives of Psychiatric Nursing, 23*(5), 351–358.

Hirota, T., Schwartz, S., & Correll, C. U. (2014). Alpha-2 agonists for attention deficit/hyperactivity disorder in youth: A systematic review and meta-analysis of monotherapy and add-on trials to stimulant therapy. *Journal of the American Academy of Child and Adolescent Psychiatry, 53*(2), 153–173.

Humphreys, K. L., Eng, T., & Lee, S. S. (2013). Stimulant medication and substance use outcomes: A meta-analysis. *JAMA Psychiatry, 70*(7), 740–749.

Jankovic, J., Gelineau-Kattner, R., & Davidson, A. (2010). Tourette's syndrome in adults. *Movement Disorders, 25*(11), 2171–2175.

Kanner, L. (1943). Autistic disturbances of affective contact. *Nervous Child, 2,* 217–250.

Kessler, R. C., Green, J. G., Adler, L. A., Barkley, R. A., Chatterji, S., Faraone, S. V., et al. (2010). Structure and diagnosis of adult attention-deficit/hyperactivity disorder: Analysis of expanded symptom criteria from the Adult ADHD Clinical Diagnostic Scale. *Archives of General Psychiatry, 67*(11), 1168–1178.

Kim, Y. S., Leventhal, B. L., Koh, Y. J., Fombonne, E., Laska, E., Lim, E. C., et al. (2011). Prevalence of autism spectrum disorders in a total population sample. *American Journal of Psychiatry, 168*(9), 904–912.

Kuehn, B. M. (2011). Increased risk of ADHD associated with early exposure to pesticides, PCBs. *Journal of the American Medical Association, 304*(1), 26–28.

Kuniyoshi, J. S. & McClellan, J. M. (2010). Early-onset schizophrenia. In M. K. Dulcan (Ed.), *Dulcan's textbook of child and adolescent psychiatry.* Arlington, VA: American Psychiatric Publishing.

Law, E. C., Sideridis, G. D., Prock, L. A., & Sheridan, M. A. (2014). Attention-deficit/hyperactivity disorder in young children: Predictors of diagnostic stability. *Pediatrics, 133*(4), 659–667.

Lecavalier, L. & Butter, E. M. (2010). Assessment of social skills and intellectual disability. In D. W. Nangle, D. Hansen, D. A. Erdley, & P. F. Norton (Eds.), *Practitioner's guide to empirically based measures of social skills* (pp. 179–192). New York: Springer.

Lomangino, K. (2011). Benefit for elimination diet in ADHD? *Clinical Nutrition Insight, 37*(4), 8–9, 11.

Mackie, L. & law, J. (2010). Pragmatic language and the child with emotional/behavioural difficulties (EBDP: A pilot study exploring the interaction between behaviour and communication disability. *International Journal of Language & Communication disorders, 45*(4), 397–410.

Manos, M. J., Tom-Revzon, C., Bukstein, O. G., & Crismon, M. L. (2007). Changes and challenges: Managing ADHD in a fast-paced world. *Journal of Managed Care Pharmacy, 13*(9 suppl), S2–S16.

Matthews, C. A. & Grados, M. A. (2011). Familiarity of Tourette syndrome, obsessive-compulsive disorder, and attention-deficit/hyperactivity disorder: Heritability analysis in a large sib-pair sample. *Journal of the American Academy of Child & Adolescent Psychiatry, 50*(1), 46–54.

Maulik, P. K., Mascarenhas, M. N., Mathers, C. D., Dua, R., & Saxena, S. (2011). Prevalence of intellectual disability: A meta-analysis of population-based studies. *Research in Developmental Disabilities, 32*(2), 419–436.

McCarthy, S. E., Gillis, J., Kramer, M., Lihm, J., Yoon, S., Berstein, Y., et al. (2014). De novo mutations in schizophrenia implicate chromatin remodeling and support a genetic overlap with autism and intellectual disability. *Molecular Psychiatry, 19*(6), 652–658. *doi:10.1038/mp.2014.29*

McQuade, J. D., Vaughn, A. M., Hoza, B., Murray-Close, D., Molina, B., Arnold, L. E, et al. (2014). Perceived social acceptance and peer status differentially predict adjustment in youth with and without ADHD. *Journal of Attention Disorders, 18*(1), 31–43.

Merikangas, K. R., He, J., Burstein, M., Swanson, S. A., Avenevoli, S., Cui, L., et al. (2010). Lifetime prevalence of mental disorders in U.S. adolescents: Results from the National Comorbidity Survey Replication–Adolescent supplement (NCS-A). *Journal of the American Academy of Child & Adolescent Psychiatry, 49*(10), 980–989.

Mikkelsen, E. J. (2014). Elimination disorders. In R. E. Hales, S. C. Yudofsy, & L. W . Roberts (Eds.). *The American Psychiatric Publishing Textbook of Psychiatry* (6th ed), Arlington, VA: American Psychiatric Publishing. www.psychiatryonline.org. doi:*10.1176/appi.books.978158625031.271596*

Milrod, B., Markowitz, J. C., Gerber, A. J., Cyranowski, J., Altemus, M., Shaprio, T., et al. (2014). Childhood separation anxiety and the pathogenesis and treatment of adult anxiety. American Journal of Psychiatry, 171(1), 34–43.

Molina, B. S., Hinshaw, S. P., Swanson, J. M., Arnold, L. E., Vitiello, B., Jensen, P. S., et al. (2009). The MTA at 8 years: Prospective follow-up of children treated for combined-type ADHD in a multisite study. *Journal of the American Academy of Child & Adolescent Psychiatry, 48*(5), 484–500.

Mokrova, I., O'Brien, M., Calkins, S., & Keane, S. (2010). Parental ADHD symptomology and ineffective parenting: The connecting link of home chaos. *Parenting: Science and Practice, 10*, 19–135.

Moriyama, T. S., Polanczyk, F. V., Terzi, F. S., Faris, K. M., & Rohde, L. A. (2013). Psychopharmacology and psychotherapy for the treatment of adults with ADHD-a systematic review of available meta-analysis. *CNS Spectrums, 18*(6), 296–306.

Mulder, M. J., Bos, D., Weusten, J. M., van Belle, J., van Dijk, S. C., Simen, P., et al. (2011). Basic impairments in regulating the speed-accuracy tradeoff predict symptoms of attention-deficit/hyperactivity disorder. *Biological Psychiatry, 68*(12), 1114–1149.

Murthy, P. & Chand, P. (2012). Treatment of dual diagnosis disorders. (Review). *Current Opinion in Psychiatry, 25*(3), 194–200.

Nigg, J. T., Lewis, K., Edinger, T., & Falk, M. (2012). Meta-analysis of attention-deficit/hyperactivity disorder or attention-deficit/hyperactivity disorder symptoms, restriction diet, and synthetic food color additives. *Journal of the American Academy of Child & Adolescent Psychiatry, 51*(1), 86–97.

Palcic, J. L., Jurbergs, M., & Kelley, M. L. (2009). A comparison of teacher and parent delivered consequences: Improving classroom behavior in low-income children and ADHD. *Child & Family Behavior Therapy, 31*(2), 117–133.

Parraga, H. C., Harris, K. M., Parraga, K. L., Balen, G. M., & Cruz, D. (2010). An overview of the treatment of Tourette's disorder and tics [review]. *Journal of Child & Adolescent Psychopharmacology, 20*(4), 249–262.

Pauli-Pott, U., Albayrak, O., Hebebrand, J., & Pott, W. (2010). Association between inhibitory control capacity and body weight in overweight and obese children and adolescents: Dependence on age and inhibitory control component. *Child Neuropsychology, 16*(6), 592–603.

Pelsser, L. M., Buitelaar, J. K., & Savelkoul, H. F. (2009). ADHD as a (non) allergic hypersensitivity disorder: A hypothesis. *Pediatric Allergy and Immunology, 20*(2), 107–112.

Pelsser, L. M., Frankena, K., Toormam, J., Savelkoul, H. F, Dubois, A. E., Pereira, R. R., et al. (2011). Effects of a restricted elimination diet on the behavior of children with attention-deficit hyperactivity. *The Lancet, 377*(9764), 494–503.

Pickles, T., Simonoff, E., Chandler, S., Louicas, T., & Baird, G. (2011). IQ in children with autism spectrum disorders: Data from the special Needs and Autism Project (SNAP). *Psychological Medicine, 41*(3), 619–627.

Polanska, K., Jurewicz, J., & Hanke, W. (2012). Exposure to environmental and lifestyle factors and attention-deficit/hyperactivity disorder in children-a review of epidemiological studies. *International Journal of Occupational Medicine & Environmental Health, 25*(4), 330–355.

Politte, L. C., Henry, C. A., & McDougle, C. J. (2014). Psychopharmacological interventions in autism spectrum disorder. *Harvard Review of Psychiatry, 22*(2), 76–92.

Rapp, A., Dodds, A., Walkup, J. T., & Runn, M. (2013). Treatment of pediatric anxiety disorders. *Annals of the New York Academy of Sciences, 1304*, 52–61.

Raymond, L. J., Deth, R. C. & Ralston, N. V. (2014). Potential Role of Selenoenzymes and Antioxidant Metabolism in relation to Autism Etiology and Pathology. *Autism Research and Treatment, 2014*, 164938. *doi:10.1155/2014/164938*

Reaven, J. A. (2009). Children with high-functioning autism spectrum disorders and co-occurring anxiety symptoms: Implications for assessment and treatment. *Journal of Specialists in Pediatric Nursing, 14*(3), 192–199.

Scarpinato, N., Bradley, J., Kurbjun, K., Bateman, X., Holtzer, B., & Ely, B. (2010). Caring for the child with an autism spectrum disorder in the acute care setting. *Journal of Specialists in Pediatric Nursing, 15*(3), 244–254.

Scharf, J. M., Yu, D., Mathews, C. A., Neale, B. M., Stewart, S. E., Fagerness, J. A., et al. (2013). Genome-wide association study of Tourette's syndrome. *Molecular Psychiatry, 18*(6), 721–728.

Shaw, P., Gilliam, M., Liverpool, M., Weddle, C., Malek, M., Sharp, W., et al. (2011). Cortical development in typically developing children with symptoms of hyperactivity and impulsivity: Support for a dimensional view of attention deficit hyperactivity disorder. *American Journal of Psychiatry, 168*(2), 143–151.

Stevens, L. J., Kuczek, T., Burgess, J. R., Stochelski, M. A., Arnold, L. E., & Galland, L. (2013). Mechanisms of behavioral, atopic and other reactions to artificial food colors in children. *Nutrition Reviews, 71*(5), 268–281.

Stoeckel, R. E., Colligan, R. C., Barbaresi, W. J., Weaver, A. L., Killian, J. M., & Katusci, S. K. (2013). Early speech-language impairment and risk for written language disorder: A population-based study. *Journal of Developmental and Behavioral Pediatrics, 34*(1), 38–44.

Syed, H., Masaud, T. M., Nkire, N., Iro, C., & Garland, M. R. (2010). Estimating the prevalence of adult ADHD in the psychiatric clinic: A cross-sectional study using the ADHD self-report scale (ASRS). *Journal of Psychological Medicine, 27*(4), 195–197.

The Foundation for Medical Practice Education. (2008). *ADHD rating scale*. Retrieved from http://www.fmpe.org/en/documents/appendix/Appendix%201%20-%20ADHD%20Rating%20Scale.pdf.

Toth, C. & King, B. H. (2010). Intellectual disability. In M. K. Dulcan (Ed.), *Dulcan's textbook of child and adolescent psychiatry* (pp. 151–172). Arlington, VA: American Psychiatric Publishing.

Vaishnavi, V., Manikandan, M., & Munirajan, A. K. (2014). Mining the 3'UTR of autism-implicated genes for SNPs perturbing microRNA regulation. *Genomics Proteomics Bioinformatics, 12*(2), 92–104. *doi:10.1016/j.gpb.2014.01.003*

Van der Leij, A., van Bergen, E., van Zuijen, T., de Jong, P., Maurits, N., Maassen, B. (2013). Precursors of developmental dyslexia: An overview of the longitudinal Dutch Dyslexia Programme study. *Dyslexia, 19*(4), 191–213.

Wagner, K. D. & Pliszka, S. R. (2011). Treatment of child and adolescent disorders. In A. F. Schatzberg & C. B. Nemeroff (Eds.), *The American Psychiatric Publishing textbook of psychopharmacology* (4th ed.). Arlington, VA: American Psychiatric Publishing.

Waite, R. & Ramsay, J. R. (2010). Adults with ADHD: Who are we missing? *Issues in Mental Health Nursing, 31*, 670–678.

Wang, L., Conlon, M. A., Christopherson, C. T., Sorich, M. J., & Angley, M. T. (2014). Gastrointestinal microbiota and metabolite biomarkers in children with autism spectrum disorders. *Biomarkers in Medicine, 8*(3), 331–334.

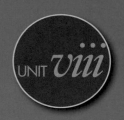

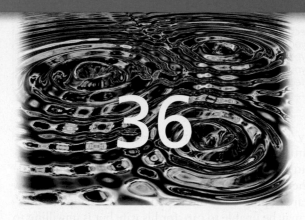

36

Mental Health Assessment of Older Adults

Peggy Healy

KEY CONCEPTS

- geropsychiatric nursing assessment
- normal aging

LEARNING OBJECTIVES

After studying this chapter, you will be able to:

1. Compare changes in normal aging with those associated with mental health problems in older adults.

2. Select various techniques in assessing older adults who have mental health problems.

3. Delineate important areas of assessment in the geropsychiatric nursing assessment.

KEY TERMS

- dysphagia • functional activities • instrumental activities of daily living • polypharmacy • xerostomia

---

The average life span in the United States has increased from 47 years in 1900 to more than 77.9 years in 2010 (National Center for Health Statistics, 2011). Health care providers will face new and increased challenges as the Baby Boomers move into the ranks of the older adult population. The older population in 2050 is projected to be twice as large as in 2010, growing from 40.2 million to 88.5 million (Vincent & Velkoff, 2010).

Normal aging is associated with some physical decline, such as decreased sensory abilities and decreased pulmonary and immune function, but many important functions do not change. Intellectual function, capacity for change, and productive engagement with life remain stable. Many myths exist about normal aging. Some people believe that "senility" is normal or that depression or hopelessness is natural for older adults. If family mem-

bers believe these myths, they will be less likely to seek treatment for their older family members with real problems. For example, although some normal cognitive changes contribute to a slower pace of learning, memory complaints are more likely related to depression than normal aging (Hurt, Burns, & Barrowclough, 2011).

The most common mental health problems in older persons are depression, anxiety disorders, and dementia (Garrido, Kane, Kaas, & Kane, 2011). Older adults with mental health problems comprise different population groups. One group consists of those with long-term mental illnesses who have reached the ranks of the older adult population. These individuals usually understand their disorders and treatments. Unfortunately, the changes associated with aging can affect a person's control of his or her chronic mental illness. Symptoms may reappear, and medications may need to be adjusted. Another group comprises individuals who are relatively free of mental health problems until their elder years. These individuals, who may already have other health problems, develop late-onset mental disorders, such as depression, schizophrenia, or dementia. For these individuals and their family members, the development of a mental disorder can be very traumatic.

Mental health problems in older adults can be especially complex because of coexisting medical problems and treatments. Many symptoms of somatic disorders mimic or mask psychiatric disorders. For example, fatigue may be related to anemia, but it also may be symptomatic of depression. In addition, older individuals are more likely to report somatic symptoms rather than psychological ones, making identification of a mental disorder even more difficult.

The purpose of this chapter is to present a comprehensive geropsychiatric–mental health nursing assessment process that serves as the basis of care for older adults. A mental health assessment is necessary when psychiatric or mental health issues are identified or when patients with mental illnesses reach their later years (usually about age 65 years). The assessment generally follows the same format as described in Chapter 10. However, the overall health care issues for older adults can be very complex, so it follows that certain components of the geropsychiatric nursing assessment are unique. Thus, the geriatric assessment emphasizes some areas that are less critical to the standard adult assessment.

> **KEYCONCEPT** **Normal aging** is associated with some physical decline, such as decreased sensory abilities and decreased pulmonary and immune function, but many important functions do not change.

TECHNIQUES FOR DATA COLLECTION

The nurse assesses the patient using an interview format that may take a few sessions to complete. He or she also may rely on self-report standardized tests, such as depression and cognitive functioning tools. A wide variety of physiologic disorders may cause changes in mental status for older adults; thus, results of laboratory tests often are significant. For example, urinalysis can detect a urinary tract infection that has affected a patient's cognitive status. Box 36.1 contains a representative listing of common physiologic causes of changes in mental status. In addition, medical records from other health care providers are useful in developing a complete picture of the patient's health status.

An important source of patient data is family members, who often notice changes that the patient overlooks or fails to recognize. A patient with memory impairment may be unable to give an accurate history. By interviewing

---

> **BOX 36.1**
>
> **Changes That Affect Mental Status in Older Adults**
>
> - Acid–base imbalance
> - Dehydration
> - Drugs (prescribed and over the counter)
> - Electrolyte changes
> - Hypothyroidism
> - Hypothermia and hyperthermia
> - Hypoxia
> - Infection and sepsis

---

family members, the nurse expands the scope of the patient assessment. Moreover, the nurse has an opportunity to evaluate the caregivers themselves to determine whether they can care for the patient adequately and how they are coping with the situation. For example, a husband may be unable to care for his wife but is unwilling to admit it. If the nurse can establish rapport with the husband, the nurse may use the assessment interview as an opportunity to help the husband to examine his wife's care requirements realistically.

BIOPSYCHOSOCIAL GEROPSYCHIATRIC NURSING ASSESSMENT

> **KEYCONCEPT** A biopsychosocial **geropsychiatric nursing assessment** is the comprehensive, deliberate, and systematic collection and interpretation of biopsychosocial data that is based on the special needs and problems of the older adult. The purpose is to determine current and past health, functional status and human responses to mental health problems, both actual and potential (Box 36.2).

At the beginning of the assessment, the nurse should determine the patient's ability to participate. A key component in a successful interview with an older adult is the formation of an atmosphere of respect for the person. Use of childlike language with the older adult signifies an ageist attitude and often results in poor communication. For example, if a patient is using a wheelchair, he or she may have physical limitations that prevent full participation in the assessment. However, physical limitations should not be assumed to indicate decreased mental capacity. The patient must be able to hear the nurse. For a patient with compromised hearing, the nurse must attend to voice projection and volume. Shouting at the older patient is unnecessary. The nurse should remember to lower the pitch of his or her voice because higher pitched sounds are often lost with presbycusis (loss of hearing sensitivity associated with aging). The nurse

BOX 36.2

Biopsychosocial Geropsychiatric Nursing Assessment

I. Major reason for seeking help _____

II. Initial information

    Name _____

    Age _____ Current marital status _____

    Gender _____ Caregiver's name _____

    Living arrangements _____

III. Level of independence:

    High (needs no help) _____

    Moderate (lives independently, but needs some help with instrumental activities) _____

    Low (relies on others for help in meeting functional and instrumental activities) _____

    Physical limitations _____

    Level of education completed _____

	Normal	Treated	Untreated
Physical functions: system review	☐	☐	☐
Activity/exercise	☐	☐	☐
Sleep patterns	☐	☐	☐
Appetite and nutrition	☐	☐	☐
Hydration	☐	☐	☐
Sexuality	☐	☐	☐
Existing physical illnesses	☐	☐	☐

    List any chronic illnesses _____

    Presence of pain (Use standardized instrument if pain is present.) No _____ Yes _____

    Score _____ Treatment of pain _____

Medication

(prescription and over-the-counter)	Dosage	Side Effects	Frequency

Significant Laboratory Tests	Values	Normal Range

IV. Responses to mental health problems

    Major concerns regarding mental health problem _____

    Major loss/change in past year: No _____ Yes _____

    Fear of violence: No _____ Yes _____

    Strategies for managing problems/disorder _____

V. Mental status examination

    General observation (appearance, psychomotor activity, attitude) _____

    Orientation (time, place, person) _____

(Continued)

BOX 36.2

Biopsychosocial Geropsychiatric Nursing Assessment (*Continued*)

Mood, affect, emotions (Geriatric Depression Scale should be used if evidence of depression)

Speech (verbal ability, speed, use of words correctly) _____

Thought processes (hallucinations, delusions, tangential, logic, repetition, rhyming of words, loose connections, disorganized) *(Describe content of hallucinations, delusions.)*

Cognition and intellectual performance *(Use standardized test scores as well as observations.)*

Attention and concentration _____

Abstract reasoning and concentration _____

Memory (recall, short-term, long-term) _____

Judgement and insight _____

VI. Significant behaviors (psychomotor, agitation, aggression, withdrawn) *(Use standardized test if behaviors are problematic.)*

_____

When did problem behavior begin? Has it gotten worse? _____

VII. Self-concept beliefs about self—body image, self-esteem, personal identity) _____

VIII. Risk assessment

Suicide: High _____ Low _____ Assault/homicide: High _____ Low _____

Suicide thoughts or ideation: No _____ Yes _____

Current thoughts or harming self _____ Plan _____

Means _____

Means available

Assault/homicide thoughts: No _____ Yes _____

What do you do when angry with a stranger? _____

What do you do when angry with family or partner? _____

Have you ever hit or pushed anyone? No _____ Yes _____

Have you ever been arrested for assault? No _____ Yes _____

Current thoughts of harming others _____

IX. Functional status *(Use standardized test such as FAQ.)* _____

X. Cultural assessment

Cultural group _____

Cultural group's view of health and mental illness _____

By what cultural rules do you try to live? _____

Special, cultural foods that are important to you _____

XI. Stresses and coping behaviors _____

Social support _____

Family members _____

Which members are important to you? _____

On whom can you rely? _____

Community resources _____

XII. Spiritual assessment _____

XIII. Economic status _____

XIV. Legal status _____

XV. Quality of life _____

Summary of significant data that can be used in formulating a nursing diagnosis:

SIGNATURE/TITLE _____ Date _____

should eliminate distracting noises, such as from a television or radio, and ensure that the patient's hearing aid is in place and turned on. Facing the patient and using distinct enunciation will help lip-reading patients understand what is being said. Sometimes deafness is mistaken for cognitive dysfunction. If a patient's hearing is questionable, the nurse should enlist the help of a speech and language specialist. Generally, the pace of the interview should mirror the patient's ability to move through the assessment. Usually, the pace will be slower than the nurse uses with younger populations.

Biologic Domain

Collecting and analyzing data for assessment of the biologic domain includes areas similar to those discussed in Chapter 10. The assessment components include present and past health status, physical examination results, physical functioning, and pharmacology review. When focusing on the biologic domain, the nurse pays special attention to the patient's general physical appearance as well as any observable manifestations of illness. The nurse should assess how all physical problems affect the patient's mental well-being. For example, pain and immobility are physical problems that can negatively affect mental health. A low energy level may be immediately apparent. Women with obvious osteoporosis are experiencing pain most of the time. Men undergoing radiation for prostate cancer worry about sexual functioning and urinary incontinence.

Present and Past Health Status

A review of the patient's current health status includes examining health records and collecting information from the patient and family members. The nurse must identify chronic health problems that could affect mental health care. For example, the patient's management of diabetes mellitus could provide clues to the likelihood of complications such as retinopathy or neuropathy, which in turn will affect the patient's ability to follow a mental health treatment regimen. The nurse must document a history of psychiatric treatment.

Physical Examination

The psychiatric nurse reviews the physical examination findings, paying special attention to recent laboratory values, such as urinalysis, white and red blood cell counts, thyroid studies, and fasting blood glucose data (see Chapter 8). Results of neurologic tests could indicate compromise of the neuromuscular systems. Many psychiatric medications lower the seizure threshold, making a history of seizures, which can cause behavior changes, an important assessment component. The nurse should

note any evidence of movement disorders, such as tremors, abnormal movements, or shuffling. If a patient has been taking conventional antipsychotics, the nurse should consider assessment for symptoms of tardive dyskinesia using one of the appropriate assessment tools (see Chapter 22 for an additional discussion of tardive dyskinesia).

The nurse should take routine vital signs during the assessment. He or she should note any abnormalities in blood pressure (i.e., hypertension or hypotension) because many psychiatric medications affect blood pressure. Generally, these medications may cause orthostatic hypotension, which can lead to dizziness, an unsteady gait, and falls. A baseline blood pressure is needed for future monitoring of medication side effects. Lying, sitting, and standing blood pressures are especially useful in assessing for orthostatic hypotension.

Physical Functions

The nurse must consider the patient's physical functioning within the context of the normal changes that accompany aging and the presence of any chronic disorders. The nurse should note the patient's use of any personal devices, such as canes, walkers, or wheelchairs; oxygen; or environmental devices, such as grab bars, shower benches, or hospital beds. Specific areas to consider are nutrition and eating, elimination, and sleep patterns.

Nutrition and Eating

Assessment of the type, amount, and frequency of food eaten is standard in any geriatric assessment. The nurse should note any weight loss of more than 10 pounds. He or she must consider such nutrition changes in light of mental health problems. For example, is a patient's weight loss related to an underlying physical problem or to the patient's belief that she is being poisoned, which makes her afraid to eat?

Eating is often difficult for older patients, who may experience a lack of appetite. The nurse must assess eating and appetite patterns because many psychiatric medications can affect digestion and may impair an already compromised gastrointestinal tract. A common problem of older adults who live in nursing homes is **dysphagia**, or difficulty swallowing. Dysphagia can lead to dehydration, malnutrition, pneumonia, or asphyxiation. People who have been exposed to conventional antipsychotics (e.g., haloperidol, chlorpromazine) may have symptoms of tardive dyskinesia, which can make swallowing difficult. Thus, the nurse should evaluate any patient who has been exposed to the older psychiatric medications for symptoms of tardive dyskinesia.

Xerostomia, or dry mouth, which is common in older adults, also may impair eating. The nurse should pay particular attention to those who are currently receiving treatment for mental illnesses, particularly with medications that have anticholinergic properties. Dry mouth is also a side effect of many other anticholinergic medications, such as cimetidine, digoxin, and furosemide. Frequent rinsing with a non–alcohol-based mouthwash will help to correct the dry condition. Observe for the frequent use of candy or sugar-based gum for these clients because dental caries and gum disease provide a portal of entry for sepsis in older adults. Decreased taste or smell is common among older adults and may reduce the pleasure of eating so that the patient may eat less. Making meal times social and relaxing experiences can help the patient compensate for some of the loss of pleasure associated with decreased taste or smell. Preparing favorite foods will also enhance the quality of meals and meal times.

The nurse also must determine the patient's use of alcohol. Alcoholism is a growing problem in the older adult population. Fifty percent of older adults in assisted-living homes have an alcohol-related problem. In 2009, 2.5 million older adults and 21% of hospital patients older than age 65 years had alcohol-related problems (Substance Abuse and Mental Health Services Administration [SAMHSA], 2011). There is a substantially increased mortality risk for heavy drinkers and a slightly reduced risk for lighter drinkers. Indications of alcohol or drug use include observable changes in sleep patterns and unusual fatigue, changes in mood, jerky eye movement, seizures, unexplained complaints about chronic pain or vision problems, poor hygiene and self-neglect, unexplained nausea or vomiting, and slurred speech (SAMHSA, 2011). Use of an assessment tool such as the CAGE questionnaire (discussed in Chapter 31) may be helpful in this area.

Elimination

The nurse must assess the patient's urinary and bowel functions. Older adults are more likely to experience constipation caused by a change in eating or activity patterns or intentional reduction in fluid intake. Medications with anticholinergic properties can cause constipation, leading to fecal impaction. Abuse of laxatives is common among older adults and requires evaluation. Although the addition of fiber is recommended for constipation, such measures may cause bloating and excessive gas production. Older patients are also more likely to experience urinary frequency because the strength of the sphincter muscles decreases. Because many older adults drink fewer fluids to manage urinary incontinence, fluid intake also becomes an important factor in assessing urinary functioning and constipation. The nurse should remember that urinary incontinence is not a normal age-related finding but a symptom of a disorder that requires follow-up and treatment.

Sleep

During the normal aging process, sleep patterns change, and patients may sleep more or less than they did when younger. The nurse must assess any recent changes in sleep patterns and evaluate whether they are related to normal aging or are symptomatic of an underlying disorder. Insomnia, the inability to fall or remain asleep throughout the night, may be the result of depression or can lead to an increased risk for depression and regular use of sleep medications. Sleep disturbances such as waking after onset of sleep and spending time in bed are associated with apathy, one of the early signs of Alzheimer's dementia (Mulin et al., 2011). Disturbed sleep patterns are also associated with interpersonal stress and loneliness (Aanes, Helland, Pallesen, & Mittelmark, 2011). If a patient reports sleep problems, the nurse should ask about the patient's use of alcohol, over-the-counter (OTC) medications, and prescription drugs, which can interfere with sleep (Box 36.3).

Pain

Older adults are more likely to experience persistent pain than younger adults because they are at increased risk for chronic illness and may be experiencing the consequences

---

BOX 36.3

Research for Best Practice: **Substance Misuse among Older Adults**

Schonfeld, L., King-Kallimani, B. L., Duchene, D. M., Etheridge, R. L., Herrera, J. R., Barry, K. L., & Lynn, N. (2010). Screening and brief intervention for substance misuse among older adults: The Florida BRITE Project. American Journal of Public Health, 100(1), 108–114.

THE QUESTION: Will the Florida Brief Intervention and Treatment for Elders (BRITE) tool effectively screen and improve substance misuse among older adults?

METHODS: Agencies in four counties conducted screenings for alcohol, medications, and illicit substance misuse among 3497 older adults. Screenings occurred in the older adults' homes, senior centers, or other selected sites. Interviews were based on questions from standardized tests for alcohol use, prescription medications, over-the-counter (OTC) medications, illicit drugs, depression, and suicide. Brief interventions involved one to five sessions delivered in the home.

FINDINGS: Prescription medication misuse was the most prevalent substance use problem followed by alcohol, OTC medications, and illicit substances. Depression was prevalent among those with alcohol and prescription problems. Those who received interventions experienced improvement in the alcohol and medication misuse and depression.

IMPLICATIONS FOR NURSING: Older adults should be screened for medication and substance misuse. Depression can also be assessed while determining misuse of substances and medications.

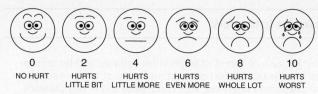

FIGURE 36.1 The Wong-Baker FACES Pain Rating Scale. Instructions: Explain to the person that each face is for a person who feels happy because he has no pain (hurt) or sad because he has some or a lot of pain. **Face 0** is very happy because he doesn't hurt at all. **Face 1** hurts just a little bit. **Face 2** hurts a little more. **Face 3** hurts even more. **Face 4** hurts a whole lot. **Face 5** hurts as much as you can imagine, although you don't have to be crying to feel this bad. Ask the person to choose the face that best describes how he is feeling. (From Hockenberry, M. J., & Wilson, D. [2009]. *Wong's essentials of pediatric nursing*, 8th ed. St. Louis: Mosby. Used with permission. Copyright Mosby.)

of a lifetime of injuries. For many older adults, chronic pain is a constant companion and contributes to unexplained behavior and personality changes. One of the most popular assessment tools, especially for acute pain, is the Wong-Baker FACES Pain Rating Scale, initially developed for children but now used for all age groups (Figure 36.1). This scale is especially useful in communicating with people whose cultures and languages are different from the nurse's.

It is important for the nurse to spend time with the patient during a pain assessment. Chronic pain assessment is more difficult because of the person's perception of pain or cognitive impairment, which interferes with communication. Older persons are often reluctant to report pain or believe that they have to be stoic about pain and "not make a big deal" about it. Older adults who are cognitively impaired and living in long-term care (LTC) institutions may not be able to use a numerical scale of pain or self-report pain intensity (Chapman, 2010). See Chapter 42 for a further discussion of pain.

Pharmacologic Assessment

One of the most important areas of the biologic domain is the pharmacologic assessment. **Polypharmacy**, the use of duplicate medications, interacting medications, or drugs used to treat adverse drug interactions, is common in older adults. The nurse must ask the patient and family to list all medications and times that the patient takes them. Asking family members to bring in all the medications the patient is taking, including OTC medications, vitamins, and herbal supplements, allows for a careful assessment of polypharmacy. Because older adults are more sensitive than younger people to medications, the possibility of drug-to-drug interactions is greater. When considering potential drug interactions, the nurse should ask the patient about his or her consumption of grapefruit juice, which contains naringin, a compound that inhibits the CYP3A4 enzyme involved in the metabolism of many

medications (e.g., antidepressants, antiarrhythmics, erythromycin, and several statins).

Psychological Domain

Assessment of the psychological domain provides the nurse with the opportunity to identify limitations, behavior symptoms, and reactions to illness. The nurse assesses many of the same areas as in other adult assessments, but again, the emphasis may be different. The following discussion focuses on the responses of older patients to mental health problems, mental status examination, behavior changes, stress and coping patterns, and risk assessments.

Responses to Mental Health Problems

Many older patients are reluctant to admit that they have psychiatric symptoms, particularly if their culture stigmatizes mental illness, and may deny having mental or emotional problems. They may also fear that if they admit to any symptoms, they may be placed outside their home. If patients do not recognize or admit to having psychiatric symptoms, their vulnerability to being taken advantage of or injured increases.

Throughout the assessment, the nurse evaluates the patient's verbal reports, obvious symptoms, and family reports. If a patient flatly denies any psychiatric symptoms (e.g., depression, mood swings, outbursts of anger, memory problems), the nurse should respectfully accept the patient's answer and avoid arguments or confrontation (Box 36.4). If the patient's family members contradict the patient's report or symptoms are obvious during the interview, the nurse can approach the issue while planning care. Nurses may need to use conflict resolution strategies in helping families and patients arrive at mutually agreed on reports.

Mental Status Examination

The areas of special interest in the mental status examination are mood and affect, thought processes, and cognitive functioning. The nurse should interpret the results in light of any accompanying physical problems, such as chronic pain, or life changes, such as loss of a spouse.

Mood and Affect

Depression in older adults is common and associated with the following risk factors: loss of spouse, physical illness, low socioeconomic status, impaired functional status, and heavy alcohol consumption. In older people, other disorders may mask depression. When symptoms are present, they may be attributed to normal aging or atherosclerosis or other age-related problems. Older patients are less likely to report feeling sad or worthless

BOX 36.4 • THERAPEUTIC DIALOGUE • Assessment Interview

Tom, 79 years old, is being seen for the first time in a geropsychiatric clinic because of recent changes in his behavior and his accusations that family members are trying to steal his house and car. He locked his wife out of the house, accusing her of being unfaithful. When Susan, the psychiatric nurse assigned to his case, is conducting the assessment interview, Tom cooperates and is very pleasant until the nurse begins to assess the psychological domain.

INEFFECTIVE APPROACH

Nurse: Have there been times when you have had problems with any members of your family?

Patient: No. (Silence)

Nurse: Have you noticed that lately you have been getting more upset than usual?

Patient: No. Who has been talking to you?

Nurse: Your wife seems to think that you may be getting a little more upset than usual.

Patient: You are just like her. She keeps telling me something is wrong with me. (Getting very agitated)

Nurse: Please, I'm trying to help you. I understand that you locked your wife out of the house last week.

Patient: Leave me alone. (Gets up and leaves)

EFFECTIVE APPROACH

Nurse: How have things been going at home?

Patient: All right.

Nurse: (Silence)

Patient: Well, my wife and I sometimes argue.

Nurse: Oh. Most husband and wives argue. Any special arguments?

Patient: No. Just the usual. I don't pick up after myself enough. I don't dress right to suit her. But, lately, she's gone a lot.

Nurse: She is gone a lot?

Patient: Yeah! A lot.

Nurse: The way you say that, it sounds like you have some feelings about her being gone.

Patient: You're damned right I do—and you would, too.

Nurse: I'm missing something.

Patient: Well, if you must know, I think she's having an affair with the man next door.

Nurse: Really? That must upset you to think your wife is having an affair.

Patient: I am devastated. I feel so bad.

Nurse: Would you say that you are depressed?

Patient: Well, wouldn't you be? Yes, I'm feeling pretty low.

CRITICAL THINKING CHALLENGE

- How do the very first questions differ in the two interviews?
- What therapeutic techniques did the nurse use in the second interview to avoid the pitfalls the nurse encountered in the first scenario?

- How did the nurse in the second scenario elicit the patient's delusion about his wife's affair?
- From the data that the second nurse gathered, how many patient problems can be identified?

---

than are younger patients. As a result, family members and primary care providers often overlook depression in older patients.

Depressive symptoms are very common. Rates vary by settings, with up to 24% in outpatient settings, 30% in acute care, and up to 43% to 85% in the LTC setting experiencing depressive symptoms (Butcher & McGonigal-Kenney, 2010). The term *late-onset depression* refers to the development of depression or depressive symptoms that impair functioning after 60 years of age.

In late-onset depression, the risk for recurrence is relatively high (Gallagher et al., 2010).

The Geriatric Depression Scale (GDS) is a useful screening tool with demonstrated validity and reliability (Hyer & Blount, 1984). The GDS was designed as a self-administered test, although it also has been used in observer-administered formats. One advantage of the test is its "yes/no" format, which may be easier for older adults than the Hamilton Rating Scale for Depression (HAM-D), which uses a scale from 0 to 4 (see Chapter 24).

BOX 36.5

Geriatric Depression Scale (Short Form)

1. Are you basically satisfied with your life?	Yes	No
2. Have you dropped many of your activities and interests?	Yes	No
3. Do you feel that your life is empty?	Yes	No
4. Do you often get bored?	Yes	No
5. Are you in good spirits most of the time?	Yes	No
6. Are you afraid that something bad is going to happen to you?	Yes	No
7. Do you feel happy most of the time?	Yes	No
8. Do you often feel helpless?	Yes	No
9. Do you prefer to stay at home rather than go out and do new things?	Yes	No
10. Do you feel you have more problems with memory than most?	Yes	No
11. Do you think it is wonderful to be alive now?	Yes	No
12. Do you feel pretty worthless the way you are now?	Yes	No
13. Do you feel full of energy?	Yes	No
14. Do you feel that your situation is hopeless?	Yes	No
15. Do you think that most people are better off than you are?	Yes	No

Score: ——/15. One point for "No" to questions 1, 5, 7, 11, 13; one point for "Yes" to other questions.

Normal	3 ± 2
Mildly depressed	7 ± 3
Very depressed	12 ± 2

From Sheikh, J. I., & Yesavage, J. A. (1986). Geriatric Depression Scale (GDS): Recent evidence and development of a shorter version. In T. L. Brink (Ed.), *Clinical gerontology: a guide to assessment and intervention* (pp. 165–173). Binghamton, NY: Haworth Press. © Haworth Press, Inc. All rights reserved. Reprinted with permission.

This tool is easy to administer and provides valuable information about the possibility of depression (Box 36.5). If results are positive, the nurse should refer the patient to a psychiatrist or advanced practice nurse for further evaluation. Among nursing home residents, the usefulness of the GDS depends on the degree of cognitive impairment. Residents who are mildly impaired may be able to answer yes/no questions; however, moderately to severely impaired patients will be unable to do the same. The best validated scale for patients with dementia is the Cornell Scale for Depression in Dementia (CSDD) (Alexopoulos, Abrams, Young, & Shamoian, 1998). The CSDD is an interview-administered scale that uses information both from the patient and an outside informant.

Anxiety is another important mood for nurses to assess in older adults because it can interfere with normal functioning. In dementia, anxiety is common (Prado-Jean et al., 2010). The Rating Anxiety in Dementia (RAID) scale was developed as a global scale to assess anxiety in patients with dementia (Shankar, Walker, Frost, & Orrell, 1999). The domains that the RAID scale assesses include worry, apprehension and vigilance, motor tension, autonomic hyperactivity, and phobias and panic attacks.

Thought Processes

Thought processes and content are critical in the assessment of older patients. Can the patient express ideas and thoughts logically? Can the patient understand questions and follow the conversation of others? If the patient shows any indication of hallucinations or delusions, the nurse should explore the content of the hallucination or delusion. If the patient has a history of mental illness, such as schizophrenia, these symptoms may be familiar to family members, who can validate whether they are old or new problems. If this is the first time the patient has experienced these abnormal thought processes, the nurse should further evaluate the content. Suspicious and delusional thoughts that characterize dementia often include some of the following beliefs:

- People are stealing my things.
- The house is not my house.
- My relative is an impostor.

Cognition and Intellectual Performance

Cognitive functioning includes such parameters as orientation, attention, short- and long-term memory, consciousness, and executive functioning. Intellectual functioning, also considered a cognitive measure, is rarely formally assessed with a standardized intelligence test in older adults. Considerable variability among individuals depends on lifestyle and psychosocial factors. Some changes in cognitive capacity may accompany aging, but important functions are spared. Normal cognitive changes during aging include a slowing of information processing and memory retrieval. Abnormalities of consciousness, orientation, judgment, speech, or language are not related to age but to underlying neuropathologic changes. Cognitive changes in older adults are associated with delirium or dementia (see Chapter 37) or with schizophrenia (see Chapter 22).

The assessment includes the number of years of education. An inverse relationship between Alzheimer's disease and the number of years of education exists. Evidence suggests that severe cognitive deterioration may occur in older adults with schizophrenia. An easy to administer and easily accessible screening tool is the SLUMS (Saint Louis University Mental Status Examination) (see Chapter 37).

Behavior Changes

Behavior changes in older adults can indicate neuropathologic processes and thus require nursing assessment.

If such changes occur, it is most likely that family members will notice them before the patient does. Apraxia (an inability to execute a voluntary movement despite normal muscle function) is not attributed to age but indicates an underlying disease process, such as Alzheimer's disease, Parkinson's disease, or other disorders. Various other behavior problems are associated with psychiatric disorders in older adults, including irritability, agitation, apathy, and euphoria. Other behaviors in older adults who are experiencing psychiatric problems include wandering and aggressive behaviors.

The Neuropsychiatric Inventory (NPI) was developed in 1994 to assess behavior problems associated with dementia. The scale assesses 10 behavior problems: delusions, hallucinations, dysphoria, anxiety, agitation or aggression, euphoria, inhibition, irritability or lability, apathy, and aberrant motor behavior (Cummings et al., 1994). This very popular tool is used in many medication clinical trials. There are two versions. The standard version is used when the patient is still at home; the second version (NPI-NH) is used when the patient is in a nursing home.

Stress and Coping Patterns

Identifying stresses and coping patterns is just as important for older patients as it is for younger adults. Unique stresses for older patients include living on a fixed income, handling declining health, losing partners and friends, and ultimately confronting death. Coping ability varies, depending on patients' unique circumstances. For example, some patients respond to stressful events with amazing adaptability, but others become depressed and suicidal.

Bereavement, a natural response to the death of a loved one, includes crying and sorrow, anxiety and agitation, insomnia, and a loss of appetite. These symptoms, although overlapping with those of major depression, do not constitute a mental disorder. Although bereavement is a normal response, the nurse must identify it and develop interventions to help the individual successfully resolve the loss. Bereavement is an important and well-established risk factor for depression. See Chapter 20.

Risk Assessment

Suicide is a major mental health risk for older adults. Suicide rates increase with age; white men over the age of 85 are at the greatest risk of suicide. (American Association of Suicidology [AAS], 2014). Unmarried, unsociable men between the ages of 42 and 77 years with minimal social networks and no close relatives have a significantly increased risk for committing suicide (Walsh, Clayton, Liu, & Hodges, 2009). White men account for more than 80% of suicide deaths in this *older* age group. Older white

men are the highest risk for suicide with a rate of approximately 31.1 suicides per 100,000 population each year (AAS, 2014).

When caring for the older patient with mental health problems, it is always important to consider the patient's potential to commit suicide. Depression is the greatest risk factor for suicide. Individuals who are suicidal often believe that they are a burden to their family who would be better off without them (Joiner & Van Orden, 2008). In assessing an older patient, the nurse should consider the following characteristics as indications of high risk for committing suicide:

- Depression
- Attempted suicide in the past
- Family history of suicide
- Firearms in the home
- Abuse of alcohol or other substances
- Unusual stress
- Burden to family
- Chronic medical condition (e.g., cancer, neuromuscular disorders)
- Social isolation

> **NCLEXNOTE** Suicide assessment is a priority for the older adult experiencing mental health problems. It is important to carefully assess recent behavior changes and loss of support.

Social Domain

Assessment of the social domain includes determining the patient's interactions with others in his or her family and community. The nurse targets social support because it is so important to the well-being of the older adult's functional status and because of the potential physical changes that can affect this area and social systems, which encompasses all community resources.

Social Support

Remaining active throughout one's life is one of the best predictors of mental health and wellness in an older patient. People obtain their sense of self-worth through their interactions with others in their environment. A sense of "who one is" is closely tied to the roles that a person plays in life. When older adults relinquish such roles because of physical disabilities, become isolated from friends and family, or begin to sense that they are a burden to those around them rather than contributing members of society, a sense of hopelessness and helplessness often follows.

The role of social support is critical to assess in this age group. Social support is a reciprocal concept, meaning that simply receiving assistance increases the person's sense of being a burden. Those older adults who believe that they contribute to the welfare of others are most likely to remain mentally healthy. For this reason, pets are often "life savers" for older adults who live alone. Nothing can be more understanding and accepting of an older adult's behavior or disabilities than a beloved pet.

The nurse should assess the patient's number of formal and informal social contacts. The nurse should ask about the frequency of contacts with others (in person and through telephone calls, letters, and cards). Determining whether these contacts are actually satisfying and supporting to the patient is essential. If family members are important to the patient's well-being, the nurse should complete a more in-depth family assessment (see Chapter 14).

The nurse can use the following questions to focus on social support:

- In the past 2 weeks, how often would you say that family members or friends let you know that they care about you?
- In the past 2 weeks, how often has someone provided you with help, such as giving you a ride somewhere or helping around the house?
- Do you have a family member or a special person you could call or contact if you needed help? Who?
- In general, other than your children, who do you consider a close friend or companion?

For patients who are isolated with few social contacts, the nurse can develop interventions to improve social support.

Functional Status

As part of a complete assessment, the nurse will need to assess the older adult's functional status. **Functional activities** or activities of daily living (ADLs) are the activities necessary for self-care (i.e., bathing, toileting, dressing, and transferring). **Instrumental activities of daily living (IADLs)** include those that facilitate or enhance the performance of ADLs (i.e., shopping, using the telephone, using transportation). These aspects are critical to consider for any older adult living alone. The most common tools used to assess functional status are the Index of Independence in Activities of Daily Living and the Instrumental Activities of Daily Living Scale (Katz & Akpom, 1976).

Social Systems

Community resources are essential to an older adult's ability to maintain mental health and wellness, as well as to his or her ability to remain at home throughout the later years. Senior centers are federally funded community resources that provide a wide array of services to the nation's older population. They provide daily balanced meals at a nominal cost. In addition, they provide opportunities for socialization, which is key to combating loneliness and social isolation. Many senior centers provide annual influenza and pneumonia vaccination clinics and education on such topics as fall prevention and recognition and prevention of elder abuse. Additional community resources that are specific to older adults include geriatric assessment clinics and adult day care centers.

During the assessment, the nurse must determine which community resources are available and if the older patient uses them. Lack of transportation to and from these community resources may be a barrier to use. Most communities have buses available for older or disabled individuals. The nurse may need to assist the older adult in accessing this important resource.

Many older citizens rely on the Social Security Administration for their monthly income. For many, this financial support, although less than adequate in most instances, is their only source of income. In addition to Social Security, the federal government provides basic health care coverage in the form of the state-administered Medicare program. Together, these programs contribute to the patient's ability to live independently and receive health care. The nurse should assess a patient's sources of financial support. Sometimes nurses are uncomfortable asking for financial information, fearing that they are invading the patient's privacy. However, such data are important for the nurse to determine whether a patient's resources adequately meet his or her needs. The source of financial support is also important. For example, a patient whose income is adequate and from personal resources is more likely to be independent than is the patient who depends on family members for income.

The nurse should ask the patient about accessible clinics, support groups, and pharmaceutical services. Information about available health care resources can provide useful data regarding the patient's ability to access services and can also provide potential referral sources. In urban areas that are likely to have adequate health care resources, cultural and language barriers may prohibit access. People who live in rural areas where health care resources are limited are less likely to enjoy the full range of health care resources than are those in urban areas. Overall, the use of mental health services by older adults with mental illnesses is low (Han, Gfroerer, Colpe, Barker, & Colliver, 2011). If older adults are married and have insurance, they are more likely to seek mental health services.

Spiritual Assessment

Spiritual needs are basic for all age groups and are requirements for establishing meaning and purpose, love and relatedness, and forgiveness. With advanced age, many people begin to reflect on their successes and failures. During such reflection, many seek out God or a higher being to make sense of the past and establish hope for the future.

The process of spiritual assessment involves active listening, thoughtful observing, and sensitive questioning. The nurse may simply ask if the person would find comfort from a visit from a spiritual leader. Many forms of religion use various rituals that are important to the person's daily routine. The nurse should explore and honor these aspects to the extent possible.

Legal Status

A growing trend in the United States is to view older adults as a special population whose rights deserve increased attention. Instances of elder abuse are far too common. Every nurse must consider him- or herself a patient advocate and be vigilant in recognizing the signs of neglect or abuse, such as unexplained injuries. At times, abuse can take the form of another individual usurping the rights of the older person. Unless the older person is determined to be incompetent, he or she has the same rights to personal decision making as any other adult, including the right to refuse treatment.

Quality of Life

A sense of quality of life is closely tied to values and beliefs. For many older adults, quality of life is not reflected in material possessions or physical health. At this stage, quality of life is connected more with contentment over how the person has lived life and the extent to which his or her life has had meaning and purpose. Keeping close personal contacts with friends and family and having the opportunity to shares stories of lifetime experiences are essential to maintaining mental health and wellness for older adults. For older adults, physical illnesses may affect the quality of life more than psychiatric disorders. The assessment of quality of life becomes especially important when assessing a patient living in a nursing home or isolated in his or her own home. The assessment of quality of life of older adults is similar to that for younger adults (see Chapter 10).

SUMMARY OF KEY POINTS

- Normal aging is associated with some physical decline, but most functions do not change. Intellectual functioning, capacity for change, and productive engagement with life remain stable.

- Mental health assessments are necessary when older patients face psychiatric or mental health issues. The biopsychosocial geropsychiatric nursing assessment examines many sources of data, including self-reports, laboratory test results, and reports from family members.

- The biopsychosocial geropsychiatric nursing assessment is based on the special needs and problems of the older adult. This assessment examines current and past health, functional status, and human responses to mental health problems.

- Assessment of the biologic domain involves collecting data about past and present health status, physical examination findings, physical functions (i.e., nutrition and eating, elimination patterns, sleep), pain, and pharmacologic information.

- Assessment of the psychological domain includes the patient's responses to mental health problems, mental status examination, behavioral changes, stress and coping patterns, and risk assessment.

- When conducting an assessment, the nurse may find several tools useful. For patients with possible depression, the Geriatric Depression Scale (GDS) may be helpful. For patients with anxiety, nurses can use the Rating Anxiety in Dementia (RAID) scale.

- Coping with the stresses of aging varies among patients. Determining stresses and coping skills for dealing with stresses is important.

- Social support is critical to patients in this age group and requires assessment.

- Determination of the patient's ability to perform functional and instrumental activities of daily living is critical in the assessment of the older adult.

- Social systems, spiritual assessment, legal information, and quality of life are components within the social domain that the nurse should consider.

CRITICAL THINKING CHALLENGES

1. The director of your church's senior center has asked you to be the guest speaker at the monthly meeting of the Retired Active Citizens group. The subject is to be "Maintaining Your Mental Health After Retirement." What key points will you touch on in your presentation? What activities or handouts will you use to highlight your talk?

2. When asking about current illnesses, a patient begins telling you her whole life story. What approach would you take to elicit the most important needed to develop an individualized plan of care for your older patient?

3. A caregiver tells you that her mother has become suspicious of the neighbors and other family members. How would you assess this perceptual experience? What other data should you gather from this patient?

4. A caregiver brings a sack of medications to the patient's assessment interview. What information should you obtain from the caregiver regarding the patient's use of these medications?

5. A woman brings her father, who has a long history of frequent psychiatric hospitalizations for depression, to the clinic. The patient's wife recently died, and the daughter fears that her father is becoming depressed again. What approach would you use in assessing for changes in mood?

6. Obtain a listing of the social services available in your community. Examine the list for areas of duplication and omission of services needed by an older adult living alone in his or her own home.

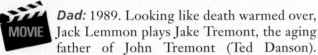

Dad: 1989. Looking like death warmed over, Jack Lemmon plays Jake Tremont, the aging father of John Tremont (Ted Danson). Always proud of being able to fend for himself, Lemmon despises being dependent on others, but his increasingly frequent periods of confusion do not allow him his old independence. For his part, Danson resents having to care for his dad as he would for an infant. To make matters even worse, Lemmon is diagnosed with cancer. As the reality of his imminent death strikes everyone around him, Lemmon retreats into fantasy, recalling the past happy events of his life as though they're happening here and now. The rest of the family humors their dying dad, and in so doing draws closer together than they've been in years.

VIEWING POINTS: Identify the physical impairments that are obvious throughout the movie. Identify specific memory problems that Jake experiences. Are these problems part of normal aging? If you were Jake Tremont's nurse, what key assessment areas would you explore?

References

Aanes, M. M., Hetland, J., Pallesen, S., & Mittlemark, M. B. (2011). Does loneliness mediate the stress-sleep quality relation? The Hordaland Health Study. *International Psychogeriatrics, 23*(1), 1–9.

Alexopoulos, G. S., Abrams, R. C., Young, R. C., & Shamoian, C. A. (1998). Cornell Scale for Depression in Dementia. *Biological Psychiatry, 23,* 271–284.

American Association of Suicidology (2014). *Elderly suicide fact sheet.* Retrieved from http://www.suicidology.org/web/guest/stats-and-toos/fact-sheets. Retrieved on May 28, 2014.

Butcher, H. K., & McGonigal-Kenney, M. (2010). Living in the doldrums: The lived experience of dispiritedness in later life. *Research in Gerontological Nursing, 3*(3), 148–161.

Chapman, S. (2010). Managing pain in the older person. *Nursing Standard, 25*(11), 35–39.

Cummings, J. L., Mega, M., Gray, K., Rosenberg-Thompson, S., Carusi, D. A., & Gornbein, J. (1994). The Neuropsychiatric Inventory: Comprehensive assessment of psychopathology in dementia. *Neurology, 44*(12), 2308–2314.

Gallagher, D., Mhaolain, A. N., Greene, E., Walsh, C., Denihan, A., Bruce I., Golden, J., Conroy, R. M., Kirby, M., & Lawlor, B. A. (2010). Late life depression: A comparison of risk factors and symptoms according to age of onset in community dwelling older adults. *International Journal of Geriatric Psychiatry, 25*(10), 981–987.

Garrido, M. M., Kane, R. L., Kaas, M., & Kane, R. A. (2011). Use of mental health care by community-dwelling older adults. *Journal of the American Geriatrics Society, 59*(1), 50–56.

Han, B., Gfroerer, J. C., Colpe, L. J., Barker, P. R., & Colliver, J. D. (2011). Serious psychological distress and mental health service use among community-dwelling older U.S. adults. *Psychiatric Services, 62*(3), 291–298.

Hurt, C. S., Burns, A., & Barrowclough, C. (2011). Perceptions of memory problems are more important in predicting distress in older adults with subjective memory complaints than coping strategies. *International Psychogeriatrics, 22*(1), 1–10.

Hyer, L., & Blount, J. (1984). Concurrent and discriminant validities of the geriatric depression scale with older psychiatric inpatients. *Psychological Reports, 54,* 611–616.

Joiner, T. E., & Van Orden, K. A. (2008). The interpersonal-psychological theory of suicidal behavior indicates specific and crucial psychotherapeutic targets. *International Journal of Cognitive Therapy, 1*(1), 80–89.

Katz, S., & Akpom, A. (1976). A measure of primary sociobiological functions. *International Journal of Health Science, 6,* 493.

Mulin, E., Zeitzer, J. M., Friedman, L., Duff, F. L., Yesavage, J., Robert, P. H., & David, R. (2011). Relationship between apathy and sleep disturbance in mild and moderate Alzheimer's Disease: An actigraphic study. *Journal of Alzheimer's Disease,* in press.

National Center for Health Statistics (2011). *Health, United States, 2010. With special feature on death and dying.* Hyattsville, MD: Author.

Prado-Jean, A., Couratier, P., Druet-Cabanac, M., Nubukpo, P., Bernard-Bourzeix, L., Thomas, P, Dechamps, N., Videaud, H., Dantoine, T., & Clement, J. P. (2010). Specific psychological and behavioral symptoms of depression in patients with dementia. *International Journal of Geriatric Psychiatry, 25*(10), 1065–1072.

Schonfeld, L., King-Kallimani, B. L., Duchene, D. M, Etheridge, R. L., Herrera, J. R., Barry, K. L., & Lynn, N. (2010). Screening and brief intervention for substance misuse among older adults: The Florida BRITE Project. *American Journal of Public Health, 100*(1), 108–114.

Shankar, K. K., Walker, M., Frost, D., & Orrell, M. W. (1999). The development of a valid and reliable scale for rating anxiety in dementia (RAID). *Aging & Mental Health, 3*(1), 39–49.

Sheikh, J. I., & Yesavage, J. A. (1986). Geriatric Depression Scale (GDS): Recent evidence and development of a shorter version. In T. L. Brink (Ed.), *Clinical gerontology: A guide to assessment and interventions* (pp. 165–177). Binghamton, NY: Haworth Press.

Substance Abuse and Mental Health Services Administration (2010). *Targeted outreach: Development of substance use disorders in older adults.* Targeted out reach: Development of substance use disorders in older adults. *Now More than Ever, 9,* 1–6.

Vincent, G. K., & Velkoff, V. A. (2010). The next four decades. The older population in the United States: 2010–2050. *Current Population Reports.* P25–1138. Washington, DC: U.S. Census Bureau.

Walsh, S., Clayton, R., Liu, L., & Hodges, S. (2009). Divergence in contributing factors for suicide among men and women in Kentucky: Recommendations to raise public awareness. *Public Health Reports, 124*(6), 861–867.

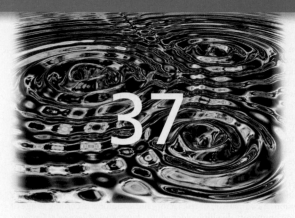

37

Neurocognitive Disorders

Mary Ann Boyd

KEY CONCEPTS

- cognition
- cognitive reserve
- delirium
- dementia
- memory

LEARNING OBJECTIVES

After studying this chapter, you will be able to:

1. Distinguish the clinical characteristics, onset, and course of delirium and dementia.

2. Integrate biologic, psychological, and social theories related to delirium and dementia.

3. Explain the important epidemiologic findings regarding delirium and dementia.

4. Discuss the primary etiologic factors of delirium and dementia.

5. Analyze human responses to delirium and dementia, with emphasis on the concepts of impaired cognition and memory.

6. Explain the primary elements involved in assessment, nursing diagnoses, nursing interventions, and evaluation of patients with delirium and dementia.

KEY TERMS

- acetylcholine (ACh) • acetylcholinesterase (AChE) • acetylcholinesterase inhibitors (AChEIs) • agnosia • amyloidosis
- aphasia • apraxia • beta-amyloid plaques • bradykinesia • catastrophic reactions • cortical dementia • disinhibition
- disturbance of executive functioning • hyperkinetic delirium • hypokinetic delirium • hypersexuality
- hypervocalization • illusions • impaired consciousness • mild cognitive impairment (MCI) • mixed variant delirium • neurocognitive disorders • neurofibrillary tangles • oxidative stress • subcortical dementia • tau

Cognition is an intellectual process of acquiring, using, or manipulating perceptions and information. Cognition involves the perception of reality and an understanding of its representations. There are a number of cognitive functions such as the acquisition and use of language, the orientation of time and space, and the ability to learn and solve problems. Cognition also is the basis of judgment, reasoning, attention, comprehension, concept formation, planning, and the use of symbols (e.g., numbers and letters used in mathematics and writing).

> **KEYCONCEPT** **Cognition** is based on a system of interrelated abilities, such as perception, reasoning, judgment, intuition, and memory that allow one to be aware of oneself and one's surroundings. Impairments in these abilities can result in a failure of the afflicted person to recognize that he or she is ill and in need of treatment.

Memory, a facet of cognition, refers to the ability to recall or reproduce what has been learned or experienced. It is more than simple storage and retrieval; it is a complex cognitive mental function that includes most areas of the brain, especially the hippocampus, which is believed to be essential to the transfer of some memories from short- to long-term storage. Defects of memory are an essential feature of many cognitive disorders, particularly dementia.

> **KEYCONCEPT** **Memory** is a facet of cognition concerned with retaining and recalling past experiences, whether they occurred in the physical environment or internally as cognitive events.

Neurocognitive disorders are characterized by a decline in cognitive function from a previous level of functioning. These disorders are acquired and have not been present since early life. The diagnosis of a neurocognitive disorder is based on deficits in the following cognitive domains: *attention* (distractibility with multiple stimuli), *executive function* (planning, decision making, working memory), *learning and memory* (recall and recognition), *language* (*expressive* including naming, work finding, fluency, grammar syntax, and *receptive language*), *perceptual-motor* (visual perception, visuoconstructional, perceptual-motor), and *social cognition deficits* (recognition of emotions, ability to consider another's mental state) (APA, 2013).

The neurocognitive disorders discussed in this chapter are delirium, a disorder of acute cognitive impairment usually caused by a medical condition (e.g., infection), substance abuse, or multiple etiologies and dementia, characterized by chronic cognitive impairments. Dementia is differentiated from delirium by underlying cause, not by symptom patterns, which are often similar. Some dementias are irreversible and progressive, such as the Alzheimer type, but not all dementias are irreversible. For example, some organic compounds and chemicals, such as lead, aluminum, manganese, and toluene (one of the toxins in glue and paint) may produce symptoms of dementia (Table 37.1). After the patient has been evaluated and treated, the symptoms of dementia can resolve in many of these disorders (e.g., endocrine disorders).

> **KEYCONCEPT** **Delirium** is a disorder of acute cognitive impairment and is caused by a medical condition (e.g., infection), substance abuse, or multiple etiologies.

> **KEYCONCEPT** **Dementia** is characterized by chronic cognitive impairments and is differentiated by underlying cause, not by symptom patterns. Dementia can be further classified as cortical or subcortical to denote the location of the underlying pathology.

Cortical dementia results from a disease process that globally afflicts the cortex. **Subcortical dementia** is caused by dysfunction or deterioration of deep gray- or white-matter structures inside the brain and brain stem. Symptoms of subcortical dementia may be more localized

Table 37.1 SELECTED COMPOUNDS AND CHEMICALS THAT MAY PRODUCE DEMENTIA

Substance	Related Symptoms
Arsenic	Headache Drowsiness Confusion
Mercury	Tremors Extrapyramidal signs Upper and lower extremity ataxia Depression Confusion
Lead	Abdominal cramps Anemia Peripheral neuropathy Encephalopathy (rare)
Manganese	Extrapyramidal symptoms Delirium
Aluminum	Myoclonus Speech disorders Seizure disorders Cognitive impairment
Toluene (methyl benzene)	Profound cognitive impairment Tremor Ataxia Loss of vision and hearing

and tend to disrupt arousal, attention, and motivation, but they can produce a variety of clinical behavioral manifestations. In this chapter, a type of cortical dementia, Alzheimer disease (AD), is highlighted because it is the most prevalent form of dementia.

DELIRIUM

Clinical Course

Delirium is a disturbance in consciousness and a change in cognition that develops over a short time. It is usually reversible if the underlying cause is identified and treated quickly. It is a serious disorder and should always be treated as an emergency.

> **EMERGENCY CARE ALERT !** Individuals who are delirious arrive in the emergency department (ED) in a state of confusion and disorientation that developed during a period of a few hours or days. If delirium is not treated in a timely manner, irreversible neurologic damage can occur. Delirium is a common complication in patients admitted to intensive care units and inpatient psychiatric units (Tang, Patel, Khubchandani, & Grossberg, 2014; Bryczkowski, Lopreiato, Yonclas, Sacca, & Mosenthal, 2014).

Diagnostic Criteria

Impaired consciousness is the key diagnostic criterion for delirium. The patient becomes less aware of his or her environment and loses the ability to focus, sustain,

Table 37.2 DIFFERENTIATING DELIRIUM FROM DEMENTIA		
Characteristics	**Delirium**	**Dementia**
Onset	Sudden	Insidious
24-h course	Fluctuating	Stable
Consciousness	Reduced	Clear
Attention	Globally disoriented	Usually normal
Cognition	Globally disoriented	Globally impaired
Hallucinations	Visual auditory	Possible
Orientation	Usually impaired	Often impaired
Psychomotor activity	Increased, reduced, or shifts	Often normal
Speech	Often incoherent; slow or rapid	Often normal
Involuntary movement	Often asterixis or coarse tremor	Rare
Physical illness or drug toxicity	One or both	Rare

Adapted from Lee, L., Weston, W. W., Heckman, G., Gagnon, M., Lee, F. J., Stoke, S. (2013). Structured approach to patients with memory difficulties in family practice. *Canadian Family Physician, 59*(3), 249–254.

and shift attention. Associated cognitive changes include problems in memory, orientation, and language. The patient may not know where he or she is, may not recognize familiar objects, or may be unable to carry on a conversation. Another important diagnostic indicator is that the problem developed during a short period (compared with dementia, which develops gradually) (American Psychiatric Association [APA], 2013). Delirium is different from dementia, but the presenting symptoms are often similar. Impaired alertness, apathy, anxiety, disorientation, and hallucinations commonly occur. Table 37.2 highlights the differences between delirium and dementia.

> **NCLEXNOTE** Delirium and dementia have similar presentations. Because delirium can be life threatening, identifying the potential underlying cause for the symptoms is a priority.

Delirium Across the Lifespan

Children

Delirium can occur in children and may be related to medications (anticholinergic agents), anesthetics, or fever. Children seem to be especially susceptible to this disorder, probably because of their immature brains. Sleep–wake disturbance, fluctuating symptoms, impaired attention, irritability, agitation, mood lability, and confusion are typical symptoms of delirium in children. However, delirium may be hard to diagnose and may be mistaken for uncooperative behavior (Dahmani, Delivet, & Hilly, 2014).

BOX 37.1

Risk Factors for Delirium

Advanced age
Preexisting dementia
Functional dependence
Endocrine and metabolic disorders
Bone fracture
Infection (pneumonia, urinary tract)
Medications (anticholinergic side effects)
Changes in vital signs (including hypotension and hyper- or hypothermia)
Electrolyte or metabolic imbalance (dehydration, renal failure, hyponatremia)
Admission to a long-term care institution
Postcardiotomy
AIDS
Pain
Acute or chronic stress
Substance use and alcohol withdrawal

Older Adults

Although delirium may occur in any age group, it is most common among older adults. In this age group, delirium is often mistaken for dementia, which in turn leads to inappropriate treatment. Patients with delirium have a reduced ability to focus, difficulty in sustaining or shifting attention, changes in cognition, or perceptual disturbances (Mattison et al., 2014).

Epidemiology and Risk Factors

Statistics concerning prevalence are based primarily on older adults in acute care settings. Estimated prevalence rates range from 10% to 50% of patients. Delirium is particularly common in older postoperative patients. In some groups, such as those with dementia, the prevalence may be nearer 90% (Flaherty, 2011).

Preexisting cognitive impairment is one of the greatest risk factors for delirium. Severe illness and age also put patients at higher risk for delirium (Voyer, Richard, Doucet, & Carmichael, 2011). Box 37.1 lists proposed risk factors for delirium, and Box 37.2 presents a vignette of a patient who experienced delirium after using an over-the-counter (OTC) sleeping medication. Box 37.3 addresses stress, which has been shown to be a risk factor in older adults.

Etiology

The etiology of delirium is complex and multifaceted. Because delirium is a fluctuating process, it is difficult to establish its onset or termination. Delirium in the older adult is associated with medications, infections, fluid and electrolyte imbalance, metabolic disturbances, or hypoxia or ischemia. The probability of the syndrome developing increases if certain predisposing factors, such as advanced

BOX 37.2
DELIRIUM

MC, a widowed 72-year-old woman living in her own home, has been having trouble sleeping. Her daughter visits her and suggests that MC try an over-the-counter (OTC) sleeping medication. MC has also been taking antihistamines for allergies and the antidepressant amitriptyline. Three nights later, a neighbor calls the daughter, concerned because she encountered MC wandering the streets, unable to find her home. When the neighbor approached MC to help her home, MC began to scream and strike out at the neighbor.

The daughter visits immediately and discovers that her mother does not know who she is, does not know what time it is, appears disheveled, and is suspicious that people have been in her home stealing the things she cannot find. MC does not recall taking any medication, but when her daughter investigates, she finds that 10 pills of the new sleeping aid have already been used. MC is irritable and refuses to go to the hospital, but over the course of a few hours, she appears to calm down, and her daughter is able to take her to see her doctor the next morning. After hearing the history, the doctor hospitalizes MC, withholds all medication, and provides intravenous hydration. Within 3 days, MC is again able to recognize her daughter, and her mental status appears to be greatly improved.

What Do You Think?
- Identify risk factors that may have contributed to MC's experiencing delirium.
- How could the addition of an OTC sleeping medication interact with the antihistamine and antidepressant to be responsible for MC's delirium?

BOX 37.3

Research For Best Practice: **Stress and Delirium in the Older Adult**

Rigney, T. (2010). Allostatic load and delirium in the hospitalized older adult. Nursing Research, 59(5), 322–330.

THE QUESTION: Is there a relationship between allostatic load (AL) and delirium in the hospitalized adult.

METHODS: Participants age 65 years and older admitted to the hospital were measured on ten parameters reflecting physiological activity across a range of regulatory systems. Separate scores were calculated for subsets of AL. Incident delirium was assessed 48 to 72 hours after admission.

FINDINGS: The incidence of delirium was 29%. The AL score derived from primary mediators, urinary cortisol, epinephrine and norepinephrine, and dehydroepiandrosterone sulfate predicted the incidence of delirium. The overall AL score were not related significantly to the incidence of delirium.

IMPLICATIONS FOR NURSING: Physiological changes may predict the development of delirium. Identifying predisposing factors such as evidence of acute or chronic stress may help prevent delirium.

---

age, brain damage, or dementia, are also present. Sensory overload or underload, immobilization, sleep deprivation, and psychosocial stress also contribute to delirium (Flaherty, 2011).

Because delirium has multiple causes, a wide variety of brain alterations may also be responsible for its development. Delirium may result from a neuroanatomic abnormality such as stroke, but the majority of cases are caused by an imbalance of key neurochemicals such as dopamine, serotonin, cortisol, acetylcholine (Ach), glutamate, and gamma-aminobutyric acid (GABA) (Caplan & Rabinowitz, 2010).

Interdisciplinary Treatment

Although delirium may be recognized and diagnosed in any health care setting, appropriate intervention usually requires that the patient be admitted to an acute care setting for rigorous assessment and rapid treatment. Priority in care is identifying the underlying cause of the delirium.

Interdisciplinary management of delirium includes two primary aspects: (1) elimination or correction of the underlying cause and (2) symptomatic and supportive measures (e.g., adequate rest, comfort, maintenance of fluid and electrolyte balance, and protection from injury).

Priority Care Issues

When developing a treatment plan for a patient in whom delirium is suspected, close attention must be paid to correcting any organic or disease-related factors. If possible, the use of all suspected medications should be stopped and vital signs monitored at least every 2 hours. Close observation of the patient with particular regard to changes in vital signs, behavior, and mental status is required. Patients are monitored until the delirium subsides or until discharge. If the delirium still exists at discharge, it is critical that referrals for postdischarge follow-up assessment and care be implemented.

NURSING MANAGEMENT: Human Response to Delirium

The best management is prevention or early recognition of delirium. If the patient is a child, the assessment process presented in Chapter 34 should be used. If the patient is an older adult, the assessment in Chapter 36 should serve as a guide. Special efforts should be made to include family members in the nursing process.

Biologic Domain

Assessment

The onset of symptoms is typically signaled by a rapid or acute change in behavior. Assessing the symptoms first requires knowing what is normal for the individual. Caregivers, family members, or significant others should be interviewed because they can often provide valuable information. Family members may be the only resource for accurate information.

Current and Past Health Status

History should include a description of the onset, duration, range, and intensity of associated symptoms. Chronic physical illness, dementia, depression, or other psychiatric illnesses should be identified. Sorting out historic information may be particularly problematic when delirium accompanies acute illness, recent surgery, or infection.

Physical Examination and Review of Systems

If the patient is cooperative, a physical examination will be conducted in the ED. Vital signs are crucial. A review of systems must be conducted in each patient suspected of having delirium or other organic mental disorders. Laboratory data, including a complete blood count, glucose, blood urea nitrogen, creatinine, and electrolyte analyses; liver function and oxygen saturation; fluid balance; signs of constipation; or a recent history of diarrhea, should be assessed in an attempt to discover an underlying cause.

Physical Functions

Functional assessment includes physical functional status (activities of daily living [ADLs]), use of sensory aids (eyeglasses and hearing aids), usual activity level and any recent changes, and pain assessment. Because sleep is often disturbed in patients with delirium, sleep patterns must be assessed, including what is typical for the individual and recent changes. Often, the sleep–wake cycle of the patient with delirium becomes reversed, with the individual attempting to sleep during the day and being awake at night. Sleep disturbances are a symptom of delirium, and sleep deprivation may add to the confusion. Restoration of a normal sleep cycle is extremely important.

Pharmacologic Assessment

A substance use history (including alcohol intake and smoking history) should be obtained (see Chapters 31 and 36). In addition, information regarding medication use must be obtained, with particular attention given to new medications or changes in dose of current medications. Table 37.3 lists some of the drugs that can cause delirium. Special attention should be given to combinations of

Table 37.3	EXAMPLES OF DRUGS THAT CAN CAUSE DELIRIUM
Class	**Specific Drugs**
Anticholinergic	Antihistamines
	Chlorpheniramine
	Antiparkinsonian drugs (e.g., benztropine [Cogentin], biperiden [Akineton], or trihexyphenidyl)
	Atropine
	Belladonna alkaloids
	Diphenhydramine
	Phenothiazines
	Promethazine
	Scopolamine
	Tricyclic antidepressants
Anticonvulsant	Phenobarbital
	Phenytoin (Dilantin)
	Sodium valproate (Depakene)
Antiinflammatory	Corticosteroids
	Ibuprofen (Motrin and Advil)
	Indomethacin (Indocin)
	Naproxen (Naprosyn)
Antiparkinsonian	Amantadine
	Carbidopa (Sinemet)
Anti-inflammatory	Levodopa (Larodopa)
	Isoniazid
	Rifampin
Analgesic	Opioids
	Salicylates
	Synthetic narcotics
Cardiac	β-Blockers
	Propranolol (Inderal)
	Clonidine (Catapres)
	Digitalis (Digoxin and Lanoxin)
	Lidocaine (Xylocaine)
	Methyldopa (Aldomet)
	Quinidine
	Procainamide (Pronestyl)
Sedative–hypnotic	Barbiturates
	Benzodiazepines
Sympathomimetic	Amphetamines
	Phenylephrine
	Phenylpropanolamine
Over-the-counter medications	Compoz
	Excedrin PM
	Sleep-Eze
	Sominex
Miscellaneous	Acyclovir (antiviral)
	Aminophylline
	Amphotericin (antifungal)
	Bromides
	Cephalexin (Keflex)
	Chlorpropamide (Diabinese)
	Cimetidine (Tagamet)
	Disulfiram (Antabuse)
	Lithium
	Metronidazole (Flagyl)
	Theophylline
	timolol ophthalmic

Source: Wynn, G. H., Oesterheid, J. R., Cozza, K. I., Armstrong, S. C. (2009). *Clinical Manual of Drug Interaction: Principles for Medical Practice*. Arlington, VA: American Psychiatric Publishing, Inc.

these medications because drug interactions can cause delirium.

Information regarding OTC medications should be included in this assessment. OTC medications are often thought of as harmless, but several, such as cold medications, taken in sufficient quantities may produce confusion, especially in older adults.

Findings from the medication assessment are integrated with findings of the physical assessment, including such things as fluid and electrolyte balance, lack of adequate pain management, or serum drug levels, if available. For example, chronic pain may lead an individual to use more medication for pain relief than has been intended. Careful monitoring of the effectiveness of pain medications may lead to the use of a different medication that is more effective with less potential for misuse. Because many classes of medications have been associated with delirium, the focus is on changes in the type and number of medications and how medications relate to other findings in the history and physical assessment.

Nursing Diagnoses for the Biologic Domain

The nursing diagnoses typically generated from assessment data are Acute Confusion, Disturbed Thought Processes, or Disturbed Sensory Perception (visual or auditory). However, an astute nurse will also use nursing diagnoses based on other indicators, such as Hyperthermia, Acute Pain, Risk for Infection, and Insomnia.

Interventions for the Biologic Domain

Important interventions for a patient experiencing an acute confusional state include providing a safe and therapeutic environment; maintaining fluid and electrolyte balance and adequate nutrition; and preventing aspiration and decubitus ulcers, which are often complications. Other interventions relate to a particular nursing diagnosis focused on individual symptoms and underlying causes (e.g., for patients with Insomnia, the Sleep Enhancement intervention is appropriate).

Safety Interventions

Behaviors exhibited by the delirious patient, such as hallucinations, delusions, illusions, aggression, or agitation (restlessness or excitability), may pose safety problems. The patient must be protected from physical harm by using low beds, guardrails, and careful supervision. Delirium management and fall prevention may be implemented for any patient at risk for falls.

Pharmacologic Interventions

No pharmacological agent is approved by the FDA for the treatment of delirium. The goal of psychopharmaco-logic management is treatment of the behaviors associated with delirium, such as symptoms of agitation, inattention, sleep disorder, and psychosis, so that the patient can be more comfortable. The decision to use medications should be based on the specific symptoms. Dosages are usually kept very low, especially with older adults. There is no consensus on the use of psychopharmacologic agents to control the symptoms of delirium, and limited studies have been conducted. Use of these medications usually relates to agitation, combativeness, or hallucinations. However, medication should be chosen in light of the potential side effects (particularly anticholinergic effects, hypotension, and respiratory suppression) and in light of making the delirium worse. There may be a limited role for antipsychotics for use among a targeted group of patients who experience hallucinations or delusions associated with delirium (Flaherty, 2011). If used, antipsychotics should be given to an "awake" patient, not one who is sedated. Benzodiazepines are also used when the delirium is related to alcohol withdrawal. In some patients, benzodiazepines may further impair cognition because of the sedation. Also, in some cases, a paradoxical agitation may develop.

Administering Medications
Patients experiencing delirium may resist taking medication because of their confusion. If medication is given, ideally, it should be oral.

Monitoring Medications and Managing Side Effects
Monitoring drug action and side effects is especially important because the cause of the delirium may not be known, and the patient may inadvertently be affected by the medication. Patients should be monitored for sedation, hypotension, or extrapyramidal symptoms. Although mental status often fluctuates during delirium, it may also be influenced by these medications, and any changes or worsening of mental status after administration of the medication should be reported immediately to the prescriber. Some side effects may also be confused with the symptoms of delirium. For example, akathisia (see Chapter 11), a side effect of antipsychotics, may appear as agitation or restlessness. The patient's physical condition and concurrent medication regimen may also influence the bioavailability, metabolism, and elimination of these medications. Adequate hydration and nutrition must be maintained. When using antipsychotic medications, closely monitor the patient for symptoms of neuroleptic malignant syndrome (see Chapter 11). The appearance of these symptoms may be missed because many may be confused with those related to delirium.

Finally, the use of antipsychotic agents or other medications for treating symptoms related to delirium should be discontinued as soon as possible. These medications should not be stopped abruptly but rather withdrawn gradually during a period of several days or weeks.

Monitoring for Drug Interactions

The etiology of delirium is often a drug–drug interaction. OTC sleeping, cold, or allergy medications may be the cause. If medication is the underlying cause, it is important to identify accurately which medications are involved before administering any other drugs. A consultation with a clinical pharmacist may also be helpful.

Teaching Points

To prevent future occurrences, provide education to the patient and family about the underlying cause of the delirium. If the delirium is not resolved before discharge, family members need to know how to care for the patient at home.

Psychological Domain

Assessment

Psychological assessment of the individual with delirium focuses on cognitive changes revealed through the mental status examination as well as the resulting behavioral manifestations. Changes in mental status must be monitored frequently for early detection of delirium, especially in older patients. In addition, other factors, such as stressors and environmental changes, may contribute to the symptoms.

Mental Status

Rapid onset of global cognitive impairment that affects multiple aspects of intellectual functioning is the hallmark of delirium. Mental status evaluation reveals several changes:

- Fluctuations in level of consciousness with reduced awareness of the environment
- Difficulty focusing and sustaining or shifting attention
- Severely impaired memory, especially immediate and recent memory

Patients may be disorientated to time and place but rarely to person. Environmental perceptions are often disturbed. The patient may believe shadows in the room are really people. Thought content is often illogical, and speech may be incoherent or inappropriate to the context. Mental status tends to fluctuate over the course of the day. During the same day, an individual with delirium may appear confused and uncooperative, but later, that person may be lucid and able to follow instructions. The cognitive status of the individual must be continually assessed throughout the day so that interventions may be modified accordingly. Whereas calculations, orientation (especially to time), and recall are most

affected in delirium, naming and registration are relatively preserved.

Behavior

Delirious patients exhibit a wide range of behaviors, complicating the process of making a diagnosis and planning interventions. At times, the individual may be restless or agitated and at other times lethargic and slow to respond. Delirium can be categorized into three types.

- **Hyperkinetic delirium** involves behaviors most commonly recognized as delirium (e.g., psychomotor hyperactivity, marked excitability, and a tendency toward hallucinations).
- **Hypokinetic delirium** is marked by lethargy, sleepiness, and apathy and a decrease in psychomotor activity; this is the "quiet" patient for whom the diagnosis of delirium often is missed.
- **Mixed variant delirium** involves behavior that fluctuates between the hyperactive and hypoactive states.

Nursing Diagnoses for the Psychological Domain

The nursing diagnosis Acute Confusion is also associated with impaired cognitive functioning. Although the underlying cause of confusion is physiologic, nursing care should focus on the psychological domain as well as the physical. Other typical nursing diagnoses related to the psychological domain include Disturbed Thought Process, Ineffective Coping, and Disturbed Personal Identity.

Interventions for the Psychological Domain

Patients with delirium need frequent interaction and support if they are confused or hallucinating. Patients should be encouraged to express their fears and discomforts that result from frightening or disconcerting psychotic experiences. Adequate lighting, easy-to-read calendars and clocks, a reasonable noise level, and frequent verbal orientation may reduce this frightening experience. If the patient wears eyeglasses or uses a hearing aid, these devices should be used. Including familiar personal possessions in the environment may also help. Interventions that may be useful for these individuals are discussed in detail later in the chapter (see the section on dementia).

Social Domain

Assessment

Discussion should be initiated with the family to determine whether the patient's behaviors are new. An assessment of living arrangements may provide information about sensory stimulation or social isolation. Cultural and educational background must be considered when the patient's mental capacity is evaluated. Individuals from certain ethnic backgrounds may not be familiar with the information used in tests of general knowledge (e.g., names of presidents, geographic knowledge) and memory (e.g., date of birth in cultures that do not routinely celebrate birthdays). Some cultural practices may involve using substances such as elixirs that contain chemicals that may exacerbate delirium. Assessment should address these practices. Assessing family interactions, support for the patient, and family members' ability to understand delirium is also important. The behaviors exhibited by the person experiencing delirium may be frightening or at least confusing for family members. Some family members may actually contribute to the patient's increased agitation. At the same time, if feasible, the family's presence may help to calm and reassure the patient.

Nursing Diagnoses for the Social Domain

Several nursing diagnoses associated with the social domain can be generated. Interrupted Family Processes, Ineffective Protection, Ineffective Role Performance, and Risk for Injury are the most typical. Risk for Injury is a high-priority diagnosis because individuals with delirium are more likely to fall or injure themselves during a confused state.

Interventions for the Social Domain

A safe environment is important to protect the patient from injury. A predictable, orienting environment will help to reestablish order to the patient's life. That is, a calendar, clocks, and other items may be provided to help orient the patient to time, place, and person. If the patient is agitated, de-escalation techniques should be used (see Chapters 10 and 19). Physical restraint should be avoided.

Families can also be encouraged to work with staff to reorient the patient and provide a supportive environment. Families need to understand that important decisions requiring the patient's input should be delayed if at all possible until the patient has recovered. Although patients may be able to participate in decision making, they may not remember the decision later; therefore, it is important to have several witnesses present.

Evaluation and Treatment Outcomes

The primary treatment goal is prevention or resolution of the delirious episode with return to previous cognitive status. Outcome measures include

---

> ## BOX 37.4
> ### *Psychoeducation Checklist:* **Delirium**
>
> When caring for the patient with delirium, be sure to include the caregivers, as appropriate, and address the following topic areas in the teaching plan:
>
> - Psychopharmacologic agents, if used, including drug action, dosage, frequency, and possible adverse effects
> - Underlying cause of delirium
> - Mental status changes
> - Safety measures
> - Hydration and nutrition
> - Avoidance of restraints
> - Decision-making guidelines

- Correction of the underlying physiologic alteration
- Resolution of confusion
- Family member verbalization of understanding of confusion
- Prevention of injury

Resolution of confusion is the primary goal; however, the nursing care provided makes important contributions to all four of these outcomes. The end result of delirium may be full recovery, incomplete recovery, incomplete recovery with some residual cognitive impairment, or a downward course leading to death.

Continuum of Care

Patients with delirium may present in a number of treatment settings (e.g., home, nursing home, ambulatory care, day treatment, outpatient setting, hospital). Patients usually are admitted to an acute care setting for rapid evaluation and treatment of the underlying etiology. An abrupt change in cognitive status can also occur while the patient is hospitalized for another reason. Delirium often persists beyond discharge from the hospital. Discharge planning should routinely include family education and referrals to community health care providers. If the patient will return to a residential long-term care setting, communication with facility staff about the patient's hospital stay and treatment regimen is crucial. For more information on caring for patients with delirium, see Box 37.4.

ALZHEIMER'S DISEASE
Clinical Course

Alzheimer's Disease (AD) is a degenerative, progressive neuropsychiatric disorder that results in cognitive impairment, emotional and behavioral changes, physical and functional decline, and ultimately death. Gradually, the patient's ability to carry out ADLs declines, although physical status often remains intact until late in the

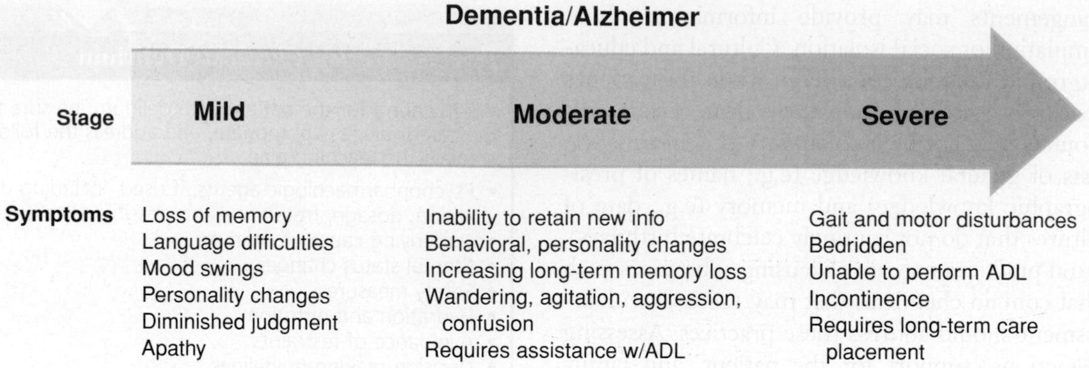

Dementia/Alzheimer

Stage	Mild	Moderate	Severe
Symptoms	Loss of memory Language difficulties Mood swings Personality changes Diminished judgment Apathy	Inability to retain new info Behavioral, personality changes Increasing long-term memory loss Wandering, agitation, aggression, confusion Requires assistance w/ADL	Gait and motor disturbances Bedridden Unable to perform ADL Incontinence Requires long-term care placement

FIGURE 37.1 Alzheimer's disease progression.

disease. Primarily a disorder of older adults, AD has been diagnosed in patients as young as age 35 years.

Two subtypes have been identified: early onset AD (age 65 years and younger) and late onset AD (age older than 65 years). Late-onset AD is much more common than early-onset AD, but early-onset AD has a more rapid progression. AD is also routinely conceptualized in terms of three stages: mild, moderate, and severe. Signs and symptoms of AD change as the patient passes from one phase of the illness to another (Figure 37.1). It is unclear whether all patients with AD pass through a specific sequence of deterioration and whether the staging of a patient at initial assessment has any prognostic implications in terms of speed of decline. Nevertheless, staging is a useful technique for determining the patient's current cognitive status and provides a sound basis for decisions in clinical management.

Diagnostic Criteria

The diagnosis of AD is made on clinical grounds, and verification is confirmed at autopsy by abnormal degenerative structures, neuritic plaques, and neurofibrillary tangles. The essential feature of AD is cognitive decline from a previous level of functioning in one or more cognitive domains (attention, executive function, learning and memory, language, perceptual-motor or social cognition) (APA, 2013). These deficits interfere with independence in daily activities. Typical deficits include **aphasia** (alterations in language ability), **apraxia** (impaired ability to execute motor activities despite intact motor functioning), **agnosia** (failure to recognize or identify objects despite intact sensory function), or a **disturbance of executive functioning** (ability to think abstractly, plan, initiate, sequence, monitor, and stop complex behavior).

Mild neurocognitive impairment (MCI) is diagnosed if there is a modest cognitive decline from a previous level of function in one or more of the cognitive domains, but the cognitive deficits do not interfere with independence in daily activities (APA, 2013). MCI is thought to be related to multiple causes and some, but not all, progress to AD (Desai & Schwarz, 2011).

Epidemiology and Risk Factors

In 2014, an estimated 5.2 million Americans had AD, one in nine older than 65 years old, and conservative projections estimate that by the year 2025, the number of cases of AD in the United States will be 7.1 million. Almost two thirds of Americans with AD are women. Dementia appears to affect all groups, but studies in the United States reveal a higher incidence in African Americans and Latinos than in whites. Currently, AD is the fifth leading cause of death among older adults in the United States (Alzheimer's Association, 2014a).

AD can run in families. Compared with the general population, first-degree biologic relatives of individuals with early-onset AD are more likely to experience the disorder. So far, studies point toward genetically related risk factors only in familial AD, which accounts for only a small proportion of cases of AD (less than 5%). The hypothesis that low educational level may increase the risk for AD remains a matter of controversy. Studies show that those with fewer years of education or those who have had a prior head injury are at higher risk of developing dementia (U.S. Department of Health and Human Services [USDHHS], 2014).

Etiology

Researchers have yet to identify a definitive cause of AD, but a combination of genetic, environmental, and lifestyle factors influence a person's risk for developing the disease. In general, the brain appears normal in the early phases of AD, but it undergoes widespread atrophy as the disease advances (USDHHS, 2014).

Beta-amyloid Plaques

One piece of the puzzle is partially explained by a leading theory that, in AD, **beta-amyloid plaques**, made up of proteins that clump together in the brain, destroy cholinergic neurons, in a manner similar to cholesterol causing atherosclerosis. Beta-amyloid is hypothesized to interfere with the process of storing memories through interrupting synaptic connection. There is also evidence that beta-amyloid is responsible for dendritic spine collapse. Neuritic plaque densities are highest in the temporal and occipital lobes, intermediate in the parietal lobes, and lowest in the frontal and limbic cortex. Symptoms such as aphasia and visuospatial abnormalities are attributable to plaque formation (USDHHS, 2011).

Current research suggests that beta-amyloid accumulate due to its overproduction or underclearance and that alterations in beta-amyloid (Aβ) may initiate the disease onset. There is evidence that **amyloidosis**, accumulation of amyloid, occurs 15 to 25 years before clinical symptoms are detected (Bateman et al., 2012). Brain imaging shows an accumulation of amyloid deposit and analyses of cerebrospinal fluid shows a decline in Aβ concentration supporting the hypothesis that there are alterations in Aβ processing that leads to Alzheimer's. This line of research is especially important because it can result in biomarkers that can be used to develop early diagnosis and new therapeutic treatments.

Neurofibrillary Tangles

Neurofibrillary tangles are made of abnormally twisted protein threads found inside the cells. The main compo-
nent of the tangles is a protein called **tau**. A healthy neuron is supported by structures of microtubules that help transport nutrients and other substances from the body of the cell to ends of the axon and back. Tau helps stabilize the microtubules. In AD, tau separates from the microtubules because excess phosphate molecules have attached to it resulting in a phosphorylation process. Loose tau proteins tangle with each other, causing the characteristic neurofibrillary tangles. The microtubules disintegrate, and the neuron's transport system collapses, resulting in cell death. The neurofibrillary tangles are initially found in the limbic area and then progress to the cortex. Neurofibrillary tangles contribute to memory disturbance and psychiatric symptoms (USDHHS, 2014) (Figure 37.2).

Cell Death and Neurotransmitters

In patients with AD, neurotransmission is reduced, neurons are lost, and the hippocampal neurons degenerate. Several major neurotransmitters are affected. **Acetylcholine (ACh)** is associated with cognitive functioning, and disruption of cholinergic mechanisms damages memory in animals and humans (see Chapter 8). Cell loss in the nucleus basalis leads to deficits in the synthesis of cortical Ach, but the number of ACh receptors is relatively unchanged. The reduced ACh is related to a

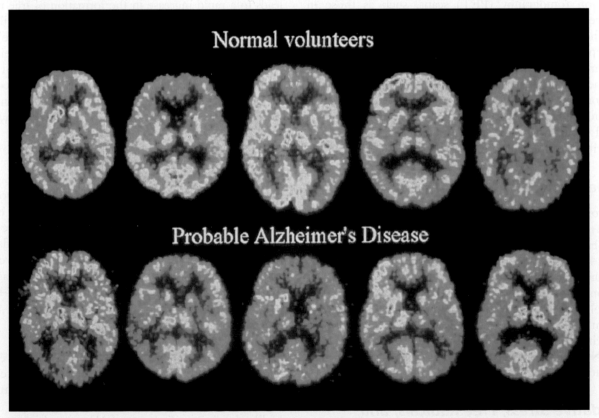

FIGURE 37.2 Series comparison of elderly control subjects (*top row*) and patients with Alzheimer's disease (AD) (*bottom row*). Although some decreases in metabolism are associated with age, in most patients with AD, there are marked decreases in the temporal lobe, an area important in memory functions. (Courtesy of Monte S. Buchsbaum, MD, The Mount Sinai Medical Center and School of Medicine, New York.)

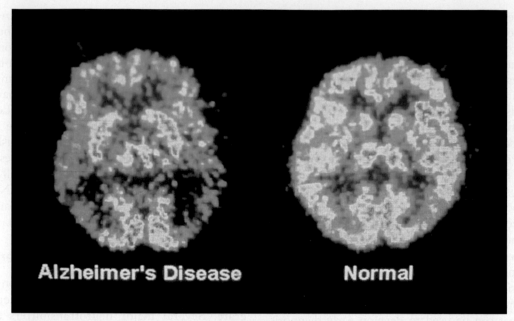

FIGURE 37.3 Metabolic activity in a subject with Alzheimer's disease (*left*) and control subject without AD (*right*). (Courtesy of Monte S. Buchsbaum, MD, The Mount Sinai Medical Center and School of Medicine, New York.)

decrease in choline acetyltransferase (a critical enzyme in the synthesis of ACh), especially in the forebrain. That is, there are fewer enzymes available to synthesize ACh, which leads to a reduction in cholinergic activity. Positron emission tomography (PET) scans, such as those in Figure 37.3, show changes in brain function.

Other neurotransmitters that are affected include norepinephrine and serotonin. Deficiencies in norepinephrine are associated with loss of cells in the locus ceruleus, and neuronal loss in the raphe nuclei leads to a loss of serotonergic activity. Other brain changes in AD include inflammation and degeneration of the brain cells that could occur in response to the neuronal malfunction or contribute to the pathology (USDHHS, 2014).

Genetic Factors

Approximately half of the cases of early-onset AD appear to be transmitted as a pure genetic, autosomal dominant trait caused by mutations in genes on chromosomes 1 and 14 (USDHHS, 2014). Mutations on chromosome 14 account for most cases of early-onset familial AD. Chromosome 21 is also associated with AD because amyloid plaques and neurofibrillary tangles accumulate consistently in older people with Down syndrome (trisomy 21) who have AD. Mutations in one of three genes (APP, PSEN1, and PSEN2) have been identified that cause alteration in the Aβ processing (Bateman et al., 2012).

Oxidative Stress, Free Radicals, and Mitochondrial Dysfunction

Oxidative stress and mitochondrial dysfunction are being studied as factors in the development of AD. The mito-

chondria, the power plants for the cell, provide the energy a cell needs to carry out its functions. It is hypothesized that in AD brains, beta-amyloid prevents the normal functioning of the mitochondria. Damage to the mitochondria leads to a rapid increase in the formation of free radicals (highly reactive molecules). If unchecked, the buildup of these free radical molecules can lead to **oxidative stress** that damages other cellular molecules such as proteins, lipids, and nucleic acid. Recently studies suggest that oxidative stress may result in changes in chromatin, (a complex of DNA and proteins) which may lead to dysfunctional gene expression (Frost, Hembuerg, Lewis, & Feany, 2014).

Inflammation

Inflammation in the brain was considered one of the causes of dementia, but research failed to support this hypothesis. Today, inflammation is again being considered as one of many factors that contribute to the development of dementia. The hypothesis is that inflammation may damage small blood vessels, initiating a cascade of pathological events related to oxidative damage and dysregulated amyloid metabolism (Marchesi, 2014).

Family Response to Disorder

Families are the first to be aware of the cognitive problem, often before the patient, who can be unaware of the extent of memory impairment. When finally confirmed, the actual diagnosis can be devastating to the family. Unlike delirium, a diagnosis of AD means long-term care responsibilities while the essence of a family member diminishes day by day. Most families keep their relative at home as long as possible to maintain contact and to avoid costly nursing home placement. The two symptoms that often result in nursing home placement are incontinence that cannot be managed and behavioral problems, such as wandering and aggression.

Especially in dementia, the needs of family members should also be considered. Caring for a family member with dementia takes its toll. Eighty percent of the home care is provided by family caregivers. Most of the caregivers are women (65%), and 21% are over the age of 65 years or older. Caregivers' health often declines and directly affects their ability to provide care (Alzheimer's Association, 2014a).

Interdisciplinary Treatment

In designing services and interventions, the interdisciplinary team must keep in mind that AD has a progressively deteriorating clinical course and that the anatomic and neurochemical changes that occur in the brain are accompanied by impairments in cognition, sensorium, affect (facial expression representing mood), behavior, and psychosocial functioning. The nature and range of services needed by patients and families throughout the illness can vary dramatically at different stages.

Initial assessment of the patient suspected of having dementia has three main objectives: (1) confirmation of the diagnosis, (2) establishment of baseline levels in a number of functional spheres, and (3) establishment of a therapeutic relationship with the patient and family that will continue through subsequent phases of the disease. Treatment efforts currently focus on managing the cognitive symptoms, delaying the cognitive decline (e.g., memory loss; confusion; and problems with learning, speech, and reasoning), treating the noncognitive symptoms (e.g., psychosis, mood symptoms, agitation), and supporting the caregivers as a means of improving the quality of life for both patients and their caregivers.

Priority Care Issues

The priority of care changes throughout the course of AD. Initially, the priority is delaying cognitive decline and supporting family members. Later, the priority is protecting the patient from injury because of lack of judgment. Near the end, the physical needs of the patient are the focus of care.

NURSING MANAGEMENT: Human Response to Alzheimer's Disease

The development and implementation of appropriate, effective, and safe nursing services for the care and support of patients with dementia and their families is a particular challenge because of the complex nature of the illness. Although AD is caused by biologic changes, the psychological and social domains are seriously affected

by this disorder. The assessment of the patient with AD should follow the geropsychiatric nursing assessment in Chapter 36.

> **NCLEXNOTE** Needs and problematic behaviors of patients with dementia vary throughout the course of the disorder. Early in the disorder, the nurse focuses on support, education, and cognitive interventions for depression. As the dementia progresses, priority care becomes safety interventions.

Biologic Domain

Assessment

The nursing assessment should include a medical history; current medication profile (prescription and OTC medications or home remedies); substance abuse history (including alcohol intake and smoking history); chronic physical or psychiatric illness; and a description of the onset, duration, range, and intensity of symptoms associated with dementia. The onset of symptoms in dementia is typically gradual, with insidious changes in behavior. To conduct a thorough assessment of the patient with dementia, the nurse needs to know what is typical for the individual; therefore, caregivers, family members, or significant others can be sources of valuable information.

Physical Examination and Review of Systems

A review of body systems must be conducted on each patient suspected of having dementia. Specific biologic assessment parameters for a patient with dementia include vital signs, neurologic status, nutritional status, bladder and bowel function, hygiene (including oral hygiene), skin integrity, rest and activity level, sleep patterns, and fluid and electrolyte balance. The neurologic function of the patient with AD is usually preserved through the early and middle stages of the disease, although seizures, gait disturbances, and tremors may occur at any time. In the later stages of the disease, neurologic signs, such as flexion contractures and primitive reflexes, are prominent features.

Physical Functions

At first, limitations may primarily involve instrumental activities, such as shopping, preparing meals, and performing other household chores. Later in the disease process, basic physical dysfunctions occur, such as incontinence, ataxia, dysphagia, and contractures. Incontinence can be a major source of stress and a considerable burden to family caregivers. Evaluation of the patient's functional abilities includes bathing, dressing, toileting, feeding, nutritional status, physical mobility, sleep patterns, and pain.

Assessment of physical functions includes ADLs, recent changes in functional abilities, use of sensory aids (glasses and hearing aids), activity level, and assessment of pain. Eyeglasses and hearing aids may need to be in place before other assessments can be made.

Self-Care

Alterations in the central nervous system (CNS) associated with dementia impair the patient's ability to collect information from the environment, retrieve memories, retain new information, and give meaning to current situations. Therefore, patients with dementia often neglect self-care activities. Periodically, biologic assessment parameters need to be reevaluated because patients with dementia may neglect activities such as bathing, eating, or skin care.

Sleep–Wake Disturbances

A variety of sleep disturbances occur in AD, such as waking up during the night, being drowsy during the day, and restless sleep. Recent evidence suggests that there is a relationship between amyloid and chronic sleep deprivation (Rothman & Mattson 2012). There is a deterioration of the circadian sleep–wake patterns. Neurotransmitter dysregulation of melatonin in the pineal gland is thought to be one of the contributing factors to the sleep disturbance. Additionally, delays in the circadian phase of core body temperature also occur. Patients with dementia have frequent daytime napping and nighttime periods of wakefulness, with little rapid eye movement (REM) sleep. Lowered levels of REM sleep are associated with restlessness, irritability, and general sleep impairment (Garcia-Alberca, Lara, Cruz, Garrido, Gris, & Barbancho, 2013).

Activity and Exercise

One of the earliest symptoms of AD is withdrawal from normal activities. Motor activity is affected in the mild stages of AD and can lead to early problems in functional performance (Alzheimer's Association, 2014a). As the disease progresses, the patient may just sit staring at a blank wall.

Nutrition

Eating can become a problem for a patient with dementia and is associated with rapid cognitive decline (Soto et al, 2012; Gomes, Martins, Fonseca, Oliveira, Resende, & Pereira, 2014). As the disease progresses, patients may lose the ability to feed themselves or recognize what is offered as food. Some patients with dementia are bulimic or hyperoral (eating or chewing almost everything possible and sometimes with an insatiable appetite). Other patients with dementia experience anorexia and have no appetite.

Pain

Assessment and documentation of any physical discomfort or pain the patient may be experiencing is a part of any geropsychiatric nursing assessment (see Chapter 36). Although AD is not usually thought of as a physically painful disorder, patients often have other comorbid physical diseases that may be painful. In the early stages of AD, the patient can usually respond to verbal questions regarding pain. Later, it may be difficult to assess objectively the comfort level, especially if the patient cannot communicate. Some patients in the end stage of dementia become hypersensitive to touch.

Pain can be assessed by obtaining vital signs, completing a physical assessment, and using one of the pain assessment scales. Sometimes laboratory tests must be conducted to help identify the source of discomfort. Subtle behavioral changes, such as lethargy, anxiety, or restlessness, or more obvious physical signs, such as pyrexia, tachypnea, or tachycardia, may be the only indications of actual or impending illness. Observing for changes in patterns of nonverbal communication, such as facial expressions, may help in identifying indicators of pain. Hypervocalizations (disturbed vocalizations), restlessness, and agitation are other possible signs of pain.

Nursing Diagnoses for the Biologic Domain

The unique and changing needs of these patients present a challenge for nurses in all settings. A multitude of potential nursing diagnoses focusing on the biologic domain can be identified for this population. A sample of common nursing diagnoses include Imbalanced Nutrition: Less (or More) Than Body Requirements; Feeding Self-Care Deficit; Impaired Swallowing; Bathing/Hygiene Self-Care Deficit; Dressing/Grooming Self-Care Deficit; Toileting Self-Care Deficit; Constipation (or Perceived Constipation); Bowel Incontinence; Impaired Urinary Elimination; Functional Incontinence; Total Incontinence; Deficient Fluid Volume; Risk for Impaired Skin Integrity; Impaired Physical Mobility; Activity Intolerance; Fatigue; Insomnia; Pain; Chronic Pain; Ineffective Health Maintenance; and Impaired Home Maintenance.

Interventions for the Biologic Domain

The numerous interventions for the biologic domain vary throughout the course of the disorder. Initially, the patient requires simple directions for self-care activities and initiation of psychopharmacologic treatment. At the end of the disorder, total patient care is required.

Self-Care Interventions

Patients should be encouraged to maintain as much self-care as possible. Promotion of self-care supports cognitive functioning and a sense of independence. In the early stages, the nurse should maximize normal perceptual experiences by making sure that the patient and family have appropriate eyeglasses and working hearing aids. If eyeglasses and hearing aids are needed but not used, patients are more likely to have false perceptual experiences (hallucinations). Ongoing monitoring of self-care is necessary throughout the course of AD. Oral hygiene can be a problem and requires excellent basic nursing care. Aging and many medications reduce salivary flow, which can lead to a painfully dry and cracking oral mucosa. Drugs that have xerostomia (dry mouth) as a side effect and are commonly prescribed for patients with progressive dementia include antidepressant, antispasmodic, antihypertensive, bronchodilator, and some antipsychotic agents. For patients with xerostomia, hard candy or chewing gum may stimulate salivary flow or modification of the drug regimen may be necessary. Glycerol mouthwash can provide as much relief from xerostomia as artificial saliva.

During later stages of dementia, bathing can be problematic for the patient and nursing staff. Bath time is a high-risk time for agitation and aggression (Whall, Hyojeong, Colling, Gwi-Ryung, DeCicco, & Antonakos, 2013). The person-centered approach focuses on personalizing care to meet residents' needs, accommodating to residents' preferences, attending to the relationship and interaction with the resident, using effective communication and interpersonal skills, and adapting the physical environment and bathing procedures to decrease stress and discomfort (Fortinsky & Downs, 2014). See Box 37.5.

Supporting Bowel and Bladder Function

Urinary or bowel incontinence affects many patients with dementia. During the middle phases of the disease, incontinence may be caused by the patient's inability to communicate the need to use the toilet or locate a toilet quickly, undress appropriately to use the toilet, recognize the sensation of fullness signaling the need to urinate or defecate, or apathy with lack of motivation to remain continent.

For the patient who is incontinent because of an inability to locate the toilet, orientation may be helpful. Signs and active training should help to modify disorientation. Displaying pictures or signs on bathroom doors provides visual cues; words should use appropriate terminology.

If the patient cannot recognize the need to void because of impaired sensory perception of fullness, increasing fluid intake can help to fill the bladder sufficiently to give a clear message of the need to urinate. In addition, getting to know the patient's habits and moods can help in identifying signals that indicate a need to void. The

BOX 37.5

Research For Best Practice: **Effects of Two Bathing Interventions**

Hoeffer, B., Talerico, K. A., Rasin, J., Mitchell, C. M., Stewart, B. J., McKenzie, D., Barrick, A. L., Rader, J., & Sloane, P. D. (2006). Assisting cognitively impaired nursing home residents with bathing: Effects of two bathing interventions on caregiving. Gerontologist, 46(4), 524–532.

THE QUESTION: Do certified nursing assistants (CNAs) who receive training in a person-centered approach with showering and with towel baths show improved caregiving behaviors (gentleness and verbal support) and experience greater preparedness (confidence and ease) and less distress (hassles) when assisting residents with bathing?

METHODS: Researchers used a crossover design and randomized 15 nursing homes into two treatment groups and a control group of five facilities each. In one treatment group, CNAs received person-centered training (showering for the first 6 weeks; towel bath for the second 6 weeks); in treatment group two, the order of the trainings was reversed. The control group used usual showering procedures without person-centered training.

FINDINGS: Data were analyzed from 37 CNAs assisting 69 residents. Compared with the control group, the treatment groups significantly improved in the use of gentleness and verbal support and in the perception of ease.

IMPLICATIONS FOR NURSING: A person-centered approach with showering and with the towel bath can improve care given to residents who become agitated and aggressive during bathing and help CNAs have a positive experience while bathing residents.

patient can then be assisted to reach the bathroom in time. Positioning the patient near the toilet or placing a portable commode nearby may help if the patient cannot reach a toilet quickly. If the patient demonstrates dressing apraxia (cannot undress appropriately), clothing can be modified with easy-to-open fasteners in place of zippers or buttons. For nocturnal incontinence, other strategies may be effective. Limiting the amount of fluid consumed after the evening meal and taking the patient to the toilet just before going to bed or upon awakening during the night should reduce or eliminate nocturia.

Indwelling urinary catheters are contraindicated in patients with dementia because they are generally not well tolerated and because hand restraints are often used to prevent them from removing the catheter. In addition, indwelling urinary catheters foster the development of urinary tract infections and may compromise the patient's dignity and comfort. Urinary incontinence can be managed with the use of disposable, adult-size diapers that must be checked regularly and changed expeditiously when soiled.

Patients with dementia often experience constipation, although they may not be able to tell the nurse about this change. Therefore, subtle signs such as lethargy, reduced appetite, and abdominal distension need to be assessed frequently. Medications, decreased food and liquid intake, lack of motor activity, and decreased intestinal motility contribute to developing constipation. In such cases, the patient's diet should be rich in fiber, including bran or whole grains, vegetables, and fruit. Adequate oral intake (minimum of 1,500 to 2,000 mL/day) helps to prevent constipation. A gentle laxative such as Milk of Magnesia (1 to 2 tablespoons every other evening) is commonly used to promote bowel elimination. Enemas and harsher chemical cathartics should be avoided because they may increase pain or discomfort. Care must be taken to ensure that the patient does not become dehydrated in the process of treating constipation.

Sleep Interventions

Disturbed sleep cycles are particularly stressful to both family caregivers and nursing staff. Disturbed sleep is difficult to manage from a behavioral perspective, and the patient's overall level of health may suffer because sleep serves a restorative function. Sedative–hypnotic agents may be prescribed for a short time for restlessness or insomnia, but they may also cause a paradoxical reaction of agitation and insomnia (especially in older adults).

Sleep hygiene interventions are appropriate for patients with dementia, although morning and afternoon naps (or rest periods for patients who do not nap) may be the most effective intervention for a patient with altered diurnal rhythms. Whereas morning naps are likely to produce REM sleep patterns and may help patients who are restless from a loss of REM sleep, afternoon naps produce deep sleep and are suitable for restlessness associated with fatigue. Rest periods (in reclining chairs) in the morning and afternoon may help to eliminate late-day confusion (sundowning) and nighttime awakenings.

Activity and Exercise Interventions

Activity and exercise are important nursing interventions for patients with dementia. To promote a feeling of success, any activity or exercise plan must be culturally sensitive and adapted to the patient's functional ability and interests. The activity or exercise must be designed to prevent excess stress (both physical and psychological), which means that it must be individualized for each patient with dementia based on his or her relative strengths and deficits. If the program of rest, activity, and exercise is truly individualized, the resultant feelings of value and competency will enhance the patient's morale and self-esteem.

Nutritional Interventions

Maintenance of nutrition and hydration are essential nursing interventions. The patient's weight, oral intake, and hydration status should be monitored carefully. Patients with dementia should eat well-balanced meals that are appropriate to their activity level and eating abilities, with special attention given to electrolyte balance and fluid intake. Hyperactive patients require frequent feedings of a high-protein, high-carbohydrate diet in the form of finger foods (which they can carry while on the go). It may be wise to secure a fanny pack around the patient's waist with an assortment of nutritious finger foods appropriate for patients who can no longer use eating utensils properly. Most patients with dementia prefer to feed themselves with their fingers rather than have someone feed them.

When swallowing is a problem for the patient, thick liquids or semisoft foods are more effective than traditionally prepared foods. If a patient is likely to choke or aspirate food, less liquid (pureed) and more semisolid foods should be included in the diet because liquid flows into the pharyngeal cavity more quickly than does solid food.

The dining environment should be calm and food presentation appealing. If the patient eats only a small portion of food at one meal, reduce the presentation of food in terms of the amount and number of choices. One-dish meals (e.g., a casseroles) are ideal. If the patient is stressed or upset, it is better to delay feeding because eating, chewing, and swallowing difficulties are accentuated.

As dementia progresses, intensive feeding efforts are needed to ensure adequate food and fluid intake. If food intake is low, vitamin and mineral supplements may be indicated. If weight loss cannot be stopped by skillful feeding or dietary adjustments, then enteral or parenteral feedings may be considered. The patient's quality of life is an important issue to consider when the family or other health care proxy must decide whether to use artificial feeding mechanisms. By inserting a feeding tube, the goal of sustaining weight can be met, but patient comfort may be jeopardized, especially if restraints are used to keep the tube in place.

The patient with dementia should be presented with food that is easy to chew (soft) and swallow and not too hot or cold. In the later stages of progressive dementia, some patients hoard food in their mouths without actually swallowing it; others swallow too rapidly or fail to chew their food sufficiently before attempting to swallow. Some patients with advanced dementia put inedible objects into their mouths, presumably because they fail to recognize the objects as nonfood items.

Watch for swallowing difficulties that place the patient at risk for aspiration and asphyxiation. Swallowing difficulties may result from changes in esophageal motility and decreased secretion of saliva.

Pain and Comfort Management

Nursing care of noncommunicative patients who have dementia and who also have pain can be challenging. Because of the difficulty in identifying and monitoring the pain, the patients are often undertreated. However, several measures may be used to assess the efficacy of pharmacologic interventions, such as decreased restlessness and agitation. Small doses of oral morphine solution appear to reduce discomfort during routine nursing procedures. The main side effect of morphine is constipation.

Relaxation

Approaching patients in a calm, confident, unhurried manner; maintaining a soothing, quiet environment; avoiding unnecessary noise or chatter around patients and lowering vocal tone and rate when addressing them; maintaining eye contact; and using touch judiciously are likely to promote a sense of security conducive to patient relaxation and comfort. Simple relaxation exercises can be used to reduce stress and should be performed by the patient.

Pharmacologic Interventions

There is no medication that cures AD. Current research is targeting the alteration in the Aβ processing to prevent or reverse the effect of amyloidosis, but the development of an effective medication is still several years away (Guo, Sha, Xing, Jiang, & Cao, 2013). Because no medication can cure AD, psychopharmacologic interventions have two goals: restoration or maintenance of cognitive function and treatment of related psychiatric and behavioral disturbances that cause discomfort for the individual, interfere with treatment, or worsen the individual's cognitive status. Doses must be kept extremely low, and individuals should be monitored closely for any side effects or worsening of cognitive status. "Start low and go slow" is the principle guiding the administration of psychopharmacologic agents in older patients.

Often, convincing the patient to take the medication is one of the biggest nursing challenges. Patients may be unwilling even though they previously agreed to take the drugs. In these cases, investigate and hypothesize the reason for the reluctance to take medication. It may be because of difficulty swallowing pills, paranoid ideas, or lack of understanding. The underlying reason for medication refusal will determine the strategy. If the patient has difficulty swallowing, most medications come in concentrate liquid form that can be easily swallowed. Some medications can also be mixed in food. If suspicion or paranoia is the reason, try to identify the conditions under which the patient feels safe to take the medication, such as for a favorite nurse or relative.

Cholinesterase Inhibitors

Acetylcholinesterase inhibitors (AChEIs) are the mainstay of pharmacologic treatment of dementia because they inhibit **acetylcholinesterase (AChE)**, an enzyme necessary for the breakdown of Ach. Inhibition of AChE results in an increase in cholinergic activity. Because these medications have been shown to delay the decline in cognitive functioning but generally do not improve cognitive function after it has declined, it is important that this medication be started as soon as the diagnosis is made. The primary side effect of these medications is gastrointestinal distress, including nausea, vomiting, and diarrhea.

Four cholinesterase inhibitors are indicated for the treatment of patients with mild to moderate AD. These drugs may help to delay or prevent symptoms from becoming worse. They include galantamine (Razadyne), donepezil (Aricept), and rivastigmine (Exelon). Aricept is also indicated for those with moderate to severe AD (Table 37.4). Because the cholinesterase inhibitors can increase

Table 37.4 CHOLINESTERASE INHIBITORS

Drug	Dose	Common Side Effects	Drug–Drug Interactions
Galantamine (Razadyne) Prevents breakdown of acetylcholine and modulates nicotinic receptors which releases acetylcholine in the brain	4 mg bid Titrate to 16–24 mg/day over 8 weeks	Nausea, vomiting, diarrhea, weight loss	Some antidepressants, such as paroxetine, amitriptyline, fluoxetine, fluvoxamine, and other drugs with anticholinergic action, may cause retention of excess Razadyne in the body. NSAIDs should be used with caution in combination with this medication.
Rivastigmine (Exelon) Prevents the breakdown of acetylcholine and butyrylcholine in the brain	1.5 mg bid Titrate to 24 mg/day by increasing 3 mg/day every 2 weeks	Nausea, vomiting, weight loss, upset stomach, muscle weakness	None observed in laboratory studies; NSAIDs should be used with caution in combination with this medication
Donepezil (Aricept) Prevents the breakdown of acetylcholine in the brain	5 mg once a day Increase after 4–6 weeks to 10 mg/day	Nausea, diarrhea, vomiting	None observed in laboratory studies. NSAIDs should be used with caution in combination with this medication

bid, twice a day; NSAID, nonsteroidal anti-inflammatory drug; qid, four times a day.
Adapted from USDHHS (2014). Alzheimer's disease medications fact sheet. Washington, DC: Alzheimer's Disease Education & Referral (ADEAR) Center, National Institute on Aging, National Institutes of Health, NIH Publication N. 08–3431. Retrieved on May 12, 2014 from http://www.nia.nih.gov/alheimers/publication/alzheimers-disease-medications-fact sheet.

the risk of stomach ulcers, the prolonged use of nonsteroidal anti-inflammatory drugs with the AChEIs should be monitored closely. The cholinesterase inhibitors are oral medications usually taken once or twice a day. The earlier in the disease process these medications are initiated, the more likely they will delay cognitive decline. There are no special monitors for these medications. With cholinesterase inhibitors, patients should not take any anticholinergic medication (USDHHS, 2014).

N-Methyl-D-Aspartate Antagonists

Overstimulation of the *N*-methyl-D-aspartate (NMDA) receptor by glutamate (excitatory neurotransmitter) is considered to have a role in AD. In dementia, it is hypothesized that there is a chronic release of glutamate that causes a permanent increased intracellular calcium concentration that leads to neuronal degeneration. Memantine (Namenda XR) is an NMDA-receptor antagonist that has been shown to improve cognition and ADLs in patients with moderate to severe symptoms of dementia (Forest Laboratories, 2014) (Box 37.6).

Antipsychotic Agents

Antipsychotic agents are often effective in reducing psychosis, agitation, or aggressive behaviors and are commonly used off-label in the moderate to severe stages of AD. Antipsychotics are not approved by the U.S Food and Drug Administration for dementia-related psychosis and have a boxed warning for their use in this population. If atypical antipsychotics are used in older adults, the dosage should be much lower than in younger adults.

Antidepressant Agents and Mood Stabilizers

A depressed mood is common in people with dementia, and they often experience a response to psychotherapeutic intervention alone (individual or group therapy) or in combination with pharmacotherapy. Although the evidence for the use of antidepressants for treating depression is inconclusive (Leong, 2014), there is limited research support for their use in reducing agitation (Porsteinsson et al., 2014).

Antianxiety Medications (Sedative–Hypnotics)

Antianxiety medications, also known as benzodiazepines, should be used with caution in older adults and, if used, should be administered on a short-term basis. An antianxiety medication may be considered in an emergency, but ideally, the patient should try a nonbenzodiazepine before being prescribed a benzodiazepine. In older adults, the benzodiazepines can cause a paradoxical reaction.

Other Medications

Clinical observations indicate that older adults with defects in the cholinergic system are more vulnerable to

---

BOX 37.6

Drug Profile: Memantine (Namenda XR)

DRUG CLASS: *N*-methyl-D-aspartate (NMDA) receptor antagonist

RECEPTOR AFFINITY: Low to moderate affinity uncompetitive (open-channel) NMDA receptor antagonist, which binds preferentially to the NMDA receptor

INDICATIONS: For treatment of moderate to severe dementia of the Alzheimer type.

ROUTES AND DOSAGE: 7, 14, 21, and 28 mg tablets; oral solution, 2 mL/mg

The recommended starting dose of Namenda XR is 7 mg once daily. The recommended target dose is 28 mg once daily. The dose should be increased in 7 mg increments to 28 mg once daily. The minimum recommended interval between dose increases is 1 week and only if the previous dose has been well tolerated. Maximum dose is 28 mg daily.

HALF LIFE (PEAK EFFECT): Terminal half-life, 60 to 80 hours (peak effect, 3–7 hours)

SELECT ADVERSE REACTIONS: Dizziness, headache, constipation; reduce dosage in patients with severe renal damage

PRECAUTIONS: Avoid use during pregnancy; effect during lactation has not been determined. May cause drowsiness or dizziness; use caution while driving and performing other activities requiring mental alertness

SPECIFIC PATIENT AND FAMILY EDUCATION: Caregivers should be instructed in the recommended administration (twice per day for doses above 5 mg) and dose escalation (minimum interval of 1 week between dose increases).

- This drug does not alter the Alzheimer's disease process, and the efficacy of the medication may decrease over time.
- Continue using other medications for dementia as prescribed by the health care provider.
- Review the Patient Information.
- Teach preparation of oral solution (attach the green cap and plastic tube to new bottles of oral solution, withdraw prescribed dose using dosing syringe, and administer the dose).
- Do not discontinue the drug or change the dose unless advised by the health care provider.
- Do not increase the dose of memantine if Alzheimer's disease symptoms do not appear to be improving or appear to be getting worse; notify the health care provider.
- Memantine may cause drowsiness or dizziness. Use caution while driving and performing other activities requiring mental alertness and coordination until tolerance is determined.
- Do not use any prescription or over-the-counter medications, dietary supplements, or herbal preparations unless advised by the health care provider.
- Follow-up visits may be required to monitor therapy and to keep appointments.

BOX 37.7

Medications With Anticholinergic Effects

Amitriptyline
Captopril (Capoten)
Codeine
Cimetidine (Tagamet)
Citalopram (Celexa)
Digoxin (Lanoxin)
Diphenhydramine
Dipyridamole (Trental)
Donepezil (Aricept)
Escitalopram (Lexapro)
Furosemide (Lasix)
Fluoxetine (Prozac)
Isosorbide (Ismotic)
Mirtazapine (Remeron)
Nifedipine (Procardia)
Oxybutynin ER
Paroxetine (Paxil)
Phenytoin (Dilantin)
Prednisolone
Ranitidine (Zantac)
Theophylline
Triamterene and hydrochlorothiazide
Tolterodine (Detrol LA)
Warfarin (Coumadin)

the effects of anticholinergic drugs that can cause confusion and amnesia. Anticholinergic medications should be avoided in patients with AD if at all possible. See Box 37.7 for examples of medications that are commonly prescribed in older adults, all of which have anticholinergic receptor activity.

Psychological Domain

Assessment

Personality changes almost always accompany dementia and can take the form of either an accentuation or a marked alteration of a patient's previous lifelong character traits. The neural substrates underlying personality change in AD are not understood, but researchers have identified two contrasting patterns. One is marked by apathy, lack of spontaneity, and passivity. The other involves growing irritability, sarcasm, self-preoccupation, and intolerance of and lack of concern for others. Assessment of the psychological domain includes sexuality and spirituality as well.

Cognitive Status

The mental status assessment can be difficult for the patient with dementia because cognitive disturbance is the clinical hallmark of dementia. The use of any of the tools discussed in Chapters 10 and 36 can be used to determine mental status. However, family members should also be a part of any assessment, especially early in

the disease process. The AD8 is a brief, sensitive measure that differentiates between those with and without dementia (Galvin et al., 2005; Galvin, Roe, Xiong, & Morris, 2006; Razavi et al., 2013). The AD8 contains eight questions asking the family member to rate any change (yes or no) in memory, problem-solving abilities, orientation, and daily activities. The higher the number of changes, the more likely dementia is present (Figure 37.4). If cognitive deterioration occurs rapidly, delirium should be suspected.

Memory

The most dramatic and consistent cognitive impairment is in memory. Patients with dementia appear mildly forgetful and repetitive in conversation. They misplace objects, miss appointments, and forget what they were just doing. They may lose track of a conversation or television story. Initially, they may complain of memory problems, but rapidly in the course of the illness, insight is lost, and they become unaware of what is lost. Sometimes they may confabulate, making what appears to be an appropriate explanation of why the information or object is missing. Eventually, all aspects of memory are impaired, and even long-term memories are affected. During the interview, short-term memory loss is usually readily evident by the patient's inability to recall three or four words given to him or her at the beginning of the assessment. Often, the earliest symptom of AD is the inability to retain new information.

Language

Language is also progressively impaired. Individuals with AD may initially have agnosia (difficulty finding a word in a sentence or in naming an object). They may be able to talk around it, but the loss is noticeable. Later, fluent aphasia develops; comprehension diminishes; and, finally, they become mute and unresponsive to directions or information.

Visuospatial Impairment

Deficits in visuospatial tasks that require sensory and motor coordination develop early, drawing is abnormal, and the ability to write may change. An inaccurate clock drawing is diagnostic of impairment in this area (Figure 37.5). Sequencing tasks, such as cooking or other self-care skills, become impaired. The individual becomes unable to complete complex tasks that require calculations, such as balancing a checkbook.

Executive Functioning

Judgment, reasoning, and the ability to problem solve or make decisions are also impaired later in the disorder, closer to the time of nursing home placement. It is hypothesized that as the disease progresses, the degeneration of neurons is spread diffusely throughout the neocortex.

Remember, "Yes, a change" indicates that there has been a change in the last several years caused by cognitive (thinking and memory) problems.	Yes, A change	No, No change	N/A, Don't know
1. Problems with judgment (e.g., problems making decisions, bad financial decisions, problems with thinking)			
2. Less interest in hobbies/activities			
3. Repeats the same things over and over (questions, stories, or statements)			
4. Trouble learning how to use a tool, appliance, or gadget (e.g., VCR, computer, microwave, remote control)			
5. Forgets correct month or year			
6. Trouble handling complicated financial affairs (e.g., balancing checkbook, income taxes, paying bills)			
7. Trouble remembering appointments			
8. Daily problems with thinking and/or memory			

The final score is a sum of the number of items marked "Yes, A change".

Based on clinical research findings from 995 individuals included in the development and validation samples, the following cut points are provided:
• 0-1: Normal cognition
• 2 or greater: Cognitive impairment is likely to be present

Interpretation of the AD8 (Adapted from Galvin, JE et al, The AD8, a brief informal interview to detect dementia, Neurology 2005; 58: 589-364)

Scores in the impaired range (see below) indicate a need for further assessment. Scores in the "normal" range suggest that a dementing disorder is unlikely, but a very early disease process cannot be ruled out. More advanced assessment may be warranted in cases where other objective evidence of impairment exists.

FIGURE 37.4 AD8 tool. (Used with permission from James E. Galvin, MD, MSc, Assistant Professor, Director of the Memory Diagnostic Center, Washington University School of Medicine, St. Louis.)

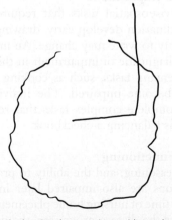

FIGURE 37.5 Clock drawing by a patient with moderate Alzheimer's disease. The patient was asked to draw a clock at 3:00 PM.

Psychotic Symptoms

Delusional thought content and hallucinations are common in people with dementia. These psychotic symptoms differ from those of schizophrenia.

Suspiciousness, Delusions, and Illusions

During the early and middle stages of dementia, many patients are aware of their cognitive losses and compensate with hyperalertness. In a hyperalert state, one becomes aware of many environmental stimuli that are not readily understood. Suspiciousness is a variant of the hyperalert or hypervigilant state in which stimuli are interpreted as dangerous. **Illusions**, or mistaken perceptions, also occur commonly in patients with dementia. For example, a woman with dementia mistakes her husband for her father. He resembles her father in that he is roughly her father's age when he was last alive. If an illusion becomes a false fixed belief, it is a delusion.

As the disease progresses, delusions develop in 34% to 50% of the people with dementia. These characteristic delusions are different from those discussed in the psychotic disorders. Common delusional beliefs include the following:

• Belief that his or her partner is engaging in marital infidelity
• Belief that other patients or staff are trying to hurt him or her
• Belief that staff or family members are impersonators
• Belief that people are stealing his or her belongings
• Belief that strangers are living in his or her home
• Belief that people on television are real

Hallucinations

Hallucinations occur frequently in dementia and are usually visual or tactile (they can also be auditory, gustatory, or olfactory). Visual, rather than auditory, hallucinations are the most common in dementia. A frequent complaint is that children, adults, or strange creatures are entering the house or the patient's room. These hallucinations may not seem unusual to the patient. If possible, the content and form of hallucination should be ascertained because this information may suggest a treatable disorder. For example, an auditory hallucination commanding the patient to commit suicide may be caused by a treatable depression, not dementia. In some cases, hallucinations may be pleasant, such as children being in the room, or they may be frightening and uncomfortable.

Mood Changes

Recognition of coexisting (and often treatable) psychiatric disorders in patients with dementia is often ignored. A depressed mood is common, but major depression and AD appear to be separate disorders (Verdelho et al., 2013) A number of people with AD experience one or more depressive episodes with symptoms such as psychomotor retardation, anxiety, feelings of guilt and worthlessness, sadness, frequent crying, insomnia, loss of appetite, weight loss, and suicidal rumination. Depressive symptoms are most prevalent in the early stages of dementia, which may be attributed to the patient's awareness of cognitive changes, memory loss, and functional decline. However, dysphoric symptoms can occur at any stage even in the most disoriented older patients. In more advanced stages of dementia, assessment of depression depends more on changes in behavior than on verbal complaints.

Anxiety

Moderate anxiety is a natural reaction to the fear engendered by gradual deterioration of intellectual function and the realization of impending loss of control over one's life. Failure to complete a task once regarded as simple creates a source of anxiety in patient with AD. As patients with AD become unsure of their surroundings and the expectations of others, they frequently react with fear and distress. It is thought that anxious behavior occurs when the patient is pressed to perform beyond his or her ability.

Catastrophic Reactions

Catastrophic reactions are overreactions or extreme anxiety reactions to everyday situations. Catastrophic responses occur when environmental stressors are allowed to continue or increase beyond the patient's threshold of stress tolerance. Behaviors indicative of catastrophic reactions typically include verbal or physical aggression, violence, agitated or anxious behavior, emotional outbursts, noisy behavior, compulsive or repetitive behavior, agitated night awakening, and other behaviors in which the patient is cognitively or socially inaccessible. Factors that contribute to catastrophic responses in patients with progressive cognitive decline include fatigue, a change in routine (pace or caregiver), demands beyond the patient's ability, overwhelming sensory stimuli, and physical stressors (e.g., pain or hunger).

Behavioral Responses

Apathy and Withdrawal

Apathy, the inability or unwillingness to become involved with one's environment, is common in AD, especially in the moderate to late stages. Apathy leads to withdrawal from the environment and a gradual loss of empathy for others. The lack of empathy is very difficult for families and friends to understand.

Restlessness, Agitation, and Aggression

Restlessness, agitation, and aggression are relatively common in the moderate to later stages of dementia. Restlessness should be further evaluated to determine its underlying cause. If the restlessness occurs during medication change or adjustment, side effects should be suspected.

Agitation and aggressive physical contacts are among the most dangerous behavior management problems encountered in any setting. They often result in placement of a family member in a nursing home. Careful evaluation of the antecedents of the agitated behavior enable planning nursing care that prevents future occurrences.

Aberrant Motor Behavior

Symptoms such as fidgeting, picking at clothing, wringing hands, loud vocalizations, and wandering may all be signs of such underlying conditions as dehydration, medication reaction, pain, or infection (suggesting delirium). One of the most difficult behaviors for which to determine an underlying cause is **hypervocalization**, the screams, curses, moans, groans, and verbal repetitiveness that are common in the later stages of disease in cognitively impaired older adults, often occurring during a hospitalization or nursing home placement. In the assessment of these hypervocalizations, it is important to identify when the behavior is occurring; antecedents of the behavior; and any related events, such as a family member leaving or a change in stimulation.

Disinhibition

One of the most frustrating symptoms of AD is **disinhibition**, acting on thoughts and feelings without exercising appropriate social judgment. In AD, the patient may decide that he or she is more comfortable naked than with clothes. Or the patient may not be able to find his or her clothes and may walk into a room of people without any clothes on. This behavior is extremely disconcerting to family members and can also lead to nursing home placement.

Hypersexuality

A closely related symptom is **hypersexuality**, inappropriate and socially unacceptable sexual behavior. The patient begins talking and behaving in ways that are uncharacteristic of premorbid behavior. This behavior is very difficult for family members and nursing home staff.

Stress and Coping Skills

Patients with dementia seem extremely sensitive to stressful situations and often do not have the coping abilities to deal with the situation. A careful assessment of the triggers that precede stressful situations will help in understanding a provoking event.

Nursing Diagnoses for the Psychological Domain

A multitude of potential nursing diagnoses can be identified for the psychological domain of this population. A sample of common nursing diagnoses includes Impaired Memory; Disturbed Thought Processes; Chronic Confusion; Disturbed Sensory Perception; Impaired Environmental Interpretation Syndrome; Risk for Violence: Self-Directed or Directed at Others; Risk for Loneliness; Risk for Caregiver Role Strain; Ineffective Sexuality Patterns; Ineffective Individual Coping; Hopelessness; and Powerlessness.

Interventions for the Psychological Domain

The therapeutic relationship is the basis for interventions for the patient and family with dementia. Care of the patient entails a long-term relationship needing much support and expert nursing care. Interventions should be delivered within the relationship context.

Interventions for Cognitive Impairment

Person-Centered Care

As with any other patient, the person with dementia should be the center of the decision-making process. Individuals with Alzheimer's dementia maintain self-awareness and continue to have the ability to identify their own needs well into the progression of the illness. They should be involved in developing their own plan of care. The plan should include educational and supportive programs individualized for the person's self-identified needs. Ideally, plans should be designed to support self-awareness, self-esteem, maintenance of abilities, and management of behavioral symptoms and health promotion (Fortinsky & Downs, 2014).

Memory Enhancement

Interventions for progressive memory impairment should always be a part of the treatment plan. The sooner patients begin taking AChE inhibitors, the slower the cognitive decline. However, pharmacologic agents are only a small part of the intervention picture. The nursing goal is to maintain memory functioning as long as possible. When caring for a patient with AD, a concerted effort should be made to reinforce short- and long-term memory. For example, reminding patients what they had for breakfast, which activity was just completed, or who their visitors were a few hours ago will reinforce short-term memory. Encouraging patients to tell the stories of their earlier years will help bring long-term memories into focus. In the earlier stages of AD, there is considerable frustration when the patient realizes that he or she has short-term memory loss. In a matter-of-fact manner, help "fill in the blanks" and then redirect to another activity. Pictures of familiar people, places, and activities are also important tools in memory retrieval. Using scents (perfume, shaving lotions, spices, different foods) to stimulate memory retrieval and asking patients to relate their memories are also useful. Formalized reminiscence groups also help patients relive their earlier experiences and support long-term memories.

Orientation Interventions

To enhance cognitive functioning, attempts should be made to remind patients of the day, time, and location. However, if the patient begins to argue that he or she is really at home or that it is really 1992, the patient need not be confronted by facts. Any confrontation could easily escalate into an argument. Instead, either redirect the patient or focus on the topic at hand (Box 37.8).

BOX 37.8 • THERAPEUTIC DIALOGUE • The Patient With Dementia of the Alzheimer Type

Lois's daughter has told the home health agency nurse that on several occasions, Lois has been found cowering and fearful under the kitchen table, saying she was hiding from voices. The nurse also knows that Lois denies having any difficulty with her memory or her ability to care for herself.

INEFFECTIVE APPROACH

Nurse: I'm here to see you about your health problems.

Patient: I have no problems. Why are you here?

Nurse: I'm here to help you.

Patient: I do not need any help. I think there is a mistake.

Nurse: Oh, there is no mistake. Your name is Ms. W, isn't it?

Patient: Yes, but I don't know who you are or why you are here. I'm very tired, please excuse me.

Nurse: OK. I will return another day.

EFFECTIVE APPROACH

Nurse: Hello, my name is Susan Miller. I'm the home health nurse, and I will be spending some time with you.

Patient: Oh, alright. Come in. Sit here.

Nurse: Thank you.

Patient: There is nothing wrong with me, you know.

Nurse: Are you wondering why I am here? (Open-ended statement)

Patient: I know why you are here. My children think that I cannot take care of myself.

Nurse: Is that true? Can you take care of yourself? (Restatement)

Patient: Of course I can care for myself. When people get older, they slow down. I'm just a little slower now, and that upsets my children.

Nurse: You are a little slower? (Reflection)

Patient: I sometimes forget things.

Nurse: Such as . . . (open-ended statement)

Patient: Sometimes I cannot remember a telephone number or a name of a food.

Nurse: Does that cause problems?

Patient: According to my children, it does!

Nurse: What about you? What causes problems for you?

Patient: Sometimes the radio says terrible things to me.

Nurse: That must be frightening. (Acceptance)

Patient: It's terrifying. Then, my daughter looks at me as if I am crazy. Am I?

Nurse: It sounds like your mind is playing tricks on you. Let's see if we can figure out how to control the radio. (Validation)

Patient: Oh, OK. Will you tell my daughter that I am not crazy?

Nurse: Sure, I would be happy to meet with both you and your daughter if you would like. (Acceptance)

CRITICAL THINKING CHALLENGE

• How did the nurse's underlying assumption that the patient would welcome the nurse in the first scenario lead to the nurse's rejection by the patient?

• What communication techniques did the nurse use in the second scenario to open communication and set the stage for the development of a sense of trust?

Maintaining Language

Losing the ability to name an object (agnosia) is frustrating. For example, the patient may describe a flower in terms of color, size, and fragrance but never be able to name it a flower. When this happens while interacting with a patient, immediately say the name of the item. This reinforces cognitive functioning and prevents disruption in the interaction. Referral to speech therapists may also be useful if the language impairment impedes communication.

Supporting Visuospatial Functioning

The patient with visuospatial impairments loses the ability to sequence automatic behaviors, such as getting dressed or eating with silverware. For example, patients often put their clothes on backward, inside out, or with undergarments over outer garments. After they are dressed, they become confused as to how they arrived at their current state. If this happens, it may help to place clothes for dressing in a sequence for the patient so they patient can move from one article to the next in the correct sequence. This same technique can be used in other situations, such as eating, bathing, and toileting.

Interventions for Psychosis

Patients who are experiencing psychosis usually are prescribed an antipsychotic agent. Interventions associated with antipsychotic therapy were presented in earlier chapters.

Managing Suspicions, Illusions, and Delusions

Patients' suspiciousness and delusional thinking must be addressed to be certain that they do not endanger themselves or others. Often, delusions are verbalized when patients are placed in a situation they cannot master cognitively. The principle of nonconfrontation is most important in dealing with suspiciousness and delusion formation. No efforts should be made to ease the patient's suspicions directly or to correct delusions. Efforts should be directed at determining the circumstances that trigger suspicion or delusion formation and creating a means of avoiding these situations.

Frequent causes of suspicion are changes in daily routine and strangers. The common accusations that "Someone has entered my room," or "Someone has changed my room" can be managed by asking, "Do you want to see if anything is missing?" Such accusations usually arise when a patient cannot remember what the room looked like or when the room was rearranged or cleaned.

Patients with dementia often hide or misplace their belongings and later complain that the item is missing. It is helpful if nurses and other caregivers pay attention to the patient's favorite hiding places and communicate this so that objects can be more easily retrieved. An outburst of delusional accusations after a social outing or other activity may indicate that the activity was too long, the setting was too stimulating, there was too much activity, or the pace was too fast for the patient. All of these elements can be modified, or it may be necessary to exclude or significantly diminish the delusional patient's participation in overstimulating activities.

Patients with dementia have delusions that a spouse, child, or other significant person is an impostor. If this situation occurs, it is important to assert in a matter-of-fact manner, "This is your wife Barbara" or "I am your daughter Jenny." More vigorous assertions, such as offering various types of proof, tend to increase puzzlement as to why a person would go so far to impersonate the spouse or child.

When patients experience illusions, find the source of the illusion and remove it from the environment if possible. For example, if a patient is watching a television program featuring animals and then verbalizes that the animal is in the room, switch the channel and redirect the conversation. Some patients with dementia may no longer recognize the reflections in the mirror as themselves and become agitated, thinking that a stranger is staring at them. Potentially misleading or disturbing stimuli, such as mirrors or art work, can be easily covered or removed from the environment.

Managing Hallucinations

Reassurance and distraction may be helpful for the hallucinating patient. For example, an 89-year-old patient with AD in a residential care facility would get up each night, walk to the nursing station, and whisper to the nurses, "There's a man in my bed who won't let me sleep. You should patrol this place better!" If the hallucination is not too disturbing for the patient, it can often be dismissed calmly with diversion or distraction. Because this patient did not seem too concerned by the man in her bed, the nurse may gently respond by saying, "I'm sorry you have to put up with so much. Just wait here (or come with me) and I'll make sure your room is ready for you." The nurse should then take the patient back to her room and help her into bed.

Frightening hallucinations and delusions usually require antipsychotic medications to dampen the patient's emotional reactions, but they can also be dealt with by optimizing perceptual cues (cover mirrors or turn off the television) and by encouraging patients to stay physically close to their caregivers. For example, one patient complained to her visiting nurse that she was being poisoned by deadly bugs that crawled up and down her arms and legs while she tried to sleep at night. Antipsychotic medication may help this patient sleep at night, and she would also likely benefit from reassurance and protection. Patients benefit more if given a specific intervention to help the hallucination, such as applying moisturizing lotion to her legs and arms to repel the bugs at night. It is not necessary to agree with the patient's hallucination or delusion, but do let the patient know that the feelings are justified based on the patient's perception of the threat.

Interventions for Mood Changes

Managing Depression

Psychotherapeutic nursing interventions for depression that accompanies dementia are similar to interventions for any depression. It is important to spend time alone with patients and to personalize their care as a way of communicating the patient's value. Encouraging expression of negative emotions is helpful because patients can talk honestly to a nonjudgmental person about their feelings.

Although depressed patients with dementia are likely to be too disorganized to commit suicide, it is wise to remove potentially harmful objects from the environment.

Do not force depressed patients to interact with others or participate in activities but do encourage activity and exercise. One of the psychogenic aspects of depression is a sense of lowered worth related to the patient's actual decreased competence to work and to deal with the problems of daily living. Therefore, it may be helpful to involve the person in a simple repetitive task or project (e.g., folding linens or setting the table), especially one that involves helping someone else. Assist the patient to meet self-care needs while encouraging independence when possible.

Managing Anxiety

Cognitively impaired patients are particularly vulnerable to anxiety. Patients with dementia become unsure of their surroundings or of what is expected of them and then tend to react with fear and distress. They may feel lost, insecure, and left out. Failure to complete a task once regarded as simple creates anxiety and agitation. Often, they cannot explain the source of their anxiety. The difficulty in developing interventions for the anxious patient with dementia is that the symptoms may also be a sign of underlying illnesses, such as depression, pain, infection, or other physical illnesses.

In many cases, lowering the demands, or perceived demands, on the patient is conducive to promoting comfort. Although maintaining autonomy in any remaining function is a high priority in nursing care of the patient with dementia, it may decrease the patient's anxiety or stress level to have things done for him or her at certain points along the illness continuum. In addition, being sensitive to the pronounced startle reflexes and potential hypersensitivity to touch also helps reduce stress.

The threshold for stress is progressively lowered in individuals with AD and other progressive dementias. Whereas a healthy person frequently uses cognitive coping strategies when under stress, a person with dementia can no longer use many of these strategies. Effective nursing interventions include simplifying routines, making routines as consistent and predictable as possible, reducing the number of choices the patient must make, identifying areas in which control can be maintained, and creating an environment in which the patient feels safe. With any of the therapeutic interventions discussed, remember that each patient has relative strengths and weaknesses and that sound nursing judgment must be used in each situation.

Commonly used therapeutic approaches may exacerbate anxiety in a patient with dementia. For example, reality orientation is usually an effective intervention for acutely confused patients. Reality orientation is contraindicated in dementia because it is possible that the patient's disoriented behavior or language has inherent meaning. If the disoriented behavior or language is continuously neglected or corrected, the patient's sense of isolation and anxiety may increase.

Another therapeutic intervention that may (or may not) be contraindicated in patients with dementia is providing the patient with information before a difficult or painful procedure. Anticipatory preparation for nonroutine events may produce anxiety because the patient is unable to retain information, use reasoning skills, or make sound judgments. Telling the patient that he or she is scheduled for an upcoming diagnostic test only communicates, on an emotional level, that something distressing is about to happen. A simple explanation immediately before the event may be more helpful.

Managing Catastrophic Reactions

If a patient reacts catastrophically, remain calm, minimize environmental distractions (quiet the environment), get the patient's attention, and softly assure the patient that he or she is safe. Give information slowly, clearly, and simply, one step at a time. Let the patient know that you understand the fear or other emotional response, such as anger or anxiety.

As nursing skills are developed in identifying antecedents to the patient's catastrophic reactions, it becomes possible to avoid situations that provoke such reactions. Patients with AD respond well to structure but poorly to change. Attempts to argue or reason with them will only escalate their dysfunctional responses.

Interventions for Behavior Problems

Managing Apathy and Withdrawal

As the patient withdraws and becomes more apathetic, it becomes more challenging to engage the patient in meaningful activities and interactions. Providing this level of care requires knowing the premorbid functioning of the patient. Close contact with family helps provide ideas about meaningful activities.

Managing Restlessness and Wandering

Restlessness and wandering are major concerns for caregivers, especially in the community (home) or long-term care setting. The principal means of dealing with restless patients who wander into other patients' rooms or out the door is to have an adequate number of staff (or caregivers in the home setting) to provide supervision, as well as electronically controlled exits. Wandering behavior may be interrupted in more cognitively intact patients by distracting them verbally or visually. Patients who are beyond verbal distraction can be distracted by physically joining them on their walk and then interrupting their course of action and gently redirecting them back to the house or facility. Many times, wandering is a result of a patient's inability to find his own room or may represent other agenda-seeking behaviors.

Managing Agitated Behavior

Agitated behavior is likely to occur when patients are pressed to assist in their own care. A calm, unhurried, and undemanding approach is usually most effective. Attempts at reasoning may only aggravate the situation and increase the patient's resistance to care. If unable to determine the source of the patient's anxiety, the patient's restless energy can often be channeled into activities such as walking. Relaxation techniques also can be effective for reducing behavioral problems and anxiety in patients with dementia.

Managing Aberrant Behavior

When patients are picking in the air or wringing hands, simple distraction may work. Hypervocalizations are another story. Direct care staff tend to avoid these patients, which only makes the vocalizations worse. In reality, these vocalizations may have meaning to the patient. Instead, develop strategies to try to reduce the frequency of vocalizations (Table 37.5).

Reducing Disinhibition

Anticipation of disinhibiting behavior is the key to nursing interventions for this problem. Disinhibition can take many forms, from undressing in a public setting to touching someone inappropriately to making cruel but factual statements. This behavior can usually be viewed as normal by itself but abnormal within its social context. Keen behavioral assessment of the patient increases the ability to anticipate the likely socially inappropriate behavior and redirect the patient or change the context of the situation. If the patient starts undressing in the dining room, offering a robe and gently escorting him or her to another part of the room might be all that is needed. If a patient is trying to fondle a staff member, having the staff member leave the immediate area or redirecting the patient may alleviate the situation.

Social Domain

Assessment

Dementia interferes with a person's ability to interact socially as much as it disrupts intellectual functioning. The social domain assessment should include the areas explained in Chapter 36, including functional status, social systems, spiritual assessment, legal status, and quality of life (see Chapter 10).

The patient's whole social network is affected by dementia, and the primary caregiver of a person with dementia (usually the partner or offspring in a community setting) is often considered a copatient. It is important to assess the family caregiver's ability to use supportive mechanisms to maintain his or her own integrity throughout the disease process.

The extent of the primary caregiver's personal, informal, and formal support systems must also be assessed, as well as personal resources, skills, and stressors. The assessment of the social domain provides objective data on the patient's social circumstances and impressions of the patient's family structure, sociocultural beliefs, attitudes toward health and disease, myths about dementia, patterns of communication, and degree of psychopathology (e.g., potential for abuse). If the patient still resides in the community, a home visit will prove useful because it provides information about the patient in the natural environment. From this assessment, the situational and psychosocial stressors that affect the family and patient can be identified, and interventions to strengthen coping strategies, including the ability to seek help from appropriate community resources, can be developed.

Nursing Diagnoses for the Social Domain

Typical nursing diagnoses for the social domain are Deficient Diversional Activity, Impaired Social Interaction, Social Isolation, Risk for Loneliness, Caregiver Role Strain, Ineffective Coping, Hopelessness, and Powerlessness. Outcomes are determined according to nursing diagnoses.

Interventions for the Social Domain

Safety Interventions

One of the primary concerns in social interventions is patient safety. In the early stages of the illness, safety may not seem to be a prime issue because the individual is cognitively intact. However, early behaviors suggesting dementia are often related to safety, such as the patient getting lost while driving or going the wrong way on the highway. Patients may be prevented from driving even though they can continue to live at home. Safety continues to be an issue in the home when patients engage in unsupervised cooking, cleaning, or household tasks. Day care centers provide a structured yet safe environment for these individuals. Family members should be encouraged to assess continually the abilities of members to live at home safely.

During hospitalizations or nursing home care, the safety issues are different. Most geropsychiatric units are locked, and in a dementia unit, there often is an electronic alarm system to alert staff of patients attempting to leave the secured floor. Staff and visitors need to be vigilant for perilous situations.

Environmental Interventions

The need for stimulation can also be an antecedent to catastrophic reactions. The need for stimulation varies from individual to individual and can change, depending

Table 37.5	MESSAGES, MEANINGS, AND MANAGEMENT STRATEGIES
Possible Underlying Meanings	**Related Management Strategies**
"*I hurt!*" (e.g., from arthritis, fractures, pressure ulcers, degenerative joint disease, cancer)	• Observe for pain behaviors (e.g., posture, facial expressions, and gait in conjunction with vocalizations). • Treat suspected pain judiciously with analgesics and nonpharmacologic measures (e.g., repositioning, careful manipulation of patient during transfers and personal care, warm or cold packs, massage, relaxation).
"*I'm tired.*" (e.g., sleep disturbances possibly related to altered sleep–wake cycle with day–night reversal, difficulty falling asleep, frequent night awakenings)	• Increase daytime activity and exercise to minimize daytime napping and promote nighttime sleep. • Promote normal sleep patterns and biorhythms by strengthening natural environmental cues (e.g., provide light exposure during the day; avoid bright, artificial lights at night), provide large calendars and clocks. • Establish a bedtime routine. • Reduce night awakenings: avoid excess fluids, diuretics, caffeine at bedtime, minimize loud noises, consolidate nighttime care activities (e.g., changing, medications, treatments).
"*I'm lonely.*"	• Encourage social interactions between patients and their family, caregivers, and others. • Increase time the patient spends in group settings to minimize time in isolation. • Provide opportunity to interact with pets.
"*I need . . .*" (e.g., food, a drink, a blanket, to use the toilet, to be turned or repositioned)	• Anticipate needs (e.g., assist the patient to toilet soon after breakfast when the gastrocolic reflex is likely). • Keep the patient comfort and safety in mind during care (e.g., minimize body exposure to prevent hypothermia).
"*I'm stressed.*" (e.g., Inability to tolerate sensory overload)	• Promote rest and quiet time. • Minimize "white noise" (e.g., vacuum cleaner) and background noise (e.g., televisions and radios). • Avoid harsh lighting and busy, abstract designs. • Limit patient's contacts with other agitated people. • Reduce behavioral expectations of patient, minimize choices, and promote a stable routine.
"*I'm bored.*" (e.g., lack of sensory stimulation)	• Maximize hearing and visual abilities (e.g., keep external auditory canals free from cerumen plugs, ensure that glasses and hearing aids are worn, provide reading material of large print, soften lighting to reduce glare). • Play soft classical music for auditory stimulation. • Offer structured diversions (e.g., outdoor activities).
"*What are you doing to me?*" (e.g., personal boundaries are invaded)	• Avoid startling patients by approaching them from the front. • Always speak before touching the patient. • Inform patients what you plan to do and why before you do it. • Allow for flexibility in patient care.
"*I don't feel well.*" (e.g., a urinary or upper respiratory tract infection, metabolic abnormality, fecal impaction)	• Identify the etiology through patient history, examination, possible tests (e.g., urinalysis, blood work, chest radiography, neurologic testing). • Treat underlying causes.
"*I'm frustrated—I have no control.*" (e.g., loss of autonomy)	• When possible, allow patient to make their own decisions. • Maximize patient involvement during personal care (e.g., offer the patient a washcloth to assist with bathing). • Treat patients with dignity and respect (e.g., dress or change patients in private).
"*I'm lost.*" (e.g., memory impairment)	• Maintain familiar routines. • Label the patient's room, bathroom, drawers, and possessions with large name signs. • Promote a sense of belonging through displays of familiar personal items, such as old family pictures.
"*I feel strange.*" (e.g., side effects from medications that may include psychotropics, corticosteroids, beta-blockers, NSAIDs)	• Minimize the overall number of medications; consider nondrug interventions when possible. • Begin new medications one at a time; start with low doses and titrate slowly. Suspect a drug reaction if the patient's behavior (e.g., vocal) changes. • Educate caregivers about the patient's medications.
"*I need to be loved!*"	• Provide human contact and purposeful touch. • Acknowledge or verify the patient's feelings. • Encourage alternative, nonverbal ways to express feelings, such as through music, painting, or drawing. • Stress a sense of purpose in life, acknowledge achievement, and reaffirm that the patient is still needed.

NSAID, nonsteroidal anti-inflammatory drug.
From Clavel, D. S. (1999). Vocalizations among cognitively impaired elders. *Geriatric Nursing, 20*, 90–93. Reprinted with permission from Elsevier.

on many factors, including cognitive intactness, alertness, emotional state, and physical state. The amount of stimulation received also influences each patient's behavior. Lack of stimulation or intense stimulation may cause emotional distress and aggression. Generally speaking, the more severe the dementia, the less stimulation can be integrated. The nurse should attempt to determine each patient's optimal level of stimulation at various times of the day. It may be that stimulating environments can be tolerated early in the morning but not in the afternoon when the patient is tired.

Socialization Activities

Overlearned social skills are rarely lost in patients with AD. It is not unusual for patients with dementia to respond appropriately to a handshake or smile well into the disease process. Even patients who are no longer able to communicate coherently will carry on long discussions with people who are willing to listen and respond (to language that does not make sense). There is a strong risk for social isolation in patients with dementia because of communication difficulties. Reinforcing social remarks and gestures, such as eye contact, smiling, greetings, and farewells, can promote a sense of competency and self-esteem. Pet therapy and "stuffed animal" therapy can also enhance social interaction in cognitively impaired individuals. It is important to remember that patients with dementia do not lose their ability to laugh and play, and the psychosocial benefits of humor are well known.

When engaging a patient with dementia in an activity, (1) avoid confronting the patient with the disability, (2) allow the level of autonomy best tolerated by the patient, (3) simplify activities and directions to the point that they can be mastered (e.g., avoid directions such as "use right or left arm" because the patient may be unable to distinguish one from the other), (4) provide adequate structure or directions, and (5) recognize that instructions may not be carried out correctly. It is important to monitor the length of time, crowding, and noise level when the patient participates in a group activity because all of these factors may increase the patient's stress level.

Activities that elicit pleasant memories from an earlier time in the patient's life (reminiscence) may produce a soothing effect. Eliciting pleasant memories may be enhanced by gentle stimulation of the patient's senses, for example, viewing and discussing photo albums, looking at personal memorabilia, providing a favorite food item, playing a musical instrument, or listening to music the person preferred in younger years. It may be useful to incorporate movement or dance along with a singing exercise.

If the patient with dementia resists structured exercise, it may be because of a fear of falling or injury or of demonstrating to others that his or her health is failing. Patients with dementia often forget how to move or how

to coordinate their movements in relation to objects. Therefore, exercise should be light and enjoyable. Encourage the patient to take rest periods at intervals throughout the activity in an effort to minimize stress.

Home Visits

The goal of in-home and community-based long-term care services is to maintain patients in a self-determining environment that provides the most home-like atmosphere possible, allows maximum personal choice for care recipients and caregiver, and encourages optimal family caregiving involvement without overwhelming the resources of the family network. All services for patients with dementia and their families must be provided within a context of continuity of care, a concept that mandates access to a variety of health and supportive services over an unpredictable and changing clinical course.

Community Actions

Nurses working with patients with dementia are especially knowledgeable about all aspects of the illness and care. These nurses are often involved in local organizations, such as the Alzheimer's Association. Issues of care and safety and reimbursement of services often require professional expertise and influence.

Family Interventions

Caregivers are faced with extreme pressures and often feel isolated, frustrated, and trapped. The potential for patient abuse is significant, especially if agitated and aggressive behaviors are present in the relative. It is important to recognize the need of the caregivers for support and relief from the 24-hour responsibility. Determining availability of family members or friends to assist with personal care of the patient should be included in the assessment. Caregivers should be encouraged to attend support groups and carve out personal time. Educational and training programs may help in understanding the complex nature of the disorder (Boxes 37.9 and 37.10). Community resources, such as day care centers, home health agencies, and other community services, can be an important aspect of nursing care for the patient with dementia.

Evaluation and Treatment Outcomes

The objectives of nursing interventions are to help the patient with dementia remain as independent as possible and to function at the highest cognitive, physical, emotional, spiritual, and social levels. The maximum level of functional ability can be promoted when nursing care is related to and based on the remaining abilities of the patient. Patients who receive diagnoses of AD or other

Psychoeducation Checklist: Tips for Caregivers

When caring for the patient with dementia, be sure to include the caregivers, as appropriate, and address the following topic areas in the teaching plan:

- Psychopharmacologic agents, if used, including drug action, dosage, frequency, and possible adverse effects
- Rest and activity
- Consistency in routines
- Nutrition and hydration
- Sleep and comfort measures
- Protective environment
- Communication and social interaction
- Diversional measures
- Community resources

types of dementia have a wide and varying range of functional abilities. As cognitive decline progresses, there is a tendency for caregivers to perform more and more tasks for the patient. It is essential to assess for strengths and to assist in the maintenance of existing skills. Adaptive and appropriate behaviors continue to some degree in people with dementia even in the presence of increasing cognitive decline. It is important for nursing interventions to focus on more than the maintenance of optimal physical

BOX 37.10

Research For Best Practice: Easing the Burden of Caregivers

Lewis, M., Hobday, J. V., & Hepburn, K. W. (2011). Internet-based program for dementia caregivers. American Journal of Alzheimer's Disease & Other Dementias, 25(8), 674–679.

THE QUESTION: Will a face-to-face psychoeducation program for caregivers be effective as an internet program to provide caregivers the knowledge, skills, and outlook to undertake and succeed in the caregiving role?

METHODS: The Internet-Based Savvy Caregiver Program merged an effective psychoeducation intervention with the access and interactivity of the Internet to make available this beneficial service. Content from four modules were selected for the program, including (1) the effects of dementia on thinking, (2) taking charge and letting go, (3) providing practical help, and (4) managing daily care and difficult behavior. Each of the storyboard documents were between 30 and 50 pages in length. A total of 47 family caregivers participated in a pilot project that was based on qualitative analysis of open ended questions.

FINDINGS: The participants provided positive ratings for the program and endorsed the program's acceptability and usability.

IMPLICATIONS FOR NURSING: The Internet format is acceptable and another option for caregivers who have a computer access. Nurses should consider encouraging caregivers to participate in quality Internet-based psychoeducation programs.

Clinical Vignette

BOX 37.11
A NURSE'S DILEMMA

It is 8 o'clock, and you are working as a nurse on an inpatient general medical unit of a large urban hospital. A 72-year-old man is admitted to your unit with symptoms of disorientation to time and place, and he is intermittently exhibiting signs of agitation. He thinks you are his child, and he falls asleep while you ask him questions about his symptoms. When you ask him to sign a consent form and hand him a pen, he looks at you as if he didn't understand your request.

The patient's wife tells you that he has had trouble with his memory for the past 3 or 4 years but that her husband has been "acting strange for the past 4 days." The patient's wife denies any history of substance abuse or head injury but states that her husband has been recently diagnosed as having dementia of the Alzheimer type.

What Do You Think?
- What assessment techniques would you use to determine whether this patient has dementia, delirium, or both?
- What nursing diagnosis would be included in the patient's plan of care?
- What nursing interventions would promote comfort and safety for this patient?

functional ability; interventions also must focus on meeting the psychological, social, and spiritual needs of patients with dementia. See Box 37.11.

Nurses can maintain quality of life if they protect a patient's overall well-being by balancing physical, mental, social, and spiritual health. Figure 37.6 illustrates the

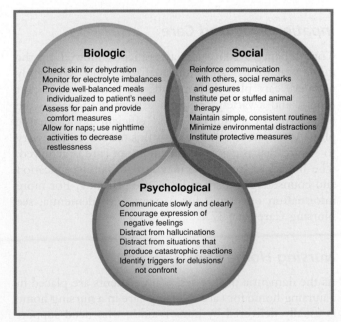

FIGURE 37.6 Biopsychosocial interventions for patients with dementia.

truly biopsychosocial aspects of the treatment of individuals with dementia by summarizing potential outcomes of nursing care.

Continuum of Care

Community Care

It is estimated that more than 60% to 70% of older adults with AD live at home. Almost 80% of home care is provided by family and friends. Unpaid caregivers provide $202 billion economic worth (Alzheimer's Association, 2014a). Use of community-based services (e.g., home health aides, home-delivered meals, adult day cares, respite care, caregiver support groups) often extends the amount of time an individual with AD or a related disorder can safely remain in the home. However, the progressive impairment associated with dementia often culminates with placement in a long-term care facility. The nurse working in a physician's office or ambulatory setting may provide ongoing information about management and problem solving. The public health nurse may provide intermittent assessment and ongoing case management. Nurses working in programs designed specifically for patients with dementia, such as adult day cares, also practice the role of educator. A nurse who is simply a neighbor or family member is often asked to advise about care of the person with dementia. The complex and interrelated problems often observed in patients with neuropsychiatric disorders will increasingly demand the attention of nurses in all health care settings. Cooperation among health care providers of different disciplines and in various settings is needed to meet the highly individualized needs of patients with neuropsychiatric deficits.

Inpatient-Focused Care

Comprehensive admission assessment followed by the development of an individualized (and constantly updated) care plan that involves the patient, significant others, and a variety of health care professionals is the foundation of an effective and efficient postdischarge plan. Attention to all aspects of this process is necessary to ensure that the goal of continuity of care is achieved. The hospital-based nurse may initiate family education and counseling as part of discharge planning. For more information on caring for patients with dementia, see Nursing Care Plan 37.1.

Nursing Home Care

As the dementia progresses, many patients are placed in a nursing home for care. Nursing care in a nursing home is usually delivered by nurses' aides, who need support and direction. Interestingly, people with dementia require complex nursing care, but the skill level of people caring for these individuals often is minimal. Education and support of the direct caregiver is the focus of most nursing homes.

Mental Health Promotion

> **KEYCONCEPT** **Cognitive reserve** refers to the brain's capacity to cope with brain damage in order to minimize symptomatology (Morbelli & Nobili, 2014).

The emerging understanding of cognitive reserve provides direction for mental health promotion strategies. Cognitive reserve is associated with white matter integrity in healthy older adults. In individuals with AD, there is a negative association between their cognitive reserve and white matter integrity (Arenaza-Urquijo et al., 2011). Cognitive reserve focuses on the protective potential of the structure of the brain such as brain size, neural density, and synaptic connectivity and its function including the efficiency of the neural networks. It is hypothesized that some factors influence the development of cognitive reserve that range from early social and material environments through inputs of education, occupation, socioeconomic environment to physical health, health behaviors, and degree of engaged lifestyle activity (Seo et al., 2011).

Certain lifelong activities help build and maintain cognitive reserve. Physical exercise, nutrition, stress management, and social engagement with family and friends are associated with positive cognitive outcomes. Levels of education and literacy are repeatedly shown to be related to higher cognitive functioning (Meng & D'Arcy, 2012; Farina, Tabet, & Rusted, 2014). Mental health promotion includes helping patients develop awareness of the importance of engaging in a lifestyle that supports the development of cognitive reserve.

OTHER DEMENTIAS

Dementia symptoms may occur as a result of a number of disorders and underlying etiologies. The subsequent sections provide a brief description of some of the dementias listed in the *DSM-5*. In each case, the classic symptoms of dementia (e.g., memory impairment with a number of other cognitive deficits) must be present. Nursing interventions for all dementias are similar to those described for individuals with AD.

Vascular Neurocognitive Disorder

Vascular neurocognitive disorder (also known as *multi-infarct dementia*) is a decline in thinking skill caused by

NURSING CARE PLAN 37.1

The Patient With Dementia

LW is a 76-year-old widow who lives independently. Recently, her children have noticed that she is becoming more forgetful and seems to have periods of confusion. She has agreed to have someone help her during the day. Her oldest son lives with her and is with her during the evening and night. LW refuses to see a health care provider but did agree to go in for a routine checkup. Her daughter helped her get dressed and took her to the primary care office.

Setting: Primary Care Office

Baseline Assessment: A well-groomed woman is accompanied by her daughter. LW says there is nothing wrong, but her daughter disagrees. A review of body systems reveals poor hearing and vision but is otherwise unremarkable. LW's Mini-Mental Status Examination score is 19. Her daughter reports that LW has become very suspicious of her neighbors and has changed her locks several times.

Associated Psychiatric Diagnosis	Medications
Probable Alzheimer Disease	Galantamine (Razadyne) 4 mg twice a day (bid); titrate to 8 mg bid over 4 weeks.

Nursing Diagnosis 1: Impaired Memory

Defining Characteristics	Related Factors
Inability to recall information Inability to recall past events Observed instances of forgetfulness Forgets to perform daily activities (grooming)	Neurocognitive changes associated with dementia

Outcomes

Initial	Long-term
Maintain or improve current memory	Delay cognitive decline associated with dementia

Interventions

Interventions	Rationale	Ongoing Assessment
Develop memory cues in home. Have clocks and calendars well displayed. Make lists for the patients	Maintaining current level of memory involves providing cues that will help the patient recall information.	Contact family members for the patient's ability to use memory cues.
Teach the patient and family about taking an acetylcholinesterase inhibitor. Review expected effects, side effects, and adverse effects. Develop a titration schedule with the family to decrease the appearance of side effects.	Confidence and self-esteem improve when a person looks well-groomed.	Monitor response to suggestions.
Observe patient for visuospatial impairment. If present, sequence habitual activities such as eating, dressing, bathing, and so on.	Visuospatial impairment is one of the symptoms of dementia.	Observe for appropriate dress, bathing, eating, and so on.

Evaluation

Outcomes	Revised Outcomes	Interventions
LW did have some improvement in memory. Suspiciousness and behavioral symptoms improved.	Continue maintaining memory.	Continue with memory cues and galantamine.

conditions that block or reduce blood flow to the brain and the second most common type of dementia. Slightly more men than women are affected. Vascular dementia results when a series of small strokes damage or destroy brain tissue. These are commonly referred to as "ministrokes" or transient ischemic attacks (TIAs), and several TIAs may occur before the affected individual becomes aware of the symptoms of vascular dementia. Most often, a blood clot or plaques (fatty deposits) block the vessels that supply blood to the brain, causing a stroke. However, a stroke can also occur when a blood vessel bursts in the brain (Alzheimer's Association, 2014b).

The primary causes of stroke include high blood cholesterol levels, diabetes, heart disease, and high blood pressure. Of these, high blood pressure is the greatest risk factor for vascular dementia. It is essential that anyone who demonstrates symptoms of dementia or who has a history of stroke should have a complete physical examination that includes neurologic and neuropsychological evaluation, diet and medication history, review of recent stressors, and an array of laboratory tests. Damage to the brain in vascular dementia is usually apparent using computed tomography scans or magnetic resonance imaging. At autopsy, multifocal lesions may be found rather than the more generalized cortical atrophy characteristic of AD.

The behavior changes that result from vascular dementia are similar to those found in AD, such as memory loss, depression, emotional lability or emotional incontinence (including inappropriate laughing or crying), wandering or getting lost in familiar places, bladder or bowel incontinence, difficulty following instructions, gait changes such as small shuffling steps, and problems handling daily activities such as money management. However, these symptoms usually begin more suddenly rather than developing slowly, as is the case in AD. Often, the neurologic symptoms associated with a TIA are minimal and may last only a few days, including slight weakness in an extremity, dizziness, or slurred speech. Thus, the clinical progression is often described as intermittent and fluctuating or of steplike deterioration, with the patient's cognitive and functional status improving or plateauing for a period of time followed by a rapid decline in function after another series of small strokes.

Treatment aims to reduce the primary risk factors for vascular dementia, including hypertension, diabetes, and additional strokes. Interventions that reduce the tendency of the blood to clot and of platelets to aggregate include using medications and lifestyle changes, such as diet, exercise, and smoking cessation to control hypertension, high cholesterol, heart disease, and diabetes. Increasingly, physicians are recommending drugs such as aspirin to help prevent clots from forming in the small blood vessels. Occasionally, surgical procedures such as carotid endarterectomy may be needed to remove blockages in the carotid artery.

Dementia Caused by Parkinson's Disease

Parkinson's disease is a neurologic syndrome of unknown etiology that manifests as a disorder of movement with a slow and progressive course. Clinical manifestations of Parkinson's disease are **bradykinesia** (the slowing of body movements), rigidity, resting tremor, and postural changes. The person's gait is unstable, which results in frequent falls. Parkinson's disease may appear at any time after a person reaches 30 years of age, but the median age of onset is about 70 years of age. In individuals with Parkinson's, 75% will develop neurocognitive dementia (APA, 2013). Although investigators do not know why, there is considerable pathologic overlap between Parkinson's disease and AD. Medical treatment of people with Parkinson's disease typically is with anticholinergics and dopamine agonists. It is important to know that in patients with dementia caused by Parkinson's disease, anticholinergic medications are likely to increase cognitive impairment (Katzenschlager, Sampaio, Costa, & Lees, 2009).

Dementia Caused by Huntington's Disease

Huntington's disease is a progressive, genetically transmitted autosomal dominant disorder characterized by choreiform movements and mental abnormalities. The onset is usually between the ages of 30 and 50 years, but onset occurs before 5 years of age in the juvenile form or as late as 85 years of age in the late-onset form. The disease affects men and women equally. A person with Huntington's disease usually lives for approximately 15 years after diagnosis (APA, 2013). The dementia syndrome of Huntington's disease is characterized by insidious changes in behavior and personality. Typically, the dementia is frontal, which means that the person demonstrates prominent behavioral problems and disruption of attention.

FRONTOTEMPORAL NEUROCOGNITIVE DISORDER

Progressive development of behavioral and personality change and/or language impairment characterizes frontotemporal neurocognitive disorder which has distinct patterns of brain atrophy and distinctive neuropathology. Individuals with this disorder have varying degrees of apathy or disinhibition. They may lose interest in socialization, self-care, and personal responsibilities. Family members report socially inappropriate behaviors, but the individuals show little insight. The cognitive deficits are typically in the area of planning, organization, and judgments. They are easily distracted (APA, 2013).

Population prevalence of frontotemporal neurocognitive disorder is 2 to 10 per 100,000 (APA, 2013). Approximately 20% to 25% of cases occur in individuals over the age of 65. This disorder usually develops between the age of 30 and 70. The disease is progressive with survival of 5 to 11 years after symptoms (APA, 2013).

NEUROCOGNITIVE DISORDER WITH LEWY BODIES

Progressive cognitive decline with visual hallucination, rapid eye movement sleep disorder, and spontaneous Parkinsonism characterizes dementia with Lewy bodies, a major neurocognitive disorder. Cognitive symptoms occur several months before motor symptoms. These symptoms fluctuate and may resemble delirium. These individuals are at high risk for falls because of periods of syncope and transient episodes of consciousness. Orthostatic hypotension and urinary incontinence may occur. The etiology is unknown, but there is evidence of a genetic component (Bruni, Conidi, & Bernardi, 2014). The pathology involves Lewy bodies found in the cortical location in the brain which are thought to be responsible for the disorder.

The estimated prevalence of this dementia ranges from 0.1% to 5% of the general elderly population with men slightly more affected (APA, 2013). This onset of disorder is typically in the sixth to ninth decade and is progressive with a 5- to 7-year survival. These individuals are more functionally impaired than those with other types of dementia such as Alzheimer's and are very sensitive to psychotropic medication, especially antipsychotics.

NEUROCOGNITIVE DISORDER DUE TO PRION DISEASE

Neurocogntive disorder due to prion is a group of spongiform encephalopathies including Creutzfeldt–Jakob disease, a rare, rapidly fatal brain disorder, and "mad cow disease". A prion is a small infectious particle composed of abnormally folded protein that causes progressive neurodegeneration. Many of the symptoms seen in Creutzfeldt–Jakob disease are similar to those found in AD and other dementias. However, changes in the brain tissue are different in Creutzfeldt–Jakob disease and are best differentiated by surgical biopsy or on autopsy (APA, 2013). Common symptoms include fluctuating fever, difficulty swallowing, incontinence, tremors, seizures, and sensitivity to touch and environmental noise.

At present, there is no effective treatment for the disease, and nothing has been found to slow progression of the illness, although antiviral drug studies are ongoing. Because of its rapid clinical course, an important nursing role is assisting family members to understand and come to terms with the illness and to make decisions related to treatment setting and life-sustaining treatments. Creutzfeldt-Jakob disease progresses much more rapidly than most dementias, and death usually occurs within 1 year after onset, although some evidence suggests that extensive changes in the brain may be present before symptoms appear (APA, 2013).

Person-to-person transmission of Creutzfeldt-Jakob disease is rare (but possible), and it can be transmitted from people to animals and between animals. Evidence indicates that the virus can be introduced into the nervous system of healthy patients during medical procedures, such as corneal transplantation, implantation of contaminated electrodes in the brain, and injection of contaminated growth hormones (a few health care workers exposed to the virus, probably through blood and spinal fluids, have experienced the disease). Because of the transmissible nature of Creutzfeldt-Jakob disease and because the virus is not easily destroyed, strict criteria for the handling of infected tissues and other contaminated materials have been developed.

NEUROCOGNITIVE DISORDER DUE TO TRAUMATIC BRAIN INJURY

Traumatic brain injury (TBI) affects about 1.4 to 1.7 million people in the United States each year resulting in a variety of symptoms including neurological, cognitive, behavioral, and emotional impairments (APA, 2013; Lee, Hou, Lee, Hsu, Huang, & Su, 2013). Repeated concussions can lead to brain injury with long-tem TBI. Evidence suggests that even mild TBI is a significant risk factor of developing dementia (Lee et al., 2013).

SUBSTANCE/MEDICATION-INDUCED NEUROCOGNITIVE DISORDER

If dementia results from the persisting effects of a substance (e.g., drugs of abuse, a medication, or exposure to toxins), substance-induced neurocognitive disorder is diagnosed. Other causes of dementia (e.g., dementia caused by a general medical condition) must always be considered even in a person with a dependence on or exposure to a substance. For example, head injuries often result from substance use and may be the underlying cause of the neurocognitive changes (APA, 2013).

Drugs of abuse are the most common toxins in young adults, and prescription drugs are the most common toxins in older adults. In older patients, dementia results from use of long-acting benzodiazepines, barbiturates, meprobamate (Equanil), and a host of other drugs, depending on their dose and the length of time they have been used. Drugs such as flurazepam (Dalmane), with a half-life of more than 120 hours, accumulate rapidly in a person's body. Other drugs accumulate more slowly or require relatively high doses for toxicity to develop. A toxic etiology should be suspected in every patient with a probable diagnosis of dementia. The nurse should inquire about exposure to drugs and toxins (exposure to toxins at work sites, medication use, and recreational drug use) for each patient with dementia, and any substances known to be potentially injurious to the nervous system should be withdrawn if at all possible.

Most of the neurocognitive disorders in this category are related to chronic alcohol abuse. Understanding the cognitive deficits associated with chronic alcohol consumption is complicated. Alcoholic dementia is directly related to the toxic effects of alcohol, although the vitamin deficiencies associated with alcoholism (thiamine and niacin) are also known to be etiologically related to dementia. Individuals with alcoholism also have a high incidence of systemic illnesses that can affect cognition (e.g., cirrhosis, cardiomyopathy), and they are susceptible to repeated head injuries, which carry cognitive consequences of their own.

Much of our knowledge about cognitive deficits in individuals with alcoholism comes from the study of patients with Korsakoff's syndrome, which is a profound deficit in the ability to form new memories and is associated with a variable deficit in recall of old memories despite a clear sensorium. Further careful examination reveals a flattening of drives, unconcern about incapacity, and profound apathy.

Chemicals and organic compounds that impair functioning of the CNS usually have their primary effects on other body systems, including the gastrointestinal, renal, hepatic, blood-forming, and peripheral nervous systems. For example, metal poisonings generally produce gastrointestinal symptoms and peripheral neuropathy. Cognitive changes with poisoning tend to be more characteristic of delirium than dementia, with altered levels of consciousness a prominent feature. Refer to Table 37.1 for a list of some of the organic compounds or chemicals that can cause symptoms of dementia. Related distinguishing symptoms are also included.

Many adolescents and indigent adults engage in the act of "huffing" because the cost of purchasing spray paint, hair spray, glue, and other aerosol products is relatively inexpensive (compared with illicit street drugs). The nurse is reminded to evaluate people who abuse drugs for signs of cognitive impairment because neural and cognitive symptoms tend to appear before permanent brain damage occurs. It is also important to realize that the patient's cognitive status may not immediately improve after discontinuation of use of the offending agent. The effects of drugs taken for a long period may be long lasting, and improvement may follow discontinuation of drug use only slowly. For example, in dementia associated with chronic alcoholism, cognition may improve only after many months of abstinence.

SUMMARY OF KEY POINTS

- Neurocognitive disorders are characterized clinically by significant deficits in cognition or memory that represent a clear-cut change from a previous level of functioning. In some disorders, the loss of cognitive function is progressive, such as in AD. It is important to recognize the differences because the interventions and expected outcomes of the two syndromes are different.

- Delirium is characterized by a disturbance in consciousness and a change in cognition that develops over a short period of time. It requires rapid detection and treatment.

- Nursing assessment is critical in determining the onset of the confusion and disorientation. A thorough nursing assessment includes recent health status changes and practices such as OTC medications.

- Usually, delirium is caused by a combination of precipitating factors. The most commonly identified causes are medications, infections (particularly urinary tract and upper respiratory tract infections), fluid and electrolyte imbalance, and metabolic disturbances such as electrolyte imbalance or poor nutrition. Other important predisposing factors include advanced age, brain damage, preexisting dementia, and biopsychosocial stressors.

- The primary goal of treatment of individuals with delirium is prevention or resolution of the acute confusional episode with return to previous cognitive status and interventions focusing on (1) elimination or correction of the underlying cause and (2) symptomatic and safety and supportive measures.

- Dementia is characterized by the gradual onset of decline in cognitive function, especially memory, usually accompanied by changes in behavior and personality. There are numerous causes of the symptoms of dementia, some of which are reversible, such as hypoxia, carbon monoxide poisoning, and vitamin deficiencies.

- AD is an example of a progressive, degenerative dementia. Treatment efforts currently focus on reduction of cognitive symptoms (e.g., memory loss; confusion; and problems with learning, speech, and reasoning) in attempts to improve the quality of life for both patients and their caregivers.

- Research efforts continue to focus on understanding the relationship among the development of the beta-amyloid plaques, neurofibrillary tangles, and cell death.

- Nursing care of a person with dementia depends on the stage of the disease and the availability of family caregivers.

- Some of the psychosocial stressors known to precipitate delirium and contribute to worsening dementia include sensory overload or underload, immobilization, sleep deprivation, fatigue, pain or hunger, a change in routine (pace or caregiver), or demands beyond the patient's ability.

- Educating and supporting families and caregivers through the progressive cognitive decline and behavior changes is essential to ensuring proper care.

- Several mental health strategies (exercise, education, cognitive stimulation) support and protect a person's cognitive reserve. A healthy cognitive reserve is thought to be protective against neuropathologic insults.

- Other neurocognitive disorders may be related to specific brain changes (Lewy bodies), infections (prion disease), genetic diseases (Huntington's), and substances/medications.

CRITICAL THINKING CHALLENGES

1. What factors should be considered in differentiating AD from vascular dementia?

2. Describe three ways in which medical disease can disrupt brain functioning and relate these mechanisms to the neurocognitive disorders presented in this chapter.

3. Suggest reasons that older adults are particularly vulnerable to the development of neurocognitive disorders.

4. Compare the nursing care of a person with delirium versus one with dementia. What are the similarities and differences in the care?

5. The physical environment is particularly important to the patient with dementia. Every effort should be made to modify the physical environment to compensate for the cognitive and functional impairment associated with AD and related disorders, including safety measures and the avoidance of misleading stimuli. Visualize your last experience in a health care setting (hospital, nursing home, day care program, or home care setting). Identify environmental factors that could be misleading or stress producing to a person with impaired cognition (dementia), and identify ways to modify this environment to alleviate some of the stressors or misleading stimuli.

6. Mr. J. has been recently diagnosed with mild AD and is asking for advice about deciding on his care in the future. His wife and daughter believe that he does not have the ability to make these decisions and asks for the nurse's advice. How should the nurse respond? Explain the rationale.

Iris: 2001. This film tells the story of British novelist Iris Murdoch (played by Judi Dench and Kate Winslet) and her relationship with her husband John Bayley (played by Jim Broadbent and Huh Bonneville) during the last 5 years of her life. Based on Bayley's memoir, *Elegy for Iris*, the film depicts Ms. Murdoch's decline into dementia and the stress associated with caregiving. This wonderful movie shows the suffering of AD but also shows the strength of relationships. The film contrasts the start of their relationship when Iris was an outgoing, dominant individual and John was a timid, shy scholarly partner with the two older adults who created a loving bond that provided the fabric of the last days of Iris' life.

VIEWING POINTS: Identify the symptoms of the progressive illness throughout the film. Were there any "breaking points" for the caregiver? Were there aspects of Iris' personality that were sustained throughout the course of her life that were evident at the end? What nursing interventions would have been helpful to support her cognitive functioning?

MOVIE viewing GUIDES related to this chapter are available at http://thePoint.lww.com/Boyd5eUpdate.

References

Alzheimer's Association. (2014a). *2014 Alzheimer's disease facts and figures.* Chicago: Alzheimer's Association.

Alzheimer's Association. (2014b). Vascular dementia. http://www.alz.org/dementia/vascular-dementia-symptoms.asp. Retrieved May 10, 2014.

American Psychiatric Association. (2013). *Diagnostic and statistical manual of mental disorders* (5th ed.). Arlington, VA: American Psychiatric Association.

Arenaza-Urquijo, E. M., Bosch, B., Sala-Llonch, R., Sole-Padulles, C., Junque, C., Fernandez-Espejo, D., et al. (2011). Specific anatomic associations between white matter integrity and cognitive reserve in normal and cognitively impaired elders. *American Journal of Geriatric Psychiatry, 19*(1), 33–42.

Bateman, R. J., Xiong, C., Benzinger, T. L., Fagan, A. M., Goate, A., Fox, N. C., et al. (2012). Clinical and biomarker changes in dominantly inherited Alzheimer' Disease. *The New England Journal of Medicine, 367*(9), 795–804.

Bruni, A. C., Conidi, M. E., & Bernardi, L. (2014). Genetics in degenerative dementia: Current status and applicability. *Journal of Alzheimer Disease & Associated Disorders*, PMID 24905970.

Bryczkowski, S. B., Lopreiato, M. C., Yonclas, P. P., Sacca, J. J., & Mosenthal, A. C. (2014). Delirium prevention program in the surgical intensive care unit improved the outcomes of older adults. *Journal of Surgical Research, 190*(1), 280–288. *doi:10.1016/j.jss.2014.02.044.*

Caplan, J. P. & Rabinowitz, R. (2010). An approach to the patient with cognitive impairment: Delirium and dementia. *Medical Clinics of North America, 94*(6), 1103–1116.

Clavel, D. S. (1999). Vocalizations among cognitively impaired elders. *Geriatric Nursing, 20*, 90–93.

Dahmani, S., Delivet, H., & Hilly, J. (2014). Emergence delirium in children: An update. *Current Opinion, 27*(3), 309–315.

Desai, A. K. & Schwarz, L. (2011). Subjective cognitive impairment: When to be concerned about "senior moments." *Current Psychiatry, 10*(4), 31–44.

Garcia-Alberca, J. M., Lara, J. P., Cruz, B., Garrido, V., Gris, E., & Barbancho, M. A. (2013). Sleep disturbances in Alzheimer's disease are associated with neuropsychiatric symptoms and antidementia treatment. *Journal of Nervous & Mental Disease. 201*(3), 251–257.

Farina, N., Tabet, J., & Rusted, J. (2014). Habitual physical activity (HPA) as a factor in sustained executive function in Alzheimer-type dementia: A cohort study. *Archives of Gerontology and Geriatrics, 59*(1), 91–97. http://dx.doi.org/10.1016/j.archger.2014.016

Flaherty, J. H. (2011). The evaluation and management of delirium among older persons. *Medical Clinics of North America, 95*(3), 555–577.

Forest Laboratories. (2014). *Namenda XR prescribing information.* Retrieved May 9, 2014, from http://www.namenda.com/Prescribing.aspx.

Fortinsky, R. H. & Downs, M. (2014). Optimizing person-centered transitions in the dementia journey: A comparison of national dementia strategies. *Health Affairs, 33*(4), 566–573.

Frost, B., hemberg, M., Lewis, J., & Feany, M. B. (2014). Tau promotes neurodegeneration through global chromatin relaxation. *Nature Neuroscience, 17*(3), 357–366. doi:10.1038/nn.3639

Galvin, J. E., Roe, C. M., Powlishta, K. K., Coats, M. A., Muich, S. J., Grant, E., et al. (2005). The AD8: A brief informant interview to detect dementia. *Neurology, 65*(4), 559–564.

Galvin, J. E., Roe, C. M., Xiong, C., & Morris, J. C. (2006). Validity and reliability of the AD8 informant interview in dementia. *Neurology, 67*(11), 1942–1948.

Gomes, S., Martins, I., Fonseca, A. C., Oliveira, C. R., Resende, R., & Pereira, C. M., (2014). Protective effect of leptin and ghrelin against toxicity induced by amyloid-β oligomers in a hypothalamic cell line. *Journal of Neuroendocrinology, 26*(3), 176–185.

Guo, W., Sha, S., Xing, X., Jiang, T., & Cao, Y. (2013). Reduction of cerebral Abeta burden and improvement in cognitive function in Tg-APPswe/PSEN1dE9 mice following vaccination with a multivalent Abeta3–10 DNA vaccine. *Neuroscience Letters, 549*, 109–115.

Katzenschlager, R., Sampaio, C., Costa, J., & Lees, A. (2009). Anticholinergics for symptomatic management of Parkinson's disease. *The Cochrane Database of Systematic Reviews,* (2), CD003735.

Lee, Y., Hou, S., Lee, C., Hsu, C., Huang, Y., & Su, Y. (2013). Increased risk of dementia in patients with mild traumatic brain injury: A nationwide cohort study. *PLoS One, 8*(5), e62422. *doi:10.1371/journal.pone.0062422*

Leong, D. (2014). Antidepressants for depression in patients with dementia: A review of the literature. *The Consultant Pharmacist, 29*(4), 254–263.

Lewis, M., Hobday, J. V., & Hepburn, K. W. (2011). Internet-based program for dementia caregivers. *American Journal of Alzheimer's Disease & Other Dementias, 25*(8), 674–679.

Marchesi, V. T. (2014). Alzheimer's disease and CADASIL are heritable, adult-onset dementias that both involve damaged small blood vessels. *Cellular & Molecular Life Sciences, 71*(6), 949–955.

Mattison, M. L., Catic, A., Davis, R. B., Olveczky, D., Moran, J., Yang, J., et al. (2014). A standardized, bundled approach to providing geriatric-focused acute care. *Journal of the American Geriatrics Society, 62*(5), 936–942. *doi: 10.1111/jgs.12780*

Meng, X. & D'Arcy, C. (2012). Education and dementia in the context of the cognitive reserve hypothesis: A systematic review with meta-analyses and qualitative analyses. *PLoS One, 7*(6), 1–16.

Morbelli, S. & Nobili, F. (2014). Cognitive reserve and clinical expression of Alzheimer's disease: Evidence and implications for baring PET imaging. *American Journal of Nuclear medicine and Molecular Imaging. 4*(3), 239–247.

Porsteinsson, A. P., Drye, L. T., Pollock, B. F., Devannand, D. P., Grangakis, C., Ismail, Z., et al. (2014). Effect of citalopram on agitation in Alzheimer disase: The CitAD randomized clinical trial. *JAMA, 311*(7), 682–691.

Razavi, M., Tolea, M., Margrett, J., Martin, P., Oakland, A., Tscholl, D. W., et al. (2013). Comparison of 2 informant questionnaire screening tools for dementia and mild cognitive impairment AD8 and IQCODE. *Alzheimer Disease Association Disorders, 28*(2), 156–161. doi:10.1097/WAD.0000000000000008. www.alzheimerjournal.com

Rothman, S. M. & Mattson, M. P. (2012). Sleep Disturbances in Alzheimer's and Parkinson's Diseases *Neuromolecular Medicine, 14*(3), 194–204. doi:10.1007/s12017-012-8181-2

Seo, S. W., Im, K., Lee, J. M., Kim, S. T., Ahn, H. J., Go, S. M., et al. (2011). Effects of demographic factors on cortical thickness in Alzheimer's disease. *Neurobiology of Aging, 32*(2), 200–209.

Soto, M. E., Secher, M., Gillette-Guyonnet, S., van, Kan, G. A., Andrieu, S., Nourhashemi, F., et al. (2012). Weight loss and rapid cognitive decline in community-dwelling patients with Alzheimer's disease. *Journal of Alzheimer's Disease, 28*(3), 647–654.

Tang, S., Patel, P., Khubchandani, J., & Grossberg, G. T. (2014). The psychogeriatric patient in the emergency room: Focus on management and disposition. *ISRN Psychiatry, doi:10.1155/2014/413572*

U.S. Department of Health and Human Services. (2014). *2012–2013 Progress report on Alzheimer's disease: Translating new knowledge.* Washington, DC: Alzheimer Disease Education & Referral (ADEAR) Center, National Institute on Aging, National Institutes of Health. Retrieved April 29, 2011, from http://www.nia.nih.gov/Alzheimers/Publications/ADProgress2009.

Verdelho, A., Madureira, S., Moleiro, C., Ferro, J. M., O'Brien, J. T., Poggesi, A., et al. (2013). Depressive symptoms predict cognitive decline and dementia in older people independently of cerebral white matter changes: the LADIS study. *Journal Neurology, Neurosurgery, & Psychiatry, 84*(11), 1250–1254.

Voyer, P., Richard, S., Doucet, L., & Carmichael, P. H. (2011). Factors associated with delirium severity among older persons with dementia. *Journal of Neuroscience Nursing, 43*(2), 62–69.

Whall, A. L., Hyojeong, K., Colling, K. B., Gwi-Ryung, H., DeCicco, B., & Antonakos, C. (2013). Measurement of aggressive behaviors in dementia. *Research in Gerontological Nursing, 6*(3), 171–177.

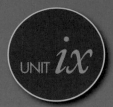

CARE OF SPECIAL POPULATIONS

UNIT *ix*

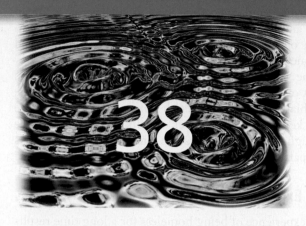

38

Caring for Persons Who Are Homeless and Mentally Ill

Ruth Beckmann Murray and Richard Yakimo

KEY CONCEPT

• homelessness

LEARNING OBJECTIVES

After studying this chapter, you will be able to:

1. Define the meaning of homelessness to the person and family.

2. Describe risk factors for becoming homeless.

3. Differentiate characteristics of various populations who are homeless.

4. Discuss personal and societal attitudes and beliefs about homelessness.

5. Describe assessment of people who are homeless and mentally ill.

6. Formulate some nursing diagnoses relevant to the homeless population.

7. Summarize interventions and discharge plans for people who are homeless and have psychiatric disorders.

8. Discuss trends that target improvement of services to people who are homeless and experiencing psychiatric disorders.

KEY TERMS

• Assertive Community Treatment (ACT) • case management • continuum of care • day treatment
• deinstitutionalization • Housing First • Safe Havens • Section 8 housing • Shelter Plus Care Program
• supportive housing • transitional housing

Children, adults, and families can become homeless from encountering a natural disaster, home fire, some situational crisis or unexpected overwhelming life situation, or economic hardship. Others find themselves homeless because of problems related to substance use or mental illness. Children or adolescents may be abandoned or may not be in parental or guardian custody.

> **KEYCONCEPT** **Homelessness** is lacking "a fixed permanent nighttime residence or living in nighttime residences that are temporary shelters, welfare hotels, transitional housing for the mentally ill, or any public or private place not designated as sleeping accommodations for human beings" (Interagency Council on the Homeless, 1994, p. 22).

BOX 38.1

Characteristics of People Who Are Mentally Ill and Homeless

- Seriously mentally ill people are at greater risk for homelessness than the general population.
- Mental health problems increase with the duration of time the person is homeless.
- They have at least one psychiatric service encounter annually, usually in an emergency department rather than inpatient or outpatient units.
- They are homeless for longer periods, often years, than are those who are homeless and not mentally ill or substance abusing.
- They are more likely to be in poor physical health than other homeless people.
- They have more contacts with the legal system than other homeless or housed people.
- They are more likely to encounter employment barriers and less likely to benefit from societal economic growth.
- They are less likely to have contact with family or friends, especially if they come from higher-income households.
- Most are eligible for, but have difficulty obtaining, income maintenance such as Social Security Disability Insurance, Veterans Affairs disability benefits, or other benefits.
- Most are willing to accept treatment after basic survival needs are met and a therapeutic relationship has been established.

Source: National Coalition for the Homeless (2009c). *Who is homeless? NCH fact sheet #3.* Available at http://www.nationalhomeless.org.

Box 38.1 lists characteristics of people who are homeless and mentally ill. This chapter explores issues relevant to individuals who are homeless and who are also experiencing mental health problems. It presents nursing care measures and suggests ways to improve services for the homeless population.

HOMELESSNESS

Homelessness is a word that evokes images and feelings in everyone. Without a consistent dwelling place, meeting basic needs is difficult. Homelessness means carrying all of one's possessions in a car, suitcase, bag, or shopping cart or storing necessities in a bus station locker or under the bed of a night shelter. It means no chest for treasured objects, no closet for next season's clothing, no pantry with food to eat, no place to entertain friends or have solitude, and no place for a child to play.

People who are homeless tend to be ignored or not seen by the general population who hurry on their own way. Homeless people who also have learning disabilities are virtually unnoticed as such (Trueland, 2009) because the demonstrated behaviors are similar to the negative stereotypes about people who are homeless.

Persons who have been or are homeless and have mental illnesses can become resilient because they have typically have endured and coped with constraints or problems with extremes stressors or catastrophes and negative life events. Deprivation of needs, the sense of isolation and stigma, and the lack of accessible resources may be of short- or long-term duration. In turn, self-confidence and sense of competence can be eroded (Fitzpatrick, 2009; Howard, 2009). Yet many people who experience homelessness maintain hope and a positive attitude, which in turn helps them to reach out to help, take advantage of opportunities, and become part of the housed population.

The key to developing resilience is to reframe the event or experience and to receive support from others. Psychiatric and mental health nurses have been and are in a key position to foster development of resilience through counseling, education, and mentoring of clients (Fitzpatrick, 2009).

The Experience of Being Homeless

The experience of being homeless for a long time results in a sense of depersonalization and fragmented identity; a loss of self-worth and self-efficacy and a stigma of being "nothing," "a bum," "lazy," and "stupid." However, most people who are homeless describe themselves as resourceful, independent, proud, and survivors (Murray, 1996).

Some people wrongly associate all homelessness with mental illness, violence, and alcohol or drug addiction. A person who is homeless for the first time or for a few months is more likely to have a more positive outlook than a person who has been homeless for a long time because the chances of recovering economic and social status are greater (Kirkpatrick & Byrne, 2009). Biographies and research describe the tragedy and nightmare of being homeless (Boydell, Goering, & Morrell-Bellai, 2000; Kirkpatrick & Byrne, 2009; Meadows-Oliver, 2005; Murray, 1996; Sullivan, Burnam, Koegel, & Hollenberg, 2000).

The person who is homeless is often engaged in hunting for shelter, food, and clothing and lacks consistent ways to meet basic needs. This lifestyle, plus grinding poverty and victimization, especially if the person is mentally ill, leave little energy for change or reentrance into mainstream society. Panhandling, hustling, doing odd jobs, and selling plasma or aluminum cans are common sources of income, although some people who are homeless receive Social Security or veterans or pension benefits.

Victims of immediate circumstances—hunger, cold, or assault—the choices and strategies that persons who homeless pursue are affected by their need to subsist and to overcome fear, loss of freedom and privacy, resignation, loneliness, and depression. The longer a person is homeless, the more likely the person is to experience mental illness or engage in substance use (Finfgeld-Connett, 2010; Hoff, Hallisey, & Hoff, 2009; North, Eyrich-Garg, Pollio, & Thirthalli, 2010).

The healthiest survivors seek support from others, maintain hope for the future, and strive to have valued lives and selves. They believe they are resourceful, can handle uncertainty, and can maintain health. Homeless women who have children have described the need to keep going for the sake of and to avoid losing their children. They cite the importance of spiritual beliefs in developing inner resources, reducing distress, and enhancing the connection to themselves, others, and powers beyond themselves (Carlton, Young, & Kelly, 2010) Huribut, Robbins, & Hoke, 2011; Washington, Moxley, Garriott & Weinberger, 2009).

Historical Perspectives

Homelessness has not always been widespread in the United States. Housing was affordable for most people and was provided for the ill. The phenomenon of many mentally ill people living on the street began in the mid-1900s. A public outcry followed a photographic essay in 1946 by *Life* magazine about deplorable conditions in state hospitals for those with mentally illnesses. The introduction of chlorpromazine (Thorazine) in 1954 provided a simple means of reducing symptoms of psychosis, and the Mental Retardation Facilities and Community Mental Health Centers Construction Act of 1963 initiated **deinstitutionalization** of the population (release of those confined to mental institutions for long periods of time into the community for treatment, support, and rehabilitation; see Chapter 1). The stigma against people with mentally illnesses became greater as cities faced real social and financial consequences. Furthermore, people who were both homeless and severely mentally ill experienced fear, suspicion, caution, and disorganized thinking, which interfered with their ability to access available services and promoted a homeless lifestyle (National Coalition for the Homeless, 2009a).

Deinstutionalization occurred again in the mid-1990s, when the Veterans Administration (VA) Hospitals reduced inpatient and expanded outpatient treatment sites to increase access for essential care to veterans. Veterans returning from the wars in the Middle East evidenced an increased rate of psychiatric disorders and consequent homelessness. More veterans returning from Iran experienced psychiatric disorders, and of these veterans, 12% were homeless. Major barriers to mental health care and general health care were access (living more than 50 miles from a VA hospital) and financial constraints (Zeber, Copeland, McCarthy, Bauer, & Kilbourne, 2009).

McKinney-Vento Homeless Assistance Act

The McKinney-Vento Homeless Assistance Act (Public Law 100–77, first passed in 1987 as the McKinney Act) was named in 2000 for Representatives Stewart B. McKinney and Bruce Vento, who worked passionately on behalf of people who are homeless (McKinney Act renamed, 2000). This landmark legislation reflected concern in the United States about people who are homeless and provided the first comprehensive federal funding program targeted specifically to address the health, education, and welfare needs of the homeless population. It allocated money for crises and community services for people with chronic mental illness, alcohol and drug detoxification and treatment programs, psychosocial rehabilitation, families with children at risk for emotional disturbance because of homelessness, long-term case management, supportive housing, training of service providers, and research (Interagency Council on the Homeless, 1994).

Subsequent revisions to the McKinney Act incorporated a **continuum of care** approach, including emergency shelter, transitional or rehabilitative services, and permanent housing or supportive living arrangements. Because of the gap in services for people who are homeless and mentally ill, amendments were made to the McKinney Act in 1992 that included a provision for the creation of **Safe Havens**, which are a form of supportive housing that serves hard-to-reach people with severe mental illness (Center for Mental Health Services, 1997). The **Shelter Plus Care Program**, also a continuum of care program, allows for various housing choices and a range of supportive services funded by other sources (U.S. Department of Housing and Urban Development [HUD], 1998). The federal Health Care for the Homeless Program, a program to assist persons who are homeless and have acquired immunodeficiency syndrome (AIDS), expanded the focus of the original Act by providing refuge in shelters for victims of domestic violence and for children in homeless families (Sullivan et al., 2000).

The McKinney-Vento Act Homeless Assistance Program of 2002 provides for (1) the Emergency Shelter Grants Program; (2) the Supportive Housing Program, which includes Transitional Housing, Supportive Housing, Supportive Services, and Safe Haven; (3) the Shelter Plus Care Program, which provides long-term rental assistance for people who are homeless with mental illness, substance dependence, or human immunodeficiency virus (HIV)/ AIDS; (4) rental assistance through the Single Room Occupancy (SRO) and SRO/Section 8 Housing Program (discussed later); and (5) an emphasis on ensuring educational rights and protective measures to children and adolescents experiencing homelessness (McKinney-Vento Homeless Assistance Act, 2002).

Bipartisan legislation (S709/HR1471), known as the Services for Ending Long-Term Homelessness Act (SELHA), authorized federal funding through HUD to finance permanent supportive housing targeted for chronically homeless people. This legislation complements housing funded under the McKinney-Vento Homeless Assistance Act (Shelter Plus Care and Subsidized Housing Program) and President Bush's "Samaritan Initiative," which centered on redirecting resources toward the development of permanent supportive housing. The focus continues to provide coordinated, flexible, "wrap-around" services to housed individuals that lead to recovery from severe, persistent mental illness and co-occurring disorders and then reintegration into community life.

Bringing Home America Act

The Bringing Home America Act (HR 4347), reintroduced by Julia Carson (D-IN) and nine cosponsors in November 2006, was based on research data, reported experiences of people who have been homeless, and presented information from service providers for the homeless. The Act includes housing development, support for living income, rental assistance (no more than 30% of income to be spent on housing by low-income families or individuals), job training opportunities, civil rights (including the right to vote) protection for persons without housing, emergency funds to prevent homelessness, and increased access to health care for this population (Bringing America Home, 2005).

This legislation continues the work of the National Housing Trust Fund and Affordable Housing Trust Funds established in major U.S. cities to build and preserve 1.5 million units of rental housing for the lowest income and homeless families by 2010 to 2015. These efforts are in response to the data showing that, on average, U.S. families must earn $18.44 hourly, more than 2.5 times the minimum wage, to afford a two-bedroom apartment at fair market value. In contrast, the estimated median wage among U.S. private sectors workers is only $16.01 (National Low Income Housing Coalition, 2010).

The Affordable Care Act

The Affordable Care Act, passed in 2010, focuses on preventive care coverage. In the first year of the implementation of the Act, all newly sold insurance plans are required to pay for prevention and wellness with no cost sharing by the person. There are no deductibles in the insurance plan. Thus, many financial barriers are removed for many Americans in relation to physical health, such as mammograms, colonoscopies, and immunizations. Legislation is needed to remove financial barriers to mental health care.

In July 2010, under the American Recovery and Reinvestment Act of 2009, $96 million was appropriated to the Human Resources and Services Administration, the primary federal agency responsible for improving access to health care for people who are uninsured, isolated, or medically vulnerable (all characteristics of the homeless population). These funds support education of the nation's health care workforce, including nurses. Such funding and education should have a positive influence on mental

---

BOX 38.2

General Causes of Homelessness

- Poverty; history of childhood family instability
- Lack of affordable housing; doubling up with relatives or friends until the situation is intolerable
- Mental illness or substance abuse and lack of needed services
- Low-paying jobs; unemployment
- Domestic violence; flight from a violent home or abandonment; youth aging out of services
- Eviction for not paying rent; multiple movers
- Limited life coping skills; disturbing behavior
- Changes or reductions in public assistance programs
- Veteran status
- Prison release; having no money, job, or place to go

---

health care as well as physical health care. In April 2011, the McKinney-Vento Homeless Assistance Grants program received a $40 million increase over fiscal year 2010, bringing total funding to $1.9 billion.

Etiology and Risk Factors for Homelessness

Homelessness has no single cause. People prefer to have a home and to be part of a family or social group. People do not choose or purposefully maintain homelessness and living on the streets. Many factors—unemployment, lack of skills, mental illness, substance abuse, domestic violence—typically combine, with time, to cause the person or family to lose permanent housing (Box 38.2). The series of events that results in having no home is the culmination of individual and environmental factors, including factors in the mental health system, society, and family or community (Box 38.3).

Homeless Populations

The homeless population includes people of all ages, economic levels, racial and cultural backgrounds, and geographic areas. Gentrification, upgrading of inner-city property so that it is affordable only to people who have the resources of upper-middle or upper economic levels, is increasingly a factor in creating homelessness among urban residents. Middle-class and upper middle-class professionals, mostly whites, are relocating to the inner city. Thus, abandoned or substandard buildings are demolished to build modern condominiums or "lofts." People who lived in the abandoned structures or empty houses are being displaced to the streets to become homeless (Hoff et al., 2009). People who are homeless are often chronically ill, jobless, or have recently lost all financial resources. Long-term homeless people may have lived in poverty for years with no home site. Among homeless people, educational level varies greatly, from less than an eighth-grade education to doctoral degrees.

BOX 38.3

Risk Factors for Homelessness Among People With Serious Mental Illness

INDIVIDUAL RISK FACTORS

- Symptoms of mental illness, including unpredictable behavior; an inability to manage everyday affairs; and an inability to communicate needs, which results in conflicts with family, employers, landlords, and neighbors
- Concurrent mental illness and substance abuse disorders in youth and adults with behaviors that place them at high risk for eviction, arrest, and incarceration in jails or repeated admissions and short stays in mental hospitals
- Coexisting HIV or AIDS with severe persistent mental illness, chemical use, or both
- Coexisting demographic and societal factors of poverty; single-parent family (usually female headed); dependent child; child in foster home; racial or ethnic minority; veteran status; single men and women; ex-offender released from jail or prison
- Coexisting physical illness or developmental disability
- Exposure to traumatic events repeatedly, resulting in posttraumatic stress disorder and deficits in independent living skills
- Exposure to victimization (physical and sexual abuse), especially if a family member was the perpetrator
- Inability to cope with or manage the requirements of family, community, or group living home
- Lack of high school education or equivalence
- History of war veteran

ENVIRONMENTAL RISK FACTORS

Mental Health System Factors

- Inadequate discharge planning with a lack of appropriate housing, treatment, and support services

- Lack of funding for community-based services
- Lack of integrated community-based treatment and support services for individual and group therapy, medication monitoring, and case management
- Lack of community-based crisis alternatives for housing, health care, and respite care for families with risk for rehospitalization and loss of residence
- Lack of attention to consumer preferences for autonomy, privacy, and integrated regular housing
- Changing environment, such as loss of home caused by natural or human-made disaster

Societal and Family Factors

- Lack of affordable housing; affluent economic times have caused housing prices to soar out of reach, to reduce construction of low-cost housing, and to create a tight rental market
- Insufficient disability benefits; Social Security income recipients are below the federal poverty level
- Lack of coordination between mental health and substance abuse systems
- Waiting lists to receive a subsidy that requires the person to pay only 30% of income for rent and utilities
- Lack of job opportunities for disabled people
- Stigma and discrimination; resistance to community housing for people with mentally illnesses is widespread
- Poor family relationships; willingness to help the ill person is exhausted as relatives cope with frightening or disturbing behavior and receive insufficient help from the community or medical profession

Sources: Carlton et al., 2010; Marshall, Bell, & Moules, 2010; National Coalition for the Homeless, 2009a, 2009d; North et al., 2010; Zeber et al., 2009.

Personal, social, and economic deprivations contribute to homelessness and sometimes to crime in an effort to survive. Deprivation exists among people living in North American urban, ghetto, and rural areas; on the reservations that are home to North American native people; among migrant farmers in the United States of America; and in the shanty towns and ghettoes in the Southern Hemisphere (Hoff et al., 2009).

Prevalence

There is no easy way to determine how many people are homeless in the United States. It is estimated that the homeless population increased by about 20,000 people from 2008 to 2009 (Sermons & Witte, 2011). Counting the homeless population is understandably difficult, given their mobility. In most cases, homelessness is a temporary circumstance, not a permanent condition. Studies of homelessness are complicated by problems of definition and methodology. For example, counting the number of people who are in shelters does not take into account those who live on the streets or in unsafe housing situations, such as abandoned buildings. Others without a

personal home but temporarily living with relatives or friends also may not be counted as homeless (National Coalition for the Homeless, 2009b).

The latest statistics on homelessness come from HUD's July 2010 *Annual Homeless Assessment Report to Congress*. Estimates include both point prevalence (snapshot) and period prevalence (within a period of time) and include people who are both sheltered and living on the street. For period prevalence, on a single night in January 2009, there were an estimated 643,067 sheltered and unsheltered people who were homeless throughout the United States. More than 60% were in emergency shelters or transitional housing programs; the remainder were on the street or living in places unsafe for habitation (U.S. HUD, 2010). Estimates of point prevalence have remained fairly consistent over the past 3 years, with a smaller proportion of people remaining unsheltered. This may reflect better counts of those living on the street but also indicates the increasing success of communities in moving people into shelters or transitional housing programs.

Of those experiencing homelessness, 63% were single, and 37% were part of a family (a family was defined as a person 18 years of age or older with at least one child).

Family members were less likely than individuals to remain unsheltered (21%). The number of people chronically homeless has dropped from 124,135 in 2008 to 110,917 in 2009. (Chronic homelessness was defined as continually homeless for 1 year or more or has had at least four episodes of homelessness in the past 3 years.) Geographically, homelessness tends to occur in the large coastal states with high costs of living, with California, New York, and Florida accounting for 39% of the total. States with the highest concentrations of homeless people were Nevada (0.85%) followed by Oregon, Hawaii, California, and Washington. The lowest concentrations of homeless people were reported by Kansas, South Dakota, and West Virginia (U.S. HUD, 2010).

For annual period prevalence, nearly 1.56 million people used an emergency shelter or transitional housing during October 2008 through September 2009. More than 170,000 families were admitted to shelters in 2009, a 30% increase since 2007. This is probably attributable to recent economic downturns and job loss resulting in loss of home. The typical sheltered person was a man with minority status, middle aged, and single. Only 2.8% of the sheltered homeless population is age 62 years or older. More than two-thirds of sheltered homeless adults have a mental or physical disability (U.S. HUD, 2010).

Among people who are mentally ill and homeless, those who became homeless before becoming mentally ill have the highest levels of disadvantage and disruption and the lowest General Assessment of Function scores. Those who became homeless after becoming mentally ill have a higher prevalence of alcohol abuse. Mental illness may be a factor in initiating homelessness for some people, but other risk factors are also involved (Moe, 2007). See also Box 38.3.

An increasing number of people who are homeless are youth, women, and families headed by single parents. In rural areas, single mothers and children are the largest group of people who are homeless; people who are white, American Indian, and immigrants are also more likely to be among the rural homeless population. Fifty percent of all women and children who experience homelessness are fleeing from domestic violence. Studies show that men tend to report that their homelessness is caused by unemployment, alcohol and drug abuse, or imprisonment (National Coalition for the Homeless, 2009b). See Box 38.4 for more information about incidence.

Diverse Groups

Homelessness occurs in many groups of people. People with severe mental illness are at much higher risk for poverty and homelessness than are others. Symptoms of mental illness, such as impulsivity, hypersexuality, and poor judgment, also may be related to risky sexual behaviors. Sexual risk-taking behaviors and drug use practices,

---

BOX 38.4

Incidence of Homelessness

The population who is homeless is estimated to consist of:
- Single men, 41%
- Families with children, 40%
- Families headed by single parent, 73%
- Single women, 14%
- Unaccompanied minors, 5%
- Adults, 25–34 years of age, 25%
- Adults, 55–64 years of age, 6%
- African Americans, 49%
- White, non-Hispanics, 35%
- Hispanics or Latinos, 13%
- American Indians, 2.9%
- Asians, 1%
- Veterans, 41% of homeless men; 10% of homeless population

Sources: Homelessness Resource Center, 2009; National Coalition for the Homeless, 2009a, 2009b.

---

such as sharing needles, contribute to a high rate of HIV infection among homeless people. Poverty also contributes to unsafe sexual behaviors because of unavailable condoms, shared sleeping sites, unplanned sexual contacts, and trading sex for other perceived needs (money, food, place to stay, illicit drugs). Furthermore, substance abuse or co-occurring substance use (cocaine, alcohol, other substances) with mental illness are stronger predictors than the sole presence of mental illness for HIV exposure risk (North et al., 2010).

Adolescents and runaway youths can become homeless because of strained family relationships, family dissolution, and instability of residential placements (Nyamathi, Marfisee, Slagle, Greengold, Liu, & Leake, 2010). Homeless young people may resort to drug trafficking and prostitution to support themselves. They are at risk for physical and mental health problems, including substance abuse, HIV infection or AIDS, pregnancy, and suicidal behaviors. Because of their high rates of exposure to violence, they are more likely to experience posttraumatic stress disorder (PTSD) and depression. To compound their problems, they are less likely than other people who are homeless to use shelters because few available shelters will accept them, and they often distrust and fear providers. Furthermore, they have poor tenant skills and often little income, so they cannot obtain rental housing (Cleverley & Kidd, 2010).

More homeless people than sheltered people have been arrested or incarcerated. In one study, 16% of the inmates were homeless (Buck, Brown, & Hickey, 2011). When released, ex-offenders are cut off from their communities and are less likely to reestablish themselves after their release. They are at high risk for homelessness. Others with criminal records may have turned to crime after they became homeless to support themselves. Another group that has arrest records are mentally ill people who have been inappropriately jailed because of inadequacies in the mental health treatment system (Buck et al., 2011).

Several other groups are at risk for homelessness or may experience homelessness at some point. About 10% to 12% of veterans who have been in combat are homeless and suffer PTSD (acute or delayed), anxiety disorders, and major depression. They experience difficulty with reentry into civilian life and employment (National Coalition for the Homeless, 2009c). New immigrants come to a specific location with the intention of setting up permanent residence. Economic problems or conflicts with the sponsoring family may jeopardize housing. Refugees are poor; they are involuntarily living outside their home countries because of persecution related to race, religion, nationality, social group membership, or political opinion. Mental health problems arise because of torture experiences, losses suffered in the country of origin, and culture shock and scapegoating experienced in the United States. Posttraumatic stress is common in this group; their physical health problems are often complex (Andrews & Boyle, 2007; Hollander, Bruce, Burström, & Ekblad, 2011).

Migrant workers and their families lack residential stability as they move from one geographic region to another for 6 to 9 months of the growing and harvest season. These laborers and their families may be U.S. citizens or foreign born. They are poor and typically lack adequate living quarters and health care. Physical health problems and depression are common in these families. After farm labor is completed, family members may be homeless until they can return to their place of origin or to a relative's home (Hollander et al., 2011; Revollo, Qureshi, Collazos, Valero, & Casa, 2011).

Family Response to Homelessness

Family homelessness, whatever its cause, has an especially adverse effect on children (Sermons & Witte, 2011). The poorest children move two or three times within the year before becoming homeless and moving into a shelter. Homeless children are generally school aged or younger. These children have high rates of both acute and chronic health problems and are more likely than children who are not homeless to be hospitalized, have delayed immunizations, and have elevated lead blood levels. In addition, they are at risk for developmental delays and emotional and behavioral difficulties. School attendance is disrupted frequently, and they are vulnerable to violence, either as victims or witnesses. Children who are homeless are more likely to experience homelessness in adulthood (Carlton, Young, & Kelly, 2010; Rew, Grady, Whittaker, & Bowman, 2008).

Living in shelters is stressful for families for several reasons. Many shelters exclude men and adolescent boys

older than 12 years; thus, family members are separated. Overcrowding prevents privacy and promotes loss of personal control. Stressors of poverty and reduced social support compound the trauma of these experiences.

A history of abuse and assault is common among homeless mothers (Marshall, Bell, & Moules, 2010; Moe, 2007). Homeless mothers have high lifetime rates of major depressive disorder, PTSD, and substance-related disorders. In addition, they have high rates of attempted suicide. Homeless women who have a social network, some cash assistance such as Social Security or welfare, or a housing subsidy are more likely to become and remain housed (Marshall et al., 2010).

NURSING MANAGEMENT: CARE OF INDIVIDUALS AND FAMILIES WHO ARE HOMELESS

A holistic perspective is essential for assessing any person or family unit who is homeless because people and homelessness are complex and multifaceted. Avoid looking at people who are homeless as deficient. Rather, look at the unique individual, the person's or family's transactions with the environment, and the client's strengths.

The fast-paced, time-focused approach of the traditional health care system is unlikely to gather the needed information to intervene. In fact, the person may leave rather than be subjected to more depersonalization. Use the principles of a therapeutic relationship and therapeutic communication described in Chapter 9 to establish rapport and trust.

Self-awareness on the part of the nurse is important. Often people do not know how to respond to a person who is homeless and who asks for food, money, or interpersonal communication because they hold common stereotypical beliefs about homelessness. Nurses and teachers, for example, who are accustomed to caring for others and giving attention to people who ask for it may find themselves considering various myths when approached by a person who is homeless (Box 38.5). To respond appropriately, one must first examine these myths and one's own feelings about people who are homeless and mentally ill. Relating to people who are homeless requires a gentle and compassionate approach.

Assessment

Assessment of the Biologic Domain

The assessment begins at the point of the person's need; often, it is a physical need or health problem (Box 38.6). Because of negative past experiences with the health care system or providers or because of mental illness or substance use, the person may not allow a thorough physical

BOX 38.5

Myths and Facts About Homeless People With Psychiatric Disorders

MYTH: People who are homeless are all alike.

FACT: People who are homeless come from all walks of life. Those with and without psychiatric illness share some characteristics. Being homeless is a leveling experience in that it is a sufficiently disabling condition in itself to cause altered adaptation. Those with chronic substance abuse may have more difficulty in meeting basic needs than do those who are chronically mentally ill.

MYTH: Most people who are homeless are lazy, passive, and do not want to work.

FACT: People who are homeless and who loiter may be actively trying to survive by avoiding extreme weather, seeking monetary or other assistance, or trying to feel a part of mainstream society. Most desire work even when physical or mental disabilities interfere.

MYTH: People who are homeless prefer being alone.

FACT: Peer relations with trusted people are preferred and essential to survival and meeting needs.

MYTH: People who are homeless are stupid and do not know how to manage life.

FACT: People who are homeless must be creative to secure resources and constantly change life ways to survive. However, the ability to think clearly is threatened under stress and in hostile environments.

MYTH: People who are homeless refuse to stay in a shelter because they are ill.

FACT: People who are homeless, including those with mental illness, do not use shelters for the following reasons: lack of shelter beds in an accessible area, difficulty in reaching the shelter, overcrowded or unpleasant conditions

in specific shelters, restrictions on length of stay or criteria for admission, and availability of alternatives (Murray, 1996).

MYTH: Street dwellers are unwilling to accept services.

FACT: Most people who are homeless recognize the need for help; however, survival needs take priority over need for mental health treatment. Nontraditional approaches may be necessary to work with people who are homeless and mentally ill.

MYTH: Most people who are homeless require acute, inpatient psychiatric care.

FACT: About 5% to 7% of adults who are mentally ill and homeless need inpatient care.

MYTH: Most people who are homeless, especially those who are mentally ill, are dangerous.

FACT: The high visibility of this population lends itself to frequent reporting of minor crimes, such as loitering; panhandling; public misconduct; minor shoplifting; or efforts to protect oneself from dangerous others, which can result in a fight.

MYTH: Most people who are homeless are mentally ill or substance abusing.

FACT: Of the people who are homeless, about 33% are mentally ill, and 32% are substance abusing.

MYTH: Homelessness is a monolithic problem that affects millions of people in the United States.

FACT: About 110,000 people are estimated to be chronically homeless; most people are homeless for a relatively short period of time.

Sources: Hoff et al., 2009; Kim, Ford, Howard, & Bradford, 2010; McNiel et al., 2005; National Coalition for the Homeless, 2009a, 2009b, 2009c, 2009d.

examination or may refuse to answer questions about history at the first visit.

Provide privacy for any examination. Be gentle. Avoid hurry. Explain the need for examination. The person may feel very embarrassed about his or her physical appearance or body odor if there has been no opportunity for physical hygiene or clothing change. Observation of mucous membrane and skin integrity, including the face, torso, limbs, and feet, is essential. Explain your concern about the person's health status and the need to remove clothing, including shoes and socks, and to pull down underwear.

Realize that many people who are homeless consider themselves well as long as they can get where they need to go. The individual may believe that refusing to admit illness is adaptive behavior. Be aware of the many health problems that may be present (Box 38.7). Children and adolescents who are homeless may experience any of those listed, plus diseases that are specific to their age group. If a homeless woman is pregnant, assess indications that she is at high risk for maternal or fetal complications.

The homeless person is likely to describe health and health care needs in a holistic way. In a study in Canada, urban homeless participants reported their concerns about physical illness, mental health, addictions, and stress. They reported that shelter life promoted spread of disease and afforded no privacy. Violence on the streets and in the shelter caused constant fear. Social exclusion and the depersonalization conveyed by others caused emotional distress. The homeless participants wanted to work and be housed (Daiski, 2007). The population that is homeless in the urban areas of the United States report the same concerns and desires.

Baseline and follow-up data for 7,213 homeless clients in a multisite program found 43.6% of the sample had need for medical care. Lack of medical care correlated with a lower educational level, depressive and psychotic symptoms, and a high number of competing needs. The main factor in 36% of the clients receiving medical services during a 3-month period was a strong therapeutic alliance with the case manager (Desai & Rosenheck,

BOX 38.6

Assessment Tips for the Biologic Domain

- Use unobtrusive observation as a part of physical assessment. Some conditions will be immediately obvious. Other conditions may become apparent during the interview.
- Examine—look, touch, palpate, auscultate—the person to the extent that he or she allows. The person may resist anything more than a superficial conversation and observation. The nurse may need to perform initial palpation of the abdomen or auscultation of the lung through several layers of clothes. If the patient perceives the health care provider as too intrusive, the patient may leave the setting even though he or she is desperate for care.
- Listen carefully to what the patient does *not* say and pay attention to nonverbal as well as verbal expressions. Avoid unnecessary directness and probing. Give the person time to answer questions. The blood test or urine screen may have to wait; a patient, nonintrusive manner may ensure that the person returns for needed tests or screening.
- Determine whether the person has been prescribed medications in the past. Often, the person who is homeless is not taking medications, even if they are prescribed and essential. The person may have difficulty keeping pills dry and easily retrievable or paying for medications. A daily insulin injection, for example, may not seem practical. Or the person may have been mugged by another homeless person seeking to quiet addictive urges or to sell drugs for cash.

2005). People who are homeless are at higher risk of becoming ill, and age-adjusted mortality rates among the homeless population are 3.5 times higher than those of the general population because of lack of health screening and early or adequate treatment of disease (Baggett, O'Connell, Singer, & Rigotti, 2010).

BOX 38.7

Common Physical Health Problems Experienced by Homeless People

- Injuries, fractures, epistaxis, or edema from trauma, falls, burns, assault, gunshot wounds
- Influenza, colds, bronchitis, asthma, shortness of breath
- Hypothermia, hyperthermia
- Arthritis, musculoskeletal disorders, headaches, fatigue
- Diabetes mellitus
- Hypertension
- Cardiovascular and peripheral vascular diseases
- Malnutrition
- Pulmonary tuberculosis
- Infestations, such as lice or scabies
- Dermatitis, sunburn or frostbite, bruises
- Foot injury, blisters, calluses
- Sexually transmitted diseases
- Hypothyroidism or hyperthyroidism
- Kidney or liver disease
- Cancer
- Epilepsy
- Impaired vision, glaucoma, cataracts
- Impaired hearing
- Dental caries, periodontal disease

Assessment of the Psychological Domain

Behavior that looks like a mental illness may in reality be an expression of normal emotional or social needs. The person who is homeless may manifest the need to feel safe, secure, and respected and to be treated as a unique and valued person with overt distancing or aggressive behavior. Ask how long the person has been homeless and in what context (shelter, street, relatives); such variables can considerably affect behavior, feelings, and psychological function.

People who experience homelessness have their own way of being in the world. They may feel

- A heightened awareness of being labeled, on display, and judged or stigmatized by outer appearance
- That they are nothing, they own nothing, and health care providers and authorities expect certain behavior
- Anxiety about having to be at a certain place at preset times to meet their daily needs
- A sense of community with other homeless and ill people as they go through rituals of waking, eating, lining up, and sharing facilities, space, and resources
- A sense of humor, amusement, aloofness, and optimism or faith about their ability to cope with a complicated lifestyle and to be hurt as little as possible (Hoff et al., 2009; Howard, 2009)

Just as the physical examination may be incomplete, so may the mental status examination have to be done in part or over several visits. See Box 38.8 for information related to psychological assessment. Symptoms of schizophrenia may be difficult to differentiate from emotional responses to the stressors of a homeless lifestyle. Required hypervigilance may augment suspicion or paranoid beliefs. The need for constant awareness of possibilities for meeting basic needs can augment self-preoccupation. Blunted affect, lack of communication, loose associations, ambivalence, isolation, and uncertainty may be the result of life on the streets and living in various places. Such symptoms or behaviors may be part of the homeless experience and reflect healthy coping mechanisms and creative survival techniques rather than pathology.

Substance abuse must be ruled out because it is common among people who are homeless, including people with mental illnesses. Because people who are homeless, especially those with psychiatric disorders, are often victims of crime and violence, the incidence of PTSD among them may be higher than in the general population. Homeless women are especially in danger of being assaulted, abused, and raped.

When a child or adolescent is homeless, ask about the educational history, if the youth is enrolled in school, and about perceived progress. Homeless children often have difficulty with school; the school district may change every time the parent changes shelters or moves from a

---

BOX 38.8

Assessment Tips for the Psychological Domain

- Observe for behavior that indicates hallucination and try to validate.
- Listen for delusions or denial over time; try to sense what purpose these serve.
- Observe and listen for what the person defines as a problem and potential solution and what he or she considers to be a strength or coping strategy; validate and reinforce when applicable.
- View the person and his or her situation from the individual's perspective; be a patient, nonthreatening listener. Such an approach encourages the person to return regularly; the nurse can then observe the patterns of behavior.
- Determine the extent of stability or integration of the person's sense of self, cognitive appraisals, and overt behavior. Lack of integration or stability indicates the need for continued monitoring and therapy.

BOX 38.9

Assessment Tips for the Social Domain

- Ask about support systems, people who could be helpful, and what services have been or could be used.
- Determine whether the person is isolated from the family, and if so, if it is by personal choice rather than by family choice.
- Respect that the person who feels isolated may avoid talking about his or her biologic family.
- Explore if the patient views a homeless peer, local pastor, counselor, or another health care provider as "family" or as a support system.
- Convey genuine interest in the person and convey that others may also care. Questions may be the catalyst to reestablishing family ties.

---

temporary residence. Determine whether the child has behavioral or emotional problems and whether he or she needs special education services.

Homelessness places parents and children at risk for mental health problems; maternal depression may affect the mother–child relationship and create child behavior problems. Homeless mothers and children also have great resilience. Homeless mothers are not necessarily depressed, nor do they have inadequate coping skills. Many homeless women, having made the decision to free themselves of a noxious relationship, are competent and resilient.

Assessment of the Social Domain

Social and Family Assessment

Cultural value differences exist between people who are homeless and people in the dominant American culture, to which most providers of health care subscribe. Thus, providers and the person who is homeless and needs health care may experience cultural conflict in their norms of health and illness, basic value systems and priorities, and perceptions about health care. Health care providers expect patients, including those who are homeless and mentally ill or chemically dependent, to problem solve, become more independent, and be future oriented. These values affect assessment, treatment, and interactions with the person and can interfere with the nursing process and patient response to the health care system (Andrews & Boyle, 2007). Consider how the homeless ill patient perceives his or her everyday life and vary the assessment and therapy approach accordingly.

Homelessness is an expression of and response to certain family, societal, or environmental conditions, as well as to individual factors. See Box 38.9 for factors included in the social and family assessment. It is also important to

consider that childhood abuse and prior trauma may be continuing to affect the person as a stressor or contribute to interpersonal crises (Box 38.10).

Spiritual Assessment

Listen for expressions that convey a spiritual faith, a connection to a transcendent being, or a belief system that helps the person endure. Questions about the spiritual dimension may convey an invitation to talk about an aspect of life that is often ignored but that may be very important to the beliefs, and preferred practices will help determine relevant therapy approaches.

BOX 38.10

Research for Best Practice: Assessing Trauma, Substance Abuse, and Mental Health in a Sample of Homeless Men

Kim, M. M., Ford, J. D., Howard, D. L., & Bradford, D. W. (2010). Assessing trauma, substance abuse, and mental health in a sample of homeless men. Health and Social Work, 35(1), 39–48.

THE QUESTION: What is the impact of physical and sexual trauma on homeless men?

METHODS: A sample of 239 homeless men completed a survey about demographic data, exposure to psychological trauma, physical and mental health status, and substance abuse. Data were statistically analyzed.

FINDINGS: A history of traumatic events was significantly associated with mental health problems but not with alcohol or drug abuse in adulthood. Abuse and victimization that began in childhood added to the long-term effects of current stressors.

IMPLICATIONS FOR NURSING: Homeless men need long-term continuity-of-care services that assess effects of prior abuse experiences as well as sporadic or current crises. Such long-term assessment fosters interventions to prevent further health problems and care needs. This study may also have implications for assessment and care of homeless women.

Nursing Diagnoses for All Domains

Nursing diagnoses related to physical health status include Impaired Dentition, Hypothermia or Hyperthermia, Imbalanced Nutrition, Fatigue, Ineffective Health Maintenance, Acute or Chronic Pain, Impaired Skin Integrity, Disturbed Sleep Patterns, Risk for Alcohol Use or Drug Use, and Risk for Sexually Transmitted Diseases. Nursing diagnoses related to emotional health status include Anxiety, Impaired Verbal Communication, Decisional Conflict, Risk for Loneliness, Powerlessness, Chronic Low Self-esteem, and Risk for Self-Mutilation or Suicide. Nursing diagnoses related to social health status include Compromised Family Coping, Impaired Social Interaction, Self-Care Deficit, and Social Isolation. Nursing diagnoses related to cognitive status include Decisional Conflict, Disturbed Thought Processes, Disturbed Sensory Perceptions, Hopelessness, and Deficient Knowledge (NANDA International [NANDA-I], 2009). The nursing diagnosis Spiritual Distress (NANDA-I, 2009), may also be expressed. Yet, many homeless people encountered by the authors have expressed a consistent and deep faith in God as their protector.

Interventions for All Domains

Interventions are to be directed at the social system, as well as at the individual or family level. Interventions should take advantage of community resources and the inner resources and support systems of the individual or family. Box 38.11 describes findings about factors that promote satisfaction with care.

Overcoming Barriers to Care

Cost and lack of insurance are the biggest barriers to health and hospital care for homeless people. Another barrier is the inability of this population to carry out treatment recommendations; survival is their first priority. Compliance with medication and treatment regimens is difficult because successful treatment requires collaboration, monitoring, time for medication and other measures to be effective, and a secure place to keep medication. Mentally ill people who are homeless often cannot routinely get prescriptions filled. Medicine may be stolen. It is necessary for the person or family unit to have a place to keep medications that can be reached at the necessary times and to have access to primary care services for regular check-ups, assessment for adverse drug responses, and necessary blood monitoring.

In a study of 439 people about utilization of mental health services in Montreal and Quebec, Canada, 36% of the participants were homeless, and 48% of the study group had been homeless previously. Barriers to use of mental health services included economic factors (poverty)

BOX 38.11

Interventions for People Who Are Homeless

- Stabilize physical health status.
- Provide a list with addresses and telephone numbers of shelters and luncheon sites that provide food; discourage rooting through dumpsters and panhandling.
- Provide a list of facilities that are safe, including shelters that provide clothing, a safe place to sleep, and opportunity for basic hygiene and laundry.
- Give information on city ordinances that forbid sleeping on park benches, in building doorways, on sidewalk grates, at bus or train stations, in vacant buildings, or in viaducts.
- Explore sources of income, such as gathering and selling aluminum cans or engaging in temporary day labor. Discourage selling blood or plasma.
- Assist the person directly or by referral to pursue entitlements, such as Social Security, veterans, or other benefits.
- Explore how to stay safe. Even in a night shelter, the person who is homeless may not be safe from assault. It is difficult for the person who is homeless to know who is trustworthy; carrying a bag or case is usually considered a marker for being robbed on the streets.
- Explore how to secure privacy, which is difficult to achieve, and how to cope with loneliness, which can be overwhelming.
- Give a list of names, addresses, and telephone numbers of agencies that offer services and socialization, such as the local mental health agency, the local chapter of National Alliance on Mental Illness, or the local Emotions Anonymous group.
- Give information about meetings of Alcoholics Anonymous, Narcotics Anonymous, or Cocaine Anonymous if the person is using substances.

---

and several demographic characteristics (gender, age, health status, lack of support system). Utilization of mental health services was related to female gender, youth, no prior homeless experience, presence of antisocial personality within the prior year, past or current alcohol-related disorders, hospitalization before the preceding year, and presence of a support system (Bonin, Fournier, & Blais, 2007).

The traditional mental health care system has been considered paternalistic; clients often lack opportunities for meaningful participation in decision making and policy planning. Mentally ill homeless individuals will visit and participate in a self-help center, if available. Clients may engage in the roles of managers and leaders in a comfortable setting and meeting place (Fountain House model) (Swarbrick, Schmidt, & Pratt, 2009). The drop-in center in this study, using the Fountain House model, fostered socialization and a sense of empowerment, personal development, authority, satisfaction with services, and thereby recovery, as well as cohesiveness in and quality of relationships among clients. Clients described that therapeutic social or environmental structure and control were important (Swarbrick et al., 2009).

Improving Quality of Life

Interventions that improve quality of life include providing food, clothing, and assistance with housing; addressing physical health problems; promoting safety and self-esteem; and educating the person to decrease the risk of victimization (Hoff et al., 2009; Sullivan et al., 2000). A trusting relationship with the care provider and ongoing follow-up care are also necessary (Christensen, 2009).

People who have been homeless for several years have greater difficulty readjusting to stability and need more time for healing, depending on illness severity, comorbidity, and available support system (Christensen, 2009; Murray, 1996). People who are homeless, including those with psychiatric disorders, become creative at surviving on the streets. Explore resources with the individual or family (see Box 38.11 for appropriate interventions). The psychiatric street outreach program to homeless people in Jacksonville, Florida, is another example of a nontraditional intervention approach to severely impaired and medically underserved individuals. The main objectives of the outreach are to foster relationship, reconnection, and recovery through a transdisciplinary team (Christensen, 2009).

Meeting Spiritual Needs

Depending on the person's beliefs, the nurse may explore ways to meet spiritual needs. In one study, respondents listed the following as ways to meet spiritual needs: pray and put trust in God, hope that things will get better, obtain strength from religious beliefs and say these beliefs to self daily, seek a religious worker and attend religious services, talk about the meaning of the life situation with someone who is understanding and caring, and read devotional material (e.g., the Bible or the Koran) (Murray, 1996).

Planning for Discharge

A crucial time for intervention occurs at discharge from inpatient or medical treatment. At this time, the nurse can assist in the patient's transition from institutional to community living by providing practical and emotional support. Nurses are in a key position to help patients reestablish family and other supportive relationships. Women who are homeless are likely to engage their children as a main social support; parents and other family members were perceived as unlikely to help (Meadows-Oliver, 2005). People with mental illness who have been homeless need assistance in using available resources, such as medical, psychiatric, substance abuse, emergency department (ED) treatment, and other outpatient psychiatric services. Adequate discharge planning includes linkages with intensive case management services. Sustained case management in the community can improve housing and mental health outcomes (Kasprow & Rosenheck, 2007).

In preparation for discharge, the nurse should make arrangements for transfer to transitional housing, if available. Provide the person with telephone numbers and directions for emergency shelters, lunch sites, day treatment programs, mental health hotlines, crisis lines (abuse, suicide), appropriate self-help or support groups, and relevant toll-free numbers. Some states fund cities to provide a Supportive Community Living Program that assists people who are mentally ill or substance abusing to receive funding for housing and utilities. Other services may also be available. Predischarge planning involves providing options to promote independent living. Whatever information is given should be legible; concise; able to fit in a pocket, purse, shoe, or boot; and as portable as possible. Bulky brochures or three-ring binders are impractical. The nurse must never assume the person's literacy level; the person may not admit inability to read. If the person is illiterate, the nurse must take the time to help him or her memorize essential information. Utilization of an Assertive Community Treatment (ACT) Program can be effective.

Evaluation and Treatment Outcomes

There are two outcomes for people who are homeless. Recovery from a mental disorder and living in a housing of choice are primary. In some instances, after the mental disorder is treated and in remission, housing, a job, and positive interpersonal relationships follow. In other instances, finding housing sets the stage for strengthening coping skills to address the mental disorder.

TRENDS FOR IMPROVING SERVICES

Diverse services and integrated systems are essential to address all aspects of the life situations of people who are homeless and experiencing psychiatric disorders. Essential components include Safe Havens or stable shelters or residences, accessible outreach, integrated case management, accessible and affordable housing options, treatment and rehabilitation services, general health care services, vocational training and assistance with employment, income support, and legal protection. The agencies that provide these services must develop a physical and emotional atmosphere that conveys a sense of caring and community. Often, community agencies are located at one site, much like a shopping mall, so that the person or family does not have to travel to numerous separately located agencies to get their needs met.

Emergency Services

Some agencies provide a street or mobile outreach program. As part of this program, a van travels the streets to areas where people who are homeless are found outdoors. Food, warm coffee, hygiene kits, and blankets are the first steps in building trust between staff and homeless persons. The person who is homeless may accept an offer to be driven to a local shelter for the night. Follow-up the next day by van or bicycle provides a way to recontact the individual and invite him or her to the agency programs or take him or her to other social service or health care services. Luncheon sites for homeless people are a basic step in emergency services. Some agencies have a health clinic on site for treatment of minor problems.

Integrating crisis intervention with physical and medical care is essential for psychotic individuals being treated in the ED. The ED is likely to emphasize triage and rapid disposition while administering essential care. The physical orientation supersedes care for the emotional status of the person. Chemical stabilization of the person should be supplemented by crisis intervention techniques (Hoff et al., 2009). The developmental level of the person, regardless of age, should also be considered. Emergency shelters typically provide refuge at night along with an evening meal and morning coffee. Shelters for homeless women and children usually allow them to remain during daytime hours as well. The child leaves the shelter for school; the mother may attend educational classes, counseling, day treatment, rehabilitation, or employment programs. Box 38.12 suggests additional ways to improve shelters.

Housing Services

The United States has a renewed commitment to ensure that everyone has a roof over his or her head, can engage in an independent lifestyle, and has the opportunity to become employed. Policy makers at all governmental levels and leaders from the private sector are working together to end homelessness. This **Housing First** approach places people who are homeless, usually also experiencing severe mental illness, substance abuse, or release from prison, into affordable housing, including Section 8 housing units. Case management, living skills

> ### BOX 38.12
> ### How Emergency Shelters Can Improve Services
>
> - Offer flexible hours to accommodate those who have temporary employment on days or evenings (i.e., earlier admission during evening, stay later in morning).
> - Maintain cleanliness and control pests.
> - Have adequate helpful staff.
> - Provide effective security inside and outside the shelter.
> - Provide a safe place to store belongings.
> - Network with other agencies for services such as transportation to employment, health care providers, clothing.
> - Have flexible policies for length of stay at shelters for those actively participating in recovery or employment programs.
>
> Adapted from Murray, R. B. (1996). Needs and resources: The lived experience of homeless men. *Journal of Psychosocial Nursing, 34*(5), 18–24.

classes, and other services are provided as "wrap-around" interventions as needed. There is a direct relationship between the safety and security provided by the Housing First program and a decrease in psychiatric symptoms and chronic homelessness, with an increased in a sense of independence, choice, and mastery of living skills (Hoff et al., 2009; Robbins, Callahan, & Monahan, 2009).

Transitional housing may consist of a halfway house, a short-stay residence or group home, or a room at a hotel designated for people who are homeless. Some agencies have a transitional home and stabilization center where the atmosphere and staff are a model for residents, who work on specific goals and a treatment plan. Sharing housekeeping tasks; obtaining psychiatric stabilization; and attending residence group meetings, social skills and budgeting classes, day treatment programs, and vocational training are steps to independent housing and employment. A holistic program reduces readmission to the hospital and reentry to street dwelling.

The continuum of care approach to homelessness, sponsored by HUD, includes both the Safe Havens and Shelter Plus Care Programs mentioned at the beginning of this chapter. A Safe Haven, in addition to serving hard-to-reach people with severe mental illness who are on the streets and have been unwilling or unable to participate in traditional supportive services, meets the following criteria: it provides 24-hour residence for an unspecified duration, it provides private or semiprivate accommodations, and it limits overnight occupancy to 25 persons (U.S. HUD, 2010). Shelter Plus Care provides long-term housing and supportive services for people who are homeless with disabilities, primarily those with serious mental illness, chronic problems with alcohol or drug use, or AIDS or related diseases (U.S. HUD, 2010).

Other housing options are also available that emphasize a self-help, communal-living setting created to foster recovery in persons who are alcohol and substance abusing.

The residents assume full responsibility for daily maintenance of the residence and for personal lifestyles and treatment management. Residents are expected to be employed, to be reducing need for government subsidies, and to engage in relapse prevention (Swarbrick et al., 2009).

Section 8 housing has been helpful to this population for many years. Section 8 federally subsidized housing units are supervised or operated by the state or city, for which tenants are responsible for paying one third of the monthly income (e.g., Supplemental Security Income or Social Security Disability Insurance) toward rent. The difference between the tenant payment and the maximum fair market rental price is calculated as the federal Section 8 Housing contribution to the housing provider. Congress has been appropriating more of the McKinney-Vento Act funds for permanent supportive housing for people who are homeless and disabled. The emphasis in Congress and HUD is on establishing housing programs that are supported by the community (Hoff et al., 2009). **Supportive housing**, permanently subsidized housing with attendant social services, was previously considered too expensive. However, such programs for people who are mentally ill and homeless are a good investment. The person who is safely housed is less likely to use other acute care and publicly funded services, such as shelters, although case management services are needed. Use of acute psychiatric and medical services is reduced, and the person is less likely to be arrested or incarcerated. For example, in St. Louis, Missouri, housing retention rates remain at an average of 70% for the first year after housing placement through an agency with wrap-around services. Altogether, such an approach provides a healthier and more humane alternative. The National Alliance on Mental Illness (NAMI) has also collaborated actively with governmental and private agencies to establish quality housing for people who are homeless and mentally ill. Cost of cutting services is higher in the long term than the cost of providing them in the first place (North et al., 2010).

Case Management

Case management involves systematic assessment, planning, goal setting, counseling and other interventions, coordination of services, referral as necessary, and monitoring of the person's or family's needs and progress. It enhances self-care capability and quality of care along the continuum of care, decreases fragmentation, provides for cost containment, and reduces unnecessary duplication of services or hospitalization. The case manager is the gatekeeper and facilitator who may at first network with services on the person's or family's behalf and then encourage them to deal directly with other service providers to obtain bus passes and transportation, children's services and supplies, medical or obstetric care, or housing. The nurse is the ideal team member or case manager because of knowledge about both psychiatric and physical diseases and the ability to develop therapeutic relationships and stay connected with persons or families who are homeless and with the health care system.

Rehabilitation and Education
Day Treatment Programs

Day treatment provides a bridge between institutional and community care for severely mentally ill and substance-abusing people. Participation in structured day treatment programs can provide emotional and practical support and strengthen ties to community services and potentially to family and friends. A day treatment program can provide legal assistance, help with finding employment and independent housing, and a mailing address for people who are homeless. It can provide case management, assistance with goal setting and problem solving, and psychiatric or medical care. The day treatment program may incorporate adult basic education classes to increase literacy and survival skills, GED classes for those who want a high school diploma, and computer skills to improve employment options. A Living Skills Program typically includes content in nutrition, budgeting, parenting, household and family management, tenant responsibilities and rights, and employment readiness. Such classes are especially useful to women who will no longer be receiving welfare benefits. The person can receive assistance applying for government benefits, if qualified, and obtaining identification, such as a birth certificate, if needed. The informal environment of day treatment programs promotes a feeling of camaraderie, self-confidence, trust in staff, and aspirations to independent living.

Alcohol and Drug Treatment

The structure of some day treatment programs follows the 12-step model of Alcoholics Anonymous (AA) for people who abuse substances or have a dual diagnosis. Sobriety is the goal; the person attends daily meetings, receives necessary psychiatric and medical treatment, and participates in all of the other activities and services available at the day treatment program. No one is terminated for relapse; the person is referred to more intensive services, including hospitalization, if necessary.

Employment Services

Job placement is most likely when an employment program teaches basic job-seeking skills (e.g., resume writing; interview skills; appropriate attire, hygiene, and behavior; and computer skills) and offers job training in settings that prepare the person for the real world and real jobs.

Case management during employment training can increase self-confidence, teach budgeting skills and methods of coping with the stresses of regular employment, and link the person with community resources. It can also help to teach various skills for job retention and career development. The employment service should periodically follow up with both the employee and his or her employer to ensure a successful record and movement to independence.

Integrated Services

Assertive Community Treatment (ACT) programs focus on service delivery to the homeless and mentally ill population by a transdisciplinary team of 10 to 12 specialists with a 1:10 staff–client ratio. A single, integrated, mobile staff team uses outreach, case management, practical assistance and support, and rehabilitation services to maximize the possibility that the most disabled consumers will live independently in the community and have a good quality of life. The team provides counseling and advocacy; monitors the person's management of housing, income, medication use, and leisure activities; and provides opportunities for employment if appropriate. Substance abuse management and physical health care are provided as needed.

Research studies of more than 25 controlled trials link ACT programs to significant reduction in psychiatric symptoms, hospitalizations, and disability. Client and family satisfaction ratings have been high. Cost analysis reveals that the ACT model is no more expensive than standard care because of the above outcomes, consequent improved quality of life, and integration of the client into the community (Carlton et al., 2010). ACT staff members are often perceived as more supportive than family or friends. Further, these relationships can be perceived as better than relationships before or during homelessness, which in turn, foster the person's integration into the community (Carlton et al., 2010). The ACT Program is an effective way to implement two recommendations by Daiski (2007): (1) reduce or eliminate health problems through safe, affordable housing and (2) integrate the person into the community through job counseling, treatment of addictions, and employment.

Ongoing social support groups; membership in day treatment programs; attendance at meetings of AA, Narcotics Anonymous, or Cocaine Anonymous; or the local NAMI or Mental Health Association can help the person who was severely mentally ill or substance abusing to remain in the community and live independently or with family. Support groups foster peer socialization and problem solving, enhance self-esteem, and offer many activities (e.g., art and recreation therapy, legal assistance). An example of a support group is an Alumni Club for the "alumni" of a job-training center. The evening mental

health, after-care program is attended by those who have become psychiatrically stabilized, are employed, and are living independently. A club-like setting provides a safe, friendly, substance-free environment for 7 evenings each week, year round. Case management, individualized treatment plans, and counseling continue for 6 months or longer. AA meetings, self-improvement classes, and other educational opportunities are integrated with case management. Socialization, fun, and effective leisure activities result (Box 38.13).

For a number of years, the Substance Abuse and Mental Health Services Administration and the Center for Substance Abuse Treatment have funded treatment programs for women and young children. Long-term stays have been found to predict positive treatment outcomes, including lower rates of drug use, criminal behavior, and unemployment. Improved parenting and mother–child relationships, less child abuse and neglect, improved developmental outcomes in children, and lowered costs for mother and infant health are other benefits.

Advocacy

Nurses can share experiences and research findings with the local chapter or national headquarters of NAMI and with state legislators and members of Congress who are involved in developing legislation and policies related to people who are homeless, mentally ill, and substance abusing. Continued advocacy is essential to convey the perceptions and needs of this population, to influence allocations for needed programs and services, and to end the social injustice of chronic homelessness.

SUMMARY OF KEY POINTS

■ People who are homeless are a heterogeneous, diverse group, some of whom are mentally ill or abusing substances.

■ There are many risks for being homeless.

■ People do not want to be homeless.

■ The nursing assessment must be holistic; the nurse must listen to the person's perceptions and observe carefully.

■ People who are mentally ill or substance abusing and homeless may have various physical health problems.

■ Intervention must be oriented to the person's or family's perceived needs, culturally sensitive, and compassionate.

■ People who are mentally ill and homeless may avoid traditional health care services.

■ Nurses must incorporate new trends in providing and improving services for health care and social integration.

CRITICAL THINKING CHALLENGES

1. How do the effects of mental illness, substance abuse, and homelessness interact with one another?

2. What factors might interfere with the ability of the person who is mentally ill to participate in treatment?

3. What barriers to communication might the nurse experience when relating to the person who is homeless and mentally ill?

The Homeless Home Movie: 1997. This video profiles several different people who are homeless who struggle with homelessness during 1 year. They include a pregnant 15-year-old runaway, a couple that lives in their car, a Vietnam veteran who lives outside all year, and a man bankrupted after his daughter's long fight with leukemia. (This video is available for purchase at faculty and student rates from Media Visions, Inc., 11626 SW 6th Lane, Gainesville, Florida 32607, 352-215-0656. Information is also available online.)

VIEWING POINTS: Identify the similarities and differences in the lives of those who are homeless. Does your view of homelessness change after seeing this documentary?

West 47th Street: 2001, 2003. This documentary describes services offered by Fountain House, the original clubhouse for persons who are homeless and mentally ill, through the eyes of four clubhouse members. Fountain House has celebrated 50 years of providing services and is the model for more than 300 clubhouses nationwide. (This video is available for purchase from Lichtenstein Creative Media, 617-682-3700. Information is also available online.)

VIEWING POINTS: Discuss the range of services needed for people who are homeless and mentally ill. Visit a clubhouse program in your community and compare the services with those of Fountain House.

References

Andrews, M., & Boyle, J. (2007). *Transcultural concepts in nursing care* (5th ed.). Philadelphia: Lippincott Williams & Wilkins.

Baggett, T. P., O'Connell, J. J., Singer, D. E., & Rigotti, N. A. (2010). The unmet health care needs of homeless adults: A national study. *American Journal of Public Health,100*(7), 1326–1333.

Bonin, J. P., Fournier, I., & Blais, R. (2007). Predictors of mental health service utilization by people using resources for homeless people in Canada. *Psychiatric Services, 58*(7), 936–941.

Boydell, K., Goering, P., & Morrell-Bellai, T. (2000). Narratives of identity: Re-presentation of self in people who are homeless. *Qualitative Health Research, 10*(1), 26–38.

Bringing America Home (2005, November). Bill to end homelessness in America introduced in Congress. Retrieved on May 14, 2006, from http://www.bringingamericahome.org.

Buck, D. S., Brown, C. A., & Hickey, J. S. (2011). The Jail Inreach Project: Linking homeless inmates who have mental illness with community health services. *Psychiatric Services, 62*(2), 120–122.

Carlton, A. D., Young, M. S., & Kelly, K. M. (2010). Changes in sources and perceived quality of social supports among formerly homeless persons receiving assertive community treatment services. *Community Mental Health Journal, 46*(2), 156–163.

Center for Mental Health Services and Office of Special Needs Assistance Programs (1997). *In from the cold: A tool kit for creating safe havens for homeless people on the street.* Washington, DC: U.S. Department of Housing and Urban Development.

Christensen, R. C. (2009). Psychiatric street outreach to homeless people: Fostering relationships, reconnection, and recovery. *Journal of Health Care for the Poor and Underserved, 20*(4), 1036–1040.

Cleverley, K., & Kidd, S. A. (2010). Resilience and suicidality among homeless youth. *Journal of Adolescence,* in press.

Daiski, I. (2007). Perspectives of homeless people on their health and health needs priorities. *Journal of Advanced Nursing,58*(3), 273–281.

Desai, M. M., & Rosenheck, R. A. (2005). Unmet need for medical care among homeless adults with serious mental illness. *General Hospital Psychiatry, 27,* 418–425.

Finfgeld-Connett, D. (2010). Becoming homeless, being homeless, and resolving homelessness among women. *Issues in Mental health Nursing, 31*(7), 461–469.

Fitzpatrick, J. (2009). Resilience. *Archives of Psychiatric Nursing,23,* 341–342.

Hoff, L. A., Hallisey, B., & Hoff, M. (2009). *People in crisis: Clinical and diversity perspectives* (6th ed.). New York: Routledge, Taylor & Francis Group.

Hollander, A. C., Bruce, D., Burström, B., & Ekblad, S. (2011). Gender-related mental health differences between refugees and non-refugee immigrants—A cross-sectional register-based study. *BMC Public Health, 11,* 180.

Homelessness Resource Center (2009). Current statistics on the prevalence and characteristics of people experiencing homelessness in the United States. Washington, DC: Substance Abuse and Mental Health Administration, Department of Health and Human Services. Available at http://homeless.samhsa.gov/Resource/Current-Statistics-on-the-Prevalence-and-Characteristics-of-People-Experiencing-Homelessness-in-the-United-States-48841.aspx.

Howard, B. (2009, November, December). The secrets of resilient people. *AARP Magazine, 32, 34, 36.*

Huribut, J. B. Robbins, L. K. & Hoke, M. M. (2011). Correlations between spirituality and health-promoting behaviors among sheltered homeless women. *Journal of Community Health Nursing,28*(2), 81–91.

Interagency Council on the Homeless (1994). *Priority: Home! The federal plan to break the cycle of homelessness.* (HUD Publication No. 1454-CPD). Washington, DC: Author.

Kasprow, W. J., & Rosenheck, R. A. (2007). Outcomes of critical time intervention case management of homeless veterans after psychiatric hospitalization. *Psychiatric Services, 58*(7), 929–935.

Kim, M. M., Ford, J. D., Howard, D. L., & Bradford, D. W. (2010). Assessing trauma, substance abuse, and mental health in a sample of homeless men. *Health and Social Work, 35*(1), 39–48.

Kirkpatrick, H., & Byrne, C. (2009). A narrative inquiry: Moving on from homelessness for individuals with a major mental illness. *Journal of Psychiatric Mental Health Nursing, 16*(1), 68–75.

Marshall, A., Bell, J. M., & Moules, N. J. (2010). Beliefs, suffering, and healing: A clinical practice model for families experiencing mental illness. *Perspectives in Psychiatric Care, 46*(3), 197–208.

McKinney Act renamed (2000, November 17). *Housing Assistance Council News, 29*(23). Retrieved on April 9, 2003, from *http://216.92.48.246/infoNews.php.*

McKinney-Vento Homeless Assistance Act (2002, March 12). *Homes & communities.* Washington, DC: U.S. Department of Housing and Urban Development (p. 1). Available at http://www.hud.gov:80/offices/cpd/homeless/rulesandregs/laws/index.cfm.

Meadows-Oliver, M. (2005). Social support among homeless and housed mothers: An integrative review. *Journal of Psychosocial Nursing and Mental Health Services, 43*(2), 40–47.

Moe, A. M. (2007). Silenced voices and structured survival: Battered women's help seeking. *Violence Against Women, 13*(7), 676–699.

Murray, R. B. (1996). Needs and resources: The lived experience of homeless men. *Journal of Psychosocial Nursing, 34*(5), 18–23.

NANDA International (2009). *NANDA Nursing Diagnoses: Definition and classification: 2009–2011.* West Sussex, UK:John Wiley & Sons.

National Coalition for the Homeless (2009a). *Why are people homeless? NCH fact sheet #1.* Available at http://www.nationalhomeless.org.

National Coalition for the Homeless (2009b). *How many people experience homelessness? NCH fact sheet #2.* Available at http://www.nationalhomeless.org.

National Coalition for the Homeless (2009c). *Who is homeless? NCH fact sheet #3.* Available at http://www.nationalhomeless.org.

National Coalition for the Homeless (2009d). *Mental illness and homelessness. NCH fact sheet #5.* Available at www.nationalhomeless.org.

National Low Income Housing Coalition (2010). *2010 Advocates' guide to community housing and community development policy.* Retrieved on August 6, 2010, from http://www.nlihc.org/doc/2010-ADVOCATES-GUIDE.pdf.

North, C. S., Eyrich-Garg, K. M., Pollio, D. E., & Thirthalli, J. (2010). A prospective study of substance use and housing stability in a homeless population. *Social Psychiatry & Psychiatric Epidemiology,46*(11), 1955–1962.

Nyamathi, A., Marfisee, M. Slagle, A., Greengold, B., Liu, Y., & Leake, B. (2010). Correlates of depressive symptoms among homeless young adults. *Western Journal of Nursing Research*, in press.

Revollo, H. W., Qureshi, A., Collazos, F., Valero, S., & Casa, M. (2011). Acculturative stress as a risk factor of depression and anxiety in the Latin American immigrant population. *International Review Psychiatry, 23*(1), 84–92.

Rew., L., Grady, M., Whittaker, T. A., & Bowman, K. (2008). Interaction of duration of homelessness and gender on adolescent sexual health indicators. *Journal of Nursing Scholarship, 40*(2), 109–115.

Robbins, P. C., Callahan, L., & Monahan, J. (2009). Perceived coercion to treatment and housing satisfaction in housing-first and supportive housing programs. *Psychiatric Services, 60*(9), 1251–1253.

Sermons, M. W., & Witte, P. (2011). *On homelessness. An in-depth examination of homeless counts, economic indicators, demographic drivers, and changes at the state and national level.* Washington, DC: National Alliance to End Homelessness.

Sullivan, G., Burnam, A., Koegel, P., & Hollenberg, J. (2000). Quality of life of homeless persons with mental illness: Results from the course-of-homelessness study. *Psychiatric Services, 51*(9), 1135–1141.

Swarbrick, M., Schmidt, L., & Pratt, C. (2009). Consumer operated self-help centers. *Journal of Psychosocial Nursing, 47*(7), 41–46.

Trueland, J. (2009). People with learning disabilities hidden among the homeless. *Learning Disability Practice, 12*(2), 18–20.

U.S. Department of Housing and Urban Development (2010). *The 2009 annual homeless assessment report to Congress.* Washington DC: Office of Community Planning and Development. Available at http://www.huduser.org/portal/publications/povsoc/ahar_5.html.

Washington, O. G., Moxley, D. P., Garriott, L., & Weinberger, J. P. (2009). Five dimensions of faith and spiritually of older African American women transitioning out of homelessness. *Journal of Religion & Health, 48*(4), 431–444.

Zeber, J., Copeland, L., McCarthy, J., Bauer, M., & Kilbourne, A. (2009). Perceived access to general medical and psychiatric care among veterans with bipolar disorder. *American Journal of Public Health, 99*(4), 720–727.

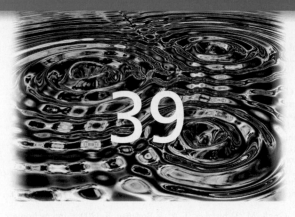

39

Caring for Persons With Co-occurring Mental Disorders

Mary Ann Boyd

KEY CONCEPTS

- co-occurring disorders (COD)
- relapse cycle

LEARNING OBJECTIVES

After studying this chapter, you will be able to:

1. Define the term *co-occurring disorders*.
2. Describe the cycle of relapse in co-occurring disorders.
3. Discuss the epidemiology of co-occurring disorders.
4. Discuss patterns of substance abuse and other mental disorders.
5. Analyze barriers to the treatment of patients with co-occurring disorders.
6. Discuss the significance of an integrated treatment approach to co-occurring disorders.
7. Describe nursing management of persons with co-occurring disorders.

KEY TERMS

- Assertive Community Treatment (ACT) • engagement • integrated treatment • motivational interventions
- quadrants of care • relapse prevention • recovery • self-medicate

> **KEYCONCEPT** The term **co-occurring disorders** (COD) refers to the presence of comorbid mental illness and a substance use disorder in the same person.

Mental illness and substance use disorder are each a primary mental disorder even though they do not necessarily appear at the same time. A diagnosis of COD means that at least one disorder of each type can be established independently. However, the person's experience, symptoms, and outcomes are influenced by the interaction of the two illnesses, not just the discrete disorders.

The goal of treatment for patients with COD is a comprehensive recovery plan for the complex problems presented—one that offers the patient a way out of what can be a downward spiral of debilitation. Effective treatment of COD requires an integrated approach based on both an understanding of mental illness and addiction.

Integrated treatment, coordinated substance abuse and mental health interventions, requires modifying traditional approaches to both the mental illness and addiction (SAMSHA, 2014a).

This chapter presents the epidemiology and etiological patterns of COD and discusses specific mental illnesses and the adverse effects of concurrent substance use. It highlights methods of assessing COD and offers treatment strategies and nursing interventions to address this complex yet common presentation in psychiatric and substance use treatment settings. A complete discussion of related substance use disorders is provided in Chapter 31.

OVERVIEW OF CO-OCCURRING DISORDERS

The problem of COD was inadvertently magnified during the community mental health reform movement when there was a rational movement toward deinstitutionalization of people with mentally illnesses (see Chapter 1). Large numbers of persons with mental illnesses were left homeless, lost to local and state mental health systems. Their long-standing mental illnesses and protected life in a state hospital increased their vulnerability to exploitation by others, particularly the more astute and streetwise addicts. Along with homelessness came the increased use of drugs and alcohol (Goldstein, Luther, Haas, & Gordon, & Appelt, 2009).

It is impossible to make any meaningful distinction between simple recreational use of a substance and actual substance use with this population because even small amounts of alcohol or other drugs can be damaging to people who have concurrent psychiatric problems. Substances of abuse exert profound effects on mental states, perception, psychomotor function, cognition, and behavior. The specific neurochemical and other biologic mechanisms that evoke these psychological features are discussed in Chapter 31. Table 39.1 lists the psychological effects of substances of abuse.

Clinical Course and Relapse

Although two types of disorders are diagnosed independently, people with COD respond to the interaction of two psychiatric illnesses, not just two discrete disorders. In many instances, the use of substances serves as a coping strategy for dealing with psychiatric symptoms. Without alternative, effective coping behaviors, the patient will continue to **self-medicate** (using medication, usually over-the-counter medications, or substances without professional prescription or supervision, to alleviate an illness or condition). Persons with COD have poorer outcomes, such as higher rates of HIV infection, relapse, rehospitalization, depression, and suicide risk (Farren, Snee, Daly, & McElroy, 2013; Effinger & Stewart, 2012).

A frequent problem of this group is relapse, which leads to repeated hospitalizations or the "revolving door" phenomenon. When symptoms of the mental disorder are stabilized, the hospitalized patient is discharged. Once in the community, the patient fails to follow the therapeutic regimen and resumes the use of alcohol or drugs. Reappearance of symptoms leads to another episode of hospitalization (Botha et al., 2010). The relapse cycle is characterized by a pattern of decompensation, hospitalization, stabilization, discharge, and then decompensation (Figure 39.1).

KEYCONCEPT   In the **relapse cycle**, reemerging psychiatric symptoms lead to ineffective coping strategies, increased anxiety, substance use to avoid painful feelings, adverse consequences, and attempted abstinence until psychiatric symptoms reemerge and the cycle repeats itself.

Table 39.1	PSYCHOLOGICAL EFFECTS OF SUBSTANCES OF ABUSE
Substance	**Psychological Effects**
Alcohol	Alcohol amnestic syndrome; dementia. Agitation, anxiety disorders, sleep disorders. Ataxia, slurred speech. Withdrawal symptoms, which may include hallucinations, confusion, illusions, delusions; protracted withdrawal delirium can occur. Depression, increased rate of suicide, disinhibition
Cocaine	Anxiety, agitation, hyperactivity, sleep disorders, delusions, paranoia, euphoria, internal sense of interest and excitement. Rebound withdrawal symptoms, such as prolonged depression, somnolence, anhedonia
Amphetamines	Similar to cocaine but more prolonged. Hyperactivity, agitation, anxiety, increased energy
Hallucinogens (MDMA, Ecstasy) and phencyclidine	Hallucinations, delusions, paranoia, confusion. Withdrawal can produce severe depression, somnolence. Hallucinations, illusions, delusions, perceptual distortions, paranoia, rage, anxiety, agitation, confusion
Marijuana	Acute reactions: panic, anxiety, paranoia, sensory distortions, rare psychotic episodes; patients with schizophrenia use these reactions to distance themselves from painful symptoms and to gain control over symptoms. Antimotivational syndrome: apathy, diminished interest in activities and goals, poor job or school performance, memory and cognitive deficits
Opiates	Confusion, somnolence. Withdrawal can produce anxiety, irritability, and depression and can trigger suicidal ideation
Sedative–hypnotics	Confusion, slurred speech, ataxia, stupor, sleep disorders, withdrawal delirium, dementia, amnestic disorder, sleep disorders
Volatile solvents	Hallucinations, delusions, hyperactivity, sensory distortions, dementia

Adapted from Beauchamp, J. K., & Olson K. R. (2000). Drug overdoses and dependence. In R. M. Wachter, L. Goldman, & H. Hollander (Eds.), *Hospital medicine*. Philadelphia: Lippincott Williams & Wilkins.

Epidemiology

The pattern of alcohol and illicit drug use by those with a mental disorder varies, but it is estimated that as many as 8.9 million adults have both disorders (depending on definitions and methodologies). The drug most commonly used substance is alcohol followed by marijuana and cocaine. Prescription drugs such as tranquilizers and sleeping medicines may also be abused (SAMSHA, 2014b, 2014c).

The risk for substance abuse varies among the mental disorders (Table 39.2). Antisocial personality disorders; bipolar depression; and disorders of childhood, including

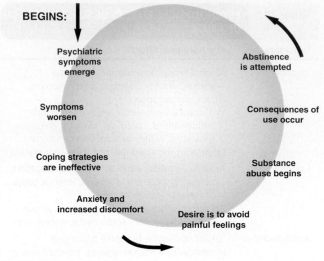

BEGINS:

Psychiatric symptoms emerge

Symptoms worsen

Coping strategies are ineffective

Anxiety and increased discomfort

Desire is to avoid painful feelings

Substance abuse begins

Consequences of use occur

Abstinence is attempted

FIGURE 39.1 Relapse cycle.

conduct disorders, oppositional-defiant disorders, and attention deficit disorders, are strongly associated with substance abuse disorders (Swendsen et al., 2010).

Etiology

There is no one model that explains why mental disorders and substance abuse occur together so frequently. In one pattern of occurrence, the mental disorder precedes the substance abuse. As adolescents with emerging mental disorders are exposed to drug use, their disinhibition and impulsivity lead to drug experimentation. Substances of abuse are used to self-medicate the underlying mental disorders. In the second pattern, the substance abuse disorder appears first and leads to the mental disorder. For example, LSD (lysergic acid diethylamide) or cocaine use may change the neurotransmission in the brain that results in panic attacks or psychosis. In the third pattern, there are common causes, either genetic or environmental, that lead to the onset or persistence of both disorders.

Table 39.2	MAJOR PSYCHIATRIC DISORDERS AND RISKS FOR SUBSTANCE ABUSE	
Psychiatric Disorder	**Increased Risk for Substance Abuse (%)**	
Antisocial personality disorder	15.5	
Manic episode	14.5	
Schizophrenia	10.1	
Panic disorder	4.3	
Major depressive episode	4.1	
Obsessive-compulsive disorder	3.4	
Phobias	2.4	

© Mental Health America. Dual Diagnosis. Retrieved May 15, 2011, from http://www.mentalhealthamerica.net/index.cfm?objectid=C7DF9405-1372-4D20-C89D7BD2CD1CA1B9.

Current research is beginning to offer an explanation for the pattern in which the symptoms of the mental disorder generally appear first followed by the substance use and abuse. Psychiatric symptoms have long been associated with dysregulation of the monoamines and neuropeptides. Drugs of abuse (cocaine, alcohol, marijuana) temporarily potentiate neurotransmission in the brain's reward system, relieving the depression and anxiety for a short period of time. Self-administration of drugs of abuse temporarily masks or suppresses the aversive psychological effects of the dysregulated neuronal systems (see Chapter 31).

BARRIERS TO TREATMENT

High morbidity rates point to the need for effective treatment of individuals with COD. Only 7.4% individuals with COD receive treatment for both disorders and 55.8% receive no treatment at all (SAMSHA, 2014b). Although it was recognized that integrated treatment should be the standard of care, these patients often face major barriers in obtaining proper treatment. There are many well-documented barriers such as regulatory prohibitions, funding barriers, and lack of staff (Knudsen, Abraham, & Oser, 2011). The following discussion highlights some other barriers. See also Box 39.1 for challenges related to health care for people with COD.

BOX 39.1

Research For Best Practice: **Challenges and Struggles with Co-occurring Disorders**

Villena, A. L. D., & Chesla, C. A. (2010). Challenges and struggles: Lived experiences of individuals with co-occurring disorders. Archives of Psychiatric Nursing, 24(2), 76–88.

THE QUESTION: What are the social and structural barriers that individuals with co-occurring disorders (COD) of mental illness, substance abuse, and general medical conditions encounter related to their health care?

METHODS: A purposive sampling of 20 individuals with COD (11 men, nine women; 65% African American) were recruited and interviewed from community treatment centers and supportive house sites using an interpretive study approach.

FINDINGS: Three realms of social and structural barriers were identified, including: (1) developing interpersonal relationships with health care providers, (2) negotiating a complex health care system, and (3) trying to manage health conditions while living in an unstable shelter.

IMPLICATIONS FOR NURSING: Nurses working with this population need to carefully reflect on their ability to provide positive, therapeutic relationships with people who have difficulty in the interactions with health care providers. Additionally, nurses need to provide guidance and support as people with COD negotiate the health care system.

Nature of Co-occurring Disorders

Patients often deny a problem with substances and do not seek treatment because they do not view themselves as needing it. They do not fully understand their mental illness or the effect of substance use on their mood or behavior. Even those who recognize their disorders are often reluctant to seek mental health treatment. It is confusing to be expected to abstain from alcohol and illicit drugs yet be prescribed medication that also affects their thoughts and feelings. If they take the substance of choice, they experience fleeting moments of joy and escape even though doing so will prompt a decline in overall function and worsen psychiatric symptoms. If they accept prescribed treatments, including medications, they will have higher levels of functioning and better treatment outcomes, but they lose their moments of joy and escape.

Staff Attitudes

Mental health professionals in psychiatric treatment programs are often frustrated in their efforts to assist substance-abusing patients. Behavior often associated with addiction, such as denial of substance use, manipulative behavior, and nonadherence with health-related protocols, is often regarded as a sign of treatment failure. This type of behavior can provoke hostility from the staff and can make planning for mental health recovery difficult.

Mental health professionals may have difficulty understanding the compelling nature of drug or alcohol cravings, may not understand differences in drug use patterns and behaviors associated with particular drugs of abuse, and may overdiagnose personality disorders in those who take drugs and commit crimes (Howard & Holmshaw, 2010). In addition, patients or their therapists may excuse substance use because of the patients' psychiatric symptoms.

Stigma

Drug-dependent patients may have the additional stigma of being regarded as criminals because they commit illegal acts every time they purchase, use, or distribute illicit drugs. Strong public feelings about alcohol-related motor vehicle accidents, negative experiences with family members or friends with drinking problems, and cultural biases against public intoxication can prejudice interactions with patients who are alcohol dependent (Anton, 2010).

Health Issues

Numerous health hazards are associated with alcohol and drug abuse (see Chapter 31). Patients with COD are more likely than others to use emergency departments (EDs) for primary health care, waiting until they can no longer ignore physical illness. They are more likely to be uncertain about the medical plan they need to follow and to be nonadherent with health care directives. The use of alcohol and illicit substances in addition to medications prescribed for mental illness can lead to drug interactions and may exacerbate side effects of these medications. Homelessness can increase these patients' medical problems with inadequate nutrition, poor hygiene, and the adverse effects of exposure to the elements adding to their difficulties. Health care providers often become frustrated with patients' nonadherence and with what they see as behaviors that are difficult to manage. Their frustration may negatively affect the way they treat patients with COD. Because of the confusion about what is the primary and most immediate problem to treat, these patients are often underserved and only partially treated.

STAGES OF INTERDISCIPLINARY TREATMENT

Treatment programs designed for people whose problems are primarily substance abuse are generally not recommended for people who also have a mental illness. These programs tend to be confrontational and coercive, and most people with severe mental illnesses are too fragile to benefit from them. Heavy confrontation, intense emotional jolting, and discouragement of the use of medications tend to be detrimental. These treatments may produce levels of stress that exacerbate symptoms or cause relapse.

The **quadrants of care** model is a conceptual framework that classifies patients according to symptom severity, not diagnosis (Figure 39.2). The quadrant can guide an individual's treatment and site of delivery of care. In an integrated treatment model, treatment for both disorders is combined in a single session or interaction or series of interactions.

Patients with COD enter treatment at various stages of recovery. Flexible treatment programs that can meet each patient's needs are the most effective. **Recovery** is sought through commonly recognized stages of treatment, including engagement, persuasion or motivation, active treatment, and relapse prevention. This recovery involves much more than avoiding alcohol and drugs. Individuals must believe that life can be better without drinking, but typically, they test the alternatives before they adopt lengthy remissions (Xie et al., 2010). An integrated interdisciplinary team is needed in order to move patients to recovery.

Engagement

Engagement entails establishing a treatment relationship and enhancing motivation to make behavior changes and a commitment to treatment. Research has shown

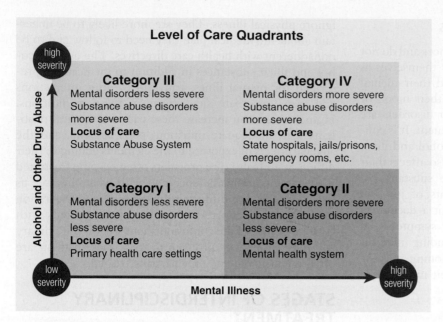

Level of Care Quadrants

high severity

Alcohol and Other Drug Abuse

Category III
Mental disorders less severe
Substance abuse disorders
more severe
Locus of care
Substance Abuse System

Category IV
Mental disorders more severe
Substance abuse disorders
more severe
Locus of care
State hospitals, jails/prisons,
emergency rooms, etc.

Category I
Mental disorders less severe
Substance abuse disorders
less severe
Locus of care
Primary health care settings

Category II
Mental disorders more severe
Substance abuse disorders
less severe
Locus of care
Mental health system

low severity

high severity

Mental Illness

FIGURE 39.2 Level of care quadrants. (From Center for Substance Abuse Treatment. [2014]. Definition, terms and classification systems for co-occurring disorders. *SAMHSA/CSAT treatment improvement protocols.* Rockville, MD: Substance Abuse and Mental Health Services Administration. Retrieved from http://www.ncbi.nlm.nih.gov/books/NBK25692.)

that engaged patients are more likely to stay in treatment and have positive outcomes (Brown, Bennett, Li, & Bellack, 2011). Patients who are abusing substances may experience repeated cycles of detoxification and relapse. Mentally ill patients may have prolonged cycles of "revolving-door" admissions and persistent medication nonadherence before acknowledging the need to engage in continuous treatment (Botha et al., 2010). Each admission is a "window of opportunity." Relapse does not mean that a treatment intervention, the health care provider, or the patient has failed. Readmission and clear, realistic goals can further the patient's engagement in the treatment process. Effective programs emphasize a combination of empathic, long-term relationship building and the use of leverage and possible confrontation by family, other caregivers, or the legal system.

Engaging patients with COD in treatment presents two main challenges. The first is developing relationships with people who tend to have difficulties in their relationships and with trusting authority figures. The second is patients' lack of motivation and the need to encourage them to enter drug and alcohol treatment programs.

Engagement in treatment is a process that may take many contacts with a patient and requires patience. Patients who struggle with authority and control issues must be convinced that the treatment team members have something to offer and are worth listening to before they will begin to trust them. The engagement process is enhanced if staff can deal with presenting crises concretely (e.g., provide help in avoiding legal penalties and obtaining food, housing, entitlements, relief from psychiatric symptoms, vocational opportunities, recreation, and socialization). Harm reduction may be a first step toward a goal of abstinence.

The process of engagement is often characterized by approach–avoidance behavior by the patient. Intake and assessment procedures may discourage the patient from engagement or be intolerable if they are protracted and begin with asking the patient numerous pointed personal questions. These procedures may have to be adjusted to tailor treatment and accommodate the needs or reactions of the patient with COD.

Motivation

Motivational interventions are useful with COD patients (see Chapter 31). Typically, these interventions consist of one to several sessions delivered within a few weeks or less during which the patient is motivated to become involved in treatment. One goal of this intervention is to increase engagement in treatment and help the patient identify his or her own goals (Xie et al., 2010).

Active Treatment: Assertive Outreach

There are two models of assertive outreach that have been shown to be effective in reducing substance use (Bukstein & Horner, 2010). In the case management model, case managers are responsible for conducting outreach activities, linking patients with direct services, monitoring patients' progress through various milieus, educating patients about psychiatric and substance use disorders, reiterating treatment recommendations, and coordinating treatment planning across programs. In this model, case managers represent different disciplines and emphasize an interdisciplinary team approach. Team members carry their own individual caseloads but discuss their patients and review cases together.

In **Assertive Community Treatment (ACT)**, the delivery of services is in the community (rather than a clinic), with shared caseloads, 24-hour responsibilities for patients, and direct provision of most services. This model was developed for patients with severe mental illness who do not use outpatient services, are prone to frequent relapses and rehospitalization, and have severe psychosocial impairment. This approach may be superior to case management in those settings characterized by high hospitalization use (de Vet, van Luijtelaar, Brilleslijper-Kater, Vanderplasschen, Beijersbergen, & Wolf, 2013).

Relapse Prevention

Persons with COD are highly prone to relapse even after they have achieved full remission. Although many relapse factors are the same for those with mental disorders as with the general population such as interpersonal problems, negative emotions, social stresses, lack of involvement in more satisfying activities, and attempts to escape from painful experiences, there are additional factors that affect this population. Symptoms of the mental illness recur, and there are inadequate treatment resources in many settings. Many people with mental illness live in extreme poverty, which forces them into high-crime, drug-infested neighborhoods, which makes them easy targets for crimes. Employment rates are low for this population even though many want to work. Finally, the same neurobiologic dysfunctions may underlie both substance abuse and mental illness (Xie et al., 2010).

Because persons with mental disorders face more challenges, emerging evidence suggests that **relapse prevention** for this population should be different than for the general population (Xie et al., 2010). Relapse prevention needs to account for the pervasive cognitive and social dysfunctions that are inherent in many people with COD. Patients usually need assistance in finding and maintaining housing and employment. Learning new skills may be difficult because of cognitive impairments that reduce the effectiveness of learning new skills. Social deficits can lead to isolation and victimization (Xie et al., 2010). Relapse prevention for COD involves the following:

- Living situations that provide meaningful opportunities and the acquisition of supports and skills
- Help in making fundamental changes, such as finding meaningful jobs and abstinent friends
- Long-term supports and relationships (new friendships with people who do not abuse substances)
- Specific and individualized treatments for specific problems
- Support for meeting spiritual needs and finding a sense of meaning in life

- Economic and political support in creating appropriate and decent housing (Xie et al., 2010).

NURSING MANAGEMENT: Care for Persons with Co-occurring Disorders

It is crucial for patients with COD to be thoroughly assessed for responses to both psychiatric and substance use disorders (SAMSHA, 2014a). In some cultural groups, recognition of psychiatric and substance abuse disorders is difficult because of the lack of access and stigma associated with COD. Nurses in nonpsychiatric, community settings may be the only health care professional contact that some groups have. Assessment should include determination of the patient's willingness to change or level of motivation for treatment.

It is important to delineate the relative contribution of each diagnosis to the severity of the current responses presented and to establish priorities accordingly. Because patients with COD often make unreliable historians or distort the reality of their mental health problems and the severity of their substance use, obtaining objective data is especially important. Ideally, one should obtain an objective history of the patient from family, significant others, board and care operators, other health care providers, or anyone familiar enough with the patient to provide an accurate history. Box 39.2 lists basic assessment tools and methods used for patients with COD. The following concepts are paramount when assessing persons with COD:

- Psychiatric and substance use disorders can coexist.
- Responses (psychosis, agitation) to both disorders can be similar.
- Substance use can mask other symptoms and syndromes.
- Psychiatric behaviors can mimic alcohol and other drug use problems.

> **NCLEXNOTE**   Patients with both mental illness and substance abuse disorders have responses to both disorders. Prioritizing nursing care depends on the immediate issue, but responses to both disorders should be assessed.

Assessment and Care for Specific Co-occurring Disorders

Thought Disorders and Substance Use

Research shows that a high percentage estimated 50% of persons with schizophrenia will have a substance abuse disorder during their lifetime. After tobacco and caffeine,

---

BOX 39.2

Assessment of Co-occurring Disorders

Obtain a history and physical examination and laboratory tests (e.g., liver function tests, complete blood count) to confirm medical indicators related to substance use and also to rule out medical disorders with psychiatric presentations

- Obtain substance use history and severity of consequences, and physical symptoms.
- Identify core cultural values; explore meaning of the symptoms.
- Assess mental status examination and severity of symptoms (e.g., suicidal, homicidal, florid psychosis).
- Explore social context—socioeconomic, environment, literacy, and support system.

Interview with and assess family members to verify or determine (1) the accuracy of the patient's self-reported substance use or mental health history; (2) the patient's history of past mental health problems during periods of abstinence; and, if possible, (3) the sequence of the diagnoses (i.e., what symptoms appeared first).

- Conduct interviews with the patient's partner, friends, social worker, and other significant people in the patient's life.
- Review court records, medical records, and previous psychiatric and substance use treatment.
- Perform urine and blood toxicity screens; use a breath analyzer to test the patient's blood alcohol level.

Revise initial assessment by observation of the patient in the clinical setting; full assessment of the underlying psychiatric problem may not be possible until there is a long (up to 6 months) period of total abstinence.

- Observe the patient for reappearance of psychiatric symptoms after a period of sobriety.
- Assess the patient's motivation to seek treatment, desire to change behavior, and understanding of diagnoses.

---

alcohol, cannabis, and cocaine are the most common substances of abuse (Thoma & Daum, 2013). There are a number of possible explanations for the high rate of substance abuse in individuals with this disorder. Individuals with COD (substance abuse and schizophrenia) score higher on measures of sensation seeking and impulsivity than those without the co-occurring disorder. Stress reduction, symptom reduction, and relaxation are also offered as explanations. A neurobiologic model suggests that a dysregulated dopamine-mediated mesocorticolimbic network in patients with schizophrenia may also underlie substance use. Whereas all people are vulnerable to experiencing psychotic episodes from the use of various drugs, one psychotic episode increases susceptibility to subsequent episodes (Thoma & Daum, 2013).

Assessing the needs of people with schizophrenia who are also chemically dependent is complicated by the changing interaction among psychotic symptoms, the antipsychotic effects of medications, and the side effects of medications. A patient with a psychotic disorder may have an altered thought process or delusional thinking and may experience auditory hallucinations. He or she

may also be cognitively impaired and have poor memory. These patients can have negative symptoms, such as poor motivation and poor hygiene. They often have low self-esteem and poor social skills and may have a general sense of not belonging to a community. Their sense of self in relation to the world may be altered.

As with all of the CODs, a multifaceted, integrated treatment approach is needed. Atypical antipsychotics continue to be the primary pharmacological agent for the treatment of patients with comorbid schizophrenia with substance use. Not only do these agents treat the symptoms of schizophrenia, but they also appear to reduce cue-trigger cravings of the substances and prevent relapse (Murthy & Chand, 2012). While monitoring side effects of antipsychotics, the nurse's attention needs to focus on liver functioning because drugs and alcohol are also metabolized by the liver. Relapse is frequently secondary to medication nonadherence, especially if patients experience side effects associated with the use of antipsychotics. Nursing interventions that focus on medication compliance may reduce the chances of relapse.

A confrontational interactive approach does not benefit this population and could even alienate patients. A more supportive approach is appropriate in which relapses are treated as an expected part of the recovery process. Addressing relapse risk is part of treatment planning. Focus on examining behavior, feelings, and the thinking process that led to the relapse. The nurse must avoid blame and guilt-inducing statements.

Social skills training is needed to help the patient learn ways of avoiding peer pressure and social situations that could lead to substance use. The goal is to successfully interact in a sober living situation, develop problem-solving skills, and refine behaviors.

Mood Disorders and Substance Use

Substance use in patients with bipolar disorders may also contribute to treatment nonadherence and less positive outcomes (Gao et al., 2010). Mood disorders may be more prevalent among patients using opiates than among other drug users. Many who use substances self-medicate an underlying mood disorder. Because many of the symptoms of substance use are the same as those of mood disorders, it is difficult to differentiate between them. This is especially true in the case of stimulant use and bipolar disorder. It is often impossible to determine the presence of an underlying mood disorder until there has been a period of abstinence.

Screening for suicide ideation is a priority during the assessment of these individuals. Both mood disorders and substance abuse are related to suicide (see Chapters 24, 25, and 31). Depression during withdrawal from alcohol, cocaine, opiates, and amphetamines also puts patients at severe risk for suicide. A person's presenting behaviors

Table 39.3	DRUGS THAT PRECIPITATE OR MIMIC MOOD DISORDERS	
Mood Disorders	During Use (Intoxication)	After Use (Withdrawal)
Depression and dysthymia	Alcohol, benzodiazepines, opioids, barbiturates, cannabis, steroids (chronic use), stimulants (chronic use)	Alcohol, benzodiazepines, opioids, barbiturates, cannabis, steroids (chronic use), stimulants (chronic use)
Mania and cyclothymia	Stimulants, alcohol, hallucinogens, inhalants, steroids (chronic and acute use)	Alcohol, benzodiazepines, barbiturates, opiates, steroids (chronic use)

may not have included depression, but depression may develop as the withdrawal syndrome unfolds. Hyperactivity often appears with stimulant use and at times with alcohol abuse. Patients may be treated for hypomania or bipolar disorder when they are actually hyperactive. Symptoms usually improve as the person maintains abstinence.

Determining whether mood disorders are the cause or the effect of protracted substance use is difficult (Table 39.3). One important nursing assessment is to determine how drug use relates to mood states. Patients may be attempting to alleviate uncomfortable symptoms, such as depression or agitation, or to enhance a mood state (e.g., hypomania). Symptoms that persist during periods of abstinence are a clue to the degree that the mood disorder contributes to the presenting symptoms.

There is little research regarding pharmacological interventions for comorbid mood disorders and substance abuse. Consequently, treatment is similar to that of mood disorders without substance use or abuse. When a pharmacological agent is selected, attention is paid to its interaction with drugs and alcohol and its potential for abuse. The selective serotonin reuptake inhibitors (SSRIs) are frequently used for co-occurring depression. Higher doses may be required because of the possibility that alcohol use may induce hepatic microsomal activity. In the bipolar disorders, mood stabilizers are used.

Treatment for bipolar disorders and chemical dependency should be individualized to accommodate the specific needs, personal goals, and cultural perspectives of these individuals in different stages of change. Using interventions centered on examining cognitive distortions (e.g., "I'll never get better; no one likes me; alcohol is my only friend") and cognitive therapy techniques can help improve mood. Use of positive self-talk can be helpful for both the depression and the substance use disorders.

Anxiety Disorders and Substance Use

Research is scant regarding the relationship of anxiety disorders to substance abuse. Because there are a variety of anxiety disorders with differing clinical symptoms and numerous substances of abuse, it is difficult to develop studies addressing all of the anxiety disorders. Posttraumatic stress disorder (PTSD) is of particular concern because it has been shown to increase the risk of substance use relapse and is associated with poor treatment outcomes (McCarthy & Petrakis, 2010).

The symptoms of anxiety may result from an anxiety disorder, such as panic attack, or may be secondary to drug or alcohol use as part of a withdrawal syndrome. Symptoms are so subjectively disturbing that they can lead to drug or alcohol abuse as self-medication for the emotional pain; therefore, they require prompt evaluation and treatment. There are many unanswered questions regarding the relationship of the anxiety symptoms, stress, and changes in the hypothalamic–pituitary–adrenal axis response to substance use. More research is sorely needed in this area.

Pharmacological treatment of patients with anxiety is difficult because the traditional medications used, the benzodiazepines, are themselves addicting. Long-term treatment of the anxiety disorders, particularly PTSD, with the SSRIs maintains and improves quality of life. For PTSD, other medications such as the atypical antipsychotics, non-SSRI antidepressants, and mood stabilizers also appear to result in improvements (see Chapter 26).

Comorbid anxiety disorders and substance abuse require psychosocial interventions along with pharmacological treatment. Patients with anxiety disorders should also pay particular attention to their physical health. Regular, balanced meals; exercise; and sleep are ways to decrease and manage stress levels. Patients should avoid excessive consumption of caffeine and sugars. If the patient has a fear of crowds, he or she may benefit from gradual desensitization techniques.

Personality Disorders and Substance Use

Personality disorders are frequently present in those who abuse alcohol and other substances. Antisocial personality and borderline disorders carry a high risk of having a comorbid substance abuse problem (Kelly, Daley, & Douaihy, 2012). The assessment of persons with comorbid personality disorders and substance abuse focuses on the problems related to the particular personality disorder as well as the substance use. Individuals with antisocial personality disorder are likely to have a family history of other psychiatric disorders and problems with hostility. Interventions should be individualized according to the disorder and are discussed in the next section.

Interventions for Persons With Co-occurring Disorders

The nurse who provides care to patients with COD faces numerous challenges. Nurses implement interventions according to their level of practice and knowledge. Comprehensive planning within a multidisciplinary team approach is highly successful in the care of such patients. The entire system is organized to care for persons with COD (SAMSHA, 2014a). Community organizations are valuable sources of support as well. Many of the interventions that are indicated for persons with COD are discussed in previous chapters (see Unit VI). The following discussion highlights interventions that are modified because of the special needs of this population.

Medication Management

One essential feature of COD treatment is medication management. Medication for a known mental disorder should never be discontinued on the grounds that the patient is using substances. Nonadherence with prescribed medications is associated with increased behavior problems after discharge and is a direct cause of relapse and rehospitalization. Impulsive behavior in response to transient exacerbations of psychotic symptoms, depressed mood, or anxiety symptoms may lead to relapse.

Treating a patient with COD can be as complex as the presenting symptoms. Errors in treatment can include treating temporary psychiatric symptoms resulting from withdrawal as if they were a permanent feature of the individual, withholding needed medication for a psychiatric disorder, or setting arbitrary limits on medication based on a belief that medication for all psychiatric symptoms should be suspended for a time. Overall, patients need ongoing help with adhering to a prescribed medication regimen.

Collaboration between the patient's prescriber and other treatment providers is important to minimize the possible misuse or abuse of prescription drugs such as forging prescriptions, acquiring drugs from nonmedical sources, frequent visits to EDs, or seeking multiple prescribers. In addition, caution is essential in prescribing medications that can increase the patient's potential for relapse into abusing the drug of choice. The patient in recovery is often reluctant to use potentially mind-altering drugs, and the nurse should explore any concerns.

Substance Abuse Counseling

With the COD patient, substance abuse counseling is slower and less confrontational than in many traditional substance abuse programs. Content needs to be repeated frequently and motivation for treatment continually assessed (Xie et al., 2010).

Cognitive Behavioral Interventions

Cognitive behavioral interventions help patients to (1) analyze which situations are most likely to trigger relapses; (2) examine cognitive, emotional, and behavioral components of high-risk situations; and (3) develop cognitive, behavioral, and effective coping strategies and environmental supports. Role-playing ways out of high-risk situations is a technique that these groups often use. Homework assignments help patients create relapse prevention plans that address new coping strategies for these high-risk situations.

Patient Education

Patient education is an essential element in treating COD. Patients need to learn about their specific mental disorder, substance use and abuse, and their effects. Relapse prevention and recovery should be highlighted. Education can be conducted in individual sessions, but group sessions encourage interaction among patients. Sharing their experiences with their peers, patients can enhance these presentations.

Topics should be clear; relevant to the group members; and illustrated with charts, handouts, or appropriate films. Each session should be relatively short and not contain too many new or difficult concepts. Reinforcing and reviewing previous discussions can be helpful to remind patients of particularly relevant concepts. Box 39.3 lists some suitable topics for nurse-led discussion groups. Individual patient education can focus on areas of knowledge deficits and reinforce topics discussed in group settings. Group sessions can also assist patients in learning interpersonal skills (e.g., assertiveness) and problem-solving skills and in relapse prevention planning.

Mutual Self-Help Groups

Several mutual self-help groups are appropriate for many patients with COD. Peer-led self-help approaches specifically for persons with COD are being tried with some success. The most common groups are 12-step programs, such as Alcoholics Anonymous (AA) and Narcotics Anonymous (NA) (see Chapter 31). The advisability of a patient enrolling in a 12-step program needs to be evaluated on an individual basis. A health care provider familiar with 12-step concepts can often facilitate patients' attempts to use these programs. The numerous advantages of self-help groups make them a potentially powerful support for continued recovery. Alternative mutual self-help programs similar to 12-step programs are available in some geographic areas. Rational Recovery and Secular Organization for Sobriety are groups that downplay the concept of powerlessness and the spiritual aspects associated with 12-step programs.

Family Support and Education

The families of patients with COD need education and support. Family psychoeducation interventions address mental illnesses, substance abuse, and their interactions. The focus of family support groups, such as those under the auspices of the National Alliance for the Mentally Ill, has been both to educate and to help the family cope with a mentally ill relative. AA and NA take a similar approach to providing peer support to families of substance users. These self-help groups aid family members in balancing confrontation of the problem, detachment from forcing a solution to it, and support of the treatment process.

Evaluation and Treatment Outcomes

Evaluation of the patient's ability to deal with both the substance abuse and mental disorder is an ongoing process. Because the goal of recovery is to have quality of life in the community of choice, treatment outcomes should be evaluated in terms of quality of life as well as management of two disorders.

CONTINUUM OF CARE

An integrated approach that combines mental health and substance abuse interventions at the clinical site has been shown to be the most effective. In an integrated system, the same team provides coordinated mental health and substance abuse interventions and guides the patient toward learning to manage these intertwined disorders. When the mental health and substance abuse systems are truly integrated, patient outcomes are positive (Mueser et al., 2012).

When Hospitalization Is Necessary

Often, patients with COD can be treated effectively in community mental health settings if their symptoms are stable, they are following their treatment plan, they are compliant with the use of psychiatric medications, and they remain alcohol and drug free. Patients are hospitalized when they have a need for detoxification, exacerbation of comorbid psychiatric or medical disorders, suicide or homicidal ideation, or an illness that prevents abstinence or outpatient treatment.

Crisis Stabilization

Setting priorities is essential for hospitalized patients with COD. The first priorities are gathering data from a physical examination and nursing assessments, stabilizing psychiatric symptoms, and treating withdrawal symptoms (see Chapter 31). After these issues are addressed, the patient enters the rehabilitation phase of treatment for both diagnoses. Rehabilitative therapy is appropriate if the patient (1) can participate in a group process, (2) can focus attention on groups or reading material, (3) does not engage in behavior that is detrimental to the group process, (4) can listen to and receive feedback from others, and (5) can benefit from the group process.

Early Stages of Recovery From Substance Use

Many patients seeking alcohol or drug abuse treatment experience transitory cognitive impairment, which usually resolves within the first month of abstinence. Patients often experience difficulties with disorientation, clouding of consciousness, incoherent thoughts, memory loss, and delirium, which may hinder their ability to learn new concepts. These problems are a result of the neurobiologic insult on the brain by these substances and psychosocial factors such as fear of legal or relationship difficulties, depression, grief, and feelings of guilt and shame. However, if Wernicke's syndrome, a reversible alcohol-induced amnestic disorder caused by a thiamine-deficient diet, or

Korsakoff's psychosis, characterized by a loss of recent memory and confabulation (or filling in the blanks in memory by making up facts to cover this deficit), are present, cognitive problems may last longer. Patients with this condition are highly suggestible, have poor judgment, and cannot reason critically. Korsakoff's psychosis often follows Wernicke's encephalopathy and is also associated with prior peripheral neuropathy (see Chapter 31).

Psychological testing and other methods of assessment determine the patient's level of cognitive functioning in order to select the appropriate treatment. It is also important to determine the extent of the mental disorder and the substance abuse. The nurse assesses the patient's abilities for self-care, independent living, impulse control, control of assaultiveness, direction taking, and development of new responses to new situations and ideas. The nurse must also evaluate changes in mental status during the past 6 months and examine previous treatment outcomes.

Clear, direct, simple interventions that avoid extraneous issues and theoretical discussion may be useful for patients with cognitive or memory impairment such as the following:

- Reading material that is relevant to recovery and that can be referred to in short study sessions
- First-person accounts of addiction and recovery found in AA and NA literature
- Basic concepts of recovery, such as those in AA slogans and on patients' need for continuing care after discharge
- Films with scenes illustrating relevant family problems or other problems related to substance use; movies can be more effective than lectures

Social interaction skills and coping skills learned in treatment need to be reinforced in community settings to create or enhance a stable living situation and possible vocational opportunities. Active planning and intervention are needed for housing and employment or deterioration may occur despite gains made during hospitalization.

Recovery

To move toward recovery, establishing a positive social network is critical. Isolation and alienation from prior sources of support is a problem that most people with comorbid mental disorders and substance use share. Some patients relate poorly to their families, others are overly dependent on their families, and others have difficulty establishing and maintaining social relationships. Some patients' only "families" are peers within the drug subculture who reinforce substance-abusing behavior.

Compliance with an agreed-on treatment plan is integral to recovery. Box 39.4 presents features of a COD outpatient program. Opportunities to socialize, access to

---

BOX 39.4

Features of a Co-occurring Disorders Outpatient Program

- *Community meeting and goal setting:* Patients set small, realistic goals for themselves for the day, which aids them in their ultimate goal of better living in recovery.
- *Anger management and social communication:* Patients learn appropriate ways to express anger and how to socialize with others.
- *Group therapy:* Patients discuss interpersonal issues, get feedback from their peers, and learn problem-solving skills.
- *Dual recovery anonymous meetings:* Patient-run meetings (a modified Alcoholics Anonymous meeting) address the specific needs of patient with co-occurring disorders.
- *Leisure planning:* Patients learn skills to enjoy leisure involving clean and sober fun.
- *Gardening, art therapy, music therapy, swimming:* These methods provide alternatives to the use of alcohol and other drugs.
- *Health education:* Patients learn about the effects of drugs and alcohol on the body and about other relevant medical topics.
- *Medication education:* Patients learn about psychiatric medications, their uses, their side effects, and interactions with drugs or alcohol.
- *Relapse prevention planning:* Patients talk about their last relapse; triggers, feelings, and stresses that contributed to the relapse; and the consequences and formulate relapse prevention plans.
- *Individual counseling:* Patients receive individual counseling to develop goals and work on problem-solving techniques.
- *Psychiatric consultation:* Patients are evaluated and followed up for medication and other psychiatric interventions.

Note: Patients are *not* discharged from the program if they are intoxicated. They are asked not to come to the program intoxicated but to return when they are sober to continue work on their recovery.

---

positive recreational activities, and a supportive peer group are stabilizing influences on patients who may otherwise drop out of treatment altogether. Part of a comprehensive relapse prevention plan is to establish or reinforce the patient's social support network so that he or she can obtain (1) opportunities for substance-free socializing, (2) crisis counseling to prevent readmission to a hospital, and (3) support for sobriety.

Supportive housing is also essential for patients with COD. Supportive housing is especially crucial for patients who are being discharged from the hospital because the risk for relapse is greatest during the first few months after discharge. Halfway houses for substance users may deemphasize medication compliance, and housing designed for chronically mentally ill individuals may not emphasize abstinence enough. Thus, an important part of the multidisciplinary team approach to discharge planning for patients with COD is to help them find the best possible living situation.

Younger patients with severe mental illness may want and expect to find appropriate employment, but some of these patients may be unrealistic about potential professions. However, this desire can be a significant motivator and a useful tool in a treatment program. Referring patients to halfway houses or residential substance use treatment programs that stress vocational skill training can be beneficial. Use of community vocational rehabilitation services and of educational opportunities can be an important part of a discharge plan.

SUMMARY OF KEY POINTS

- In co-occurring mental illness and substance use disorder, each disorder is considered a primary disorder. They should be treated concurrently with an integrated approach.

- People with co-occurring disorders (COD) are at high risk for relapse. The relapse cycle repeats itself without treatment.

- There is no one model that explains why mental disorders and substance abuse occur together so frequently. The most common pattern is the onset of the mental disorder followed by the problems with substance use leading to abuse. It appears that the substance use is an attempt to self-medicate the psychiatric symptoms.

- Barriers for treatment include homelessness, unemployment, and lack of social support. Other barriers include the complexity of the COD, staff attitudes, stigma, and health issues that interfere with treatment.

- Interdisciplinary treatment is through an integrated approach. Patients are moved toward recovery through engagement, motivation, assertive outreach and treatment, and relapse prevention.

- Recovery through commonly recognized stages of treatment—engagement, persuasion or motivation, active treatment, and relapse prevention—involves much more than avoiding alcohol and drugs.

- Nursing assessment of COD often depends on objective data obtained from interviews with family members, reviews of court records, laboratory test results, and physical examination findings. Assessment should include a determination of the willingness to change and motivation for treatment.

- Treatment and nursing care need to be individualized within the context of the specific mental disorder and substances used.

- Interventions that are tailored to the special needs of the patient with a COD are medication management, substance abuse counseling, cognitive behavioral interventions, patient education, and family support and education. Participation in peer-led self-help groups has had some success.

- An ideal continuum of care is an integrated approach with one team coordinating the mental health and substance abuse interventions. Patients should not have to negotiate treatment with two separate systems. Hospitalization may be required during periods of crises. Most treatment occurs in the community, where recovery is the goal.

CRITICAL THINKING CHALLENGES

1. An 18-year-old patient, newly diagnosed with schizophrenia, is relatively compliant with his medication and treatment. He was recently at a social event where he was experimenting with alcohol and marijuana. Develop a teaching plan for him that includes the risks of developing a substance abuse disorder.

2. A nurse in an emergency department recommends AA for every patient who is admitted for detoxification. Is that an appropriate referral for a person with comorbid mental disorder and substance abuse?

3. A community health nurse wants to refer a young woman who lives in a poor rural area to an integrated treatment program several miles away. Discuss the likelihood of the patient's actually being able to access services. What barriers would she face, and how could she have access to the care she needs?

4. How would you respond to a patient with COD who states, "Once my medication is stable, I will be able to drink again."

5. Compare traditional substance abuse approaches to an integrated treatment program.

6. A patient with a COD tells the nurse, "All chemicals are bad for you. I do not want to take my medication." Develop a response to this statement that reflects the use of engagement.

7. Discuss the differences in behavior of a person with schizophrenia who uses cocaine and a person with a mood disorder who uses marijuana.

8. Which COD concepts should be included in patient education?

 Born on the Fourth of July: 1989. This wrenching but true account shows the experiences of Ron Kovic, played by Tom Cruise. Ron was a patriotic teen from a small town who volunteered to serve in Vietnam. During the war, he was shot in the spine, which left him paralyzed from the chest down. He returned home, bitterly alienated from his family, friends, and community. He faced a long and slow rehabilitation process. His depression and abuse of substances only compounded his physical problems. This movie depicts depression, PTSD, and substance dependence coexisting with major physical disabilities.

Viewing Points: How does Ron express his depression? Is he using, abusing, or dependent on alcohol and drugs? How are you feeling throughout this movie? Do your feelings about the character change?

References

Anton, R. (2010). Substance abuse is a disease of the human brain: Focus on alcohol. *The Journal of Law, Medicine & Ethics, 38*(4), 735–744.

Botha, U. A., Koen, L., Joska, J. A., Parker, J. S., Horn, N., Hering, L. M., & Oosthuizen, P. P. (2010). The revolving door phenomenon in psychiatry: Comparing low-frequency and high-frequency users of psychiatric inpatient services in a developing country. *Social Psychiatry Psychiatric Epidemiology, 45*(4), 462–468.

Brown, C. H., Bennett, M. E., Li, L., & Bellack, A. S. (2011). Predictors of initiation and engagement in substance abuse treatment among individuals with co-occurring serious mental illness and substance use disorders. *Addictive Behaviors, 36*(5), 439–447.

Bukstein, O. G., & Horner, M. S. (2010). Management of the adolescent with substance use disorders and comorbid psychopathology. *Child & Adolescent Psychiatric Clinics of North America, 19*(3), 609–623.

de Vet, R., van Luijtelaar, M. J., Brilleslijper-Kater, S. N., Vanderplasschen, W., Beijersbergen, M. D., & Wolf, J. R. (2013). Effectiveness of case management for homeless persons: A systematic review. *American Journal of Public Health, 103*(10), e13–e26.

Effinger, J. M. & Stewart, D. G. (2012). Classification of co-occurring depression and substance abuse symptoms predicts suicide attempts in adolescents. *Suicide & Life-threatening Behavior, 42*(4), 353–358.

Farren, C. K., Snee, L., Daly, P., & McElroy, S. (2013). Prognostic factors of 2-year outcomes of patients with comorbid bipolar disorder or depression with alcohol dependence: Importance of early abstinence. *Alcohol and Alcoholism, 48*(1), 93–98.

Gao, K., Kemp, D. E., Wang, A. et al. (2010). Predictors of non-stabilization during the combination therapy of lithium and divalproex in rapid cycling bipolar disorder: A post-hoc analysis of two studies. *Psychopharmacology Bulletin, 43*(1), 23–38.

Goldstein, G., Luther, J. F., Haas, G. L., & Gordon, A. J., & Appelt, C. (2009). Comorbidity between psychiatric and general medical disorders in homeless veterans. *Psychiatric Quarterly, 80*(4), 199–212.

Howard, V., & Holmshaw, J. (2010). Inpatient staff perceptions in providing care to individuals with co-occurring mental health problems and illicit substance use. *Journal of Psychiatric Mental Health Nursing, 17*(10), 862–877.

Kelly, T. M., Daley, D. C., & Douaihy, A. B. (2012). Treatment of substance abusing patients with comorbid psychiatric disorders (Review). *Addictive Behaviors, 37*(1), 11–24.

Knudsen, H. K., Abraham, A. J., & Oser, C. B. (2011). Barriers to the implementation of medication-assisted treatment for substance use disorders: The importance of funding policies and medical infrastructure. *Evaluation and Program Planning*, in press.

McCarthy, E., & Petrakis, I. (2010). Epidemiology and management of alcohol dependence in individuals with post-traumatic stress disorder. *CNS Drugs, 24*(12), 997–1007.

Mueser, K. T., Glynn, S. M., Cather, C., Xie, H., Zarate, R., Smith, L. F., et al. (2012). A randomized controlled trial of family intervention for co-occurring substance use and severe psychiatric disorders. *Schizophrenia Bulletin, 39*(3), 658–672.

Murthy, P. & Chand, P. (2012). Treatment of dual diagnosis disorders. (Review). *Current Opinion in Psychiatry, 25*(3), 194–200.

Substance Abuse and Mental Health Services Administration (SAMSHA). (2014a). Screening and assessment. http://media.samhsa.gov/co-occurring/topics/screening-and-assessment/index.aspx. Retrieved on May 29, 2014.

Substance Abuse and Mental Health Services Administration (SAMSHA). (2014b). Office of Applied Studies, National Survey on Drug Use and Health, 2008 and 2009 http://media.samhsa.gov/co-occurring/

Substance Abuse and Mental Health Services Administration (SAMSHA). (2014c). *The TEDS Report: Gender Differences in Primary Substance of Abuse across Age Groups.* Rockville, MD. http://www.samhsa.gov/data/2k14/TEDS077/sr077-gender-differences-2014.pdf

Swendsen, J., Conway, K. P., Degenhardt, L., Glantz, J., Jin, R., Merikangas, K. R., Sampson, N., & Kessler, R. C. (2010). Mental disorders as risk factors for substance use, abuse and dependence: Results from the National Comorbidity Survey. *Addiction, 105*(6), 1117–1128.

Thoma, P. & Daum, I. (2013). Comorbid substance use disorder in schizophrenia: A selective overview of neurobiological and cognitive underpinnings. *Psychiatry and Clinical Neuroscience, 67*(6), 367–383.

Villena, A. L. D., & Chesla, C. A. (2010). Challenges and struggles: Lived experiences of individuals with co-occurring disorders. *Archives of Psychiatric Nursing, 24*(2), 76–88.

Xie, H., Drake, R. E., McHugo, G. J., Xie, L., Mohandas, A. (2010). The 10-year course of remission, abstinence, and recovery in dual diagnosis. *Journal of Substance Abuse Treatment, 39*(2), 132–140.

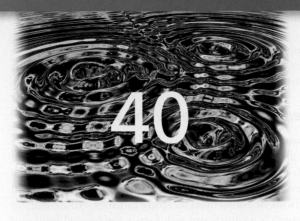

40

Caring for Survivors of Violence

Beverly Baliko, Mary R. Boyd, and Stephanie Burgess

KEY CONCEPTS

- intimate partner violence
- psychological abuse
- sexual assault

LEARNING OBJECTIVES

After studying this chapter, you will be able to:

1. Describe types of violence and abuse, including intimate partner violence, stalking, rape and sexual assault, child abuse, and elder abuse.

2. Describe selected theories of violence.

3. Analyze the reasons some people become abusive and why some victims remain in violent relationships.

4. Describe consequences of and responses to violence for the survivor.

5. Formulate nursing care plans for survivors of violence and abuse.

6. Describe treatment for perpetrators of abuse.

KEY TERMS

- child abuse - child neglect - cyberstalking - cycle of violence - elder abuse - intergenerational transmission of violence - rape - revictimization - self-esteem - stalking

Violence in the form of abuse of intimate partners, children, and elders is a national health problem. This type of violence permanently changes the survivor's reality and meaning of life. It wounds deeply, endangering core beliefs about self, others, and the world. It can damage or destroy the survivor's self-esteem.

Nurses encounter survivors of violence and abuse in all health care settings. For this reason, being knowledgeable about abuse risk factors, indicators, causes, assessment techniques, and effective nursing interventions is a must. This chapter presents evidence that can shape contemporary nursing practice in caring for persons and families who survive violence and abuse.

TYPES OF VIOLENCE AND ABUSE

The most common type of abuse occurs as a result of domestic (family) violence; that is, the perpetrator is or once was a loved and trusted partner or family member.

When this kind of violence occurs, the world and home are no longer safe in the eyes of the survivor, people seem dangerous, and life may become a tortured existence of warding off ever-present threats.

Intimate Partner Violence

Intimate partner violence (IPV) is a significant public health problem in the United States, and across the globe. Behaviors that constitute IPV include physical and sexual violence, threats of violence, and emotional abuse. Costs of billions of dollars annually are associated with acute and chronic medical and mental health needs of survivors, lost productivity, and with lives lost due to IPV-related homicide (Centers for Disease Control and Prevention [CDC], 2013a).

> **KEYCONCEPT** **Intimate partner violence** involves psychological, physical, or sexual harm perpetrated by a current or former spouse or partner (CDC, 2013b).

In the United States, approximately one in four women and one in seven men are victims of severe physical violence by an intimate partner at some point in their lives (CDC, 2013a). Many sustain multiple assaults. Aside from injuries that directly result from physical violence, IPV is associated with many physiologic and psychological problems. These are reviewed later in this chapter. IPV occurs on a continuum from psychological abuse to lethal violence. In 2011, 61% of female murder victims were killed by current or former intimate partners (Violence Policy Center, 2013). The majority of murder–suicides involve intimate partners, and perpetrators are far more likely males (Violence Policy Center, 2012). In addition to homicide, a history of IPV is associated with suicide in both victims and perpetrators. Fortunately, rates of intimate partner homicides have been falling since 1993, particularly for male victims. The greater availability of resources for survivors may have contributed to this decline, including resources to help more women find a way out of violent relationships (Campbell, Webster, & Glass, 2009).

Many women are afraid or reluctant to identify their abusers, fearing retaliation against themselves or their children. Often, they continue to hold strong feelings for their partners despite the abuse. When medical care is required, women may attribute their injuries to other causes, and health care providers may be reluctant to inquire about abuse. Provision of assistance to women who are involved in violent intimate relationships can pose unique problems in that seeking support can be dangerous to the women if their activities are discovered by the abusive partner. Therefore, the challenge for health care providers is twofold—ensuring that support is both available and safely accessible.

Although females are disproportionately affected by IPV, its impact on the millions of male survivors should not be discounted. Men are sometimes hesitant to report victimization or may not consider behaviors such as shoving or slapping "abuse." Others, even health care providers, may minimize the impact of abuse on men or not take their victimization seriously, believing that men could defend themselves if they wanted to.

IPV in same-sex couples occurs with at least the same frequency as in heterosexual relationships, but individuals with same-sex partners have not historically been offered the same support or access to resources (National Coalition of Antiviolence Programs, 2013). After much congressional debate, the Violence Against Women Act (VAWA, signed into law in 1994 and expiring in 2012) was reauthorized in 2013 and reworded to be more inclusive of underserved populations (National Network to End Domestic Violence, 2014). The law now prohibits anyone from being refused services on the basis of sexual orientation or gender identity and expands protection for lesbian, gay, bisexual, and transgender (LGBT) individuals, as well as Native Americans and immigrants.

Violence and Abuse During Pregnancy

Estimates of the prevalence of IPV battering during pregnancy and the postpartum period vary from 4% to as high as 22% (Sharps, Laughon, & Giangrade, 2007). Differences in prevalence rates may be attributed to differences in definitions of abuse used by study authors. Abuse during pregnancy is a significant risk factor for several fetal and maternal complications, including low birth weight, low maternal weight gain, infections, and anemia as well as miscarriages (Morland, Leskin, Block, Campbell, & Friedman, 2008). Moreover, abuse of women often results in their use of alcohol and other drugs (AODs), which in turn may harm unborn children (Duke & Cunradi, 2011). Pregnancy is a window of opportunity for health care providers to screen women for IPV and refer them to the appropriate services.

Psychological Abuse

Although much of the preceding discussion has centered on physical abuse, it is important to remember that psychological, or emotional, abuse can be just as harmful. In a recent national survey, nearly half of both female and male respondents reported having experienced psychological aggression by an intimate partner during their lifetime, and even more men (18%) than women (14%) reported experiencing it during the year prior to the survey (Black et al., 2011).

> **KEYCONCEPT** **Psychological abuse** includes behaviors such as criticizing, insulting, humiliating, or ridiculing someone in private or in public. It can also involve actions such as destroying another's property, threatening or harming pets, controlling or monitoring spending and activities, or isolating a person from family and friends.

Whereas physical violence may be episodic, psychological abuse is frequently more unrelenting. Over time, psychological abuse is devastating to an individual's self-esteem and can lead to depression, anxiety, substance abuse, and other psychological disorders as well as other physical illnesses (CDC, 2013a). The varieties of abuse used to exert power and control over romantic partners are represented in Figure 40.1.

Risk Factors for Intimate Partner Violence

IPV crosses all ethnic, racial, and socioeconomic lines. Evidence suggests that younger, single, divorced, and separated women may actually be at greater risk for abuse than are married women (Burgess & Tavakoli, 2005). This group is at particularly high risk for severe violence because abusive ex-partners often exhibit obsessive threatening behavior after their relationships end and pose significant dangers to women. This information is important for health care providers, who frequently pressure women to end abusive relationships.

Rates of IPV vary among women of different racial backgrounds. Asian and Pacific Islander women report the lowest rates of IPV, and African American and Native American and Alaska Native women report the highest rates (Black, et al., 2011). However, a more significant risk factor is low income, which is associated with a multitude of stressors that can contribute to violence. Additionally, individuals who lack financial resources, education, and job skills often find it more difficult to leave an abusive relationship (Duke & Cunradi, 2011). Although rates of IPV are similar across rural and urban areas, fewer resources are available in rural areas and, rural victims of IPV face numerous obstacles and safety risks that their urban counterparts do not, including geographic isolation, fewer local police services, and lack of anonymity within small communities (Eastman, Bunch, Williams, & Carawan, 2007). Most intimate partner deaths are preceded by IPV, which further emphasizes the importance of early intervention in family violence (Catalano, Smith, Snyder, & Rand, 2009). Individuals are sometimes so used to being in an abusive situation that they do not recognize the degree of danger they may actually be facing, or do not have adequate resources to maintain their own safety when attempting to leave a dangerous relationship and risks for escalated violence increase.

Children of Intimate Partner Violence Victims: Secondary Victimization

Children who witness IPV are often overlooked as abuse victims unless they demonstrate evidence of physical or sexual abuse themselves. Witnessing violence puts children at risk for developing depression and PTSD, and they may become fearful for their own and their abused parent's lives (Child Welfare Information Gateway, 2013). In addition, children who grow up in violent families experience living with secrecy and relocations. These children who witness violence may begin to accept it as a normal part of relationships and a way to deal with problems. Fortunately, there is increasing awareness within legal systems of risks to child witnesses of family violence. As of 2012, half of the states in the United States have statutes that acknowledge these risks and individuals who engage in IPV in the presence of children may face stiffer penalties (Child Welfare Information Gateway,

2013). Despite these changes, a history of IPV within families is frequently not considered in family court decisions. When a parent is separated from an abusive partner, custody and visitation can provide a context for batterers to continue to control and victimize their former partners and their children.

Teen Partner Abuse

Teens and adults are often not aware of the frequency in which teen dating violence occurs. In a recent national survey, over 9% of teens reported being struck or physically hurt on purpose by a boyfriend or girlfriend in the 12 months prior to the survey (Black et al., 2011). Conflict or relationship problems with parents and peers may be predictors of teen partner abuse. Teens who experience violence in intimate relationships are more likely to develop problems such as depression, substance abuse, eating disorders, and thoughts of suicide (CDC, 2012). School performance may suffer. Teens, like adults, may be afraid or embarrassed to tell anyone what is happening to them and may even mistake early signs of abuse (e.g., jealousy, teasing) as affection or normal relationship behavior. It is critical to intervene when teen partner violence occurs, because it also increases the risk that a teenager will be a victim or perpetrator of physical, sexual, or psychological abuse as an adult.

Stalking

Stalking is a pattern of repeated unwanted contact, attention, and harassment that often increases in frequency. Stalking is a crime of intimidation. Stalkers harass and terrorize their victims through behavior that causes fear or substantial emotional distress. Stalking may include such behaviors as following someone, showing up at the person's home or workplace, vandalizing property, or sending unwanted gifts. **Cyberstalking** is the use of the Internet, e-mail or other telecommunications technology to harass or stalk another person.

In a recent survey, 1 in 6 females and 1 in 19 males reported having been stalked so that they feared for their safety (Black et al., 2011). People at greatest risk were 18 to 24 years old. Although media attention has focused on stalking of celebrities by fans or admirers, offenders are most often ex-intimates or acquaintances of the victim. Although celebrity stalkers tend to have delusions about their victims or fantasized relationships with their victims, stalking is more likely to occur in response to attempts by the victim to end a relationship. The most common reasons victims perceive for the stalking are retaliation, anger, spite, and a desire to control the victim (Baum, Catalano, Rand, & Rose, 2009).

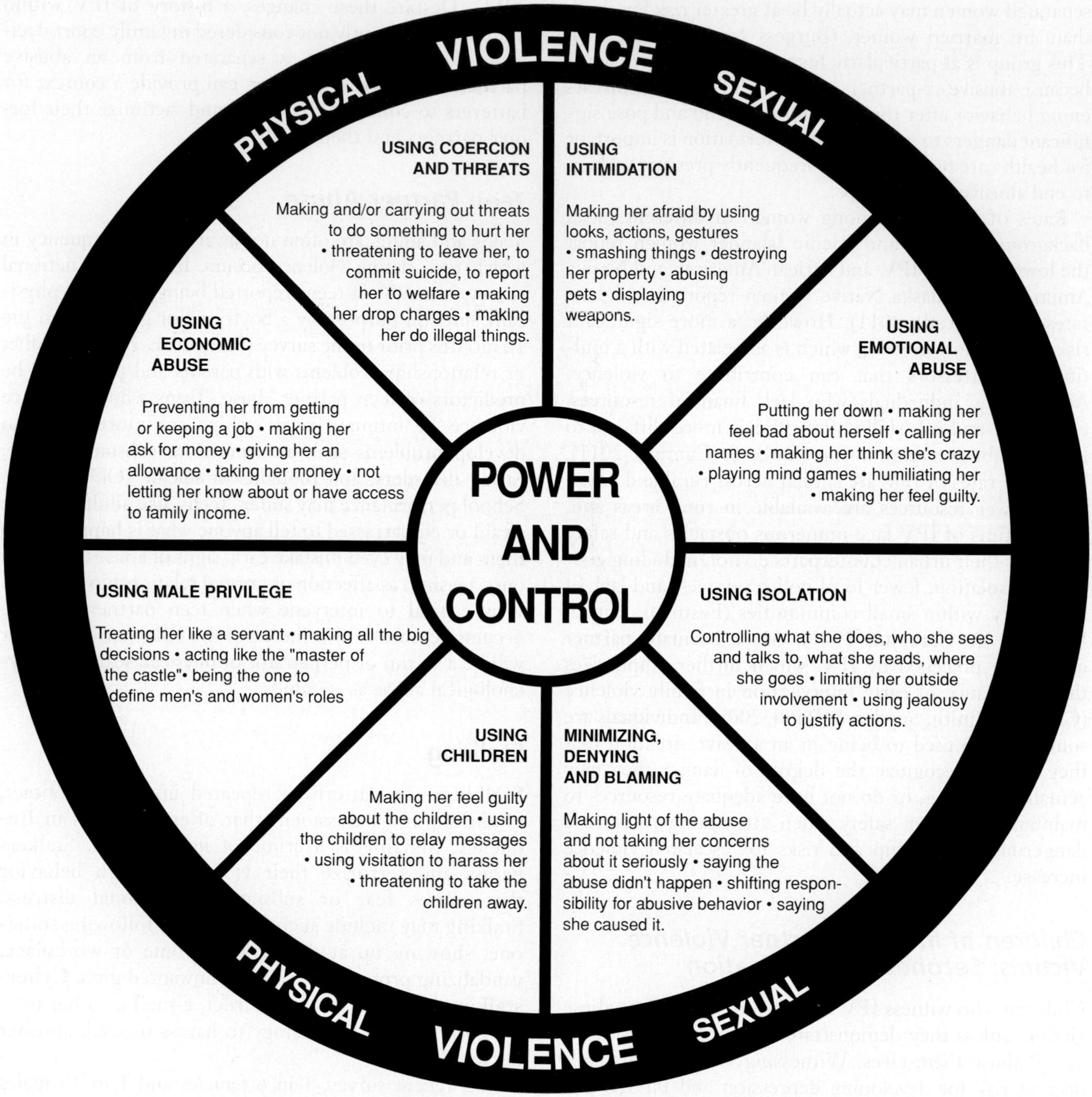

FIGURE 40.1 Power and control wheel. (Courtesy of Domestic Abuse Intervention Programs, 202 East Superior Street, Duluth, MN.)

Rape and Sexual Assault

> **KEYCONCEPT** **Sexual assault** includes any form of non-consenting sexual activity, ranging from fondling to penetration.

Rape and sexual assault are common in the United States; however, prevalence rates are difficult to determine because of underreporting. The definition of *rape*, the most severe form of sexual assault, was recently revised to cover a broader range of situations. **Rape** is defined as "the penetration, no matter how slight, of the vagina or anus with any body part or object, or oral penetration by a sex organ of another person, without the consent of the victim" (US Department of Justice, 2013). This definition includes victims and perpetrators of either gender, penetration beyond actual intercourse, and circumstances in which the victim is unable to give consent because of age, mental status, or impairment. Physical resistance is not required to constitute rape, so instances of coercion or threats of harm would be applicable. The broadened definition changes the way rape is reported, and more accurately reflects the scope of the experience. However, the challenge remains to change societal attitudes about rape and rape victims, and improve law enforcement and criminal justice responses to reports of rape and other sexual assaults.

Anyone of any age can be a victim of sexual assault; however, in 93% of reported rapes, the victim is a woman. In a recent national study 18% of women reported that they had been raped (Black et al., 2011). More than half of the perpetrators were intimate partners, and another 40% were acquaintances. Adolescents and young adults were most vulnerable to rape and sexual assault. Native American or Alaska native and multiracial women experienced higher rates of rape and other forms of sexual assault than women of other races.

Less than half of rapes and sexual assaults against women are reported. Victims do not report sexual assault for the same reason that IPV is underreported—embarrassment, shame, concern about not being believed, and fear of being blamed for the assault. Knowing the attacker may be a factor that inhibits reporting. Approximately two-thirds of women are raped by people they know—spouses, boyfriends, friends, or acquaintances. Among young women, about 50% of rapes are date rapes. In some cases, perpetrators use drugs or alcohol to subdue the victim, compromising his or her ability to consent to sexual activity. When substances are ingested voluntarily, resulting in impairment, victims and others may be more likely to blame themselves for the assault. Additionally, rape and sexual assault can occur in the context of IPV. Marital rape, which was first prosecuted as a crime in the mid 1970s, is probably one of the most underreported types of rape and is frequently accompanied by severe violence (Catalano, Smith, Snyder, & Rand, 2009; Schafran, Lopez-Boy, & Davis, 2008).

Men are even less likely than women to report rape or sexual assault, partly because of the stigma of what may be perceived as a homosexual attack. However, just as with women, male rape is an act of domination and violence. Although some perpetrators are gay men who commit assaults on partners, as in date rape, other perpetrators are heterosexual men who use rape as a means to humiliate or degrade other men. About 3% of American men have been victims of rape or attempted rape (Catalano et al., 2009).

Rape is a crime of violence. Rapists use sexuality as a weapon to dominate, intimidate, and humiliate another person. Rapists can be classified into three categories: the power rapist, the anger rapist, and the sadistic rapist (Pardue & Arrigo, 2008). Power rapists account for 55% of sexual assaults. They often attack people their own age and use intimidation and minimal physical force to control their victims. Their assaults are generally premeditated. Anger rapists account for 40% of sexual assaults. These rapists tend to target either very young or old victims. They may use extreme force and restraint that results in

physical injury to the victim. Sadistic rapists account for 5% of sexual assaults; however, they are the most dangerous. Their crimes are premeditated, and they often torture and kill their victims. Sadistic rapists derive erotic gratification from their victims' suffering.

Men compose the majority of perpetrators of rape and sexual assault, although women can also be perpetrators. Female offenders are more likely to engage in sexual assault of children, or statutory offenses, as in highly publicized cases involving teacher–student sexual relationships. Alarmingly, recent years have brought a trend in cases of juvenile girls charged with sex offenses (USDOJ, 2007).

Child Abuse

Child abuse can take several forms, and the definition of each type varies by state. All forms of child abuse rob children of rights they should have. Those rights include the rights to be and behave like a child; to be safe and protected from harm; and to be fed, clothed, and nurtured so that the child can grow, develop, and fulfill his or her unique potential.

The actual prevalence of child abuse is unknown. The most recent information based on Child Protective Services data indicates that children are victimized at a rate of 9.3 per 1000 children, equaling nearly 693,174 confirmed cases (U.S. Department of Health and Human Services [USDHHS], 2010). Of the total number of reported child abuse cases, estimates are that 78.3% represent neglect, 17.8% physical abuse, 9.5% sexual abuse, 7.6% psychological maltreatment, and 2.4% medical neglect. An additional 9% suffered "other" injury such as abandonment, threats of harm, or congenital drug addiction. In 2007, an estimated 1760 children died as a result of neglect, physical abuse, or both (USDHHS, 2010). The most vulnerable children were those younger than the age of 4 years and children with mental, physical, or emotional disabilities.

Risk for abuse tends to decrease with age. Perpetrators of fatal child abuse are most likely to be caregivers who are young, poorly educated, and living at or below the poverty level. Individuals with mental health or substance abuse problems or who have difficulty coping are at highest risk to abuse their children. Whereas mothers are responsible for the majority of fatalities related to child neglect, fathers and other male caregivers cause most deaths resulting from physical abuse. Family situations that are chaotic or stressful increase the likelihood that abuse or neglect will occur. Some individuals who abuse or neglect their children are thought to be either victims or perpetrators of IPV, but the actual incidence is unknown (Sedlak et al., 2010).

Children who are abused or neglected are at risk for numerous physical, emotional, and behavioral problems. Their cognitive development may be impaired, and they may exhibit academic difficulties. They may have problems getting along with or trusting others. They are at risk for depression, anxiety, low self-esteem, and substance abuse (Joshi, Daniolos, & Salpekar, 2010).

Child Neglect

Child neglect is failure to provide for a child's physical, emotional, health care, or educational needs; failure to adequately supervise a child; or intentionally exposing a child to a dangerous environment. Child neglect is the most common form of child abuse reported (USDHHS, 2010). There are several types of neglect. *Physical neglect* includes failure to provide food, clothing, and shelter. *Medical neglect* is failure to provide for the child's medical needs, including failure to seek appropriate care or to comply with prescribed treatments. *Educational neglect* is not enrolling a child in school or permitting truancy. Other types of neglect are leaving young children alone without adequate supervision; exposing them to unsanitary household conditions or hazards such as poisons, weapons, or drugs; and not using car safety restraints. Neglect is not as easy to identify as more obvious types of abuse. Cues for nurses to further investigate are observing a child who chronically wears soiled, ill-fitting clothing; always seems to be hungry; has poor hygiene; exhibits signs of inadequate medical or dental care; or reports frequently being left alone or caring for younger children.

Child Physical Abuse

Physical abuse may include severe spanking, hitting, kicking, shoving, or any other type of physical action directed toward the child that results in non-accidental injury. Injuries to children caused by physical abuse range from mild to severe and life threatening. Types of injuries include skin and soft tissue injuries; internal injuries; dislocations and fractures; tooth loss; burns; abrasions or bruises made by fists or belts; hair loss from pulling the hair; wounds from guns, knives, razors, or other sharp objects; retinal hemorrhage; and conjunctival hemorrhage. Often, clothing hides these injuries, and practitioners must look for other signs of abuse, such as fear, aggressive or withdrawn behavior, poor social relations, learning problems, delinquent behavior, and wearing clothing that is meant to cover injuries but is inappropriate for the weather. In addition, when treating a child with such injuries, professionals should suspect abuse when explanations are implausible and inconsistent with injuries, involved parties give different versions of the incident, or treatment seeking is delayed.

Child Psychological Abuse

The child who is emotionally or psychologically abused does not have visible injuries to alert others. Nevertheless, psychological abuse severely affects a child's self-esteem and often leaves permanent emotional scars. For many survivors of childhood abuse, emotional abuse is worse than physical abuse. Psychological abuse frequently co-occurs with other types of abuse and can take various forms.

The most obvious form is verbal abuse, which can include behaviors such as frequent ridiculing, name calling, bullying, threatening, or shaming the child. Other, more subtle forms include rejecting or ignoring the child by refusing to acknowledge the child's worth or respond to his or her needs and isolating the child by preventing the child from forming friendships and hindering the development of social skills. At times, the abuse takes the form of creating a climate of fear by intentionally frightening or bullying the child or by setting up rigid expectations that are almost impossible for the child to meet. Teaching or forcing the child to engage in self-destructive and antisocial behaviors (e.g., stealing, prostitution, using substances) that interfere with healthy social development is also a form of psychological abuse.

Child Sexual Abuse

Behaviors that constitute child sexual abuse range from mild, covert behaviors to overt sexual acts. Examples of sexual abuse include exhibitionism, voyeurism, and touching the child's sexual organs, as well as oral, anal, and vaginal penetration. Child sexual abuse can take within the family by a parent, stepparent, sibling, or other relatives and can also occur outside the family by a friend or neighbor. This type of abuse is reported up to 80,000 times per year, but the incidence is much greater (American Academy of Child & Adolescent Psychiatry [AACAP], 2008). The children are afraid to tell what is happening. Children age 5 years and older who know the abuser are conflicted between affection and loyalty for the person and the sense that sexual activities are wrong. Sexual abuse by someone that the child knows and trusts causes more severe trauma. The child abused by a family member experiences a devastating breach of trust, loss of a safe home, and threats to fundamental survival requirements (Boyd & Mackey, 2000).

No child is psychologically prepared to cope with repeated sexual stimulations. A victim of prolonged sexual abuse will develop low self-esteem, a feeling of worthlessness, and a distorted view of sex. The child may become withdrawn, distrustful, or suicidal. Other characteristics of children who have been sexually abused include an unusual interest or avoidance of sexually related content, seductiveness, refusal to go to school, delinquency, secretiveness, and unusual aggressiveness (AACAP, 2008).

Elder Abuse

Elder abuse is abuse or neglect of adults older than age 60 years. There are six types of elder abuse, including physical (injury by hitting, kicking, pushing, slapping, burning, and so on), sexual (unconsented sexual act), emotional (harm of self-worth or emotional well-being), neglect (failure to meet the older adult's basic needs of shelter, food, and so on), abandonment (leaving an older adults alone and no longer providing care), and financial (illegally misusing money, property, or assets) (CDC, 2013c).

Elder abuse is increasingly recognized as a serious problem in the United States and other countries. As the population continues to age, it is likely that the problem will worsen. The violence usually occurs at the hands of a caregiver or a person the older adult trusts, but is also a significant problem in nursing homes and assisted living facilities (National Council on Elder Abuse [NCEA], n.d.).

There is relatively little information about the prevalence of elder abuse, but in a 2008 study, 1 in 10 elderly people reported having experienced some type of abuse or neglect in the past year (Acierno et al., 2010). Individuals who are isolated, have poor support systems, or have mental or physical impairments that foster dependency on others are more vulnerable to harm. Older people may be reluctant to report maltreatment by those they love or upon whom they are dependent, or cognitive deficits may prevent them from being able to articulate their situation. In addition to the obvious physical problems (e.g., injuries, pressure sores, malnutrition) that can result from abuse or neglect, older adults can experience worsening of existing medical conditions and emotional problems such as depression, anxiety, and fearfulness (CDC, 2013c). Costs of medical care related to abuse and neglect are estimated to be well over $5 billion annually, and losses to elderly individuals associated with financial exploitation are similarly alarming (NCEA, n.d.). High-risk factors for those who are more likely to abuse older adults include using drugs or alcohol, high levels of stress, lack of social support, high emotional or financial dependence on the older adult, lack of training in taking care of older adults, and depression (CDC, 2013c). Caring for a dependent older adult can be overwhelming. It is important for the nurse to listen to and assess both older adults and their caregivers to help prevent abuse and neglect in this population.

THEORIES OF VIOLENCE

Many theories attempt to explain IPV and other types of violence in the family. In all likelihood, family violence is truly a biopsychosocial phenomenon that no one theory can fully explain (Figure 40.2).

Neurologic Problems

Neurologic abnormalities are found in some persons who exhibit aggressive behavior (see Chapter 19). It is unclear how these abnormalities affect specific cognitive and affective processes, especially how they might be related to violence directed at intimate partners, children, and older adults. Head injury in particular has been associated with IPV. Head injury is associated with changes in per-

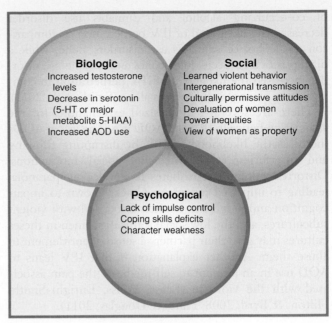

FIGURE 40.2 Biopsychosocial etiologies for violent behavior.

sonality, irritability, rage, and reduced impulse control, all of which may increase the risk of aggressive behavior (Ali & Naylor, 2013).

Alcohol and Other Drug Use

There is a strong association of AOD use and IPV. The relationship between AOD use and IPV may be reciprocal and cyclical in nature. That is, AOD abuse increases the probability of perpetration and being the victim of violence which then increases the use of AOD to self-medicate emotional and physical sequelae of violence (Ali & Naylor, 2013). AOD abuse plays a role in both perpetration of violence and in being a victim of violence. Women may be particularly vulnerable to victimization when under the influence of AOD (Ali & Naylor, 2013).

In a large, representative sample of the United States noninstitutionalized adult population, researchers found that among perpetrators of violence, alcohol use disorders were the most prevalent (21.7%) followed by cannabis use disorders (21.7%), cocaine use disorders (2.1%), and opioid use disorders (1.5%) (Smith, Homish, Leonard, & Cornelius, 2012). Among victims of IPV, alcohol use disorders were also the most prevalent (24.6%), followed by cannabis use disorders (7.4%), cocaine use disorders (2%), and opioid use disorders (2.4%) (Smith et al., 2012). When specifically examining the effects of AOD on perpetration of violence, cocaine and alcohol use disorders were most strongly associated with IPV perpetration. Cannabis and opioid use disorders were strongly associated with being a victim of IPV. Marijuana was associated with increased perpetration of violence by women and with victimization for both men and women (Smith et al., 2012). A diagnosis of co-occurring alcohol and cannabis use disorder decreased the likelihood of IPV perpetration in comparison to alcohol or cannabis use disorders alone, while a diagnosis of a co-occurring alcohol and cocaine use disorder increased the likelihood of IPV perpetration in comparison to alcohol use disorders alone (Smith et al., 2012).

There are several hypothesized explanations for the association between IPV and AOD use. The use of AODs increases the likelihood of IPV by disrupting thinking and interfering with processing social interactions. Distorted thinking contributes to developing paranoia, leading to impaired judgment. Crack, known to impair cognition and judgment, is often associated with violent subcultures, and the low social status of women in theses cultures may give their partners a sense of entitlement to abuse them. Another explanation is that IPV leads to AOD use in an attempt to self-medicate the pain associated with the violence (Ernst, Weiss, Enright-Smith, Hilton, & Byrd, 2008; Hines & Douglas, 2011).

Psychopathology

Men who batter women are psychologically a heterogeneous group (Babcock, Green, & Webb, 2008; Mauricio & Lopez, 2009). Three types of perpetrators have been identified according to their severity of violence, use of violence, and degree of psychopathology. The first group of family-only perpetrators engage in lower severity violent behaviors and exhibit the lowest levels of psychopathology. Next, those with borderline personality disorder characteristics or dysphoria engage in moderate to severe violence and demonstrate the highest levels of emotional volatility, dependency, and psychological distress. These perpetrators have a heightened sensitivity to emotional displays that predisposes them to interpret social situations as threatening and to respond with emotional dysregulation, verbal attacks, and physical violence. One study of husbands with these characteristics found that these men had diminished sensitivity to their wives' expressions of happiness (Marshall & Holtzworth-Munroe, 2010). They frequently interpreted expressions of happiness as disgust or rejection and then became violent toward their wives.

Finally, the perpetrators who are generally violent and engage in moderate to severe violence, both inside and outside of the home, tend to meet criteria for antisocial personality disorder and are likely to have an extensive history of criminal behavior (Babcock et al., 2008). These perpetrators become aggressive when they misinterpret neutral and positive emotional cues as negative and when they are unable to identify expressions of fear (Marshall & Holtzworth-Munroe, 2010). This typology has been validated in later research conducted with psychiatric patients and found to be pertinent to both male and female perpetrators (Walsh, O'Connor, Shea, Swogger, Schonbrun, & Stuart, 2010).

Attachment styles are also used to explain violent behavior. According to attachment theory, the *attachment avoidance* style is characterized by pervasive discomfort with intimate closeness and a strong orientation toward being excessively self-reliant or socially withdrawn. Similar to those with antisocial personality disorder, they may be narcissistic, self-centered, and lack empathy for others, making them more prone to violence in intimate relationships.

An *attachment anxiety* style is characterized by low self-esteem, pervasive fears of partner rejection and abandonment, and either highly dependent or conflicted and disorganized relationship behaviors. Adults with anxious attachment who experience their partners as unavailable and have intense abandonment anxiety may respond with hostile, overt expressions of anger similar to those with borderline or dysphoric characteristics described above (Mauricio & Lopez, 2009).

Social Learning Theory (Intergenerational Transmission of Violence)

Violent families create an atmosphere of tension, fear, intimidation, and confusion about intimate relationships. Children in violent homes often learn that violent behavior is an approved and legitimate way to solve problems and to cope with difficulty. Social learning or **intergenerational transmission of violence** theory posits that children who witness or experience violence in their homes often perpetuate violent behavior Harsh physical discipline has also been implicated in future IPV. The same study found that being the recipient of physical forms of childhood punishment (being spanked, hit, or slapped) increased the odds of perpetrating IPV by 2.06 times (Franklin & Kercher, 2012). Research also supports the relationship between witnessing and/or experiencing childhood violence and being the victim of IPV. Franklin and Kercher (2012) found that those who witnessed their parents' use of violence against each other were 1.96 times more likely to report being the victim of IPV in adulthood, and those who received physical punishment as children were 2.20 times more likely to report being victims of adult IPV (Franklin & Kercher, 2012). Age, employment, and marital status significantly impacted victimization risk with those who are older, employed, and married having decreased odds of experiencing adult IPV (Franklin & Kercher, 2012).

Implicit Theories Held by Perpetrators

Implicit theories held by perpetrators of IPV are thoughts, core beliefs, or world views that support their offending behavior (Pornari, Dixon, & Humphreys, 2013; Weldon & Gilchrist, 2012). Researchers have identified the following seven implicit theories held by male and female perpetrators of IPV: (1) opposite sex is dangerous refers to emotions and beliefs that the opposite gender is deceitful, manipulative, controlling, and demanding; (2) general entitlement beliefs refer to beliefs that perpetrators consider themselves to be superior to others and that they are entitled to special privileges; (3) relationship entitlement beliefs are beliefs that one is superior to their partner and view their own needs as more important. Individuals with these beliefs expect their partners to behave according to their demands; (4) normalization of relationship violence is a belief that violence between partners is a normal and effective way of solving problems and dealing with undesired behavior of a partner. Additionally, individuals with this belief believe that the battered partner exaggerates the extent of the violence; (5) normalization of violence refers to beliefs that violence is acceptable, justifiable, and effective in solving conflicts and achieving personal goals, and controlling others outside of the intimate relationship; (6) it's not my fault refers to beliefs that they deny responsibility for violence and attribute it to external factors such as alcohol and other drugs or attribute blame to the abused partner; (7) I am the man refers to stereotypical beliefs that men are superior to women in all aspects, that men are strong, dominant, authoritative, assertive, controlling, and aggressive and women are passive, dependent, and emotional (Pornari et al., 2013). Modification of these beliefs may be an important focus for treatment of IPV perpetrators.

Economic Disadvantage, Community Disorganization, and Attitudes Supportive of Violence

Most theories of violence focus on person-centered factors. However, factors at the community level also contribute to violence within and outside of the family. Organized neighborhoods share common values that foster social cohesion. Neighborhoods that are more socially cohesive are more intolerant of deviant behavior. The presence of concentrated economic disadvantage (i.e. neighborhoods with the lowest incomes, high unemployment, and institutional disinvestment), racial or ethnic heterogeneity, and community instability is associated with community disorganization and weak social control, which leads to increased levels of crime and IPV. Within these disadvantaged communities, institutions that normally foster social control, such as churches, schools, and other community organizations, lose their ability to exercise social control over the community. Community disorganization, crime, and weak social control also foster individual acceptance of violence, which in turn is associated with increased rates of IPV, child abuse, and elder abuse (Button, 2008; Li, Kirby, Sigler, Hwang, & LaGory, 2010).

Imbalances in Relationship Power

Another body of literature suggests that IPV is a manifestation of gender-based imbalances in relationship power.

Usually, this perspective explains IPV as violence against women by their male romantic partner related to issues of gender, inequality, power and privilege, patriarchy, and the subordination of women (Hunnicutt, 2009; McPhail, Busch, Kulkarni, & Rice, 2010). Patriarchal systems exist at the macro level (government, bureaucracies, religion) and at the micro level (families), and both have gender inequities (Hunnicutt, 2009). Within a patriarchal society, men often hold traditional gender role beliefs. For example, men are head of households and provide for their families, and women are homemakers and mothers. If these beliefs are threatened, such as when a woman enters the work force and earns more than her partner, men may feel threatened and respond with violence (Kwesiga, Bell, Pattie, & Moe, 2007).

However, data suggest that women engage in IPV as often (or more often) than men but that women are more likely than men to sustain injuries as a result of aggression (Duke & Cunradi, 2011). Women's acts of aggression put them at higher risk for retaliation. One qualitative study of male and female migrant farm workers found that changing gender roles within household with regard to wage earning, household maintenance, and child rearing were frequent sources of conflict, which would sometimes result in IPV (Grzywacz, Rao, Gentry, Marin, & Arcury, 2009). Furthermore, violence between parents (no matter the gender of the perpetrator) is likely to be psychologically harmful to their children. It is not understood why teen girls experience or stay in relationships where they experience partner abuse, but some researchers theorize that it may occur from inexperience in negotiating intimate relationships. Others report inequities or differences in race, ethnicity, geographic area, sexual orientation, or disability status (CDC, 2012).

Cycle of Violence

Many cases of IPV reflect a recognized **cycle of violence**. The cycle consists of three recurring phases that often increase in frequency and severity. The cycle is fully described in Figure 40.3.

Factors Influencing Leaving Versus Staying in a Violent Relationship

Victims who leave violent relationships do so for many reasons. They may be young and blame their partners rather than themselves for the violence. The victims may have previously attempted to leave their relationships and are finally successful in seeking help from shelters, the health care system, or the legal system; they may have protection orders against the perpetrators. Economic independence, or the ability to support oneself and one's children, is one of the most influential factors enabling women to leave violent relationships. Seeking,

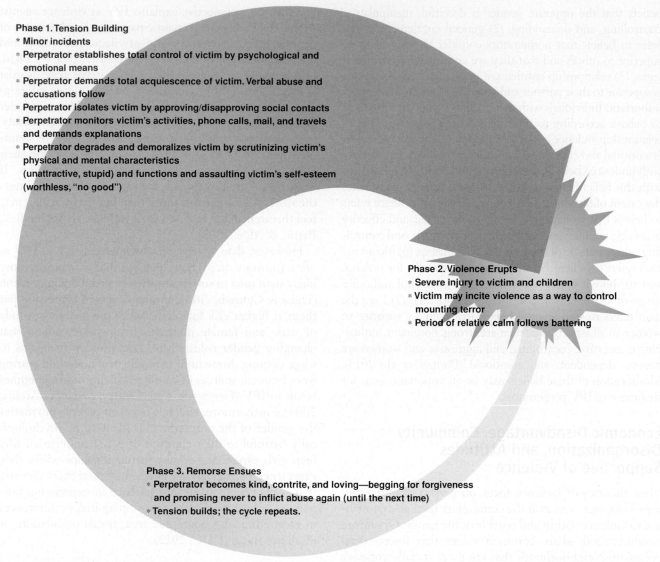

Phase 1. Tension Building
* Minor incidents
* Perpetrator establishes total control of victim by psychological and emotional means
* Perpetrator demands total acquiescence of victim. Verbal abuse and accusations follow
* Perpetrator isolates victim by approving/disapproving social contacts
* Perpetrator monitors victim's activities, phone calls, mail, and travels and demands explanations
* Perpetrator degrades and demoralizes victim by scrutinizing victim's physical and mental characteristics (unattractive, stupid) and functions and assaulting victim's self-esteem (worthless, "no good")

Phase 2. Violence Erupts
* Severe injury to victim and children
* Victim may incite violence as a way to control mounting terror
* Period of relative calm follows battering

Phase 3. Remorse Ensues
* Perpetrator becomes kind, contrite, and loving—begging for forgiveness and promising never to inflict abuse again (until the next time)
* Tension builds; the cycle repeats.

FIGURE 40.3 The cycle of violence.

but not receiving, external support is an important factor in women's decisions to remain in the relationship. Women who leave violent relationships are less likely to be problem drinkers; are less likely to experience a longer duration of psychological abuse; and are more likely to have experienced severe physical or sexual abuse (Koepsell, Kernic, & Holt, 2006; Shurman, 2006). More research is needed regarding men's reasons for leaving abusive relationships.

Victims are also more likely to leave violent relationships if the perpetrator is behaving in an overly negative or contemptuous manner, has pathological personality traits, keeps weapons in the home, stalks the victim, refuses to participate in batterer intervention programs, refuses to change, and abuses alcohol.

Victims are more likely to stay in the relationship if they love their partner, are satisfied with the relationship, are emotionally attached, and are committed to their partner (Rhatigan, Street, & Axsom, 2006). Another important factor in the deciding whether to leave or to

stay in a violent relationship is recognizing that leaving may not stop the violence. Often perpetrators escalate their violence, stalk their partners, and may even kill their partners if they threaten to leave or actually do leave the relationship.

Victims or survivors may leave and return several times as they are learning new coping skills. Initially, they seem to endure and manage the violence while disconnecting from others. As they acknowledge the abuse, they may reframe it ("If only I had not been late . . .") and eventually begin to counteract it and focus on their own needs.

SURVIVORS OF VIOLENCE AND ABUSE

People who suffer violence and abuse experience a variety of responses and consequences. It is important for the psychiatric nurse to understand the range of responses and appropriate nursing management for these individuals.

Survivor Responses to Trauma from Violence

The experience of violence and abuse is overwhelming for most survivors and often has devastating long-term biopsychosocial consequences.

Biologic Responses

Victims of violence experience mild to severe physical consequences. Mild injuries may include bruises and abrasions of the head, neck, face, trunk, and extremities (Wu, Huff & Bhandari, 2010). Severe injuries include multiple traumas, major fractures, major lacerations, and internal injuries (including chest and abdominal injuries and subdural hematomas) (Wu et al., 2010). Loss of vision and hearing can result from blows to the head. Physical or sexual violence may result in head injuries that can produce changes in cognition, affect, motivation, and behavior. Victims of sexual abuse may have vaginal and perineal trauma. Anorectal injuries may also be present, including disruption of anal sphincters, retained foreign bodies, and mucosal lacerations. The following section covers the most common biologic responses to violence and abuse:

Physical Problems Associated with Intimate Partner Violence

Numerous adverse health outcomes are associated with having experienced violence. Some conditions are a direct result of the abuse, such as bruises, abrasions, broken bones, and knife wounds. Other problems, such as headaches, chronic pain, neck and back problems, and traumatic brain injury, can also be linked to past injuries. Studies have demonstrated a relationship between abuse and negative health consequences. Female survivors of IPV for example are more likely than others to perceive their overall health as poor (Dutton, Green, Kaltman, Roesch, Zeffiro, & Krause, 2006). The trauma associated with chronic abuse, both physical and psychological, can lead to impairment of the immune system and other physical symptoms. Common somatic complaints of women who have experienced IPV include insomnia, musculoskeletal pain, fibromyalgia, respiratory problems, hypertension, chest pain, pelvic pain, irritable bowel syndrome, and other gastrointestinal symptoms (Breiding, Black, & Ryan, 2008; Crofford, 2007; Leserman & Drossman, 2007). Gynecologic symptoms and sexually transmitted infections (STDs) are associated with a history of sexual abuse. Because health problems are not always obviously linked to current or past abuse, it is important for clients to be routinely screened for exposure to violence. Primary care and women's health settings offer opportunities for ongoing therapeutic relationships with providers that can increase clients' comfort with disclosure of abuse.

Mental Health Consequences of Violence

The most prevalent mental health sequelae for survivors are mood disorders (depression), anxiety disorders (PTSD), and alcohol and other drug disorders (Afifi, MacMillan, Cox, Asmundson, Stein, & Sareen, 2010). Physical, emotional, and sexual IPV are associated with depressive symptoms, suicidality, and PTSD symptoms. Being a victim of emotional IPV and alcohol abuse increases the risk for depressive symptoms, and being a victim of sexual abuse increases the risk of both depression and PTSD symptoms (Duke & Cunradi, 2011).

Depression, PTSD, and AOD disorders cause significant distress and have profound effects on functioning and quality of life with role functioning impairment in the areas of relationships, emotional behavior, work, and recreation (Pirkola et al., 2009; Saarni et al., 2007). Individuals may self-medicate anxiety and mood disorders with AOD use (Afifi et al., 2010; Bolton, Robinson, & Sareen, 2009). Recent studies found that among those with anxiety disorders, 22% self-medicated with alcohol or drugs, and among those with mood disorders, 24% self-medicated with alcohol or drugs (Bolton et al., 2009). These studies also found that those who self-medicate have significantly more distress and more suicide attempts than those who do not self-medicate.

Co-occurring disorders are often more severe, more chronic, more difficult to treat, and require more service utilization (Lipsky, Krupski, Roy-Byrne, Lucenko, Mancuso, & Huber, 2010). Individuals with more than one disorder may have difficulty managing treatment. Higher levels of burden associated with multiple disorders are associated with lower levels of retention in treatment programs and with gaining fewer benefits from treatment (Lipsky et al., 2010). Importantly, having any psychiatric disorder may make it much more difficult to leave an abusive relationship.

Psychological Responses

Fear

Living with an abusive partner, parent, or caregiver means living with constant fear and uncertainly. Because victims never know what might precipitate an incident of violence, they are constantly hypervigilant and fearful. The back-and-forth nature of the relationship, that is, alternating between loving and violent behavior, is confusing, and the survivor may try to do everything possible to please the abuser to try to prevent another episode of violence. Many victims, particularly women, fear for their lives and believe they will be killed in the next violent episode (Scheffer & Renck, 2008).

Low Self-Esteem

Being the victim of abuse is devastating to a healthy **self-esteem,** or feelings of self-acceptance, self-worth, self-love, and self-nurturing. Emotional abuse may be particularly devastating. Victims are criticized, rejected, devaluated, and ignored. Feeling stupid was a recurring theme in a qualitative study of women who had left abusive relationships. Women consistently labeled themselves stupid for not recognizing abusive behaviors, allowing their partners to abuse them, and staying in an abusive relationship (Enander, 2010). Low self-esteem has been linked to physical and mental health problems, problems with relationships, and even with decreased economic success (Finzi-Dottan & Karu, 2006; Trzesniewski, Donnellan, Moffitt, Robins, Poulton, & Caspi, 2006).

Low self-esteem may also be one factor contributing to a victim's reluctance to disclose abuse or to leave an abusive relationship. Because of low self-esteem, battered victims, even many who are successful outside the home, underestimate their ability to do anything about the abuse (Boyd & Mackey, 2000).

Guilt and Shame

A history of abuse is often associated with guilt and shame. Survivors are ashamed of being manipulated and violated and for having put themselves in such a situation. Abusive partners tell the survivors that the abuse is their fault, and many victims believe them. Feelings of humiliation and shame prevent survivors from seeking medical care and other forms of support and reporting abuse to authorities. The experience of being battered is so degrading and humiliating that survivors are often afraid to disclose it to anyone. Many fear that they will not be taken seriously or will be blamed for inciting the abuse or for staying with their abusers. Keeping their circumstances secret and maintaining a front of normality places enormous tension and pressure on survivors (Boyd & Mackey, 2000; Scheffer & Renck, 2008).

Social and Interpersonal Responses

Problems with Intimacy

Abused children, especially those who have experienced child sexual abuse, experience intrusion, abandonment, devaluation, or pain in the relationship with the abuser instead of the closeness and nurturing that are normal for intimate relationships (AACAP, 2008). Consequently, intimacy is associated with shame and fear rather than warmth and caring and with concerns about dominance and submission rather than mutuality. Shame in turn is associated with being submissive, feeling devalued, and the desire to retaliate against a person who is seen as the source of humiliation. In adulthood, unresolved feelings

of shame as well as symptoms of PTSD or depression may disrupt the development of intimacy and lead to relationships characterized with dissatisfaction and poor relationship quality (Fering, Simon, & Cleland, 2009).

On the other hand, some survivors of child abuse and child sexual abuse may engage in risky sexual behavior such as early sexual activity (before age 15 years), promiscuity, and prostitution. These behaviors place survivors at risk for developing STDs and HIV. Survivors who engage in this type of behavior may have learned that sexual activity is a means for securing affection, intimacy, or material rewards such as money or drugs (Wilson & Widom, 2008).

Revictimization

Many survivors who experienced childhood trauma are revictimized later in life. Rates of **revictimization,** or reoccurrence of violence toward the survivor, range from 15% to 79%. Numerous factors are related to revictimization, including PTSD symptoms, dissociation, use of AODs, boundary issues, and role reversal with both mothers and fathers (Cole, Logan, & Shannon, 2008; Enander, 2010).

People with abuse histories frequently have difficulty with boundaries. During childhood abuse, they experienced frequent boundary violations and associate those violations with intimate relationships. Role reversal in childhood in which a child takes care of one or both parents may lead to difficulty with boundaries and may be associated with intrusiveness, boundary dissolution with a partner, and risk of IPV in adulthood (Enander, 2010).

Abuse of AODs places survivors of abuse at risk for revictimization as they socialize with others who also use and therefore have an increased likelihood of entering into a relationship with someone who also uses (Cole et al., 2008). In addition, victims who use are more vulnerable and less able to defend themselves.

NURSING MANAGEMENT: Human Response to Violence

Nurses encounter survivors of violence and abuse in many health care settings. The percentage of emergency department (ED) visits that are attributed to domestic violence ranges up to 12% with an estimated prevalence rate from 36% to 54% (Houry, Kemball, Click, & Kaslow, 2007). Approximately 33% to 52% of female patients admitted to psychiatric facilities are victims of either child or adult abuse (Meade, Kershaw, Hansen, & Sikkema, 2009). Other settings in which battered women and men are encountered include teen clinics, primary care settings, obstetrics and gynecology settings, pediatric units, well-child clinics, geriatric units, and nursing homes.

Unfortunately, few nurses ask about abuse because doing so is often uncomfortable. It requires nurses to acknowledge evil in human nature and their own vulnerability to that evil. Protection and recovery from abuse requires survivors to remember and discuss terrible events. However, secrecy and silence protect perpetrators and seriously endanger survivors. Nurses communicate a powerfully disturbing message with their silence: that the most traumatic event of a patient's life is too upsetting for others to hear. If nurses do not empower survivors to tell their stories, the abuse experiences will continue to haunt patients, often manifesting as symptoms of mental disorders.

The pediatric ED provides a unique opportunity to identify and respond to child survivors as well as battered mothers. As many as 40% to 50% of mothers of child abuse victims are battered women, and child abuse occurs disproportionately in homes with IPV (McDonald, Touriles, Tart, & Minze, 2009). Identifying battered mothers may be the most important means of identifying child abuse. Conversely, when child abuse is suspected, the possibility cannot be ignored that a parent or caregiver is also a victim. Identifying children who are traumatized by witnessing the battering of their parents also is essential. However, despite the opportunity the pediatric ED affords, disturbingly few battered victims are screened or identified. Health care providers in pediatric EDs have reported several obstacles to identification, including lack of training, time constraints, powerlessness, lack of effective interventions, lack of comfort, lack of control over the victim's circumstances, and fear of offending the patient (Baig, Shadigian, & Heisler, 2006).

Similar to other forms of abuse, nurses may encounter elder abuse in virtually any setting. Examples include EDs, medical–surgical units, psychiatric units, and homes during home care visits. In addition, elder abuse may occur in nursing homes. Events such as unnecessary chemical (medications) or physical restraints used to control an older adult's behavior may be abusive and should be investigated (Yaffe, 2010).

Although some aspects of care are specific to adult, child, or older adult survivors of abuse, many elements are common in the nursing management of all survivors regardless of age or setting. The goals of all nursing interventions in cases of violence are to prevent injury, stop the violence, and ensure the survivor's safety (Burgess & Tavakoli, 2005; Lindhorst, Meyers, & Casey, 2008; Rabin, Jennings, Campbell, Bair-Merritt, 2009; Yaffe, 2010). Victimization removes all power and control from a survivor of IPV, child abuse, or elder abuse. Therefore, as appropriate for age and ability, all nursing interventions should empower survivors to act on their own behalf and must be done in a collaborative partnership. To that end, nurses must be willing to offer support and information and not impose their own values on survivors by encouraging them to leave abusive relationships (Campbell et al., 2009). Strong psychological and economic bonds tie many survivors to their perpetrators. Moreover, adult survivors

who are capable of making decisions are the experts on their situations. They are the best judges to determine the appropriate time to leave a relationship.

However, removing children and older adults from their families or caregivers often is necessary to ensure their immediate safety (Thackarey, Hibbard, & Dowd, 2010). If the home of an abused or neglected child or older adult cannot be made safe, the nurse must facilitate other professionals involved in placing the child or older adult in a foster or nursing home (Jacobi, Dettmeyer, Banaschak, Brosig, & Herrman, 2010). Still, intervening in cases of elder abuse is not a clear-cut issue (Laumann, Leitsch, & Waite, 2008). When an older adult's decision making is not impaired (*competence* is the legal term), he or she must be allowed an appropriate degree of autonomy in deciding how to manage the problem even if he or she chooses to remain in the abusive situation (Laumann et al., 2008). Forcing someone to do something against his or her wishes is itself a form of victimization and denies autonomous decision making.

Intervention strategies for older adults depend on whether the individual accepts or refuses assistance and whether he or she can make decisions. If the person refuses treatment, it is important to remain nonjudgmental and provide information about available services and emergency numbers. The nurse must contact the adult protective & Oxford, services department (APS) if mandated to do so by state law. If the older adult appears incapable of making decisions, contact APS and assist in making arrangements for guardianship, foster care, nursing home placement, or court proceedings as needed (Laumann et al., 2008).

Biologic Domain

Assessment

Research indicates that health care providers often fail to respond therapeutically to survivors of violence. In many instances, they neglect to identify violence as the cause of traumatic injuries or mental health problems (Lindhorst Meyers & Casey, 2008; Rhodes, Frankel, Levinthal, Prenoveau, Bailey, & Levinson, 2007). Even more damaging, many health care professionals treat abuse survivors derogatorily, blaming them for the abuse or for staying in abusive situations. For example, nursing staff may revictimize survivors with borderline personality disorder. Often these individuals have been severely traumatized, and their behavior is difficult and disruptive. In some cases, caregivers react negatively, labeling this behavior attention seeking and manipulative. When nurses react to the patient in a negative, punitive manner, they retraumatize the survivor. It is common to see this behavior punished by staff avoidance, time in seclusion rooms, and overmedication. Borderline personality disorder symptoms should be interpreted as ineffective coping strategies developed in response to severe trauma rather than as deliberate attempts to manipulate staff (Sansone, McLean, & Wiederman, 2008).

To improve providers' responses, the American Nurses Association (ANA) recommends instruction for all nurses and health care providers in the skills necessary to prevent violence and manage the treatment of survivors. Moreover, the ANA recommends that nurses assess all women for abuse in every setting. That recommendation should be expanded to include all people, both women and men, no matter what age or presenting problem. If suspected abuse is never assessed, it will never be uncovered.

Establishing a Nurse–Patient Relationship

Establishing a trusting nurse–patient relationship is one of the most important steps in assessing any type of violence. Survivors are unlikely to disclose sensitive information unless they perceive the nurse to be trustworthy and nonjudgmental. Important considerations in establishing open communication are ensuring confidentiality and providing a quiet, private place in which to conduct assessment. The law mandates that nurses report child and elder abuse to the authorities, and nurses must make that responsibility clear before beginning the assessment. Child abuse is usually reported to the department of social services (DSS), and elder abuse is reported to APS. In states that mandate reporting intimate partner abuse, the nurse must also inform women of that responsibility before assessment. Mandatory reporting is controversial because it may act as a barrier to disclosure, especially in cases in which the woman fears that the abuser will retaliate (Wooldredge & Thistlethwaite, 2006).

Conducting a Lethality Assessment First

The most important assessment conducted is a lethality assessment. Therefore, it should also be the first assessment in order to ascertain whether the survivor is in danger for his or her life, either from homicide or suicide and, if children are in the home, whether they are in danger (Salari, 2007). If so, take immediate steps to ensure the survivor's safety. Those steps may include reporting to police, DSS, or APS. In the case of suspected child abuse assessed in a health care agency, an interdisciplinary team consisting of physicians, psychologists, nurses, and social workers usually makes this decision. In other settings, the nurse may be the person to make the decision. Nurses do not have to obtain proof of abuse; they only need a reasonable suspicion. The Danger Assessment Screen developed by Jacquelyn Campbell and colleagues is a useful tool for assessing the risk that either an adult survivor or perpetrator will commit homicide (Campbell & Humphries, 1993) (Box 40.1).

BOX 40.1

Danger Assessment

Several risk factors have been associated with homicides (murders) of both batterers and victims in research that has been conducted after the killings have taken place. We cannot predict what will happen in your case, but we would like you to be aware of the danger of homicide in situations of severe battering and to see how many of the risk factors apply to your situation.

1. Has the physical violence increased in frequency during the past year?
2. Has the physical violence increased in severity during the past year or has a weapon or threat with weapon been used?
3. Does your partner ever try to choke you?
4. Is there a gun in the house?
5. Has your partner ever forced you to have sex when you did not wish to do so?
6. Does your partner use drugs? By drugs, I mean "uppers" or amphetamines, speed, angel dust, cocaine, "crack," street drugs, heroin, or mixtures.
7. Does your partner threaten to kill you, or do you believe he or she is capable of killing you?
8. Is your partner drunk every day or almost every day? (In terms of quantity of alcohol.)
9. Does your partner control most or all of your daily activities? For instance, does he or she tell you who you can be friends with, how much money you can take with you shopping, or when you can take the car?
10. Has your partner ever beaten you while you were pregnant? (If never pregnant by him, check here—.)
11. Is your partner violently and constantly jealous of you? (For instance, does he or she say, "If I can't have you, no one can.")
12. Have you ever threatened or tried to commit suicide?
13. Has he ever threatened or tried to commit suicide?
14. Is your partner violent toward the children?
15. Is your partner violent outside the home?

TOTAL YES ANSWERS: _____

Thank you. Please talk to your nurse, advocate, or counselor about what the danger assessment means in terms of your situation.

Adapted from Campbell, J., & Humphreys, J. (Eds.) (1993). *Nursing care of survivors of family violence* (p. 259). St. Louis: Mosby.

Screening for Violence and Abuse

Most survivors do not report violence to health care workers without being asked specifically about it. Only 1% to 12% of women seen in the ED or primary care settings after a battering incident either told or were asked by staff about abuse (Chen et al., 2007). Survivors may be reluctant to report abuse because of shame and fear of retaliation, especially if the victim depends on the abuser as caregiver. In addition, children may be afraid that they will not be believed. Asking specific abuse screening questions has been shown to increase the detection of abuse substantially (from 3% to 46%). For that reason, nurses must develop a repertoire of age-appropriate, culturally sensitive abuse-related questions (Burgess & Tavakoli, 2005; Chen et al., 2007).

BOX 40.2
Abuse Assessment Screen

1. Have you ever been emotionally or   YES   NO
   physically abused by your partner or
   someone important to you?
2. Within the past year, have you been   YES   NO
   hit, slapped, kicked or otherwise physically hurt by someone?
   If YES, by whom: _____
   Number of times: _____
   Mark the area of injury on body map.
3. Within the past year, has anyone forced   YES   NO
   you to have sexual activities?
   If YES, who: _____
   Number of times: _____
4. Are you afraid of your partner or any-   YES   NO
   one you listed above?

Appropriate questions to ask in assessing abuse are found in the Abuse Assessment Screen (Box 40.2) and in the Burgess-Partner Abuse Scale for Teens (Box 40.3). Other questions that might be useful in eliciting disclosure are: "When there are fights at home, have you ever been hurt or afraid?" "It looks like someone has hurt you. Tell me about it." "Some women have described problems like yours. If this is happening to you, can we talk about it?" When survivors are disclosing abuse, they need privacy and time to tell their story. They need to know that the nurse is listening, believes them, and is concerned for their safety and well-being (Eddy, Kilburn, Chang, Bullock, & Sharps, 2008; Lindhorst et al., 2008; Rhodes et al., 2007; Salari, 2007).

Most survivors are not offended when health care providers ask about abuse directly as long as they conduct the interview nonjudgmentally (Chen et al., 2007; Eddy

BOX 40.3
Burgess-Partner Abuse Scale for Teens

Directions: During the past 12 months, you and one of your partners may have had a fight. Below is a list of things one of your partners may have done to you. Please circle the number of how often this partner did these things to you. This is not a test and there are no right or wrong answers. Remember, having a partner(s) does not mean you are having sex with the partner(s).

If you have not had a partner in the past 12 months, do not fill this form out.

	Never	Once	A few times	More than a few times	Routinely or a lot
1. My partner doesn't let me go out with my friends	0	1	2	3	4
2. My partner tells me what to wear	0	1	2	3	4
3. My partner says if I don't have sex with him/her then I don't love him/her	0	1	2	3	4
4. My partner says he/she will hurt me if I talk to another guy/girl	0	1	2	3	4
5. My partner calls me bad names like bitch	0	1	2	3	4
6. My partner says he/she will hurt me with a weapon	0	1	2	3	4
7. My partner forces me to have sex	0	1	2	3	4
8. My partner tells me I am stupid or dumb		1	2	3	4
9. My partner follows me when I do things with my friends or family	0	1	2	3	4
10. My partner hits or kicks something when he/she gets mad at me	0	1	2	3	4
11. My partner kicks me	0	1	2	3	4
12. My partner says he/she can have sex with other people even though he/she said I can't	0	1	2	3	4
13. My partner gives me sex infections	0	1	2	3	4
14. My partner hurts me using a weapon	0	1	2	3	4
15. My partner forces me to use drugs even though I don't want to	0	1	2	3	4
16. My partner beats me up so bad	0	1	2	3	4
17. My partner says he/she will hurt my family if I don't do what he/she says	0	1	2	3	4
18. My partner tells me what school activities I can and can't do	0	1	2	3	4
19. My partner tells me what friends I can hang out with	0	1	2	3	4
20. My partner chokes me if he/she gets mad at me	0	1	2	3	4
21. My partner yells at me if he/she doesn't know where I am	0	1	2	3	4
22. My partner says we can't break up even though I want to	0	1	2	3	4

How many partners have you had in the past 12 months?_____

Copyright, 2002 & 2003 Stephanie E. Burgess Permission is granted for use in research or clinical settings. Burgess, S., & Tavakoli, A. (2005). Psychometric assessment of the Burgess-Partner Abuse Scale for Teens (B-PAST). *Aquichan, 5*, 96–107.

et al., 2008; Rabin et al., 2009). Survivors may perceive failure of the nurse or other provider to ask about abuse as evidence of lack of concern, adding to feelings of entrapment and helplessness. The high prevalence of abuse and the reluctance of survivors to volunteer information about abuse or domestic violence mandate routine screening of every patient for abuse by explicit questioning. Perhaps even more important is that such screening is completed in privacy away from the partner; the child's parents or legal guardians; and the older adult's relative, companion, or caregiver. If a partner, parent, other relative, or companion accompanies the patient to the health care facility, protocols should be in place to separate the patient from these individuals until assessment is completed. One approach is to ask the other person to wait in the reception area, explaining that assessments are always done in private.

After assessment is completed in a health care agency and abuse is evident, the nurse should offer the adult survivor use of the telephone. This may be the only time that the survivor can make calls in private to family, who might offer support, or to the police, lawyers, or shelters. Scheduling future appointments may provide the survivor with a legitimate reason to leave the perpetrator and continue to explore options.

History and Physical Examination

All survivors who report or for whom abuse is suspected should receive a complete history and physical examination. Throughout, the nurse must remain nonjudgmental and communicate openly and honestly (Chen et al., 2007; Eddy et al., 2008; Rabin et al., 2009; Rhodes et al., 2008). It is not the nurse's responsibility to judge any situation, whether that is a woman's decision to remain in an abusive relationship, the abusive actions of a children's parents, or abuse perpetrated by caregivers of an older adult. Therefore, it is imperative to continually monitor personal feelings toward the abuser and survivor, especially in cases of child abuse. Working with child survivors often causes distress and feelings of anger and inadequacy. Seeking value clarification by the nurse may prevent negative feelings from influencing the nurse–patient relationship that could lead to a nontherapeutic interaction and perhaps retraumatize the survivor.

The patient's history should include past and present medical history, psychosocial history, family history, ADLs, and social and financial support. The nurse should obtain a detailed history of how injuries occurred. As with any history, begin with the complaint that brought the patient to the health care facility and assess whether the explanation for the injuries or symptoms is plausible, given their nature. Discrepancies between the history and physical examination findings may suggest abuse or neglect. Move from safe to more sensitive topics; for example, asking

about the nature of the injuries involves asking the survivor to describe the first incident remembered, the most recent incident, the worst incident, and a typical incident. This series of questions is designed to elicit a complete picture of the cycle of violence and its progression. If a child is too young or an older adult is too impaired to give a history, interview one or both parents of the child or the caregiver of the older adult. If the survivor is a child or dependent older adult who cannot describe what happened or make decisions about personal safety and care, the health care team may take steps to place the survivor in protective custody and defer additional assessment to the appropriate agency (DSS or APS).

The physical examination should include a complete history and physical with a neurologic examination, radiographs to identify any old or new fractures, and examination for sexual abuse. Typically, examination for sexual abuse, acute or chronic events, may require referral to a trained registered nurse in sexual assault, known as SANE (sexual assault nurse examiner) (Cole & Logan, 2008). See Box 40.4 for additional considerations.

When assessing older adults, be familiar with normal aging and signs and symptoms of common illnesses to distinguish those conditions from abuse (Sandmoe & Kirkevold, 2010). Similarly, healthy child development and deviations that may be related to abuse or neglect are critical components of the nursing assessment. For children, assessing developmental milestones, school history, and relationships with siblings and friends are important (Holmbeck et al., 2008). Any discrepancies between the history and physical examination and implausible explanations for injuries and other symptoms should be an alert to the possibility of abuse. Box 40.5 lists indicators of actual or potential abuse that need to be thoroughly assessed for all survivors.

Thoroughly document all findings. Injuries should be photographed if possible, but this can be done only with written permission from an adult survivor or one of the child's parents or guardians. If the survivor will not permit photographing, document the injuries on a body map. Documentation should include size, shape, color, location, and discharge. Survivors may need assurance that their medical records will not be released to anyone without written permission and that documentation of injuries will be important if legal action is taken. If the survivor does not admit abuse, abuse cannot be noted in the record. However, it can be documented that the description of injuries is inconsistent with the injury pattern.

Biologic indicators, such as elevated pulse and blood pressure, sleep and appetite disturbances, exaggerated startle responses, flashbacks, and nightmares, may suggest PTSD or depression. Signs and symptoms of dissociation include memory difficulties, a feeling of unreality about oneself or events, a feeling that a familiar place is

BOX 40.4

Special Concerns for Victims of Sexual Assault

ASSESSMENT FOCUS

The history and physical examination of the survivor of sexual assault differ significantly from other assessment routines because the evidence obtained may be used in prosecuting the perpetrator. Therefore, the purpose is twofold:

- To assess the patient for injuries
- To collect evidence for forensic evaluation and proceedings

Usually, someone with special training, such as a nurse practitioner who has taken special courses, examines a rape or sexual assault victim. Generalist nurses may be involved in treating the injuries that result from the assault, including genital trauma, such as vaginal and anal lacerations, and extragenital trauma, such as injury to the mouth, throat, wrists, arms, breasts, and thighs.

KEY INTERVENTIONS

Nursing intervention to prevent short- or long-term psychopathology after sexual assault is crucial. Psychological trauma after rape and sexual assault includes immediate anxiety and distress and the development of PTSD, depression, panic, and substance abuse.

Key interventions include:

- Early treatment because initial levels of distress are strongly related to later levels of posttraumatic stress disorder, panic, and anxiety
- Supportive, caring, and nonjudgmental nursing interventions during the forensic rape examination are also crucial. This examination often increases survivors' immediate distress because they must recount the assault in detail and submit to an invasive pelvic or anal examination.
- Anxiety-reducing education, counseling, and emotional support, particularly in regard to unwanted pregnancies and sexually transmitted infections, including HIV. All survivors should be tested for these possibilities. Treatment may include terminating a pregnancy; administering medications to treat gonorrhea, chlamydia, trichomoniasis, and syphilis; and administering medications that may decrease the likelihood of contracting HIV infection.
- Interventions that are helpful for survivors of domestic violence; these also apply to survivors of sexual assault.

---

strange and unfamiliar, auditory or visual hallucinations, and evidence of having done things without remembering them. If any of these signs or symptoms is present, the survivor requires a thorough diagnostic workup for PTSD and dissociative identity disorder (DID). The nurse should assess every adult or adolescent who discloses victimization for substance abuse. See Chapters 26 and 31.

Nursing Diagnoses for the Biologic Domain

Selected nursing diagnoses for the biologic domain may include Post-Trauma Syndrome, Delayed Growth and Development, Impaired Memory, and Rape-Trauma Syndrome.

Interventions for the Biologic Domain

Restoring health is a primary concern for survivors of abuse. When injuries are severe and surgery is required, the survivor may require hospital admittance.

Treating Physical Symptoms

Treatment of trauma symptoms may include cleaning and dressing burns or other wounds and assisting with casting of broken bones. Malnourished and dehydrated children and older adults may require nursing interventions such as intravenous therapy or nutritional supplements that alleviate the alteration in nutrition and fluid and electrolyte balance. Victims of sexual assault require additional considerations (see Box 40.5).

> **NCLEXNOTE** Individuals who are experiencing IPV need their basic needs met (safety, housing, food, child care) before their psychological traumas can be addressed.

Promoting Healthy Daily Activity

Teaching sleep hygiene (practices conducive to healthy sleep patterns) and promoting exercise, leisure time, and nutrition will help battered survivors regain a healthy physical state and self-care activities. Taking care of themselves may be difficult for survivors who have spent years trying to separate themselves from their bodies (dissociate) to survive years of abuse. Techniques such as going to bed and arising at consistent times, avoiding naps and caffeine, and scheduling periods for relaxation just before retiring may be useful in promoting sleep (Pigeon, May, Perlis, Ward, Lu, & Talbot, 2009). Aerobic exercise is a useful technique for relieving anxiety and depression and promoting sleep.

Administering and Monitoring Medications

Survivors with a comorbid mood or anxiety disorder, including PTSD, may require pharmacologic interventions. Although only nurses with advanced preparation and prescriptive authority may prescribe medications, all nurses must be familiar with medications used to treat mood and anxiety disorders, including the side effects of these drugs. Of special concern are medications that are used cautiously or are contraindicated for young and older adult survivors. See Chapters 24 to 26.

Managing Care of Patients with Co-occurring Alcohol and Drug Disorders

Survivors who have a comorbid AOD disorder need referral to a treatment center for AOD disorders. The treatment center should have programs that address the special needs of survivors. Alcohol- and drug-dependent

BOX 40.5

History and Physical Findings Suggestive of Abuse

PRESENTING PROBLEM
- Vague information about cause of problem
- Delay between occurrence of injury and seeking of treatment
- Inappropriate reactions of significant other or family
- Denial or minimizing of seriousness of injury
- Discrepancy between history and physical examination findings

FAMILY HISTORY
- Past family violence
- Physical punishment of children
- Children who are fearful of parent(s)
- Father or mother (or both) who demands unquestioning obedience
- Alcohol or drug abuse
- Violence outside the home
- Unemployment or underemployment
- Financial difficulties or poverty
- Use of older adult's finances for other family members
- Finances rigidly controlled by one member

HEALTH AND PSYCHIATRIC HISTORY
- Fractures at various stages of healing
- Spontaneous abortions
- Injuries during pregnancy
- Multiple visits to the emergency department
- Elimination disturbances (e.g., constipation, diarrhea)
- Multiple somatic complaints
- Eating disorders
- Substance abuse
- Depression
- Posttraumatic stress disorder
- Self-mutilation
- Suicide attempts
- Feelings of helplessness or hopelessness
- Low self-esteem
- Chronic fatigue
- Apathy
- Sleep disturbances (e.g., hypersomnia, hyposomnia)
- Psychiatric hospitalizations

PERSONAL AND SOCIAL HISTORY
- Feelings of powerlessness
- Feelings of being trapped
- Lack of trust
- Traditional values about home, partner, and children's behavior
- Major decisions in family controlled by one person
- Few social supports (isolated from family, friends)
- Little activity outside the home
- Unwanted or unplanned pregnancy
- Dependency on caregivers
- Extreme jealousy by partner
- Difficulties at school or work
- Short attention span
- Running away
- Promiscuity
- Child who has knowledge of sexual matters beyond that appropriate for age
- Sexualized play with self, peers, dolls, toys
- Masturbation
- Excessive fears and clinging in children
- Verbal aggression
- Themes of violence in artwork and school work
- Distorted body image

- History of chronic physical or psychological disability
- Inability to perform activities of daily living
- Delayed language development

PHYSICAL EXAMINATION FINDINGS
General Appearance
- Fearful, anxious, hyperactive, hypoactive
- Watching partner, parent, or caregiver for approval of answers to questions
- Poor grooming or inappropriate dress
- Malnourishment
- Signs of stress or fatigue
- Flinching when approached or touched
- Inappropriate or anxious nonverbal behavior
- Wearing clothing inappropriate to the season or occasion to cover body parts

Vital Statistics
- Elevated pulse or blood pressure
- Other signs of autonomic arousal (exaggerated startle response, excessive sweating)
- Underweight or overweight

Skin
- Bruises, welts, edema, or scars
- Burns (cigarette, immersion, friction from ropes, pattern like an electric iron or stove)
- Subdural hematoma
- Missing hair
- Poor skin integrity: dehydration, decubitus ulcers, untreated wounds, urine burns or excoriation

Eyes
- Orbital swelling
- Conjunctival hemorrhage
- Retinal hemorrhage
- Black eyes
- No glasses to accommodate poor eyesight

Ears
- Hearing loss
- No prosthetic device to accommodate poor hearing

Mouth
- Bruising
- Lacerations
- Missing or broken teeth
- Untreated dental problems

Abdomen
- Abdominal injuries during pregnancy
- Intraabdominal injuries

Genitourinary System or Rectum
- Bruising, lacerations, bleeding, edema, tenderness
- Untreated infections

Musculoskeletal System
- Fractures or old fractures in various stages of healing
- Dislocations
- Limited range of motion in extremities
- Contractures

Neurologic System
- Difficulty with speech or swallowing
- Hyperactive reflexes
- Developmental delays
- Areas of numbness
- Tremors

(Continued)

BOX 40.5

History and Physical Findings Suggestive of Abuse (*Continued*)

Mental Status
- Anxiety, fear
- Depression
- Suicidal ideation
- Difficulty concentrating
- Memory loss

Medications
- Medications not indicated by physical condition
- Overdose of drugs or medications (prescribed or over the counter)
- Medications not taken as prescribed

Communication Patterns and Relations
- Verbal hostility, arguments
- Negative nonverbal communication, lack of visible affection
- One person answers questions and looks to other person for approval
- Extreme dependency of family members

survivors frequently stop treatment and return to AOD abuse if their violence-related problems are not addressed appropriately (Klostermann, 2006; Resnick, Acierno, Amstadter, & Self-Brown, 2007).

Survivors, especially those with AOD problems, are at high risk for HIV infection and AIDS. If survivors do not know their HIV status, they should be encouraged to get tested. Those with positive test results should initiate appropriate medication (to include antivirals) as prescribed by their provider and receive counseling. Regardless of their HIV status, all sexually active patients need to be educated about the high-risk behaviors for HIV infection and how to protect themselves from contracting or transmitting HIV infection (Pinkerton, Bogart, Howerton, Snyder, Becker, & Asch, 2009).

Psychological Domain

Assessment

A mental status evaluation should be part of every health assessment. Symptoms such as anhedonia, difficulties concentrating, feelings of worthlessness or guilt, and thoughts of death or suicide suggest depression or PTSD. A thorough assessment of suicidal or homicidal intent is essential to the evaluation.

Nursing Diagnoses for the Psychological Domain

Selected nursing diagnoses for the psychological domain may include Ineffective Coping, Hopelessness, Chronic Low Self-Esteem, Anxiety, Risk for Self-Directed Violence, and Risk for Other-Directed Violence.

Interventions for the Psychological Domain

Assisting with Psychotherapy or Counseling

Psychotherapy may include individual, group, family, or marital therapy. Only psychiatric nurse specialists (advanced practice nurses) at the master's or doctoral levels who have

had training in these therapeutic methods may conduct psychotherapy. In addition, the nurse therapist should have training in conducting therapy specifically with survivors of abuse. That training should include management of PTSD, DID, depression, and AOD disorders. The goal of therapy is to integrate the patient's traumatic memories with the remainder of the patient's personal history and identity, manage painful affect and anxiety, and restructure the meaning of the traumatic experiences (Roy-Byrne et al., 2010). The ultimate goal is for the survivor to integrate the trauma in memory as a past event that no longer has the power to terrorize.

Family or marital therapy may be unwise unless the perpetrator of abuse has obtained individual therapy and demonstrated change. Otherwise, survivors are placed in a very difficult situation. If they disclose abuse in family or marital therapy, perpetrators may retaliate with violence, but if they do not disclose the abuse, the crucial issue will not be addressed (Eddy et al., 2008; Lindhorst Meyers, & Casey 2008; Rhodes et al., 2008; Salari, 2007).

Several issues must be addressed for all survivors in psychotherapy or counseling. All nurses can implement these interventions using skills appropriate to their educational level and training. They include addressing the guilt, shame, and stigmatization that survivors experience. These issues can be approached in several ways. Assisting survivors to verbalize their experience in an accepting, non-judgmental atmosphere is a first step. Directly challenging attributions of self-blame for the abuse and feelings of being dirty and different is another. Helping survivors to identify their strengths and validating thoughts and feelings may help to increase their self-esteem.

Working with Children

Children may need to learn a "violence vocabulary" that allows them to talk about their abuse and assign responsibility for abusive behavior. Children also need to learn that violence is not okay, and it is not their fault (Thackarey et al., 2010). Allowing children to discuss their abuse in the safety of a supportive, caring relationship may alleviate anxiety and fear (Thackarey et al., 2010).

Reenacting the abuse through play is another technique that may be helpful in assisting children to express and work through their anxiety and fear. Play therapy uses dolls, human or animal figures, video games, or puppets to work through anxiety or fears (Ceranoglu, 2010; Van Breemen, 2009). Other techniques include reading stories about recovery from abusive experiences (literal or metaphoric), using art or music to express feelings, and psychodrama. In addition, teaching strategies to manage fear and anxiety, such as relaxation techniques, coping skills, and imagery, may give the child an added sense of mastering his or her fear (Ceranoglu, 2010; Van Breemen, 2009).

Managing Anger

Anger and rage are part of the healing process for survivors. Expression of intense anger is uncomfortable for many nurses. However, anger expression should be expected from the survivor, and it is necessary to develop comfortable ways to respond. Moreover, an important nursing intervention is teaching and modeling anger expression appropriately. Inappropriate expressions of anger might drive supportive people away. Anger management techniques include appropriately recognizing and labeling anger and expressing it assertively rather than aggressively or passive-aggressively (Son & Choi, 2010). Assertive ways of expressing anger include owning the feeling by using "I feel" statements and avoiding blaming others (Nidich et al., 2009). Teaching anger management and conflict resolution may be especially important for children who have seen nothing but violence to resolve problems (Puskar, Ren, Bernardo, Haley, & Stark, 2008).

Teaching Skills and Clarifying Identity

Other nursing interventions include teaching self-protection skills, healthy relationship skills, and healthy sexuality. Again, this teaching may be especially important for children who have no role models for healthy relationships. Children also need to know what constitutes controlling and abusive behavior and how to get help for abuse.

Children who have been sexually abused may become confused about their sexuality. They may regard sex as dirty and as something that can be used against other people. Discussions about healthy sexuality and feelings about sex may help these children regain a healthy perspective on sex-related matters (Habigzang, Stroeher, Hatzenberger, Cunha, Ramos, & Koller, 2009; Harvey & Taylor, 2010).

Group therapy with survivors offers a powerful method to counter self-denigrating beliefs and to confront issues of secrecy and stigmatization (Habigzang et al., 2009; Harvey & Taylor, 2010). Moreover, one of the therapeutic factors in group therapy, universality or the discovery

that others have had similar experiences, may be a tremendous relief, especially to child survivors.

Providing Education

Education is a key nursing intervention for survivors (Box 40.6). As appropriate to age or condition, survivors must understand the cycle of violence and the danger of homicide that increases as violence escalates or the survivor attempts to leave the relationship. Survivors also need information about resources, such as shelters for battered women, legal services, government benefits, and support networks. Before giving the survivor any written material, first discuss the possibility that if the perpetrator were to find the information in the survivor's possession, he or she might use it as an excuse for battering.

Survivors also need education appropriate for age and cognitive ability about the symptoms of anxiety, depression, dissociation, and PTSD. They must understand that these symptoms are common in anyone who has sustained significant stressors and are not signs of being "crazy" or weak. If survivors require medication for these symptoms, they must know how to monitor symptoms so that the effectiveness of pharmacologic management can be determined. One of the most important teaching goals is to help survivors develop a safety plan. The first step in developing such a plan is helping the survivor recognize the signs of danger. Changes in tone of voice, drinking and drug use, and increased criticism may indicate that the perpetrator is losing control. Detecting early warning signs helps survivors to escape before battering begins (Burgess & Tavakoli, 2005; Walton et al., 2009).

The next step is to devise an escape route. This involves mapping the house and identifying where the battering usually occurs and what exits are available. The survivor needs to have a bag packed and hidden but readily accessible that has what is needed to get away. Important things to pack are clothes, a set of car and house keys,

---

BOX 40.6

Psychoeducation Checklist: **Abuse**

When caring for the patient who has been abused, be sure to address the following topics in the teaching plan:

- Cycle of violence
- Access to shelters
- Legal services
- Government benefits
- Support network
- Symptoms of anxiety, dissociation, and posttraumatic stress disorder
- Safety or escape plan
- Relaxation
- Adequate nutrition and exercise
- Sleep hygiene
- HIV testing and counseling

bank account numbers, birth certificate, insurance policies and numbers, marriage license, valuable jewelry, important telephone numbers, and money. The survivor must carefully hide the bag so the perpetrator cannot find it and use it as an excuse for assault. If children are involved, the adult survivor should make arrangements to get them out safely. That might include arranging a signal to indicate when it is safe for them to leave the house and to meet at a prearranged place. A safety plan for a child or dependent elder might include safe places to hide and important telephone numbers, including 911 and those of the police and fire departments and other family members and friends.

Finding Strength and Hope

Providing hope and a sense of control is important for survivors of trauma (Kanter, Rusch, Landes, Holman, Whiteside, & Sedivy, 2009). Help survivors find hope by assisting them to identify specific strengths and aspects of their lives that are under their control. This type of intervention may empower survivors to find options to remaining in an abusive relationship.

Using Behavioral Interventions

Treatment for depression, anxiety, and PTSD symptoms can be divided into two categories: exposure therapy and anxiety management training. Only professionals trained in exposure therapy techniques can use them; however, it is important to be familiar with this approach. The goal of exposure therapy, which includes flooding and systematic desensitization, is to promote the processing of the traumatic memory by exposing the survivor to the traumatic event through memories or some cue that reactivates trauma memories. Through repeated exposure, the event loses its ability to cause intense anxiety. See Chapter 26.

Teaching Coping with Anxiety

Anxiety management is a crucial intervention for all survivors. There is a high comorbidity among trauma, PTSD, and anxiety disorders (Back, 2010; Hien et al., 2010). During treatment, survivors experience situations and memories that provoke intense anxiety and must know how to soothe themselves when they experience painful feelings. Moreover, most survivors struggle with control issues, especially involving their bodies. Anxiety management skills offer one way to maintain some control over their bodies (Back, 2010; Hein et al., 2010).

Anxiety management training may include progressive relaxation, deep breathing, imagery techniques, and cognitive restructuring. Progressive relaxation entails systematically tensing and then relaxing the major muscle groups. Visualization consists of imagining a scene that is especially relaxing (e.g., spending a day at the beach) while practicing relaxation and deep breathing. Any interventions that reduce dysphoric symptoms can help survivors feel more in control of their situation.

Anxiety disorders, including PTSD, and depression are associated with cognitive distortions that cognitive therapy techniques can challenge (Back, 2010; Hein et al., 2010). Self-defeating thoughts in anxiety disorders involve perceptions of threat and danger, and those in depression involve negative self-perceptions. Nurses can teach survivors how to identify and challenge these self-defeating thought patterns. Cognitive therapy techniques may be especially useful in helping survivors to stop blaming themselves for their abuse.

Nurses must become accustomed to measuring gains in small steps when working with survivors. Making any changes in significant relationships has serious consequences and can be done only when the adult survivor is ready. It is easy to become angry or discouraged with survivors, so it is important to not to communicate these feelings. Discussing such feelings with other staff provides a way of dealing with them appropriately. In such discussions with supervisors or other staff, it is a must to protect the patient's confidentiality by discussing feelings around issues, not particular patients. The nurse should frame the discussion in such a way that individual patients cannot be identified.

Social Domain

Assessment

An evaluation of social networks and daily activities may provide additional clues of psychological abuse and controlling behavior (Burgess & Tavakoli, 2005). When a nurse assesses social isolation, evaluating the reasons behind it is crucial. Many perpetrators isolate their family from all social contacts, including other relatives. Some survivors isolate themselves because they are ashamed of the abuse or fear nonsupportive responses. An evaluation of social support is important for other reasons. Having supportive family or friends is crucial in short-term planning for developing a safety plan and is also important to long-term recovery. A survivor cannot leave an abusive situation if there is nowhere to go. Supportive family and friends may be willing to provide shelter and safety.

Nurses can assess restrictions on freedom that may suggest abuse and control by asking such questions as: "Are you free to go where you want?" "Is staying home your choice?" and "Is there anything you would like to do that you cannot?"

The degree of dependency on the relationship is another important variable to assess. Women who have young children and are economically dependent on the perpetrator may believe that they cannot leave the abusive relationship. Those who are emotionally dependent on the perpetrator may experience an intense grief reaction that further complicates their leaving (Ford-Gilboe, Wuest, Varcoe, Davies, & Merritt-Gray, 2009). Older adults and children are often dependent on the abuser and cannot leave the abusive situation without alternatives.

Nursing Diagnoses for the Social Domain

Selected nursing diagnoses for the social domain may include Hopelessness, Powerlessness, and Ineffective Role Performance.

Interventions for the Social Domain

Teaching for Abusive Families

Family interventions in cases of child abuse focus on behavioral approaches to improve parenting skills. A behavioral approach has multiple components. *Child management skills* help parents manage maladaptive behaviors and reward appropriate behaviors. *Parenting skills* teach parents how to be more effective and nurturing with their children. *Leisure skills* training is important to reduce stress in the household and promote healthy family time. *Household organization* training is another way to reduce stress by teaching effective ways to manage the multiple tasks that families have to perform. Such tasks include meal planning, cooking, shopping, keeping providers' (e.g., dental, health visits, counseling) appointments, and planning family activities (Arnold, Doctoroff, Ortiz, & Zeljo, 2008; Boonstra, 2009; Boster & Strom, 2007).

Anger control and stress management skills are important parts of behavioral programs for families. Anger control programs teach parents to identify events that increase anger and stress and to replace anger-producing thoughts with more appropriate ones. Parents learn self-control skills to reduce the expression of uncontrolled anger. Stress-reduction techniques include relaxation techniques and methods for coping with stressful interactions with their children (Arnold et al., 2008; Boonstra, 2009; Boster & Strom, 2007). These skills may be especially important in families in which elder abuse is occurring. Both caregivers and the abused individual may need to learn assertive ways to express their anger and healthy ways to manage their stress. Helping caregivers obtain some relief from their caregiving burdens may be crucial in reducing abuse that comes from exhaustion in trying to manage multiple roles. Examples include identifying agencies that offer respite care or agencies that offer day care for older adults and support groups in which caregivers can share experiences and gain support from others dealing with similar issues.

Community Involvement

Nurses may be involved in interventions to reduce violence at the community level. Many abusive caregivers and parents and guardians as well as battered partners, older adults, and children are socially isolated. Developing support networks may help reduce stress and therefore reduce abuse. Community contacts vary for each abuser and survivor but might include crisis hot lines, support groups, and education classes (Casey & Beadnell, 2010; Henderson, Rowe, Dakof, Hawes, & Liddle, 2009; Leggatt, 2007; Morton, Tong, Howard, Snelling, & Webster, 2010).

Nurses may also make home visits. Home visits provide support to families and provide them with knowledge about stress and management (Barnet, Liu, DeVoe, Duggan, Gold, & Pecukonis, 2009; Cutchin, Coppola, Talley, Syihula, Catellier, & Shank, 2009; Karande, Kumbhare, Kulkarni, & Shah, 2009). Abuse of any kind is a volatile situation, and nurses may place themselves or the survivor in danger if they make home visits. Carefully assess this possibility before proceeding. If necessary, arrange a safe place to meet the survivor instead.

Evaluation and Treatment Outcomes

Evaluation and outcome criteria depend on the setting for interventions. For instance, if a survivor is encountered in the ED, successful outcomes might be that injuries are appropriately managed and the patient's immediate safety is ensured. For long-term care, outcome criteria and evaluation might center on ending abusive relationships. Examples of other outcome criteria that would indicate successful nursing interventions are recognizing that one is not to blame for the violence, demonstrating knowledge of strengths and coping skills, and reestablishing social networks.

Evaluation of nursing care for abused children depends on attaining goals mutually set with the parents or guardians. An end to all violence is the optimal outcome criterion; however, attainment of smaller goals indicates progress toward that end. Outcomes such as increased problem-solving and communication skills within the family, increased self-esteem in both children and parents, and increased use of nonphysical forms of discipline may all indicate progress toward the total elimination of child abuse.

Follow-up efforts are important in evaluating the outcomes of elder abuse. The optimal outcome is to end all abuse and keep the older adult in his or her own living environment, if appropriate. Although the abuse may have been resolved temporarily, it may flare up again. Ongoing support for the caregiver and assistance with caregiving tasks may be necessary if the older adult is to remain at home. Nursing home or assisted living may be the most desirable option if the burden is too great for the family and the likelihood of ongoing abuse or neglect is high.

Another important outcome of nursing intervention with survivors is appropriate treatment of any disorder resulting from abuse (e.g., ASD, PTSD and other anxiety disorders, DID, major depression, substance abuse). Follow-up nursing assessments should monitor symptom reduction or exacerbation, adherence to any medication regimen, and side effects of medication. The ultimate outcome is to end violence and enable the survivor to return to a more productive, safe, and nurturing life without being continually haunted by memories of the abuse.

TREATMENT FOR THE ABUSER

Participants in programs that treat abusers are usually there because the court has mandated the treatment. Programs are often outpatient groups that meet weekly for an extended period of time, often 36 to 48 weeks. Some programs advocate longer programs, believing that chronic offenders require from 1 to 5 years of treatment to change abusive behavior.

Groups often use cognitive behavioral techniques or a psychoeducational, skill-building approach (Eckhardt, Murphy, Black, & Suhr, 2006). This approach helps the abuser to understand that violent acts are not uncontrollable outbursts but rather foreseeable behavior patterns that can be interrupted. Cognitive behavioral interventions target three elements: (1) what the batterer thinks about before a battering incident, (2) the batterer's physical and emotional response to these thoughts, and (3) the batterer's actions that progress to violence (yelling, throwing things). The group teaches members to recognize and interrupt negative feelings about their partners and to reduce physiologic arousal through relaxation techniques.

Similar to topics in the model Duluth Curriculum, group psychoeducational topics may include nonviolence and nonthreatening behavior, respect, support, trust, honesty, accountability, sexual respect, partnership, negotiation, and fairness (Levesque, Driskell, Prochaska, & Prochaska, 2008). If the problem were simply a deficit in skills, the abuser would be dysfunctional in work or relationships outside the family. Abusers need resocialization that convinces them that they do not have the right to abuse their partners. Other programs add a moral aspect by taking a value-laden approach against violence and confronting the batterer's behavior as unacceptable and illegal.

Accountability for violent acts is an important early goal in treating batterers (Eckhardt et al., 2006; Levesque et al., 2008). Most batterers deny responsibility for their actions and refuse to look at violence and abuse as a choice. Therefore, it is important that the individuals become accountable for their actions. Interventions aim at getting abusers to acknowledge their violence across the full range of abusive acts that they have committed (e.g., verbal abuse,

intimidation, controlling behavior, and sexual abuse). The person may use several tactics to avoid accountability, and all must be addressed. Tactics include denying the abuse ever happened ("I never touched her"); minimizing the abuse by downplaying the violent acts or underestimating its effects ("It was just a slap" or "she bruises easily"); and blaming the abuse on the victim ("she pushed me too far"), alcohol or other drugs ("I was high"), or other life circumstances ("I had too many pressures at work").

States vary on requiring that treatment programs for abusers contact partners (CDC, 2013a). Because abusers typically minimize or deny their violent behavior, it is often necessary to interview the survivor to gain a complete picture of the abuser's behavior. A trained victim advocate usually contacts partners. There are other reasons for contacting partners. This may be the first contact the partner has had with professionals, and he or she may benefit by telling her or his story. Many partners do not know that services are available to them, and this is an opportunity to communicate what is available. In addition, advocates often explain the treatment program and emphasize that it takes a long time and requires the abuser to take responsibility for violent behavior. Partners need to hear that many abusers are not willing to change their behavior. Another important point that partners need to know and discuss with professionals is that abusers often use entry into treatment as a justification for pressuring partners to remain in the relationship but that this behavior is a good indicator that abuse will continue (Stalans & Magnus, 2007).

Interventions must be culturally competent. Many factors can affect violence against others, including socioeconomic status, racial or ethnic identity, country of origin, and sexual orientation, and those differences must be addressed. Another factor that must be addressed is AOD use. Intervention programs may require abusers to undergo substance abuse treatment concurrently, and patients are required to remain sober and submit to random drug testing.

Treatment programs alone are not sufficient to stop many abusers (Eckhardt et al., 2006). To be effective, programs must operate within a comprehensive intervention effort that includes criminal justice support (Coulter & Vandeweerd, 2009). The criminal justice response includes arrest, incarceration, adjudication, and probation supervision that includes issuing a warrant if the abuser does not attend the treatment program or supervision. The combination of criminal justice response and treatment may convey a more powerful message to the abuser about the seriousness of his or her actions than an abuser program alone. Unfortunately, many offenders never show up for intervention, and arrests for violation of probation may be rare because of overload and staffing shortages. Inaction by the criminal justice system is serious; it sends the message that there is little concern for violence against intimate partners and that abusers can escape accountability.

Several approaches to intervention exist. Anger management attributes physical abuse to out-of-control anger and teaches anger management techniques. There are several arguments against this approach. It does not address the real issue—abusers' desire to control their partners. Abusers are able to control their behavior in other difficult situations but choose anger and intimidation to control their partners. Anger management may merely teach abusers nonviolent methods to exert control. Couples counseling may endanger the survivor, who will not be free to disclose, and any disclosures may give the abuser reason to retaliate. Self-help groups modeled on Alcoholics Anonymous are inappropriate for initial intervention for several reasons. Without trained facilitators who will confront denial and excuses, abusers may never accept accountability for their violence. On the other hand, an untrained facilitator may use an excessively confrontational approach that is abusive and models antagonistic behavior.

How effective is treatment for abusers? Results from an extended follow-up of court-ordered intervention programs show that many men continue to be assaultive during or on completion of treatment. Studies have shown only small effects of intervention programs on preventing future abuse (Eckhardt et al., 2006).

SUMMARY OF KEY POINTS

- The abuse of intimate partners, teens, children, and older adults is a national health problem that requires awareness and sensitivity from nurses.

- Intimate partner abuse may be physical, emotional and psychological, or social.

- Child abuse may be neglectful, physical, psychological, or sexual. Other forms of abuse include witnessing abuse of their mothers or significant caregivers.

- Elder abuse may be physical, emotional, neglectful, or financial.

- Among the many theories that have been proposed to explain violence are neurologic problems, psychopathology, alcohol and other drug abuse, intergenerational transmission of violence, and economic and community factors. There are also feminist theories specific to violence toward women.

- A well-documented cycle of violence consists of three phases of increasing frequency and severity.

- Responses to violence include depression, acute stress disorder (ASD), posttraumatic stress disorder (PTSD), and dissociative identity disorder (DID).

- Child abuse leaves many scars that can lead to such problems in adulthood as depression, anxiety, self-destructive behavior, poor self-esteem, and lack of trust.

- Nurses need to be familiar with signs and symptoms of abuse and to be vigilant when assessing patients.

- Nurses can help victims of abuse to view themselves as survivors.

- Treatment for those who abuse others requires multiple approaches with a strong motivation from the individual to change behavior.

CRITICAL THINKING CHALLENGES

1. Abuse is a pervasive problem, and anyone can be a victim (women, men, children, older adults, gays, lesbians). Why do so few nursing units and nurses make it routine to ask questions about abuse?

2. Abuse is not just a "women's issue." The prevalence of abuse might decrease if men make it a "men's issue" as well. What is preventing this from happening?

3. What are your thoughts and feelings about women who are victims of violence in which both partners (victim and perpetrator) abuse alcohol and other drugs?

4. What are your thoughts and feelings about women who will not leave an abusive relationship?

5. What are some reasons that people remain in abusive relationships?

6. Why do some survivors become involved in more than one abusive relationship?

7. How do you handle your feelings toward abusive parents or relatives who abuse older adults?

8. What are the issues in mandatory reporting of violence toward women, particularly violence?

9. Would your thoughts, feelings, and ability to intervene change if the violent relationship is between same sex partners?

Once Were Warriors: 1994. A mother of five reevaluates her 18-year marriage to her alcoholic, hot-tempered husband when his bar-room violence tragically encroaches into their home life. Produced and filmed in New Zealand, this film also presents how urbanization has undermined the culture and strength of the indigenous Maori people.

VIEWING POINTS: What evidence can you find in this film that may reflect intergenerational transmission of violence? In what ways do you think that culture can influence attitudes toward abuse (both positive and negative)? What are positive and negative cultural influences in this film?

Sybil: 1976. Sally Field plays Sybil, a woman who experiences dissociative identity disorder after suffering horrible abuse during childhood. Help from a psychiatrist (Joanne Woodward) uncovers the memories that have led to the splitting of Sybil's personality. The movie contains harrowing scenes of the abuse Sybil experienced.

VIEWING POINTS: What symptoms does Sybil show in the film? How does the psychiatrist work with Sybil's different personalities in this film?

Enough: 2002. Jennifer Lopez stars as a blue-collar beauty (Slim Hiller) who marries the really wrong guy. Eventually, she discovers his philandering and spends the rest of the movie in a nomadic flight from his hot-tempered brutality. Bankrolled by her estranged father, she protects her young daughter. Knowing she must face the inevitable showdown, she turns to self-defense courses for empowerment.

VIEWING POINTS: When did Slim and Mitch's relationship turn destructive? What are the characteristics of an abused partner displayed by Slim? What were Mitch Hiller's primary motives in stalking Slim?

References

Acierno, R., Hernandez, M. A., Amstadter, A. B., Resnick, H. S., Steve, K., Muzzy, W., et al. (2010). Prevalence and correlates of emotional, physical, sexual, and financial abuse and potential neglect in the United States: The National Elder Mistreatment Study. *American Journal of Public Health, 100*(2), 292–297.

Afifi, T. O., MacMillan, H., Cox, B. J., Asmundson, G. J. G., Stein, M. B., & Sareen, J. (2010). Mental health correlates of intimate partner violence in marital relationships in a nationally representative sample of males and females. *Journal of Interpersonal Violence, 24*(8), 1398–1417.

Ali, P. A., & Naylor, P. B. (2013). Intimate partner violence: A narrative review of the biological and psychological explanations for its causation. *Aggression and Violent Behavior, 18*, 373–382.

American Academy of Child & Adolescent Psychiatry. (2008). Facts for families. *No.9.* Retrieved from http://www.aacap.org/galleries/FactsFor-Families/09_child_sexual_abuse.pdf

Arnold, D., Doctoroff, G., Ortiz, C., & Zeljo, A. (2008). Parent involvement in preschool: Predictors and the relation of involvement to pre-literacy development. *School Psychology Review, 37*(1):74–90.

Babcock, J. C., Green, C. E., & Webb, S. A. (2008). Decoding deficits of different types of batterers during presentation of facial affect slides. *Journal of Family Violence, 23*(5), 295–302.

Back, S. (2010). Toward an improved model of treating co-occurring PTSD and substance use disorders. *American Journal of Psychiatry, 167*(1), 11–13.

Baig, A., Shadigian, E., & Heisler, M. (2006). Hidden from plain sight: Residents' domestic violence screening attitudes and reported practices. *Journal of General Internal Medicine, 21*(9), 949–954.

Barnet, B., Liu, J., DeVoe, M., Duggan, A., Gold, M., & Pecukonis, E. (2009). Motivational intervention to reduce rapid subsequent births to adolescent mothers: A community-based randomized trial. *Annals of Family Medicine, 7*(5), 436–445.

Baum, K., Catalano, S., & Rand, M., & Rose (2009). Stalking victimization in the United States. National crime victimization survey. *Bureau of Justice Statistics: Special report.* Washington, DC: Office of Justice Programs, U.S. Department of Justice. Retrieved from http://www.ncvc.org/src/AGP.Net/Components/DocumentViewer/Download.aspxnz?DocumentID=45862.

Black, M. C, Basile, K. C., Breiding, M. J., Smith, S. G., Walters, M. L., Merrick, M. T., et al. (2011). *The National Intimate Partner and Sexual Violence Survey (NISVS): 2010 Summary Report.* Atlanta, GA: National Center for Injury Prevention and Control, Centers for Disease Control and Prevention. Retrieved from http://www.cdc.gov/Violence Prevention/pdf/NISVS_Report2010-a.pdf

Bolton, J. M., Robinson, J., & Sareen, J. (2009). Self-medication of mood disorders with alcohol and drugs in the National Epidemiologic Survey on Alcohol and Related Conditions. *Journal of Affective Disorders, 115*, 367–375.

Boonstra, H. (2009). Home visiting for at-risk families: A primer on a major Obama administration initiative. *Guttmacher Policy Review, 12*(3).

Boster, F., & Strom, R. (2007). Dropping out of high school: A meta-analysis assessing the effect of messages in the home and in school. *Communication Education, 56*(4), 433–452.

Boyd, M. R., & Mackey, M. (2000). Alienation from self and others: The psychosocial problem of rural alcoholic women. *Archives of Psychiatric Nursing, 14*(3), 134–141.

Breiding, M. J., Black, M. C., & Ryan, G. W. (2008). Chronic disease and health risk behaviors associated with intimate partner violence—18 U.S. states/territories, 2005. *Annals of Epidemiology, 18*(7), 538–544.

Burgess, S., & Tavakoli, A. (2005). Psychometric Assessment of the Burgess-Partner Abuse Scale for Teens (B-PAST). *Aquichan, 5*(1), 96–107.

Button, D. M. (2008). Social disadvantage and family violence: Neighborhood effects on attitudes about intimate partner violence and corporal punishment. *American Journal of Criminal Justice, 33*(1), 130–147.

Campbell, J. & Humphreys, J. (Eds). (1993). *Nursing care of survivors of family violence.* St. Louis: Mosby.

Campbell, J. C., Webster, D. W., & Glass, N. (2009). The danger assessment: Validation of a Lethality Risk Assessment Instrument for intimate partner femicide. *Journal of Interpersonal Violence, 24*(4), 653–674.

Casey, E., & Beadnell, B. (2010). The structure of male adolescent peer networks and risk for intimate partner violence perpetration: Findings from a national sample. *Journal of Youth & Adolescence, 39*(6), 620–633.

Catalano, S., Smith, E., Snyder, H., & Rand, M. (2009). *Female victims of violence. Bureau of Justice Statistics: Selected findings.* Washington, DC: U.S. Department of Justice, Office of Justice Programs. Retrieved from http://bjs.ojp.usdoj.gov/content/pub/pdf/fvv.pdf

Centers for Disease Control and Prevention (2012). *Understanding teen dating violence. Fact sheet.* Washington, DC: National Center for Injury Prevention and Control, Division of Prevention. Retrieved from http://www.cdc.gov/violenceprevention/pdf/teendatingviolence2012-a.pdf

Centers for Disease Control and Prevention (2013a). *Intimate partner violence: Consequences.* Washington, DC: National Center for Injury Prevention and Control, Division of Prevention. Retrieved from http://www.cdc.gov/violenceprevention/intimatepartnerviolence/consequences.html

Centers for Disease Control and Prevention (2013b). *Intimate partner violence: Definitions.* Washington, DC: National Center for Injury Prevention and control, Division of Prevention. Retrieved from http://www.cdc.gov/ViolencePrevention/intimatepartnerviolence/definitions.html

Centers for Disease Control and Prevention (2013c). *Understanding elder abuse. Fact sheet 2013.* Washington, DC: National Center for Injury Prevention and Control, Division of Prevention. Retrieved from http://www.cdc.gov/violenceprevention/pdf/em-factsheet-a.pdf

Ceranoglu, T. A. (2010). Star Wars in psychotherapy: Video games in the office. *Academy of Psychiatry, 34*(3), 233–236.

Chen, P., Rovi, S., Washington, J., Jacobs, A., Vega, M., Pan, K., et al. (2007). Randomized comparison of 3 methods to screen for domestic violence in family practice. *Annals of Family Medicine, 5*(5), 430–435.

Child Welfare Information Gateway (2013). *Child witnesses to domestic violence.* Washington, DC: U.S. Department of Health and Human Services, Children's Bureau.

Cole, J., & Logan, T. K. (2008). Negotiating the challenges of multidisciplinary responses to sexual assault victims: Sexual assault and victim advocacy programs. *Research in Nursing and Health, 31*(1), 76–85.

Cole, J., Logan, T. K., & Shannon, L. (2008). Women's risk for revictimization by a new abusive partner: For what should we be looking? *Violence & Victims, 23*(3), 315–330.

Crofford, L. J. (2007). Violence, stress, and somatic syndromes. *Trauma, Violence, & Abuse, 8*(3), 299–313.

Coulter, M., & VandeWeerd, C. (2009). Reducing domestic violence and other criminal recidivism: effectiveness of a multilevel batterers intervention program. *Violence & Victims, 24*(2), 139–152.

Cutchin, M., Coppola, S., Talley, V., Syihula, J., Catellier, D., & Shank, K. (2009). Feasibility and effects of preventive home visits for at-risk older people: design of a randomized controlled trial. *BMC Geriatrics, 9*, 54.

Duke, J. R., & Cunradi, C. B. (2011). Measuring intimate partner violence among male and female farmworkers in San Diego County, CA. *Cultural Diversity and Ethnic Minority Psychology, 17*(1), 59–67.

Dutton, M. A., Green, B. L., Kaltman, S. I., Roesch, D. M., Zeffiro, T. A., & Krause, E. D. (2006). Intimate partner violence, PTSD, and adverse health outcomes. *Journal of Interpersonal Violence, 21*(7), 955–967.

Eastman, B. J., Bunch, S. G., Williams, A. H., & Carawan, L. W. (2007). Exploring the perceptions of domestic violence service providers in rural localities. *Violence Against Women, 13*(7), 700–716.

Eckhardt. C., Murphy, C., Black, D., & Suhr, L. (2006). Intervention programs for perpetrators of intimate partner violence: Conclusions from a clinical research perspective. *Public Health Report, 121*(4), 369–381.

Eddy, T., Kilburn, E., Chang, C., Bullock, L., & Sharps, P. (2008). Facilitators and barriers for implementing home visit interventions to address intimate partner violence: Town and gown partnerships. *Nursing Clinics North America, 43*(3), 419–435.

Enander, V. (2010). "A fool to keep staying": Battered women labeling themselves stupid as an expression of gendered shame. *Violence Against Women, 16*(1), 5–31.

Ernst, A. A., Weiss, S. J., Enright-Smith, S., Hilton, E., & Byrd, S. C. (2008). Perpetrators of intimate partner violence use significantly more methamphetamine, cocaine, and alcohol than victims: A report by victims. *American Journal of Emergency Medicine, 2*(5), 592–596.

Fering, C., Simon, V. A., & Cleland, C. M. (2009). Childhood sexual abuse, stigmatization, internalizing symptoms, and the development of sexual difficulties and dating aggression. *Journal of Consulting and Clinical Psychology, 77*(1), 127–137.

Finzi-Dottan, R., & Karu, T. (2006). From emotional abuse in childhood to psychopathology in adulthood: A path mediated by immature defense mechanisms and self-esteem. *Journal of Nervous and Mental Disorders, 194*(8), 616–621.

Ford-Gilboe, M., Wuest, J., Varcoe, C., Davies, L., & Merritt-Gray, M. (2009). Modelling the effects of intimate partner violence and access to resources on women's heath in the early years after leaving an abusive partner. *Social Science & Medicine, 68*(6), 1021–9.

Franklin, C. A., & Kercher, G. A. (2012). The intergenerational transmission of intimate partner violence: Differentiating correlates in a random community sample. *Journal of Family Violence, 27*, 187–199.

Grzywacz, J. G., Rao, P., Gentry, A., Marin, A., & Arcury, T. A. (2009). Acculturation and conflict in Mexican immigrants' intimate partnerships: The role of women's labor force participation. *Violence Against Women, 15*(10), 1194–1212.

Habigzang, L., Stroeher, F., Hatzenberger, R., Cunha, R., Ramos, S., & Koller, S. (2009). Cognitive behavioral group therapy for sexually abused girls. *Review Saude Publica, 43*(suppl 1), 70–78.

Harvey, S., & Taylor, J. (2010). A meta-analysis of the effects of psychotherapy with sexually abused children and adolescents. *Clinical Psychology Review, 30*(6), 749–767.

Henderson, C., Rowe, C., Dakof, G., Hawes, S., & Liddle, H. (2009). Parenting practices as mediators of treatment effects in an early-intervention trial of multidimensional family therapy. *American Journal of Drug and Alcohol Abuse, 35*(4), 220–226.

Hien, D., Jiang, H., Campbell, A., Hu, M., Miele, M., Cohen, L., et al. (2010). Do treatment improvements in PTSD severity affect substance use outcomes? A secondary analysis from a randomized clinical trial in NIDA's Clinical Trials Network. *American Journal of Psychiatry, 167*(1), 95–101.

Hines, D. A., & Douglas, E. M. (2011). Alcohol and drug abuse in men who sustain intimate partner violence. *Aggressive Behavior, 38*, 31–46.

Holmbeck, G., Thill, A., Bachanas, P., Garber, J., Miller, K., Abad, M., et al. (2008). Evidence-based assessment in pediatric psychology: Measures of psychosocial adjustment and psychopathology. *Journal of Pediatric Psychology, 33*(9), 958–980.

Houry, D., Kemball, R., Click, L., & Kaslow, N. (2007). Development of a brief mental health screen for intimate partner violence victims in the emergency department. *Academy of Emergency Medicine, 14*(3), 202–209.

Hunnicutt, G. (2009). Varieties of patriarchy and violence against women. *Violence Against Women, 15*(5), 553–573.

Jacobi, G., Dettmeyer, R., Banaschak, S., Brosig, B., & Herrmann, B. (2010). Child abuse and neglect: Diagnosis and management. *Deutsches Ärzteblatt International, 107*(13), 231–240.

Joshi, P. T., Daniolos, P. T., & Salpekar, J. A. (2010). Child abuse & neglect. In M. K. Dulcan (Ed.), *Dulcan's textbook of child and adolescent psychiatry.* Arlington, VA: American Psychiatric Publishing.

Kanter, J., Rusch, L., Landes, S., Holman, G., Whiteside, U., & Sedivy, S. (2009). The use and nature of present-focused interventions in cognitive and behavioral therapies for depression. *Psychotherapy, 46*(2), 220–223.

Karande, S., Kumbhare, N., Kulkarni, M., & Shah, N. (2009). Anxiety levels in mothers of children with specific learning disability. *Journal of Postgraduate Medicine, 55*(3), 165–170.

Klostermann, K. (2006). Substance abuse and intimate partner violence: Treatment considerations. *Substance Abuse Treatment Prevention Policy, 1*, 24.

Koepsell, J. K., Kernic, M. A., & Holt, V. L. (2006). Factors that influence battered women to leave their abusive relationships. *Violence & Victims, 21*(2), 131–147.

Kwesiga, E., Bell, M. P., Pattie, M., & Moe, A. M. (2007). Exploring the literature on relationships between gender roles, intimate partner violence, occupational status, and organizational benefits. *Journal of Interpersonal Violence, 22*(3), 312–326.

Laumann, E., Leitsch, S., & Waite, L. (2008). Elder mistreatment in the United States: Prevalence estimates from a nationally representative study. *Journal of Gerontology, 63*(4), S248–S254.

Leggatt, M. (2007). Minimising collateral damage: Family peer support and other strategies. *Medical Journal of Australia, 187*(7 suppl), S61–S63.

Leserman, J. & Drossman, D. A. (2007). Relationship of abuse history to functional gastrointestinal disorders and symptoms: Some possible mediating mechanisms. *Trauma, Violence & Abuse, 8*(3), 331–43.

Levesque, D., Driskell, M., Prochaska, J. & Prochaska, J. (2008). Acceptability of a stage-matched expert system intervention for domestic violence offenders. *Violence & Victims, 23*(4), 432–445.

Li, Q., Kirby, R. S., Sigler, R. T., Hwang, S., & LaGory, M. E. (2010). A multilevel analysis of individual, household, and neighborhood correlates of intimate partner violence among low-income pregnant women in Jefferson County, Alabama. *American Journal of Public Health, 3*, 531–539.

Lindhorst, T., Meyers, M. & Casey, E. (2008). Screening for Domestic Violence in Public Welfare Offices: An Analysis of Case Manager and Client Interactions. *Violence against Women, 14*(5), 5–28.

Lipsky, S., Krupski, A., Roy-Byrne, P., Lucenko, B., Mancuso, D., & Huber, A. (2010). Effects of co-occurring disorders and intimate partner violence on substance abuse treatment. *Journal of Substance Abuse Treatment, 38*(3), 231–244.

Marshall, A. D., & Holtzworth-Munroe, A. (2010). Recognition of wives' emotional expressions: A mechanism in the relationship between psychopathology and intimate partner violence. *Journal of Family Psychology, 24*(1), 21–30.

Mauricio, A. M., & Lopez, F. G. S. (2009). A latent classification of male batterers. *Violence & Victims, 24*, 419–438.

McDonald, R., Jouriles, E., Tart, C., & Minze, L. (2009). Children's adjustment problems in families characterized by men's severe violence toward women: Does other family violence matter? *Child Abuse & Neglect, 33*(2), 94–101.

McPhail, B. A., Busch, N. B., Kulkarni, S., & Rice, G. (2010). An integrative feminist model: The evolving feminist perspective on intimate partner violence. *Violence Against Women, 13*(8), 817–841.

Meade, C., Kershaw, T., Hansen, N., & Sikkema, K. (2009). Long-term correlates of childhood abuse among adults with severe mental illness: Adult victimization, substance abuse, and HIV sexual risk behavior. *AIDS Behavior, 13*(2), 207–216.

Morland, L. A., Leskin, G. A., Block, C. R., Campbell, J. C., & Friedman, M.J. (2008). Intimate partner violence and miscarriage: Examination of the role and physical and psychological abuse and posttraumatic stress disorder. *Journal of Interpersonal Violence, 23*(5), 652–669.

Morton, R., Tong, A., Howard, K., Snelling, P., & Webster, A. (2010). The views of patients and carers in treatment decision making for chronic kidney disease: Systematic review and thematic synthesis of qualitative studies. *British Medical Journal*, in press.

National Coalition of Antiviolence Programs (2013). *2012 Report on lesbian, gay, bisexual, transgender, queer, and HIV-affected intimate partner violence.* Retrieved from http://www.avp.org/storage/documents/ncavp_2012_ipvreport.final.pdf

National Council on Elder Abuse (n.d.). *Frequently asked questions.* Retrieved from www.nced.aoa.gov/faq/index.aspx

National Network to End Domestic Violence (2014). *The Violence Against Women Reauthorization Act.* Retrieved from http://nnedv.org/policy/issues/vawa.html.

Nidich, S. I., Rainforth, M. V., Haaga, D. A., Hagelin J., Salerno J. W., Travis F, et al. (2009). A randomized controlled trial on effects of the transcendental mediation program on blood pressure, psychological distress, and coping in young adults. *American Journal of Hypertension, 22*(12), 1326–1331.

Pardue, A., & Arrigo, M. (2008). Power, anger, and sadistic rapists: Toward a differentiated model of offender personality. *International Journal of Offender Therapy and Comparative Criminology, 52*(4), 378–400.

Pigeon, W., May, P., Perlis, M., Ward, E., Lu, N., & Talbot, N. (2009). The effect of interpersonal psychotherapy for depression on insomnia symptoms in a cohort of women with sexual abuse histories. *Journal Trauma Stress, 22*(6), 634–648.

Pinkerton, S., Bogart, L., Howerton, D., Snyder, S., Becker, K., & Asch, S. (2009). Cost of OraQuick oral fluid rapid HIV testing at 35 community clinics and community-based organizations in the USA. *AIDS Care, 21*(9), 1157–1162.

Pirkola, S., Saarni, S., Suvisaari, J., Elovainio, M., Partonen, T., Aalto, A., et al. (2009). General health and quality-of-life measures in active, recent, and comorbid mental disorders: A population-based health 2000 study. *Comprehensive Psychiatry, 50*(2), 108–114.

Pornari, C. D., Dixon, L., & Humphreys, G. W. (2013). Systematically identifying implicit theories in male and female intimate partner violence perpetrators. *Aggression and Violent Behavior, 18*, 496–505.

Puskar, K., Ren, D., Bernardo, L., Haley, T., & Stark, K. (2008). Anger correlated with psychosocial variables in rural youth. *Issues in Comprehensive Pediatric Nursing, 31*(2), 71–87.

Rabin, R., Jennings, M., Campbell, J., & Bair-Merritt, M. (2009). Intimate partner violence screening tools. *American Journal Preventive Medicine, 36*(5), 439–445.

Resnick, H., Acierno, R., Amstadter, A., & Self-Brown, S. (2007). An acute post-sexual assault intervention to prevent drug abuse: Updated findings. *Addictive Behaviors, 32*(10), 2032–2045.

Rhatigan, D. L., Street, A. E., & Axsom, D. K. (2006). A critical review of theories to explain violent relationship termination: Implications for research and intervention. *Clinical Psychological Review, 26*, 321–345.

Rhodes, K., Frankel, R., Levinthal, N., Prenoveau, E., Bailey, J., & Levinson, W. (2007). "You're not a victim of domestic violence, are you?" Provider–patient communication about domestic violence. *Annals of Internal Medicine, 147*(9), 620–627.

Roy-Byrne, P., Craske, M., Sullivan, G., Rose, R., Edlund, M., Lang, A., et al. (2010). Delivery of evidence-based treatment for multiple anxiety disorders in primary care: a randomized controlled trial. *Journal of the American Medical Association, 303*(19), 1921–1928.

Saarni, S., Suvisaari, J., Sintonen, H., Pirkola, S., Koskinen, S., Aromaa, A., et al. (2007). Impact of psychiatric disorder on health-related quality of life: General population study. *British Journal of Psychiatry, 190*(4), 326–332.

Salari, S. (2007). Patterns of intimate partner homicide suicide in later life: Strategies for prevention. *Journal of Clinical Interventions in Aging, 2*(3), 441–452.

Sandmoe, A., & Kirkevold, M. (2010). Nurses' clinical assessments of older clients who are suspected victims of abuse: An exploratory study in community care in Norway. *Journal of Clinical Nursing, 20*(1–2), 94–102.

Sansone, R., McLean, J., & Wiederman, M. (2008). The relationship between medically self-sabotaging behaviors and borderline personality disorder among psychiatric inpatients. *Prim Care Companion Journal of Clinical Psychiatry, 10*(6), 448–452.

Schafran, L. H., Lopez-Boy, S., & Davis, M. R. (2008). Making marital rape a crime: A long road traveled, a long way to go. *Washington Coalition of Sexual Assault Programs.* Retrieved from http://www.wcsap.org/pdf/makingmartialrapeacrime.pdf.

Scheffer, L., & Renck, B. (2008). It is still so deep-seated, the fear: Psychological stress reactions as consequences of intimate partner violence. *Journal of Psychiatric and Mental Health Nursing, 15*(3), 219–228.

Sedlak, A. J., Mettenburg, J., Basena, M., Petta, I., McPherson, K., Greene, A., et al. (2010). *Fourth National Incidence Study of Child Abuse and Neglect (NIS–4): Report to Congress.* Washington, DC: U.S. Department of Health and Human Services, Administration for Children and Families.

Sharps, P. W., Laughon, K., & Giangrande, S. K. (2007). Intimate partner violence and the childbearing year: maternal and infant health consequences. Trauma Violence Abuse, 8(2), 105–116.

Shurman, L. A. (2006). Cognitive-affective predictors of women's readiness to end domestic violence relationships. *Journal of Interpersonal Violence, 21*(11), 1417–1439.

Smith, P. H., Homish, G. G., Leonard, K. E., & Cornelius, J. R. (2012). Intimate partner violence and specific substance use disorders: Findings from the National Epidemiologic Survey on Alcohol and Related Conditions. *Psychology and Addictive Behavior, 26*(2), 236–245.

Son, J., & Choi, Y. (2010). The effect of an anger management program for family members of patients with alcohol use disorders. *Archives of Psychiatric Nursing, 24*(1), 38–45.

Stalans, L. J., & Magnus, S. (2007). Indentifying subgroups at high risk of dropping out of domestic batterer treatment. *Journal of Offender Therapy and Comparative Criminology, 51*(2), 151–169.

Thackarey, J., Hibbard, R., & Dowd, M. D. (2010). Intimate partner violence: The role of the pediatrician. *Pediatrics, 125*(5), 1094–1100.

Trzesniewski, K. H., Donnellan, M. B., Moffitt, T. E., Robins, R. W., Poulton, R., & Caspi, A. (2006). Low self-esteem during adolescence predicts poor health, criminal behavior, and limited economic prospects during adulthood. *Developmental Psychology, 42*(2), 381–390.

U.S. Department of Health and Human Services, Administration for Children and Families, Administration on Children, Youth and Families, Children's Bureau (2010). *Child maltreatment 2009.* Retrieved from http://www.acf.hhs.gov/programs/cb/stats_research/index.htm#can.

U.S. Department of Justice (2007). *Female sex offenders.* Retrieved from http://www.csom.org/pubs/female_sex_offenders_brief.pdf.

U.S. Department of Justice (2013). *Reporting rape in 2013.* Retrieved from http://www.fbi.gov/about-us/cjis/ucr/recent-program-updates/reporting-rape-in-2013.

Van Breemen, C. (2009). Using play therapy in paediatric palliative care: Listening to the story and caring for the body. *International Journal of Palliative Nursing, 15*(10), 510–514.

Violence Policy Center (2012). *American roulette: Murder suicide in the United States* (4th ed). http://www.vpc.org/studies/amroul2012.pdf

Violence Policy Center (2013). *When men murder women: An analysis of 2011 homicide data.* Retrieved from www.vpc.org/studies/wmmw2013.pdf

Walsh, Z., O'Connor, B. P., Shea, M. T., Swogger, M. T., Schonbrun, Y. C. & Stuart, G. L. (2010). Subtypes of partner violence perpetrators among male and female psychiatric patients. *Journal of Abnormal Psychology, 119*(3), 563–574.

Walton, M., Murray, R., Cunningham, R., Chemack, S., Barry, K., Booth, B., et al. (2009). Correlates of intimate partner violence among men and women in an inner city emergency department. *Journal of Addiction Disorders, 28*(4), 366–381.

Weldon, S., & Gilchrist, E. (2012). Implicit theories in intimate partner violence offenders. *Journal of Family Violence, 27*, 761–772.

Wilson, H. W., & Widom, C. S. (2008). An examination of risky sexual behavior and HIV in victims of child abuse and neglect: A 30-year follow-up. *Health Psychology, 27*(2), 149–158.

Wooldredge, J., & Thistlethwaite, A. (2006). Changing marital status and desistance from intimate assault. *Public Health Report, 121*(4), 428–434.

Wu, V., Huff, H. & Bhandari, M. (2010). Pattern of physical injury associated with intimate partner violence in women presenting to the emergency department: a systematic review and meta-analysis. *Trauma, Violence & Abuse, 8*(3), 331–43.

Yaffe, M. (2010). Detection and reporting of elder abuse. *Family Medicine, 42*(2), 481–486.

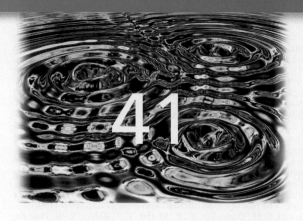

41

Caring for Persons With Mental Illness and Criminal Behavior

Rhonda Kay Wilson

KEY CONCEPTS

- early recognition
- fairness
- forensic

LEARNING OBJECTIVES

After studying this chapter, you will be able to:

1. Describe the mentally ill populations in forensic settings.

2. Discuss the stigma of mental illness and criminality.

3. Describe legal outcomes for persons with mental illness in forensic systems.

4. Assess personal attitudes in caring for persons with mental illness who have committed crimes.

5. Identify the nursing challenges in criminal justice systems.

6. Discuss rehabilitation and recovery after the mentally ill person no longer needs the forensic system.

KEY TERMS

- conditional release • court process counseling • fitness to stand trial • forensic examiner • guilty but mentally ill (GBMI) • not guilty by reason of insanity (NGRI) • probation • unfit to stand trial (UST)

The term *forensic* has its roots in the Latin word "forensics," pertaining to forum. In ancient Rome, the forum was a marketplace where people gathered to purchase things and conduct business, including legal affairs. Today the term *forensic* refers to courts of law and legal proceedings.

> **KEYCONCEPT** In mental health, the term **forensic** pertains to legal proceedings and mandated treatment of persons with a mental illness.

As the number of state hospitals was dramatically reduced beginning in the 1960s, the number of persons with mental illness incarcerated in jails and prisons increased. A large number of persons with mental illness are confined to U.S. prisons and jails. More than half of all prison and jail inmates have (or have had) a mental health problem (Thompson, 2011). It is estimated that approximately 705,600 state prison inmates, 78,800 federal prisoners, and 479,900 inmates in local jails have mental health problems (Thompson, 2011).

Individuals with mental illnesses are at higher risk for arrest than the general population (Fisher et al., 2011) and are more likely to have encounters with the criminal justice system and be convicted of a crime than those without a mental illness (Bradley-Engen, Cuddeback, Gayman, Morrissey, & Mancuso, 2010). After they enter the corrections system, female offenders are more likely than male offenders to received mental health services, and African American offenders receive significantly less mental health treatment than similar non–African Americans (Thompson, 2011).

Most of the crimes committed by persons with mental illness are misdemeanors against person and property and crimes against public decency. Other charges include drug-related offenses and assault and battery crimes on police officers (Fisher et al., 2011). There is a higher risk of serious violence (homicide) for those with a first-episode psychosis who have not yet been treated than for those who have previously received treatment (Nielssen, Yee, Millard, & Large, 2011). Despite the large number of people with mental illnesses that commit crimes, the majority of the encounters with the justice system occur when individuals with mental illness are victims of crime (Ascher-Svanum, Nyhuis, Faries, Ball, & Kinon, 2010).

Forensic patients are treated in a variety of settings, including county jails, correctional facilities, psychiatric hospitals, and the community. Inpatient services in most state hospitals now focus on those individuals who commit crimes or who are charged with an offense. The number of admissions to state psychiatric hospitals is increasing for the first time since the 1970s because of an increase of forensic patients (Manderscheid, Atay, & Crider, 2009).

Treatment and psychiatric nursing care are regulated by the mental health and legal systems, two complex systems that are sometimes in conflict with each other. Nursing care is challenging because the rules of the criminal justice system are often at odds with nursing practice standards. This chapter discusses criminal judicial processes related to mental illness, nursing management issues in forensic care, and transition for patients from a forensic setting into the community.

PERSPECTIVES ON MENTAL ILLNESS AND CRIMINAL BEHAVIOR

There are different views of mental illness and criminal behavior. Some people believe that people with mental illness commit criminal acts, and it is their mental illness that causes their actions. For example, patients with certain mental illnesses, such antisocial personality disorders or traits, are more likely to come into contact with the legal system or commit criminal acts. Others believe that people who engage in criminal behavior may also happen to be mentally ill. A third view is that, after being committed to jail, the person may develop or have an exacerbation of a mental illness such as depression and intermittent explosive disorder.

Forensic patients suffer the combined effects of the stigma of mental illness and criminality. Although stigma is an issue for all persons with a mental illness, it is magnified for those who have committed a crime. There is often reluctance on the part of mental health professionals to treat these patients, especially if murder and childhood sexual abuse are involved. Even if the worry is unfounded, clinicians express safety concerns for themselves and other patients and may refuse to care for these patients.

Stigma affects treatment and discharge of forensic patients as well. Delivery of coordinated mental health care services within a humane treatment network can be interrupted by conflict between the inpatient facility and the community. When nonforensic patients receive the maximum benefit from hospitalization, they are normally

---

BOX 41.1

The Stigma of Mental Illness: Nowhere to Call Home

"But the insane criminal has nowhere to call home: no age or nation has provided a place for him. He is everywhere unwelcome and objectionable. The prisons thrust him out; the hospitals are unwilling to receive him; the law will not let him stay at his house; and the public will not permit him to go abroad. And yet humanity and justice, the sense of common danger, and a tender regard for a deeply degraded brother-man, all agree that something should be done for him . . . " (Edward Jarvis, (pg. 195). 1857).

---

discharged into the community. For stigmatized forensic patients, the community often wants a more stringent discharge threshold and unrealistically expects the hospital to guarantee compliance with community rules and structure. These conflicting views can result in patients being discharged into community settings in a poorly coordinated fashion that sets them up for failure and another trip through the system (Box 41.1).

CRIMINAL JUDICIAL PROCESSES

There are two sides in any arrest and conviction: one side presented by the attorney of the accused and the other by the prosecution. It is important that the accused is represented by an attorney. Fairness is a basic concept underlying the criminal judicial process.

> **KEYCONCEPT** **Fairness** means that the individual who is charged with a crime should know the legal rules and be able to explain the events surrounding the alleged crime or be "fit to stand trial."

Initiation of forensic psychiatric care ideally begins at the time of arrest. If the mental illness is recognized during the arrest, the forensic mental health system becomes involved before trial. If the mental illness is not recognized, the individual may be sentenced to prison without treatment. Once in a correctional facility, if a mental illness is diagnosed, prisoners are treated in prison or transferred to a mental hospital for treatment and then returned to prison to complete their sentences.

A **forensic examiner** is a key person in the legal process. The examiner is a mental health specialist, usually a psychiatrist or psychologist, who is certified as a forensic examiner and assigned by the judge to assess and testify to the patient's competency and responsibility for the crime, including the person's mental state at the time of an offense. This testimony is based on interviews with the offender and a review of available records. The testimony directly influences the verdicts, judgments, sentencing, and damages of the defendant. For sex offenders, the examiner assesses the likelihood of recidivism and competence to stand trial.

Fitness to Stand Trial

After a mental illness is diagnosed, the person's **fitness to stand trial** is determined. Fitness means that a person is able to consult with a lawyer with a reasonable degree of rational understanding of the facts of the alleged crime and of the legal proceedings as spelled out in the court case of *Dusky vs. U.S.* of 1960 (Beran & Tommey, 1979, p. 12). A defendant is presumed to be fit to stand trial or to plead and be sentenced. A defendant is found **unfit to stand trial (UST)** if, because of mental or physical condition, he or she is unable to understand the nature and purpose of the proceedings or to assist in the defense (West, 2010).

In most states, when a mentally ill individual is found UST, hospitalization in a forensic mental health facility follows. The goal of this hospitalization is to help the person become "fit" to stand trial, not to treat the mental illness. Sometimes the patient's mental illness has to be treated to attain fitness. Simply stated, to be fit to stand trial, the person must be able to communicate with counsel and assist in the defense; be able to appreciate his or her presence in relation to time, place, and things; be able to understand that he or she is in a court of justice charged with a criminal offense; show an understanding of the charges and their consequences, as well as court procedures and the roles of the judge, jury, prosecutor, and defense attorney; and have sufficient memory to relate the circumstances surrounding the alleged criminal offense. When fitness is attained, the court is notified, and a hearing is held. If the court agrees that the individual is fit to stand trial, the case then goes to trial. If it is the court's opinion that the individual is still unfit, the individual is returned to the hospital.

An individual cannot be "unfit" forever. If fitness cannot be attained within 1 year, a hearing must be held, during which the facts of the alleged crime are presented to a judge who rules on the case. If the charges are dismissed, the judge could order a civil commitment (see Chapter 4). If there is sufficient evidence to convict, the individual could be sent back to the hospital for further treatment to attain fitness. The maximum length of this additional treatment is based on the severity of the charge. For those accused of sexual-related offenses (because of mental disorder), states usually have special statutes for hospitalization and discharge (e.g., registration and community notification).

Not Guilty by Reason of Insanity

A possible outcome or disposition of a hearing or trial is **not guilty by reason of insanity (NGRI)**. The accused

is judged to not know right from wrong or to be unable to control his or her actions at the time of the crime. The rationale underlying this ruling is one of fairness. It is unfair to hold a person responsible if that individual does not know that the action is wrong or does not have control over his or her behavior.

After a finding of NGRI, the individual is ordered to a forensic facility for a psychiatric evaluation, and the treatment recommendations are submitted to the court. Nearly all of those individuals found NGRI are also subject to involuntary commitment in a "secure" setting. Periodic reports of the individual's progress are sent back to the court. The patient cannot leave hospital grounds without court approval, and only the committing court can discharge these individuals from the hospital.

There are many misconceptions about the insanity plea. One is that the insanity defense provides a loophole through which criminals can escape punishment for illegal acts. In reality, the insanity defense is extremely difficult to use even in the cases of severely ill individuals. As a result, despite popular belief, the insanity defense is used in fewer than 1% of criminal cases (Box 41.2).

Countless newspaper articles, talk shows, and news commentaries concerning the insanity defense have bombarded the public. Some of the cases have been highly publicized. One such case was that of John Hinckley, who attempted to assassinate President Ronald Reagan in 1981 and who was found NGRI. On psychiatric examination, Hinckley was found to be living in a "fantasy world with magical and grandiose expectations of impressing and winning over" his love, actress Jodie Foster (Goldstein, 1995, p. 309). Hinckley attempted to commit a historic deed that would make him famous and unite him with the love object of his delusions. His acquittal stimulated public cries for reform of the insanity defense. Within 2.5 years of John Hinckley's acquittal, 34 states changed their insanity

---

BOX 41.2

The Case of Andrea Yates

In March 2002, Andrea Yates, age 37 years, was convicted of murder for drowning her five children. She was sentenced to life in prison despite past treatment for postpartum depression and psychosis, four hospitalizations, and two suicide attempts. Andrea Yates was found guilty because in her testimony to the police, she stated that she knew the criminal justice system would punish her for her actions, implying that she knew the acts were wrong in the eyes of the law. Texas law does not recognize that for someone as ill as Andrea Yates, mental illnesses can create more powerful hierarchies of right and wrong than societal law. In July 2006, Andrea was granted a retrial because the previous verdict was overturned on appeal because of erroneous testimony. At the second trial, Andrea was found not guilty by reason of insanity. She was committed to a state mental hospital with periodic hearings before a judge to determine whether she should be released (FoxNews, 2006).

defense statutes to limit its use or to prevent the premature release of dangerous people.

Despite its rarity, there continues to be a variety of strongly held opinions over whether the insanity defense is a way to "beat the rap" or results in unfair, lengthy hospitalizations for those stigmatized as "bad and mad." Many believe that hospitalizations are shorter than prison sentences. In reality, it is nearly certain that after an individual is judged NGRI, more time is spent in a mental hospital than if the person had been sentenced to a correctional facility.

A person sentenced NGRI is given a date that is equal to the time or sentence to be served if he or she had been guilty of the crime. Most mental health facilities are reluctant to release a patient before the expiration of his or her Thiem date (date marking the end of the maximum period of sentencing). After the Thiem date expires, the forensic hospital will do an assessment, and if the patient is still a threat to him- or herself or others, the hospital will petition the court for involuntary commitment.

Guilty but Mentally Ill

Different from NGRI, in which "not guilty" individuals are committed to the mental health system, **guilty but mentally ill (GBMI)** is a criminal conviction, and the person is sent to the correctional system. Mental illness is considered a factor in the crime but not to the extent that the individual is incapable of knowing right from wrong or controlling their actions. The sentence for the GBMI is the same type of determinate sentence any inmate receives. Before release, every effort is made to ensure that patients will receive proper follow-up care in the community and close monitoring by parole staff.

Both NGRI and GBMI persons are treated for their mental disorders, but one is treated in jail and the other in a hospital. The conditions of release are different. Whereas individuals with a GBMI are subject to the correctional system's parole decisions, those with an NGRI are discharged from the hospital through the courts upon recommendations of the forensic mental health professionals.

Probation

Probation is a sentence of conditional or revocable release under the supervision of a probation officer for a specified time. For individuals with a mental illness who have committed minor offenses, probation is sometimes used instead of jail as long as care in a treatment facility can be arranged. If treatment and rehabilitation are successful, criminal charges may be dropped and a prison record avoided. Probation is also used when a criminal has served time and continued monitoring is needed after being released from the correctional facility.

Probation often includes requirements such as a mental health evaluation and an order to follow through with any recommended forms of treatment. It may include

restrictions on certain activities such as the use of alcohol and other drugs, monetary fines, or mandatory community service. Successful completion of a probationary sentence for a person with a mental illness almost certainly depends on the ability and the willingness of a community mental health clinician to work cooperatively with the court and the assigned probation officer. Forensic assertive community treatment programs are becoming more common and decrease the likelihood of recidivism (Lamberti, Deem, Weisman, & LaDuke, 2011).

Forensic Conditional Release Program

In some states, patients who are judicially committed and found to be NGRI, incompetent to stand trial, or mentally disordered sex offenders are discharged through a forensic conditional release program. Patients whose psychiatric symptoms have been stabilized and are no longer considered a danger qualify for this program, which is very similar to parole for inmates released from a correctional facility. In **conditional release**, patients are discharged but are monitored on an ongoing basis by the court and must follow established conditions and criteria to maintain their discharged status. In states that do not have this program, the patient will remain an inpatient until the date expires or until the court grants them some form of conditional release. If the patient is granted a conditional release, the court will dictate the conditions of the release.

NURSING MANAGEMENT ISSUES IN FORENSIC CARE

Forensic mental health professionals who have been providing treatment of the mentally ill forensic patients have just begun publishing evidence-based practice standards (Bowring-Lossock, 2006). These areas are addressing the skills, competence, challenges, interventions, and areas needing further research for defining the role of the forensic mental health nurse in providing care and handling the challenges of the forensic patient (Mason, Coyle, & Lovell, 2008). Self-awareness on the part of the nurse is essential. Assessment, care, medication, documentation, and interventions are targeted at the patient's specific legally relevant behaviors and issues that are the basis for their involuntary treatment. For the best possibility of recovery, it is believed that the sequencing of the interventions is the key to successful rehabilitation and recovery of the forensic patient (Glorney et al., 2010).

Self-Awareness

Self-assessment is an ongoing process in which the nurse examines personal beliefs and attitudes about patients and crimes. It is the first step toward being an effective psychiatric nurse in a forensic setting. It is essential for

BOX 41.3

Perceptions of Diagnostic Labels

One of the major barriers in recovery-oriented care is the stigma associated with persons with mental illnesses who have committed crimes. One study showed that the diagnostic label of a personality disorder further influences nurses' perception of the patient. When patients have a personality disorder, nurses are more likely to see them as needing management strategies (security and safety) than clinical interventions, which are not considered to be effective. However, the management approach does not support patients' recovery and should be recognized as ineffective (Mason, Caulfield, Hall, & Melling, 2010).

the nurse to be aware of personal feelings about patients' crimes and to identify and recognize any bias toward these patients. A positive attitude toward people with mental illnesses, including those who have committed a crime, is basic to psychiatric nursing practice. At no time is it appropriate to convey a personal negative feeling toward the patient (Box 41.3).

If there is a negative attitude toward patients, the nurse should develop a plan to deal with the underlying feelings. In the mental health treatment environment, there are many skilled clinicians such as psychiatrists, social workers, and peers who can help the nurse talk through feelings and thoughts and assist the nurse to begin to work around or through the negativity. The nurse must want to change or explore this area in order to successfully resolve any issues he or she may have.

Some nurses have found that it is not necessary to know the details of the crime in order to work effectively with the forensic patient. The legal status and dangerousness of patients are important data, but it is not essential to know the actual crimes that patients committed.

Whereas some nurses develop biases against the patients, other nurses become too involved with patients in forensic facilities. It is essential to maintain professional boundaries, and the nurse should seek assistance if he or she is unable to maintain these professional boundaries. The supervisor should be notified if the nurse finds him- or herself in a situation in which professional boundaries have been broken. Together the employee and supervisor will decide the best course of action. In some cases, the nurse will be relocated or change job assignments to avoid future contact with the patient; be referred to an Employee Assistance Program for counseling; or if the breach of professionalism is too great, the employee may be encouraged to seek other employment for his or her safety and professional integrity.

Assessment

The nursing assessment should be completed according to accepted standards (see Chapter 10). Essential assessment

considerations for the forensic patient include development of rapport, assessment of risk, and early recognition of aggressive behavior.

Development of Rapport

The development of rapport and trust are important for a successful nursing assessment. Forensic patients may be uncomfortable discussing their crimes for fear of rejection by the nursing staff and treatment team. They may also be reluctant to disclose personal information if they perceive themselves to be at risk for further prosecution if information about prior criminal activity is leaked to the district attorney's office. The nurse should reassure the patient that the focus of the assessment is mental health issues and behaviors but not specific details of the crimes.

Risk Assessment

Risk assessment is an important determination to maintain the safety of the patient and others. Upon admission to a mental health treatment facility, the staff performs a risk assessment. Patients' current level and history of dangerousness are reviewed, and a safety plan is developed. Some state mental health facilities perform a risk assessment screening to determine placement. The patient may be sent to a maximum secure mental health treatment facility based on this risk assessment. The data obtained in the risk assessment, including the patient's known history, habits, legal status, and triggers, are used to develop an individualized treatment plan.

Early Recognition

KEYCONCEPT **Early recognition** (anticipating aggressive behavior) is based on the premise that even though behavior is idiosyncratic, it is reconstructable, similar to a "signature." After being reconstructed, the signature behavior can be used to detect early signs of deterioration and thus prevent violent behavior (Fluttert, Van Meijel, Webster, Nijman, Bartels, & Grypdonck, 2008).

Early recognition is approached from examining the antecedent, deteriorating behavior. Special attention is paid to the social and interpersonal factors related to the individual behaving violently. Subjective thoughts, feelings, and behavior underlying the aggression are precursors to violence. These early warning signs can indicate the onset of aggression, and early recognition of these warning signs can help prevent such deterioration. The aviation metaphor of a "black box" is used to emphasize the importance of attention to early warning signs. People draw upon their previous experiences (i.e., their own black box) to gain insight into their violent behavior and the warning signals for this. The goal is cooperation between the patient and the nurse in the creation of an "early recognition plan" aimed at preventing and enhancing the patient's self-management skills and thereby increasing his or her capacity to recognize the early stages of behavioral deterioration. The early recognition method provides an approach in which patients and nurses also gradually attune their perspectives on the early warning signs for aggression rather than the actual aggressive reactions in incidents. This concept is important because it enables patients to control their own behavior. Early recognition has strong practical implications for forensic nurses because it allows them to attenuate aggression by assisting patient with the detection of early warning signs (Fluttert et al., 2008).

Informed Consent

Informed consent is necessary before initiation of pharmacological treatment of forensic patients. The nursing staff collaborates with the psychiatrist to educate patients about their medications and the need to take them. The nurse also collaborates with the psychiatrist to obtain informed written or verbal consent from the patient to take medication. The informed consent is the legal responsibility of the physician, but the nurse often assists in obtaining the consent.

Forensic patients can refuse medication just as any other patient can. If patients refuse to take medication and then become a threat to themselves or others, the nurse may administer medications on an emergency basis under the direction and orders of the treating psychiatrist. The treating psychiatrist must then petition the court for a court enforced medication order if further medication or treatment is warranted. Only after a court order is obtained is medication allowed to be administered to someone who has not consented to it after the initial emergency enforce medication order period. (However, there are issues involving court ordered medication; see Box 41.4). If patients are not a threat to themselves or others, it is unlikely that the court will order medication administration. In these situations, the rights of the patient are respected, but it is often at the expense of the patient receiving the best treatment available.

BOX 41.4

Issues Regarding Court Ordered Medication

One of the biggest issues regarding enforced medication is that there is not a large variety of psychiatric medication available in the injectable form. Most injectable medications are psychotropic medications that work well for patients whose diagnoses involve psychosis or delusions. Unfortunately, a large number of forensic patients have mood disorders and issues with violence, and the medications that best treat these disorders are not available in an injectable form.

Documentation

Documentation is essential when caring for a patient with a mental illness in a forensic setting. Accurate and frequent recording of changes in mental condition, responses to treatment, and effectiveness of medication is useful information for the treatment team and the legal advocates. It is crucial that moods, behaviors, and overall mental health state are monitored and documented on a regular basis. Nursing interventions and the patient's response to the nursing care should always be documented. In addition, the patient's medical condition and the nursing care associated with these physical problems should be recorded.

Specific Interventions

Court Process Counseling

An understanding of the legal proceedings is essential for any person charged with crimes. **Court process counseling** educates mentally ill patients about impending legal procedures and prepares them for courtroom appearances. This intervention is used for all forensic patients, including those preparing for their fitness to stand trial hearing as well as those preparing for discharge. Factual information such as roles and functions of key courtroom personnel, potential pleas that might be offered in court, and the nature of the legal process are basic to this intervention. Fitness issues are discussed as appropriate.

Patients also have an opportunity to develop skills for interacting in a courtroom through mock trials and court process games. Groups and classes are often held for patients who are UST. These group sessions or class sessions teach the patient about fitness issues for the psychiatrist, forensic examiner, and the court to find them fit. These groups and classes usually test the patient's knowledge of the court by giving a written examination that the patient must pass before being found fit.

Physical Management of Aggression

Forensic patients frequently come from violent backgrounds and are often physically aggressive. Confined to living with others who are also aggressive, these patients are easily provoked into verbal and physical aggression. Management of aggressive behavior is a priority and involves structuring of the physical environment, de-escalation techniques, and pharmacological interventions.

Forensic mental health facilities focus on providing a safe and secure environment. Furniture and decorations are minimal, and patient rooms are routinely inspected for any objects that can be used to cause injury to the patient or others. Patient movement and daily activities are carefully overseen and are very structured so the staff knows the whereabouts of the patients and their activities at all times.

BOX 41.5

Sensory Modulation and Integration Activities

GROUNDING PHYSICAL ACTIVITIES
Holding
Weighted blankets
Arm massages
Aerobic exercise
Sour or fireball candies

CALMING SELF-SOOTHING ACTIVITIES
Hot shower or bath
Drumming
Decaffeinated tea
Rocking in a rocking chair
Beanbag tapping
Yoga
Wrapping in a heavy quilt

COMFORT ROOMS
The comfort room is a room that provides sanctuary from stress or can be a place for persons to experience feelings within acceptable boundaries. The comfort room is set up to be physically comfortable and pleasing to the eye, including a recliner chair, walls with soft colors and murals, and colorful curtains.

De-escalation techniques are commonly used in the forensic mental health setting. The primary goal of de-escalation is to resolve angry or violent conflicts in nonviolent ways (see Chapter 19). Most forensic mental health facilities use a nonviolent crisis intervention model that is based on the assumption that patients should not be further provoked if they are already in a state of agitation. These patients should be given space and time to calm down. They should be addressed in a calm, reasonable, and nonthreatening tone. For staff safety, agitated patients should be de-escalated by more than one staff member. Other de-escalation techniques include distraction, active listening, and sensory modulation and integration activities (Box 41.5). At all times, the patient should be involved in the decision-making process, and their wishes and preferences for de-escalation techniques should be considered and honored if possible. For example, some patients may ask to talk to someone, and others may want to be left alone. As a last resort, physical holds, seclusion, or restraints to protect patients from harming themselves or others can be applied.

Antianxiety medications, mood stabilizers, or antipsychotic medications can be given to assist agitated patients in calming down. Antipsychotic medications are used for patients with psychosis and mania. The disadvantage of antipsychotic medication is the risk of side effects such as acute muscular spasms and potentially irreversible tardive dyskinesia. Antianxiety and hypnotic medications such as lorazepam (Ativan) and diphenhydramine (Benadryl) are used for as-needed management of aggressive episodes that occur despite taking antipsychotic medication as prescribed. Other medications that have been found to be helpful in managing symptoms underlying aggressive

behavior are the mood stabilizers (lithium, carbamazepine, valproic acid) and β-blockers (propranolol, metoprolol).

Promotion of Medication Adherence

Medication administration presents unique challenges for the nursing staff. Patients frequently do not believe they have mental illnesses or do not believe or trust the staff to properly treat their mental illnesses. When patients do not trust the staff, they often refuse to take their medications as prescribed. Nursing staff should always be vigilant and observe patients carefully to ensure that they are taking their medications and not spitting, cheeking (hiding medication in their cheeks to avoid swallowing), hiding, or throwing away their medications. At the same time, nurses need to work on developing a trusting therapeutic relationship with their patients. As nurses gain the trust of their patients, patients often agree to try the medication.

Issues Specific to a Correctional Setting

Correctional facilities are regulated by the judicial system, not by state departments of mental health. Nursing care in these facilities is held to the same standard of care as in any setting, but the circumstances are different. For example, medications are administered through a window or opening in the bars in the cell house and are usually crushed and dissolved in water before giving them to the patient. If an inmate refuses medication, the authorities take the necessary steps to enforce compliance.

The nursing care in the corrections setting is conducted in a call line system. Any inmate who becomes ill or has a medical complaint notifies the guard, who in turn contacts the nurse, who checks the inmate and administers first aid if indicated. After the assessment, the nurse may place the inmate on the sick call line, which is either medical or psychiatric. The inmate will then be seen by the nurse or physician during office hours. If indicated, medications will be ordered. After being seen, the inmate returns to the cell house. If physically ill, the patient may be admitted to the health care unit for medical treatment until the illness is resolved. If psychiatric problems persist despite medication, the patient may be transferred to a psychiatric treatment facility within the correctional system.

Rehabilitation and Recovery

To successfully rehabilitate a forensic patient, the treatment team must provide many interventions timed appropriately that will teach and prepare the patient to live, work, and excel upon discharge. The biggest challenge is to balance the concept of recovery and human rights while maintaining safety, risk assessment, and security (Timmons, 2010). The forensic patient with a mental illness has a new hope that exists today because of acceptance of the recovery model; the patient can realize the potential to lead a "normal" life, possibly for the first time in his or her life. The areas to be addressed in the rehabilitation or teaching phase of care include education, risk-reduction strategies, interpersonal skills training, occupational training, violence prevention skills or plan development, physical health education and maintenance care plans, cultural and spiritual needs, living skills training, development of connections for a support group to foster hope, and planning on how to coordinate and continue all of these areas upon discharge (Glorney et al., 2010).

TRANSITIONING TO THE COMMUNITY AFTER DISCHARGE OR RELEASE
Public Safety on Release

The issue of public safety is often raised regarding the care and discharge of patients with psychiatric disorders. The reality is that patients with psychiatric problems are more likely victims than perpetrators of criminal activity. For patients who are admitted to treatment facilities because they have committed a crime, the development of sound conditional release programs (discussed earlier) is one approach many states use. The authority to release from hospitalization or to monitor and enforce mandatory outpatient treatment varies considerably across jurisdictions. The fate of the forensic patient may lie with a legal agent (court), a clinical agent (hospital staff), or a special administrative panel (clinical review board or psychiatric security review board).

Often social and political considerations influence judges and clinicians toward conservative placement and release decisions. Judges risk adverse publicity if they release a patient who again becomes violent in the community. Clinicians, on the other hand, may be fearful of malpractice litigation for wrongful imprisonment. In reality, the treatment team's release decision is based on a variety of factors, including the patient's potential for future violence, the current political climate, and skillfulness of the attorney who portrays the patient as having no potential for violence.

Services to Facilitate Transition

Providing quality services to persons with mental illness who are involved with the legal system can be a long and complicated process. There are many opportunities for an individual to "fall through the cracks" and miss receiving services that are needed to live successfully in the community. Sometimes critical services are not available, and sometimes service planners, family members, and the individuals do not know how to access available services. Some mental health agencies are unwilling to serve an "ex-offender." Patients discontinue treatment and services for a variety of reasons, including medication side effects, substance abuse, long waiting lists, lack of services, lack of

money for medication, and a lack of sufficient parole staff to monitor and encourage compliance. When individuals do not receive the services they need, for whatever reason, their chances for repeat hospitalizations or legal difficulties are high.

In addition to mental health services, these patients need a wide range of other services, including medical and dental care, housing, food, and clothing. Financial and legal services along with support services such as self-help groups and spiritual and recreational opportunities are also needed. Rehabilitation services, including education, training, and employment, are needed.

SUMMARY OF KEY POINTS

- There are special legal terms and considerations for individuals who have mental disorders and commit crimes. Those determined to be *unfit to stand trial* are mentally incompetent and unable to understand the proceedings against them or assist in their own defense. These patients are committed to a mental health facility for treatment until they achieve fitness. Those determined to be *not guilty by reason of insanity* are those who demonstrate that they had no understanding of their actions and no control over them when they committed the crime. These patients are committed to a mental health facility for treatment and then discharged after treatment.

- *Guilty but mentally ill* applies to those who demonstrate that they knew the wrongfulness of their actions and had the ability to act otherwise. These patients enter the correctional system and receive treatment for their disorder but are returned after treatment to serve their sentences. For mentally disordered sex offenders, states usually have special statutes for hospitalization and discharge. Prisoners who develop mental illness while in prison are transferred to a mental hospital, treated, and returned to prison to complete their sentences.

- In caring for the forensic patient, the nurse focus is on assessment, communication, developing a trusting relationship, and compliance with treatment.

- The role of the nurse in managing the forensic patient is to pharmacologically treat symptoms underlying aggression and at times use seclusion or restraints to manage physical aggression. The nurse needs to build a trusting therapeutic relationship with the patient to help the patient make informed choices about being compliant with his or her desired treatment plan. Another nursing intervention is to ensure that the teaching needs of the patient are met. These needs include medication education, court process education, and rehabilitation skills.

■ After the decision to release the forensic patient from the inpatient setting is made, often the community providers have felt reluctant to accept recipients who have been involved with the criminal justice system. They express fears about the person's level of dangerousness, protection of staff and peers, and potential liability.

■ The goal is to coordinate mental health services and to provide the forensic patient with a wide range of services that will help him or her successfully live within his or her community.

CRITICAL THINKING CHALLENGES

1. Describe the differences between UST, NGRI, and GBMI.

2. What are the criteria to be met by patients who are UST before they are determined to be fit to stand trial?

3. Under what circumstances should a person in a forensic setting no longer have the right to refuse medication? Keep in mind the patient's right for informed consent.

4. A patient has schizoaffective disorder and has been violent with injuries to both patients and staff. The patient has been ordered court-enforced medication as a result of his violence and psychosis. The intramuscular psychotropic enforced medication is not improving the patient's delusions or his violence. The court has ordered valproic acid medication, and it has improved the patient's violence in the past, but it does not come in an intramuscular injectable form. Discuss feasible strategies for administering the medication.

5. If you were responsible for a caseload at a community mental health center, would you be fearful of accepting a patient with a criminal background?

MOVIES *Sling Blade:* 1996. Sling Blade is a drama set in rural Arkansas starring Billy Bob Thornton, who plays a man named Karl Childers who is released from a psychiatric hospital where he has lived since committing murder at 12 years of age. He is a very simple man who thinks in concrete terms. He befriends a young boy and begins a friendship with the boy's mother. He then finally confronts the mother's abusive boyfriend. This film won many awards.

VIEWING POINTS: If Karl had been successfully rehabilitated, how would he have handled his rage? Does this film perpetuate the myth that people with mental illness are dangerous? Was the murder justified?

Inside/Outside Video: 2004. This video was developed by and stars consumers who have all reached recovery.

The video envisions the patient on a journey to recovery and parallels Theo's primary focus is to give the consumers hope for the future, encouraging them to take responsibility for themselves and their actions and to try to seek recovery.

VIEWING POINTS: How does this video realize the components of recovery components? How would you use this film to instill hope in a person who has a mental illness and is incarcerated in prison?

References

Ascher-Svanum, H., Nyhuis, A. W., Faries, D. E., Ball, D. E., & Kinon, B. J. (2010). Involvement in the U.S. criminal justice system and cost implications for persons treated for schizophrenia. *BMC Psychiatry, 10,* 11.

Beran, N. J., & Tommey, B. G. (1979). Mentally ill offenders and the criminal justice system. In *Issues in forensic services* (p. 1–23). New York: Proeger Publishers, Proeger Special Studios.

Bowring-Lossock, E. (2006). The forensic mental health nurse—A literature review. *Journal of Psychiatric and Mental Health Nursing, 13*(6), 780–785.

Bradley-Engen, M. S., Cuddeback, G. S., Gayman, M. D., Morrissey, J. P., & Mancuso, D. (2010). Trends in state prison admission of offenders with serious mental illness. *Psychiatric Services, 61*(12), 1263–1265.

Fisher, W. H., Simon, L., Roy-Bujnowski, K., Grudzinskas, A., Wolff, N., Crockett, E. & Banks, S. (2011). Risk of arrest among public mental health services recipients and the general public. *Psychiatric Services, 62*(1), 67–72.

Fluttert, F., Van Meijel, B., Webster, C., Nijman, H., Bartels, A., & Grypdonck, M. (2008). Risk management by early recognition of warning signs in patients in forensic psychiatric care. *Archives of Psychiatric Nursing, 22*(4), 208–216.

FOXNews.com. (July, 2006). *Jury finds Andrea Yates not guilty of murdering her children.* Retrieved December 12, 2010, from http://www.foxnews.com/printer_friendly_story/0,3566,205696,00.html.

Glorney, E., Perkins, D., Adshead, G., McGauley, G., Murray, K., Noak, J., & Sichau, G. (2010). Domains of need in a high secure hospital setting: A model for streamlining care and reducing length of stay. *International Journal of Forensic Mental Health, 9*(2), 138–148.

Goldstein, R. (1995). Paranoids in the legal system: The litigious paranoid and the paranoid criminal. *Psychiatric Clinics of North America, 18*(2), 303–315.

Jarvid, E (1857). Criminal insane. Insane transgressors and insane convicts. *American Journal of Insanity, 13*(3), 198–231.

Lamberti, J. S., Deem, A., Weisman, R. L., & LaDuke, C. (2011). The role of probation in forensic assertive community treatment. *Psychiatric Services, 62*(4), 418–421.

Manderscheid, R. W., Atay, J. E., & Crider, R. A. (2009). Changing trends in state psychiatric hospital use from 2002 to 2005. *Psychiatric Services, 60*(1), 29–34.

Mason, T., Caulfield, M., Hall, R., & Melling, K. (2010). Perceptions of diagnostic labels in forensic psychiatric practice: A survey of differences between nurses and other disciplines. *Issues in Mental Health Nursing, 31*(5), 336–344.

Mason, T., Coyle, D., & Lovell, A. (2008). Forensic psychiatric nursing: Skills and competencies: II: Clinical aspects. *Journal of Psychiatric and Mental Health Nursing, 15*(2), 131–139.

Nielssen, O. B., Yee, N. L., Millard, J. M., & Large, J. J. (2011). Comparison of first-episode and previously treated persons with psychosis found NGMI for a violent offense. *Psychiatric Services, 62*(7), 759–764.

Timmons, D. (2010). Forensic psychiatric nursing: a description of the role of the psychiatric nurse in a high secure psychiatric facility in Ireland. *Journal of Psychiatric and Mental Health Nurse, 17*(7), 636–646.

Thompson, M. (2011). Gender, race, and mental illness in the criminal justice system. *Corrections & mental health: An update of the National Institute of Corrections.* National Institute of Corrections. Retrieved from http://community.nicic.gov/blogs/mentalhealth/archive/2011/03/02/gender-race-and-mental-illness-in-the-criminal-justice-system.aspx.

West, T. (Ed.). (2010). *West Illinois criminal law and procedure, 2010 edition* (pp. 640–641). Chicago, IL: Thompson Reuters.

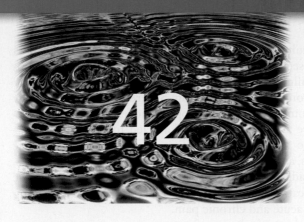

42

Caring for Medically Compromised Persons

Gail L. Kongable

KEY CONCEPT

- chronic pain

LEARNING OBJECTIVES

After studying this chapter, you will be able to

1. Identify medically ill populations at risk for psychosocial problems.

2. Discuss the impact of having both a mental disorder and a medical problem on patients and their families.

3. Discuss the psychosocial impact of pain, especially for those experiencing chronic pain.

4. Describe assessment and nursing care for patients who are experiencing mental health problems associated with HIV/AIDS, trauma, or central nervous system disorders.

5. Discuss biopsychosocial interventions that promote mental health for patients with medical disorders.

6. Discuss the importance of integrating the medical aspects of care into psychiatric care for patients with mental health problems.

KEY TERMS

- acute pain • allodynia • comorbidity • endorphins • gate-control theory • HIV-associated neurocognitive disorder (HAND) • hyperalgia • hyperesthesia • ischemic cascade • nociceptors • plasticity • prostaglandins • self-efficacy • substance P • traumatic brain injury (TBI)

A mental health problem often occurs with physical illness and has a significant impact on the person. This **comorbidity** (presence of a disorder simultaneously with and independently of another disorder) of medical and mental health conditions impairs functioning and contributes to disabilities in children and adults (Anesetti-Rothermel & Sambamoorthi, 2011; El-Mallakh, Howard, & Inman, 2010). People who have chronic medical illnesses have higher rates of psychiatric disorders than people who are healthy (Benton, Staab, & Evans, 2007).

Mood, bipolar, anxiety, and substance-related disorders are the most prevalent psychiatric conditions of patients with chronic or terminal illnesses. Increasing clinical evidence suggests that the presence of these psychiatric disorders may be an independent risk factor for increased morbidity and mortality, particularly in conditions such as chronic pain, acquired immunodeficiency syndrome (AIDS), acute trauma, cerebrovascular accident (stroke),

and cancer. Additionally, because most medically ill people are older, changes in biologic, psychological, and social function may place them at even greater risk for mental illness and increased morbidity and mortality (Moussavi, Chatterji, Verdes, Tandon, Patel, & Ustun, 2007).

OVERVIEW OF CONNECTIONS BETWEEN MENTAL HEALTH AND MEDICAL DISORDERS

Even though the pathologies of medical and psychiatric disorders are intertwined, they are often treated separately. Mental health providers may not recognize medical illness, and medical providers may not screen for mental health problems. By not recognizing the connection between the medical and mental disorders, care is fragmented and inconsistent with a holistic, recovery-oriented approach as well as *Healthy People 2020* (U.S. Department of Health and

Human Services, 2010). Consequently, medical and mental illnesses are inadequately treated and result in higher rates of morbidity and mortality (Benton et al., 2007).

Mental health problems and psychiatric symptoms may be masked by physical symptoms or remain a secondary concern when managing a medical problem. Some treatment regimens contribute to psychosocial dysfunction because many medications prescribed for chronic illness alter mood and thought processes. Health care providers may consider a patient's depressed mood or anxiety as a normal response to loss of health when in fact a mental health problem exits. When psychosocial dysfunction is not examined closely and is not treated, it can affect the course and outcome of associated medical illness. Mental health problems may precede or occur during acute hospitalization and continue after discharge and apparent physical recovery. The presence of mental health problems may diminish the motivation for self-care, impair symptom reporting, and delay treatment. As a result, hospitalization for medical problems may be prolonged and recovery delayed or impaired at increased emotional and financial cost to the patient and the family (Zhu, Zhao, Ye, Marciniak, & Swindle, 2009). In severe cases, mood disorders associated with medical illness predict morbidity and mortality (Benton et al., 2007). Therefore, careful assessment and treatment of co-occurring mental illness is required.

A related area of concern is the common comorbidity of physical disorders among people who require primary psychiatric care. Acute psychiatric settings, residential treatment settings, and psychiatric home health programs are reporting increasing numbers of patients with primary or secondary physical and medical problems (Fagiolini & Goracci, 2009). Factors associated with increased hospital stays for psychiatric patients include physical disabilities and medical illnesses (Zhu et al., 2009). Mental health professionals must carefully evaluate and monitor changes in coexisting medical conditions to prevent their exacerbation or serious complications.

This chapter reviews the psychosocial disturbances associated with chronic pain, human immunodeficiency virus (HIV), trauma, neurologic disorders, stroke, and chronic medical illnesses such as heart disease and cancer. These medical conditions were chosen because they are associated with mental health problems. Additionally, medical conditions common in those with mental disorders are discussed.

PAIN

Despite major advances in treatments that lessen its force, pain remains one of the most powerful and complex of human experiences. Assessing and treating pain is difficult because the pain response is subjective and the degree of pain cannot be observed directly and may be difficult to localize. In addition, the person's discomfort may seem out of proportion to the observed conditions or influenced by disordered emotions, personality, or environmental conditioning. Severe or chronic pain may affect mentally healthy people in adverse ways. The prevalence and impact of pain have led to numerous therapeutic approaches, including the use of antipsychotic drugs, antidepressants, antianxiety agents, and stimulants. Considerable evidence suggests that these psychiatric medications and interventions can be effective in treating both acute and chronic pain.

The Pain Response

Physiologic pain is a protective response to noxious stimuli that serves as a warning of tissue injury, inflammation, and pathologic processes that lower the threshold of sensitization. As the leading explanation of pain, the gate-control theory led to the recognition that there is not a single pain mechanism but that the processing of pain occurs on at least three levels—peripheral, spinal, and supraspinal. The **gate-control theory** holds that there are neurologic gates that can either inhibit or allow pain signals to be transmitted to the brain. At the site of the tissue injury, pain receptors (**nociceptors**) cause of release of **prostaglandins** (an unsaturated fatty acid that helps control smooth muscle contraction, blood pressure, inflammation, and body temperature) and **substance P** (a peptide found in body tissues, especially nervous tissue, that is involved in the transmission of pain and in inflammation), as well as potassium, histamine, leukotrienes (short-range chemical messengers that help regulate the state of blood vessels and airways and influence the activities of some white blood cells), and bradykinin (chemical that dilates blood vessels). These function as transmitters of a relay signal sent to the dorsal horn of the spinal cord that in turn increases the flow of impulses relayed to the brain (Box 42.1). The excitability of this pathway can be altered by inhibitory interneurons at the site of the dorsal horn, closing the gate. No pain. If the cytokines or projection neurons are released, they sensitize and stimulate central pain receptors to spread the pain experience and activate areas of the brain responsible for memory, emotion, and personality (Figure 42.1). As these ascending pathways signal higher centers, descending noradrenergic and serotonergic pathways are activated and inhibit the release of substance P, which closes the gate and thereby reduces the pain (Bartsch & Goadsby, 2011; DeLeo, 2006). See Figure 42.2.

A common question for nurses is how pain response can vary so much from person to person. There is not an easy answer, but physiologically, during pain, serotonin causes the release of **endorphins**, neurotransmitters that exhibit opioid-like behavior and produce an inhibitory effect at opioid receptor sites. This causes a muffling of the pain and, in some instances, relief. Both serotonin and endorphins are probably responsible for pain tolerance, but they may also influence emotion (limbic area), mood (medial frontal lobes), and behavioral response to pain (motor and sensory areas) (Basbaum & Julius, 2006). The interpretation of pain is personal and a result of the physical, emotional, and cognitive perception of pain interacting with cultural, social, and environmental influences.

Acute Versus Chronic Pain

Acute pain is one of the most common symptoms of patients in emergency and acute care settings. It can result from a variety of physiologic abnormalities and trauma. It is characterized by a sudden, severe onset of symptoms at

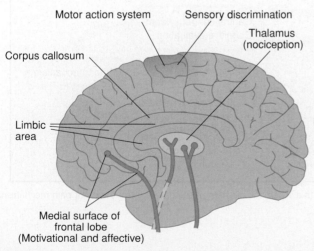

FIGURE 42.1 Pain stimuli activate regions of the brain that influence memory, emotion, and personality.

the time of injury or illness and generally subsides as the associated condition subsides or the injury heals. For example, postoperative incisional pain is an iatrogenic (treatment-induced) tissue injury most often seen in medical settings. Careful assessment and treatment of acute pain have a great impact on healing and recovery.

> **KEY CONCEPT** **Chronic pain**, defined as pain on a daily basis or pain that is constant for more than 6 months, can be related to a variety of pathologies and takes the form of syndromes such as headache, temporomandibular pain disorders, back pain, and arthritis.

Chronic pain is associated with the clinical syndromes of neoplasia (cancer), thalamic stroke (central pain), diabetes mellitus (neuropathy), and reflex sympathetic dystrophy (Box 42.2). Nervous tissue injury leads to neuropathic pain, described as burning, aching, or pricking. This central or neuropathic pain is the underlying mechanism for most chronic pain and leads to **hyperalgia** (increased sensation of pain), **allodynia** (pain unrelated to noxious stimuli, lowered pain threshold), and **hyperesthesia** (increased nociceptor sensitivity). Permanent change in central pain interpretation (**plasticity**) frequently results in abnormal physiologic, biochemical, cellular, and molecular responses that misinterpret nonpainful sensations as painful (Bartsch & Goadsby, 2011). This neural plasticity also contributes to the development of errant firing and the pain syndromes of referred pain (pain felt in a body part other than where it was produced) and phantom pain (pain sensation in a missing [amputated] limb).

Psychosocial Aspects of Chronic Pain

Chronic pain has a devastating impact on one's quality of life. When pain persists for an extended period, mood, coping skills, interpersonal relations, and financial and social resources are affected. Preoccupation with pain becomes a daily burden. Demoralization, sadness, loss of interest in life, feelings of worthlessness, self-reproach, excessive guilt, indecisiveness, and suicidal ideation are associated with chronic pain (Humphreys, Cooper, & Miaskowski, 2010).

Mood and anxiety disorders are prevalent among people with chronic pain (Casucci, Villani, & Finocchi, 2010; Tragesser, Bruns, & Disorbio, 2010). Chronic pain may precipitate major depressive or manic episodes, generalized anxiety, or panic episodes. The severity and duration of chronic pain have been shown to increase the severity of depression (Humphreys et al., 2010). Substance abuse disorders may arise as the person self-medicates in search for relief through overuse of drugs that lessen the pain sensation. Anorexia, sleep disturbance, and agitation or psychomotor retardation may occur (Humphreys et al., 2010).

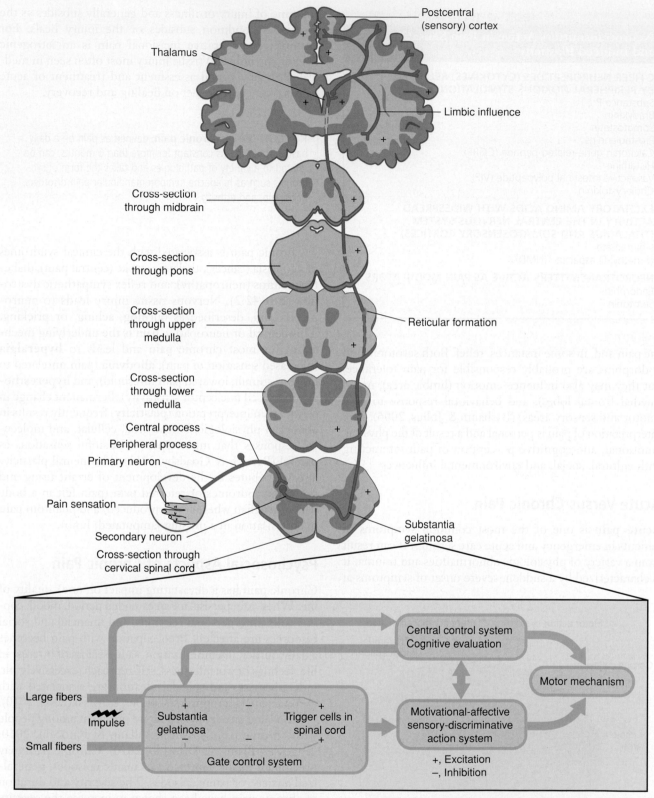

FIGURE 42.2 Ascending sensory pathways: anterior spinothalamic tract with a schematic diagram of the gate-control theory of pain mechanism.

BOX 42.2

Pain Syndromes Seen in the Primary Care Setting

- *Migraine headache:* a cerebrovasomotor disorder in which a focal reduction of cerebral blood flow initiates an ischemic headache. It may be preceded by a visual aura and followed by nausea, vomiting, and incapacitating head pain.
- *Low back pain:* pain arising from the vertebral column or surrounding muscles, tendons, ligaments, or fascia. Causes range from simple muscle strain to arthritis, fracture, or nerve compression from a ruptured disk.
- *Chronic benign orofacial pain:* temporomandibular joint pain, trigeminal neuralgia
- *Rheumatoid arthritis:* more than 100 different types of joint disease produce inflammation of the joints. Associated with varying degrees of pain and stiffness and eventual loss of use of the affected joints.
- *Reflex sympathetic dystrophy:* a painful burning syndrome that occurs after peripheral nerve injury. Associated with hyperesthesia, vasomotor disturbances, and dystrophic changes caused by sympathetic hyperactivity.
- *Cancer pain:* pain from malignant tumors that is caused by local infiltration or metastatic spread involving specific organs, bones, peripheral or cranial nerves, or the spinal cord. Pain therapy is aimed at providing sufficient relief to allow maximum possible daily functioning and a relatively pain-free death.

- *Neuropathic pain*
  - *Polyneuropathy:* neuropathy involving multiple peripheral nerves
  - *Diabetic neuropathy:* neuropathy caused by diabetes mellitus; marked by diminished sensation secondary to vascular changes
  - *Inflammatory neuropathy:* neuropathy related to the presence of chemical or microorganic pathogens
  - *Traumatic neuropathy:* neuropathy caused by avulsion or compression
  - *Plexopathy:* neuropathy involving a peripheral nerve plexus
  - *Peripheral or central neuralgia:* abrupt, intense, paroxysmal pain caused by intrinsic nerve injury or extrinsic nerve compression
  - *Herpetic neuralgia:* pain associated with the dermatomal rash of acute herpes zoster
  - *Radiculopathy:* pain radiating along a peripheral nerve tract, such as sciatica
- *Vasoocclusive pain:* thrombotic crisis of sickle cell anemia in joints and peripheral muscles that is caused by ischemia
- *Myofascial pain:* pain in palpable bands (trigger points) of muscle; associated with stiffness, limitation of motion, and weakness

Interdisciplinary Treatment and Recovery

The treatment of pain is complex and multifaceted. A thorough discussion of the treatment of pain is outside the scope of this chapter, but approaches to pain are summarized in Box 42.3. Patients' responses to individual drugs vary, and many agents at different doses may be tried before pain relief is achieved. The use of physical and psychological modulation techniques as well as pharmacotherapy or physical therapy is more successful than medical therapies alone. Alternatives to traditional medical intervention are increasingly used as adjunct therapy in patients with pain related to cancer, neuropathy, and degenerative disorders. Natural and herbal therapies, therapeutic massage, zero balancing, thought-field therapy, imaging, prayer, and meditation have all been found to be useful in easing the mental and physical discomfort of patients with medical illnesses. Also, these therapies are more satisfying to patients who otherwise must receive toxic medications as part of their conventional medical treatment.

Combination treatment often improves mood and reduces anxiety. Patients trained to use cognitive strategies such as biofeedback, a positive emotional state, relaxation, physical therapy or exercise, meditation, guided imagery, suggestion, hypnosis, placebos, and positive self-talk are able to tolerate higher levels of pain than patients without specific coping strategies. Most of these techniques involve redirecting the patient's attention away from the pain and helping the person learn strategies of **self-efficacy** (self-care effectiveness).

There are many barriers to effective pain management (Box 42.4). Reluctance to acknowledge the pain on the part of health professionals and the patient may contribute to persistent pain, which ultimately can adversely affect the patient's quality of life. Maladaptive coping leads to a fear of pain and a negative attitude about the pain and its daily effects. Non-adherence with sequential

FAME & FORTUNE

John Fitzgerald Kennedy (1917–1963)
President of the United States

PUBLIC PERSONA

As the very popular 35th president of the United States, John Kennedy promoted the civil rights movement in the United States, was instrumental in the space program, and successfully averted war with the Soviet Union over nuclear missiles placed in Cuba.

PERSONAL REALITIES

On a day-to-day basis, however, Kennedy maintained mental health despite suffering with severe pain most of his adult life. Three fractured vertebrae caused by osteoporosis gave him so much pain that he could not put a sock or a shoe on his left foot without help. He also had persistent digestive problems and Addison's disease. He took several medications a day and often received injections of procaine in his back in order to carry out his leadership duties.

BOX 42.3

Treatment Approaches to Pain

PRINCIPLES OF PAIN TREATMENT
- Establish the correct diagnosis.
- Recognize that pain reduction, rather than complete pain control, is a reasonable goal.
- Control other symptoms besides pain. This includes treating the symptoms that were present before treatment (e.g., depression and anxiety) and the adverse effects associated with the pain therapy.
- Treat physical conditions that may initiate or exacerbate the pain.

FIRST STEP
Analgesics for treatment of pain and:
Nonsteroidal antiinflammatory drugs (NSAIDs)
  Acetaminophen
  Acetylsalicylic acid
  Ibuprofen
  Ibuprofen
  Oral local anesthetics
  Flecainide
  Mexiletine
  Tocainide
Topical agents
  Capsaicin
  EMLA
  Lidocaine gel
  Baclofen
  Neuroleptics
  Pimozide
  Corticosteroids
  Calcitonin
  Benzodiazepines
  Clonazepam
Drugs for sympathetically maintained pain
  Nifedipine
  Phenoxybenzamine
  Prazosin
  Propranolol

SECOND STEP
Antidepressants, TENS, and psychosocial support, and/or:
Tricyclic and tetracyclic antidepressants
  Amitriptyline
  Clomipramine
  Desipramine
  Doxepin
  Imipramine
  Maprotiline
  Nortriptyline
  Mirtazapine
Selective and nonselective serotonin reuptake inhibitors
  Bupropion
  Citalopram
  Escitalopram
  Fluoxetine
  Fluvoxamine
  Nefazodone
  Olanzapine
  Paroxetine
  Sertraline
  Trazodone
  Venlafaxine

Serotonin–norepinephrine or dopamine reuptake inhibitors
  Desvenlafaxine
  Duloxetine
  Ziprasidone
Anticonvulsants
  Carbamazepine
  Divalproex
  Neurontin
  Phenytoin
Opioid analgesics
  Codeine
  Meperidine
  Morphine
Monoamine oxidase inhibitors
  Isocarboxazid
  Phenelzine sulfate
  Selegiline
  Tranylcypromine
  Methylphenidate
Herbal and alternative medicines
  SAMe
  Ginseng
  Swedish massage
  Acupressure
  Acupuncture
  Zero balancing
  Reflexology
  Meditation
  Prayer

Note: Treat the adverse effects of all the agents used

THIRD STEP
Adrenergic agents, TENS, and psychosocial support, and/or:
Clonidine naloxone infusion, and/or:
Other agents (mexiletine, diphenhydramine)

Note: Add the third-step agents to partially helpful agents used in first step or use alone and treat the adverse effects of all the agents used.

PROCEDURES FOR SELECTED PATIENTS
Neuroblockade
- Trigger point injection (TPI)
- Epidural steroid injection (ESI)
- Facet joint injection (FJI)
- Nerve root blocks
- Medial branch blocks
- Peripheral nerve block
- Sympathetic nerve block

Spinal Cord Stimulation
- Neurostimulator implants
- TENS
- Thalamic stimulation implants

TENS, transcutaneous electrical nerve stimulation
Note: If the patient has failed to experience response to all standard pharmacologic treatments, psychiatric evaluation for underlying problems (e.g., severe depression and risk for suicide) should be emphasized.

BOX 42.4

Barriers to Pain Management

PROBLEMS OF HEALTH CARE PROFESSIONALS
- Inadequate knowledge and experience with pain management
- Poor assessment of pain
- Concern about regulation of controlled substances
- Fear of patient tolerance and addiction
- Concern about side effects of analgesics

PROBLEMS OF PATIENTS
- Reluctance to report pain
- Concern about primary treatment of underlying disease
- Fear that pain means the disease is worse
- Concern about being a good patient and not a complainer
- Reluctance to take pain medications
- Fear of tolerance and addiction, fear of "addict" label
- Fear of unmanageable side effects

PROBLEMS OF HEALTH CARE SYSTEM
- Cost or inadequate reimbursement
- Restrictive regulation of controlled substances
- Problems with availability of treatment or access to it

---

prescription changes and combined treatments can be problematic as well. Strategies to assess adherence are regular self-report, assessment of behavioral change, biochemical assay, clinical improvement, and outcome assessment.

Assessment of Patients with Chronic Pain

Appropriate diagnosis and treatment of pain begins with a comprehensive history and physical examination. In discussing pain, a patient will not only describe its characteristics, location, and severity but also provide information about possible psychosocial and behavioral factors that are influencing the pain experience (Box 42.5). A direct relationship between the severity or extent of detectable disease and the intensity of the patient's pain may not be evident during the first interaction. Pain assessment instruments can aid in evaluation; however, using an instrument designed to measure acute pain, such as asking the patient to rate pain on a scale of 1 to 10, is inadequate for assessing chronic pain because the pain may always be a 3 or 4, but the chronic nature of the pain is the problem (Haefeli & Effering, 2006). Even when the cause of the pain is known, a comprehensive assessment of chronic pain is needed to determine the degree to which physical and psychosocial factors impact the person's life.

Nursing Interventions for Responses to Chronic Pain

The nurse has an important role in the helping the patient manage chronic pain. Listening and acknowledging the pain is important because others may ignore or invalidate the impact of the pain. The nurse can help the patient identify circumstances when the pain was diminished and use this information to develop strategies. Encouraging healthy behaviors such as diet and exercise is also important. If the patient is taking medications, the nurse should closely monitor therapeutic and untoward effects. Nurses should provide education to the patient and family about managing chronic pain and approaches to pain control.

Biologic, psychological, and sociocultural outcome measures for the patient with chronic pain control are depicted in Figure 42.3.

BOX 42.5

Assessing Patients Who Report Pain

QUESTIONS TO ASSESS PAIN
The following questions can guide the nurse in reflecting on the significance of the chronic pain to the individual and family:
- What is the extent of the patient's disease or injury (physical impairment)?
- What is the magnitude of the illness? That is, to what extent is the patient suffering, disabled, and unable to enjoy usual activities?
- Does the person's behavior seem appropriate to the disease or injury, or is there any evidence of amplification of symptoms for any of a variety of psychological or social reasons or purposes?
- How often and for how long does the patient perform specific behaviors, such as reclining, sitting, standing, and walking?
- How often does the patient seek health care and take analgesic medication (frequency and quantity)?

PAIN BEHAVIOR CHECKLIST
Pain behaviors have been characterized as interpersonal communications of pain, distress, or suffering. Pain behavior may be a more accurate indication of intensity and tolerance than verbal reports. Check the box of each behavior you observe or infer from the patient's comments.
- Facial grimacing, clenched teeth
- Holding or supporting of affected body area
- Questions such as, "Why did this happen to me?"
- Distorted gait, limping
- Frequent shifting of posture or position
- Requests to be excused from tasks or activities; avoidance of physical activity
- Taking of medication as often as possible
- Moving extremely slowly
- Sitting with a rigid posture
- Moving in a guarded or protective fashion
- Moaning or sighing
- Using a cane, cervical collar, or other prosthetic device
- Requesting help in ambulation; frequent stopping while walking
- Lying down during the day
- Irritability

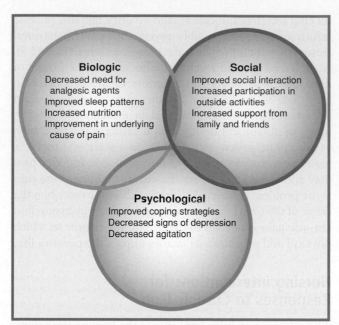

FIGURE 42.3 Biopsychosocial outcome measures for patients with pain control.

PSYCHOLOGICAL COMPLICATIONS OF HIV-ASSOCIATED NEUROCOGNITIVE DISORDER

Acquired immunodeficiency syndrome (AIDS) is characterized by multiple opportunistic infections and is associated with malignancy. People with AIDS are often overwhelmed by devastating illnesses that cause profound fatigue, insomnia, anorexia, emaciation, pain, and disfigurement. The psychological impact of AIDS is considerably worsened by the social stigma associated with the infection and the special affinity of HIV for brain and central nervous system (CNS) tissue.

Cognitive and Motor Changes in HIV-Associated Neurocognitive Disorder

HIV-associated neurocognitive disorder (HAND), one of the most common CNS manifestations of HIV, is a chronic neurodegenerative condition characterized by cognitive, central motor, and behavioral changes. HAND can affect any psychologic domain, but the most commonly reported deficits are in attention and concentration, psychomotor speed, memory and learning, information processing, and executive function. Language and visuospatial abilities are relatively unaffected. HAND is classified as a subcortical dementia (see Chapter 37) with deficits in the working memory (i.e., ability to remember information over a brief period) and executive function (e.g., planning, cognitive flexibility, abstract thinking) occurring early in the course that are present early on

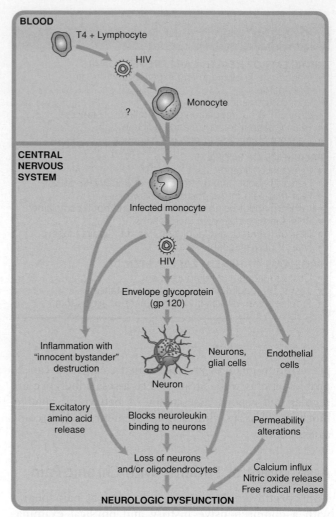

FIGURE 42.4 Possible pathologic progression of HIV neuronal injury.

(Singer, Valdes-Sueiras, Commins, & Levine, Commins, & Levine, 2010). Figure 42.4 shows the possible pathologic invasion and progression of HIV neuronal injury through inflammation, neuronal invasion, and neuronal destruction.

HIV can have profound effects on the pyramidal and extrapyramidal systems. Milder forms of extrapyramidal symptoms include ataxia, motor slowing, loss of coordination, and tremor. They can progress to disabling weakness, spasticity, and paraparesis (Singer et al., 2010). These symptoms are improved after treatment with antiretrovirals. Some studies have shown that psychostimulants (methylphenidate) improve the neurocognitive symptoms (Singer et al., 2010).

Psychological Changes Associated with HIV-Associated Neurocognitive Disorder

Apathy, irritability, and psychomotor retardation are characteristic of the behavioral changes that occur in HAND.

These changes overlap with the symptoms of depression, which occurs at a very high rate in HAND. Co-occurring conditions such as addiction to alcohol or drugs, brain damage, chronic illness, hypoxia related to pneumonia, infections, space-occupying brain lesions, and systemic reactions to medications may contribute to the progression of mental changes associated with AIDS. The psychological influences of stress and sleep and sensory deprivation can further contribute to the altered perception and mentation.

Psychiatric disorders contribute to the course of AIDS in several ways. Depression and bipolar disorder are linked to biologic changes in HIV/AIDS that may contribute to disease progression and mortality. Abnormalities in the hypothalamic–pituitary–adrenal (HPA) axis and hypercortisolemia associated with physiologic and psychological distress may alter immune response and diminish host defense in people with low CD4 counts (Cole, 2008). The neuropathology associated with the presence of HIV then may also contribute to poor adherence to antiretroviral treatment, progression of the disease, and deterioration. AIDS-associated psychopathology is frequently unrecognized, misdiagnosed, and incorrectly treated. The diagnosis can be difficult when risk factors are not known or when cognitive or psychiatric symptoms precede the onset of other manifestations of HIV/AIDS infection.

Early CNS involvement is detected through neuropsychological testing and magnetic resonance imaging. The degree of cognitive dysfunction may not be a valid indication of the degree of organic involvement. Also, diagnostic findings on computed tomography scanning such as cerebral atrophy and prominent basal ganglia calcification may not correlate with the severity of the patient's dementia (Singer et al., 2010).

Assessment of Patients with HIV-Associated Neurocognitive Disorder

Early recognition of psychiatric disorders associated with HIV/AIDS is important to enhance the understanding of the behavior of people with HIV/AIDS. Mental status changes and altered affect should be investigated through formal neurologic and psychological testing to determine the extent of impairment. Successful coping and cognitive adaptation are often further hindered by the presence of psychiatric disorders associated with HIV/AIDS (Box 42.6). These mental illnesses include mood disorders, adjustment disorders, anxiety disorders, substance use disorders, and personality disorders.

A mood disorder may be characterized by symptoms of a major depressive or manic episode. The depressed mood, feelings of guilt, anhedonia, and hopelessness can be accompanied by insomnia or hypersomnia, psychomotor retardation, or agitation and suicidal ideation. Low self-esteem, feelings of worthlessness and hopelessness,

---

BOX 42.6

Psychiatric Disorders Associated With HIV Infection

Organic mental disorder
HIV dementia or AIDS–dementia complex
Dementia associated with opportunistic infection
  Fungal
    Cryptococcoma
    Cryptococcal meningitis
    Candidal abscesses
  Protozoal
    Toxoplasmosis
  Bacterial
    Mycobacterium avium–intracellulare
  Viral
    Cytomegalovirus
    Herpesvirus
    Papovavirus progressive multifocal
    Leukoencephalopathy
Dementia associated with cancer
    Primary cerebral lymphoma
    Disseminated Kaposi's sarcoma
Delirium
Organic delusional disorder
Organic mood disorder
  Depression
  Mania
  Mixed
Affective disorders
  Major depression
  Dysthymic disorder
Adjustment disorders
  Adjustment disorder with depressed mood
  Adjustment disorder with anxious mood
Substance abuse disorder
Borderline personality disorder
Antisocial personality disorder
Bereavement
Anxiety disorders
  Generalized anxiety
  Obsessive-compulsive disorder
  Panic disorder

---

and impaired thinking or concentration are other common findings. It is important to differentiate between major depression and complicated or uncomplicated grieving over the loss of health or of significant others to premature death caused by HIV/AIDS.

Nursing Interventions for Responses to HIV-Associated Neurocognitive Disorder

Treatment of patients with HAND often includes include individual and family therapy, as well as psychotropic medications in a manner similar to the treatment of primary psychiatric disorders. Early diagnosis and treatment are imperative to maximize the patient's adherence to risk-reduction regimens and to prevent the transmission of infection. Treatment plans can be very complicated, requiring intervention for multiple problems. Ongoing psychiatric intervention can often be tailored to meet the needs of the patient and family. The consultation–liaison psychiatric professional can recommend appropriate multidisciplinary interventions to meet the challenge of HIV/AIDS with compassion and dignity.

Antiviral agents, such as non-nucleoside reverse transcriptase inhibitors, nucleoside/nucleotide reverse transcriptase inhibitors, protease inhibitors, entry/fusion inhibitors, integrase inhibitors, and multiclass fixed-dose combination therapy (i.e., highly active antiretroviral therapy [HAART]) combinations cross the blood–brain barrier and achieve adequate anti-HIV concentrations in cerebrospinal fluid after systemic administration.

When a patient receives the diagnosis of AIDS, he or she may withdraw into social isolation, delaying treatment because of mistrust of unfamiliar and perhaps ineffective treatments and the prospect of premature death. Interventions should focus on encouraging early and ongoing treatment with antiretroviral formulations and treatment of specific conditions, as well as maintaining health.

Stigma and discrimination are challenges for the person with HIV (Sowell & Phillips, 2010). Depression is a major problem for many diagnosed with HIV and is associated with impaired cognition (Fazeli, Marceaux, Vance, Slater, & Long, 2011). Nursing care should be empathic in approach and based on the recognition that persons with HIV often fear social consequences and want to keep their infection a secret. The nurse should help the patient problem solve to identify the best time and circumstances for self-disclosure.

In addition, it is important to provide the patient and the patient's family, friends, and caregivers with emotional and educational support. The behavioral changes are difficult for family members, particularly if they are still adjusting to the diagnosis of HIV and are now seeing profound behavior changes in their loved one. Those close to the patient may especially need psychotherapy if the patient is young (Kelly, 2010).

PSYCHOLOGICAL ILLNESS RELATED TO TRAUMA

Physiologic trauma activates the overall stress response of the autonomic nervous system. Massive catecholamine release causes certain cardiovascular, muscular, gastrointestinal, and respiratory symptoms that release energy stores and support survival. Tissue destruction, musculoskeletal pain, physical disability, and body image changes all contribute to the physiologic and psychological stress response, which continues long after the traumatic experience. The overwhelming behavioral responses are hypervigilance, fear, and anxiety. Psychological sequelae may include social isolation; agitation; personality disorders; posttraumatic stress disorder (PTSD); depression; and in extreme cases, dissociative identity disorders.

Biologic Basis of the Trauma Response

The neurotransmitters responsible for behavioral responses to fear and anxiety are usually held in balance to maintain a level of arousal appropriate for environmental threat. Information from the sensory processing areas in the thalamus and cortex alerts the amygdala (the lateral and central nucleus). Events that are appraised as threatening activate HPA axis, which releases adrenal steroids initiating the generalized stress response (see Chapter 18). When the perceived threat is sustained, complex neurochemical processes involving norepinephrine, gamma-aminobutyric acid (GABA), dopamine, and serotonin are overwhelmed, leading to a general dysregulation of the HPA axis. Inappropriate and prolonged secretion of high levels of catecholamines results (Radley, Williams, & Sawchenko, 2008). Chronic stress is linked to increased susceptibility to diseases of immunosuppression, such as certain cancers, as well as infection, myocardial disease, and neurologic degenerative disorders (Dhabhar, 2009).

Adaptation to trauma is related to such factors as the severity of the trauma, the person's maturity and age when the trauma occurs, available social support, and the person's ability to mobilize coping strategies (Alderfer, 2010). During adaptation to prolonged stress, the patient's cognitive thought processes and coping behaviors cause dopamine and serotonin to be released in the prefrontal cortex of the brain. These noradrenergic systems are presumed to play a major role in physiologic and emotional coping responses, storage of the trauma experience into memory, and possibly the development of PTSD (Radley et al., 2008).

Psychological Response to Trauma

An individual's psychological response to trauma depends on the extent of endocrine and autonomic activity that occurs during stress coupled with prior experience, developmental history, and physical status. Psychological manifestation of sustained stress and trauma may be manifested as flashbacks, intrusive recurring thoughts, panic or anxiety attacks, paranoia, inappropriate startle reactions, nightmares, or the extreme of PTSD (see Chapter 26). The patient may become so withdrawn and depressed that he or she stops participating in activities of daily living (ADLs). Toward the other extreme, the patient may become agitated and combative, perceiving any treatment as a continued threat.

Assessment of Patients Experiencing Trauma

Complete physical assessment after physical traumatic injury is imperative in life-threatening circumstances. Multiple trauma and head injuries are the major causes of death and disability in young adults in society as well as in military deployment. Highly trained emergency and intensive care providers look for signs and symptoms of physiologic injury and intervene to stabilize primary and secondary trauma in the general medical setting.

After physical stabilization, the patient should be examined for psychological injury through observation and interview to determine prevalent signs and symptoms of accompanying psychological disorders (Gray, Elhai, Owen, & Monroe, 2009). This process includes evaluating the patient's adjustment and coping skills, his or her personal way of dealing with the trauma, social circumstances, and environmental and life stressors. Assessment must be ongoing to help the patient deal with disfigurement, sudden disability, and changes in self-care. The evaluation should include assessment of the patient's perception of experienced stress, feelings related to the stress, dominant mood, cognitive functioning, defense and coping mechanisms, and available support systems. In addition, assessment of the risk for self-inflicted injury or suicide is critical.

Nursing Interventions for Responses to Trauma

Psychiatric clinicians provide an important aspect of emergency care. Interventions that establish trust, reduce anxiety, promote adaptive coping, and cultivate a sense of control help the patient to begin recovery and maintain emotional health. Crisis intervention methods, stress management, cognitive behavioral therapies, psychotherapy, and psychotropic medications, alone or in combination, may be useful in achieving the best possible outcome.

Traumatic death is sudden and unexpected, and the victim is often young. When trauma causes the patient's death, the family must be informed of the death and allowed to grieve to prevent the development of a pathologic or prolonged grief response. Surviving family members may have a severe emotional reaction to the death. Dysfunctional family dynamics may become evident during this period. Ideally, the psychiatric–mental health liaison nurse can use family intervention strategies to enhance or improve relationships while the family's motivation to do all that is possible is high.

PSYCHOLOGICAL ILLNESS RELATED TO CENTRAL NERVOUS SYSTEM DISORDERS

Neurologic impairment is most often related to brain cell (neuron) destruction. The primary causes of neuronal damage are traumatic injury, ischemia, infarction (cerebrovascular accident), abnormal neuron growth (brain tumor), and metabolic poisoning associated with systemic disease. Brain cell loss may also be the result of degenerative processes, such as those that occur in Alzheimer's or Parkinson's disease. Psychiatric disorders are often complications of these neurologic diseases and may be difficult to distinguish from the neuropathology itself. Therefore, appropriate intervention depends on skilled assessment to discriminate and detect mental status changes related to organic brain injury as well as disorders of mood and thought.

An injury to the brain can destroy brain cells directly or initiate a cascade of cell breakdown from ischemia. This **ischemic cascade** begins with hypoxia and is followed by paralysis of the ion exchange across the cell membrane, edema, calcium influx, free radical production, and lipid peroxidation (oxidative degradation of lipids). The severity of brain injury is related to the degree and duration of ischemia. Complete ischemia results in brain cell death or infarction, commonly known as stroke. The resulting neurologic impairment is related to the size and location of the affected brain area. More eloquent areas of the brain, such as the internal capsule, are extremely sensitive to ischemia. They are typically injured first and contribute to more generalized impairment, such as memory loss or altered judgment (Endres, Dirnagl, & Moskowitz, 2009).

Traumatic Brain Injury

Traumatic brain injury (TBI) is an intracranial injury that occurs when an outside force traumatically injures the brain. TBI is a major cause of disability in U.S. wounded soldiers (Bombardier, Fann, Temkin, Esselman, Barber, & Dikmen, 2010). Even though the focus of recovery is on physical and cognitive rehabilitation, a significant portion of the disability is psychological. Depression is estimated to occur in up to 53% of those with TBI and is thought to be a result of the changes in the autonomic and endocrine systems after a cerebral assault (Bombardier et al., 2010). Poorer cognitive functioning, aggression and anxiety, greater functional disability, poorer recovery, higher rates of suicide attempts, and greater health care costs are thought to be associated with TBI depression (Bombardier et al., 2010). Depressed mood may become evident in the acute recovery phase or during rehabilitation and often negatively affects survival and recovery. It impedes progress throughout the rehabilitation process and ultimately prevents an optimal outcome. Early evaluation assists in the detection of mental illness after brain injury.

Ischemic Stroke

Depressive disorder is a frequent complication of ischemic stroke. The incidence of stroke can range from 10% to 50% of stroke patients in the acute period (3 months) (Johnson, Minarik, Nyström, Bautista, & Gorman, 2006). The mood changes are not only a result of the changes in

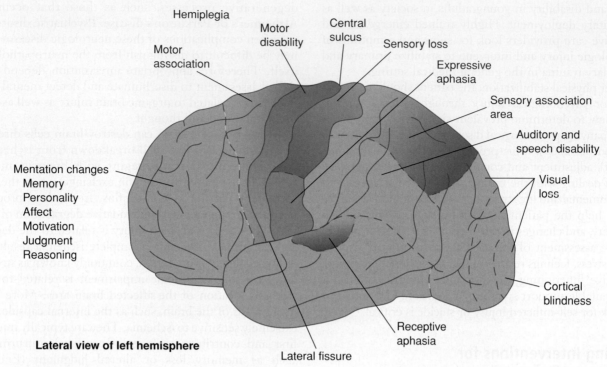

Hemiplegia

Motor
association

Motor
disability

Central
sulcus

Sensory loss

Expressive
aphasia

Sensory association
area

Auditory and
speech disability

Visual
loss

Cortical
blindness

Receptive
aphasia

Lateral fissure

Mentation changes
Memory
Personality
Affect
Motivation
Judgment
Reasoning

Lateral view of left hemisphere

FIGURE 42.5 Functional cerebral anatomy and stroke.

the autonomic and endocrine systems but also a result of the breakdown of biogenic amines after ischemia and brain cell death. Recent studies show that in some parts of the brain, there is actually atrophy (Hudak, Warner, Marquex de la Plata, Moore, Harper, & Diaz-Arrastia, 2010). See Figure 42.5. Other symptoms, such as sleep disturbances, cognitive dysfunction, poor concentration, difficulty making decisions, somatic discomfort, poor appetite, social withdrawal, and fatigue or agitation, often accompany the mood disturbance (Gurr, 2011).

Minor and moderate depression may go unrecognized and undiagnosed when patients with stroke describe somatic symptoms and demonstrate lack of motivation in ADLs. There is no one risk factor for the development of mood disorders. Depression is more likely to develop in stroke patients if they have altered speech or aphasia, severe hemiparesis, or both. Age and severity of stroke are also associated with poststroke depression (Gurr, 2011).

Parkinson's Disease

In Parkinson's disease and other neuromuscular diseases, there is degeneration in the motor pathways with a loss of dopamine secretion. This dysregulation affects other neurotransmitters. About 35% of patients with Parkinson's disease experience depression that contributes to impairment in daily functioning possibly as much as the underlying disease (Reijnders, Ehrt, Weber, Aarsland, & Leentjens,

2008). Depression negatively affects quality of life and is a source of distress for the patient, family, and caregivers. Evidence suggests that altered serotonergic function may be responsible, at least in part, for the depressive symptoms in Parkinson's disease and that altered noradrenergic function may underlie some of the associated anxiety symptoms (Kano, Ikeda, Cridebring, Takazawa, Yoshi, & Iwasaki, 2011).

Assessment of Psychological Responses to Central Nervous System Disorders

A thorough neurologic examination is important in determining the location and degree of disability but is even more critical in establishing the locus of retained function. Cognitive functioning, mood, and functionality are key assessment areas. Many scales exist that accurately assess these areas, are easy to administer, and are generally accepted as reliable tools to detect the degree and limitations of disability. Cognition can be measured using the Saint Louis University Mental Status (SLUMS) Examination (see Chapter 37), and functionability for self-care can be measured using the Barthel Index (Mahoney & Barthel, 1965). Evaluation of mood using the Center for Epidemiological Studies Depression Scale (CES-D) or the Beck Depression Inventory (Beck, Ward, Mendelson, Mock, & Erbaugh, 1961) provides important information for designing intervention strategies for the at-risk neurologic patient. Findings of depressive symptoms indicate the need for a more definitive neuro-psychological referral.

Nursing Interventions for Responses to Central Nervous System Disorders

Isolation, lack of companionship, bereavement, and poverty are associated with depressive symptoms in the general population and compound the relative risk of depression developing after brain damage. In addition, a history or family history of major depression increases the risk for depressed mood. Prevention strategies should be used as early as possible for patients known to have these risks. These strategies include (1) the assessment and provision of social support resources while the patient is hospitalized and as an important component of discharge planning to rehabilitation services; (2) early identification of potential mental health problems with a referral for complete evaluation; (3) education of patient and family about the mental health complications of CNS disorders so they will know when to seek medical attention and treatment to avert major problems; (4) encouragement to seek treatment for mental health problems, including pharmacologic strategies; and (5) enhancement of competence in performing ADLs, with a focus on the use of retained function rather than on adaptation to disabilities only.

MENTAL HEALTH PROBLEMS RELATED TO ACUTE AND CHRONIC MEDICAL ILLNESS

Systemic medical illness is associated with a higher prevalence of concurrent mental health problems. Conditions such as cancer, heart disease, endocrine abnormalities, and organ failure are often associated with more functional disability than most chronic medical illnesses and may be the basis of medically unexplained somatic symptoms. Among the psychiatric disorders, substance abuse disorders, anxiety, and depressive disorder occur most frequently in patients with chronic medical illnesses. Emerging evidence suggests that anxiety disorders rival depression in terms of risk, comorbidity, and outcomes in medical illnesses (Roy-Byrne, 2008).

Biologic Aspects of Mental Illness Related to Medical Disease

Mental health problems can occur during the course of these medical illnesses and in some instances may contribute to the genesis of them. A psychiatric disorder may be the first manifestation of a primary disease, such as depressive syndrome in Huntington's chorea, multiple sclerosis, Parkinson's disease, HIV, Cushing's disease, and systemic

Table 42.1	MEDICAL ILLNESSES ASSOCIATED WITH SYMPTOMS OF DEPRESSION
Endocrinopathies	Hypothyroidism and hyperthyroidism; Hypoparathyroidism and hyperparathyroidism; Cushing's syndrome (steroid excess); Adrenal insufficiency (Addison's disease); Hyperaldosteronism
Malignancies	Abdominal carcinomas, especially pancreatic; Brain tumors (temporal lobe); Breast cancer; Gastrointestinal cancer; Lung cancer; Prostate cancer; Metastases
Neurologic disorders	Ischemic stroke; Subarachnoid hemorrhage; Parkinson's disease; Normal-pressure hydrocephalus; Multiple sclerosis; Closed head injury; Epilepsy
Metabolic imbalance	Serum sodium and potassium reductions; Vitamin B_{12}, niacin, vitamin C deficiencies; iron deficiency (anemias); Metal intoxication (thallium and mercury); Uremia
Viral or bacterial infection	Infectious hepatitis; Encephalitis; Tuberculosis; AIDS
Hormonal imbalance	Premenstrual, premenopausal, postpartum periods
Cardiopulmonary	Acute myocardial infarction; Post–cardiac arrest; Post–coronary artery bypass graft; Post–heart transplantation; Cardiomyopathy
Inflammatory disorders	Rheumatoid arthritis

lupus erythematosus. In particular, depressive symptoms are an intrinsic part of the primary pathophysiology of endocrine disorders, metabolic disturbances, malignancies, viral infections, inflammatory disorders, and cardiopulmonary conditions. Table 42.1 lists medical conditions associated with depression. Endocrine system pathologies involve abnormal HPA axis function, affecting neurotransmitter balance. Depression and anxiety are often present in patients with hyperthyroidism and hypothyroidism, Cushing's disease (hyperadrenalism), and Addison's disease (hypoadrenalism), complicating the clinical picture in up to 40% of cases (Arogones, Pinol, & Labad, 2007). Depression has been shown to be an independent risk factor for type 2 diabetes, and the early onset of vascular disease, multiple infections, and disability are associated with increased depressive symptoms (Benton et al., 2007).

Malignancies have also been associated with anxiety and depression. Depressive syndromes have been associated with cancer in up to 50% of cancer cases, and biologic relationships between the two disorders may exist such that the onset of depression may herald undetected carcinoma. Diagnoses range from major depression to adjustment disorder with depressed mood. Depression might also be a consequence of antineoplastic therapy (Saini et al., 2009) and consequently lead to poor adherence to cancer prevention behavior (e.g., smoking cessation). Available evidence strongly suggests that depression in the patient with cancer responds to selective serotonin reuptake inhibitors (SSRIs) and mirtazapine. Psychosocial interventions also have been shown to reduce depressive and anxiety symptoms and result in longer survival (Zebrack, 2011).

Up to 40% of patients with systemic infections and generalized inflammatory disorders such as rheumatoid arthritis experience mental health problems, usually depression (Margaretten et al., 2009). In addition, renal, pancreatic, and hepatic transplant recipients, who are artificially immunosuppressed because of treatment with prophylactic anti-infectious agents, experience primary neuropsychiatric symptoms related to metabolic imbalances and neuropsychiatric side effects from treatment. Diagnosing depression and anxiety in medically ill patients is not straightforward. For example, shared symptoms such as fatigue and weight loss can impede recognition in these patients by masking underlying pathology. Failure to diagnose and treat depressed mood or anxiety can result in a failure to heal, prolonged illness, and hospitalization.

In addition, some drugs used to treat chronic disease are known to cause agitation, anxiety, and depression as a side effect (Table 42.2). The pharmacologic activity of these medications may exacerbate normal physiologic effects to levels that are uncomfortable or unexpected. All medically ill patients should be considered at risk for developing mental health problems, and special attention should be given to medication side effects. In addition, medically ill older adults are particularly susceptible to medication effects at lower doses. When a drug is suspected of causing mental changes, the recommended course of action is to withdraw the drug and find an effective alternative. When an adequate substitute is not available, the dosage should be decreased to an effective level at which symptoms resolve.

Cardiac disease deserves special attention because it has been associated with precipitated depressive syndromes in 20% to 50% of patients and anxiety disorders in up to 80%. The fact that more than 70% of patients who have an acute myocardial infarction (MI) remain depressed for up to 1 year after the event indicates that the mental illness may not be simply an adjustment disorder. The incidence of depression is similar in cardiac transplant recipients (54%) but is much lower in cardiac

Table 42.2	MEDICATIONS ASSOCIATED WITH MENTAL ILLNESS IN MEDICALLY ILL PATIENTS
Analgesics and NSAIDs	Ibuprofen
	Indomethacin
	Opiates
	Pentazocine
	Phenacetin
	Phenylbutazone
Antihypertensives	Clonidine
	Hydralazine
	Methyldopa
	Propranolol
	Reserpine
Antimicrobials	Ampicillin (gram-negative agents)
	Clotrimazole
	Cycloserine
	Griseofulvin
	Metronidazole
	Nitrofurantoin
	Streptomycin
	Sulfamethoxazole (sulfonamides)
Neurologic agents	L-Dopa
	Levodopa
Antiparkinsonism drugs	Amantadine
Anticonvulsants	Carbamazepine
	Phenytoin
Antispasmodics	Baclofen
	Bromocriptine
Cardiac drugs	Digitalis
	Guanethidine
	Lidocaine
	Oxprenolol
	Procainamide
Psychotropic drugs	Benzodiazepines
Stimulants and sedatives	Amphetamines
	Barbiturates
	Chloral hydrate
	Chlorazepate
	Diethylpropion
	Ethanol
	Fenfluramine
	Haloperidol
Steroids and hormones	Adrenocorticotropic hormone
	Corticosteroids
	Estrogen
	Oral contraceptives
	Prednisone
	Progesterone
	Triamcinolone
Antineoplastic drugs	Bleomycin
	C-Asparaginase
	Trimethoprim
	Vincristine
Other miscellaneous drugs	Anticholinesterases
	Cimetidine
	Diuretics
	Metoclopramide

NSAID, nonsteroidal antiinflammatory drug.

bypass surgery patients (6%–15%) (Lesperance, Frasure-Smith, Talajic, & Bourassa, 2002). Risk of cardiac death in the 6 months after an acute MI is approximately four times greater in patients with depression than in nondepressed patients. Depressive and anxiety-related symptoms may actually have an additive effect on challenges to patient function, well-being, and recovery when combined with medical illness.

Psychological Aspects of Medical Illness

It is natural for patients to respond to the loss of health with hopelessness, particularly when the illness is demoralizing, life threatening, and without a clear prognosis. People who are chronically ill are distressed by loss of function and limitations on their daily activities. They are often forced to comply with treatments that add discomfort but no apparent benefit. Medical patients commonly experience weight loss, insomnia, and motor retardation but perhaps not to the degree of "conspicuous" psychiatric illness. In addition, chronic life stress and mental illness may have set into motion a series of biologic processes ultimately resulting in the medical disorder, which may be further exacerbated by the stress of hospitalization. A vicious cycle of medical and mental disorders may arise.

Mental illness in medically ill people is potentially lethal because stable moods and cognitive functioning may be essential to recovery and compliance with the medical treatment plan. In addition, the use of excessive analgesics and reluctance to perform self-care and rehabilitative activities hinder recovery and expose the person to other potential complications. The detection and diagnosis of any secondary mental illnesses in patients with medical illnesses is critical. The physiologic and pharmacologic factors that contribute to the mental illness must be explored and ruled out before effective intervention can begin.

Clinical Features of Special Significance

Two problems of special significance, psychosis and suicidal thoughts, are related in that patients with delusions or hallucinations tend to be at greater risk for suicide attempts and more likely to resist treatment (e.g., to refuse to eat or take medication) for their medical condition. It is important to distinguish between a mentally competent patient's right to refuse lifesaving medical treatment and a depressed patient's desire to die. A clinical evaluation of the effect of depression on the patient's capacity to make competent decisions is imperative. If optimal medical and psychiatric treatments have been provided and the patient has been found competent enough to make decisions about further medical care for a fatal disease, it may be appropriate to honor the patient's desire to die. Patients

with primary mental illness and comorbid chronic medical illness may pose similar problems in psychiatric hospitals when their medical condition fails. The use of advance directives helps in addressing these problems.

Assessment of Patients with Medical Illness

Unfortunately, when evaluating a medically ill patient in whom psychiatric symptoms develop, it may be very difficult for the clinician to ascertain whether these symptoms are the result of direct psychobiologic changes brought about by the illness. A brief mental health assessment as part of the admission process helps in detecting stress, risks, and symptom relapse. This assessment should include mood level, presence of disproportionate fear and anxiety, and motivation for self-care to provide the minimum information needed for each patient. This information is useful in determining relevant nursing diagnoses and developing the plan of care.

People at obvious risk have a family or personal history of mental illness or were experiencing psychological problems before symptoms of the medical illness were present. The main challenge for the clinician is to determine which signs and symptoms are part of the medical illness and its treatment and which signify the presence of a psychological disorder.

A complete health and mental health assessment and physical examination help determine the severity and priority of symptoms and interventions. All patients with chronic medical illnesses are at risk for psychological distress and should be approached with this understanding. Clinicians should include a general cognitive-affective status evaluation in their assessment of all medically ill patients and make appropriate psychiatric liaison consultation to offset the negative impact of mental illness on recovery (Katon et al., 2010).

In some instances, the primary disorder may be depression, although the symptoms may be similar to those of medical illness (e.g., insomnia, weight loss). Factors to be considered in assessing mental health problems in medical patients are outlined in Box 42.7. Several important cognitive-affective symptoms best differentiate the effects of depression from those of medical illness. These include feelings of failure, low self-esteem, guilt feelings, loss of interest in people, feelings of being punished, suicidal ideation, dissatisfaction, difficulty with decisions, and crying (Evans et al., 2005). The severity of these symptoms generally increases with the severity of the depressive disorder as well as the severity of the medical illness. Decreased appetite, sleep disturbances, and loss of energy are not considered indicators of depression in medically ill patients because these symptoms are common in medical illness as well. The Beck Depression Inventory and the CES-D are easy to administer and provide some indication of whether a psychiatric liaison referral is needed.

Assessment of anxiety and depression is ongoing, and crisis intervention with psychotherapy may be necessary to reduce the severity of mental distress. Physiologic symptoms, such as an increased heart rate, blood pressure, and respiration, and signs of restlessness and sadness, such as tearfulness, can be measured to determine the effectiveness of the intervention.

Nursing Interventions for Responses to Medical Illness

It is essential to provide optimal treatment of patients' medical illnesses without neglecting their mental distress. Ideally, a multidisciplinary team of care providers that includes a psychiatric liaison nurse should work closely together to deliver optimum treatment of complex medical and mental illness. When available, stress management training, systematic relaxation, supportive education, and stress monitoring should be built into the plan of care regardless of the medical diagnosis. Cognitive and behavioral strategies have a place in the treatment regimen and offer the practitioner an opportunity to expand the boundaries of traditional patient-oriented practice in effective ways.

Most reports suggest that clinicians should be more aggressive in the pharmacologic treatment of mental illness in medically ill patients. The basic rules for medicating patients include using the minimum dose initially, advancing the dose slowly, and performing frequent blood level monitoring if appropriate. The doses required to achieve therapeutic blood levels may be lower or even half the usual therapeutic dose and take longer to titrate. It is important to understand the pharmacokinetics (absorption, distribution, metabolism, and elimination) of the treatment of choice to prevent further systemic effects. SSRIs and serotonin–norepinephrine reuptake inhibitors are used equally as the treatment for depression in the medically ill patient population. Because the side effects of psychopharmacologic agents can be especially troublesome in medically ill people, treatment must be changed or stopped if drug or illness interactions occur or if treatment of the mental illness appears to be unsuccessful. SSRIs are increasingly popular in treating medically ill patients because their side effect profile is more tolerable within a wider therapeutic range. Most patients respond to antidepressant therapy with a decrease in the severity of their symptoms in 4 to 8 days.

Both supportive individual psychotherapy and family therapy are helpful. Assisting the patient and family in understanding the nature and relationship of the medical and psychiatric diagnoses may strengthen the support system, alter the perception of caregiver burden, and identify appropriate coping strategies. Mutually agreed-upon goals and therapy actively involve the patient in progress toward recovery. At some point, the clinician may need to help the patient identify psychodynamic conflicts and maladaptive coping strategies that may be contributing to his or her distress. Cognitive intervention should address the areas of the patient's life that can be controlled, despite major lifestyle changes, to reinforce a feeling of competence. Also, it is important to convey the fact that although medical and mental illness are difficult to prevent, they are often treatable (Katon et al., 2010; McEvoy & Barnes, 2007).

Secondary mental illness (mental disorders caused by a medical problem) can be approached using the same strategies that are effective for primary mental dysfunction. Interventions apply across criteria and all interventions provide some element of supportive therapy or social support.

PHYSICAL ILLNESSES IN PERSONS WITH MENTAL DISORDERS

Persons served by state mental health agencies die 25 years younger than the general population; men are likely to die at age 53 years and females at age 59 years (Manderscheid, 2009). Two factors are responsible for the early death of individuals with mental illness. Chronic physical disabilities account for 15 to 20 years of the difference, and mental factors such as suicide account for 5 to 10 years (Manderscheid, 2009). According to these data, life expectancy estimates appear shorter in 2006 than in 1986.

Patients with primary mental illness in need of medical care are at particular risk when somatic complaints are viewed as part of the primary process. Undiagnosed pathophysiologic processes may progress to advanced stages while being attributed to somatization. A thorough medical history and physical examination with complementary laboratory evaluation are standard practice for these patients in all settings. Many psychiatric care settings are limited in the ability to manage mentally ill patients who are acutely and critically ill and appropriately transfer them to a medical unit for medical treatment.

Ideally, psychiatric mental health liaison clinicians are consulted to see patients with psychiatric conditions in all phases of their medical illness, from acute hospitalization and treatment to rehabilitation and return to the community. The consultation–liaison psychiatric professional can recommend appropriate multidisciplinary interventions to meet the challenges of mental illness associated with medical illness for optimal outcomes.

SUMMARY OF KEY POINTS

- Psychiatric disorders are more common in people with systemic or chronic medical illnesses than in the healthy population. Comorbid depression is common in several medical diseases, including endocrine and metabolic disturbances, viral infections, inflammatory disorders, and cardiopulmonary diseases.

- Psychiatric illness that accompanies medical illness is seldom recognized and treated. Psychiatric symptoms may precede the onset of disease symptoms, and it may be difficult to distinguish between the symptoms of the two conditions.

- Mental illness in medically ill people is potentially lethal because normal affective-cognitive function may be critical to recovery and compliance with the medical treatment plan. Therefore, it is imperative that mental health is included in the standard health assessment of all medically ill persons and that appropriate referrals be made.

- Premature death among individuals cared by state mental health agencies is 25 years earlier than the general population.

CRITICAL THINKING CHALLENGE

1. You are caring for a patient who is recovering from a stroke and refuses breakfast and a morning bath. Applying what you know about the neurologic damage caused by stroke and the frequency of depression in stroke patients, develop a care plan addressing the patient's biopsychosocial needs.

2. As you care for a patient with HAND, you notice that his partner is pacing and hyperventilating. Using your knowledge of relationships, systems, and the interconnectedness of physical and psychological illness, how would you approach the patient's partner?

3. Discuss the pain syndromes you may see in the primary care setting.

4. A patient is being seen for chronic pain. Discuss how you would go about assessing barriers to pain management with this patient.

5. You are a psychiatric–mental health liaison nurse and have been asked to prepare a program for the

medical–surgical nursing staff on psychiatric aspects of medical illnesses. What topics would you include, and what would be your rationale for including each?

References

Alderfer, M. A., Long, K. A., Lown, E. A., Marsland, A. L., Ostrowski, N. L., Hock, J. M., & Ewing, L. J. (2010). Psychosocial adjustment of siblings of children with cancer: A systematic review. *Psycho-Oncology*, 19(8), 789–805.
Anesetti-Rothermel, A., & Sambamoorthi, U. (2011). Physical and mental illness burden: disability days among working adults. *Population Health Management*, in press.
Arogones, E., Pinol, J. L., & Labad, A. (2007). Depression and physical comorbidity in primary care. *Journal of Psychosomatic Research*, 63, 107–111.
Basbaum A. I., & Julius, D. (2006). Pain control. *Scientific American*, 294(6), 60–67.
Bartsch, T., & Goadsby, P. J. (2011). Central mechanisms of peripheral nerve stimulation in headache disorders. *Progress in Neurologic Surgery*, 24, 16–26.
Beck, A. T., Ward, C. H., Mendelson, M., Mock, J., & Erbaugh, J. (1961). An inventory for measuring depression. *Archives of General Psychiatry*, 4, 561–656.
Benton, T., Staab, J., & Evans, D. L. (2007). Medical co-morbidity in depressive disorders. *Annals of Clinical Psychiatry*, 19(4), 289–303.
Bombardier, C. H., Fann, J. R., Temkin, N. R., Esselman, P. C., Barber, J., & Dikmen, S. S. (2010). Rates of major depressive disorder and clinical outcomes following traumatic brain injury. *Journal of the American Medical Association*, 303(19), 1938–1945.
Casucci, G., Villani, V., & Ginocchi, C. (2010). Therapeutic strategies in migraine patients with mood and anxiety disorders: Physiopathological basis. *Neurologic Sciences*, 31(suppl 1), S99–S101.
Cole, S. W. (2008). Psychosocial influences on HIV-1 disease progression: Neural, endocrine, and virologic mechanisms. *Psychosomatic Medicine*, 70(5), 562–568.
DeLeo, J. A. (2006). Basic science of pain. *The Journal of Bone and Joint Surgery*, 88(2), 58–62.
Dhabhar, F. D. (2009). Enhancing versus suppressive effects of stress on immune function: Implications for immunoprotection and immunopathology. *Neuroimmunomodulation*, 16(5), 300–317.
El-Mallakh, P., Howard, P.B., & Inman, S.M. (2010). Medical and psychiatric comorbidities in children and adolescents: A guide to issues and treatment approaches. *Nursing Clinics of North America*, 45(4), 541–554.
Endres, M., Dirnagl, U., & Moskowitz, M. A. (2009). The ischemic cascade and mediators of ischemic injury. *Handbook of Clinical Neurology*, 92, 31–41.
Evans, D. L., Charney, D. S., Lewis, L., Golden, R. N., Gorman, J. M., Krishnan, K. R. R., et al. (2005). Mood disorders in the medically ill: Scientific review and recommendations. *Journal of Biological Psychiatry*, 58, 175–189.
Fagiolini, A., & Goracci, A. (2009). The effects of undertreated chronic medical illnesses in patients with severe mental disorders. *Journal of Clinical Psychiatry*, 70(suppl 3), 22–29.
Fazeli, P. L., Marceaux, J. C., Vance, D. E., Slater, L., & Long, C. A. (2011). Predictors of cognition in adults with HIV: Implications for nursing practice and research. *Journal of Neuroscience Nursing*, 43(1), 36–50.
Gray, M. J., Elhai, J. D., Owen, J. R., & Monroe, R. (2009). Psychometric properties of the Trauma Assessment for Adults. *Depression & Anxiety*, 26(2), 190–195.
Gurr, B. (2011). Stroke mood screening on an inpatient stroke unit. *British Journal of Nursing*, 20(2), 94–100.
Haefeli, M., & Elfering, A. (2006). Pain assessment. *European Spine Journal*, 15(suppl 1), S17–S24.
Hudak, A., Warner, M., Marquex de la Plata, C., Moore, C., Harper, C., & Diaz-Arrastia, R. (2011). Brain morphometry changes and depressive symptoms after traumatic brain injury. *Psychiatry Research Neuroimaging*, 191(3), 160–165.
Humphreys, J., Cooper, B. A., & Miaskowski, C. (2010). Differences in depression, posttraumatic stress disorder, and lifetime trauma exposure in formerly abused women with mild versus moderate to severe chronic pain. *Journal of Interpersonal Violence*, 25(12), 2316–2338.
Johnson, L. J., Minarik, P. A., Nyström, K. V., Bautista, C., & Gorman, M. J. (2006). Post-stroke depression incidence and risk factors: An integrated literature review. *Journal of Neurologic Nursing*, 38(4), 316–327.

Kano, O., Ikeda, K., Cridebring, D., Takazawa, T., Yoshi, Y., & Iwasaki, Y. (2011). Neurobiology of depression and anxiety in Parkinson's disease. *Parkinson's Disease*, in press.

Katon, W. J., Lin, E. H., VonKorff, M., Ciechanowski, P., Ludman, E., Young, B., Peterson, D., Rutter, C. M., Mcgregor, M., & McCulloch, D. (2010). Collaborative care for patients with depression and chronic illness. *New England Journal of Medicine, 363*, 2611–2620.

Kelly, A. (2010). Lost the feel for the game: Meanings of onset and diagnosis of AIDS dementia for significant others. *Qualitative Health Research, 20*(4), 531–540.

Lesperance, F., Frasure-Smith, N., Talajic, M., & Bourassa, M. G. (2002). Five-year risk of cardiac mortality in relation to initial severity and one-year changes in depression symptoms after myocardial infarction. *Circulation, 105*, 1049–1053.

Mahoney, F. T., & Barthel, D. W. (1965). Functional evaluation: Barthel index. *Maryland Medical Journal, 14*, 61–65.

Manderscheid, R. W. (2009). Premature death among state mental health agency consumers: Assessing progress in addressing a quiet tragedy. *International Journal of Public Health, 54*(suppl 1), 7–8.

Margaretten, M., Yelin, E., Imboden, J., et al. (2009). Predictors of depression in a multiethnic cohort of patients with rheumatoid arthritis. *Arthritis & Rheumatism, 61*(11), 1586–1591.

McEvoy, P., & Barnes, P. (2007). Using the chronic care model to tackle depression among older adults who have long term conditions. *Journal of Psychiatric Nursing, 14*, 233–238.

Moussavi, S., Chatterji, S., Verdes, E., Tandon, A., Patel, V., & Ustun, B. (2007). Depression, chronic disease and decrements in health: Results from the World Health Surveys. *Lancet, 370*, 851–858.

Radley, J. J., Williams, B., & Sawchenko, S. (2008). Noradrenergic innervation of the dorsal medial prefrontal cortex modules hypothalamo-pituitary-adrenal responses to acute emotional stress. *Journal of Neuroscience, 28*(22), 5806–5816.

Reijnders, J., Ehrt, U., Weber, W., Aarsland, D., & Leentjens, A. (2008). A systematic review of prevalence studies of depression in Parkinson's disease. *Movement Disorders, 23*(2), 183–189.

Roy-Byrne, P. P., Davidson, K. W., & Kessler, R. C., et al. (2008). Anxiety disorders and comorbid medical illness. *Focus, 6*(4), 467–485.

Saini, A., Ostacoli, L., Gorzegno, G., et al. (2009). Risk of depressive events in long-term surviving patients affected by hormone-related cancer according to time after diagnosis. *Journal of Clinical Oncology, 27*(25), 91–92.

Singer, E. J., Valdes-Sueiras, M., Commins, D. & Levine, A. (2010). Neurologic presentations of AIDS. *Neurologic Clinics, 28*(1), 235–275.

Sowell, R. L., & Phillips, K.D. (2010). Understanding and responding to HIV/AIDS stigma and disclosure: An international challenge. *Issues in Mental Health Nursing, 31*(6), 394–402.

Tragesser, S. L., Bruns, D., & Disorbio, M. J. (2010). Borderline personality disorder features and pain: The mediating role of negative affect in a pain patient sample. *Clinical Journal of Pain, 26*(4), 348–353.

U.S. Department of Health and Human Services (2010). *Healthy people 2020.* Retrieved from http://www.healthypeople.gov.

Zebrack, B. J. (2011). Psychological, social, and behavioral issues for young adults with cancer. *Cancer, 117*(10 suppl), 2289–2294.

Zhu, B., Zhao, A., Ye, W., Marciniak, M. D., & Swindle, R. (2009). The cost of comorbid depression and pain for individuals diagnosed with generalized anxiety disorder. *The Journal of Nervous and Mental Disease, 197*(2), 136–139.

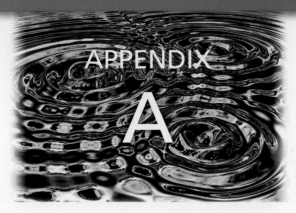

APPENDIX A

Brief Psychiatric Rating Scale

DIRECTIONS: Place an X in the appropriate box to represent level of severity of each symptom.

	Not Present	Very Mild	Mild	Moderate	Mod. Severe	Severe	Extremely Severe
SOMATIC CONCERN—preoccupation with physical health, fear of physical illness, hypochondriasis.	☐	☐	☐	☐	☐	☐	☐
ANXIETY—worry, fear, overconcern for present or future, uneasiness.	☐	☐	☐	☐	☐	☐	☐
EMOTIONAL WITHDRAWAL—lack of spontaneous interaction, isolation deficiency in relating to others.	☐	☐	☐	☐	☐	☐	☐
CONCEPTUAL DISORGANIZATION—thought processes confused, disconnected, disorganized, disrupted.	☐	☐	☐	☐	☐	☐	☐
GUILT FEELINGS—self-blame, shame, remorse for past behavior.	☐	☐	☐	☐	☐	☐	☐
TENSION—physical and motor manifestations of nervousness, overactivation.	☐	☐	☐	☐	☐	☐	☐
MANNERISMS AND POSTURING—peculiar, bizarre unnatural motor behavior (not including tic).	☐	☐	☐	☐	☐	☐	☐
GRANDIOSITY—exaggerated self-opinion, arrogance, conviction of unusual power or abilities.	☐	☐	☐	☐	☐	☐	☐
DEPRESSIVE MOOD—sorrow, sadness, despondency, pessimism.	☐	☐	☐	☐	☐	☐	☐
HOSTILITY—animosity, contempt, belligerence, disdain for others.	☐	☐	☐	☐	☐	☐	☐
SUSPICIOUSNESS—mistrust, belief others harbor malicious or discriminatory intent.	☐	☐	☐	☐	☐	☐	☐
HALLUCINATORY BEHAVIOR—perceptions without normal external stimulus correspondence.	☐	☐	☐	☐	☐	☐	☐
MOTOR RETARDATION—slowed weakened movements or speech, reduced body tone.	☐	☐	☐	☐	☐	☐	☐
UNCOOPERATIVENESS—resistance, guardedness, rejection of authority.	☐	☐	☐	☐	☐	☐	☐
UNUSUAL THOUGHT CONTENT—unusual, odd, strange, bizarre thought content.	☐	☐	☐	☐	☐	☐	☐
BLUNTED AFFECT—reduced emotional tone, reduction in formal intensity of feelings, flatness.	☐	☐	☐	☐	☐	☐	☐
EXCITEMENT—heightened emotional tone, agitation, increased reactivity.	☐	☐	☐	☐	☐	☐	☐
DISORIENTATION—confusion or lack of proper association for person, place, or time.	☐	☐	☐	☐	☐	☐	☐
Global Assessment Scale (Range 1–100)	☐	☐	☐	☐	☐	☐	☐

From Overall, J. E. & Gorham, D. R. (1962). The brief psychiatric rating scale. Psychological Reports, 10: 799–812. Used with permission.

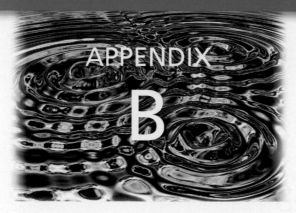

APPENDIX B

Abnormal Involuntary Movement Scale (AIMS)

		None	Minimal	Mild	Moderate	Severe
Facial and Oral Movements	1: **Muscles of facial expression:** e.g., movements of forehead, eyebrows, periorbital area, cheeks; include frowning, blinking, smiling, grimacing	0	1	2	3	4
	2: **Lips and perioral area:** e.g., puckering, pouting, smacking	0	1	2	3	4
	3: **Jaw:** e.g., biting, clenching, chewing, mouth opening, lateral movement	0	1	2	3	4
	4: **Tongue:** Rate only increase in movement both in and out of mouth, *not* the inability to sustain movement	0	1	2	3	4
Extremity Movements	5: **Upper (arms, wrists, hands, fingers):** Include choreic movements (i.e., rapid, objectively purposeless, irregular, spontaneous), athetoid movements (i.e., slow, irregular, complex, serpentine); *do not* include tremor (i.e., repetitive, regular, rhythmic)	0	1	2	3	4
	6: **Lower (legs, knees, ankles, toes):** e.g., lateral knee movement, foot tapping, heel dropping, foot squirming, inversion and eversion of foot	0	1	2	3	4
Trunk Movements	7: **Neck, shoulders, hips:** e.g., rocking, twisting, squirming, pelvic gyrations	0	1	2	3	4
Global Judgment	8: **Severity of abnormal movements overall**	0	1	2	3	4
	9: **Incapacitation caused by abnormal movements**	0	1	2	3	4
	10: **Patient's awareness of abnormal movements:** Rate only patient's report					

No awareness	0
Aware, no distress	1
Aware, mild distress	2
Aware, moderate distress	3
Aware, severe distress	4

Dental Status	11: Current problems with teeth or dentures	No	0
		Yes	1
	12: Does patient usually wear dentures?	No	0
		Yes	1

Examination Procedure for AIMS

Either before or after completing the examination procedure, observe the patient unobtrusively, at rest (e.g., in the waiting room). The chair to be used in this examination should be a hard, firm one without arms.

1: Ask the patient whether there is anything in his or her mouth (e.g., gum, candy) and if there is, to remove it.

2: Ask the patient about the *current* condition of his or her teeth. Ask the patient if he or she wears dentures. Do teeth or dentures bother the patient *now*?

3: Ask the patient whether he or she notices any movements in the mouth, face, hands, or feet. If yes, ask to describe and to what extent they *currently* bother patient or interfere with his or her activities.

4: Have the patient sit in the chair with his or her hands on knees, legs slightly apart, and feet flat on floor. (Look at the entire body for movements while in this position.)

5: Ask the patient to sit with his or her hands hanging unsupported. If male, between legs, if female and wearing a dress, hanging over knees. (Observe hands and other body areas.)

6: Ask the patient to open his or her mouth. (Observe the tongue at rest within the mouth.) Do this twice.

7: Ask the patient to protrude his or her tongue. (Observe the tongue at rest within the mouth.) Do this twice.

*8: Ask the patient to tap his or her thumb, with each finger, as rapidly as possible for 10–15 seconds; separately with the right hand and then with the left hand. (Observe facial and leg movements.)

9: Flex and extend the patient's left and right arms (one at a time). (Note any rigidity and rate on NOTES.)

10: Ask the patient to stand up. (Observe in profile. Observe all body areas again, hips included.)

*11: Ask the patient to extend both arms outstretched in front with the palms down. (Observe trunk, legs, and mouth.)

*12: Have the patient walk a few paces, turn, and walk back to the chair. (Observe hand and gait.) Do this twice.

---

*Activated movements.
Reprinted from Guy, W. (1976). *ECDEU: Assessment manual for psychopharmacology* (DHEW Publ No 76–338). Washington, DC: Department of Health, Education, and Welfare, Psychopharmacology Research Branch.

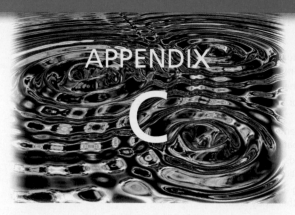

APPENDIX C

Simplified Diagnosis for Tardive Dyskinesia (SD-TD)

The following instructions accompany the Dyskinesia Identification System: Condensed User Scale (DISCUS). See Box 22.5.

PREREQUISITES.—The three prerequisites are as follows. Exceptions may occur.
1. A history of at least 3 months' total cumulative neuroleptic exposure. Include amoxapine and metoclopramide in all categories below as well.
2. **SCORING/INTENSITY LEVEL.** The presence of a **TOTAL SCORE OF FIVE (5) OR ABOVE.** Also be alert for any change from baseline or scores below five which have at least a "moderate" (3) or "severe" (4) movement on any item or at least two "mild" (2) movements on two items located in different body areas.
3. Other conditions are not responsible for the abnormal involuntary movements.

DIAGNOSES.—The diagnosis is based upon the current exam and its relation to the last exam. The diagnosis can shift depending upon: (a) whether movements are present or not, (b) whether movements are present for 3 months or more (6 months if on a semiannual assessment schedule), and (c) whether neuroleptic dosage changes occur and effect movements.

- **NO TD.**—Movements **are not** present on this exam **or** movements are present, but some other condition is responsible for them. The last diagnosis must be NO TD, PROBABLE TD, or WITHDRAWAL TD.
- **PROBABLE TD.**—Movements **are** present on this exam. This is the first time they are present or they have never been present for 3 months or more. The last diagnosis must be NO TD or PROBABLE TD.
- **PERSISTENT TD.**—Movements are present on this exam **and** they have been present for 3 months or more with this exam or at some point in the past. The last diagnosis can be any except NO TD.
- **MASKED TD.**—Movements **are not** present on this exam **but** this is due to a neuroleptic dosage increase or reinstitution after a prior exam when movements were present. Also use this conclusion if movements are not present due to the addition of a non-neuroleptic medication to treat TD. The last diagnosis must be PROBABLE TD, PERSISTENT TD, WITHDRAWAL TD, or MASKED TD.
- **REMITTED TD.**—Movements **are not** present on this exam **but** PERSISTENT TD has been diagnosed and neuroleptic dosage increase or reinstitution has occurred. The last diagnosis must be PERSISTENT TD or REMITTED TD. If movements re-emerge, the diagnosis shifts back to PERSISTENT TD.
- **WITHDRAWAL TD.**—Movements **are not seen while** receiving neuroleptics or at the last dosage level **but are seen within** 8 weeks following a neuroleptic reduction or discontinuation. The last diagnosis must be NO TD or WITHDRAWAL TD. If movements continue for 3 months or more after the neuroleptic dosage reduction or discontinuation, the diagnosis shifts to PERSISTENT TD. If movements do not continue for 3 months or more after the reduction or discontinuation, the diagnosis shifts to NO TD.

INSTRUCTIONS
1. The rater completes the Assessment according to the standardized exam procedure. If the rater also completes Evaluation items 1–4, he/she must also sign the preparer box. The form is given to the physician. Alternatively, the physician may perform the assessment.
2. The physician completes the Evaluation section. The physician is responsible for the entire Evaluation section and its accuracy.
3. IT IS RECOMMENDED THAT THE PHYSICIAN EXAMINE ANY INDIVIDUAL WHO MEETS THE THREE PREREQUISITES OR WHO HAS MOVEMENTS NOT EXPLAINED BY OTHER FACTORS. NEUROLOGICAL ASSESSMENTS OR DIFFERENTIAL DIAGNOSTIC TESTS WHICH MAY BE NECESSARY SHOULD BE OBTAINED.
4. File form according to policy or procedure.

OTHER CONDITIONS (partial list)
1. Age
2. Blind
3. Cerebral Palsy
4. Contact Lenses
5. Dentures/No Teeth
6. Down Syndrome
7. Drug Intoxication (specify)
8. Encephalitis
9. Extrapyramidal Side-Effects (specify)
10. Fahr's Syndrome
11. Heavy Meta Intoxication (specify)
12. Huntington's Chorea
13. Hyperthyroidism
14. Hypoglycemia
15. Hypoparathyroidism
16. Idiopathic Torsion Dystonia
17. Meige Syndrome
18. Parkinson's Disease
19. Stereotypies
20. Sydenham's Chorea
21. Tourette's Syndrome
22. Wilson's Disease
23. Other (specify)

Sprague, R. L., & Kalachnik, J. E. (1991). Reliability, validity, and a total score cutoff for the Dyskinesia Identification System, Condensed User Scale (DISCUS) with mentally ill and mentally retarded populations. *Psychopharmacology Bulletin*, 27(1), 51–58.

Glossary

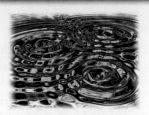

ABCDE An acronym for the basic framework of rational emotive behavior therapy.

ABCs of psychological first aid Focusing on A (arousal), B (behavior), and C (cognition).

absorption Movement of drug from the site of administration into plasma.

abuse Use of alcohol or drugs for the purpose of intoxication or, in the case of prescription drugs, for purposes beyond the intended use.

accreditation Process by which a mental health agency is recognized or approved in accordance with established standards to be providing acceptable quality of care.

acculturation Act or process of assuming the beliefs, values, and practices of another, usually dominant culture.

acetylcholine (ACh) The primary cholinergic neurotransmitter. Found in the greatest concentration in the peripheral nervous system, ACh provides the basic synaptic communication for the parasympathetic neurons and part of the sympathetic neurons, which send information to the central nervous system. An important neurotransmitter associated with cognitive functioning; disruption of cholinergic mechanisms damages memory in animals and humans.

acetylcholinesterase (AChE) Key enzyme that inactivates the neurotransmitter acetylcholine. AChE is found in high concentrations in the brain and is one of two cholinesterase enzymes capable of breaking down ACh.

acetylcholinesterase inhibitors (AChEI) Mainstay of pharmacologic treatment of dementia; these drugs inhibit AChE, resulting in an enhancement of cholinergic activity.

activating event The "A" in the ABCDE framework of rational emotive behavior therapy. It represents an external or internal stimulus. Not necessarily an actual event, it may be an emotion, or thought or expectation that is interpreted according to a set of beliefs.

active listening Focusing on what the patient is saying in order to interpret and respond to the message in an objective manner while using techniques such as open-ended statements, reflection, and questions that elicit additional responses from the patient.

acute pain A sudden, severe onset of pain symptoms at the time of injury or illness that generally subsides as the associated condition subsides or the injury heals.

acute stress disorder (ASD) A mental disorder characterized by persistent, distressing stress-related symptoms that last between 2 days and 1 month and that occur within 1 month after a traumatic experience.

adaptation A person's capacity to survive and flourish as it affects health, psychological well-being, and social functioning.

adaptive behavior Behavior that is composed of three skill types: conceptual, social, and practical skills.

addiction A condition of continued use of substances (or reward-seeking behaviors) despite adverse consequences.

adherence An individual's compliance to a therapeutic routine.

advance care directives Treatment directives (living wills) and appointment directives (power of attorney or health proxies) that apply only if the individual is unable to make his or her own decisions because the patient is incapacitated or, in the opinion of two physicians, is otherwise unable to make decisions for himself or herself.

advanced practice psychiatric–mental health nurse A licensed registered nurse who is educationally prepared at the graduate level and is nationally certified as a specialist by the American Nurses Credentialing Center (ANCC).

adverse reactions (adverse effects) Unwanted medication effects that may have serious physiologic consequences.

affect An expression of mood manifest in a person's outward emotional expression; varies considerably both within and among different cultures.

affective instability Rapid and extreme shifts in mood, erratic emotional responses to situations, and intense sensitivity to criticism or perceived slights; one of the core characteristics of borderline personality disorder.

affective lability Abrupt, dramatic, unprovoked changes in the types of emotions expressed.

affinity Degree of attraction or strength of the bond between a drug and its biologic target.

aggression Overt behavior intended to hurt, belittle, take revenge, or achieve domination and control; can be verbal or physical. Behaviors or attitudes that reflect rage, hostility, and the potential for physical or verbal destructiveness; usually occurs if the person believes someone is going to do him or her harm.

agitation Inability to sit still or attend to others accompanied by heightened emotions and tension.

agnosia Failure to recognize or identify objects despite intact sensory function.

agonists Substances that initiate the same response as the chemical normally present in the body.

agoraphobia Fear of open spaces; commonly occurs with panic disorder.

agranulocytosis Dangerously low level of circulating neutrophils.

akathisia An extrapyramidal side effect characterized by the inability to sit still or restlessness; more common in middle-aged patients. Sometimes misdiagnosed as agitation or an increase in psychotic symptoms.

Alcoholics Anonymous The first 12-step, self-help program; a worldwide fellowship of people with alcoholism who provide support, individually and at meetings, to others who seek help.

alcohol withdrawal syndrome A syndrome that occurs after the reduction of alcohol consumption or when abstaining from alcohol after prolonged use, causing changes in vital signs, diaphoresis, and other adverse gastrointestinal and central nervous system side effects.

alexithymia Difficulty identifying and expressing emotion.

allodynia Pain unrelated to noxious stimuli; lowered pain threshold.

allostasis The dynamic regulatory process that maintains homeostasis through a process of adaptation.

allostatic load (AL) An increase in the number of abnormal biological parameters as a consequence of wear and tear on the body and brain; leads to ill health.

alogia Reduced fluency and productivity of thought and speech. Brief, empty verbal responses; often referred to as *poverty of speech*.

ambivalence Presence and expression of two opposing feelings, leading to inaction.

amino acids Building blocks of proteins that have different roles in intraneuronal metabolism. Amino acids function as neurotransmitters in as many as 60% to 70% of synaptic sites in the brain.

anger An internal affective state, usually temporary rather than an enduring negative attitude, that may or may not be expressed in overt behavior. If expressed, anger behavior can be constructive or destructive.

anger management A psychoeducational intervention for persons whose anger behavior is dysfunctional in some way (i.e., interfering with success in work or relationships) but *not violent.*

anhedonia Inability to experience pleasure.

anorexia nervosa A life-threatening eating disorder characterized by a mixture of biopsychosocial symptoms, including significantly low body weight, intense fear of gaining weight or becoming fat, and a disturbance in experiencing body weight or shape.

anorgasmia The inability to achieve an orgasm.

antagonists Chemicals blocking the biologic response at a given receptor site.

antisocial personality disorder A disorder characterized by a marked pattern of disregard for, and violation of, the rights of others.

anxiety Energy that arises when expectations that are present are not met (Peplau). An uncomfortable feeling of apprehension or dread that occurs in response to internal or external stimuli and can result in physical, emotional, cognitive, and behavioral symptoms.

apathy Reactions to stimuli that are decreased along with a diminished interest and desire.

aphasia Alterations in language ability.

appraisal The process whereby all aspects of a given event or situation are considered—the demands, constraints, and resources are balanced with personal goals and beliefs.

apraxia Impaired ability to execute motor activities despite intact motor functioning.

Asperger syndrome Formerly named Asperger syndrome, it is now diagnosed as autism spectrum disorder with persistent difficulty in social communication and interaction. It appears to be a milder form of autism.

assault The threat of unlawful force to inflict bodily injury on another. The threat must be imminent and cause reasonable apprehension in the individual.

assertive community treatment A model that calls for a multidisciplinary clinical team approach to providing 24-hour, intensive community-based services to help patients meet the requirements of community living during reintegration.

assessment The deliberate and systematic collection and interpretation of biopsychosocial information or data to determine current and past health, functional status, and human responses to mental health problems, both actual and potential.

assortative mating Tendency for individuals to select mates who are similar in genetically linked traits such as intelligence and personality styles.

asylum Safe haven.

attachment Emotional bond formed between children and their and parental figures at an early age; attaining and retaining interpersonal connection to a significant person, beginning at birth.

attachment disorganization A consequence of extreme insecurity that results from feared or actual separation from the attached figure. Infants appear to be unable to maintain the strategic adjustments in attachment behavior.

attention A complex mental process that involves concentrating on one activity to the exclusion of others, as well as sustaining interest over time.

attention deficit hyperactivity disorder (ADHD) A persistent pattern of inattention, hyperactivity, and impulsiveness; typically diagnosed based on teacher and parent reports and direct observation of the behavior patterns described.

atypical antipsychotics Newer antipsychotics that are equally or more effective than conventional antipsychotics but have fewer side effects.

augmentation A strategy of adding another medication to enhance effectiveness.

autism spectrum disorders Disorders characterized by neurodevelopmental delays that are typically diagnosed in childhood. Children with autism spectrum disorders may or may not have an intellectual disability, but they commonly show an uneven pattern of intellectual strengths and weaknesses.

autistic thinking Thinking restricted to the literal and immediate so that the individual has private rules of logic and reasoning that make no sense to others.

autonomic nervous system Part of the nervous system that regulates involuntary vital functions including cardiac muscle, smooth muscles, and glands. It is composed of the sympathetic and parasympathetic systems.

autonomy Concept that each person has the fundamental right of self-determination.

avoidant personality disorder A disorder characterized by avoiding social situations in which there is interpersonal contact with others. Individuals appear timid, shy, and hesitant; fear criticism; and feel inadequate. They are extremely sensitive to negative comments and disapproval and appraise situations more negatively than others do.

avolition Withdrawal and inability to initiate and persist in goal-directed activity.

basal ganglia Subcortical gray matter areas in both the right and the left hemisphere that contain many cell bodies or nuclei.

behaviorism A paradigm shift in understanding human behavior that was initiated by Watson, who theorized that human behavior is developed through a stimulus–response process rather than through unconscious drives or instincts.

behavior modification A specific therapy technique that can be applied to individuals, groups, or systems. The aim of behavior modification is to reinforce desired behaviors and extinguish undesired ones.

behavior therapy Interventions that reinforce or promote desirable behaviors or alter undesirable ones.

belief system The "B" in the ABCDE framework of rational emotive behavior therapy. Beliefs underlying thoughts and emotions are shaped by rationality, which is self-constructive, and irrationality, which is self-defeating.

beneficence The health care provider uses knowledge of science and incorporates the art of caring to develop an environment in which individuals achieve maximum health care potential.

bereavement The process of mourning and coping with the loss of a loved one. It begins immediately after the loss, but it can last months or years.

beta-amyloid plaques Dense, mostly insoluble deposits of protein and cellular material outside and around neurons; pathology of Alzheimer's disease.

bibliotherapy The use of provider-assigned books and other reading materials to help individuals gain therapeutic benefit.

binge eating Rapid, episodic, impulsive, and uncontrollable ingestion of a large amount of food during a short period of time, usually 1 to 2 hours, usually followed by feelings of guilt that result in purging.

binge-eating disorder A newly identified eating disorder in its infancy relative to research; individuals binge in the same way as those with bulimia nervosa but do not purge or compensate for binges through other behaviors.

bioavailability Amount of a drug that actually reaches the systemic circulation unchanged.

biogenic amines Small molecules manufactured in the neuron that contain an amine group. These include dopamine, norepinephrine, and epinephrine (all synthesized from the amino acid tyrosine) and serotonin (from tryptophan).

biologic markers Physical indicators of disturbances within the central nervous system that differentiate one disease state from another; found using diagnostic testing.

biopsychosocial model An organizational model consisting of three separate but interdependent domains: biologic, psychological, and social. Each domain has an independent knowledge and treatment focus but can interact and be mutually interdependent with the other dimensions.

biosexual identity   Anatomic and physiologic state of being male or female that results from genetic and hormonal influences.

biotransformation   Metabolism of a drug or substance; the process by which the drug is altered and broken down into smaller substances, known as metabolites.

bipolar disorders   Mood disorders that are characterized by periods of mania or hypomania that alternate with depression. These disorders can be further designated as bipolar I, bipolar II, and cyclothymic disorder depending on the severity of the manic and depressive symptoms.

bipolar I   A type of bipolar disorder that is diagnosed when at least one manic episode or mixed episode.

bipolar II   A type of bipolar disorder that has less dramatic symptoms than bipolar I. Hypomania (mild mania) and a major depressive episode are characteristic symptoms.

blood alcohol level   The level of alcohol in the blood; used to determine intoxication.

board-and-care homes   Facilities that provide 24-hour supervision and assistance with medications, meals, and some self-care skills but in which individualized attention to self-care skills and other activities of daily living is generally not available.

body dissatisfaction   A sense of dissatisfaction and low self esteem when one's own body is perceived to fall short of an ideal.

body dysmorphic disorder   Disorder in which there is a preoccupation with an imagined or slight defect in appearance, such as a large nose, thinning hair, or small genitals.

body image   How each individual perceives his or her own body, including such dimensions as size and attractiveness.

body image distortion   Extreme discrepancy between one's perception of one's own body image and others' perceptions of one.

borderline personality disorder   A disorder characterized by a disruptive pattern of instability related to self-identity, interpersonal relationships, and affects combined with marked impulsivity and destructive behavior.

boundaries   Limits in which a person may act or refrain from acting within a designated time or place. Invisible barriers with varying permeabilities that surround family subsystems.

boxed warning   Serious adverse effects that can occur with the use of a specific medication; noted in issued warning in the package insert.

bradykinesia   An extrapyramidal condition characterized by a slowness of voluntary movement and speech.

brain stem   Area of the brain containing the midbrain, pons, and medulla, which continues beneath the thalamus.

breach of confidentiality   Release of patient information without the patient's consent in the absence of legal compulsion or authorization to release information.

brief intervention   A negotiated conversation between professional and patient designed to reduce alcohol and drug use; any short-term intervention.

bulimia nervosa   An eating disorder in which the individual engages in recurrent episodes of binge eating and compensatory behavior to avoid weight gain through purging methods such as self-induced vomiting or use of laxatives, diuretics, enemas, or emetics or through non-purging methods such as fasting or excessive exercise.

bullying   Repeated, deliberate attempts to harm someone that are usually unprovoked. An imbalance in strength is a part of the pattern, with most victims having difficulty defending themselves.

carrier protein   A membrane protein that transports a specific molecule across the cell membrane.

case finding   Identifying people who are at risk for suicide to initiate proper treatment. Identification of depression and risk factors associated with suicide.

case management   Service model in which a case manager locates services, links the patient with these services, and then monitors the patient's receipt of these services.

cataplexy   Bilateral loss of muscle tone triggered by a strong emotion such as laughter. This muscle atonia can range from subtle (drooping eyelids) to dramatic (buckling knees). Respiratory muscles are not affected. Cataplexy usually lasts only seconds. Individuals are fully conscious, oriented, and alert during the episode. Prolonged episodes of cataplexy may lead to sleep episodes.

catastrophic reactions   Overreactions or extreme anxiety reactions to everyday situations.

catatonic excitement   Hyperactivity characterized by purposeless activity and abnormal movements like grimacing and posturing.

catharsis   A Freudian concept meaning release of feelings, as in the venting of anger.

cerebellum   Part of the brain that is responsible for controlling movement and postural adjustments; it receives information from all parts of the body.

chemical restraint   Use of medication to control patients or manage behavior.

child abuse   Any action that robs children of rights they should have including the rights to be and behave like a child; to be safe and protected from harm; and to be fed, clothed, and nurtured so the child can grow, develop, and fulfill his or her unique potential.

child neglect   A form of child abuse defined as failure to provide for a child's physical, emotional, health care, or educational needs; failure to adequately supervise a child; or intentionally exposing a child to a dangerous environment.

chronic pain   Pain on a daily basis or pain that is constant for more than 6 months.

chronic syndromes   Symptom patterns that last for long periods of time. Medication-related movement disorders that develop from longer exposure to antipsychotic drugs.

chronobiology   Study and measure of time structures or biologic rhythms.

chronopharmacotherapy   Resetting the biologic clock by using short-acting hypnotics to induce sleep.

circadian cycle   A biologic system that has a 24-hour cycle.

circadian rhythm   Physiologic and psychological functions that fluctuate in a pattern that repeats itself in a 24-hour cycle.

circumstantiality   Extremely detailed and lengthy discourse about a topic.

clang association   Repetition of word phrases that are similar in sound but in no other way, for example, "right, light, sight, might."

classical conditioning   A learning situation in which an unconditioned stimulus initially produces an unconditioned response; over time, a conditioned response is elicited for a specific stimulus (Pavlov).

clearance   Total amount of blood, serum, or plasma from which a drug is completely removed per unit of time.

clinical reasoning   Using critical thinking and reflection to address patient problems and interventions.

closed group   A group in which all the members begin at one time. New members are not admitted after the first meeting.

codependence   An "enabling" method of coping in which an individual in a relationship with a person who abuses alcohol inadvertently reinforces the drinking behavior of the other person.

cognition   A high level of intellectual processing in which perceptions and information are acquired, used, or manipulated; for Beck, verbal or pictorial events in the stream of consciousness. A person's ability to think and know. An internal process of perception, memory, and judgment through which an understanding of self and the world is developed.

cognitive behavioral therapy   A highly structured psychotherapeutic method used to alter distorted beliefs and problem behaviors by identifying and replacing negative inaccurate thoughts and changing the rewards for behaviors.

cognitive distortions   Automatic thoughts generated by organizing distorted information or inaccurate interpretation of a situation.

cognitive interventions or cognitive therapy   Interventions or psychotherapy that aims to change or reframe an individual's automatic thought patterns that develop over time and that interfere with the ability to function optimally.

cognitive reserve   The brain's ability to operate effectively even when there is disruption in functioning.

cognitive schema   Patterns of thoughts that determine how a person interprets events. Each person's cognitive schema screen, code, and evaluate incoming stimuli.

cognitive theory   An outgrowth of different theoretic perspectives, including the behavioral and the psychodynamic, that attempts to link internal thought processes with human behavior.

cognitive triad   Thoughts about oneself, the world, and the future.

cohesion   The ability of a group to stick together.

co-leadership   When two people share responsibility for leading a group.

commitment to treatment statement   Statement in which a patient verbally or in writing agrees to seek treatment or access emergency services if needed.

communication blocks   Interruptions in the content flow of communication that can be identified in process recordings as such changes in topic that either the nurse or patient makes.

communication disorders   Disorders that involve speech or language impairments.

communication triad   A technique used to provide a specific syntax and order for patients to identify and express their feelings and seek relief. The "sentence" consists of three parts: (1) an "I" statement to identify the prevailing feeling, (2) a nonjudgmental statement of the emotional trigger, and (3) a statement of what the person would like differently or what would restore comfort to the situation.

communications pathways   An aspect of group interaction based on interaction patterns related to who is most liked in the group, who occupies a position of power, what subgroups have formed, and who is isolated from the group.

comorbidity (comorbid)   Presence of a disorder simultaneously with and independently of another disorder.

competence The degree to which the patient is able to understand and appreciate the information given during the consent process; the patient's cognitive ability to process information at a specific time; the patient's ability to gather and interpret information and make reasonable judgments based on that information to participate fully as a partner in treatment.

complicated grief A reaction to the loss of a loved one in which a person is frozen or stuck in a state of chronic mourning.

compliments Affirmations of the patient.

comprehensive family assessment The collection of all relevant data related to family health, psychological well-being, and social functioning to identify problems for which the nurse can generate nursing diagnoses.

compulsions Behaviors that are performed repeatedly, in a ritualistic fashion, with the goal of preventing or relieving anxiety and distress caused by obsessions.

concrete thinking Lack of abstraction in thinking in which people are unable to understand punch lines, metaphors, and analogies.

conditional release Discharge of patients whose psychiatric symptoms have been stabilized and are no longer considered a danger to the community. Patients are monitored on an ongoing basis by the court and must follow established conditions and criteria to maintain their discharged status.

conduct disorder A disorder characterized by more serious violations of social norms, including aggressive behavior, destruction of property, and cruelty to animals.

confabulation Telling a plausible but imagined scenario to compensate for memory gaps.

confidentiality An ethical duty of nondisclosure; the patient has the right to disclose personal information without fear of it being revealed to others.

conflict resolution A specific type of counseling in which the nurse helps the patient resolve a disagreement or dispute.

confrontation Presenting evidence of inconsistencies in a person's thoughts, feelings, and actions.

confused speech and thinking Symptoms of schizophrenia that render the patient unable to respond accurately to the ordinary signs and sounds of daily living.

connections Mutually responsive and enhancing relationships.

constraints Limitations that are both personal (internalized cultural values and beliefs) and environmental (finite resources such as money and time).

containment The process of providing safety and security; involves the patient's access to food and shelter.

content themes Repetition of concerns or feelings that occur within the therapeutic relationship. Themes may emerge as symbolic representations of fears.

continuum of care Providing care in an integrated system of settings, services (physical, psychological, and social), and care levels appropriate to the individual's specific needs in a continuous manner over time, with channels of communication among the service providers.

conventional antipsychotics Also known as typical antipsychotics, "older" medications used to treat psychotic disorders with more side effects than "newer" atypical antipsychotics.

conversion disorder (functional neurological symptom disorder) When severe emotional distress or unconscious conflict is expressed through physical symptoms.

co-occurring disorders (COD) Refers to the presence of comorbid mental illness and a substance use disorder in the same person.

coordination of care The integration of appropriate services so that individualized care is provided. When several agencies are involved, this allows a person's needs to be met without duplication of services.

coping A deliberate, planned, and psychological effort to manage stressful demands.

cortex Outermost surface of the cerebrum of the mature brain.

cortical dementia A type of dementia that is characterized by amnesia, aphasia, apraxia, and agnosia. Results from a disease process that globally affects the cortex.

counseling (counseling interventions) Specific time-limited interactions between a nurse and a patient, family, or group experiencing intermediate or ongoing difficulties related to their health or well-being.

countertransference The therapist or nurse's reactions to a patient that are based on interpersonal experiences, feelings, and attitudes. It can significantly interfere with the nurse–patient relationship.

court process counseling An approach that educates mentally ill patients about the impending legal procedures and prepares them for courtroom appearances.

craving The urge or desire to engage in a behavior such as drinking.

crisis A time-limited event that triggers adaptive or non-adaptive responses to maturational, situational, or traumatic experiences; results from stressful events for which coping mechanisms fail to provide adequate adaptive skills to address the perceived challenge or threat.

crisis intervention A specialized short-term (usually no longer than 6 hours) goal-directed therapy designed to assist patients in an immediate manner; focuses on stabilization, symptom reduction, and prevention of relapse requiring inpatient services.

Crisis Intervention Teams (CIT) Teams that train police officers to recognize and intervene in crisis situations in the community and determine whether emergency psychiatric services are needed.

Critical Time Intervention (CTI) A "bridge" between inpatient and outpatient treatment by coordinating care between staff in these settings.

cue elimination Emotional and environmental cues are identified and alternative responses are suggested, tried, and reinforced. When a cue or stimulus leads to a dysfunctional or unhealthy response, the response can be eliminated or an alternate, healthier response to the cue can be substituted, tried, and then reinforced.

cultural brokering Act of bridging, linking, or mediating between groups or individuals of different cultural systems for the purpose of reducing conflict or producing change. Cultural competence is a set of academic and interpersonal skills that are respectful of and responsive to the health belief practices and cultural and linguistic needs of diverse patients to bring about positive health care outcomes.

cultural competence A set of academic and interpersonal skills that allows individuals to increase their understanding and appreciation of cultural differences and similarities within, among, and between groups.

cultural identity A set of cultural beliefs with which one looks for standards of behavior; many consider themselves to have multiple cultural identities.

cultural idiom of distress A linguistic term, phrase, or a way of talking about suffering among individuals of a cultural group (*DSM-5*).

cultural syndrome A cluster or group of co-occurring symptoms found in a specific cultural group, community, or context.

culture Any group of people who identify or associate with each other on the basis of some common purpose, need, or similarity of background; the set of learned, socially transmitted beliefs, values, and behaviors that arise from interpersonal transactions among members of the cultural group.

cyberstalking Use of the Internet, e-mail, or other telecommunications technology to harass or stalk another person.

cycle of violence A three-phase pattern of tension, abuse, and kindness in which the abuser engages first in abuse and then in seemingly sincere expressions of love, contrition, and remorse.

cyclothymic disorder Chronic fluctuating mood disturbance. Does not meet criteria for hypomania or depressive disorder.

cytochrome P-450 (CYP450) system A set of microsomal enzymes (usually hepatic) referred to as CYP1, CYP2, and CYP3.

day treatment A bridge between institutional and community care for severely mentally ill and substance-abusing people. Participation in structured day treatment programs provides emotional and practical support and strengthens ties to community services and potentially to family and friends.

debriefing The reconstruction of the traumatic events by the victim as a psychological intervention.

de-escalation An interactive process of calming and redirecting a patient who has an immediate potential for violence directed at others or self.

defense mechanisms Coping styles; the automatic psychological process protecting the individual against anxiety and creating awareness of internal or external dangers or stressors.

deinstitutionalization Release of patients with severe and persistent mental illness from state mental hospitals into the community for treatment, support, and rehabilitation as the result of a national movement that began in the 1960s.

delayed ejaculation (DE) Delay or absence of ejaculation.

delirium A disorder of acute cognitive impairment that can be caused by a medical condition (e.g., infection) or substance abuse, or it may have multiple etiologies.

delirium tremens An acute symptom of alcohol withdrawal syndrome that is characterized by autonomic hyperarousal, disorientation, hallucinations, and tremors or grand mal (tonic–clonic) seizures.

delusions Erroneous fixed, false beliefs that cannot be changed by reasonable argument. They usually involve a misinterpretation of experience and are unchanged by reasonable arguments.

delusional disorder A psychotic disorder characterized by delusions that occur in the absence of other psychiatric disorders; includes several subtypes: erotomania, grandiose, jealous, somatic, mixed, and unspecified. Individual can function fairly well and abnormal behavior is not observable.

demands Pulls put on an individual's resources that are generated by physiologic and psychological needs. Includes external pulls (crowding, crime, noise, pollution) imposed by the physical environment and internal pulls (behavior and role expectations) imposed by the social environment.

dementia From the Latin *de* (from or out of) and *mens* (mind); characterized by chronic cognitive impairments. It is differentiated from delirium by underlying cause, not by symptom patterns.

denial The patient's inability to accept loss of control over substance use or the severity of the consequences associated with substance abuse.

dependence The state of being psychologically or physiologically dependent on a drug after a prolonged period of use.

dependent personality Person who clings to others in a desperate attempt to keep them close. Their need to be taken care of is so great that it leads to doing anything to maintain the closeness, including total submission and disregard for self.

depersonalization A nonspecific experience in which the individual loses a sense of personal identity and feels strange or unreal.

depression The primary mood of depressive disorders defined as an overwhelming state of sadness, loss of interest or pleasure, feelings of guilt, disturbed sleep patterns and appetite, low energy, and an inability to concentrate.

depression not otherwise specified A category that includes disorders with depressive features that do not meet strict criteria for major depressive disorder.

depressive disorders Also referred to as unipolar depression, a specific subset of mood disorders consisting of major depression, dysthymia, and depression not otherwise specified (NOS).

derealization Feelings of unreality.

desensitization A rapid decrease in drug effects that may develop within a few minutes of exposure to a drug.

desynchronized Two or more circadian rhythms reaching their peaks at different times.

deteriorating relationship A type of nontherapeutic relationship with several defined phases during which the patient and nurse feel very frustrated and keep varying their approach with each other in an attempt to establish a meaningful relationship.

detoxification Process of safely and effectively withdrawing a person from an addictive substance, usually under medical supervision.

developmental crisis A significant maturational event, such as leaving home for the first time, completing school, or accepting the responsibility of adulthood.

developmental delay An impairment of normal growth and development that may not be reversible. Delays slow a child's progress and can interfere with the development of self-esteem.

dialectical behavior therapy (DBT) An important biosocial approach to treatment that combines numerous cognitive and behavior therapy strategies. It requires patients to understand their disorders by actively participating in formulating treatment goals by collecting data about their own behavior, identifying treatment targets in individual therapy, and working with the therapists in changing these target behaviors.

diathesis A genetic predisposition that increases susceptibility to developing a disorder.

dichotomous thinking Evaluating experiences, people, and objects in terms of mutually exclusive categories (e.g., good or bad, success or failure, trustworthy or deceitful), which informs extreme interpretations of events that would normally be viewed as including both positive and negative aspects.

dietary restraint Instituting severe dieting (e.g., setting rules such as no sweets, no fats) to eliminate out-of-control feelings related to binge eating.

differentiation of self An individual's resolution of attachment to his or her family's emotional chaos. It involves an intrapsychic separation of thinking from feelings and an interpersonal freeing of oneself from the chaos.

difficult temperament Characterized by withdrawal from stimuli, low adaptability, and intense emotional reactions. Four key behaviors are present in a difficult temperament: aggression, inattention, hyperactivity, and impulsivity.

diminished emotional expression One of the core negative symptoms of schizophrenia.

direct leadership The leader controls the interaction of the group by giving directions and information and allowing little discussion.

disaster A sudden overwhelming catastrophic event that causes great damage and destruction that may involve mass casualties and human suffering that requires assistance from all available resources.

disconnections Lack of mutually responsive and enhancing relationships.

disinhibition A concept borrowed from physics and biology and based on the idea of a dynamic, self-regulatory model of equilibrium in which equilibrium is defined (Piaget) as compensation for external disturbance; a mechanism for providing the self-regulation by which intelligence adapts to internal and external changes. A symptom of Alzheimer's disease in which a patient acts on thoughts and feelings without exercising appropriate social judgment.

disorganized symptoms Symptoms of schizophrenia that make it difficult for the person to understand and respond to the ordinary sights and sounds of daily living. These include confused speech and thinking and disorganized behavior.

dissociation A disruption in the normally occurring linkages among subjective awareness, feelings, thoughts, behavior, and memories (i.e., a person is physically present but mentally in another place).

distraction   The purposeful focusing of attention away from undesirable sensations.

distribution   The amount of a drug that may be found in various tissues at the site of the drug action for which it is intended.

disturbance of executive functioning   Problems in the ability to think abstractly, plan, initiate, sequence, monitor, and stop complex behavior.

dopamine   An excitatory neurotransmitter found in distinct regions of the central nervous system involved in cognition, motor, and neuroendocrine function.

dosing   Administration of medication over time so that therapeutic levels may be achieved or maintained without reaching toxic levels.

drive for thinness   A characteristic of anorexia nervosa in which individuals experience an intense physical and emotional drive to be thinner that overrides all physiologic body cues.

drug–drug interaction   Reaction of two or more drugs with each other; may cause unexpected side effects. Can occur if one substance inhibits an enzyme system.

DSM-5   Abbreviation for the *Diagnostic and Statistical Manual of Mental Disorders*, Fifth Edition, which provides revised diagnostic criteria for mental disorders.

DSM-IV-TR   Abbreviation for the *Diagnostic and Statistical Manual of Mental Disorders*, Fourth Edition, text revision; contains criteria for the diagnosis of mental disorders.

dual process model   A model of bereavement where a person adjusts to loss by oscillating between loss-orientated coping that includes preoccupation with the deceased and restoration-oriented coping in which the bereaved is preoccupied with stressful events as a result of the death.

dyad   A group of only two people who are usually related, such as a married couple, siblings, or parent and child.

dysfunctional   The state of a group, such as a family, whose interactions, decisions, or behaviors interfere with the positive development of the group as a whole and its individual members.

dysfunctional consequences   Part of the "C" in the ABCDE framework of rational emotive behavior therapy. The result of the interaction between A (an activating event) and B (the person's belief system) that follows from absolute, rigid, irrational beliefs.

dyslexia   Significantly lower score for mental age on standardized test in reading that is not caused by low intelligence or inadequate schooling.

dyspareunia   Pain during sexual intercourse.

dysphagia   Difficulty swallowing.

dysphoric (mood)   Depressed, disquieted, or restless.

dysthymic disorder   A milder but more chronic form of major depressive disorder that is diagnosed when the depressed mood is present for most days for at least 2 years with 2 or more of the following symptoms: poor appetite or overeating, insomnia or oversleeping, low energy or fatigue, low self-esteem, poor concentration or difficulty making decisions, and feelings of hopelessness.

dystonia   An impairment in muscle tone that is generally the first extrapyramidal symptom to occur, usually within a few days of initiating an antipsychotic. Dystonia is characterized by involuntary muscle spasms, especially of the head and neck muscles.

early intervention programs   Community outreach efforts designed to work with infants and preschool-aged children and their caretakers to foster healthy physical, psychological, social, and intellectual development.

early recognition   Anticipating aggressive behavior based on the premise that even though behavior is idiosyncratic, it is reconstructable and therefore can provide early signs when violent behavior is likely.

echolalia   Repetition of another's words that is parrot-like and inappropriate.

echopraxia   Involuntary imitation of another person's movements and gestures.

efficacy   Ability of a drug to produce a response.

egocentric thinking   A type of thinking in which children naturally view themselves as the center of their own universe.

egocentrism   Tendency to view the world as revolving around oneself. A preoccupation with one's own appearance, behavior, thoughts, and feelings.

elation   Feeling "high," "ecstatic," "on top of the world," or "up in the clouds."

elder abuse   Abuse or neglect of adults older than 60 years of age.

elder mistreatment   Actions (or inaction) by caregivers or trusted persons that cause harm or the possibility of harm to a vulnerable older adult.

elevated mood   A mood that is expressed as euphoria (exaggerated feelings of well-being) or elation (feeling "high," "ecstatic," "on top of the world," or "up in the clouds.")

e-mental health   The use of electronics and the Internet to provide assessment and interventions.

emotions   Psychophysiologic reaction that defines a person's mood and can be categorized as negative (anger, fright, anxiety guilt, shame, sadness, envy, jealousy, and disgust), positive (happiness, pride, relief, and love), borderline (hope, compassion, empathy, sympathy, and contentment), or non-emotions (confidence, awe, confusion, excitement).

emotional cutoff If a member cannot differentiate from his or her family, that member may flee from the family either by moving away or avoiding personal subjects of conversation. A brief visit from parents can render these individuals helpless.

emotional dysregulation Inability to control emotion in social interactions.

emotional vulnerability Sensitivity and reactivity to environmental stress.

emotion-focused coping A type of coping in which a person reduces stress by reinterpreting the situation to change its meaning.

empathic linkage Ability to feel in oneself the feelings being expressed by another person or persons.

empathy The ability to experience, in the present, a situation as another did at some time in the past; the ability to put oneself in another person's circumstances and feelings.

empty nest A home devoid of children and caregiving responsibilities.

encopresis Soiling clothing with feces or depositing feces in inappropriate places.

endorphins Neurotransmitters that have opiate-like behavior and produce an inhibitory effect at opioid receptor sites; probably responsible for pain tolerance.

engagement Establishing a treatment relationship and enhancing motivation to make behavior changes and a commitment to treatment.

enmeshment An extreme form of intensity in family interactions that results in low individual autonomy in a family.

enuresis Involuntary excretion of urine after the age at which a child should have attained bladder control.

enzymes Any of numerous proteins that act as catalysts for physiologic reactions and can be targets for drugs.

epidemiology The study of patterns of disease distribution and determinants of health within populations; contributes to the overall understanding of the mental health status of population groups, or aggregates, and associated factors.

erectile dysfunction Inability of a man to achieve or maintain an erection sufficient for completion of sexual activity.

erotomanic Subtype of delusional disorder characterized by the delusional belief that the person is loved intensely by the "loved object," who is usually married

and of a higher socioeconomic status or otherwise unattainable.

ethnopsychopharmacology The study of cultural variations and differences that influence the effectiveness of pharmacotherapies used in mental health; includes genetics and psychosocial factors.

euphoria An exaggerated feeling of well-being.

euphoric (mood) An elated mood.

euthymic (mood) A normal mood.

evidence-based practice The use of current best evidence in making decisions; the search for and appraisal of the most relevant evidence to answer a clinical question.

exception questions Questions used to help the patient identify times when whatever is bothering him or her is not present or is present with less intensity based on the underlying assumption that during these times the patient is usually doing something to make things better.

excitement Phase of the human sexual response cycle marked by erotic feelings that lead to penile erection in men and vaginal lubrication in women. Heart rate and respirations also increase.

excretion The removal of drugs from the body either unchanged or as metabolites.

expansive mood A mood characterized by inappropriate lack of restraint in expressing one's feelings and frequently overvaluing one's own importance. Expansive qualities include an unceasing and indiscriminate enthusiasm for interpersonal, sexual, or occupational interactions.

exposure therapy The treatment of choice for agoraphobia in which the patient is repeatedly exposed to real or simulated anxiety-provoking situations until he or she becomes desensitized and anxiety subsides.

extended family Several nuclear families who may or may not live together and who function as one group.

external advocacy system Organizations that operate independently of mental health agencies and serve as advocates for the treatment and rights of mental health patients.

externalizing disorders Disorders that are characterized by acting-out behavior.

extinction The loss of a learned conditioned emotional response after repeated presentations of the conditioned fear stimulus without a contiguous traumatic event.

extrapyramidal motor system Collection of neuronal pathways that provides significant input in involuntary motor movements; a bundle of nerve fibers connecting the thalamus to the basal ganglia and cerebral cortex.

extrapyramidal side effects See extrapyramidal syndromes.

extrapyramidal symptoms (EPS) Acute abnormal movements developing early in the course of treatment with antipsychotic agents. Include dystonia, pseudoparkinsonism, and akathisia.

factitious disorder A type of psychiatric disorder characterized by somatization in which the person intentionally causes an illness for the purpose of becoming a patient.

factitious disorder on another Sometimes called Munchausen's by proxy; involves a person who inflicts injury on another person in order to gain the attention of a health care provider (i.e., a mother who inflicts injury on her child).

fairness In the criminal judicial process, a term meaning that the individual who is charged with a crime should know the legal rules and be able to explain the events surrounding the alleged crime or be "fit to stand trial."

family A group of people connected by birth, adoption, or marriage who have a shared history and future.

family development A broad term that refers to all the processes connected with the growth of a family, including changes associated with work, geographic location, migration, acculturation, and serious illness.

family dynamics The patterned interpersonal and social interactions that occur within the family structure over the life of a family.

family life cycle A process of expansion, contraction, and realignment of relationship systems to support the entry, exit, and development of family members.

family preservation Efforts made by professionals to preserve the family unit by preventing the removal of children from their homes through parental support and education and through work to facilitate a secure attachment between the child and parent.

family projection process In a triangulated family situation, the triangulated member becomes the center of family conflicts.

family structure According to Minuchin, the organized pattern within which family members interact.

fear conditioning A type of classic conditioning that occurs when a neutral stimulus (the conditioned stimulus [CS]) is paired with an aversive unconditioned stimulus (US) that elicits an unconditioned fear response (UR). After repeated pairing, the CS alone will elicit the fear response, which is now the conditioned response (CR).

fetal alcohol syndrome A syndrome that occurs in infants whose mothers abuse alcohol during pregnancy; includes symptoms such as permanent brain damage, often resulting in mental retardation.

fetishism When an object such as women's undergarments or foot apparel is used for sexual arousal.

fidelity Faithfulness to obligations and duties.

first-pass effect Metabolism of part of oral drugs after being absorbed from the gastrointestinal tract and carried through the portal circulation to the liver. Only part of the drug dose reaches systemic circulation.

fitness to stand trial Ability to consult with a lawyer with a reasonable degree of rational understanding of the facts of the alleged crime and of the legal proceedings.

flight of ideas Repeated and rapid changes in the topic of conversation, generally after just one sentence or phrase.

flooding A technique used to desensitize the patient to the fear associated with a particular anxiety-provoking stimulus. Desensitizing is done by presenting feared objects or situations repeatedly without session breaks until the anxiety dissipates.

forensic In mental health, a term that pertains to legal proceedings and mandated treatment of persons with a mental illness.

forensic examiner A mental health specialist, usually a psychiatrist or psychologist, who is certified as a forensic examiner and assigned by the judge to assess and testify to the patient's competency and responsibility for the crime, including the mental state at the time of an offense.

formal group roles The designated leader and members of a group.

formal operations The ability to use abstract reasoning to conceptualize and solve problems.

formal support system Large organizations that provide care to individuals, such as hospitals and nursing homes.

frontal, parietal, temporal, occipital lobes Lobes of the brain located on the lateral surface of each hemisphere.

frotteurism A paraphilia characterized by sexually arousing urges, fantasies, and behaviors resulting from touching or rubbing one's genitals against the breasts, genitals, or thighs of a nonconsenting person.

functional activities Activities of daily living necessary for self-care (i.e., bathing, toileting, dressing, and transferring).

functional consequences Part of the "C" in the ABCDE framework of rational emotive behavior therapy. The results of the interaction between A (an activating event) and B (a person's belief system) that follow from flexible, rational beliefs.

functional imaging The aspect of neuroimaging that visualizes processing of information.

functional neurologic symptoms   New name recommended to replace conversion disorder in the *Diagnostic and Statistical Manual of Mental Disorders*, 5th Edition (*DSM-5*), for when severe emotional distress or unconscious conflict is expressed through physical symptoms.

functional status   Extent to which a person has the ability to carry out independent personal care, home management, and social functions in everyday life in a way that has meaning and purpose.

GABA   Gamma-aminobutyric acid, the primary inhibitory neurotransmitter for the central nervous system (CNS). The pathways of GABA exist almost exclusively in the CNS, with the largest GABA concentrations in the hypothalamus, hippocampus, basal ganglia, spinal cord, and cerebellum.

gambling disorder   (also referred to as pathologic gambling) Persistent and recurrent gambling leading to clinically significant impairment or distress.

gate-control theory   The leading explanation of pain; holds that neurologic gates can either inhibit or allow pain signals to be transmitted to the brain. Led to the recognition that there is not a single pain mechanism but that the processing of pain occurs on at least three levels—peripheral, spinal, and supraspinal.

gender, culture, and ethnic differences   Factors that must be taken into consideration before planning interventions; for example, when considering interventions for the expression of anger, cultural norms should be understood.

gender dysphoria   Incongruence between an individual's experienced/expressed gender and assigned gender.

gender identity   A sense of self as being male or female.

gender identity disorders   A category of dysfunction in which there is a persistent cross-gender identification with accompanying discomfort about one's assigned sex.

genetic susceptibility   A concept that suggests that an individual may be at increased risk for a psychiatric disorder based on genetic transmission.

genogram   A multigenerational schematic diagram that lists family members and their relationships.

geropsychiatric nursing assessment   The comprehensive, deliberate, and systematic collection and interpretation of biopsychosocial data that is based on the special needs and problems of older adults.

gerotranscendence   A concept of Erikson; continued growth in dimensions such as spirituality and inner strength during old age.

glutamate   The most widely distributed excitatory neurotransmitter; the main transmitter in the associational areas of the cortex.

grandiosity   Elevated self-esteem.

grief   An intense, biopsychosocial response that often includes spontaneous expressions of pain, sadness, and desolation, such as with the loss of a loved one.

group   Two or more people who are in develop interactive relationships and share at least one common goal or issue.

group dynamics   All of the verbal and nonverbal interactions within groups.

group process   The culmination of the session-to-session interactions of the members that move the group toward its goals.

group themes   The collective conceptual underpinnings of a group that express the members' underlying concerns or feelings, regardless of the group's purpose.

groupthink   The tendency of many groups to avoid conflict and adopt a normative pattern of thinking that is often consistent with the group leader's ideas.

guided imagery   The purposeful use of imagination to achieve relaxation or direct attention away from undesirable sensations.

guilty but mentally ill (GBMI)   Persons with a mental illness who demonstrate they knew the wrongfulness of their actions and had the ability to act otherwise.

half-life   The time required for plasma concentrations of a drug to be reduced by 50%.

hallucinations   Perceptual experiences that occur in the absence of actual external sensory stimuli and may be auditory, visual, tactile, gustatory, or olfactory.

hallucinogen   A class of drug that produces euphoria or dysphoria, altered body image, distorted or sharpened visual and auditory perception, confusion, uncoordination, and impaired judgment and memory.

harm reduction   A community health intervention designed to reduce the harm of substance use to the individual, the family, and society that has replaced a moral or criminal approach to drug use and addiction.

hippocampus   Subcortical gray matter embedded within each temporal lobe of the brain that may be involved in determining the best way to store information, especially the emotions attached to a memory.

histamine   A neurotransmitter derived from the amino acid histidine that originates predominantly in the hypothalamus and projects to all major structures in the cerebrum, brain stem, and spinal cord. Its functions are not well known, but it appears to have a role in autonomic and neuroendocrine regulation.

histrionic personality   Type of person who could be described as "attention seeking," "excitable," and "emotional," with an insatiable need for attention and approval. Also tend to be highly dependent on others, making them overly trusting and gullible. They are moody and experience helplessness when others are disinterested in them. They are also sexually seductive in attempts to gain attention are often uncomfortable within a single relationship.

HIV-associated neurocognitive disorder (HAND) One of the most common CNS manifestations of HIV, it is a chronic neurodegenerative condition characterized by cognitive, central motor, and behavioral changes. HAND can affect any psychologic domain, but the most commonly reported deficits are in attention and concentration, psychomotor speed, memory and learning, information processing, and executive function.

homelessness State of being without a consistent residence or living in nighttime residences that are temporary shelters or any place not designated as sleeping accommodations.

homeostasis The body's tendency to resist physiologic change and hold bodily functions relatively consistent, well-coordinated, and usually stable. Introduced as a concept by Walter Cannon in the 1930s.

home visits Delivery of nursing care in a patient's living environment.

hopelessness A belief that nothing positive will happen or negative events will occur.

hostile aggression Aggression that is intended solely to inflict injury or pain on the victim with no reward or advantage to the aggressor.

Housing First A mental health approach that places people who are homeless, usually also experiencing severe mental illness, substance abuse, or release from prison, into affordable housing.

human sexual response cycle A theory of sexual response described by Masters and Johnson (1966) as consisting of four phases: excitement, plateau, orgasm, and resolution.

hyperactivity Excessive motor activity, movement, or utterances that may be either purposeless or aimless.

hyperalgia Increased sensation of pain.

hyperesthesia Increased nociceptor sensitivity.

hyperkinetic delirium A type of delirium in which the patient demonstrates behaviors most commonly recognized as delirium, including psychomotor hyperactivity, marked excitability, and a tendency toward hallucinations.

hypersexuality Inappropriate and socially unacceptable sexual behavior.

hypervigilance Sustained attention to external stimuli as if expecting something important or frightening to happen.

hypervocalization Screams, curses, moans, groans, and verbal repetitiveness that are common in the later stages of cognitively impaired older adults, often occurring during a hospitalization or nursing home placement.

hypnagogic hallucinations Intense dream-like images that occur when an individual is falling asleep and usually involve the immediate environment.

hypnotic Medication that causes drowsiness and facilitates the onset and maintenance of sleep.

hypochondriasis When individuals are fearful of developing a serious illness based on their misinterpretation of body sensations.

hypofrontality Reduced cerebral blood flow and glucose metabolism in the prefrontal cortex.

hypokinetic delirium A type of delirium in which the patient is lethargic, somnolent, and apathetic and exhibits reduced psychomotor activity.

hypomania A mild form of mania.

hypomanic episode A less intense manic episode in which there is little impairment in social or occupational functioning and normal judgment is mostly intact.

identity diffusion Occurs when parts of a person's identity are absent or poorly developed; a lack of consistent sense of identity.

illness anxiety disorder A preoccupation with having or acquiring a serious, undiagnosed medical illness, but somatic symptoms are not present or, if present, only mild.

illusions Disorganized perceptions that create an oversensitivity to colors, shapes, and background activities, which occur when the person misperceives or exaggerates stimuli in the external environment.

imagery rehearsal therapy A technique in which patients change the endings of the nightmares while awake.

impaired consciousness Less environmental awareness and loss of the ability to focus, sustain, and shift attention. Associated cognitive changes include problems in memory, orientation, and language.

implosive therapy A provocative technique useful in treating agoraphobia in which the therapist identifies individual phobic stimuli for the patient and then presents highly anxiety-provoking imagery in a dramatic, vivid fashion.

impulse-control disorders A disorder than often coexists with other disorders. Characterized by an inability to resist an impulse or temptation to complete an activity that is considered harmful to oneself or others.

impulsiveness The tendency to act on urges, notions, or desires without adequately considering the consequences.

impulsivity Acting without considering the consequences of the act or alternative actions.

incidence A rate that includes only new cases that have occurred within a clearly defined time period.

incompetent A person is legally determined not to be able to understand and appreciate the information given during the consent process.

indirect leadership Leader who primarily reflects the group members' discussion and offers little guidance or information to the group.

individual roles Group roles that either enhance or detract from the group's functioning but have nothing to do with either the group task or maintenance.

inducer Drugs or substances that speed up metabolism, which in turn increases the clearance of the substrate and decreases its plasma level.

informal caregivers Unpaid individuals who provide care.

informal group roles Positions within the group with implicit rights and duties that can either help or hinder the group's process. These positions are not formally sanctioned.

informal support systems Family members, friends, and neighbors who can provide care and support to an individual.

informed consent The right mandated by state laws for a patient to determine what shall be done with one's own body and mind. To provide informed consent, the patient must be given adequate information on which to base decisions about care and actively participate in the decision-making process.

inhalants Organic solvents, also known as volatile substances, that are central nervous system depressants and when inhaled cause euphoria, sedation, emotional lability, and impaired judgment.

inhibited grieving A pattern of repetitive, significant trauma and loss together with an inability to fully experience and personally integrate or resolve these events.

inhibitor Drugs or substances that slow down metabolism, which in turn decreases the clearance of the substrate and elevates its plasma level.

in-home mental health care The provision of skilled mental health nursing care under the direction of a psychiatrist or physician for individuals in their residences. Emphasizes personal autonomy of patient.

insight The ability of the individual to be aware of his or her own thoughts and feelings and to compare them with the thoughts and feelings of others.

insomnia (initial) Difficulty falling asleep.

institutionalization The forced confinement of individuals for long periods of time in large state hospitals.

This was the primary treatment for people with mental illness in the period from 1900 to 1955.

instrumental activities of daily living (IADLs) Activities that facilitate or enhance the performance of activities of daily living (e.g., shopping, using the telephone, transportation); these aspects are critical to consider for any older adult living alone.

instrumental aggression Aggression that provides some reward or advantage to the aggressor, is premeditated, and is unrelated to the person's pain.

integrated treatment Treatment for both mental illness and substance use disorders is combined in a single session or interaction or series of interactions.

intellectual disability Limitations in intellectual functioning and adaptive behavior that develops before the age of 18 years. The term is currently used interchangeably with *mental retardation*.

intensive case management An approach targeted for adults with serious mental illnesses or children with serious emotional disturbances. Managers of such cases have fewer caseloads and higher levels of professional training than do traditional case managers.

intensive outpatient program Program focused on continued stabilization and prevention of relapse in vulnerable individuals who have returned to their previous lifestyle (i.e., job or school), usually with sessions running 2 to 3 days per week and lasting 3 to 4 hours per day.

intensive residential services Intensively staffed residential care and mental health services that may include medical, nursing, psychosocial, vocational, recreational, or other support services. May be short or long term.

intergenerational transmission of violence Social learning theory concept that explains the process of violence being transmitted from one generation to the next. Children who witness violence in their homes often perpetuate violent behavior in their families as adults.

intermittent explosive disorder Impulse-control disorder characterized by episodes of uncontrolled aggressiveness that result in assault or destruction of property; the severity of aggressiveness is out of proportion to the provocation.

internal rights protection system Patient protective mechanisms developed by the U.S. mental health care system's organizations to help combat any violation of mental health patients' rights, including investigating any incidents of abuse or neglect.

internalizing disorders Disorders of mood, such as anxiety disorders and depression, in which the symptoms tend to be within the individual.

interoceptive awareness The sensory response to emotional and visceral cues, such as hunger.

interoceptive conditioning Pairing a somatic discomfort, such as dizziness or palpitations, with an impending panic attack.

interpersonal functioning Ability to relate to others with empathy or intimacy.

interpersonal relations Characteristic interaction patterns that occur between human beings that are the basis of human development and behavior and the health or sickness of one's personality.

intervention fit Finding and implementing interventions that are appropriate to a patient's particular needs and circumstances.

intimate partner violence (IPV) Defined by the Centers for Disease Control and Prevention (2009) as psychological, physical, or sexual harm perpetrated by a current or former spouse or partner.

intrinsic activity The ability of a drug to produce a biologic response when it becomes attached to its receptor.

introspective The self-examination of personal beliefs, attitudes, and motivations.

intrusion Thoughts, memories, or dreams of traumatic events occur involuntarily, especially when there are cues that symbolize or resemble the events, causing psychological and sometimes physiological distress.

invalidating environment A highly personal social situation that negates the individual's emotional responses and communication.

invincibility fable An aspect of egocentric thinking in adolescence that causes teens to view themselves as immune to dangerous situations and death.

involuntary commitment The confined hospitalization of a person without his or her consent but with a court order (because the person has been judged to be a danger to him- or herself or others).

inwardly directed anger Anger that is stifled despite strong arousal.

irritable mood Being easily annoyed and provoked to anger, particularly when wishes are challenged or thwarted.

ischemic cascade Cell breakdown resulting from brain cell injury.

judgment The ability to reach a logical decision about a situation and to choose a course after looking at and analyzing various possibilities.

justice Duty to treat all fairly, distributing the risks and benefits equally.

kleptomania A disorder in which the patient is unable to resist the urge to steal and independently steals

items that he or she could easily afford. These items are not particularly useful or wanted. The underlying issue is the act of stealing.

Korsakoff's amnestic syndrome An amnestic syndrome associated with alcoholism in which there is a problem acquiring new information and retrieving memories and involving the heart and vascular and nervous systems; considered to be the chronic stage of Wernicke-Korsakoff syndrome.

label avoidance Type of stigma that occurs when an individual avoids treatment or care in order not to be labeled as being mentally ill.

labile (lability of mood) Changeable mood.

late adulthood The period of life beginning at age 65 years; divided into three chronological groups: young-old, middle-old, and old-old.

learning disorder A discrepancy between actual achievement and expected achievement that is based on a person's age and intellectual ability.

least restrictive environment The patient has the right to be treated in the least restrictive environment possible for the exercise of free will; an individual cannot be restricted to an institution when he or she can be successfully treated in the community.

lethality The probability that a person will successfully complete suicide, determined by the seriousness of the person's intent and the likelihood that the planned method of death will succeed.

libido The energy or psychic drive associated with the sexual instinct that resides in the id, literally translated from Latin to mean "pleasure" or "lust."

life events Major times or experiences such as marriage, divorce, and bereavement.

limbic system (limbic lobe) A "system" of several small structures within the brain that work in a highly organized way. These structures include the hippocampus, thalamus, hypothalamus, amygdala, and limbic midbrain nuclei.

linguistic competence The ability to communicate in a way that is easily understood by diverse audiences.

living will An advanced care directive that states what treatment should be omitted or refused in the event that a person is unable to make those decisions because of incapacitation.

locus ceruleus A tiny cluster of neurons that fans out and innervates almost every part of the brain, including most of the cortex, the thalamus and hypothalamus, the cerebellum, and the spinal cord.

loose associations Absence of the normal connectedness of thoughts and ideas; sudden shifts without apparent relationship to preceding topic.

loss-oriented coping   Part of the dual process model of bereavement that includes preoccupation with the deceased.

luminotherapy   Light therapy used to manipulate the circadian system.

maintenance roles   The informal role of group members that encourages the group to stay together.

major depressive episodes   A depressed mood or a loss of interest or pleasure in nearly all activities for at least 2 weeks. Four of seven additional symptoms must be present: disruption in sleep, appetite (or weight), concentration, or energy; psychomotor agitation or retardation; excessive guilt or feelings of worthlessness; and suicidal ideation.

maladaptive anger   Excessive outwardly directed anger or suppressed anger; linked to psychiatric conditions, such as depression, as well as medical conditions.

malingering   To produce illness symptoms intentionally with an obvious self-serving goal such as being classified as disabled or avoiding work.

mania   A symptoms of bipolar disorder that is primarily characterized by an abnormally and persistently elevated, expansive, or irritable mood.

manic episode   A distinct period during which there is an abnormally and persistently elevated, expansive, or irritable mood.

maturation   Healthy development of the brain and nervous system during childhood and adolescence.

medical battery   Intentional and unauthorized (without informed consent) treatment that is harmful or offensive.

memory   One aspect of cognitive function; an information storage system composed of short-term memory (retention of information over a brief period of time) and long-term memory (retention of an unlimited amount of information over an indefinite period of time); the ability to recall or reproduce what has been learned or experienced.

mental disorders   Health conditions characterized by alterations in thinking, mood, or behavior. They are associated with distress or impaired functioning.

mental health   The emotional and psychological well-being of an individual who has the capacity to interact with others, deal with ordinary stress, and perceive one's surroundings realistically.

mental health recovery   A journey of healing and transformation enabling a person with a mental health problem to live a meaningful life in a community of his or her choice while striving to achieve his or her full potential.

mental status examination   An organized systematic approach to assessment of an individual's current psychiatric condition.

metabolism   Biotransformation, or the process by which a drug is altered and broken down into smaller substances, known as metabolites.

metabolites   Result when drugs are altered and broken down into smaller substances by metabolism. Substance necessary for or taking part in a particular metabolic process.

methadone maintenance   The treatment of opioid addiction with a daily, stabilized dose of methadone.

metonymic speech   Use of words with similar meanings interchangeably.

middle-age adulthood   A term used to describe adults approximately ages 45 to 65 years.

middle-old   A term used to describe adults ages 75 to 84 years.

mild cognitive impairment (MCI)   A transitional state between normal cognition and Alzheimer's disease.

milieu therapy   An approach that provides a stable and coherent social organization to facilitate an individual's treatment; often used interchangeably with *therapeutic environment*. The design of the physical surroundings, structure of patient activities, and promotion of a stable social structure and cultural setting enhance the setting's therapeutic potential.

miracle questions   Patients are asked to use their imagination in crafting their response to very specific questions about a scenario.

mixed episode   When mania and depression occur at the same time, which leads to extreme anxiety, agitation, and irritability.

mixed variant delirium   Behavior that fluctuates between the hyperactive and hypoactive states.

modeling   Pervasive imitation; one person trying to be similar to another person.

mood   The prominent, sustained, overall emotions that a person expresses and exhibits; influences one's perception of the world and how one functions.

mood disorder   Recurrent disturbances or alterations in mood that cause psychological distress and behavioral impairment.

mood episode   A severe mood change that lasts at least 2 weeks that causes clinically significant distress or impairment.

mood lability   The rapid shifts in moods that often occur in patients with bipolar disorder with little or no change in external events.

moral treatment An approach to curing mental illness, popular in the 1800s, that was built on the principles of kindness, compassion, and a pleasant environment.

motivation A goal-oriented attitude that propels action for change and can help sustain the development of new activities and behaviors.

motivational interventions One to several sessions delivered within a few weeks or less during which a patient is motivated to become involved in treatment.

motivational interviewing A method of therapeutic intervention often used with those with substance abuse that seeks to elicit self-motivational statements from patients, supports behavioral change, and creates a discrepancy between the patient's goals and his or her continued alcohol and other drug use.

motor tics Usually quick, jerky movements of the eyes, face, neck, and shoulders, although they may involve other muscle groups as well.

multigenerational transmission process The transmission of emotional processes from one generation to the next.

multiple sleep latency test (MSLT) A standardized procedure that measures the amount of time a person takes to fall asleep during a 20-minute period.

Munchausen's syndrome Term (no longer used) used to describe the most severe form of factitious disorder characterized by fabricating a physical illness, having recurrent hospitalizations, and going from one provider to another.

narcissistic personality Person who could be described as grandiose, with an inexhaustible need for admiration. Beginning in childhood, they believe themselves to be superior, special, and unique, and want recognition for such. They also lack empathy.

negative symptoms A lessening or loss of normal functions, such as restriction or flattening in the range of intensity of emotion; reduced fluency and productivity of thought and speech; withdrawal and inability to initiate and persist in goal-directed activity; and inability to experience pleasure.

negligence A breach of duty of reasonable care for a patient for whom the nurse is responsible that results in personal injuries. A clinician who does get consent but does not disclose the nature of the procedure and the risks involved is subject to a negligence claim.

neologisms Words that are made up that have no common meaning and are not recognized.

neurocircuitry The complex neural functional networks that link brain structures, including the prefrontal cortex, striatum, hippocampus, and amygdala. Research indicates that a dysfunctional neurocircuitry underlies most psychiatric disorders.

neurocognitive impairment An impairment in memory, vigilance, verbal fluency, and executive functioning that exists in schizophrenia. May be independent of positive and negative symptoms.

neurodevelopmental delay When a child's development in attention, cognition, language, affect, and social or moral behavior is outside the norm. It is manifested by delayed socialization, communication, peculiar mannerisms, and idiosyncratic interests.

neurofibrillary tangles Fibrous proteins, or *tau proteins*, that are chemically altered and twisted together and spread throughout the brain, interfering with nerve functioning in cholinergic neurons. It is hypothesized that formation of these neurofibrillary tangles are related to the apolipoprotein E_4 (apoE_4).

neurohormones Hormones produced by cells within the nervous system, such as antidiuretic hormone (ADH).

neuroleptic malignant syndrome A life-threatening condition that can develop in reaction to antipsychotic medications. Patients develop severe muscle rigidity with elevated temperature and a rapidly accelerating cascade of symptoms. (occurring during the next 48 to 72 hours), which can include two or more of the following: hypertension, tachycardia, tachypnea, prominent diaphoresis, incontinence, mutism, leukocytosis, changes in level of consciousness, and laboratory evidence of muscle injury.

neuromodulators Chemical messengers that make the target cell membrane or postsynaptic membrane more or less susceptible to the effects of the primary neurotransmitter.

neuron Nerve cells responsible for receiving, organizing, and transmitting information. Each neuron has a cell body, or soma, which holds the nucleus containing most of the cell's genetic information.

neuropeptides Short chains of amino acids that exist in the central nervous system and have a number of important roles, including as neurotransmitters, neuromodulators, or neurohormones.

neuroplasticity The continuous process of modulation of neuronal structure and function in response to the changing environment.

neurosis A category used by Freud and his followers to define those with less severe mental illness but who were often distressed about their problems.

neurotransmitters Small molecules that directly and indirectly control the opening or closing of ion channels.

night terrors   Episodes of screaming, fear, and panic while sleeping, causing clinical distress or impairing social, occupational, or other areas of functioning.

nociceptors   Pain receptors.

nonbizarre delusions   Beliefs that are characterized by adherence to possible situations that could appear in real life and are plausible in the context of the person's ethnic and cultural background.

nonmaleficence   The duty to cause no harm, both individually and for all.

non–rapid eye movement sleep (NREM)   A sleep cycle state of non–rapid eye movement that occurs about 90 minutes after falling asleep.

nontherapeutic relationship   A nontrusting relationship between the nurse and patient. Both feel very frustrated and keep varying their approach with each other in an attempt to establish a meaningful relationship.

nonverbal communication   The gestures, expressions, and body language used in communications.

norepinephrine   An excitatory neurochemical that plays a major role in generating and maintaining mood states. Heavily concentrated in the terminal sites of sympathetic nerves, it can be released quickly to ready the individual for a fight-or-flight response to threats in the environment.

normal aging   Changes that occur with age associated with some physical decline, such as decreased sensory abilities and decreased pulmonary and immune function, but many important functions do not change.

normalization   Teaching families what are normal behaviors and expected responses.

not guilty by reason of insanity (NGRI)   Persons who demonstrate they had no understanding of their actions and no control over them when they committed the crime.

nuclear family   Two or more people related by blood, marriage, or adoption.

nuclear family emotional process   Patterns of emotional functioning in a family within single generations.

nurse–patient relationship   A dynamic, time-limited interpersonal process that can be viewed in steps or phases with characteristic behaviors during each phase for both the patient and the nurse.

nursing diagnosis   A clinical judgment about the individual, family, or community response to actual or potential health problems and life processes. It provides the basis for the selection of interventions and outcomes.

nursing interventions   Nursing actions or treatment, selected based on clinical judgment, that are designed to achieve patient, family, community outcomes; can be direct or indirect.

nursing process   The basis of clinical decision making and an evidence base for practice.

object relations   The psychological attachment to another person or object.

obsessive-compulsive personality disorder (OCPD)   Persons with OCPD do not demonstrate obsessions and compulsions but rather a pervasive pattern of preoccupation with orderliness, perfectionism, and control. They attempt to maintain control by careful attention to rules, trivial details, procedures, and lists.

obsessions   Excessive, unwanted, intrusive, and persistent thoughts, impulses, or images that cause anxiety and distress and are incongruent with the patient's usual thought patterns.

oculogyric crisis   A medication side effect resulting from an imbalance of dopamine and acetylcholine in which the muscles that control eye movements tense and pull the eyeball so that the patient is looking toward the ceiling; may be followed by torticollis or retrocollis.

off-label   Use of medication for a condition that is not approved by the Food and Drug Administration.

old-old   A term used to describe adults ages 85 years and older.

open communication   Staff and patient willingly share information about relevant topics.

open group   A group in which new members can join at any time, and old members may leave at different sessions.

operant behavior   A type of learning that is a consequence of a particular behavioral response, not a specific stimulus.

opioid   Any substance that binds to an opioid receptor in the brain to produce an agonist action.

oppositional defiant disorder   A disruptive behavior disorder characterized by a persistent pattern of disobedience; argumentativeness; angry outbursts; low tolerance for frustration; and tendency to blame others for misfortunes, large and small.

orgasmic disorder   The inability to reach orgasm or reduced intensity by any means.

orgasmic phase   Phase in the human sexual response cycle that includes ejaculation of semen for men and rhythmic contractions of the vaginal muscles for women.

orientation phase   The first phase of the nurse–patient relationship in which the nurse and the patient get to know each other. During this phase, the patient develops a sense of trust.

oscillation   Part of the dual process model of bereavement that involves a person moving between the process of confronting (loss-oriented coping) and avoiding (restoration-oriented coping) the stresses associated with bereavement.

outcomes   A patient's response to care received; the end result of the process of nursing.

outpatient detoxification   A specialized form of partial hospitalization for patients requiring medical supervision during withdrawal from alcohol or other addictive substances, with or without use of a 23-hour bed during the initial withdrawal phase.

outwardly directed anger   Anger expression particularly the hostile, attacking forms.

oxidative stress   A condition of increased oxidant production in cells characterized by the release of free radicals and resulting in cellular degeneration.

package insert   The approved Food and Drug Administration product labeling that includes approved indications for the medication, side effects, adverse effects, contraindications, and other important information.

panic   A normal but extreme overwhelming form of anxiety often experienced when an individual is placed in a real or perceived life-threatening situation.

panic attacks   Sudden, discrete periods of intense fear or discomfort that are accompanied by significant physical and cognitive symptoms.

panic control treatment   Intentional exposure through exercise to panic-invoking sensations such as dizziness, hyperventilation, tightness in chest, and sweating.

panicogenic   Substances that produce panic attacks.

paranoia   Suspiciousness and guardedness that are unrealistic and often accompanied by grandiosity.

paranoid personality   Marked by traits including long-standing suspiciousness and mistrust of persons in general, a refusal to assume personal responsibility for one's own feelings, and avoidance of relationships in which the person is not in control or loses power.

paraphilias   Problematic sexual behaviors characterized by recurrent, intense sexual urges, fantasies, or behaviors involving unusual objects, activities, or situations. These cause significant distress to the individual or impair social or occupational functioning.

parasuicidal behavior   Deliberate self-injury with intent to harm oneself.

parasuicide   Deliberate, apparent attempt at suicide, commonly called a suicidal gesture, in which the aim is not death (e.g., taking a sublethal drug); also called *parasuicidal behavior.*

partial agonist   A drug that has some intrinsic activity (although weak) to initiate the same response in the body as a chemical that is normally present.

partial hospitalization   A time-limited (usually full- or half-day), ambulatory, active treatment program that offers therapeutically intensive, coordinated, and structured clinical services for patients with acute psychiatric symptoms who are experiencing a decline in social or occupational functioning, who cannot function autonomously on a daily basis, or who do not pose imminent danger to themselves or others. The aim is patient stabilization without hospitalization or a reduced length of inpatient care.

passive listening   A nontherapeutic mode of interaction that involves sitting quietly and allowing the patient to talk without focusing on guiding the thought process; includes body language that communicates boredom, indifference, or hostility.

paternalism   The belief that knowledge and education authorizes professionals to make decisions for the good of the patient.

patient observation   The ongoing assessment of the patient's mental status to identify and subvert any potential problem.

peak marriage age   An age when the person is most likely to have a successful marriage; currently between the ages of 23 and 27 years.

pedophilia   Sexual activity with a child usually 13 years of age or younger by an individual at least 16 years of age or 5 years older than the child.

peer assistance programs   Programs developed by state nurses' associations to offer consultation, referral, and monitoring for nurses whose practice is impaired or potentially impaired because of the use of drugs or alcohol or a psychological or physiological condition.

perfectionism   Setting high personal standards for oneself combined with concern over mistakes and their consequences for self-worth and others' opinions.

persecutory delusions   Delusions in which the person believes that he or she is being conspired against, cheated, spied on, followed, poisoned, drugged, maliciously maligned, harassed, or obstructed in the pursuit of long-term goals.

personal identity   Knowing "who I am" formed through the numerous biologic, psychological, and social challenges and demands faced throughout the stages of life.

personality A complex pattern of psychological characteristics, largely outside a person's awareness, that comprise the individual's distinctive pattern of perceiving, feeling, thinking, coping, and behaving.

personality disorder An enduring pattern of inner experience and behavior that deviates markedly from the expectations of the individual's culture, is pervasive and inflexible, has an onset in adolescence or early adulthood, is stable over time, and leads to distress or impairment.

personality traits Prominent aspects of personality that are exhibited in a wide range of social and personal contexts; intrinsic and pervasive, personality traits emerge from a complicated interaction of biologic dispositions, psychological experiences, and environmental situations that ultimately comprise a distinctive personality.

person–environment relationship The interaction between the individual and the environment that changes throughout the stress experience.

pharmacodynamics The study of the biologic actions of drugs on living tissue and the human body in general.

pharmacogenomics Blends pharmacology with genetic knowledge; understanding and determining an individual's specific CYP450 makeup and then individualizing medications to match the person's CYP450 profile.

pharmacokinetics The process by which a drug is absorbed, distributed, metabolized, and eliminated by the body.

phenotype Observable characteristics or expressions of a specific trait.

phobia Persistent, unrealistic fears of situations, objects, or activities that often lead to avoidance behaviors.

phonic tics Tics that typically include repetitive throat clearing, grunting, or other noises but may also include more complex sounds, such as words; parts of words; and in a minority of patients, obscenities.

phonologic processing Thought to be the cause of reading disability; a process that involves the discrimination and interpretation of speech sounds. Reading disability is believed to be caused by some disturbance in the development of the left hemisphere.

phototherapy Also known as *light therapy;* involves exposing the patient to an artificial light source during winter months to relieve seasonal depression.

pineal body Located in the epithalamus; contains secretory cells that emit the neurohormone melatonin (as well as other substances), which has been associated with sleep and emotional disorders and modulation of immune function.

plasticity Permanent change in central pain interpretation.

plateau Phase of the human sexual response cycle that is represented by sexual pleasure and increased muscle tension, heart rate, and blood flow to the genitals.

polypharmacy Using more than one group from a class of medications at one time.

polysomnography A special procedure that involves the recording of the electroencephalogram throughout the night. This procedure is usually conducted in a sleep laboratory.

polyuria Excessive need to urinate.

population genetics The study of the inheritance of illness or traits from generation to generation.

positive self-talk Countering fearful or negative thoughts by using preplanned and rehearsed positive coping statements.

positive symptoms An excess or distortion of normal functions, including delusions and hallucinations.

posttraumatic stress disorder A mental disorder characterized by persistent, distressing symptoms lasting longer than 1 month after exposure to an extreme traumatic stressor.

potency The dose of drug required to produce a specific effect.

power of attorney As it relates to health care, an advanced care directive through which a proxy, usually a relative or trusted friend, is appointed to make health care decisions on behalf of an individual if that person is incapacitated.

premature ejaculation (PE) The inability to control ejaculation before or shortly after penetration.

pressured speech Speaking as if the words are being forced out.

privacy The part of an individual's personal life that is not governed by society's laws and governmental intrusion.

proband A person who has a genetic disorder or a trait of a mental disorder.

probation A sentence of conditional or revocable release under the supervision of a probation officer for a specified time.

problem-focused coping A type of coping in which a person attacks the source of stress and solves the problem (eliminating it or changing its effects), which changes the person–environment relationship.

process recording A verbatim transcript of a verbal interaction usually organized according to the nurse–patient interaction. It often includes analysis of the interaction.

prodromal An early symptom indicating the development of a disease or syndrome.

prostaglandins An unsaturated fatty acid that helps control smooth muscle contraction, blood pressure, inflammation, and body temperature. One of the most common nociceptive transmitters.

protective factors Characteristics that reduce the probability that a person will develop a mental health disorder or problem or decrease the severity of existing problems.

protective identification A psychoanalytic term used to describe behavior of people with borderline personality disorder when they falsely attribute to others their own unacceptable feelings, impulses, or thoughts.

protein binding The degree to which a drug binds to plasma proteins.

pseudologia fantastica Fascinating but false stories of personal triumph. Stories that are not entirely improbable and often contain a matrix of truth and falsehood.

pseudoparkinsonism Sometimes referred to as *drug-induced parkinsonism;* presents identically as Parkinson's disease without the same destruction of dopaminergic cells.

psychiatric–mental health nurse A registered nurse who demonstrates specialized competence and knowledge, skills, and abilities in caring for persons with mental health issues and problems and psychiatric disorders.

psychiatric–mental health nursing A specialized area of nursing practice committed to promoting mental health through the assessment, diagnosis, and treatment of human responses to mental health problems and psychiatric disorders.

psychiatric rehabilitation programs Programs that are focused on reintegrating people with psychiatric disabilities back into the community through work, educational, and social avenues while also addressing their medical and residential needs.

psychoanalysis The Freudian treatment of choice; therapy focused on repairing the trauma of the original psychological injury through the process of accessing the unconscious conflicts that originate in childhood and then resolving the issues with a mature adult mind. Includes attempts to reconstruct the personality by examining free associations (spontaneous, uncensored verbalizations of whatever comes to mind) and the interpretation of dreams.

psychoeducation An educational approach used to enhance knowledge and shape behavior by adapting teaching strategies to a patient's disorder-related deficits.

psychoeducational programs A form of mental health intervention in which basic coping skills for dealing with various stressors are taught.

psychological abuse Emotional abuse that includes behaviors such as criticizing, insulting, humiliating, or ridiculing someone in private or in public. It can also involve actions such as destroying another's property, threatening or harming pets, controlling or monitoring spending and activities, or isolating a person from family and friends.

psychoneuroimmunology The study of relationships among the immune system, nervous system, and endocrine system and our behaviors, thoughts, and feelings.

psychopath Also called a sociopath, a person with a tendency toward antisocial and criminal behavior with little regard for others; a term often used by the general public to refer to persons with an antisocial personality disorder.

psychosis A category used by Freud and his followers to define those with severe mental illness that impaired daily functioning. Today, the term is used to describe a state in which the individual is experiencing hallucinations, delusions, or disorganized thoughts, speech, or behavior.

psychosomatic Term traditionally used to describe, explain, and predict the psychological origins of illness and disease.

public stigma Type of stigma that occurs after individuals are publicly "marked" as being mentally ill.

pyromania Irresistible impulses to start fires.

quadrants of care A conceptual framework that classifies patients according to symptom severity, not diagnosis.

rape The most severe form of sexual assault; the penetration of any bodily orifice by the penis, fingers, or an object.

rapid cycling In bipolar disorder, the occurrence of four or more mood episodes that meet criteria for a manic, mixed, hypomanic, or depressive episode during the previous 12 months.

rapid eye movement sleep (REM) A sleep cycle state of rapid eye movement.

rapport Interpersonal harmony characterized by understanding and respect that is established through interpersonal warmth, a nonjudgmental attitude, and a demonstration of understanding.

rational emotive behavior therapy (REBT) A psychotherapeutic approach that proposes that unrealistic and irrational beliefs cause many emotional problems. Its primary emphasis is on changing irrational beliefs into thoughts that are more reasonable and rational.

reappraisal Appraisal after coping that provides feedback about the outcomes and allows for continual adjustment to new information.

receptors Proteins that receive released neurotransmitters. Each neurotransmitter has a specific receptor, or protein, for which it and only it will fit; serves a physiologic regulatory function.

recovery Recovery from mental disorders and/or substance use disorders is a process of change through which individuals improve their health and wellness, live a self-directed life, and strive to reach their full potential.

referential thinking Belief that neutral stimuli have special meaning to the individual, such as a television commentator speaking directly to the individual.

referral Act of sending an individual from one clinician to another or from one service setting to another for care or consultation.

reflection Continual self-evaluation through observing, monitoring, and judging nursing behaviors with the goal of providing ideal interventions.

regressed behavior Behaving in a manner of a less mature life stage; childlike and immature.

reintegration A term used to describe the process of the return and acceptance of a person as a fully participating member of a community through work, educational, and social avenues.

relapse Recurrence or marked increase in severity of the symptoms of the disease, especially after a period of apparent improvement or stability; the recurrence of alcohol- or drug-dependent behavior in an individual who has previously achieved and maintained abstinence for a significant time beyond the period of detoxification.

relapse cycle When reemerging psychiatric symptoms lead to ineffective coping strategies, increased anxiety, substance use to avoid painful feelings, adverse consequences, and attempted abstinence until psychiatric symptoms reemerge and the cycle repeats itself.

relapse prevention An approach that focuses on preventing recurrence of symptoms.

relational aggression A type of bullying, more commonly used by girls, that involves disrupting peer relationships by excluding or manipulating others and spreading rumors.

relationship questions Questions used to amplify and reinforce positive responses to the other questions.

relaxation training A variety of procedures to reduce somatic arousal, such as progressive muscle relaxation, autogenic training, and biofeedback.

religiousness The participation in a community of people who gather around common ways of worshiping.

reminiscence Thinking about or relating past experiences.

repetitive transcranial magnetic stimulation Noninvasive, painless method to stimulate the cerebral

cortex, which activates inhibitory and excitatory neurons.

residential services A place for people to reside during a 24-hour period or any portion of the day on an ongoing basis.

resilience Ability to recover readily from illness, depression, adversity, or the like. The ability to recover or adjust to challenges over time. Attaining good mental health despite the presence of risk factors and genetic predisposition.

resolution The termination phase of the nurse–patient relationship that lasts from the time the problems are resolved to the close of the relationship. Also, in regards the human sexual response cycle, the gradual return of the organs and body systems to the unaroused state.

restoration-oriented coping Part of the dual process model of bereavement during which the bereaved person is preoccupied with stressful events as a result of the death (financial issues, new identity as a widow[er]).

restraint The use of any manual, physical, or mechanical device or material that when attached to the patient's body (usually to the arms and legs) restricts the patient's movements.

retrocollis The neck muscles pull back the head.

revictimization A reoccurrence of violence toward the survivor.

rhythm Movement with a cadence. A measured flow that occurs at regular intervals, with a cycle of coming and going, ebbing and rising, to return at the start point and begin again.

risk factors Characteristics, conditions, situations, or events that increase the patient's vulnerability to threats to safety or well-being.

Safe Havens A form of supportive housing that serves hard-to-reach people with severe mental illness.

sandwich generation People with caregiving responsibilities toward the elder generation above and two generations of children below them.

scaling questions Questions that quantify exceptions noted in intensity and in tracking change over time using a scale of 1 to 10.

schema A cognitive structure, or an individual's life rules, that act as a filter that screens, codes, and evaluates the incoming stimuli through which the individual interprets events.

schizoaffective disorder (SAD) A disorder characterized by periods of intense symptom exacerbation alternating with quiescent periods, during which psychosocial functioning is adequate. This disorder is at times marked by symptoms of schizophrenia; at other times, it appears to be a mood disorder. In other cases, both psychosis and pervasive mood changes occur concurrently.

schizoid personality   Personality trait characterized as being expressively impassive and interpersonally unengaged.

schizotypal personality disorder   A disorder characterized by a pattern of social, interpersonal deficits, and impairments in capacity for close relationships. Perceptual distortions are usually present.

schizotypy   Traits that are similar to the symptoms of schizophrenia but less severe. Cognitive perceptual symptoms are a primary characteristic and include magical beliefs (similar to delusions) and perceptual aberrations (similar to hallucinations). Other common symptoms include referential thinking (interpreting insignificant events as personally relevant) and paranoia (suspicious of others).

school phobia   Anxiety in which the child refuses to attend school in order to stay at home and with the primary attachment figure. School phobia is a common presenting complaint in child psychiatric clinics and is diagnosed as a separation anxiety disorder.

seclusion   Solitary confinement in a full protective environment for the purpose of safety or behavior management.

Section 8 housing   Federally subsidized housing units that are supervised or operated by the state or city; tenants are responsible for paying one third of the monthly income toward rent.

sedative–hypnotics   Medications that induce sleep and reduce anxiety.

sedatives   Medications that reduce activity, nervousness, irritability and excitability without causing sleep, but if given in large enough doses, they have an hypnotic effect.

selectivity   The ability of a drug to be specific for a particular receptor, interacting only with specific receptors in the areas of the body where the receptors occur and therefore not affecting tissues and organs where these receptors do not occur.

self-awareness   Being cognizant of one's own beliefs, thoughts, motivations, biases, physical and emotional limitations and the impact one may have on others.

self-care   The ability to perform activities of daily living (ADLs) successfully.

self-concept   The sum of beliefs about oneself, which develops over time. Includes three interrelated dimensions: body image, self-esteem, and personal identity.

self-determinism   Being empowered or having the free will to make moral judgments. Includes the right to choose one's own health-related behaviors, which at times differ from those recommended by health professionals.

self-disclosure   The act of revealing personal information about oneself.

self-efficacy   Self-effectiveness; a person's belief in his or her own abilities.

self-esteem   Attitude about oneself. Healthy self-esteem includes feelings of self-acceptance, self-worth, self-love and self-nurturing.

self harm   Deliberate self-injurious behavior with the intent to hurt oneself.

self-identity   The development of a separate and distinct personality.

self-medicate   Using medication, usually over-the-counter or substances without professional prescription or supervision, to alleviate an illness or condition.

self-monitoring   Observing and recording one's own information, usually behavior, thoughts, or feelings.

self-stigma   Type of stigma that occurs when negative stereotypes are internalized by people with mental illness.

self-system   An important concept in Peplau's model. Drawing from Sullivan, Peplau defined the self as an "anti-anxiety system" and a product of socialization.

sensate focus   A method of sex therapy in which partners learn what each finds arousing and how to communicate those preferences.

separation anxiety disorder   Developmentally inappropriate fear and anxiety around separation from home or attachment figure.

separation-individuation   A normal developmental process during which the child develops a sense of self, a permanent sense of significant others (object constancy), and an integration of both bad and good as a component of the self-concept.

serotonin   Also called 5-hydroxytryptamine or 5-HT, this is primarily an excitatory neurotransmitter that is diffusely distributed within the cerebral cortex, limbic system, and basal ganglia of the central nervous system. Serotonergic neurons also project into the hypothalamus and cerebellum. Plays a role in emotions, cognition, sensory perceptions, and essential biologic functions (e.g., sleep and appetite).

serotonin syndrome   A potentially life-threatening side effect that occurs as a result of an overactivity of serotonin or an impairment of the serotonin metabolism. Symptoms include mental status changes (hallucinations, agitation, and coma), autonomic instability (tachycardia, hyperthermia, changes in blood pressure), neuromuscular problems (hyperreflexia, incoordination), and gastrointestinal disturbance (nausea, vomiting, diarrhea).

sex role identity   Outward expression of gender.

sex therapist   A therapist who blends education and counseling with psychotherapy and specific sexual exercises.

sexual arousal   A state of mounting sexual tension characterized by vasoconstriction and myotonia.

sexual assault   Any form of nonconsenting sexual activity, ranging from fondling to penetration.

sexual desire   Ability, interest, or willingness to receive or a motivational state to seek sexual stimulation.

sexual disorders   Called sexual dysfunction in the *DSM-5*. A disturbance in sexual desire or sexual response or pain associated with intercourse.

sexuality   Basic dimension of every individual's personality encompassing all that is male or female, undergoing periods of growth and development, and influenced by biologic and psychosocial factors.

sexual maturation   The aspect of sexual development that encompasses biosexual identity, gender identity, sex role identity, and sexual orientation.

sexual orientation (sexual preference)   An individual's feelings of sexual attraction and erotic potential.

sexual sadism   The real act of experiencing sexual excitement from causing physical or psychological suffering of another individual.

Shelter Plus Care Program   A continuum of care program that allows for various housing choices and a range of supportive services.

sibling position   The relative social status of the children in the family based on birth order.

side effects   Unintended effects of medications.

simple relaxation techniques   Interventions that encourage and elicit relaxation to decrease undesirable signs and symptoms.

situational crisis   A crisis that occurs whenever a specific stressful event threatens a person's biopsychosocial integrity and results in some degree of psychological disequilibrium.

skills groups   An integral part of dialectical behavior therapy; skills are taught in group settings in which patients practice emotional regulation, interpersonal effectiveness, distress tolerance, core mindfulness, and self-management skills.

sleep architecture   A predictable pattern during a night's sleep that includes the timing, amount, and distribution of REM and NREM stages.

sleep debt   Interruption of basic restoration after recurrent long-term sleep deprivation.

sleep diary   A written account of the sleep experience.

sleep disorders   Ongoing disruptions of normal waking and sleeping patterns that lead to excessive daytime sleepiness; inappropriate naps; chronic fatigue; and the inability to perform safely or properly at work, school, or home.

sleep efficiency   Expressed as the ratio of total sleep time to time in bed.

sleepiness   The urge to fall asleep.

sleep latency   Amount of time it takes for an individual to fall asleep. It is the time period measured from "lights out," or bedtime, to initiation of sleep.

sleep paralysis   Being unable to move or speak when falling asleep or waking.

sleep restriction   Deliberately spending less time in bed and avoiding napping.

sleep–wake cycle   The biphasic 24-hour cycle that makes up the patterned activity of sleep.

slow-wave sleep   Deepest state of sleep.

social change   The structural and cultural evolution of society.

social distance   Degree to which the values of a formal organization and its primary group members differ.

social functioning   Performance of daily activities within the context of interpersonal relations and family and community roles.

social network   Linkages among a defined set of people, among whom there are personal contacts.

social skills training   A psychoeducational approach that involves instruction, feedback, support, and practice with learning behaviors that helps people interact more effectively with peers and children with adults.

social support   Positive and harmonious interpersonal interactions that occur within social relationships.

sociopath   Also called a psychopath, a person with a tendency toward antisocial and criminal behavior with little regard for others; a term often used by the general public to refer to persons with an antisocial personality disorder.

solubility   Ability of a drug to dissolve.

solution-focused brief therapy   A cognitive therapy approach that differs from other cognitive approaches in its de-emphasis on the patient's "problems," or symptoms, and an emphasis on what is functional and healthful.

somatic symptom disorder (SSD)   Multiple current, somatic symptoms that are distressing and disruptive of daily life. Individuals report all aspects of their health as poor. Physical symptoms may last 6 to 9 months.

somatization Experiencing multiple physical symptoms that are distressing and disruptive of daily life.

somnambulism Sleep walking.

speed–accuracy shift A type of mental processing in which an older adult focuses more on accuracy than speed in responding.

spirituality Beliefs and values related to hope and meaning in life.

spiritual support Assisting patients to feel balance and connection within their relationships; involves listening to expressions of loneliness, using empathy, and providing patients with desired spiritual articles.

splitting Defense mechanism in which the person views the world in absolutes, alternately categorizing people as all good or all bad; also used to describe a person manipulating one group against another.

stabilization Short-term care, usually lasting fewer than 7 days, with a symptom-based indication for hospital admission. Primary focus is on control of precipitating symptoms with medications, behavioral interventions, and coordination with other agencies for appropriate after care.

stalking A pattern of repeated unwanted contact, attention, and harassment that often increases in frequency.

standardized nursing language Language readily understood by all nurses to describe care in order to provide a common means of communication.

standards of practice Standards that guide nursing practice. These are organized around the nursing process and include assessment, diagnosis, outcome identification, planning, implementation, and evaluation.

steady state Absorption equals excretion and the therapeutic level plateaus.

stereotypic behavior Repetitive, driven, nonfunctional, and potentially self-injurious behavior, such as head banging, rocking, and hand flapping, seen in autistic disorder, with an extraordinary insistence on sameness.

stereotypy Repetitive, purposeless movements that are idiosyncratic to the individual and to some degree outside of the individual's control.

stigma A mark of shame, disgrace, or disapproval that results in an individual being shunned or rejected by others.

stilted language Overly and inappropriately artificial formal language.

stimulus control A technique used when the bedroom environment no longer provides cues for sleep but has become the cue for wakefulness. Patients are instructed to avoid behaviors in the bedroom that are incompatible with sleep.

stress A transactional process arising from real or perceived internal or external environmental demands that are appraised as threatening or benign.

stress response Physiologic, behavioral and cognitive reaction to an appraised threatening person–environment event.

structural imaging The aspect of neuroimaging that visualizes the structure of brain and allows diagnosis of gross intracranial disease and injury.

structured interaction Purposeful interaction that allows patients to interact with others in a useful way.

subcortical dementia Dementia that is caused by dysfunction or deterioration of deep gray or white matter structures inside the brain and brain stem.

substance P A peptide found in body tissues, especially nervous tissue, that is involved in the transmission of pain and in inflammation. It is the most common nociceptive transmitter that is released and transported along the central and peripheral pain synapses in the presence of noxious stimuli.

substrate The drug or compound that is identified as a target of an enzyme.

subsystems A systems term used by family theorists to describe subgroups of family members who join together for various activities.

sudden sniffing death Sudden death for inhalant users when the inhaled fumes take the place of oxygen in the lungs and central nervous system, causing the user to suffocate.

suicidal behavior The occurrence of persistent thought patterns and actions that indicate a person is thinking about, planning, or enacting suicide.

suicidal ideation Thinking about and planning one's own death without actually engaging in self-harm.

suicidality All suicide-related behaviors and thoughts of completing or attempting suicide and suicide ideation.

suicide The act of killing oneself voluntarily.

suicide attempt A nonfatal, self-inflicted destructive act with explicit or implicit intent to die.

suicide contagion Suicide behavior that occurs after the suicide death of a known other (i.e., a friend, acquaintance, or idolized celebrity). Also called *cluster suicide*.

supportive housing Permanently subsidized housing with attendant social services.

symbolism The use of a word or a phrase to represent an object, event, or feeling.

synaptic cleft A junction between one nerve and another; the space where the electrical intracellular signal becomes a chemical extracellular signal.

synchronized Two or more circadian rhythms reaching their peak at the same time.

syndrome A set of symptoms that cluster together that may have multiple causes and may represent several different disease states that have not yet been defined.

systematic desensitization A method used to desensitize patients to anxiety-provoking situations by exposing the patient to a hierarchy of feared situations. Patients are is taught to use muscle relaxation as levels of anxiety increase through multi-situational exposure.

tangentiality When the topic of conversation changes to an entirely different topic that is within a logical progression but causes a permanent detour from the original focus.

tardive dyskinesia A late-appearing extrapyramidal side effect of antipsychotic medication that involves irregular, repetitive involuntary movements of the mouth, face, and tongue, including chewing, tongue protrusion, lip smacking, puckering of the lips, and rapid eye blinking. Abnormal finger movements are common as well.

target symptoms Specific measurable symptoms expected to improve with treatment for which psychiatric medications are prescribed. Examples include hallucinations, delusions, paranoia, agitation, assaultive behavior, bizarre ideation, social withdrawal, disorientation, catatonia, blunted affect, thought blocking, insomnia, and anorexia.

task roles The group role of an individual that is concerned about the purpose of the group and keeps the focus on the task of the group.

tau A protein that is the main component found in neurofibrillary tangles inside the cells.

temperament A person's characteristic intensity, activity level, rhythmicity, adaptability, energy expenditure, and mood.

therapeutic communication The ongoing process of interaction in which meaning emerges; may be verbal or nonverbal.

therapeutic foster care The placement of patients in residences of families specially trained to handle individuals with mental illnesses. Indicated for patients in need of a family-like environment and a high level of support.

therapeutic index A ratio of the maximum nontoxic dose to the minimum effective dose.

thought stopping A practice in which a person identifies negative feelings and thoughts that exist together, says "stop," and then engages in a distracting activity.

thymoleptic Mood stabilizing.

tics Sudden, rapid, repetitive, stereotyped motor movements or vocalizations.

token economy The application of behavior modification techniques to multiple behaviors. In a token economy, patients are rewarded with tokens for selected desired behaviors that they can then redeem for special privilege or similar.

tolerance A gradual decrease in the action of a drug at a given dose or concentration in the blood. The ability to ingest an increasing amount of alcohol before a "high" and cognitive and motor effects are experienced.

torticollis The neck muscles pull the head to the side.

Tourette's disorder The most severe tic disorder. Defined by multiple motor and phonic tics for at least 1 year.

toxicity The point at which concentrations of a drug in the bloodstream become harmful or poisonous to the body.

transaction Transfer of value between two or more individuals.

transfer The formal shifting of responsibility for the care of an individual from one clinician to another or from one care unit to another.

transference The unconscious assignment to a therapist or nurse of a patient's feelings and attitudes that were originally associated with important figures such as parents or siblings.

transitional housing Temporary housing such as a halfway house, short-stay residence or group home, or a room at a hotel designated for people who are homeless and looking for permanent housing.

transition times Times of addition, subtraction, or change in status of family members.

traumatic brain injury (TBI) An intracranial injury that occurs when an outside force traumatically injures the brain.

traumatic crisis A crisis initiated by unexpected, unusual events in which people face overwhelming hazards that entail injury, trauma, destruction, or sacrifice. May affect an individual or a multitude of people at once.

traumatic grief A difficult and prolonged grief.

triad A group consisting of three people.

triangles A three-person system and the smallest stable unit in human relations.

trichotillomania Chronic, self-destructive hair pulling that results in noticeable hair loss, usually in the crown, occipital, or parietal areas, and sometimes of the eyebrows and eyelashes.

23-hour observation A short-term treatment that serves the patient in immediate but short-term crisis. This type of care admits individuals to an inpatient setting for as long as 23 hours during which time services are provided at a less-than-acute care level.

uncomplicated grief Grief that is painful and disruptive within normal expectations after the loss of a loved one.

unconditional positive regard A nonjudgmental caring for a client.

unfit to stand trial (UST) Persons who are determined to be unable to understand the proceedings against them or assist in their own defense because of mental or physical condition.

uptake receptors See *carrier proteins*.

use The drinking of alcohol or the swallowing, smoking, sniffing, or injecting of a mind-altering substance.

vaginismus Condition characterized by a psychologically induced spastic, involuntary constriction of the perineal and outer vaginal muscles fostered by imagined, anticipated, or actual attempts at vaginal penetration.

validation A process that affirms patient individuality and reflects the staff member respect for a patient in any interaction.

veracity The duty to tell the truth.

verbal communication The use of the spoken word, including its underlying emotion, context, and connotation.

verbigeration Purposeless repetition of words or phrases.

violence (violent behavior) An extreme form of aggression involving the physical act of force intended to cause harm to a person or an object.

voluntary admission (voluntary commitment) The legal status of a patient who has consented to being admitted to the hospital for treatment, during which time he or she maintains all civil rights and is free to leave at any time even if it is against medical advice.

vulnerable child syndrome A phenomenon that occurs when family members view a child as sickly despite current good health and as a result are overprotective of the child.

waxy flexibility Posture held in an odd or unusual fixed position for extended periods of time.

Wernicke's encephalopathy An alcohol-induced degenerative brain disorder caused by a thiamine deficiency and characterized by vision impairment, ataxia, hypotension, confusion, and coma.

Wernicke-Korsakoff syndrome An alcohol-induced amnestic disorder that includes an acute phase of Wernicke's encephalopathy and a chronic phase of Korsakoff's amnestic syndrome.

withdrawal The adverse physical and psychological symptoms that occur when a person ceases to use a substance.

word salad A string of words that are not connected in any way.

working memory An important aspect of the brain's frontal lobe function, including the ability to plan and initiate activity with future goals in mind.

working phase The second phase of the nurse–patient relationship in which patients can examine specific problems and learn new ways of approaching them.

xerostomia Dry mouth.

young adulthood A term used to describe adults ages 18 to 44 years.

young-old A term used to describe adults ages 65 to 74 years.

Zeitgebers Specific events that function as time givers or synchronizers and that result in the setting of biologic rhythms.

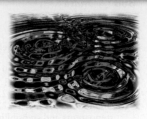

Index

A

ABCDE, framework for REBT, 189–190, 189b
ABCs of psychological first aid, 311
Aberrant behavior, 740
Aberrant motor behavior, 735–736
Abnormal Involuntary Movement Scale (AIMS), 128, 167, 346, 347, 360, 360b, 836–837
Absolute thinking, 190
Absorption, pharmacokinetics, 157t
Abstract nursing theories, 73
Abstract reasoning and comprehension, 132
Abuse, 781–782. *See also* Substance-related disorders
 adult abuser, 62
 alcohol and other drugs (AODs), 787–788
 alcohol and substance, 257
 biological responses to
  co-occurring disorders, 791
  effects on functioning and quality of life, 791
  mental health sequelae for survivors, 791
  mood disorders (depression) and anxiety disorders (PTSD), 791
  physical consequences, 791
 child, 246, 785–786, 794
  neglect, 786
  physical, 786
  prevention, 236
  psychological, 786
  risk factors for, 235
  sexual, 786
  signs of physical and sexual abuse, 235b
  telephone hotlines for, 308
  verbal, 786
 comorbid substance, 44
 cyberstalking, 783
 elder, 786
  prevalence of, 787
  risk factors for, 787
  types of, 786–787
 evaluation and treatment outcomes, 802–803
 history and physical findings suggestive of, 796–797, 798b–799b
  older adults, 796
  questions in, 796
 intervention strategies
  for abuser, 803–804
  anger management, 800
  anxiety management, 801
  behavioral interventions, 801
  community involvement, 802
  education, 800–801
  family interventions, 802
  finding strength and hope, 801
  group therapy, 800
  healthy daily activity, promotion of, 797
  medications administration, 797
  for patients with AOD disorder, 797, 799
  physical symptoms, treatment of, 797
  psychotherapy, 799
  teaching skills, 800
  working with children, 799–800

intimate partner violence (IPV), 781–782
 and AOD use, 788
 children of victims of, 783
 cycle of violence, 789, 790f
 lethality of, 782
 physical problems associated with, 791
 prevalence of, during pregnancy, 782
 psychological abuse, 782
 risk factors for, 782–783
and negative health consequences, 791
nursing diagnoses
 for biologic domain, 797
 for psychological domain, 799
 for social domain, 802
during pregnancy, 782
psychological responses to
 fear, 791
 guilt and shame, 792
 low self-esteem, 792
rape and sexual assault, 784–785
reporting of, 794
screening for, 794–796, 795b
social and interpersonal responses to
 problems with intimacy, 792
 revictimization, 792
special concerns for victims of sexual assault, 797
stalking, 783
teen partner, 783
theories of violence, 787
 alcohol and drug use, 787–788
 attachment theory, 788
 community disorganization, 789
 economic disadvantage, 789
 imbalances in relationship power, 789–790
 implicit theories held by perpetrators, 788–789
 neurologic problems, 787
 psychopathology, 788
 social learning theory, 788
treatment for abusers, 803–804
victims in pediatric ED, 793
Abuse Assessment Screen, 795b
Abused substances, effects of, 588t–589t
Accountability issues
 lawsuits in psychiatric health care, 33
 legal liability in psychiatric nursing practice, 33
 nursing documentation, 33–34
Accreditation, 30
Acculturation, 19
Accumulated beliefs, 187
Acetylcholine (ACh), 88, 90, 90f, 725
Acetylcholinesterase (AChE), 731
Acetylcholinesterase inhibitors (AChEIs), 731, 736
Aches and pains, 22
Acquired immunodeficiency syndrome (AIDS), 824
 assessment, 825
 cognitive and motor changes, 824
 depression in, 825, 826

extrapyramidal symptoms, 824
hypothalamic-pituitary-adrenal axis in, abnormalities in, 825
nursing interventions, 825
 antiviral agents, 826
 emotional and educational support, 826
 psychiatric intervention, 825–826
paraparesis in, 824
psychiatric disorders and, 825, 825b
 adjustment disorders, 825
 agitation and suicidal ideation, 825
 anxiety disorders, 825
 mood disorders, 825
 personality disorders, 825
 substance use disorders, 825
psychological changes, 824–825
psychological sequelae, 826
social consequences, 826
spasticity in, 824
trauma
 assessment, 826–827
 nursing interventions
 response to, 826, 827
Acrophobia, 472b
Acting-out behaviors, 112, 113t
Action for Mental Health, 8
Activating event, 189–190
Active listening, 107, 107t
Activities of daily living (ADLs), 40, 128, 139, 256, 713, 720, 723, 728, 732, 796, 826, 828, 829
Activity and exercise interventions, 128, 139, 141, 203, 245, 248, 249, 260, 261, 276, 351, 407–408, 454–455, 728, 730, 739
ACT model, 41–42
Acupressure, 595
Acute dystonia, 165
Acute dystonic reaction. *See* Dystonia
Acute extrapyramidal symptoms, 164–166
Acute inpatient care, 38–39
Acute pain, 819
Acute Panic Inventory, 459b
Acute stress disorder (ASD), 485–486
AD. *See* Alzheimer's disease (AD)
Adaptation, 275f
 health, 274–275
 psychological well-being, 275
 social functioning, 275
Adaptation model, 75
Adaptive behavior, 678
Adaptive function, 678
Addiction, 585
 behaviors in, 302b
 effective treatment, principles of, 610b
Addison's disease, 98
Adherence, 182–183, 183b
Adherence to treatment, 182–183, 183b, 353, 385, 413, 416, 431, 436, 522, 803, 814
Adler, Alfred, 63
Adler's foundation for individual psychology, 63
Adolescents, 233–234
 attachment behaviors, 228
 childhood problems, mental health

Adolescents (*cont.*)
  adolescent risk-taking behaviors, 233–234
  bullying, 232
  death and grief, 228–229, 228t, 230f
  physical illness, 232–233
  separation and divorce, 229–231, 231t
  sibling relationships, 232, 232f
  stepparents and stepsiblings, 230
  vulnerable child syndrome, 233
  homeless, 756
  intervention approaches, 237–239, 238b, 239f
    bibliotherapy, 238–239
    early intervention programs, 238
    normalization, 238
    psychoeducational programs, 238
    social skills training, 238
  learning disorders, 689
  preventing child abuse and neglect, 235–236
  sexual behaviors in, 641
Adoption studies, 95
β-Adrenergic blockers, 166
α₂–Adrenergic receptor agonist clonidine
    (Catapres), 694
Adrenocorticotropic hormone (corticotropin),
    271
AD8 tool, 733, 734f
Adult abuser, 62
Adult Children of Alcoholics (ACOA), 236
Adulthood
  challenges, mental health
    caring for others, 243–244
    changes in family structure, 243, 243t
    unemployment, 243
  sexual behaviors in, 641–642
Advance care directives, 28
Advanced practice psychiatric–mental health
    nurse, 55
Advanced Practice Psychiatric-Mental Health
    Registered Nurses (PMH-APRN), 53, 54
Advanced sleep phase type, 634
Adverse outcome, 289, 291
Adverse reactions, psychiatric medications, 151
Advocacy services, for homelessness, 765–766
Aerosols, 600, 748
Affective lability, 362
Affinity, receptors, 153
Affordable Care Act, 46
Affordable Care Act, 2010, 754
Affordable Housing Trust Fund, 754
African Americans, 21, 21b
African Americans, culture of
  access to mental health services, 22
  eating disorder, 561
  and family life cycle, 214–216
  family networks, 21
  men attitudes, 21b
  and racial discrimination, 21
  rates of IPV, 783
  and stresses of double stigma, 21
  subcultural and individual differences, 21
  suicide behavior, 415
  women's attitudes, 21b
AFSP. *See* American Foundation for Suicide
    Prevention (AFSP)
Age of onset
  in anorexia nervosa, 560–561
  in antisocial personality disorder, 515
  in bipolar disorder, 426
  in bulimia nervosa, 575
  in delusional disorder, 391
  in depressive disorder, 402
  in schizoaffective disorder, 379
  in schizophrenia, 338
  in somatic symptom disorder, 538
  in substance-related disorder, 585–586

Age-related groups, 204, 205b
Aggression, 337
Aggression and violence, 287
  assessment for
    characteristics predictive of, 289
    impaired communication, 290
    milieu and environmental factors, 290, 290f
    physical condition, 290
    social factors, 290
  behavioral theories, 288
  biologic theories, 287–288, 288b
  evaluation and treatment outcomes, 295
  general aggression model (GAM), 288–289,
    289f
  influencing factors, 287
  nursing diagnoses for, 290
  promoting safety, interventions for
    administering and monitoring PRN
      medications, 294
    cognitive, 291–292, 292b
    communication and development of
      therapeutic nurse-patient relationship,
      290–291
    de-escalation, 293–294, 294f
    environmental interventions, 292–293,
      293b
    milieu intervention, 292–293, 293b
    seclusion and restraint, avoiding use of,
      294–295
  psychoanalytic theories, 288
  research and policy initiatives, 297
  responding to assault on nurses, 296–297, 296t
  social learning theory, 288
Aggression-related gene, 287
Agitated behavior, 740
Agitation, 337
Agnosia, 724, 733, 737
Agnosticism, 24t
Agonists, 151, 153f
Agoraphobia, 471, 472b
Agoraphobia Cognitions Questionnaire, 459b
Agranulocytosis, 164, 356–357
AIDS–related dementia, 93
Ailurophobia, 472b
AIMS. *See* Abnormal Involuntary Movement
    Scale (AIMS)
Akathisia, 166, 355
Alanine aminotransferase (ALT; SGPT),
    serum, 130t
Al-Anon, 41, 236
Alateen, 41
Alcohol, 587–593
  alcohol-induced amnestic disorders, 587–589
  blood alcohol level, 587, 589t
  detoxification, 590
  long-term abuse, effects of, 587
  prolonged use, 588t
  promotion of health and, 592–593
  psychological effects of, 769b
  relapse prevention, 592
  tolerance to, 587
Alcohol abuse
  case vignette, 604–606
  effects of, 588t
    long-term, 587
  medical complications of, 590b
  withdrawal syndromes of, 588t
Alcohol and substance abuse, 257
Alcoholic dementia, 748
Alcoholics Anonymous (AA), 41, 204, 221,
    612–613, 613b, 764, 765, 776
Alcohol-induced amnestic disorders, 587–589
Alcoholism, 20, 748
  case vignette, 604–606
  characteristics of person with, 603, 610b

Alcohol withdrawal syndrome, 590, 590t
Aldridge, Lionel, 337
Alexithymia, 539
Algophobia, 472b
Allodynia, 819
Allostasis, 272
Allostatic load (AL), 272, 272f, 273b
Alprazolam (Xanax), 174, 457b
Alumni Club, 765
Alzheimer's disease (AD), 82, 717
  assessment
    of biologic domain, 727–728
    of psychological domain, 733–736
    of social domain, 740
  clinical course, 723–724
  clinical vignette, 743b
  continuum of care, 744
  diagnostic criteria, 724
    agnosia, 724
    aphasia, 724
    apraxia, 724
    disturbance of executive functioning,
      724
    mild cognitive impairment (MCI), 724
  early-onset, 724
  epidemiology and risk factors, 724
  etiology, 724–726
    beta-amyloid plaques, 724–725
    cell death and neurotransmitters, 725–726
    free radicals, 726
    genetic factors, 726
    inflammation, 726
    neurofibrillary tangles, 725, 725f
    oxidative stress and mitochondrial
      dysfunction, 726
  evaluation and treatment outcomes,
    742–744
  family response to, 726–727
  interdisciplinary treatment, 727
  interventions
    for biologic domain, 728–733
    for psychological domain, 736–740
    for social domain, 740–742
  late-onset, 724
  mental health promotion, 744
  nursing diagnoses
    for biologic domain, 728
    for psychological domain, 736
    for social domain, 740
  nursing management, 727
    biologic domain, 727–733
    psychological domain, 733–740
    social domain, 740–742
  priority care issues, 727
  progression, 724f
Ambivalence, 363
Ambulatory services, 42t
Amenorrhea, 560
American Foundation for Suicide Prevention
    (AFSP), 317
American Healthcare Association, 29
American Hospital Association, 29
American Managed Behavioral Healthcare
    Association (AMBHA), 47
American Nurses Association (ANA), 2, 139
American Nurses Credentialing Center
    (ANCC), 54
American Psychiatric Association (APA), 285
American Psychiatric Nurses Association
    (APNA), 55
American Public Health Association, 30
American Recovery and Reinvestment Act of
    2009, 32, 754
Americans With Disabilities Act of 1990 (ADA),
    28–29